C O N T E M P O R A R Y

ORAL AND MAXILLOFACIAL SURGERY

CONTEMPORARY

ORAL AND MAXILLOFACIAL SURGERY

SENIOR EDITOR

LARRY J. PETERSON, D.D.S., M.S.
Professor and Chairman, Oral and Maxillofacial Surgery
College of Dentistry, The Ohio State University
Columbus, Ohio

ASSOCIATE EDITORS

EDWARD ELLIS III, D.D.S., M.S.
Professor, Oral and Maxillofacial Surgery
University of Texas Southwestern Medical Center
Dallas, Texas

JAMES R. HUPP, D.M.D., M.D., J.D., F.A.C.S.
Professor and Chair, Oral and Maxillofacial Surgery
University of Maryland
Baltimore, Maryland

MYRON R. TUCKER, D.D.S.
Adjunct Clinical Professor, Oral and Maxillofacial Surgery
University of North Carolina at Chapel Hill
Chapel Hill, North Carolina
Private Practice
Charlotte, North Carolina

THIRD EDITION

with 1072 *illustrations*

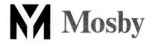

St. Louis Baltimore Boston Carlsbad Chicago Minneapolis New York Philadelphia Portland
London Milan Sydney Tokyo Toronto

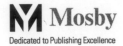

Mosby
Dedicated to Publishing Excellence

Publisher: John Schrefer
Editor: Penny Rudolph
Project Manager: Mark Spann
Production Editor: Beth Hayes
Book Design Manager: Judi Lang
Designer: TSI Graphics
Manufacturing Manager: Karen Boehme
Cover Art: GW Graphics

THIRD EDITION

Printed in the United States of America
Composition by Graphic World, Inc.
Lithography/color film by Graphic World, Inc.
Printing/binding by Von Hoffman Press

Mosby–Year Book, Inc.
11830 Westline Industrial Drive
St. Louis, Missouri 63146

Library of Congress Cataloging-in—Publication Data

Contemporary oral and maxillofacial surgery / senior editor, Larry J. Peterson ; associate
   editors, Edward Ellis III, James R. Hupp, Myron R. Tucker. — 3rd ed.
      p.   cm.
   Includes bibliographical references and index.
   ISBN 0-8151-6699-0
   1. Mouth—Surgery.   2. Maxilla—Surgery.   3. Face—Surgery.
   I. Peterson, Larry J., 1942—   .
   [DNLM: 1. Surgery, Oral. 2. Maxilla—surgery. 3. Face—surgery.
WU 600 C761 1998]
RK529.C66   1998
617.5′22059—dc21
DNLM/DLC
for Library of Congress   97-14848
                                                                               CIP

99   00   01   02 / 9 8 7 6 5 4 3 2

CONTRIBUTORS ⎯⎯⎯⎯⎯◇

M. Franklin Dolwick, DMD, PhD
Professor
Oral and Maxillofacial Surgery
College of Dentistry
University of Florida
Gainesville, Florida

Peter E. Larsen, DDS
Associate Professor and Program Director
Oral and Maxillofacial Surgery
College of Dentistry
The Ohio State University
Columbus, Ohio

Ed McGlumphy, DDS, MS
Associate Professor
Director of Implant Dentistry
Restorative and Prosthetic Dentistry
College of Dentistry
The Ohio State University
Columbus, Ohio

Michael Miloro, DMD, MS
Assistant Professor
Oral and Maxillofacial Surgery
College of Dentistry
The Ohio State University
Columbus, Ohio

Sterling R. Schow, DMD
Professor
Oral and Maxillofacial Surgery
Baylor College of Dentistry
Texas A & M University System
Dallas, Texas

Richard Small, JD
Small, Toth, Baldridge & Van Belkum
Attorneys and Counselors
30100 Telegraph Road, Suite 250
Bingham Farms, Michigan

Richard E. Walton, DMD, MS
Professor
Department of Endodontics
College of Dentistry
University of Iowa
Iowa City, Iowa

PREFACE

Oral and maxillofacial surgery is a rapidly changing and expanding area of health care, and a multidisciplinary approach is necessary to meet the needs of many patients. Cooperation and coordination of care between the general dentist and medical and dental specialists is essential to provide the best care for the patients.

The primary purpose of *Contemporary Oral and Maxillofacial Surgery* is to present a comprehensive description of the basic oral surgery procedures that the general practitioner performs in his or her office. A secondary goal is to provide information on advanced and complex surgical management of patients provided by the specialist in oral and maxillofacial surgery. This book is designed primarily for use as an instructional text for the dental student, but the material is sufficiently comprehensive to serve as a reference book for the general practitioner in private practice, general practice residents, and graduate students in other dental specialties. The resident as well as the specialist in oral and maxillofacial surgery will also find this text to be of value, especially the sections that relate to the medically compromised patients and to concepts of team approach in management in a variety of problems.

This textbook presents the fundamental principles of surgical and medical management of oral surgery problems. The basic techniques of evaluation, diagnosis, and medical management are described in sufficient detail to allow immediate clinical application. The discussion of surgical techniques is heavily illustrated so that the reader can understand them readily. The large amount of detail is intended to help the reader understand the biologic as well as the technical aspects of surgical procedures so that he or she can appropriately respond to surgical situations that are not "textbook cases."

The portions of the text that discuss complex oral and maxillofacial surgery procedures are written in an overview style, and no attempt has been made to describe the procedures in sufficient detail to allow one to actually learn the surgical technique.

For the third edition, the entire book was carefully reviewed and updated. Although certain chapters, such as the chapter on armamentarium, have few changes, other chapters, such as the medicolegal chapter, were entirely rewritten. A new chapter on surgical endodontics was added.

Section I has been updated to include the recent refinements in recommendations related to disease transmission, both from the surgeon to the patient and from the patient to the surgeon and his or her assistants.

In Section II, alterations have been made in the chapters on postoperative management and surgical complications. The chapter on medicolegal considerations has been completely reworked and has a significantly different format.

In Section III, the chapter on advanced preprosthetic surgery has been de-emphasized, whereas the chapter on dental implants has been upgraded.

Section IV, on infection, has been revised in light of current information on bacteria and antibiotics. Chapter 18, on endodontic surgery, was added to this section. The indication and principles for surgical intervention in the periapical region have been clearly described. Sections V and VI, concerning pathology and trauma, have been updated to reflect current philosophies of treatment.

Section VII on dentofacial deformities has undergone a rigorous revision and illustrated to reflect the refinement and nuances of orthognatic surgery.

Section VIIIs and IX have been refined and updated.

The Appendices have been updated to include current information, as available in the late 1990s.

Larry J. Peterson
Edward Ellis III
James R. Hupp
Myron R. Tucker

ACKNOWLEDGMENTS ———◇

My efforts are dedicated to my family, teachers, residents, and students, who have made my life so wonderful.

Larry J. Peterson

I dedicate my time and efforts devoted to this work to Carmen, my wife, best friend, and life-partner, to our magnificent and too-swiftly maturing kids, Jamie, Justin, Joelle, and Jordan; to my inspirational parents, Lucie and Richard; and to my accomplished sister, Judy, and her wonderful family. Thank you all for the loving support you provide me.

James R. Hupp

I dedicate my contribution to this textbook to Dr. Bill C. Terry, an inspiring mentor, colleague and close friend. I will always appreciate his tremendous contributions to the entire specialty of Oral and Maxillofacial Surgery, founded on expertise and always shared by Bill with enthusiasm.

Myron R. Tucker

I acknowledge with gratitude my mentor, Dr. James R. Hayward, for his many contributions to my chapters. I also acknowledge one of my colleagues, Dr. Richard F. Scott, for several of the clinical cases used to illustrate these same chapters. Their contributions and assistance have been of inestimable value.

Edward Ellis III

Oral and maxillofacial surgery is the specialty of *dentistry* that includes the diagnosis and surgical, and adjunctive treatment of diseases, injuries, and defects, including both the functional and esthetic aspects of the hard and soft tissues of the oral and maxillofacial regions. This definition is intentionally broad and all-inclusive, pertaining primarily to the specialty of oral and maxillofacial surgery. The surgery that general practitioners perform in the office is usually much less extensive than that practiced by specialists in oral and maxillofacial surgery.

The scope of oral and maxillofacial surgery for the general practitioner is defined by several factors. The first is the individual dentist's desire to perform surgical procedures. Some dentists have little or no interest in surgical activity, whereas other dentists quite enjoy it. The second factor is the individual dentist's training and experience in performing complex surgical procedures. A dentist may be interested in performing surgery for the removal in impacted teeth, but without adequate training and experience would be unwise to do so. The third factor defining the scope of a dentist's surgical practice is the individual dentist's level of skill. Even with a high interest level and extensive training, a dentist who has little or no skill in the surgical arena should probably not perform complex surgical procedures. On the other hand, with high levels of interest, extensive training, and sufficient skill, the general practitioner should seriously consider performing more complex surgical procedures. The fourth and final factor is the availability of specialists in the dentist's vicinity. If specialists in oral and maxillofacial surgery are geographically separated from the general practitioner by a large distance, the general practitioner may wish to perform more surgical procedures and surgery of greater complexity than if there is a specialist relatively near.

It is important to note that the scope of oral and maxillofacial surgery practice for the general practitioner of dentistry is *not* defined by state law. For the most part, state dental boards issue a single license for the practice of dentistry to both general practitioners and specialists. The general practitioner has the legal right to perform any oral and maxillofacial surgery procedure. Therefore each dentist must decide which surgical procedure to perform and which should be referred to a specialist, keeping in mind the best interests of the patient. The factors listed in the previous paragraph are those upon which such decisions should be made.

The scope of oral and maxillofacial surgery for the general practitioner usually includes several surgical procedures. Most often performed are the extraction of erupted teeth and the removal of fractured roots. On completion of dental school, every dentist should have adequate training, experience, and skill to provide this service. The dentist should be able to perform minor preprosthetic surgical procedures. This includes most procedures that can be performed with local anesthesia in an office setting. The dentist should be able to manage minor infections of the teeth and soft tissues of the mouth. Most odontogenic infections are minor and can be managed by the reasonably experienced general dentist. The dentist should be able to evaluate a patient with an oral pathologic lesion and determine if a biopsy is necessary. In many situations, the dentist should be the one who performs such a biopsy. Finally, the general dentist should have facility in managing traumatic injuries of the teeth and soft tissues of the mouth. In many situations definitive care must be provided by specialists, but initial care often can be provided by a general dentist.

The specialist in oral and maxillofacial surgery is a dentist who has had formal training in oral and maxillofacial surgery for 4 or more years after completing dental school. During this period he or she gains extensive experience in complex surgical and medical management and receives extensive training and experience in the diagnosis and surgical management of impacted teeth and the techniques of tooth extraction in patients with severe medical compromises. Important to the training of oral and maxillofacial surgeons is the acquisition of knowledge and skill in advanced and complex pain control methods, including intravenous sedation and ambulatory general anesthesia. The oral and maxillofacial surgeon also gets extensive training and experience in the initial and definitive care of the trauma patient, management of extensive odontogenic infections of the head and neck, management of oral pathologic lesions (such as cysts and tumors of the jaws), diagnosis and management of dentofacial deformities (congenital, developmental, or acquired), complex maxillofacial preprosthetic surgery (including the use of dental implants), reconstruction with bone grafts of missing portions of the jaws, and management of facial pain and temporomandibular joint disorders.

Surgery does not require technical skill alone; it is a complex discipline that includes many factors. Surgical skill is the technical portion of the total surgical activity and accounts for less than one third of a surgeon's ability. Surgical judgment is the wisdom to make decisions in managing the surgical patient. The discipline of surgery also includes the diagnosis of the surgical problem; the preparation of the patient, both psychologically and physiologically, for the procedure; the timing of the operation for the patient's maximal benefit; the adjustment and modification of standard surgical procedures to fit the individual needs of each patient; and, finally, the supportive postoperative care that is essential for an uneventful recovery from the surgical procedure.

To be excellent a surgeon must be technically skilled but must also have strong components of humanism, kindness, and compassion. It is important that he or she have a great deal of insight into the patient's concerns regarding the upcoming surgical procedure. The surgeon must take advantage of this insight and project an image of caring about these concerns, which all patients have. This humanistic approach will be the most important factor in the patient's judgment of the surgeon's overall skill. The excellent surgeon must have good surgical judgment, which is a measure of both maturity and surgical experience. Finally, the surgeon must have great respect for soft tissue as well as hard tissue. Surgeons with less respect for tissue will have patients who take longer to heal and have a higher incidence of complications.

The excellent surgeon must reflect these characteristics by knowing when operations are necessary, where anatomically to do the operation, and how technically to perform the procedure. Equally important is that the surgeon must know when *not* to operate. As the beginning surgeon enters training, he or she should watch teachers for examples of surgical maturity. He or she should look for teachers who emphasize surgical finesse over surgical force, and should observe how surgeons, be they other students or senior faculty, help anxious patients through a surgical procedure by expressing concern and interest in the patients as people, as well as in the technical portion of the surgery.

Contents ⸻◇

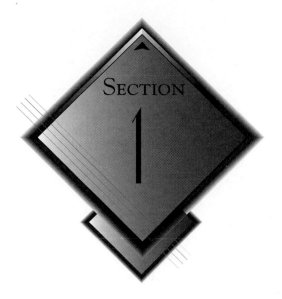

PRINCIPLES OF SURGERY

Surgery is a discipline based on principles that evolved from both basic research and centuries of trial and error. These principles pervade every area of surgery, whether it be oral and maxillofacial surgery, periodontal surgery, or open heart surgery. This section provides the reader with basic information about patient evaluation and surgical concepts, which is a necessary foundation for the discussions of the specialized surgical techniques presented in succeeding sections.

Many patients have medical conditions that affect their ability to tolerate oral and maxillofacial surgery and their wound healing. Chapter 1 discusses the process of evaluating the health status of patients. The chapter also describes methods of altering surgical treatment plans to accommodate patients with common medical problems.

Preventing medical emergencies in a patient undergoing oral and maxillofacial surgery is always easier than managing them once they occur. Chapter 2 discusses the means of recognizing and managing medical emergencies in the dental office. However, just as important, it provides information about measures to lessen the likelihood of emergencies.

Contemporary surgery is guided by a set of principles, the majority of which apply no matter where in the human body they are put into practice. Chapter 3 covers the principles of most importance to practitioners performing surgery in the oral cavity and jaws.

Surgery always leaves a wound, whether or not one was initially present. This is a statement of the obvious, but it is often forgotten by the beginning surgeon who may believe that the surgical procedure is complete once the final suture has been tied. The surgeon's responsibility to a patient does not end until the wound created during surgery has healed, so an understanding of wound healing is important for anyone who intends to create wounds surgically or treat accidental wounds. Chapter 4 presents basic wound-healing concepts, particularly as they relate to oral surgery.

The work of Semmelweiss and Lister in the 1800s made clinicians aware of the microbial origin of postoperative infections, thereby changing surgery from a last resort to a more predictably successful endeavor. The advent of antibiotics able to be used systemically further advanced surgical science, allowing completely elective surgery to be performed at low risk. However, pathogenic communicable organisms still exist that, when the epithelial barrier is breached during surgery, can cause wound infections or systemic infectious diseases. The most serious examples are the hepatitis B and the human immunodeficiency viruses. Chapter 5 describes means of minimizing the risk of significant wound contamination and the spread of infectious organisms between individuals through decontamination of the surgical instruments, the room in which surgery is performed, the operative site, and the members of the surgical team—in other words, aseptic technique.

PREOPERATIVE HEALTH STATUS EVALUATION

James R. Hupp

CHAPTER OUTLINE

The taking of a medical history and the physical and laboratory examinations of a patient requiring ambulatory dentoalveolar surgery usually differ from those that are necessary for a patient requiring hospital admission for other surgical procedures. Comprehensive histories and physical examinations of patients are best performed by a patient's primary care physician. It is impractical and of little value for the dentist to duplicate this process. However, the dental health care provider must discover the presence or history of medical problems that may have an impact on the safe delivery of care in the dental office.

Dentists are educated in the basic sciences and preclinical medical sciences particularly as they relate to the maxillofacial region. This expertise in oral medicine makes dentists valuable resources in a community's health care delivery team. The responsibility this designation carries is that dentists must be capable of recognizing and appropriately managing pathologic oral conditions. To maintain this expertise, a dentist must be informed of new developments in oral medicine, vigilant when treating patients, and prepared to communicate a thorough but succinct evaluation of the oral health of patients to other health care providers.

MEDICAL HISTORY

An accurate medical history is the most useful information the dentist can have when deciding whether a patient can safely undergo planned dental therapy. The dentist must also be prepared to interpret how a medical problem will alter a patient's response to anesthetic agents and dental surgery. The physical and laboratory examinations of a patient play relatively minor roles in the presurgical evaluation if the history is well taken. The standard format used for recording the results of medical histories and physical examinations is illustrated in Box 1-1.

The medical history interview and the physical examination should be tailored to each patient's particular needs, considering the patient's medical problems, age, intelligence, and lifestyle; the complexity of the planned procedure; and the anticipated methods of pain and anxiety control.

BIOGRAPHIC DATA

The most important information to initially obtain from a patient is biographic data. These include the patient's full name, address, age, gender, occupation, and marital status and the name of the patient's primary care physician. This information, along with an impression of the patient's intelligence and personality, is then used by the clinician to

Standard format for recording results of history and physical examinations

1. Biographic data
2. Chief complaint and its history
3. Past medical history
4. Social and family medical histories
5. Review of systems
6. Physical examination
7. Laboratory and radiographic/imaging examinations

Baseline health history database

1. Past hospitalizations, operations, traumatic injuries, and serious illnesses
2. Recent minor illnesses or symptoms
3. Medications currently or recently in use and allergies (particularly drug allergies)
4. Description of health-related habits or addictions, such as the use of ethanol, tobacco, illicit drugs, and amount and type of daily exercise
5. Date and result of last medical checkup or physician visit

assess the patient's reliability. This is important because the worth of the remainder of the medical history depends primarily on the reliability of the patient as a historian. If the identification data or patient interview gives the dentist reason to suspect that the medical history will be unreliable, alternative methods of obtaining the necessary information must be found. A reliability assessment should continue throughout the entire history interview and physical examination, with the interviewer looking for illogic, improbable, or inconsistent patient responses that might suggest the need for corroborating information.

CHIEF COMPLAINT

Every patient should be asked to state his or her chief complaint. This can be accomplished on a form the patient completes or during the initial interview the patient's answer should be transcribed into the dental record, preferably verbatim. This statement helps the clinician establish priorities during history taking and treatment planning. Also, by having patients formulate a chief complaint, they are encouraged to clarify for themselves and the clinician why they desire treatment. Occasionally, a hidden agenda may exist for the patient, either consciously or subconsciously. In such circumstances subsequent information elicited from the patient interview may reveal the true reason the patient is seeking care.

HISTORY OF THE CHIEF COMPLAINT

The patient should be asked to describe the history of the present complaint or illness, particularly its first appearance, any changes since its first appearance, and its impact on or by other factors. Descriptions of pain should include onset, intensity, duration, location, and radiation, and factors that worsen and mitigate the pain. In addition, an inquiry should be made about constitutional symptoms such as fever, chills, lethargy, anorexia, malaise, and weakness associated with the chief complaint.

This portion of the health history may be extremely straightforward (for instance, a 2-day history of pain and swelling around an erupting third molar). However, it may be relatively involved, such as a lengthy history of a painful, nonhealing extraction site in a patient who received thera-

peutic irradiation. In this case a detailed history of the chief complaint is necessary.

MEDICAL HISTORY

Most dental practitioners find health history forms (questionnaires) an efficient means of initially collecting the medical history. When a health history form is completed by a credible patient, the dentist can use pertinent answers to direct the interview. Properly trained dental assistants can flag important patient responses on the form to bring positive answers to the attention of the dentist (for example, by circling allergies to medications in red).

Health questionnaires should be written clearly, be in lay language, and should not be lengthy. To lessen the chance of patients giving incomplete or inaccurate responses, the form should include a statement that assures the patient of the confidentiality of the information. The form should also include a place for patient signature, verifying that the patient understands the questions and the accuracy of the answers. Numerous health questionnaires designed for dental patients are available from sources such as the American Dental Association, dental schools, and dental textbooks (Figure 1-1). The dentist should either choose a prepared form or formulate an individualized one.

The items listed in Box 1-2 help establish a suitable health history database for patients, collected either on a form or verbally; if the data are collected verbally, written documentation of the results of the inquiry is important.

In addition to this basic information, it is helpful to inquire specifically about relatively common medical problems that are likely to alter dental management of the patient. These problems include angina, myocardial infarction, heart murmurs, rheumatic heart disease, bleeding disorders (including anticoagulant use), asthma, lung disease, hepatitis, sexually transmitted disease, renal disease, diabetes, corticosteroid use, seizure disorder, and implanted prosthetic devices such as artificial joints or heart valves. Patients should be asked specifically about allergies to local anesthetics and penicillin. Female patients also must be asked at each visit whether they may be pregnant. A brief family history can be useful and should focus on relevant inherited diseases, such as hemo-

MEDICAL HISTORY

Name _____ M ___ F ___ Date of Birth _____

Address _____

Telephone: (Home) _____ (Work) _____ Height _____ Weight _____

Today's Date _____ Occupation _____

Answer all questions by circling either YES or NO and fill in all blank spaces when indicated.
Answers to the following questions are for our records only and are confidential.

1. My last medical physical examination was on (approximate) _____

2. The name & address of my personal physician is _____

_____

3. Are you now under the care of a physician . . . .   YES   NO

   a. If so, what is the condition being treated? _____
4. Have you had any serious illness or operation. . . . .   YES   NO

   a. If so, what was the illness or operation _____
5. Have you been hospitalized within the past 5 years . . . .   YES   NO

   a. If so, what was the problem _____
6. Do you have or have you had any of the following diseases or problems:
   a. Rheumatic fever or rheumatic heart disease . . . .   YES   NO
   b. Heart abnormalities present since birth . . . .   YES   NO
   c. Cardiovascular disease (heart trouble, heart attack, angina, stroke, high
      blood pressure, heart murmur) . . . .   YES   NO
      1) Do you have pain or pressure in chest upon exertion . . . .   YES   NO
      2) Are you ever short of breath after mild exercise . . . .   YES   NO
      3) Do your ankles swell. . . . .   YES   NO
      4) Do you get short of breath when you lie down, or do you require
         extra pillows when you sleep . . . .   YES   NO
      5) Have you been told you have a heart murmur . . . .   YES   NO
   d. Asthma or hay fever . . . .   YES   NO
   e. Hives or a skin rash . . . .   YES   NO
   f. Fainting spells or seizures . . . .   YES   NO
   g. Diabetes. . . . .   YES   NO
      1) Do you have to urinate (pass water) more than six times a day . . .   YES   NO
      2) Are you thirsty much of the time. . . . .   YES   NO
      3) Does your mouth usually feel dry . . . .   YES   NO
   h. Hepatitis, jaundice or liver disease . . . .   YES   NO
   i. Arthritis or other joint problems.   YES   NO
   j. Stomach ulcers. . . . .   YES   NO
   k. Kidney trouble . . . .   YES   NO
   l. Tuberculosis . . . .   YES   NO
   m. Do you have a persistent cough or cough up blood. . . . .   YES   NO
   n. Venereal disease. . . . .   YES   NO

   o. Other (list) _____

_____

_____

7. Have you had abnormal bleeding associated with previous extractions, surgery, or trauma . . . .   YES   NO
   a. Do you bruise easily . . . .   YES   NO
   b. Have you ever required a blood transfusion . . . .   YES   NO

   If so, explain the circumstances _____

_____

8. Do you have any blood disorder such as anemia, including sickle cell
   anemia . . . .   YES   NO
9. Have you had surgery or radiation *treatment* for a tumor, cancer, or other
   condition of your head or neck. . . . .   YES   NO

◇ Figure 1-1

Example of health history questionnaire useful for screening dental patients. *(Modified from form provided by the American Dental Association.)*

MEDICAL HISTORY—CONT'D

10. Are you taking any drug or medicine . . . .   YES   NO

    If so, what _____

11. Are you taking any of the following:
    a. Antibiotics or sulfa drugs . . . .   YES   NO
    b. Anticoagulants (blood thinners) . . . .   YES   NO
    c. Medicine for high blood pressure. . . . .   YES   NO
    d. Cortisone (steroids) (including prednisone) . . . .   YES   NO
    e. Tranquilizers. . . . .   YES   NO
    f. Aspirin . . . .   YES   NO
    g. Insulin, tolbutamide (Orinase) or similar drug . . . .   YES   NO
    h. Digitalis or drugs for heart trouble . . . .   YES   NO
    i. Nitroglycerin. . . . .   YES   NO
    j. Antihistamine . . . .   YES   NO
    k. Oral contraceptive or other hormonal therapy . . . .   YES   NO

    l. Other _____   YES   NO
12. Are you allergic or have you reacted adversely to:
    a. Local anesthetics (procaine [Novocain]). . . . .   YES   NO
    b. Penicillin or other antibiotics. . . . .   YES   NO
    c. Sulfa drugs . . . .   YES   NO
    d. Aspirin . . . .   YES   NO
    e. Iodine or xray dyes. . . . .   YES   NO
    f. Codeine or other narcotics . . . .   YES   NO

    g. Other _____   YES   NO
13. Have you had any serious trouble associated with any previous dental
    treatment. . . . .   YES   NO

    If so, explain _____

    _____

14. Do you have any disease, condition, or problem not listed above that you
    think I should know about . . . .   YES   NO

    If so, please explain _____

    _____

15. Are you employed in any situation which exposes you regularly to xrays or
    other ionizing radiation. . . . .   YES   NO
16. Are you wearing contact lenses. . . . .   YES   NO
WOMEN:
17. Are you pregnant or have you recently missed a menstrual period . . . .   YES   NO
18. Are you presently breast feeding . . . .   YES   NO

Chief dental complaint (Why did you come to the office today?): _____

_____

_____

_____

_____

Signature of Patient (verifying accuracy
of historical information)

_____

Signature of Dentist

◇ Figure 1-1, cont'd
For legend see previous page.

◇ Box 1-3 ◇

Common health conditions to inquire about verbally or on a health questionnaire

Angina

Myocardial infarction (heart attack)

Heart murmurs

Rheumatic heart disease

Bleeding disorders

Anticoagulant use

Asthma

Lung disease

Tuberculosis

Hepatitis

Sexually transmitted disease

Renal disease

Hypertension

Diabetes

Corticosteroid use

Seizure disorder

Implanted prosthetic devices

Allergies to antibiotics or local anesthetics

Pregnancy

Breast feeding

◇ Box 1-4 ◇

Routine review of head, neck, and maxillofacial regions

Constitutional: Fever, chills, sweats, weight loss, fatigue, malaise, loss of appetite

Head: Headache, dizziness, fainting, insomnia

Ears: Decreased hearing, tinnitus (ringing), pain

Eyes: Blurring, double vision, excessive tearing, dryness, pain

Nose and sinuses: Rhinorrhea, epistaxis, problems breathing through nose, pain, change in sense of smell

Temporomandibular joint area: Pain, noise, limited jaw motion

Oral: Dental pain or sensitivity, lip or mucosal sores, problems chewing, problems speaking, bad breath, loose restorations, sore throat, loud snoring

Neck: Difficulty swallowing, change in voice, pain or stiffness

philia or malignant hyperthermia (see Box 1-3). The medical history should be periodically updated, at least on an annual basis. Many dentists have their assistants specifically ask each patient at each of their checkup appointments if there has been any change in their health since their last dental visit. The dentist is alerted if a change has occurred, and changes are documented in the record.

REVIEW OF SYSTEMS

The review of systems is a sequential, comprehensive method of eliciting patient symptoms on an organ system basis. The review of systems may reveal undiagnosed medical conditions unknown to the patient. This review can be extensive when performed by a physician for a patient with complicated medical problems. However, the review of systems conducted by the dentist before oral surgery should be guided by pertinent answers obtained from the history. For example, the review of the cardiovascular system in a patient with a positive history of ischemic heart disease includes questions concern-

◇ Box 1-5 ◇

Review of cardiovascular and respiratory systems

Cardiovascular review

Chest discomfort on exertion, when eating, or at rest; palpitations; fainting; ankle edema; shortness of breath (dyspnea) on exertion; dyspnea on assuming supine position (orthopnea or paroxysmal nocturnal dyspnea); postural hypotension; fatigue; leg muscle cramping

Respiratory review

Dyspnea with exertion, wheezing, coughing, excessive sputum production, coughing up blood (hemoptysis)

ing chest discomfort (during exertion, eating, or at rest), palpitations, fainting, and ankle swelling. Such questions help the dentist decide whether to perform surgery at all or alter the surgical or anesthetic methods. If anxiety-controlling adjuncts such as intravenous (IV) and inhalation sedation are planned, the cardiovascular, respiratory, and nervous systems should always be reviewed; this can disclose previously undiagnosed problems that may jeopardize successful sedation. In the role of the oral medicine specialist, the dentist is expected to perform a quick review of the head, ears, eyes, nose, mouth, and throat on every patient, regardless of whether other systems are reviewed. Items to be reviewed are outlined in Box 1-4.

The need to review organ systems in addition to those in the maxillofacial region depends on clinical circumstances. The cardiovascular and respiratory systems commonly require evaluation before oral surgery or sedation (see Box 1-5). If no changes have occurred, the patient signs the record, indicating the lack of change (Figure 1-1).

PHYSICAL EXAMINATION ───◇

The physical examination of the dental patient focuses on the oral cavity and to a lesser degree on the entire maxillofacial region. Recording the results of the physical examination should be an exercise in accurate description rather than a listing of suspected medical diagnoses. For example, the dentist may find a chin lesion that is 2 mm in diameter, is raised and erythematous, and is painful to palpation. These physical findings should be recorded in a similarly descriptive manner; the dentist should not jump to a diagnosis and record only "pimple on chin."

Any physical examination should begin with the measurement of vital signs. This serves as both a screening device for unsuspected medical problems and as a baseline for future measurements. The techniques of measuring blood pressure and pulse rates are illustrated in Figures 1-2 and 1-3.

The physical evaluation of various parts of the body usually involves one or more of the following four primary means of evaluation: inspection, palpation, percussion, and auscultation. In the oral and maxillofacial regions, inspection should

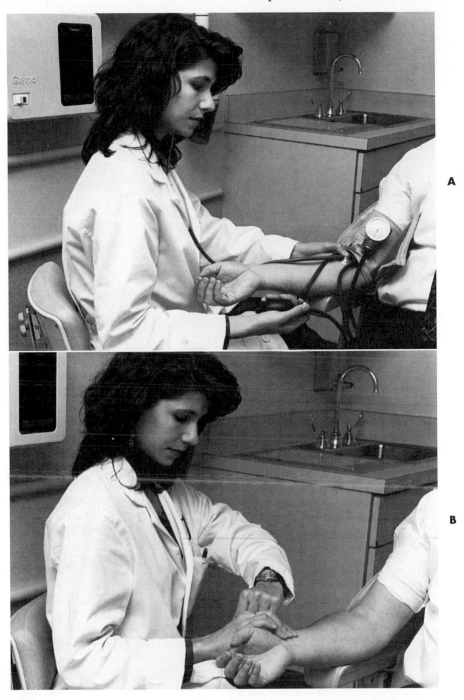

⟨ Figure 1-2

A, Measurement of systemic blood pressure. Cuff of proper size placed securely around upper arm so that lower edge of cuff lies 2 to 4 cm above antecubital fossa. Branchial artery is palpated in fossa, and stethoscope diaphragm is placed over artery and held in place with fingers of left hand. Squeeze bulb is held in palm of right hand, and valve screwed closed with thumb and index finger of that hand. Bulb is then repeatedly squeezed until pressure gauge reads approximately 220 mm Hg. Air is slowly allowed to escape from cuff by partially opening valve while dentist listens through stethoscope. Gauge reading at point when faint blowing sound is first heard is systolic blood pressure. Gauge reading when sound from artery disappears is diastolic pressure. Once diastolic pressure reading is obtained, valve is opened to deflate cuff completely. **B,** Pulse rate and rhythm most commonly evaluated by using tips of middle and index fingers of right hand to palpate radial artery at the wrist. Once rhythm has been determined to be regular, number of pulsations to occur during 30 seconds is multiplied by 2 to give number of pulses per minute. If weak pulse or irregular rhythm is discovered while palpating radial pulse, heart should be auscultated directly to determine heart rate and rhythm.

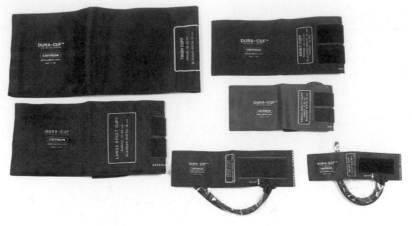

◇ Figure 1-3

Blood pressure cuffs of varying sizes for patients with arms of different diameters (ranging from infant through obese patients). Use of an improper cuff size can jeopardize the accuracy of blood pressure results. Too small a cuff causes readings to be falsely high, and too large a cuff causes artificially low readings. Blood pressure cuffs typically are labeled as to the type and size of patient for whom they are designed.

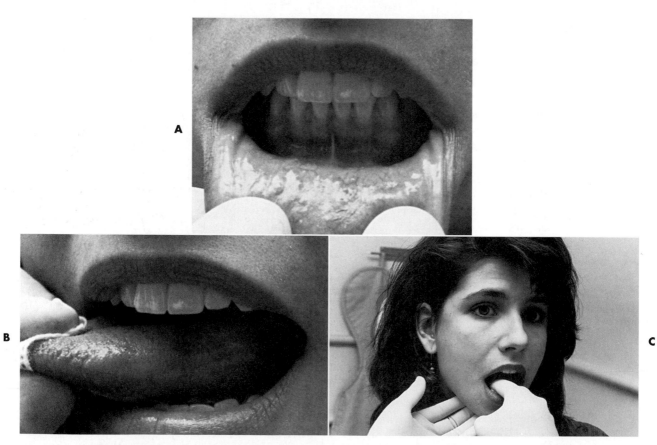

◇ Figure 1-4

A, Lip mucosa examined by everting upper and lower lips. **B,** Tongue examined by having patient protrude it. Examiner then grasps tongue with cotton sponge and gently manipulates it to examine lateral borders. Patient also asked to lift tongue to allow visualization of ventral surface and floor of mouth. **C,** Submandibular gland examined by bimanually feeling gland through floor of mouth and skin under floor of mouth.

◇ Box 1-6 ◇

Preoperative physical examination of the oral and maxillofacial surgery patient

Inspection
Head and face: General shape, symmetry, hair distribution
Ear: Normal reaction to sounds (otoscopic examination if indicated)
Eye: Symmetry, size, reactivity of pupil, color of sclera and conjunctiva, movement, test of vision
Nose: Septum, mucosa, patency
Oral: Teeth, mucosa, pharynx, lips, tonsils
Neck: Size of thyroid, jugular distention
Palpation
TMJ: Crepitus, tenderness
Paranasal: Pain over sinuses
Oral: Salivary glands, floor of mouth, lips, muscles of mastication
Neck: Thyroid size, lymph nodes
Percussion
Paranasal: Resonance over sinuses (difficult to assess)
Oral: Teeth
Auscultation
TMJ: Clicks, crepitus
Neck: Carotid bruits

◇ Box 1-7 ◇

Brief maxillofacial examination

While interviewing the patient, the dentist should visually examine the patient for general shape and symmetry of head and facial skeleton, eye movement, color of conjunctiva and sclera, and ability to hear. The clinician should listen for speech problems, TMJ sounds, and breathing ability.

Routine examination
TMJ region:
Palpate and auscultate joints.
Measure range of motion of jaw and opening pattern.
Nose and paranasal region:
Occlude nares individually to check for patency.
Inspect anterior nasal mucosa.
Mouth:
Take out all removable prostheses.
Inspect oral cavity for dental, oral, and pharyngeal mucosal lesions; look at tonsils and uvula.
Hold tongue out of mouth with dry gauze while inspecting lateral borders.
Palpate tongue, lips, floor of mouth, and salivary glands (check for saliva).
Palpate neck for lymph nodes and thyroid size. Inspect jugular veins.

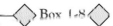 ◇ Box 1-8 ◇

American Society of Anesthesiologists (ASA) classification of physical status

ASA I: A normal healthy patient
ASA II: A patient with mild systemic disease or significant health risk factor
ASA III: A patient with severe systemic disease that is not incapacitating
ASA IV: A patient with severe systemic disease that is a constant threat to life
ASA V: A moribund patient who is not expected to survive without the operation
ASA VI: A declared brain-dead patient whose organs are being removed for donor purposes

---

always be performed. The clinician should note hair distribution and texture, facial symmetry and proportion, eye movements and conjunctival color, nasal patency and mucosal color, the presence or absence of skin lesions or discoloration, and neck or facial masses. A thorough inspection of the oral cavity is necessary, including the oropharynx, tongue, floor of the mouth, and oral mucosa (Figure 1-4).

Palpation is important when examining temporomandibular joint (TMJ) function, salivary gland size and function, thyroid size, presence or absence of enlarged or tender lymph nodes, and induration of oral soft tissues, and for determining pain or the presence of fluctuance in areas of swelling.

Percussion is commonly used by physicians during thoracic and abdominal examinations, and the dentist can use it to test teeth and paranasal sinuses. Auscultation is used by the dentist primarily for TMJ evaluation, but is also used for cardiac and pulmonary systems evaluations (Box 1-6). A brief maxillofacial examination that all dentists should perform is described in Box 1-7.

The results of the medical evaluation are used to assign a physical status classification. A few classification systems exist, but the one most commonly used is the American Society of Anesthesiologists' (ASA) physical status classification system (Box 1-8).

Once an ASA physical status class has been determined, the dentist can decide if needed treatment can be safely and routinely performed in the dental office. If a patient is not ASA class I or a relatively healthy class II patient, the practitioner

generally has the following four options: (1) modifying routine treatment plans by anxiety-reduction measures, pharmacologic anxiety-control techniques, and/or more careful monitoring of the patient during treatment (this is usually all that is necessary for ASA class II); (2) obtaining medical consultation for guidance in preparing patients to undergo ambulatory oral surgery (such as by preoperative administration of oxygen and nitroglycerin for patients with angina); (3) refusing to treat the patient in the ambulatory setting; or (4) referring the patient to an oral and maxillofacial surgeon.

◇ Box 1-9 ◇

Box 1-9

General anxiety-reduction protocol

Before appointment

Hypnotic agent to promote sleep on night before surgery (optional)

Sedative agent to decrease anxiety on morning of surgery (optional)

Morning appointment and schedule so that reception room time is minimized

During appointment

Nonpharmacologic means of anxiety control:

  Frequent verbal reassurances

  Distracting conversation

  No surprises (warn patient before doing anything that could cause anxiety)

  No unnecessary noise

  Surgical instruments out of patient's sight

  Relaxing background music

Pharmacologic means of anxiety control:

  Local anesthetics of sufficient intensity and duration

  Nitrous oxide

  Intravenous anxiolytics

After surgery

Succinct instructions for postoperative care

Patient information on expected postsurgical sequelae (for example, swelling or minor oozing of blood)

Further reassurance

Effective analgesics

Patient information on who can be contacted if any problems arise

Telephone call to patient at home during evening after surgery to check if any problems exist

---

MANAGEMENT OF PATIENTS WITH COMPROMISING MEDICAL CONDITIONS ◇
CARDIOVASCULAR PROBLEMS

ISCHEMIC HEART DISEASE

Angina pectoris. Obstruction of the arterial supply to the myocardium is one of the most common health problems dentists encounter. This condition occurs primarily in men over age 40, although it is also prevalent in postmenopausal females. The basic disease process is a progressive narrowing and/or spasm of one or more of the coronary arteries. This leads to a discrepancy between the myocardial oxygen demand and the ability of the coronary arteries to supply oxygen-carrying blood. Myocardial oxygen demand can be increased, for example, by exertion and anxiety and during digestion of a large meal. Angina is a symptom of ischemic heart disease produced when myocardial blood supply cannot be sufficiently increased to meet the increased oxygen requirements that result from coronary artery disease.* The myocardium becomes ischemic, producing a heavy pressure or squeezing sensation in the patient's substernal region that can radiate into the left shoulder and arm and into the mandibular region. The discomfort typically disappears once the myocardial work requirements are lowered or the oxygen supply to the heart muscle is increased.

The dentist's responsibility to a patient with a history of angina is to use all available preventive measures, thereby reducing the possibility that the oral surgical procedure will precipitate an anginal episode. Preventive measures begin with taking a careful history of the patient's angina. The patient should be questioned about the events that produce angina; the frequency, duration, and severity of angina; and the response to medications or diminished activity. The patient's physician can be consulted concerning the cardiac status.

If the patient's angina arises only during moderately vigorous exertion and responds readily to oral nitroglycerin, and if no recent increase in severity has occurred, ambulatory oral surgery procedures are usually safe when performed with proper precautions.

However, if anginal episodes occur after only minimal exertion, if several doses of nitroglycerin are needed to relieve chest discomfort, or if the patient has unstable angina (angina present at rest or worsening in frequency, severity, ease of precipitation, duration of attack, or predictability of response to medication), elective oral surgery should be deferred until a medical consultation is obtained. Alternatively, the patient can be referred to an oral and maxillofacial surgeon if emergency surgery is necessary.

Once the decision is made that ambulatory elective oral surgery can safely proceed, the patient should be prepared for surgery; the patient's myocardial oxygen demand should be lowered while the oxygen supply is increased. The increased oxygen demand during ambulatory oral surgery is the result primarily of patient anxiety. An anxiety-reduction protocol should therefore be used (Box 1-9). In addition, during surgery the patient should be given supplemental oxygen, premedicated with nitroglycerin (if the patient is extremely prone to angina), and have profound local anesthesia. Although some controversy exists over the use of local anesthetics containing epinephrine in angina patients, the benefits (prolonged and accentuated anesthesia) outweigh the risks. However, care should be taken to avoid excessive epinephrine administration by using proper injection techniques and giving no more than 4 mL of a local anesthetic solution with a 1:100,000 concentration of epinephrine for a total dose of 0.04 mg in any 30-minute period.

---

*The term *angina* is derived from the ancient Greek word for choking.

◇ Box 1-10 ◇

Management of patient with history of angina pectoris

1. Consult patient's physician.
2. Use anxiety-reduction protocol.
3. Have nitroglycerin tablets or spray readily available. Use nitroglycerin premedication if indicated.
4. Administer supplemental oxygen.
5. Ensure profound local anesthesia before starting surgery.
6. Consider use of nitrous oxide sedation.
7. Monitor vital signs closely.
8. Limit amount of epinephrine used (0.04 mg maximum).
9. Maintain verbal contact with patient throughout procedure to monitor status.

◇ Box 1-11 ◇

Management of patient with history of myocardial infarction

1. Consult patient's primary care physician.
2. Defer major elective surgery until 6 months after infarction.
3. Check if patient is using anticoagulants (including aspirin).
4. Use anxiety-reduction protocol.
5. Have nitroglycerin available; use prophylactically if physician advises.
6. Administer supplemental oxygen.
7. Provide profound local anesthesia.
8. Consider nitrous oxide.
9. Monitor vital signs and maintain verbal contact.
10. Limit epinephrine use to 0.04 mg.
11. Consider referral to oral and maxillofacial surgeon.

Before and during surgery, vital signs should be monitored periodically. In addition, verbal contact with the patient should be maintained. The use of N_2O or other conscious sedation methods for anxiety control in patients with ischemic heart disease should be considered. A fresh bottle of nitroglycerin tablets or a canister of nitroglycerin spray should be available at the chairside for use if necessary (Box 1-10).

Myocardial infarction.   Myocardial infarction (MI) occurs when ischemia (resulting from the oxygen demand and supply discrepancy) causes cellular death. The infarcted area of myocardium becomes nonfunctional and necrotic and is surrounded by an area of ischemic myocardium that is prone to become a focus for dysrhythmias. During the early weeks after an MI, treatment consists of limiting myocardial work requirements, increasing myocardial oxygen supply, and suppressing the production of dysrhythmias by irritable foci in ischemic tissue. In addition, if any of the primary conduction pathways are involved in the infarction, pacemaker insertion may be necessary. If the patient survives the early weeks after an MI, the necrotic area is gradually replaced with scar tissue, which is unable either to contract or properly conduct electrical signals.

The management of an oral surgical problem in a patient who has had an MI begins with a consultation with the patient's physician. Generally, it is recommended that elective major surgical procedures be deferred until at least 6 months after an infarction. This delay is based on statistical evidence that the risk of reinfarction after an MI drops to as low as it will be by about 6 months, particularly if the patient is properly supervised medically. Straightforward oral surgical procedures typically performed in the dental office may be performed less than 6 months after an MI if the procedure is unlikely to provoke significant anxiety and the patient has had an uneventful recovery from the MI.

Patients with a history of MI should be carefully questioned concerning their cardiovascular health. An attempt to elicit evidence of undiagnosed dysrhythmias or congestive heart failure (hypertrophic cardiomyopathy) should be made. Some patients who have had an MI are receiving aspirin or other anticoagulants to decrease coronary thrombogenesis; this information should be sought because it affects surgical management.

Patients requiring major elective oral surgery before 6 months have elapsed after the MI should have their primary care physician's clearance. If an emergency oral surgical condition exists, hospitalization is usually warranted. However, if more than 6 months have elapsed or physician clearance is obtained, the management of the patient who has had an MI is similar to care of the patient with angina. An anxiety-reduction program should be used, along with supplemental oxygen. Prophylactic nitroglycerin should be used only if directed by the patient's primary care physician but should be kept available. Local anesthetics containing epinephrine are safe to use if given in proper amounts using an aspiration technique. Vital signs should be monitored throughout the perioperative period (Box 1-11).

Coronary artery bypass grafting.   In general, with respect to major oral surgical care, patients who have had coronary artery bypass grafting (CABG) are treated in a manner similar to patients who have had an MI. Before major elective surgery is performed, 6 months are allowed to elapse. If major surgery is necessary before 6 months after the CABG, the patient's physician should be consulted. Patients who have had CABG usually have a history of angina, MI, or both and therefore should be managed as previously described. Routine office oral surgical procedures may be safely performed in patients less than six months after CABG surgery if their recovery has been uncomplicated and anxiety is kept to a minimum.

Coronary angioplasty.   The introduction of catheters containing balloons into narrowed coronary arteries for the purpose of reestablishing adequate blood flow is becoming commonplace. If the angioplasty has been successful (based on cardiac stress testing), oral surgery can proceed soon thereafter, with the same precautions as those used for angina patients.

Cerebrovascular accident (stroke).   Patients who have had a cerebrovascular accident are always susceptible to further neurovascular accidents. They are generally placed on anticoagulants by their physicians and, if hypertensive, are taking blood pressure–lowering agents. If such a patient requires oral surgery, treatment is best deferred until 6 months have passed and any hypertensive tendencies have been controlled. At that time, the patient should be treated by a nonpharmacologic anxiety-reduction protocol, receive supplemental oxygen, and have vital signs carefully monitored during surgery. If pharmacologic sedation is necessary, low concentrations of nitrous oxide can be used. Techniques to manage patients taking anticoagulants are discussed later in this chapter.

DYSRHYTHMIAS.   Patients who are prone to or who have cardiac dysrhythmias usually have a history of ischemic heart disease requiring dental management modifications, including limiting the total amount of epinephrine administration to 0.04 mg. However, in addition, they may have been placed on anticoagulants or have a permanent cardiac pacemaker. Pacemakers pose no contraindications to oral surgery, and no evidence exists showing the need for antibiotic prophylaxis in patients with pacemakers. Electrical equipment, such as electric cautery and microwaves, should not be used. As with other medically compromised patients, vital signs should be carefully monitored.

HEART ABNORMALITIES PREDISPOSED TOWARD INFECTIVE ENDOCARDITIS.   The internal cardiac surface, or endocardium, can be predisposed toward infection when abnormalities of its surface allow pathologic bacteria to attach and multiply. A complete description of this process and recommended means of preventing it are discussed in Chapter 16.

CONGESTIVE HEART FAILURE (HYPERTROPHIC CARDIOMYOPATHY).   Congestive heart failure occurs when a diseased myocardium is unable to deliver the cardiac output demanded by the body or when excessive demands are placed on a normal myocardium. The heart begins to have an increased end-diastolic volume that, in the case of the normal myocardium, increases contractility through the Frank-Starling mechanism. However, as the normal or diseased myocardium further dilates, it becomes a less efficient pump, causing blood to back up into the pulmonary, hepatic, and mesenteric vascular beds. This eventually leads to pulmonary edema, hepatic dysfunction, and compromised intestinal nutrient absorption. The lowered cardiac output causes generalized weakness, and impaired renal clearance of excess fluid leads to vascular overload.

Symptoms of congestive heart failure include orthopnea, paroxysmal nocturnal dyspnea, and pedal edema. Orthopnea is a respiratory disorder that manifests as shortness of breath when the patient is in the supine position. Orthopnea usually occurs as a result of the redistribution of blood pooled in the lower extremity when a patient assumes the supine position (as when sleeping). The heart's ability to handle the increased cardiac preload is overwhelmed, and blood backs up in the pulmonary circulation, producing pulmonary edema. Patients with orthopnea usually must sleep with their upper body supported on several pillows.

Paroxysmal nocturnal dyspnea is a symptom of congestive heart failure that is similar to orthopnea. The patient has respiratory difficulty 1 or 2 hours after assuming a supine position. The disorder occurs when pooled blood and interstitial fluid reabsorbed into the vasculature from the legs are redistributed centrally, overwhelming the heart and producing pulmonary edema. Patients suddenly wake shortly after laying down to sleep feeling short of breath and frequently desiring to open a window to breathe cool air.

Pedal edema is swelling of the foot and ankle caused by an increase in interstitial fluid. Usually the fluid collects as a result of any problem that increases venous pressure, forcing increased amounts of plasma to remain in the tissue spaces of the feet. Pedal edema is detected by pressing a finger into the swollen area for a few seconds; if an indentation in the soft tissue is left after the finger is removed, pedal edema is present.

Other symptoms of congestive heart failure include weight gain, dyspnea on exertion, and general weakness.

Patients with congestive heart failure who are under a physician's care usually are on low-sodium diets to reduce fluid retention and are receiving diuretics to reduce intravascular volume; cardiac glycosides, such as digoxin, to improve cardiac efficiency; and sometimes afterload-reducing drugs, such as nitrates, beta-blockers, or calcium slow-channel blockers, to control the amount of work the heart is required to do. In addition, patients with chronic atrial fibrillation caused by hypertrophic cardiomyopathy are usually prescribed anticoagulants.

Patients with congestive heart failure that is well compensated through dietary and drug therapy can safely undergo ambulatory oral surgery. The anxiety-reduction protocol and supplemental oxygen are helpful. Patients with orthopnea should not be placed supine during any procedure. Surgery for patients with uncompensated hypertrophic cardiomyopathy is best deferred until compensation is achieved or procedures can be performed in the hospital setting (Box 1-12).

PULMONARY PROBLEMS

ASTHMA.   When a patient relates a history of asthma, the dentist should first determine through further questioning whether the patient truly has asthma or has a respiratory problem such as allergic rhinitis that is less significant for dental care. True asthma involves the episodic narrowing of small airways, which produces wheezing and dyspnea as a result of chemical, infectious, immunologic, or emotional

◇ Box 1-12 ◇

> ### Management of patient with congestive heart failure (hypertrophic cardiomyopathy)
>
> 1. Defer treatment until heart function has been medically improved and physician believes treatment is possible.
> 2. Use anxiety-reduction protocol.
> 3. Administer supplemental oxygen.
> 4. Avoid supine position.
> 5. Consider referral to oral and maxillofacial surgeon.

◇ Box 1-13 ◇

> ### Management of asthmatic patient
>
> 1. Defer dental treatment until asthma is well controlled and patient has no signs of a respiratory tract infection.
> 2. Listen to chest with stethoscope to detect wheezing before major oral surgical procedures or sedation.
> 3. Use anxiety-reduction protocol, including nitrous oxide, but avoid use of respiratory depressants.
> 4. In children, consult physician about possible use of preoperative cromolyn sodium.
> 5. If patient is or has been chronically on corticosteroids, prophylax for adrenal insufficiency (see p. 16).
> 6. Keep a bronchodilator-containing inhaler easily accessible.
> 7. Avoid use of NSAIDs in susceptible patients.

stimulation or a combination of these. The patient with asthma should be questioned concerning precipitating factors, frequency and severity of attacks, medications used, and response to medications. The severity of attacks can often be gauged by the need for emergency room visits and hospital admissions. Asthmatic patients should be questioned specifically about aspirin allergy because of the relatively high frequency of this type of allergy in asthmatic patients.

Patients with asthma are placed on medications by their physicians based on the frequency, severity, and causes of their disease. Patients with severe asthma require xanthine-derived bronchodilators, such as theophylline, and corticosteroids. Cromolyn sodium may be used to protect against acute attacks, but it is ineffective once bronchospasm occurs. Many patients carry sympathomimetic amines such as epinephrine or metaproterenol in an aerosol form that can be self-administered if wheezing begins.

Oral surgical management of the patient with asthma involves recognition of the role of anxiety in bronchospasm initiation and of the potential adrenal suppression in patients receiving corticosteroid therapy (see p. 11). Elective oral surgery should be deferred if a respiratory tract infection or wheezing is present. When oral surgery is performed, an anxiety-reduction protocol is followed, and if the patient takes steroids, the patient's primary care physician should be consulted concerning the possible need for corticosteroid augmentation during the perioperative period. Nitrous oxide is safe to administer to people with asthma and is especially indicated for patients whose asthma is triggered by anxiety. The patient's own inhaler should be available during surgery, and drugs such as injectable epinephrine and theophylline should be kept in an emergency kit. The use of nonsteroidal inflammatory drugs (NSAIDs) should be avoided, because they often precipitate asthma attacks in susceptible individuals (Box 1-13).

CHRONIC OBSTRUCTIVE PULMONARY DISEASE. Chronic obstructive and restrictive pulmonary diseases are usually grouped together and called chronic obstructive pulmonary disease (COPD). In the past the terms *emphysema* and *bronchitis* were used to describe clinical manifestations of COPD, but COPD has been recognized to be a mixture of pathologic pulmonary problems. COPD is usually caused by long-term exposure to pulmonary irritants, such as tobacco smoke, that cause metaplasia of pulmonary airway tissue. Airways are disrupted, lose their elastic properties, and become obstructed because of mucosal edema, excessive secretions, and bronchospasm, leading to the clinical manifestations of COPD. Patients with COPD frequently become dyspneic during mild-to-moderate exertion. They have a chronic cough that produces large amounts of thick secretions, frequent respiratory tract infections, and barrel-shaped chests, and they may purse their lips to breathe and have audible wheezing during breathing.

Patients with significant COPD are usually placed on bronchodilators such as theophylline and, in more severe cases, on corticosteroids. Only in the most severe chronic cases is supplemental portable oxygen used.

When patients with COPD who are receiving corticosteroids are treated, the dentist should consider the use of additional supplementation before surgery. Sedatives, hypnotics, and narcotics that depress respiration should be avoided. Patients may need to be kept in an upright sitting position in the dental chair to enable them to better handle their commonly copious pulmonary secretions. Finally, supplemental oxygen during surgery should not be used in patients with severe COPD unless the physician advises it. In contrast with healthy people in whom an elevated arterial CO_2 level is the major stimulation to breathing, the patient with COPD becomes acclimated to elevated arterial CO_2 levels and comes to depend entirely on depressed arterial oxygen levels to stimulate breathing. If the arterial oxygen concentration is elevated by the administration of oxygen in a high concentration, the hypoxia-based respiratory stimulation is removed and the patient's respiratory rate may become seriously slow (Box 1-14).

RENAL PROBLEMS

RENAL DIALYSIS. Patients requiring periodic renal dialysis need special consideration during oral surgical care. Chronic dialysis treatment requires the presence of an arteriovenous shunt (a large, surgically created junction

◇ Box 1-14 ◇

Management of patient with chronic obstructive pulmonary disease (COPD)

1. Defer treatment until lung function has improved and treatment is possible.
2. Listen to chest bilaterally with stethoscope to determine adequacy of breath sounds.
3. Use anxiety-reduction protocol, but avoid use of respiratory depressants.
4. If patient is on chronic oxygen supplementation, continue at prescribed flow rate. If patient is not on supplemental oxygen therapy, consult physician before administering oxygen.
5. If patient chronically receives corticosteroid therapy, manage patient for adrenal insufficiency (see p. 16).
6. Avoid placing patient in supine position until confident that patient can tolerate it.
7. Keep a bronchodilator-containing inhaler readily accessible.
8. Closely monitor respiratory and heart rates.
9. Schedule afternoon appointments to allow for clearing of secretions.

◇ Box 1-15 ◇

Management of patients with renal insufficiency and patients receiving hemodialysis

1. Avoid the use of drugs that depend on renal metabolism or excretion. Modify the dose if such drugs are necessary.
2. Avoid the use of nephrotoxic drugs, such as NSAIDs.
3. Defer dental care until the day after dialysis has been given.
4. Consult physician concerning use of prophylactic antibiotics.
5. Monitor blood pressure and heart rate.
6. Look for signs of secondary hyperparathyroidism.
7. Consider hepatitis B screening before dental treatment. Take hepatitis precautions if unable to screen for hepatitis.

between an artery and vein), which allows easy vascular access, and heparin administration, which allows blood to move through the dialysis equipment without clotting.

Consideration should be given to the use of prophylactic antibiotics during oral surgery to prevent infection of the shunt. The shunt should not be used by the dentist for venous access except in an emergency.

Elective oral surgery is best undertaken the day after a dialysis treatment has been performed. This allows the heparin used during dialysis to disappear and the patient to be in the best physiologic state with respect to intravascular volume and metabolic by-products.

Drugs that depend on renal metabolism or excretion should be avoided or used in modified doses to prevent systemic toxicity. Drugs removed during dialysis will also need special dosing regimens. Relatively nephrotoxic drugs, such as NSAIDs, should also be avoided in patients with compromised kidneys.

Because of the higher incidence of hepatitis in renal dialysis patients, dentists should take the necessary precautions. The altered appearance of bone caused by secondary hyperparathyroidism in patients with renal failure should also be noted. Metabolic radiolucencies should not be mistaken for dental disease (Box 1-15).

RENAL TRANSPLANT OR TRANSPLANT OF OTHER ORGANS.
The patient requiring oral surgery following renal or other major organ transplantation is usually receiving a variety of drugs to preserve the function of the transplanted tissue. These patients receive corticosteroids and may need supplemental corticosteroids in the perioperative period (see p. 17).

Most of these patients also receive immunosuppressive agents that may cause otherwise self-limiting infections to become severe. Therefore more aggressive use of antibiotics and early hospitalization for infections are warranted. The patient's primary care physician should be consulted concerning the need for prophylactic antibiotics.

Cyclosporine A, an immunosuppressive drug administered after organ transplantation, may cause gingival hyperplasia. The dentist performing oral surgery should recognize this so as not to wrongly attribute gingival hyperplasia entirely to hygiene problems.

Patients who have had renal transplants occasionally have problems with severe hypertension. Vital signs should be obtained before oral surgery is performed in these patients (Box 1-16).

HYPERTENSION.
Chronically elevated blood pressure for which the etiology is unknown is called *essential hypertension.* Mild or moderate hypertension (systolic pressure of less than 200 or diastolic pressure of less than 110) is usually not a problem in ambulatory oral surgical care.

Care of the hypertensive patient includes use of an anxiety-reduction protocol and monitoring of vital signs. Epinephrine-containing local anesthetics should be used cautiously, and, after surgery, patients should be advised to seek medical care for their hypertension.

Elective oral surgery for patients with severe hypertension (systolic pressure of 200 or more or diastolic pressure of 110 or more) should be postponed until the pressure is controlled. Emergency oral surgery should be performed in the hospital to allow the pressure to be controlled acutely (Box 1-17).

HEPATIC DISORDERS
IMPAIRED LIVER FUNCTION.
The patient with severe liver damage resulting from infectious disease, ethanol abuse, or vascular or biliary congestion requires special consideration before oral surgery is performed. An alteration of dosage or avoidance of drugs that require hepatic metabolism may be necessary.

The production of vitamin K–dependent coagulation

◇ Box 1-16 ◇

Management of patient with renal transplant*

1. Defer treatment until primary care physician or transplant surgeon clears patient for dental care.
2. Avoid use of nephrotoxic drugs.
3. Consider use of supplemental corticosteroids.
4. Monitor blood pressure.
5. Consider hepatitis B screening before dental care. Take hepatitis precautions if unable to screen for hepatitis.
6. Watch for presence of cyclosporin A–induced gingival hyperplasia. Emphasize importance of oral hygiene.
7. Consider use of prophylactic antibiotics, particularly for patients on immunosuppressive agents.

*Most of these recommendations apply to patients with other transplanted organs. In patients with other transplanted organs, avoid the use of drugs toxic to that organ.

◇ Box 1-17 ◇

Management of hypertensive patient

Mild-to-moderate hypertension (systolic >140; diastolic >90)
1. Recommend that the patient seek the primary care physician's guidance for medical therapy of hypertension.
2. Monitor the patient's blood pressure at each visit and whenever administration of epinephrine-containing local anesthetic surpasses 0.04 mg during a single visit.
3. Use an anxiety-reduction protocol.
4. Avoid rapid posture changes in patients taking drugs that cause vasodilation.
5. Avoid administration of sodium-containing intravenous solutions.

Severe hypertension (systolic >200; diastolic >110)
1. Defer elective dental treatment until hypertension is better controlled.
2. Consider referral to oral and maxillofacial surgeon for emergency problems.

factors (II, VII, IX, X) may be depressed in very severe liver disease; therefore obtaining a prothrombin time (PT) or partial thromboplastin time (PTT) may be useful before surgery in patients with more severe liver disease. Portal hypertension caused by liver disease also may cause hypersplenism, a sequestering of platelets causing thrombocytopenia. This problem is revealed by finding a prolonged Ivy bleeding time. Patients with severe liver dysfunction may require hospitalization for dental surgery, because their decreased ability to metabolize the nitrogen in swallowed blood may cause encephalopathy. Finally, unless documented otherwise, a patient with liver disease should be presumed to carry hepatitis virus (Box 1-18).

◇ Box 1-18 ◇

Management of patient with hepatic insufficiency

1. Attempt to learn the cause of the liver problem; if the cause is hepatitis B, take usual precautions.
2. Avoid drugs requiring hepatic metabolism or excretion; if their use is necessary, modify dose.
3. Screen patients with severe liver disease for bleeding disorders with platelet count, PT, PTT, and Ivy bleeding time.
4. Attempt to avoid situations in which the patient might swallow large amounts of blood.

ENDOCRINE DISORDERS

DIABETES MELLITUS. Diabetes mellitus is caused by an underproduction of insulin, a resistance of insulin receptors in end-organs to the effects of insulin, or both. Diabetes commonly is divided into insulin-dependent and non–insulin-dependent diabetes. Insulin-dependent diabetes usually begins in children or teenagers. The major problem in this form of diabetes is an underproduction of insulin, which results in the inability of the patient to use glucose. The serum glucose rises above the level at which renal reabsorption of all glucose can take place, causing glucosuria. The osmotic effect of the glucose solute results in polyuria, stimulating patient thirst and causing polydipsia (frequent consumption of liquids). In addition, carbohydrate metabolism is altered, leading to fat breakdown and the production of ketone bodies. This can produce ketoacidosis and the attendant tachypnea with somnolence and eventually coma.

People with insulin-dependent diabetes must strike a balance among caloric intake, exercise, and insulin administration. Any decrease in regular caloric intake or increase in activity, metabolic rate, or insulin dose can lead to hypoglycemia and vice versa.

Patients with non–insulin-dependent diabetes usually produce insulin but in insufficient amounts because of decreased insulin activity, insulin receptor resistance, or both. This form of diabetes begins in adulthood, is exacerbated by obesity, and usually does not require insulin therapy. It is treated by weight control, dietary restrictions, and the use of oral hypoglycemics. Insulin is required only if the patient is unable to maintain acceptable serum glucose levels using the usual therapeutic measures. Severe hyperglycemia in non–insulin-dependent diabetic patients rarely produces ketoacidosis but leads to a hyperosmolar state with altered levels of consciousness.

Short-term mild-to-moderate hyperglycemia usually is not a significant problem for people with diabetes. Therefore when an oral surgical procedure is planned it is best to err on the side of hyperglycemia rather than hypoglycemia; that is, it is best to avoid an excessive insulin dose and to give a glucose source. Ambulatory oral surgery procedures should be performed early in the day, using an anxiety-reduction program. If intravenous sedation is not being used, the patient should be asked to eat a normal meal and take the usual

◇ Table 1-1. Types of insulin*

Onset and duration of action	Name	Peak effect of action (hr after injection)	Duration of action (hr)
Fast (F)	Regular	2-3	6
	Semilente	3-6	12
Intermediate (I)	Globin zinc	6-8	18
	NPH	8-12	24
	Lente	8-12	24
Long (L)	Protamine zinc	16-24	36
	Ultralente	20-30	36

*Insulin sources are pork—*F, I*; beef—*F, I, L*; beef-pork—*F, I, L*; and recombinant DNA—*F, I, L*.

morning amount of regular insulin and a half dose of NPH insulin (Table 1-1). The patient's vital signs should be monitored, and, if signs of hypoglycemia, such as hypotension, hunger, drowsiness, nausea, diaphoresis, tachycardia, or a mood change occur, an oral or intravenous supply of glucose should be administered. If the patient temporarily will be unable to eat after surgery, any delayed-action (most commonly NPH) insulin normally taken in the morning should be eliminated and restarted only after normal caloric intake resumes. The patient should be advised to monitor urine or serum glucose closely for the first 24 hours postoperatively. Some dental offices have their own serum glucose-monitoring equipment to use to quickly test diabetic patients while in the office.

If a patient must miss a meal before an oral surgical procedure, the patient should be told not to take any morning insulin until intravenous glucose in water is started in the office. One half of the usual dose of regular insulin and no NPH insulin should be used in this situation. Regular insulin should then be used, with the dose based on serum or urinary glucose monitoring and as directed by the patient's physician. Once the patient has resumed normal dietary habits, the usual insulin regimen can be restarted.

People with well-controlled diabetes are no more susceptible to infections than people without diabetes, but they have more difficulty containing infections. This is caused by altered leukocyte function, as well as by other factors that affect the body's ability to control an infection. Difficulty in containing infections is more significant in people with poorly controlled diabetes. Therefore elective oral surgery should be deferred in patients with poorly controlled diabetes until control is accomplished. However, if an emergency situation or a serious oral infection exists in any person with diabetes, consideration should be given to hospital admission to allow for acute control of the hyperglycemia and aggressive management of the infection. Many clinicians also believe that prophylactic antibiotics should be given routinely to patients with diabetes undergoing any surgical procedure. However, this position is controversial (Box 1-19).

ADRENAL INSUFFICIENCY. Adrenal insufficiency may be caused by diseases of the adrenal cortex. Symptoms of primary adrenal insufficiency include weakness, weight loss,

---

◇ Box 1-19 ◇

Management of patient with diabetes

Insulin-dependent diabetes

1. Defer surgery until diabetes is well controlled; consult physician.
2. Schedule an early morning appointment; avoid lengthy appointments.
3. Use anxiety-reduction protocol, but avoid deep sedation techniques in outpatients.
4. Monitor pulse, respiration, and blood pressure before, during, and after surgery.
5. Maintain verbal contact with patient during surgery.
6. If patient must not eat or drink before oral surgery and will have difficulty eating after surgery, instruct patient to not take the usual dose of regular or NPH insulin; start an IV with an D_5W drip at 150 mL/hr.
7. If allowed, have the patient eat a normal breakfast before surgery and take the usual dose of regular insulin but only half the dose of NPH insulin.
8. Advise patients not to resume normal insulin dosage until they are able to return to usual level of caloric intake and activity level.
9. Consult physician if any questions concerning modification of the insulin regimen arise.
10. Watch for signs of hypoglycemia.
11. Treat infections aggressively.

Non–insulin-dependent diabetes

1. Defer surgery until diabetes is well controlled.
2. Schedule an early morning appointment; avoid lengthy appointments.
3. Use an anxiety-reduction protocol.
4. Monitor pulse, respiration, and blood pressure before, during, and after surgery.
5. Maintain verbal contact with the patient during surgery.
6. If patient must not eat or drink before oral surgery and will have difficulty eating after surgery, instruct patient to skip any oral hypoglycemic medications that day.
7. If patient can eat before and after surgery, instruct him or her to eat a normal breakfast and to take the usual dose of hypoglycemic agent.
8. Watch for signs of hypoglycemia.
9. Treat infections aggressively.

---

fatigue, and hyperpigmentation of skin and mucous membranes. However, the most common cause of adrenal insufficiency is chronic therapeutic corticosteroid administration (secondary adrenal insufficiency). Patients regularly taking corticosteroids are characterized by having a "moon facies," a "buffalo hump," and thin, translucent skin. Their inability to increase endogenous corticosteroid levels in response to physiologic stress may cause them to become hypotensive, syncopal, nauseated, and feverish during complex, prolonged oral surgery.

◇ Box 1-20 ◇

Management of patient with adrenal suppression who requires major oral surgery*

If patient is currently on corticosteroids:
1. Use anxiety-reduction protocol.
2. Monitor pulse and blood pressure before, during, and after surgery.
3. Instruct patient to double usual daily dose on the day before, day of, and day after surgery.
4. On second postsurgical day, advise the patient to return to a usual steroid dose.

If the patient is not currently on steroids, but has received at least 20 mg of hydrocortisone (cortisol or equivalent) for more than 2 weeks within past year:
1. Use anxiety-reduction protocol.
2. Monitor pulse and blood pressure before, during, and after surgery.
3. Instruct patient to take 60 mg of hydrocortisone (or equivalent) the day before and the morning of surgery, or dentist should administer 60 mg of hydrocortisone (or equivalent) intramuscularly or intravenously before complex surgery.
4. On first 2 postsurgical days, dose should be dropped to 40 mg and dropped to 20 mg for 3 days thereafter. Can cease administration of supplemental steroids 6 days after surgery.

*If a major surgical procedure is planned, strongly consider hospitalizing the patient. Consult the patient's physician if any questions arise concerning the need for or the dose of supplemental corticosteroids.

If a patient with primary or secondary adrenal suppression requires oral surgery, the primary care physician should be consulted regarding the potential need for supplemental steroids. In general, minor procedures require only the use of an anxiety-reduction protocol. However, more complicated procedures in an adrenally suppressed patient usually require steroid supplementation by administration of double the usual dose just before the surgery or by administration of 60 mg of hydrocortisone presurgically with a decrease of the amount to 40 mg the first 2 days after surgery, 20 mg the next 3 days, and the usual dose thereafter (Box 1-20).

HYPERTHYROIDISM. The thyroid dysfunction of primary significance in oral surgery is thyrotoxicosis, because it is the only thyroid disease in which an acute crisis can occur. Thyrotoxicosis is the result of an excess of circulating triiodothyronine (T_3) and thyronine (T_4), which is caused most frequently by Graves' disease, a multinodular goiter, or a thyroid adenoma. The early manifestations of excessive thyroid hormone production include fine, brittle hair, hyperpigmentation of skin, excessive sweating, tachycardia, palpitations, weight loss, and emotional lability. Patients frequently, although not invariably, develop exophthalmos (a bulging of the eyes caused by increases of fat in the orbits). If hyperthyroidism is not recognized early, the patient may

◇ Box 1-21 ◇

Management of patient with hyperthyroidism

1. Defer surgery until thyroid dysfunction is well controlled.
2. Monitor pulse and blood pressure before, during, and after surgery.
3. Limit amount of epinephrine used.

develop heart failure. The diagnosis is made by the demonstration of elevated circulating thyroid hormones, using direct or indirect laboratory techniques.

Thyrotoxic patients usually are treated with agents that block thyroid hormone synthesis and release, with a thyroidectomy, or with both. However, patients left untreated or incompletely treated can develop a thyrotoxic crisis, caused by the sudden release of large quantities of preformed thyroid hormones. Early symptoms of a thyrotoxic crisis include restlessness, nausea, and abdominal cramps. Later symptoms are a high fever, diaphoresis, tachycardia, and, eventually, cardiac decompensation. The patient becomes stuporous and hypotensive, with death often following if no intervention occurs.

The dentist may be able to diagnose previously unrecognized hyperthyroidism by taking a complete medical history and performing a careful examination of the patient, including thyroid inspection and palpation. If severe hyperthyroidism is suspected from the history and inspection, the gland should not be palpated, because that manipulation alone can trigger a crisis. Patients suspected of having a thyroid abnormality should be referred for medical evaluation before any oral surgery.

Patients with treated thyroid disease can safely undergo ambulatory oral surgery. However, if a patient is found to have an oral infection, the primary care physician should be notified, particularly if the patient manifests signs of hyperthyroidism. Atropine and excessive amounts of epinephrine-containing solutions should be avoided if a patient is thought to have incompletely treated hyperthyroidism (Box 1-21).

HYPOTHYROIDISM. The dentist can play a role in the initial recognition of hypothyroidism. Early symptoms of hypothyroidism include fatigue, constipation, weight gain, hoarseness, headaches, arthralgia, menstrual disturbances, edema, dry skin, and brittle hair and fingernails. If the symptoms of hypothyroidism are mild, no modification of dental therapy is required.

HEMATOLOGIC PROBLEMS

HEREDITARY COAGULOPATHIES. Patients with inherited bleeding disorders usually are aware of their problem, allowing the clinician to take the necessary precautions before any surgical procedure. However, in many patients, prolonged bleeding after the extraction of a tooth may be the first evidence that a bleeding disorder exists. Therefore all patients should be questioned concerning coagulation following

◇ Box 1-22 ◇

Management of patient with a coagulopathy*

1. Defer surgery until a hematologist is consulted about the patient's management.
2. Obtain baseline coagulation tests as indicated (PT, PTT, Ivy bleeding time, platelet count) and a hepatitis screen.
3. Schedule the patient in a manner that allows surgery soon after any coagulation-correcting measures have been taken (that is, after platelet transfusion, factor replacement, or aminocaproic acid administration).
4. Augment clotting during surgery with the use of topical coagulation-promoting substances, sutures, and well-placed pressure packs.
5. Monitor the wound for 2 hours to ensure that a good initial clot forms.
6. Instruct the patient in ways to prevent dislodgment of the clot and in what to do should bleeding restart.
7. Avoid prescribing NSAIDs.
8. Take hepatitis precautions during surgery.

*Patients with severe coagulopathies who require major surgery should be hospitalized.

previous injuries and surgery. A history of nosebleeds, easy bruising, hematuria, heavy menstrual bleeding, and spontaneous bleeding should alert the dentist to the possible need for a presurgical laboratory coagulation screening. A prothrombin time (PT) is used to test the extrinsic pathway factors (I, II, V, VII, and X), whereas a partial thromboplastin time (PTT) is used to detect intrinsic pathway factors. Platelet inadequacy is usually manifested by easy bruising and is evaluated by a bleeding time and platelet count. If a coagulopathy is suspected, the primary care physician or a hematologist should be consulted about more-refined testing to better define the cause of the bleeding disorder and to help manage the patient in the perioperative period.

The management of patients with coagulopathies who require oral surgery depends on the nature of the bleeding disorder. Specific factor deficiencies, such as hemophilia A, B, or C or von Willebrand's disease, usually are managed by the perioperative administration of factor replacement and by the use of an antifibrinolytic agent, such as aminocaproic acid (Amicar). The physician decides the form in which factor replacement is given based on the degree of factor deficiency and on the patient's history of factor replacement. Patients who receive factor replacement sometimes contract hepatitis or the human immunodeficiency virus. Therefore appropriate staff protection measures should be taken during oral surgery.

Platelet problems may be quantitative or qualitative. Quantitative platelet deficiency may be a cyclic problem, and the hematologist can help determine the proper timing of elective surgery. Patients with a chronically low platelet count can be given platelet transfusions. Counts usually dip below 50,000 before abnormal postoperative bleeding occurs. The hematologist may wish to withhold platelet transfusion until

postoperative bleeding becomes a problem, if the platelet count is between 20,000 and 50,000. However, platelet transfusions may be given to patients with counts higher than 50,000, if a qualitative platelet problem exists. Platelet counts under 20,000 usually require presurgical platelet transfusion. Local anesthesia should be given by local infiltration rather than by field blocks to lessen the likelihood of damaging large blood vessels, which may lead to prolonged postinjection bleeding and hematoma formation. Consideration should be given to the use of topical coagulation-promoting substances in oral wounds, and the patient should be instructed in ways to avoid dislodging blood clots once they have formed (Box 1-22).

THERAPEUTIC ANTICOAGULATION. Therapeutic anticoagulation is administered to patients with thrombogenic implanted devices, such as prosthetic heart valves; with thrombogenic cardiovascular problems, such as atrial fibrillation or postmyocardial infarction; or with a need for extracorporeal blood flow, such as for hemodialysis. Patients may also take drugs with anticoagulant properties, such as aspirin, as a secondary effect.

When elective oral surgery is necessary, the need for continuous anticoagulation must be weighed against the need for blood clotting after surgery. This decision should be made in consultation with the patient's primary care physician. Drugs such as aspirin usually can be safely withdrawn temporarily to allow surgery. Generally, 1 week after aspirin is stopped, its antiplatelet effects become clinically insignificant. Patients on heparin usually can have their surgery delayed until the circulating heparin is inactive (6 hours if heparin is given intravenously, 24 hours if given subcutaneously [SC]). Protamine sulfate, which reverses the effects of heparin, also can be used if emergency oral surgery cannot be deferred until heparin is naturally inactivated.

Patients requiring Coumadin for anticoagulation who also need elective oral surgery benefit from close cooperation between the patient's physician and dentist. Coumadin has a 2- to 3-day delay in the onset of action; therefore alterations of Coumadin anticoagulant effects appear several days after the dose is changed. The PT is used to gauge the anticoagulant action of Coumadin. Most physicians allow the PT to drop to 1½ times control during the perioperative period, which usually allows sufficient coagulation for safe surgery. Patients should stop taking Coumadin 2 or 3 days before the planned surgery. On the morning of surgery, the PT should be checked; if it is between 1½ and 2 times the control level, surgery can be performed. If the PT is still greater than 2 times control, surgery should be delayed until the PT approaches 1½ times control. Surgical wounds should be dressed with thrombogenic substances, and the patient should be given instruction in promoting clot retention. Coumadin therapy can be resumed the day of surgery (Box 1-23).

NEUROLOGIC DISORDERS

SEIZURE DISORDER.
Patients with a history of seizures should be questioned about the frequency, type, duration, and

◇ Box 1-23 ◇

Management of patient who is therapeutically anticoagulated

Patients receiving aspirin or other platelet-inhibiting drugs
1. Consult physician to determine the safety of stopping the anticoagulant drug for several days.
2. Defer surgery until the platelet-inhibiting drugs have been stopped for 5 days.
3. Take extra measures during and after surgery to help promote clot formation and retention.
4. Restart drug therapy on the day after surgery if no bleeding is present.

Patients receiving warfarin (Coumadin)
1. Consult the patient's physician to determine the safety of allowing the PT to fall to 1½ times control for a few days.*
2. Obtain the baseline PT.
3. (a) If the PT is 1 to 1½ times greater than control, proceed with surgery and skip to step 6. (b) If the PT is more than 1½ times greater than control, go to step 4.
4. Stop warfarin approximately 2 days before surgery.
5. Check the PT daily, and proceed with surgery on the day when the PT falls to 1½ times control.
6. Take extra measures during and after surgery, to help promote clot formation and retention.
7. Restart warfarin on the day of surgery.

Patients receiving heparin
1. Consult the patient's physician to determine the safety of stopping heparin for the perioperative period.
2. Defer surgery until at least 6 hours after the heparin is stopped or reverse heparin with protamine.
3. Restart heparin once a good clot has formed.

*If the patient's physician feels it is unsafe to allow the PT to fall, the patient must be hospitalized for conversion from warfarin to heparin anticoagulation during the perioperative period.

◇ Box 1-24 ◇

Management of patient with a seizure disorder

1. Defer surgery until the seizures are well controlled.
2. Consider having serum levels of antiseizure medications measured if patient compliance is questionable.
3. Use anxiety-reduction protocol.
4. Avoid hypoglycemia and fatigue.

sequelae of seizures. Seizures can be the result of ethanol withdrawal, high fever, hypoglycemia, or traumatic brain damage or can be idiopathic. The dentist should inquire about medications used to control the seizure disorder, particularly about patient compliance and any recent measurement of serum levels. The patient's physician should be consulted concerning the seizure history and to establish whether there is any reason to defer oral surgery. If the seizure disorder is well controlled, standard oral surgical care can be delivered without any further precautions (except for the use of an anxiety-reduction protocol) (Box 1-24). If good control cannot be obtained, the patient should be referred to an oral and maxillofacial surgeon for treatment under deep sedation in the office or hospital.

ETHANOLISM (ALCOHOLISM). Patients volunteering a history of ethanol abuse or in whom ethanolism is suspected and then confirmed through means other than history-taking require special consideration before surgery. The primary problems ethanol abusers have in relation to dental care are hepatic insufficiency, ethanol and medication interaction, and withdrawal phenomena. Hepatic insufficiency has already been discussed (see p. 16). Ethanol interacts with many of the sedatives used for anxiety control during oral surgery. The interaction usually potentiates sedation and suppresses the gag reflex.

Finally, ethanol abusers may undergo withdrawal phenomena in the perioperative period if they have acutely lowered their daily ethanol intake before seeking dental care. This may manifest by mild agitation, tremors, seizure, diaphoresis, or, more rarely, delirium tremens with hallucinosis, marked agitation, and circulatory collapse.

Patients requiring oral surgery who manifest signs of severe alcoholic liver disease or signs of ethanol withdrawal should be treated in the hospital setting. Liver function tests, a coagulation profile, and medical consultation before surgery are desirable. In patients able to be treated on an ambulatory basis, the dosage of drugs metabolized in the liver should be altered and the patients should be monitored closely for signs of oversedation.

MANAGEMENT OF PREGNANT AND POSTPARTUM PATIENTS ◇

PREGNANCY

Although not a disease state, pregnancy is still a situation in which special considerations are necessary when oral surgery is required. The primary concern when providing care for a pregnant patient is the prevention of genetic damage to the fetus. Two areas of oral surgical management with potential for creating fetal damage are dental radiography and drug administration. It is virtually impossible to perform an oral surgical procedure properly with neither radiographs nor the administration of medications; one option therefore is to defer any elective oral surgery until after delivery, to avoid fetal risk. Frequently, temporary measures can be used to delay surgery.

However, if surgery during pregnancy cannot be postponed, efforts should be made to lessen fetal exposure to teratogenic factors. In the case of irradiation, this is accomplished by using protective aprons and taking periapical films

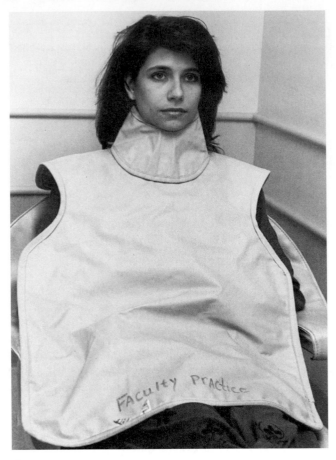

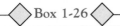

◇ Figure 1-5 ◇

Proper lead apron shielding for dental radiography. Notice use of thyroid protection.

◇ Box 1-25 ◇

Management of pregnant patients

1. Defer surgery until after delivery if possible.
2. Consult the patient's obstetrician if surgery cannot be delayed.
3. Avoid dental radiographs unless information about tooth roots or bone is necessary for proper dental care. If radiographs must be taken, use proper shielding.
4. Avoid the use of drugs with teratogenic potential. Use local anesthetics when anesthesia is necessary.
5. Use at least 50% oxygen if nitrous oxide sedation is used.
6. Avoid keeping the patient in the supine position for long periods, to prevent vena cava compression.
7. Allow the patient to take frequent trips to the rest room.

◇ Box 1-26 ◇

Dental medications to avoid in pregnant patients

Aspirin and other NSAIDs
Carbamazepine
Chloral hydrate (if chronically used)
Chlordiazepoxide
Corticosteroids
Diazepam and other benzodiazepines
Diphenhydramine hydrochloride (if chronically used)
Morphine
Nitrous oxide (if exposure is greater than 9 hr/week or O_2 is less than 50%)
Pentazocine hydrochloride
Phenobarbital
Promethazine hydrochloride
Propoxyphene
Tetracyclines

---

of only the areas requiring surgery (Figure 1-5). The list of drugs thought to pose little risk to the fetus is relatively small. For purposes of oral surgery the following drugs are believed least likely to harm a fetus when used in moderate amounts: lidocaine, bupivacaine, acetaminophen, codeine, penicillin, and erythromycin. Although aspirin is otherwise safe to use, it should not be given late in the third trimester because of its anticoagulant property. All sedative drugs are best avoided in pregnant patients. Nitrous oxide should not be used during the first trimester but if necessary can be used in the second and third trimesters as long as it is delivered with at least 50% oxygen (Boxes 1-25 and 1-26). The Food and Drug Administration (FDA) created a system of drug categorization based on the known degree of risk to the human fetus posed by particular drugs. The clinician required to give a medication to a pregnant patient should check that the drug falls into an acceptable risk category before administering it to the patient (Box 1-27).

Pregnancy can be emotionally, as well as physiologically, stressful; therefore an anxiety-reduction protocol is recommended. Patient vital signs should be obtained, with particular attention paid to any elevation in blood pressure (a possible sign of preeclampsia). A patient nearing delivery may need special positioning of the chair during care, because if the patient is placed in a nearly supine position, the uterine contents may cause compression of the inferior vena cava, compromising venous return to the heart and thereby cardiac output. The patient may need to be in a more upright position or with her trunk turned slightly to one side during surgery. Frequent breaks to allow the patient to void are commonly necessary late in pregnancy because of fetal pressure on the urinary bladder. Before performing any oral surgery on a pregnant patient, her obstetrician should be consulted.

◇ Box 1-27 ◇

Food and Drug Administration Pregnancy Drug-Risk Categories

Category A:
Controlled studies in women fail to demonstrate a fetal risk in the first trimester (and there is no evidence of risk in later trimesters), and the possibility of fetal harm appears remote.

Category B:
Either animal reproduction studies have not demonstrated a fetal risk and there are no controlled studies in pregnant women, or animal reproduction studies have shown an adverse effect (other than decreased fertility) that was not confirmed in controlled studies on women in the first trimester (and there is no evidence of a risk in later trimesters).

Category C:
Either studies in animals have revealed adverse fetal effects and there are no controlled studies in humans, or studies in women and animals are not available. Drugs in this category should only be given if safer alternatives are not available and if the potential benefit justifies the *known fetal risk(s)*.

Category D:
Positive evidence of human fetal risk exists, but benefits for pregnant women may be acceptable despite the risk, as in life-threatening or serious diseases for which safer drugs cannot be used or are ineffective. An appropriate statement must appear in the "warnings" section of the labeling of drugs in this category.

Category X:
Either studies in animals or humans have demonstrated fetal abnormalities, or there is evidence of fetal risk based on human experience, or both, and the risk of using the drug in pregnant women clearly outweighs any possible benefit. The drug is contraindicated in women who are or may become pregnant. An appropriate statement must appear in the "contraindications" section of the labeling of drugs in this category.

POSTPARTUM

Special considerations should be taken when providing oral surgical care for the postpartum patient who is breast-feeding.

◇ **Table 1-2.** Effect of dental medications in lactating mothers

No apparent clinical effects in breast-feeding infants	Potentially harmful clinical effects in breast-feeding infants
Acetaminophen	Ampicillin
Antihistamines	Aspirin
Cephalexin	Atropine
Codeine	Barbiturates
Erythromycin	Chloral hydrate
Fluoride	Corticosteroids
Lidocaine	Diazepam
Meperidine	Metronidazole
Oxacillin	Penicillin
Pentazocine	Propoxyphene
	Tetracyclines

Avoiding drugs that are known to enter breast milk and to be potentially harmful to infants is prudent. The patient's obstetrician or the infant's pediatrician can provide guidance. Information about some drugs is provided in Table 1-2. However, in general, all the drugs common in oral surgical care are safe to use in moderate doses, with the exception of corticosteroids, aminoglycosides, and tetracyclines, which should not be used.

BIBLIOGRAPHY

Gage TW, Pickett FA: *Mosby's 1997 Dental drug reference,* St Louis, 1997, Mosby.

Halstead CL et al: *Physical evaluation of the dental patient,* St Louis, 1982, Mosby.

Hupp JR, Williams TP, Vallerand WP: *The 5 Minute clinical consult for dental professionals,* Baltimore, 1996, Williams & Wilkins.

Little JW et al: *Dental management of the medically compromised patient,* ed 5, St Louis, 1997, Mosby.

Lynch MA, Brightman VJ, Greenberg MS: *Burket's oral medicine,* ed 9, Philadelphia, 1994, JB Lippincott.

Rose LF, Kaye D: *Internal medicine for dentistry,* ed 2, St Louis, 1990.

PREVENTION AND MANAGEMENT OF MEDICAL EMERGENCIES

CHAPTER 2

JAMES R. HUPP

CHAPTER OUTLINE

Medical emergencies in the dental office are, fortunately, relatively rare. The ambulatory nature of dental practice (severely ill patients are usually unable to use ambulatory facilities) is partially responsible. However, the primary reason for the limited frequency of emergencies in dental offices is the nature of dental education, which prepares practitioners to recognize potential problems and manage them before they cause an emergency. This chapter begins with a presentation of the various means of lowering the likelihood of medical emergencies in the dental office. It also details ways to prepare for emergencies and discusses the clinical manifestations and initial management of the more common emergencies.

PREVENTION

An understanding of the relative frequency of emergencies and knowledge of those likely to produce serious morbidity and mortality are important when the dentist sets priorities for preventive measures. A study by Malamed of patients in the dental school setting revealed that hyperventilation, seizures, and hypoglycemia were the three most common emergency situations occurring in patients before, during, or soon after general dental care. These were followed in frequency by vasovagal syncope, angina pectoris, orthostatic hypotension, and hypersensitivity (allergic) reactions.

The incidence of medical emergencies may be higher in patients receiving ambulatory oral surgery when compared with those receiving nonsurgical care because of the following three factors: (1) surgery is more often stress-provoking, (2) commonly, a greater number of medications is administered to patients undergoing surgery, and (3) longer appointments may be necessary when surgery is performed. These factors are well known to increase the likelihood of medical emergencies. Other factors known to increase the potential for emergencies are the age of the patient (very young and old patients being at greater risk), the ability of the medical profession to keep relatively unhealthy people ambulatory and able to seek dental care, and the increasing variety of drugs dentists are able to administer in their offices.

Prevention of medical emergencies is the cornerstone of their management. The first step is risk assessment. This begins with a careful medical evaluation that, in the dental office, primarily involves accurate taking of a medical history, including a review of systems guided by pertinent positive responses in the patient's history. Vital signs should be recorded, and a physical examination, tailored to the patient's medical history and present problem, should be performed. Techniques for this are described in Chapter 1.

Although any patient can have a medical emergency at any time, certain medical conditions predispose patients to medical emergencies in the dental office. These conditions are more liable to turn into an emergency when the patient is physiologically or emotionally stressed. The most common conditions affected or precipitated by anxiety are listed in Box 2-1. Once those patients who are likely to have medical

◇ Box 2-1 ◇

Medical emergencies commonly provoked by anxiety

Angina pectoris
Myocardial infarction
Asthmatic bronchospasm
Adrenal insufficiency (acute)
Severe hypertension

Thyroid storm
Insulin shock
Hyperventilation
Epilepsy

◇ Box 2-2 ◇

Preparation for medical emergencies

1. Personal continuing education in emergency recognition and management
2. Auxiliary staff education in emergency recognition and management
3. Establishment and periodic testing of a system to readily access medical assistance when an emergency occurs
4. Equipping office with supplies necessary for emergency care

◇ Box 2-3 ◇

Basic life support (BLS)

ABCs A Airway
     B Breathing
     C Circulation
Airway obtained and maintained by combination of:
1. Extending head at the neck by tilting forehead back with one hand and lifting neck up with other hand
2. Pushing mandible forward by pressure on the mandibular angles
3. Pulling mandible forward by pulling on anterior mandible
4. Pulling tongue forward, using suture material or instrument to grasp anterior tongue
Breathing provided by one of the following:
1. Mouth-to-mouth or mouth-to-mask ventilation
2. Resuscitation bag ventilation
Circulation provided by external cardiac compressions

emergencies are recognized, the dentist can prevent most problems from occurring by modifying the manner in which oral surgical care is provided.

PREPARATION

Preparedness is the second most important factor after prevention in the management of medical emergencies. Preparation to handle emergencies includes the following: (1) ensuring that the dentist's own education about emergency management is adequate, (2) having an auxiliary staff trained to assist in medical emergencies, (3) establishing a system to gain ready access to other health care providers able to assist during emergencies, and (4) equipping the office with supplies necessary to care for patients having serious problems (Box 2-2).

CONTINUING EDUCATION

Dentists should have received training in dental school in the ways to assess patient risk and to manage medical emergencies. However, because of the rarity of these problems, dentists should seek continuing education in this area, not only to refresh their knowledge but also to learn new ideas concerning medical evaluation and management of emergencies. An important feature of continuing education should be certification in Basic Life Support (BLS) (Box 2-3). Many have recommended that continuing education in medical emergency management be obtained by dentists on an annual basis, with BLS skills update and review obtained annually. Dentists who deliver parenteral sedatives other than nitrous

oxide should be trained in Advanced Cardiac Life Support (ACLS) and have the equipment necessary for ACLS available.

OFFICE STAFF TRAINING

The dentist must ensure that all office personnel are trained to assist in the recognition and management of emergencies. This should include reinforcement by periodic emergency simulations in the office and annual BLS skills renewal and update. The office staff should be preassigned definite responsibilities, so that in the event of a problem each person knows what will be expected during an emergency.

ACCESS TO HELP

The ease of access to other health care providers is variable. It is helpful to seek out individuals with training that would make them useful during a medical emergency. If the dental practice is located near other professional offices, prior arrangement should be made to obtain assistance in the event of an emergency. Not all physicians are well versed in the management of emergencies, and dentists must be selective in the physicians they contact for help during an emergency. Oral-maxillofacial surgeons are a good resource, as are most general surgeons. Ambulances carrying emergency medical technicians (EMTs) are useful to the dentist facing an emergency situation, and most communities now provide easy telephone access to a rapid-response EMT team. Finally, it is important to identify a nearby hospital with a well-staffed emergency care department.

Once the dentist has established who can be of assistance in the event of an emergency, the appropriate phone numbers should be kept readily available. Easily identified lists can be placed on each telephone, or numbers can be entered into the memory of an automatic-dial telephone. The numbers should be called periodically to test their accuracy and to ensure that the person to be reached is commonly available to respond.

EMERGENCY SUPPLIES AND EQUIPMENT

The final means of preparing for emergencies is by ensuring that adequate emergency drugs and equipment are available in the office. One basic piece of equipment is the dental chair, which should be capable of allowing the patient to be placed in a flat position or, even better, in a head-down, feet-raised position (Figure 2-1, *A*). In addition, the chair must be capable of being lowered close to the floor to allow BLS to be performed properly. Operatories should be large enough to allow a patient to be placed on the floor for BLS performance while still providing room for the dentist and staff to deliver emergency care. If the operatory is too small to allow placement of the patient on the floor, special plastic boards are available to be used in the office to place under the patient's thorax to allow BLS administration in the dental chair.

Other equipment frequently found necessary during emergencies is that used for respiratory assistance and the administration of injectable drugs. Equipment for respiratory assistance includes oral and nasal airways, tonsil suction tips (Figure 2-1, *B*), connector tubing that allows the use of high-volume suction, and resuscitation bags (Air Mask Bag Unit [AMBU bags]) with clear face masks (Figure 2-1, *C*).

Oral and nasal airways, laryngoscopes, and endotracheal tubes may be helpful for dentists trained in their proper use or for others called into the office to assist during an emergency.

Useful drug administration equipment includes syringes and needles, tourniquets, intravenous (IV) solutions, indwelling catheters, and intravenous tubing (Table 2-1). Although emergency kits containing a variety of drugs are commercially available (Figure 2-2), dentists may prefer to assemble their own. This allows properly educated dentists to choose only those agents they feel are likely to be most useful during an emergency. This also helps the dentist to organize the kit in a manner that is easy to use during emergency situations. If dentists have made arrangements for help from nearby professionals, they may also want to include drugs in their kits that the assisting individuals suggest may be helpful. The drugs and any equipment in the kit must be well labeled and the kit checked frequently for completeness and to ensure that no drugs are out of date. Labeling can include not only the drug name but also situations in which the drug is most commonly used. A list of drugs that should be considered for inclusion in a dental office emergency kit appears in Table 2-2.

One emergency drug already available in most dental offices is oxygen. Many dentists use oxygen supplied in a portable tank. These individuals need only to provide a means of delivering the oxygen *under positive pressure* for use by themselves if properly trained or by others called in to assist. It is important to establish a system to periodically check that a sufficient supply of oxygen is always available. Dentists who use a central oxygen system also need to have oxygen available that is portable, for use outside of the operatory, such as in the waiting room or during transport to an emergency facility.

Table 2-1. Emergency supplies for the dental office

Use	Supplies
Establishment and maintenance of IV access	Plastic indwelling (catheter)
	Metal indwelling (catheter)
	IV tubing with flow valve
	Tourniquet
	1-in-wide plastic tape
	Crystalloid solution (normal saline, D_5W)
High-volume suction	Large-diameter suction tip
	Tonsillar suction tip
	Extension tubing
	Connectors to adapt tubing to office suction
Drug administration	Plastic syringes (5 and 10 mL sizes)
	Needles (18- and 21-gauge)
Oxygen administration	Clear face mask
	Resuscitation bag (AMBU)
	Extension oxygen tubing (with and without nasal catheters)
	Oxygen cylinder with flow valve
	Oral and nasal airways*
	Laryngoscope*
	Endotracheal tube*
	Lubricating jelly*
	Demand valve oxygen mask*

*For use by dentists with appropriate training or by those called to give medical assistance.

MEDICAL EMERGENCIES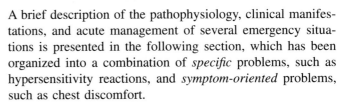

A brief description of the pathophysiology, clinical manifestations, and acute management of several emergency situations is presented in the following section, which has been organized into a combination of *specific* problems, such as hypersensitivity reactions, and *symptom-oriented* problems, such as chest discomfort.

HYPERSENSITIVITY REACTIONS

Several of the drugs administered to patients undergoing oral surgery can act as antigenic stimuli, which produce allergic reactions. Of the four basic types of hypersensitivity reactions, only type I (immediate hypersensitivity) can cause an acute, life-threatening condition. Type I allergic reactions are mediated primarily by IgE antibodies. As with all allergies, initiation of a type I response requires exposure to an antigen with which the immune system has previously come in contact. The reexposure to the antigen triggers a cascade of events, which then manifest either locally or systemically in varying degrees of severity. Table 2-3 details the manifestations and their management.

The least-severe manifestation of type I hypersensitivity is dermatologic. Skin reactions include localized areas of pruritus (itching), erythema, urticaria (wheals consisting of slightly elevated areas of skin that are erythematous, indurated, and frequently pruritic), and angioedema (large areas of swollen tissue generally with little erythema or induration). Although skin reactions are not in themselves dangerous, they may be the first indication of more serious allergic manifes-

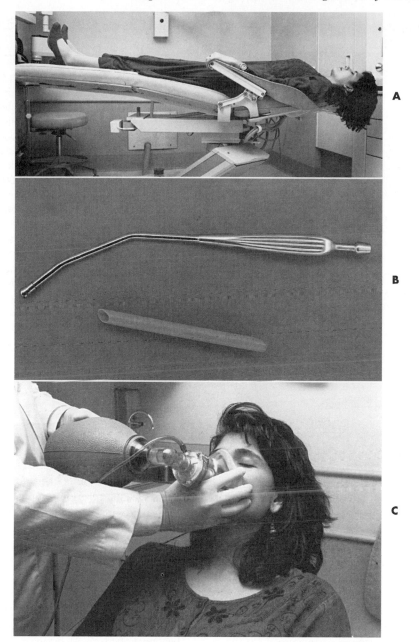

◇ Figure 2-1

A, Dental chair capable of placing patient in position such that legs are raised above level of trunk. This position is useful for emergency conditions in which increased venous return to heart is necessary or when gastric contents or foreign bodies are in upper airway. **B,** Tonsil suction tip useful for clearing fluids out of mouth and pharynx *(above)* and high-volume suction tip useful for rapidly clearing fluids and small particulate matter from mouth *(below)*. **C,** Resuscitation (AMBU) bag with clear face mask properly positioned over mouth and nose holding a good peripheral seal. Dentist's right hand is used to secure mask in place, while left hand is used to squeeze bag. Oxygen-enriched air provided by connecting the AMBU bag unit to oxygen source (note small tubing leading down from junction of bag and mask).

tations that will soon follow. Skin lesions usually take anywhere from minutes to hours to appear; however, those appearing rapidly after administration of the antigenic drug are the most foreboding.

Allergic reactions affecting the respiratory tract are more serious and require more aggressive intervention. The involvement of small airways manifests with wheezing, as constriction of bronchial smooth muscle (bronchospasm) occurs. The patient will complain of dyspnea and may eventually become cyanotic. Involvement of the larger

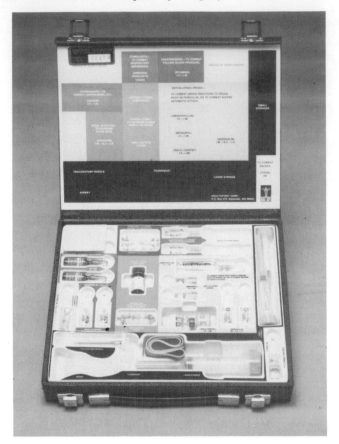

Figure 2-2

Example of commercially available emergency kit of appropriate size and complexity for dental office.

Table 2-2. Emergency drugs for the dental office

General drug group	Common examples
Parenteral preparations	
Analgesic	Morphine sulfate
Anticonvulsant	Diazepam, midazolam
Antihistamine	Diphenhydramine (Benadryl), chlorpheniramine (Chlor-Trimeton)
Antihypoglycemic	50% dextrose in water, glucagon
Corticosteroid	Methylprednisolone (Solu-Medrol), dexamethasone (Decadron), hydrocortisone (Solu-Cortef)
Narcotic antagonist	Naloxone (Narcan)
Sympathomimetic	Epinephrine
Vagolytic	Atropine
Oral preparations	
Antihistamine	Diphenhydramine (Benadryl), chlorpheniramine (Chlor-Trimeton)
Antihypoglycemic	Candy, fruit juice, sugar
Vasodilator	Nitroglycerin (Nitrostat, Nitrolingual)
Inhaled preparations	
Bronchodilator	Metaproterenol (Alupent), epinephrine bitartrate (Medihaler-Epi)
Oxygen	
Respiratory stimulant	Aromatic ammonia

airways usually first manifests at the most narrow portion of those air passages, the vocal cords in the larynx. Angioedema of the vocal cords causes partial or total airway obstruction. The patient is usually unable to speak and produces high-pitched crowing sounds (stridor) as air passes through constricted cords. As the edema worsens, total airway obstruction eventually occurs, which is an immediate threat to life.

Generalized anaphylaxis is the most dramatic hypersensitivity reaction, usually occurring within seconds or minutes following the parenteral administration of the antigenic medication; there is a more delayed onset after oral drug administration. A variety of signs and symptoms of anaphylaxis exist, but the most important with respect to early management are those resulting from cardiovascular and respiratory tract disturbances.

An anaphylactic reaction typically begins with a patient complaining of malaise or a feeling of impending doom. Skin manifestations soon appear, including flushing, urticaria, and pruritus on the face and trunk. Nausea and vomiting, abdominal cramping, and urinary incontinence may occur. Symptoms of respiratory embarrassment soon follow, with dyspnea and wheezing. Cyanosis of nail beds and mucosa will next appear if air exchange becomes insufficient. Finally, total airway obstruction occurs, which causes the patient to quickly become unconscious. Disordered cardiovascular function manifests initially with tachycardia and palpitations. Blood pressure tends to fall, and cardiac dysrhythmias appear. Cardiac output eventually may be compromised to a degree sufficient to cause loss of consciousness and cardiac arrest. Despite the potentially severe cardiovascular disturbances, the usual cause of death in patients having an anaphylactic reaction is laryngeal obstruction caused by vocal cord edema.

As with any potential emergency condition, prevention is the best therapy. During the initial interview, patients should be questioned about drugs to which they have a history of allergy. In addition, dentists should ask patients specifically about medications they intend to use during the planned oral surgical procedure. If a patient claims to have an allergy to a particular drug, the clinician should question the patient further concerning the way in which the allergic reaction manifested and the procedure that was necessary to manage the problem. Many patients will claim an allergy to local anesthetics. However, before subjecting patients to alternative forms of anesthesia, the clinician should ensure that an allergy to the local anesthetic does indeed exist, because many patients have been told they had an allergic reaction when in fact they had experienced a vasovagal hypotensive episode. If an allergy is truly in question, the patient may require referral to a physician who can perform hypersensitivity testing. After it is determined that a patient does have a drug allergy, the information should be displayed prominently on the permanent record.

Table 2-3. Manifestations and management of hypersensitivity (allergic) reactions

Manifestations	Management
Skin signs	
Delayed-onset skin signs: erythema, urticaria, pruritus, angioedema	Stop administration of all drugs presently in use Administer IM or IV Benadryl* 50 mg or Chlor-Trimeton† 10 mg Refer to physician Prescribe oral antihistamine such as Benadryl 50 mg q6h or Chlor-Trimeton 10 mg q6h
Immediate-onset skin signs: erythema, urticaria, pruritus, angioedema	Stop administration of all drugs presently in use Administer epinephrine 0.3 mL of 1:1000 SC, IM, or IV or epinephrine 3 mL of 1:10,000 IM or IV Can repeat q5min if signs progress Administer antihistamine IM or IV: Benadryl 50 mg or Chlor-Trimeton 10 mg Monitor vital signs frequently Consult patient's physician Observe in office 1 hr Prescribe Benadryl 50 mg q6h or Chlor-Trimeton 10 mg q6h
Respiratory tract signs with or without skin signs:	
Wheezing, mild dyspnea	Stop administration of all drugs presently in use Place patient in sitting position Administer epinephrine‡ Give oxygen (6 L/min) by face mask or nasally Monitor vital signs frequently Administer antihistamine Provide IV access Consult patient's physician or emergency room physician Observe in office at least 1 hr Prescribe antihistamine
Stridorous breathing (crowing sound), moderate-to-severe dyspnea	Stop administration of all drugs presently in use Sit the patient upright and have someone summon medical assistance Administer epinephrine‡ Give oxygen (6 L/min) by face mask or nasally Monitor vital signs frequently Administer antihistamine Provide IV access; if signs worsen, treat as for anaphylaxis Consult patient's physician or emergency room physician; prepare for transport to emergency room if signs do not improve rapidly
Anaphylaxis (with or without skin signs): malaise, wheezing, moderate to severe dyspnea, stridor, cyanosis, total airway obstruction, nausea and vomiting, abdominal cramps, urinary incontinence, tachycardia, hypotension, cardiac dysrhythmias, cardiac arrest	Stop administration of all drugs Position patient supine on back board or on floor and have someone summon assistance Administer epinephrine‡ Initiate BLS and monitor vital signs Consider cricothyrotomy if trained in use and if laryngospasm is not quickly relieved with epinephrine Provide IV access Give oxygen 6 L/min Administer antihistamine IV or IM Prepare for transport

*Brand of diphenhydramine.
†Brand of chlorpheniramine.
‡As described in "immediate onset" section.

Management of allergic reactions depends on the severity of the signs and symptoms. The initial response to any sign of untoward reaction to a drug being given parenterally should be to cease its administration. If the allergic reaction is confined to the skin, an antihistamine should be administered either intravenously or intramuscularly (IM). Diphenhydramine hydrochloride (Benadryl) 50 mg or chlorpheniramine maleate (Chlor-Trimeton) 10 mg are the commonly chosen antihistamines.* The antihistamine is then continued in an oral

*All dosages given in this chapter are those recommended for an average adult. Dosages will vary for children, the elderly, and for those with debilitating diseases. Consult a drug reference book for additional information.

◇ Box 2-4 ◇

Clinical characteristics of chest pain caused by myocardial ischemia or infarction

Discomfort (pain) described by patients as being:
1. Squeezing, bursting, pressing, burning, choking, and/or crushing in character (not typically sharp or stabbing in quality)
2. Substernally located, with variable radiation to left shoulder, arm, and/or left side of neck and mandible
3. Frequently associated at the onset with exertion, heavy meal, anxiety, or upon assuming horizontal posture
4. Relieved by vasodilators, such as nitroglycerin, or rest (in the case of angina)
5. Accompanied by dyspnea, nausea, weakness, palpitations, perspiration, and/or a feeling of impending doom

◇ Box 2-5 ◇

Differential diagnosis of acute-onset chest pain

Common causes
Cardiovascular system: Angina pectoris, myocardial infarction
Gastrointestinal tract: Dyspepsia (heartburn), hiatal hernia, reflux esophagitis, gastric ulcers
Musculoskeletal system: Intercostal muscle spasm
Psychologic: Hyperventilation
Uncommon causes
Cardiovascular system: Pericarditis, dissecting aortic aneurysm
Respiratory system: Pulmonary embolism, pleuritis, tracheobronchitis, mediastinitis, pneumothorax
Gastrointestinal tract: Esophageal rupture, achalasia
Musculoskeletal system: Osteochondritis, chondrosternitis
Psychologic: Psychogenic chest pain (imagined chest pain)

form (Benadryl 50 mg or Chlor-Trimeton 8 mg) every 6 to 8 hours for 24 hours. Immediate, severe urticarial reactions warrant immediate parenteral (subcutaneously [SC] or intramuscularly) administration of 0.3 mL of a 1:1000 epinephrine solution, followed by an antihistamine. The patient's vital signs should be frequently monitored for 1 hour, and, if stable, the patient should be referred to a physician or an emergency care facility for further follow-up.

If a patient begins to show signs of lower respiratory tract involvement, that is, wheezing during an allergic reaction, several actions should be initiated. Outside emergency assistance should be summoned. The patient should be placed in a semireclined position and oxygen administration begun. Epinephrine should be administered either by parenteral injection of 0.3 mL of a 1:1000 solution or with an aerosol inhaler (for example, Medihaler-Epi) (each inhalation of which delivers 0.3 mg). Epinephrine is short-acting, so if symptoms recur, the dose can be repeated within 5 minutes. Antihistamines such as diphenhydramine or chlorpheniramine are then given. The patient should be transferred to a nearby emergency facility to allow further management as necessary.

If a patient shows signs of laryngeal obstruction, that is, stridor (crowing sounds), epinephrine (0.3 mL of 1:1000 solution) should be given and oxygen administered. If a patient loses consciousness and appears to be unable to ventilate, an emergency cricothyrotomy may be required to bypass the laryngeal obstruction.† A description of the technique of cricothyrotomy is beyond the scope of this book, but this technique may be lifesaving in an anaphylactic reaction. Once an airway is reestablished, an antihistamine and further doses of epinephrine should be given. Vital signs should be monitored, and steps necessary to maintain

the patient should be taken until emergency assistance is available.

Patients who show signs of cardiovascular system compromise should be closely monitored for the appearance of hypotension, which may necessitate initiation of BLS if cardiac output falls below the level necessary to maintain viability or if cardiac arrest occurs (Table 2-3).

CHEST DISCOMFORT

The appearance of chest discomfort in a patient who may have ischemic heart disease in the perioperative period calls for rapid identification of the etiology so that appropriate measures can be taken (Box 2-4). Discomfort from cardiac ischemia is frequently described as a squeezing sensation, with a heaviness on the chest (Box 2-5). It usually begins in a retrosternal location, radiating to the left shoulder and arm. Patients with documented heart disease who have had such discomfort in the past will usually be able to confirm that the discomfort is cardiac in origin. For patients who are unable to remember such a sensation in the past or who have been assured by their physician that such discomfort does not represent heart disease, further information is useful before assuming a cardiac origin of the symptom. The patient should be asked to describe the exact location of the discomfort and any radiation, the way in which the discomfort is changing with time, and if postural position affects the discomfort. Pain resulting from gastric reflux into the esophagus because of chair position should improve when the patient sits up. Discomfort caused by costochondritis or pulmonary conditions should vary with respirations or be stimulated by pressure on the thorax. The only other common condition that can manifest with chest discomfort is anxiety, which may be difficult to differentiate from cardiogenic problems without monitoring devices not commonly present in the dental office.

If chest discomfort is suspected to be caused by myocardial

---

†Cricothyrotomy is the surgical creation of an opening into the cricothyroid membrane just below the thyroid cartilage to create a path for ventilation that bypasses the larynx.

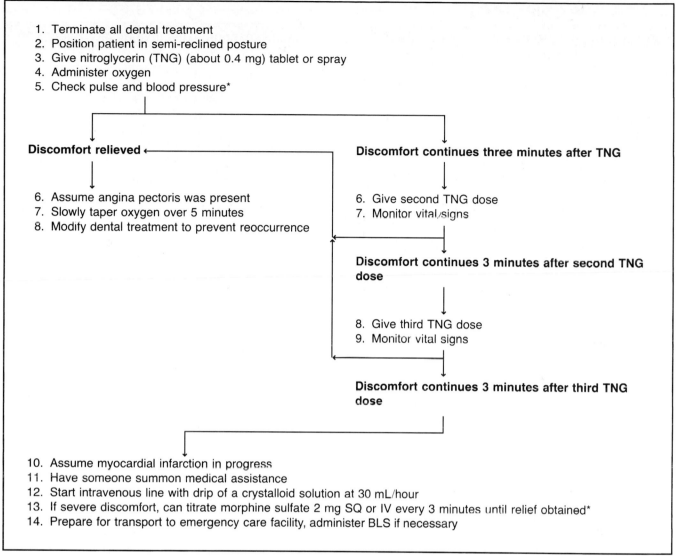

1. Terminate all dental treatment
2. Position patient in semi-reclined posture
3. Give nitroglycerin (TNG) (about 0.4 mg) tablet or spray
4. Administer oxygen
5. Check pulse and blood pressure*

Discomfort relieved

6. Assume angina pectoris was present
7. Slowly taper oxygen over 5 minutes
8. Modify dental treatment to prevent reoccurrence

Discomfort continues three minutes after TNG

6. Give second TNG dose
7. Monitor vital signs

Discomfort continues 3 minutes after second TNG dose

8. Give third TNG dose
9. Monitor vital signs

Discomfort continues 3 minutes after third TNG dose

10. Assume myocardial infarction in progress
11. Have someone summon medical assistance
12. Start intravenous line with drip of a crystalloid solution at 30 mL/hour
13. If severe discomfort, can titrate morphine sulfate 2 mg SQ or IV every 3 minutes until relief obtained*
14. Prepare for transport to emergency care facility, administer BLS if necessary

*If blood pressure ever falls below 90 systolic or 50 diastolic, withhold TNG and MS and call or wait for arrival of medical assistance.

◇ Figure 2-3

Management of patient having chest discomfort while undergoing dental surgery.

ischemia or if that possibility cannot be ruled out, measures should be instituted that decrease myocardial work and increase myocardial oxygen supply. All dental care must be stopped, even if the surgery is only partially finished. The patient should be reassured that everything is under control while vital signs are being obtained, oxygen administration is started, and nitroglycerin is being administered sublingually or by oral spray. The nitroglycerin dose should be 0.4 mg dissolved sublingually and repeated if necessary every 5 minutes as long as systolic blood pressure is at least 90 mm Hg, up to a maximum of 3 doses. If vital signs remain normal, the chest discomfort is relieved, and the amount of nitroglycerin that was required to relieve the discomfort was not more than normally necessary, the patient should be discharged with plans for future surgery to be done in an oral and maxillofacial surgery office or in a hospital (Figure 2-3).

There are circumstances for which transport to an emergency facility is indicated. If the pulse is found to be irregular, rapid, or weak or the blood pressure is found to be below baseline, outside emergency help should be summoned while the patient is placed in an almost supine position and oxygen and nitroglycerin therapy are started. Venous access should be initiated, if possible, for use by emergency personnel. Another serious situation requiring transfer to a hospital is a case in which the patient's discomfort is not relieved after 20 minutes of appropriate therapy. In this case it should be presumed that a myocardial infarction is in progress. Such a patient is especially prone to the appearance of serious cardiac dysrhythmias or cardiac arrest, so vital signs should be monitored frequently and BLS should be instituted if the patient loses consciousness. Morphine sulfate (4 to 6 mg) may be administered intramuscularly or subcutaneously to help

◇ Box 2-6 ◇

Manifestations of an acute asthmatic episode

Mild to moderate
Wheezing (audible with or without stethoscope)
Dyspnea (labored breathing)
Tachycardia
Coughing
Anxiety
Severe
Intense dyspnea, with flaring of nostrils and use of accessory muscles of respiration
Cyanosis of mucous membranes and nail beds
Minimal breath sounds on auscultation
Flushing of face
Extreme anxiety
Mental confusion
Perspiration

◇ Box 2-7 ◇

Manifestations of hyperventilation syndrome

Neurologic
Dizziness
Tingling or numbness of fingers, toes, or lips
Syncope
Respiratory
Increased rate and depth of breaths
Feeling of shortness of breath
Chest pain
Xerostomia
Cardiac
Palpitations
Tachycardia
Musculoskeletal
Myalgia
Muscle spasm
Tremor
Tetany
Psychologic
Extreme anxiety

relieve the discomfort and reduce anxiety. Morphine also provides a beneficial effect for patients who develop pulmonary edema (Figure 2-3).

RESPIRATORY DIFFICULTY

There are several situations in which patients undergoing oral surgery in the office setting may begin to have respiratory difficulty that, if not promptly treated, can be life-threatening. Many patients are predisposed to respiratory problems in the dental setting; these patients include patients with asthma, patients with chronic obstructive pulmonary disease (COPD), extremely anxious patients, patients who are atopic, and patients in whom a noninhalation sedative technique is to be used. Special precautions should be taken with these patients to help prevent the occurrence of emergencies.

ASTHMA. Patients with a history of asthma can be a particular challenge to manage safely if their respiratory problems are easily triggered by emotional stress or a variety of pharmacologic agents. Most patients with asthma are aware of the symptoms that signal the onset of bronchospasm. Patients will complain of shortness of breath and want to sit erect. Wheezing is usually audible, tachypnea begins, and patients will start using their accessory muscles of respiration. As bronchospasm progresses, patients may become cyanotic and hypoxic, with eventual loss of consciousness (Box 2-6).

Management should start with placing patients in an erect or semierect position. Patients should then administer bronchodilators, using their own inhalers or inhalers provided from the office emergency supply. The inhaler can contain epinephrine, isoproterenol, metaproterenol, or albuterol. Repeated doses should be administered cautiously to avoid giving the patient an overdose. Oxygen administration should follow, using nasal prongs or a face mask. In more severe asthmatic episodes or when aerosol therapy is ineffective, epinephrine (0.3 mL of a 1:1000 dilution) can be injected subcutaneously or intramuscularly. When patients have severe respiratory embarrassment, it may be necessary to obtain outside emergency medical assistance (Figure 2-4).

Respiratory problems caused by drug allergy may be difficult to differentiate from those resulting from asthma. Management of the respiratory problems is the same in either case.

HYPERVENTILATION. The most frequent cause of respiratory difficulty in the dental setting is anxiety that manifests as hyperventilation, which is usually seen in patients in their teens, twenties, and thirties and can frequently be prevented through anxiety control. Dentists should be attuned to the signs of patient apprehension and, through the health interview, should encourage patients to express their concerns. Patients with extreme anxiety should be managed with an anxiety-reduction protocol. In addition, pharmacologic anxiolysis may be necessary.

The first manifestation of hyperventilation syndrome is frequently a complaint by patients that they cannot get enough air. They breathe very rapidly (tachypnea) and become agitated. The rapid ventilation allows an increased elimination of CO_2 through the lungs. The patient rapidly becomes alkalotic; may complain of becoming lightheaded and of having a tingling sensation in the fingers, toes, and perioral region; and may even develop muscle twitches or convulsions. Eventually, loss of consciousness occurs (Box 2-7).

Management of a hyperventilating patient involves terminating the surgical procedure, positioning the patient in a semierect position, and providing reassurance. If symptoms of alkalosis occur, the patient should be forced to breathe into and out of a small bag (Figure 2-5). Oxygen-enriched air is not

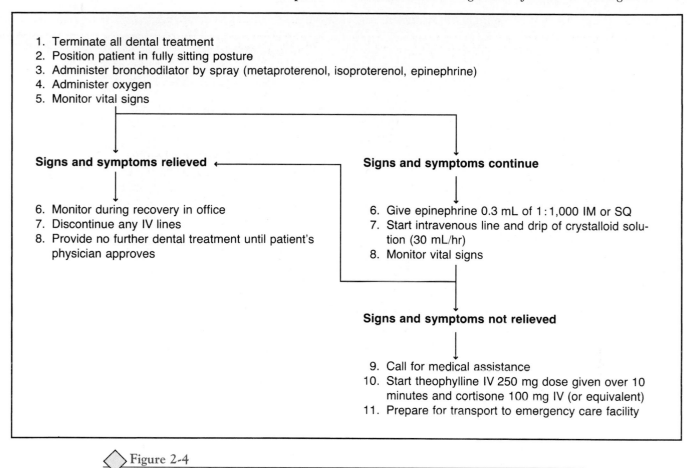

1. Terminate all dental treatment
2. Position patient in fully sitting posture
3. Administer bronchodilator by spray (metaproterenol, isoproterenol, epinephrine)
4. Administer oxygen
5. Monitor vital signs

Signs and symptoms relieved

6. Monitor during recovery in office
7. Discontinue any IV lines
8. Provide no further dental treatment until patient's physician approves

Signs and symptoms continue

6. Give epinephrine 0.3 mL of 1:1,000 IM or SQ
7. Start intravenous line and drip of crystalloid solution (30 mL/hr)
8. Monitor vital signs

Signs and symptoms not relieved

9. Call for medical assistance
10. Start theophylline IV 250 mg dose given over 10 minutes and cortisone 100 mg IV (or equivalent)
11. Prepare for transport to emergency care facility

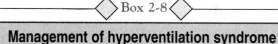

Figure 2-4

Management of acute asthmatic episode occurring during dental surgery.

indicated. If hyperventilation continues, the clinician may have to administer a sedative such as diazepam, by giving 10 mg intramuscularly or by intravenous titration of the drug until hyperventilation ceases or the patient is sedated. Once hyperventilation stops, the patient should be rescheduled, with plans to use preoperative and/or intraoperative sedation during the next visit (Box 2-8).

CHRONIC OBSTRUCTIVE PULMONARY DISEASE. Patients with well-compensated chronic obstructive pulmonary disease (COPD) can have difficulty during oral surgery. Many of these patients depend on maintaining an upright posture to breathe adequately. In addition, they become accustomed to having high arterial CO_2 levels and use a low level of blood oxygen as the primary stimulus to drive respirations. Many of these patients experience difficulty if placed in an almost supine position or if placed on high-flow nasal oxygen. Patients with COPD often rely on their accessory muscles of respirations to breathe. Lying supine interferes with the use of these accessory muscles. COPD also is accompanied by excessive lung secretions that are more difficult to clear when supine. Therefore patients will usually ask to sit up before problems resulting from positioning occur.

If excessive oxygen is administered to a patient susceptible to COPD, the respiratory rate will fall, which produces

Box 2-8

Management of hyperventilation syndrome

1. Terminate all dental treatment and remove foreign bodies from mouth
2. Position patient in chair in almost fully upright position
3. Attempt to verbally calm patient
4. Have patient breathe CO_2-enriched air, such as in and out of a small bag
5. If symptoms persist or worsen, administer diazepam 10 mg intramuscularly or titrate slowly intravenously until anxiety is relieved, or administer midazolam 5 mg intramuscularly or titrate slowly intravenously until anxiety is relieved
6. Monitor vital signs
7. Perform all further dental surgery using anxiety-reducing measures

cyanosis, and apnea may eventually occur. The treatment for such a problem is to discontinue oxygen administration. The respiratory rate should soon improve. If apnea persists and the patient loses consciousness, artificial ventilation must be initiated and emergency assistance summoned.

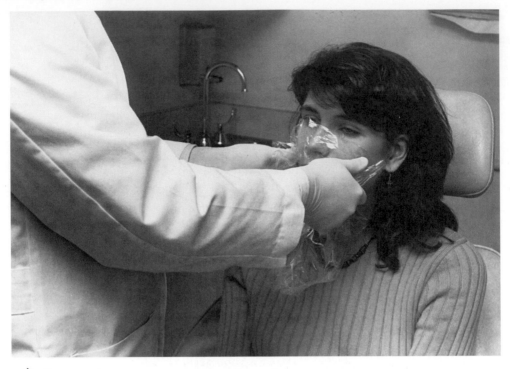

◇ **Figure 2-5**

Bag placed over nose and mouth to force rebreathing of CO_2-enriched air, reversing tendency for alkalosis caused by hyperventilation. In this case a plastic headrest cover is being used.

◇ **Box 2-9** ◇

Acute manifestations of aspiration into the lower respiratory tract

Large foreign body
Coughing
Choking sensation
Stridorous breathing (crowing sounds)
Severe dyspnea
Feeling of something caught in throat
Inability to breathe
Cyanosis
Loss of consciousness
Gastric contents
Coughing
Stridorous breathing
Wheezing or rales (cracking sound) on chest auscultation
Tachycardia
Hypotension
Dyspnea
Cyanosis

FOREIGN BODY ASPIRATION. Aspiration of foreign bodies into the airway is always a potential problem during oral surgical procedures. This is especially true if the patient is positioned supine or semierect in the chair or is sufficiently sedated to dull the gag reflex. Objects that fall into the hypopharynx are frequently swallowed and usually pass harmlessly through the gastrointestinal tract. Even if the clinician feels confident the material was swallowed, chest and abdominal radiographs should be obtained to eliminate the possibility of asymptomatic aspiration into the respiratory tract. Occasionally, the foreign object is aspirated into the larynx, where, in the lightly sedated or nonsedated patient, violent coughing will ensue that may expel the aspirated material. The patient can usually still talk and breathe. However, larger objects that are aspirated may obstruct the airway and become lodged in such a manner that coughing is ineffective, because the lungs cannot be filled with air before the attempted cough. In this situation the patient usually cannot produce any vocalizations and becomes extremely anxious. Cyanosis soon occurs, followed by loss of consciousness (Box 2-9).

The manner in which aspirated foreign bodies are managed depends primarily on the degree of airway obstruction. Patients with an intact gag reflex and a partially obstructed airway should be allowed to attempt to expel the foreign body by coughing. If the material will not come up, the patient should be given supplemental oxygen and transported to an emergency facility to allow laryngoscopy or bronchoscopy to be performed. The completely obstructed but awake patient should have abdominal thrusts (Figure 2-6, *A*) or Heimlich maneuvers (Figure 2-6, *B*) performed until successful or until consciousness is lost. If a patient has a diminished gag reflex as a result of sedation or has a completely obstructed airway and loses consciousness, abdominal thrusts should be performed with the patient in a supine position. After each volley

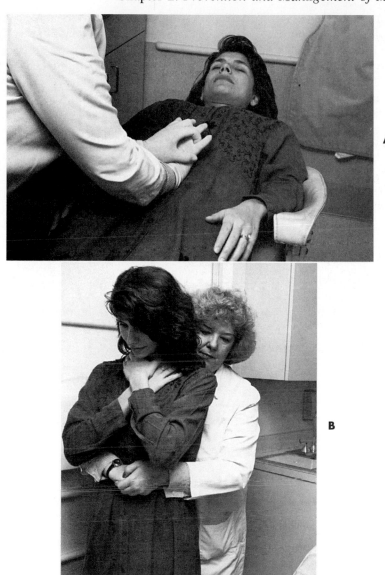

◇ Figure 2-6

A, Method of performing abdominal thrusts for unconscious patient with foreign body obstructing airway. Chair first placed in recumbent position. Heel of dentist's right palm placed on abdomen just below xiphoid process, with elbow kept locked and left hand placed over the right for further delivery of force. Arms quickly thrust into patient's abdomen, directing force down and superiorly. **B,** Proper positioning for Heimlich maneuver. Rescuer approaches patient from behind and positions hands on the patient's abdomen, just below the rib cage. Rescuer's hands are then quickly pulled into abdominal area, attempting to have any residual air in lungs dislodge obstruction from airway. Note patient's hands on throat; this is universal sign of airway obstruction.

of thrusts, the patient should be quickly turned onto the side, and the clinician should finger sweep the mouth to remove any object that may have been forced out. If the patient is not exchanging air, BLS should be started. If air cannot be blown into the lungs, additional abdominal thrusts should be attempted, followed by oral finger sweeps and BLS. Dentists trained in laryngoscopy can look into the larynx and use Magill forceps to remove any foreign material. If several attempts to relieve the obstruction fail, an emergency cricothyrotomy may be necessary (Figure 2-7).

GASTRIC CONTENTS ASPIRATION. Aspiration of gastric contents into the lower respiratory tract presents another situation that frequently leads to serious respiratory difficulties. The particulate matter in gastric contents causes physical obstruction of pulmonary airways, but it is usually the high acidity of gastric material that produces more serious problems. The low pH of gastric juice quickly necrotizes pulmonary tissue with which it comes in contact, and an adult respiratory distress syndrome soon follows, with transudation of fluid into pulmonary alveoli and a loss of functioning lung tissue. The patient with an intact gag reflex rarely aspirates gastric contents during vomiting. Rather, it is the patient with a diminished gag reflex who is at greatest risk for gastric aspiration. This may result from pharmacologic obtundation, such as with sedative agents, or from a loss of consciousness because of any of a variety of problems. The sedated or unconscious patient who aspirates a significant amount of gastric material will first show signs of respiratory difficulty, such as tachypnea and wheezing. Tachycardia and

hypotension may soon occur and, as ventilatory capability worsens, cyanosis may appear. Eventually, respiratory failure occurs that is refractory to BLS and requires both intubation and the delivery of high concentrations of oxygen.

Prevention of gastric aspiration involves the avoidance of levels of sedation that obtund the gag reflex and the instruction of patients that are to be moderately or deeply sedated to avoid eating or drinking for 8 hours before their oral surgery appointment.

A sedated or unconscious patient who begins to vomit should be immediately placed into a head-down, feet-raised position and turned onto the right side to encourage oral drainage of vomitus. Box 2-10 lists several symptoms exhibited by patients preparing to vomit. High-volume suction

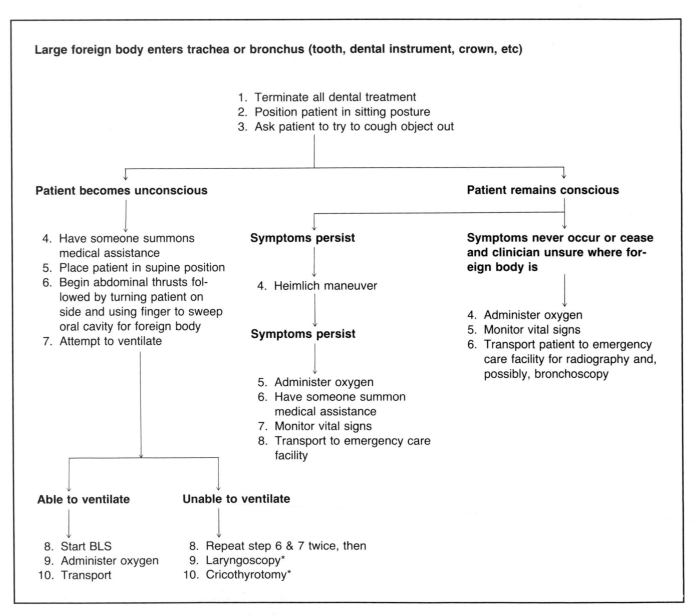

◇ Figure 2-7

Management of respiratory tract foreign body aspiration in patient undergoing dental surgery.

should be used to assist removal of vomitus from the oral cavity. If there is any suspicion that gastric material may have entered the lower respiratory tract, a call should be placed for emergency assistance. The patient should be placed on supplemental oxygen and vital signs monitored. If possible, the dentist should gain venous access (start an IV) and be prepared to administer crystalloid solution, such as normal saline, to help treat a falling blood pressure and to allow emergency technicians to administer intravenous bronchodilators if necessary. Transportation to an emergency facility is mandatory (Figure 2-8).

ALTERED CONSCIOUSNESS

An alteration in the level of consciousness of a patient may result from a large variety of medical problems. The altered state can range from lightheadedness to a complete loss of consciousness. Without attempting to include all possible causes of altered consciousness, a discussion is presented of commonly occurring conditions that may lead to an acutely altered state of consciousness while patients are undergoing oral surgical procedures.

VASOVAGAL SYNCOPE. The most common cause of a transient loss of consciousness in the dental office is vasovagal

Manifestations of patient preparing to vomit

Nausea
Frequent swallowing
Perspiration
Feeling of warmth
Feeling of anxiety
Gagging

syncope. This generally occurs because of a series of cardiovascular events triggered by the emotional stress brought on by the anticipation of or delivery of dental care. The initial event in a vasovagal syncopal episode is the stress-induced release of increased amounts of catecholamines that cause a decrease in peripheral vascular resistance, tachycardia, and sweating. The patient may complain of feeling generalized warmth, nausea, and palpitations. As blood pools in the periphery, a drop in the arterial blood pressure appears, with a corresponding decrease in cerebral

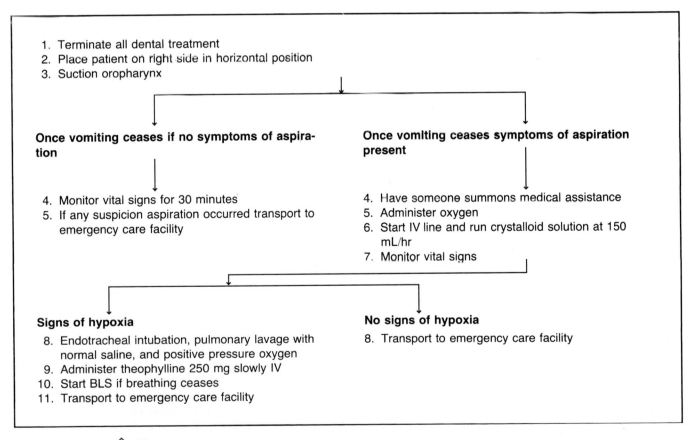

1. Terminate all dental treatment
2. Place patient on right side in horizontal position
3. Suction oropharynx

Once vomiting ceases if no symptoms of aspiration

4. Monitor vital signs for 30 minutes
5. If any suspicion aspiration occurred transport to emergency care facility

Once vomiting ceases symptoms of aspiration present

4. Have someone summons medical assistance
5. Administer oxygen
6. Start IV line and run crystalloid solution at 150 mL/hr
7. Monitor vital signs

Signs of hypoxia

8. Endotracheal intubation, pulmonary lavage with normal saline, and positive pressure oxygen
9. Administer theophylline 250 mg slowly IV
10. Start BLS if breathing ceases
11. Transport to emergency care facility

No signs of hypoxia

8. Transport to emergency care facility

◇ Figure 2-8

Management of vomiting patient and of possible aspiration of gastric contents.

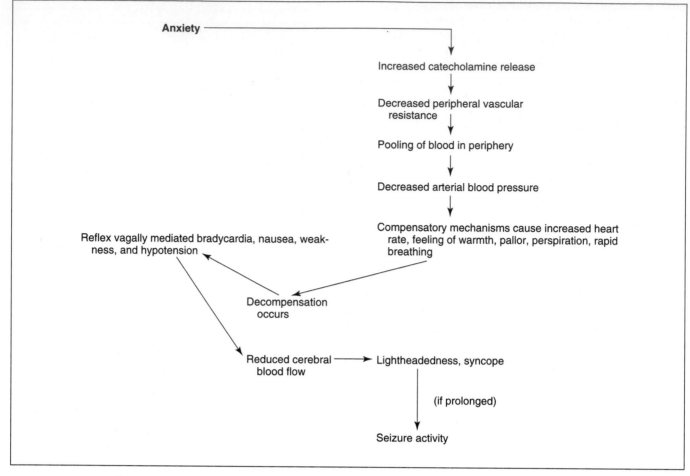

◇ Figure 2-9

Pathophysiology and manifestations of vasovagal syncope.

blood flow. The patient will then complain of feeling dizzy or weak. Compensatory mechanisms attempt to maintain adequate blood pressure, but they soon fatigue, which leads to vagally mediated bradycardia. Once the blood pressure drops below levels necessary to sustain consciousness, syncope occurs (Figure 2-9).

If cerebral ischemia is sufficiently severe, the patient may also develop seizure activity. The syncopal episode usually ends rapidly once the patient assumes or is placed in a horizontal position with the feet elevated (Figure 2-10). Once consciousness is regained, the patient may have pallor, nausea, and fatigue for several minutes to hours.

Prevention of vasovagal syncopal reactions involves proper patient preparation. The extremely anxious patient should be treated by using an anxiety-reduction protocol and, if necessary, given pretreatment anxiolytic drugs. Oral surgical care should be provided while the patient is in a semierect or supine position. Any signs of an impending syncopal episode should be quickly treated by placing the patient in a fully supine position or a position in which the legs are elevated above the level of the heart and by placing a cool moist towel on the forehead. If the patient is hypoventilating and is slow to recover consciousness, a respiratory stimulant

such as aromatic ammonia may be useful. If the return of consciousness is delayed for more than a minute, an alternative cause for depressed consciousness other than vasovagal syncope should be sought. Following early recovery from the syncopal episode, the patient should be allowed to recover in the office and then discharged with an escort. Future office visits by the patient will require preoperative sedation and/or additional anxiety-reducing measures.

ORTHOSTATIC HYPOTENSION. Another common cause of a transient altered state of consciousness in the dental setting is orthostatic (or postural) hypotension. This problem occurs because of pooling of blood in the periphery that is not remobilized quickly enough to prevent cerebral ischemia when a patient rapidly assumes an upright posture. The patient will therefore feel lightheaded or become syncopal. Patients with orthostatic hypotension who remain conscious will usually complain of palpitations and generalized weakness. Most individuals who are not hypovolemic or have orthostatic hypotension resulting from pharmacologic effects will quickly recover by reassuming the reclined position. Once symptoms disappear, the patient can generally sit up, although this should be done slowly, and sit on the edge of the chair for a few

Prodrome:

1. Terminate all dental treatment
2. Position patient in supine posture with legs raised above level of head
3. Attempt to calm patient
4. Cool towel to forehead
5. Monitor vital signs

Syncopal episode:

1. Terminate all dental treatment
2. Position patient in supine posture with legs raised
3. Check for breathing

If absent

4. Start BLS
5. Have someone summons medical assistance
6. Consider other causes of syncope including hypoglycemia, cerebral vascular accident, cardiac dysrhythmia, etc

If present

4. Crush ammonia ampule under nose, administer O_2
5. Monitor vital signs
6. Have patient escorted home
7. Plan anxiety control measures during future dental care

Figure 2-10

Management of vasovagal syncope and its prodrome.

moments before standing. Blood pressure should be taken in each position and allowed to return to normal before a more upright posture is assumed (Box 2-11).

Some patients have a predisposition to orthostatic hypotension. In the ambulatory population this is usually encountered in patients receiving the following medications: drugs that produce intravascular depletion, such as diuretics; drugs that produce peripheral vasodilation, such as most nondiuretic antihypertensives, narcotics, and many psychiatric drugs; and drugs that prevent the heart rate from increasing reflexly, such as b-sympathetic blocking medications (for example, propranolol). Patients with a predisposition to postural hypotension can usually be managed by allowing a much longer period to attain a standing position, that is, by stopping at several increments while becoming upright, to allow reflex cardiovascular compensation to occur. If the patient was sedated by using long-acting narcotics, an antagonist such as naloxone may be necessary. Patients with severe problems with postural hypotension as a result of drug therapy should be referred to their physician for alteration of their drug regimen.

SEIZURE.   Idiopathic seizure disorders manifest in many ways, ranging from grand mal seizures, with their frightening display of clonic contortions of the trunk and extremities, to the petit mal seizure, which may manifest with only episodic absences (blank stare). Although rare, some seizure disorders, such as those secondary to injury-induced brain damage or

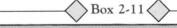

Box 2-11

Management of orthostatic hypotension

1. Terminate all dental treatment
2. Position patient in supine posture, with legs raised above the level of the head
3. Monitor vital signs
4. Once blood pressure improves, slowly return patient to sitting posture
5. Discharge to home once vital signs are normal and stable
6. Obtain medical consultation before any further dental care

caused by ethanol abuse, have known etiology. Usually the patient will have had the seizure disorder previously diagnosed and will be receiving antiseizure medications, such as phenytoin (Dilantin), phenobarbital, or valproic acid. Therefore the dentist should discover through the medical interview the amount of seizure control present to decide if oral surgery can be safely performed. The patient should be asked to describe what witnesses have said occurs just before, during, and after the patient's seizures. It is helpful to discover any factors that seem to precipitate the seizure, the patient's compliance with antiseizure drugs, and the recent frequency of seizure episodes. Patients with seizure disorders who appear to have good control of their disease, that is, infrequent

Manifestations

Isolated, brief seizure

Tonic-clonic movements of trunk and extremities, loss of consciousness, vomiting, airway obstruction, loss of urinary and anal sphincter control

Acute Management

1. Terminate all dental treatment
2. Place in supine position
3. Protect from nearby objects

After seizure

Patient unconscious

4. Have someone summons medical assistance
5. Place on side and suction airway
6. Monitor vital signs
7. Initiate BLS (if necessary)
8. Administer oxygen
9. Transport to emergency care facility

Patient conscious

4. Suction airway if necessary
5. Monitor vital signs
6. Administer oxygen
7. Consult physician
8. Observe in office for 1 hour
9. Have patient escorted home

Repeated or sustained seizure (status epilepticus)

(as above)

1. Diazepam 5 mg/min IV up to 10 mg or midazolam 3 mg/min IV or IM up to 6 mg* titrated until seizures stop
2. Have someone summons medical assistance
3. Protect from nearby objects

Once seizure ceases

4. Place on side and suction airway
5. Monitor vital signs
6. Initiate BLS (if necessary)
7. Administer oxygen
8. Transport to emergency care facility

*Total dose can be doubled if no signs of respiratory depression occur. Total dose should be halved in children and elderly patients.

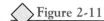

Figure 2-11

Manifestations and acute management of seizures.

episodes that are brief in duration and are not easily precipitated by anxiety, are usually able to safely undergo oral surgery in the ambulatory setting. See Chapter 1 for recommendations.

The occurrence of a seizure while a patient is undergoing care in the dental office, although usually creating great concern among the office staff, is rarely an emergency that calls for actions other than simply protecting the patient from self-injury. However, management of the patient during and after a seizure varies, based on the type of seizure that occurs. The patient's ability to exchange air must be monitored by close observation. If it appears that the airway is obstructed, measures to reopen it must be taken, for example, by placing the head in moderate extension (chin pulled away from the chest) and moving the mandible away from the pharynx. If the patient vomits or seems to be having problems keeping secretions out of the airway, the patient's head must be positioned to the side to allow obstructing materials to drain out of the mouth. If possible, high-volume suction should be used to evacuate materials from the pharynx. Brief periods of apnea may occur, which require no treatment other than ensuring a patent airway. However, apnea for more than 30 seconds demands that BLS techniques be initiated. Although frequently described as being important, the placement of objects between the teeth in an attempt to prevent tongue-biting is hazardous and therefore usually unwarranted.

◇ Table 2-4. Suggested maximum doseage of local anesthetics*

Drug	Common brand		Maximum dose mg/kg	Maximum number of 1.8 mL cartridges
Lidocaine	Xylocaine	2%	5	10
Lidocaine with epinephrine[†]	Xylocaine with epinephrine	2% lidocaine 1/10^5 epinephrine	5	10
Mepivacaine	Carbocaine	3%	5	6
Mepivacaine with levonordefrin	Carbocaine with Neo-Cobefrin	2% mepivacaine 1:20,000 levonordefrin	5	8
Prilocaine	Citanest	4%	5	6
Bupivacaine with epinephrine	Marcaine with epinephrine	0.5% bupivacaine 1:200,000 epinephrine	1.5	10
Etidocaine with epinephrine	Duranest with epinephrine	1.5% etidocaine 1:200,000 epinephrine	8	15

*Maximum doses are those for normal healthy individuals.
†Maximum dose of epinephrine is 0.2 mg per appointment.

Continuous or repeated seizures without periods of recovery between them are known as *status epilepticus*. This problem warrants notification of outside emergency assistance because it is the most common type of seizure disorder to cause mortality. Therapy includes instituting measures already described for self-limiting seizures. However, in addition, administration of a benzodiazepine is indicated. Injectable water-insoluble benzodiazepines such as diazepam must be given intravenously to allow predictability of results, which may be difficult in the seizing patient if venous access is not already available. Injectable water-soluble benzodiazepines such as midazolam provide a better alternative, because intramuscular injection will give a more rapid response. However, the doctor administering benzodiazepines for a seizure must be prepared to provide BLS, because patients may experience a period of apnea after receiving a large rapid dose of benzodiazepines.

After seizures have ceased, most patients will be left either somnolent or unconscious. Vital signs should be monitored carefully during this time, and the patient should not be allowed to leave the office until he or she is fully alert and has an escort. The patient's primary care physician should be notified to decide if medical evaluation is necessary and if ambulatory dental care is advisable in the future (Figure 2-11).

Seizures caused by ethanol withdrawal are usually preceded by tremors, palpitations, and anxiety. Therefore the appearance of these signs in a patient should warn the clinician to defer care until proper medical care for the patient's condition is instituted. Control is usually obtained by the use of benzodiazepines, which are used until the effects of abstinence from ethanol cease. Seizures that occur in ethanol-abusing patients are treated in a similar manner to other seizures.

LOCAL ANESTHETIC TOXICITY. Local anesthetics, when properly used, are a safe and effective means of providing pain control when performing dentoalveolar surgery. However, as with all medications, toxicity reactions occur if the local anesthetic is given in an amount or in a manner that produces an excessive serum concentration.

Prevention of a toxicity reaction to local anesthetics generally involves several factors. First, the dose to be used should be the least amount of local anesthetic necessary to produce the intensity and duration of pain control required to successfully complete the planned surgical procedure. The patient's age, lean body mass, liver function, and history of problems with local anesthetics must be considered when choosing the dose of local anesthesia. The second factor to consider in preventing a local anesthetic overdose reaction is the manner of drug administration. The dentist should give the required dose slowly, avoiding intravascular injection, and use vasoconstrictors to slow the entry of local anesthetics into the blood. It should be remembered that topical use of local anesthetics in wounds or on mucosal surfaces allows rapid entry of local anesthetics into the systemic circulation. The choice of local anesthetic agents is the third important factor to consider in attempting to lessen the risk of a toxicity reaction. Local anesthetics vary in their lipid solubility, vasodilatory properties, protein binding, and inherent toxicity. Therefore the dentist must be knowledgeable about the various local anesthetics available, to allow a rational decision to be made when choosing which drug to administer (Table 2-4).

The clinical manifestations of a local anesthetic overdose vary, depending on the severity of the overdose, how rapidly it occurs, and the duration of the excessive serum concentrations. Signs of a mild toxicity reaction may be limited to increased patient confusion, talkativeness, anxiety, and slurring of speech. As the severity of the overdose increases, the patient may display stuttering speech, nystagmus, and generalized tremors. Symptoms such as headache, dizziness, blurred vision, and drowsiness may also occur. The most serious manifestations of local anesthetic toxicity are the appearance of generalized tonic-clonic seizure activity and cardiac depression leading to cardiac arrest (Table 2-5).

Mild local anesthetic overdose reactions are managed by

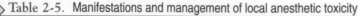

Table 2-5. Manifestations and management of local anesthetic toxicity

Manifestations	Management
Mild toxicity: talkativeness, anxiety, slurred speech, confusion	Stop administration of all local anesthetics Monitor vital signs Observe in office for 1 hr
Moderate toxicity: stuttering speech, nystagmus, tremors, headache, dizziness, blurred vision, drowsiness	Stop administration of all local anesthetics Place in supine position Monitor vital signs Administer oxygen Observe in office for 1 hr
Severe toxicity: seizure, cardiac dysrhythmia or arrest	Place in supine position If seizure, protect from nearby objects and suction oral cavity if vomiting occurs Have someone summon medical assistance Monitor vital signs Administer oxygen Start IV Administer diazepam 5-10 mg slowly or midazolam 2-6 mg slowly Institute BLS if necessary Transport to emergency care facility

monitoring vital signs, instructing the patient to hyperventilate moderately with or without administering oxygen, and gaining venous access. If signs of anesthetic toxicity do not rapidly disappear, a slow intravenous 2.5- to 5-mg dose of diazepam should be given. Medical assistance should also be summoned if signs of toxicity do not rapidly resolve or if they progressively worsen.

If convulsions occur, patients should be protected from hurting themselves. Basic life-support measures are instituted as needed and venous access gained, if possible, for administration of anticonvulsants. Medical assistance should be obtained. If venous access is available, diazepam should be slowly titrated until the seizure activity stops (5 to 25 mg is the usual effective range). Vital signs should be checked frequently.

DIABETES MELLITUS.   Diabetes mellitus is a metabolic disease in which the patient's long-term prognosis appears dependent on keeping serum glucose levels close to normal. An untreated insulin-dependent diabetic constantly runs the risk of developing ketoacidosis and its attendant alteration of consciousness, requiring emergency treatment. Although a compliant insulin-taking diabetic may suffer long-term problems because of relatively high serum glucose levels, the more common emergency situation they encounter is hypoglycemia resulting from a mismatch of insulin dose and serum glucose. Severe hypoglycemia is the emergency situation dentists are most likely to face when providing oral surgery for a diabetic patient.

Serum glucose concentration in the diabetic patient represents a balance between administered insulin, glucose placed into the serum from various sources, and glucose utilization. The two primary sources of glucose are dietary and gluconeogenesis from adipose tissue, muscle, and glycogen stores. Physical activity is the principal means by which serum glucose is lowered. Therefore serum glucose levels can fall because of any or all of the following:

1. Increasing administered insulin
2. Decreasing dietary caloric intake
3. Increasing metabolic utilization of glucose (exercise, infection, emotional stress)

Problems with hypoglycemia during dental care usually arise because the patient has acutely decreased caloric intake, an infection, or an increased metabolic rate caused by marked anxiety. If the patient has not compensated for this diminution of available glucose by decreasing the usual dose of insulin, hypoglycemia results. Although patients taking oral hypoglycemics can also have problems with hypoglycemia, their swings in serum glucose levels are usually less pronounced than those of insulin-dependent diabetics, so they are much less likely to quickly become severely hypoglycemic.

Many diabetics are well informed about their disease and are capable of diagnosing their own hypoglycemia before it becomes severe. The patient may feel hunger, nausea, or lightheadedness or may develop a headache. The dentist may notice the patient becoming lethargic, with decreased spontaneity of conversation and ability to concentrate. As hypoglycemia worsens, the patient may become diaphoretic or have tachycardia, piloerection, or increased anxiety and exhibit unusual behavior. The patient may soon become stuporous or lose consciousness (Table 2-6).

Severe hypoglycemia in diabetic patients usually can be avoided through measures designed to keep serum glucose levels on the high side of normal or even temporarily above normal. During the health history interview, the dentist should get a clear idea of how well controlled the patient's diabetes is. If patients do not regularly check their own urine or serum glucose, the physician should be contacted to determine whether routine dental care can be performed safely. Before any planned procedures, measures discussed in Chapter 1 concerning the diabetic patient should be taken.

If a diabetic patient indicates a feeling of low blood sugar or if signs or symptoms of hypoglycemia appear, the

1. Terminate all dental treatment

Signs and symptoms of mild hypoglycemia

2. Administer glucose source such as sugar or fruit juice PO
3. Monitor vital signs
4. Consult physician if unsure if or why hypoglycemia occurred before further dental care

Signs and symptoms of moderate hypoglycemia

2. Administer glucose source such as sugar or fruit juice orally
3. Monitor vital signs
4. If symptoms do not rapidly improve administer 50 mL of 50% glucose or 1 mg glucagon IV or IM
5. Consult physician before further dental care

Signs and symptoms of severe hypoglycemia

2. Administer 50 mL of 50% glucose IV or IM or 1 mg glucagon
3. Have someone summons medical assistance
4. Monitor vital signs
5. Administer oxygen
6. Transport to emergency care facility

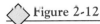

Figure 2-12

Management of acute hypoglycemia.

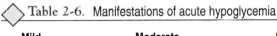

Table 2-6. Manifestations of acute hypoglycemia

Mild	Moderate	Severe
Hunger	Tachycardia	Hypotension
Nausea	Perspiration	Unconsciousness
Mood change	Pallor	Seizures
Weakness	Anxiety	
	Behavioral change: belligerence, confusion, uncooperativeness	

procedure being performed should be stopped and the patient allowed to consume a high-caloric carbohydrate, such as a few packets of sugar, a glass of fruit juice, or sugar-containing carbonated soda. If the patient fails to rapidly improve, becomes unconscious, or is otherwise unable to take a glucose source by mouth, venous access should be gained and an ampule (50 mL) of 50% glucose (dextrose) in water administered over 2 to 3 minutes. If venous access cannot be established, 1 mg of glucagon can be given intramuscularly. If 50% glucose and glucagon are unavailable, a 0.5-mL dose of 1:1000 epinephrine can be administered subcutaneously and repeated every 15 minutes as needed (Figure 2-12).

A patient who seems to have recovered from a hypoglycemic episode should remain in the office for at least 1 hour, and further symptoms should be treated with oral glucose sources. The patient should be escorted home with instructions on how to avoid a hypoglycemic episode during the next dental appointment.

THYROID DYSFUNCTION. Hyperthyroidism and hypothyroidism are slowly developing disorders that can produce an altered state of consciousness but rarely cause emergencies. The most common circumstance in which an ambulatory, relatively healthy-appearing patient develops an emergency from thyroid dysfunction is when a thyroid storm (crisis) occurs.

Thyroid storm is sudden, severe exacerbation of hyperthyroidism that may or may not have been previously diagnosed. It can be precipitated by infection, surgery, trauma, pregnancy, or any other physiologic or emotional stress. Patients predisposed to thyroid crisis frequently have signs of hyperthyroidism, such as tremor, tachycardia, weight loss, hypertension, irritability, intolerance to heat, and exophthalmos, and may have even received therapy for the thyroid disorder.

Patients with known hyperthyroidism should have their primary care physician consulted before any oral surgical procedure. A determination of the adequacy of control of excessive thyroid hormone production should be obtained from the patient's physician, and, if necessary, the patient should receive antithyroid drugs and iodide treatment preoperatively. If clearance for ambulatory surgery is given, the patient should be managed as shown in the outline in Chapter 1.

The first sign of a developing thyroid storm is an elevation of temperature and heart rate. Most of the usual signs and symptoms of untreated hyperthyroidism occur in an exaggerated form. The patient becomes irritable, delirious, or even comatose. Hypotension, vomiting, and diarrhea also occur.

Treatment of thyrotoxic crisis begins with termination of any procedure and notification of those outside the office able to give emergency assistance. Venous access should be attained, crystalloid solution started at a moderately high rate, and the patient kept as calm as possible. Attempts may be taken to cool the patient until he or she can be transported to a hospital, where antithyroid and sympathetic blocking drugs can be administered safely (Table 2-7).

ADRENAL INSUFFICIENCY. Primary adrenocortical insufficiency (Addison's disease) or other medical conditions in which the adrenal cortex has been destroyed are rare, and patients are usually well informed concerning their need

Table 2-7. Manifestations and acute management of thyroid storm

Manifestations	Management
Hyperpyrexia (fever)	Terminate all dental treatment
Tachycardia	Have someone summon medical
Nervousness and agitation	assistance
Tremor	Administer oxygen
Weakness	Monitor vital signs
Palpitations	Initiate BLS as necessary
Cardiac dysrhythmias	Start IV line with drip of crystalloid
Nausea and vomiting	solution (150 mL/hr)
Abdominal pains	Transport to emergency care facility
Partial or complete loss of consciousness	

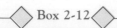
Box 2-12

Manifestations of acute adrenal insufficiency

Weakness
Feeling of extreme fatigue
Confusion
Hypotension
Nausea
Abdominal pain
Myalgias
Partial or total loss of consciousness

Table 2-8. Equivalency of commonly used glucocorticosteroids

Relative duration of action	Generic	Common brand name	Relative glucocorticoid potency	Equivalent glucocorticoid dose (mg)
Short	Cortisol (hydrocortisone)	Solu-Cortef	1	20
	Cortisone	—	0.8	25
	Prednisone	Deltasone	4	5
	Prednisolone	Delta-Cortef	4	5
	Methylprednisolone sodium succinate	Solu-Medrol	5	4
Intermediate	Triamcinolone	Kenalog	5	4
Long	Betamethasone	Celestone	25	0.6
	Dexamethasone	Decadron	30	0.75
	Methylprednisolone acetate	Depo-Medrol	5	4

for additional corticosteroid administration during stressful situations. However, adrenal insufficiency secondary to exogenous corticosteroid administration is relatively common because of the multitude of clinical conditions for which corticosteroids are given therapeutically. Patients with secondary adrenal insufficiency are frequently not informed concerning their potential need for supplemental medication and may fail to inform the dentist that they are taking corticosteroids. This is not a problem, provided the patient is not physiologically or emotionally stressed.

However, should the patient be stressed, adrenal suppression that results from exogenous corticosteroids may prevent the normal release of increased amounts of endogenous glucocorticoids needed to help the body meet the increased metabolic demands. Patients at risk for acute adrenal insufficiency as a result of adrenal suppression are generally those who take at least 20 mg of cortisol (or its equivalent) daily for at least 2 weeks any time during the year preceding the planned major oral surgical procedure (Table 2-8). However, in most straightforward oral surgical procedures done under local anesthesia or nitrous oxide and local anesthesia, administration of supplemental corticosteroids is unnecessary. If adrenal suppression is suspected, the steps discussed in Chapter 1 should be followed.

Early clinical manifestations of acute adrenal insufficiency crisis include mental confusion, nausea, fatigue, and muscle weakness. As the condition worsens, the patient develops more severe mental confusion; pain in the back, abdomen, and legs; vomiting; and hypotension. Without treatment the patient will eventually begin to drift in and out of consciousness, with coma being the preterminal stage (Box 2-12).

Management of an adrenal crisis involves stopping all dental treatment and taking vital signs. If the patient is found to be hypotensive, the head-down, feet-raised position should be assumed. Oxygen should be administered, and venous access gained. A 100-mg dose of hydrocortisone sodium succinate should be given intravenously (or intramuscularly if necessary) and medical assistance summoned. Intravenous fluids should be administered until hypotension improves. Vital signs should be measured frequently while therapeutic measures are being taken. Should the patient lose consciousness, the need for initiation of basic life-support measures should be evaluated (Box 2-13).

If any patient who needs oral surgery treatment begins to display symptoms that may be related to adrenal insufficiency, strong consideration should be given to administering a high dose of hydrocortisone before the procedure.

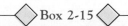

Box 2-13

Management of acute adrenal insufficiency

1. Terminate all dental treatment
2. Position patient in supine position, with legs raised above level of head
3. Have someone summon medical assistance
4. Administer corticosteroid (100 mg of hydrocortisone or its equivalent) intramuscularly or intravenously
5. Administer oxygen
6. Monitor vital signs
7. Start intravenous line and drip of crystalloid solution
8. Start BLS if necessary
9. Transport to emergency care facility

Box 2-15

Management of cerebrovascular compromise in progress*

1. Terminate all dental treatment
2. Have someone summon medical assistance
3. Position patient in supine posture, with head slightly raised
4. Monitor vital signs
5. If loss of consciousness, administer oxygen and institute BLS as necessary
6. Transport to emergency care facility

*If symptoms are present only briefly (TIA), terminate dental treatment, monitor vital signs, and consult patient's physician concerning safety of further dental care.

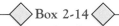

Box 2-14

Manifestations of cerebrovascular compromise in progress

Headache can range from mild to the worst the patient ever experienced

Weakness or paralysis of extremities and/or facial muscles unilaterally

Slurring of speech or inability to speak

Difficulty breathing and/or swallowing

Loss of bladder and bowel control

Seizures

Visual disturbance

Dizziness

Partial or total loss of consciousness

CEREBROVASCULAR COMPROMISE. Alterations in cerebral blood flow can be compromised in the following three principal ways: (1) embolization of particulate matter from a distant site, (2) formation of a thrombus in a cerebral vessel, or (3) rupture of a vessel. Material that embolizes to the brain comes most frequently from thrombi in the left side of the heart and the carotid region or from bacterial vegetations on infected heart surfaces. Cerebrovascular thrombi generally form in areas of atherosclerotic changes. Finally, vascular rupture can occur because of rare congenital defects in the vessel, that is, berry aneurysms.

The effect on the level of consciousness of a cerebrovascular problem depends on the severity of the cerebral lesion. If the problem rapidly resolves, such as happens with transient ischemic attacks, the symptoms of cerebral vascular compromise may last only a few seconds or minutes. However, if ischemia is severe enough, an infarction may occur in an area of the brain and leave a permanent neurologic deficit.

A transient ischemic attack (TIA) that occurs during dental care requires that the procedure be terminated. However, there is little that must be done for the patient other than reassurance, because most patients experience only a temporary numbness and/or weakness of the extremities on one side of the body. Consciousness is usually unaltered. TIAs frequently precede a cerebral infarction, so immediate physician referral is important.

Cerebrovascular compromise that results from embolism usually first manifests with a mild headache, followed by the gradual appearance of other neurologic symptoms, such as weakness in an extremity, vertigo, or dizziness. On the other hand, cerebral hemorrhage typically has the abrupt onset of a severe headache, followed in several hours by nausea, dizziness, vertigo, and diaphoresis. The patient may go on to lose consciousness (Box 2-14).

If signs or symptoms of a cerebrovascular compromise arise and are not transient, a major problem affecting the cerebral vasculature may be occurring. The procedure should be stopped and frequent monitoring of vital signs started. Medical help should be called to assist in the event the patient becomes hypotensive or unconscious. If the patient develops respiratory difficulty, oxygen should be administered. However, oxygen is otherwise contraindicated in patients with cerebrovascular insufficiency. Any narcotics that the patient has been administered should be reversed. If consciousness is lost, vital signs should be frequently monitored and cardiopulmonary resuscitation begun if necessary (Box 2-15).

BIBLIOGRAPHY

Chilo V, Borea G, Strong M: *Life threatening emergencies in dentistry,* Padova, Italy, 1988, Ishiyaku Euroamerica.

Hupp JR, Williams TP, Vallerand WP: *The 5 minute clinical consult for dental professionals,* Baltimore, 1996, Williams & Wilkins.

Malamed SF: *Handbook of medical emergencies in the dental office,* ed 3, St Louis, 1993, Mosby.

PRINCIPLES OF SURGERY

JAMES R. HUPP

CHAPTER OUTLINE ◇

H uman tissues have genetically determined properties that make their responses to injury fairly predictable. Depending on this predictability, principles of surgery that help to optimize the wound-healing environment have evolved through time. This chapter presents the prin-

ciples of surgical practice that clinicians have found most successful.

DEVELOPING A SURGICAL DIAGNOSIS ◇

Most of the important decisions concerning a maxillofacial surgical procedure are made long before the dentist administers any anesthetic. The decision to perform surgery should be the culmination of several diagnostic steps. In the analytic approach the surgeon first identifies the various signs and symptoms and relevant historical information and then, through logical reasoning and using available data, establishes the relationship between the individual problems.

The initial step in the presurgical evaluation is the collection of accurate and pertinent data. This is accomplished through patient interviews; physical, laboratory, and imaging examinations; and the use of consultants when necessary. Patient interviews and examinations should be performed in an unhurried and thoughtful fashion. The dentist should not be willing to accept incomplete data, such as a poor-quality radiograph, especially when there is a reasonable probability that additional data might change the decision concerning surgery.

For a good analysis, data must be organized into a form that allows for the testing of hypotheses; that is, the dentist should be able to consider a list of possible diseases and eliminate those that the data do not support. By using this method, along with the knowledge of which diseases have a probability of being present, the surgeon is usually able to reach a decision about whether surgery is indicated.

Clinicians also must be thoughtful observers. Whenever a procedure is performed, they should note all aspects of its outcome, to advance their surgical knowledge and to improve future surgical results. This procedure should also be followed whenever a clinician is learning about a new technique. In addition, a clinician should evaluate the purported results of any new technique by weighing the scientific merit of studies that investigate the technique. Frequently, scientific methods are violated by the unrecognized introduction of a placebo effect, observer bias, patient variability, or use of inadequate control groups.

BASIC NECESSITIES FOR SURGERY

There is little difference between the basic necessities required for oral surgery and those required for the proper performance of other aspects of dentistry. The two principal requirements are adequate visibility and assistance.

Although visibility may seem too obvious to mention as a requirement for performing surgery, it is often overlooked by clinicians. Adequate visibility depends on the following three things: adequate access, adequate light, and a surgical field free of excess blood and other fluids.

Adequate access not only requires the patient's ability to open the mouth widely but also may require surgically created exposure. Retraction of tissues away from the operative field provides much of the necessary access. (Proper retraction also protects tissues from being accidentally injured, for example, by cutting instruments.) Improved access is also gained by the creation of surgical flaps, which are discussed later in this chapter.

Adequate light is another obvious necessity for surgery. However, clinicians often forget that many surgical procedures place the surgeon or assistant in positions that block chair-based light sources. To correct this problem, the light source must continually be repositioned or the surgeon or assistant must avoid obstructing the light or use a headlight.

A surgical field free of fluids is also necessary for adequate visibility. High-volume suctioning with a small tip can remove blood and other fluids from the field quickly.

As in other types of dentistry, a properly trained assistant provides invaluable help during oral surgery. The assistant should be sufficiently familiar with the procedures being performed to anticipate the surgeon's needs. It is extremely difficult to perform good surgery with no or poor assistance.

ASEPTIC TECHNIQUE

Aseptic technique includes minimizing wound contamination by pathogenic microbes. This important surgical principle is discussed in detail in Chapter 5.

INCISIONS

Many oral and maxillofacial surgical procedures necessitate incisions. A few basic principles are important to remember when performing tissue incisions.

The first principle is that a sharp blade of the proper size should be used. A sharp blade allows incisions to be made cleanly, without unnecessary damage caused by repeated strokes. The rate at which a blade dulls depends on the resistance of tissues through which the blade cuts. Bone and ligamental tissues dull blades more rapidly than does buccal mucosa. Therefore the surgeon should change blades whenever the knife does not seem to be incising easily.

The second principle is that a firm, continuous stroke should be used when incising. Repeated, soft strokes increase both the amount of damaged tissue within a wound and the amount of bleeding, thereby impairing wound healing. Long, continuous strokes are preferred to short, interrupted ones (Figure 3-1, *A*).

The third principle is that the surgeon should carefully avoid cutting vital structures when incising. No patient's microanatomy is exactly the same. Therefore to avoid unintentionally cutting large vessels or nerves the surgeon must incise only deeply enough to define the next layer. Vessels can be more easily controlled before they are completely divided, and important nerves can usually be freed from adjacent tissue and retracted away from the area to be incised.

The fourth principle is that incisions through epithelial surfaces that the surgeon plans to reapproximate should be made with the blade held perpendicular to the epithelial surface. This angle produces squared wound edges that are both easier to reorient properly during suturing and less susceptible to necrosis of the wound edges as a result of ischemia (Figure 3-1, *B*).

The fifth principle is that incisions in the oral cavity should be properly placed. It is more desirable to incise through attached gingiva and over healthy bone than through unattached gingiva and over unhealthy or missing bone. Properly placed incisions allow the wound margins to be sutured over intact, healthy bone that is at least a few millimeters away from the damaged bone, thereby providing support for the healing wound. Incisions placed near the teeth for extractions should be made in the gingival sulcus, unless there is a specific reason to excise the marginal gingiva or to leave the marginal gingiva untouched.

FLAP DESIGN

Surgical flaps are made to gain surgical access to an area or to move tissue from one place to another. Several basic principles of flap design must be followed to prevent the complications of flap surgery, which are flap necrosis, dehiscence, and tearing.

PREVENTION OF FLAP NECROSIS

Flap necrosis can be prevented if the surgeon attends to four basic principles. First, the apex (tip) of a flap should never be wider than the base, unless a major artery is present in the base. Flaps should have sides that either run parallel to each other or, preferably, converge from the base to the apex of the flap. Second, in general, the length of a flap should be no more than twice the width of the base (Figure 3-2, *A, B,* and *C*). Strict adherence to this principle is less critical in the oral

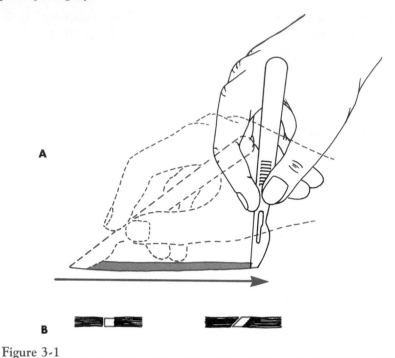

A

B

◇ Figure 3-1

A, Proper method of making incision using no. 15 scalpel blade. Note scalpel motion made by moving hand at wrist and not by moving entire forearm. **B,** When creating tissue layer that is to be sutured closed, blade should be kept perpendicular to tissue surface to create squared wound edges. Holding blade at any angle other than 90 degrees to tissue surface creates an oblique cut that is difficult to close properly and that compromises blood supply to the wound edge. *(Modified from Clark HB Jr:* Practical oral surgery, *ed 3, Philadelphia, 1965, Lea & Febiger.)*

cavity, but in this location the length of the flap should never exceed the width. Third, when possible, an axial blood supply should be included in the base of the flap. For example, a flap in the palate should be based toward the greater palatine artery (Figure 3-2, *D*). Fourth, the base of flaps should not be excessively twisted, stretched, or grasped with anything that might damage the vessel, because these maneuvers may compromise the vessels feeding the flap.

PREVENTION OF FLAP DEHISCENCE

Flap margin dehiscence (separation) is prevented by approximating the edges of the flap over healthy bone (Figure 3-3), by handling the edges of the flap gently, and by not placing the flap under tension. Dehiscence exposes underlying bone, producing pain, bone loss, and increased scarring.

PREVENTION OF FLAP TEARING

Tearing of a flap is a common complication of the inexperienced surgeon who attempts to perform a procedure using a flap that provides insufficient access. Because a properly repaired long incision heals just as quickly as a short one, it is preferable to create a flap at the onset of surgery that is large enough for the surgeon to avoid either tearing it or interrupting surgery to enlarge it. Envelope flaps are those created by incisions that produce a one-sided flap. An example is an incision made around the necks of several teeth to expose the alveolar bone without any vertical incisions. However, if an envelope flap does not provide sufficient access, another

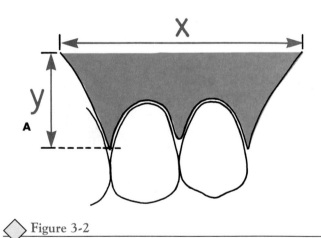

◇ Figure 3-2

A, Principles of flap design. In general, flap base dimension *(x)* must not be less than height dimension *(y),* and preferably flap should have *x = 2y.*

incision should be made to prevent it from tearing (Figure 3-4). Vertical (oblique) releasing incisions should be placed one full tooth anterior to the area of any anticipated bone removal. The incision is generally started at the line angle of a tooth or in the adjacent interdental papilla and carried obliquely apically into the unattached gingiva. It is uncommon to need more than one releasing incision when using a flap to gain surgical access.

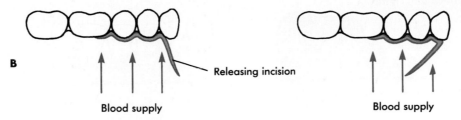

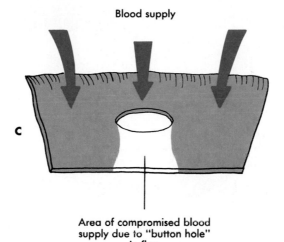

Figure 3-2, cont'd

B, When releasing, incision is used to reflect a two-sided flap; incision should be designed to maximize flap blood supply by leaving wide base. Design on left is *correct;* design on right is *incorrect.* **C,** When "buttonhole" occurs near free edge of flap, blood supply to flap tissue on side of hole away from flap base is compromised.

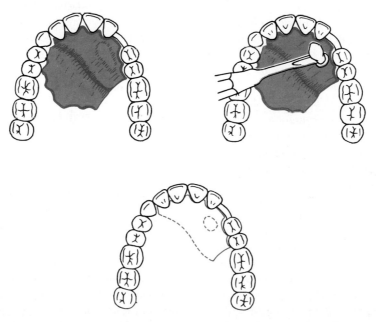

Figure 3-3

When closing wound over bony defect, make final closure rest over intact bone. This principle is illustrated here during removal of impacted canine. Incision is designed so that final suture line rests over intact bone.

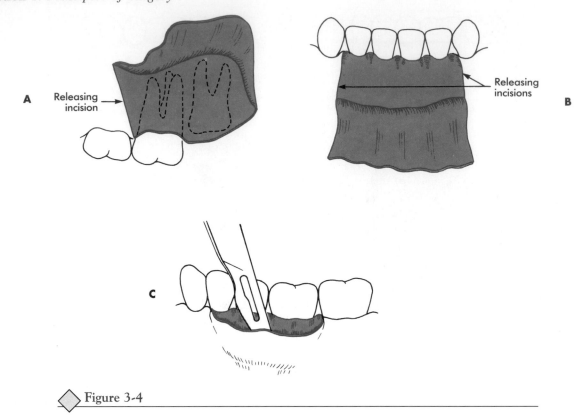

A
Releasing
incision

B
Releasing
incisions

C

◇ Figure 3-4

Three types of properly designed oral soft tissue flaps. **A,** Horizontal and single vertical incisions used to create two-sided flap. **B,** Horizontal and two vertical incisions used to create three-sided flap. **C,** Single horizontal incision used to create single-sided (envelope) flap.

Tissue Handling ────────◇

The difference between an acceptable and an excellent surgical outcome often rests on how the surgeon handles the tissues. The use of proper incision and flap design techniques plays a role; however, tissue also must be handled carefully. Tissue is easily damaged by excessive pulling or crushing, extremes of temperature, desiccation, and the use of unphysiologic chemicals. Therefore the surgeon should use care whenever touching tissue. When tissue forceps are used, they should not be pinched together too tightly. When possible, toothed forceps or tissue hooks should be used to hold tissue (Figure 3-5). Tissue should not be retracted overaggressively to gain surgical access. This includes not pulling excessively on the cheeks or tongue during surgery. When bone is cut, copious amounts of irrigation should be used to decrease the amount of bone damage from heat. Soft tissues should also be protected from frictional heat or direct trauma from drilling equipment. Tissues should not be allowed to desiccate; open wounds should be frequently moistened or covered with a damp sponge. Finally, only physiologic substances should come in contact with living tissue. For example, tissue forceps used to place a specimen into formalin during a biopsy procedure should not be returned to the wound until any contaminating formalin is thoroughly removed. The surgeon who handles tissue gently is rewarded with wounds that heal with fewer complications and grateful patients.

Hemostasis ────────◇

Prevention of excessive blood loss during surgery is important for preserving a patient's oxygen-carrying capacity. However, there are other important reasons to maintain meticulous hemostasis during surgery. One is the decreased visibility that uncontrolled bleeding creates. Even high-volume suctioning cannot keep a surgical field completely dry, particularly in the well-vascularized oral and maxillofacial regions. Another problem bleeding causes is the formation of hematomas. Hematomas place pressure on wounds, decreasing vascularity; increase tension on the wound edges; and act as culture media, potentiating the development of a wound infection.

Means of Promoting Wound Hemostasis

There are five means of obtaining wound hemostasis. The first is by assisting natural hemostatic mechanisms. This is usually accomplished by either using a fabric sponge to place pressure on bleeding vessels or placing a hemostat on a vessel. Both methods cause stasis of blood in vessels, which promotes coagulation. A few small vessels generally require pressure for only 20 to 30 seconds, whereas larger vessels require 5 to 10 minutes of continuous pressure. The surgeon and assistants should dab rather than wipe the

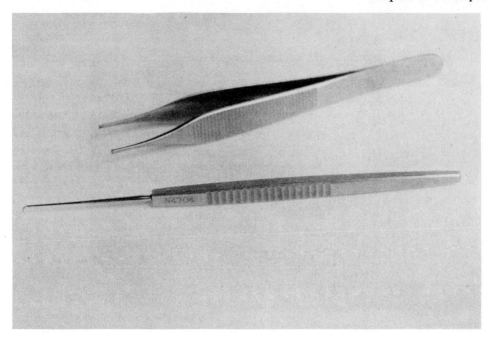

◇ Figure 3-5

Instruments used to minimize damage while holding soft tissue. *Above,* finely toothed tissue forceps (pickups); *below,* soft tissue (skin hook).

wound with sponges to remove extravasated blood. Wiping is more likely to reopen vessels that are already plugged by clotted blood.

A second means of obtaining hemostasis is by the use of heat to cause the ends of cut vessels to fuse closed (thermal coagulation). Heat is usually applied through an electrical current that the surgeon concentrates on the bleeding vessel by holding the vessel with a metal instrument, such as a hemostat, or by touching the vessel directly. Three conditions should be created for proper use of thermal coagulation. First, the patient must be grounded, to allow the current to enter the body. Second, the cautery tip and any metal instrument the cautery tip contacts cannot touch the patient at any point other than the site of the bleeding vessel. Otherwise the current may follow an undesirable path and create a burn. The third necessity for thermal coagulation is the removal of any blood or fluid that has accumulated around the vessel to be cauterized. Fluid acts as an energy sump and thus prevents a sufficient amount of heat from reaching the vessel to cause vessel closure.

The third means of providing surgical hemostasis is by suture ligation. If a vessel is already severed, each end is grasped with a hemostat. The surgeon then ties a nonabsorbable suture around the vessel (Figure 3-6, *A, B,* and *C*). If a vessel can be dissected free of surrounding connective tissue before it is cut, two hemostats can be placed on the vessel, with enough space left between them to cut the vessel. Once the vessel is severed, sutures are tied around each end and the hemostats removed (Figure 3-6, *D, E,* and *F*).

The fourth means of gaining hemostasis is by placement of a pressure dressing over the wound. This creates pressure on the small vessels that were cut, which promotes coagulation.

Care must be taken not to apply so much pressure as to compromise wound vascularity. Most bleeding from dentoalveolar surgery can be controlled by this means.

The fifth method of promoting hemostasis is by placing vasoconstrictive substances, such as epinephrine, in the wound or by applying procoagulants, such as commercial thrombin or collagen, on the wound. Epinephrine serves as a vasoconstrictor most effectively when placed in the site of desired vasoconstriction at least 7 minutes before surgery commences.

DEAD SPACE MANAGEMENT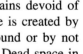

Dead space in a wound is any area that remains devoid of tissue after closure of the wound. Dead space is created by either removing tissue in the depths of a wound or by not reapproximating tissue planes during closure. Dead space in a wound usually fills with blood, which creates a hematoma with a high potential for infection.

There are four means of eliminating dead space. The first is by suturing tissue planes together to minimize the postoperative void. A second method is to place a pressure dressing over the repaired wound. The dressing compresses tissue planes together until they are bound by fibrin, are pressed together by surgical edema, or both. This usually takes about 12 to 18 hours. The third way to eliminate dead space is to place a packing into the void until bleeding has stopped and then remove the packing. This technique usually is used when the surgeon is unable to tack tissue together or to place

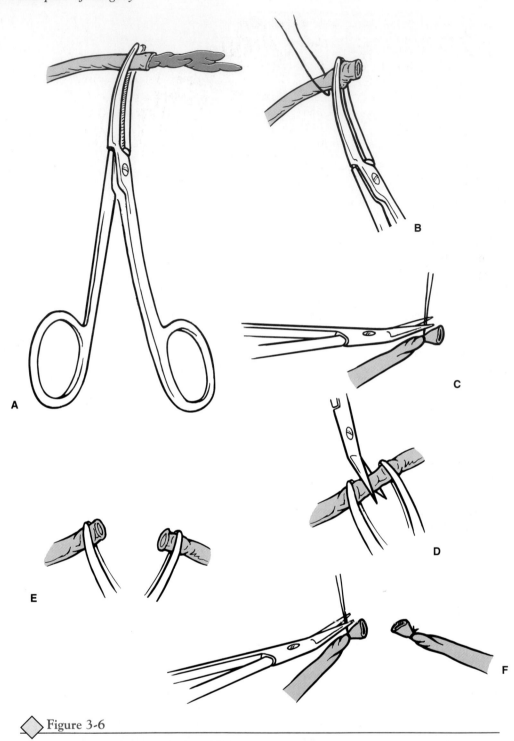

◈ Figure 3-6

Method of ligating blood vessels. **A** to **C,** Ligating cut, bleeding vessel. **A,** Hemostat clamped onto vessel, staying 2 to 3 mm short of the end. **B,** Nonresorbable suture is placed around vessel and tied tightly just under side of hemostat away from vessel's end. **C,** Free ends of suture are then cut off at knot. **D** to **F,** Dividing blood vessel. Hemostats placed on vessel to be divided, spaced about 1 cm apart. **D,** Blade or scissors is used to cut vessel cleanly between hemostats. **E,** Two clamped ends are ready for suture ligation, as in **A** to **C. F,** Sutures are tied and cut short.

pressure dressings (for example, when bony cavities are present). The packing material is usually impregnated with an antibacterial medication to lessen the chance of infection. The fourth means of preventing dead space is through the use of drains, either by themselves or in addition to pressure dressings. Suction drains continually remove any blood that accumulates in a wound until the bleeding stops and the tissues bind together and eliminate dead space. Nonsuction drains allow any bleeding to drain to the surface rather than to form a hematoma (Figure 3-7).

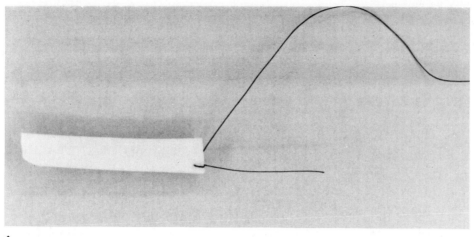

◇ Figure 3-7

Example of nonsuction drain. This is a Penrose drain and is made of flexible, rubberized material that can be placed into wound during closure or after incision and drainage of abscess to prevent premature sealing of wound before blood or pus collections can drain to surface. Draining material runs both along and through Penrose drain. In this illustration, suture has been tied to drain and drain is ready for insertion into wound. Needled end of suture will be used to attach drain to wound edge to hold drain in place.

DECONTAMINATION AND DÉBRIDEMENT ◇

Bacteria invariably contaminate all wounds that are open to the external or oral environment. Because the risk of infection rises with the increased size of an inoculum, one way to lessen the chance of wound infection is to decrease the bacterial count. This is easily accomplished by irrigating the wound during surgery and closure. Irrigation dislodges bacteria and other foreign materials and rinses them out of the wound. Irrigation can be achieved by forcing large volumes of fluid under pressure on the wound. Although solutions containing antibiotics can be used, most surgeons simply use sterile saline or sterile water.

Wound débridement is the careful removal from injured tissue of necrotic, foreign, and severely ischemic material that would impede wound healing. Débridement generally is used only during care of traumatically incurred wounds or of severe tissue damage caused by a pathologic condition.

SUTURING ◇

The final step of most surgical procedures involving an incision or laceration is to suture the wound. The material and methods used for wound closure must be selected carefully, because this important step prepares the wound for healing and, if done improperly, can prevent normal healing. Also, one of the few signs that patients use to judge the surgeon's skill is the appearance of the sutured wound.

Sutures are made of a wide variety of materials and come in several sizes, each designed for a particular purpose (Figure 3-8). The two basic types of suture material are resorbable (that is, the body is capable of easily breaking the material down) and nonresorbable. In general, resorbable sutures do not require removal, whereas nonresorbable sutures do.

RESORBABLE SUTURES

The following three types of resorbable sutures are commonly used for oral and maxillofacial surgery: gut, polyglycolic acid, and a copolymer of glycolic and lactic acids in a ratio of 9:1 (polyglactin 910). Gut is fabricated from the submucosa of sheep intestines or the serosa of beef intestines. Plain gut is susceptible to rapid digestion by proteolytic enzymes produced by inflammatory cells. For procedures requiring more prolonged suture strength, some gut is treated with basic chromium salts (chromic catgut) to provide more resistance to proteolytic enzymes. Plain gut sutures retain their strength for 5 to 7 days, whereas chromic sutures maintain strength for 9 to 14 days. However, in the oral cavity, gut suture generally lasts only 2 to 4 days and chromic sutures last approximately 3 to 5 days. Plain and chromic gut are supplied in foil packages that prevent desiccation, and the suture should be kept moist with water or saline during suturing. Polyglycolic acid and polyglactin 910 do not enzymatically break down. Rather, they undergo slow hydrolysis, eventually being resorbed by macrophages. Polyglycolic acid and polyglactin 910 sutures have the advantage of being less stiff than gut sutures. Surgeons often find it easier to tie sutures made of these materials, and the knots are more likely to remain tight. However, polyglycolic acid and polyglactin 910 sutures are more costly than gut sutures.

Resorbable sutures are highly reactive, compared with nonresorbable sutures; that is, resorbable sutures evoke an intense inflammatory reaction that may impede wound healing, occasionally to a clinically significant extent. This is the reason neither plain nor chromic gut is used for suturing the surface of a skin wound.

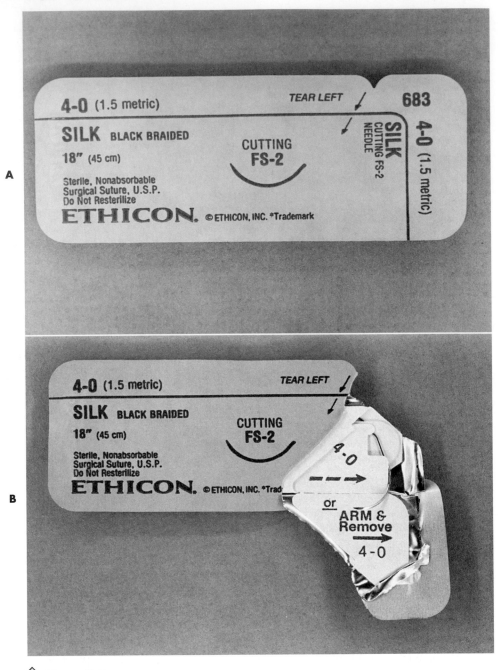

◇ Figure 3-8

Typical suture packaging. **A,** Information visible from exterior of pack includes suture diameter (4-0 [1.5 metric]), length (18 in [45 cm]), material (black braided silk, nonresorbable), and type of needle (cutting, FS-2). Approximate size and shape of needle is illustrated on package. **B,** Tearing open pack at appropriate site exposes needle ready to grasp with needle holder.

NONRESORBABLE SUTURES

The most commonly used nonresorbable sutures in oral and maxillofacial surgery are silk, nylon, polyester, and polypropylene. Although silk is classified as a nonresorbable suture material, it gradually loses its tensile strength and disappears in about 2 years if not removed.

Nonresorbable sutures are either monofilamentous, multifilamentous, or both. The multifilamentous form increases its strength but also increases suture abrasiveness and is more likely to convert contamination into infection. Silk and polyester sutures are available only in a multifilamentous form, polypropylene is produced only in a monofilamentous form, and nylon comes in both monofilamentous and multifilamentous forms (Figure 3-9, *A*).

All nonresorbable sutures have some reactivity. Of the

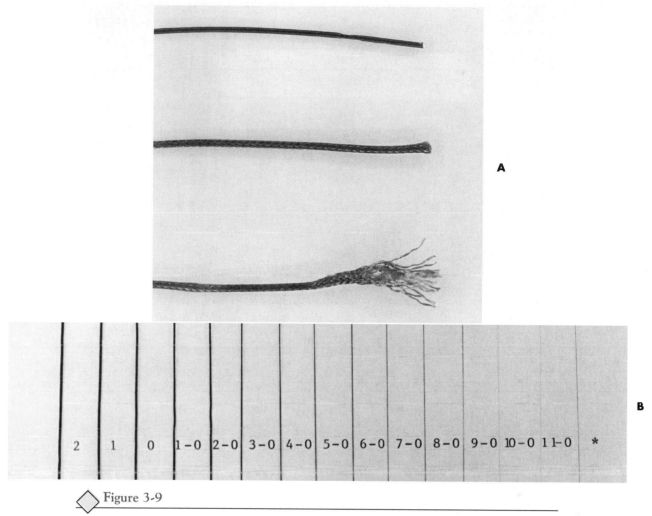

◇ Figure 3-9

A, Monofilamentous suture *(top)* compared with multifilamentous suture *(middle);* multifilamentous suture purposely frayed to demon strate multifilamentous construction *(bottom).* **B,** Available suture sizes ranging from size 2 to size 11-0 (smallest diameter); human hair included for size comparison. *Suture sizes 3 to 7 are manufactured but not included here.

commonly used nonresorbable sutures, silk evokes the most intense inflammatory response. Polyester is much less reactive than silk, nylon is less reactive than polyester, and polypropylene has the least tendency to induce inflammation. In situations in which it is important to minimize wound inflammation, such as in a facial laceration, nylon is usually the cutaneous suture of choice.

SUTURE SIZES

Sutures are available in various sizes that range from the largest size, 7, down to the extremely fine 11-0 suture. The increasing number of zeros correlates with decreasing suture diameter and strength. For example, size 1-0 suture is larger in diameter than size 2-0, size 3-0 is larger than size 7-0, and so on (Figure 3-9, *B*). Because suture material is foreign to the human body, the smallest-diameter suture sufficient to keep a wound closed properly should be employed. Generally, the size of suture is chosen to corre-

late with the tensile strength of the tissue being sutured. Most oral and maxillofacial surgical procedures require the use of a 3-0 or 4-0 suture.

SUTURE HANDLING

The ease of handling is another essential variable in choosing suture materials. The ease of knot tying and the ability of the suture to hold a knot are important. In general, multifilamentous sutures handle better than monofilamentous sutures (Figure 3-9, *A*). Most surgeons find silk the easiest suture to handle. A properly tied silk suture requires only three knotting throws. Polyester, gut, polyglactin 910, and polyglycolic acid sutures usually need four knotting throws to keep the knot secure. Polypropylene knots tend to stay tied, because the material is soft and thus provides a locking mechanism. Minimizing the number of throws is beneficial, because each throw of the suture provides another niche in which contaminating bacteria may hide.

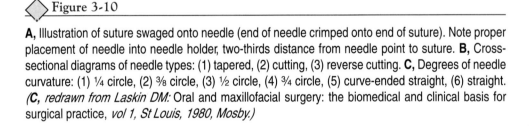

◇ Figure 3-10

A, Illustration of suture swaged onto needle (end of needle crimped onto end of suture). Note proper placement of needle into needle holder, two-thirds distance from needle point to suture. **B,** Cross-sectional diagrams of needle types: (1) tapered, (2) cutting, (3) reverse cutting. **C,** Degrees of needle curvature: (1) ¼ circle, (2) ⅜ circle, (3) ½ circle, (4) ¾ circle, (5) curve-ended straight, (6) straight. *(C, redrawn from Laskin DM:* Oral and maxillofacial surgery: the biomedical and clinical basis for surgical practice, *vol 1, St Louis, 1980, Mosby.)*

NEEDLES

Sutures are manufactured with and without needles attached. A wide variety of needles are available on those sutures with preattached needles. Sutures without attached needles are used to ligate blood vessels or to thread closed or French-eyed needles.

Most sutures used for oral and maxillofacial surgery are swaged onto needles; that is, during manufacture the suture has been placed into a hollow end of a needle and the end then slightly crimped to retain the suture (Figure 3-10, *A*). Swaging sutures onto needles simplifies handling and causes less tissue damage during suturing than is caused by closed or French-eyed needles.

Needle points also vary. The basic point types are cutting and tapered. Cutting needles have sharp edges that allow the needle to penetrate tough tissues, such as gingiva and skin. The tapered point is round and without cutting edges. It causes less tissue damage during penetration but cannot easily go through relatively firm tissue (Figure 3-10, *B*). Most oral and maxillofacial surgery is performed with a cutting needle.

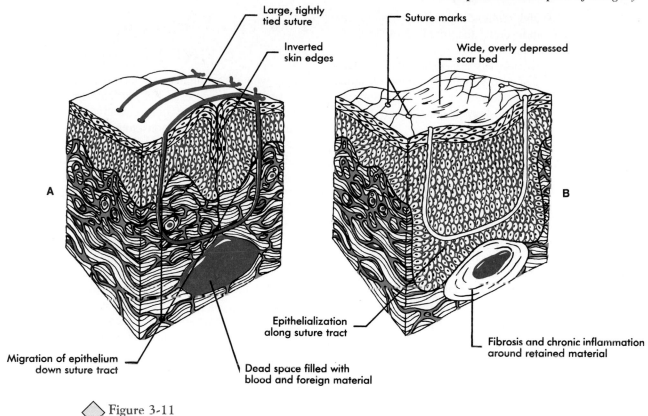

Large, tightly tied suture

Inverted skin edges

Suture marks

Wide, overly depressed scar bed

A

B

Epithelialization along suture tract

Migration of epithelium down suture tract

Dead space filled with blood and foreign material

Fibrosis and chronic inflammation around retained material

◇ Figure 3-11

A, Improper suturing technique. Excessively large suture tied too tightly, inverting wound edges, leaving dead space, and failing to remove suture early enough to prevent epithelial migration down along sutures. **B,** Poor appearance of scar is caused by wound-closure errors, as illustrated in **A.** *(From Bryant WM: CIBA-GEIGY Clin Symp, 1977.)*

Needles also differ in their curvature, diameter, and length (Figure 3-10, *C*). The dentist learns through experience which type of needle works best in his or her hands.

BASIC SUTURING TECHNIQUES

When suturing, a few basic principles should be followed. The needle should be grasped with the needle holder half to three fourths of the distance away from the point (Figure 3-10, *A*). The needle should be placed perpendicular to the surface being entered and pushed through the tissue, following the curvature of the needle, rotating the wrist only, not the arm. The needle should not be forced through the tissue, because it may bend and break. The point of the needle should never be grasped with an instrument. When suturing a mobile tissue to a relatively fixed tissue, the suture should first be placed through the movable tissue. Movable tissue should be gently grasped with a toothed forceps to stabilize it while the needle is being pushed through the tissue. While tying a suture in the facial region, the needle should be held in the palm of the hand to prevent it from entering the patient's eyes. Suture ends should be pulled together and tied only tightly enough to gently approximate the wound edges; any excessive tightness compromises the vascularity of the wound edge (Figure

3-11). The number of sutures should be limited to only those necessary to close the wound properly. An excessive number of sutures introduces more foreign material into the wound, produces more tissue injury, prolongs the procedure, and wastes suture material. Sutures that hold knots well, such as silk, but are to be buried should have all suture material above the knot removed. However, suture materials that do not hold knots well, such as chromic, but are to be buried should have the ends cut approximately 2 to 3 mm above the knot.

POSTOPERATIVE CARE OF SUTURED WOUNDS

Postoperative care of sutured wounds is important. Sutured wounds within the oral cavity should be kept clean by having the patient rinse frequently with normal saline, hydrogen peroxide diluted with saline, or fresh tap water. Sutured wounds on the vermilion of the lips or on the face should be kept free of dried blood and other debris by gentle cleansing of the wound with hydrogen peroxide on cotton applicator sticks at least twice a day. Most patients can be taught to do this themselves. Skin wounds can then be covered with a thin layer of antibiotic ointment. Nonresorbable oral sutures can usually be removed in 5 days; facial skin sutures should be removed after 4 days and replaced by adhesive strips to prevent epithelial migration down the suture tracks and to lessen wound inflammation.

Many general surgeons currently use staples to close skin wounds. Although this is feasible in facial wound closure, staples generally do not permit as precise a closure as sutures do. Tissue adhesives are being tested for suitability for wound closure but are not in general use.

EDEMA CONTROL

Edema occurs after surgery as a result of tissue injury. Edema is an accumulation of fluid in the interstitial space because of transudation from damaged vessels and lymphatic obstruction by fibrin. Two variables help determine the degree of postsurgical edema. First, the greater the amount of tissue injury, the greater the amount of edema. Second, the more loose connective tissue that is contained in the injured region, the more edema is present. For example, attached gingiva has little loose connective tissue, so it exhibits little tendency toward edema; however, the lips and floor of the mouth contain large amounts of loose connective tissue and can swell significantly.

The dentist can control the amount of postsurgical edema by performing surgery in a manner that minimizes tissue damage. Some believe that ice applied to a freshly wounded area decreases vascularity and thereby diminishes transudation. However, no controlled study has verified the effectiveness of this practice. Patient positioning in the early postoperative period is also used to decrease edema by having patients try to keep their head elevated above the rest of their body as much as possible during the first few postoperative days. Systemic corticosteroids can be administered to the patient and have an impressive ability to lessen inflammation and transudation and thus edema. However, corticosteroids are useful for edema control only if administered before tissue is damaged.

PATIENT GENERAL HEALTH AND NUTRITION

Proper wound healing depends on a patient's ability to resist infection, to provide essential nutrients for use as building materials, and to carry out reparative cellular processes. Numerous medical conditions impair a patient's ability to resist infection and heal wounds. These include conditions that establish a catabolic state of metabolism, that impede oxygen or nutrient delivery to tissues, and that require administration of drugs or physical agents that interfere with immunologic or wound-healing cells. Examples of diseases that induce a catabolic metabolic state include poorly controlled insulin-dependent diabetes mellitus, end-stage renal or hepatic disease, and malignant diseases. Conditions that interfere with the delivery of oxygen or nutrients to wounded tissues include severe chronic obstructive pulmonary disease (COPD), poorly compensated congestive heart failure (hypertrophic cardio-myopathy), and drug addictions, such as ethanolism. Diseases requiring the administration of drugs that interfere with host defenses or wound-healing capabilities include autoimmune diseases, for which long-term corticosteroid therapy is given, and malignancies, for which cytotoxic agents and irradiation are used.

The surgeon can help improve the patient's chances of having an elective surgical wound that heals normally by evaluating and optimizing the patient's general health status before surgery. For malnourished patients, this includes improving the nutritional status, so that the patient is in a positive nitrogen balance and an anabolic metabolic state.

BIBLIOGRAPHY

Peacock EE Jr: *Wound repair,* ed 3, Philadelphia, 1984, WB Saunders.

WOUND REPAIR

JAMES R. HUPP

CHAPTER OUTLINE ————————◇

A n important aspect of any surgical procedure is the preparation of the wound for healing. It is therefore mandatory that individuals intending to perform surgery possess a thorough understanding of tissue-repair processes.

Tissue injury can be caused by either pathologic or traumatic events. The dental surgeon has little control over pathologic tissue damage but can favorably or unfavorably alter the amount and severity of traumatically induced tissue injury and thereby promote or impede wound healing.

This chapter discusses the ways in which tissue injury occurs and the events normally present during the healing of soft and hard tissues.

WOUND REPAIR ————————————◇
ETIOLOGY OF TISSUE DAMAGE

Traumatic injuries can be caused by physical or chemical insults (Box 4-1). Physical methods of producing tissue damage include incision or crushing, extremes of temperature or irradiation, desiccation, and obstruction of arterial inflow or venous outflow. Chemicals able to cause injury include those with unphysiologic pH or tonicity, those that disrupt protein integrity, and those causing ischemia by producing vascular constriction or thrombosis.

EPITHELIALIZATION

Injured epithelium has a regenerative ability that allows it to reestablish its integrity through migration and a process known as *contact inhibition.* In general, a free edge of epithelium continues to migrate (by proliferation of germinal epithelial cells that push the free edge forward) until it comes into contact with another free edge of epithelium, where it is signaled to stop growing laterally. Although it is theorized that chemical mediators (released from epithelial cells that have lost contact with other epithelial cells circumferentially) regulate this process, no definitive evidence for this is yet available. Wounds in which only the surface epithelium is injured (abrasions) heal by migration of epithelium across the wound bed. Because epithelium does not normally contain blood vessels, the epithelium in wounds in which the subepithelial tissue is also damaged migrates across whatever vascularized tissue bed is available and stays under the portion of the superficial blood clot that desiccates (forms a scab) until it reaches another epithelial margin. Once the wound is fully epithelialized, the scab loosens and is dislodged.

An example of the detrimental effect of the process of contact inhibition controlling epithelialization occurs when an opening is accidentally made into a maxillary sinus. If the epithelium of both the sinus wall and the oral mucosa is injured, it begins to migrate in both areas. In this case the first free epithelial edge the sinus epithelium is likely to contact is oral mucosa, thereby creating an oroantral fistula (an epithelialized tract between the oral cavity and the maxillary sinus).

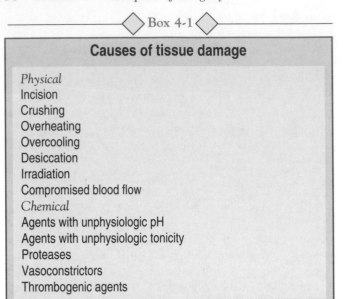

◇ Box 4-1 ◇

Causes of tissue damage

Physical
Incision
Crushing
Overheating
Overcooling
Desiccation
Irradiation
Compromised blood flow
Chemical
Agents with unphysiologic pH
Agents with unphysiologic tonicity
Proteases
Vasoconstrictors
Thrombogenic agents

The process of reepithelialization (secondary epithelialization) is sometimes used therapeutically by oral and maxillofacial surgeons during certain preprosthetic surgical procedures in which an area of oral mucosa is denuded of epithelium (unattached gingiva) and then left to epithelialize by adjacent epithelium (attached gingiva) creeping over the wound bed.

STAGES OF WOUND HEALING

Regardless of the cause of nonepithelial tissue injury, a stereotypic process is initiated that, if able to proceed unimpeded, works to restore tissue integrity. This process is called *wound healing*. The process has been divided into three basic stages (inflammatory, fibroplastic, and remodeling) that, although not mutually exclusive, take place in this sequence.

INFLAMMATORY STAGE. The inflammatory stage begins the moment tissue injury occurs and, in the absence of factors that prolong inflammation, lasts 3 to 5 days. It has two phases, vascular and cellular. The vascular events set in motion during inflammation begin with an initial vasoconstriction of disrupted vessels as a result of normal

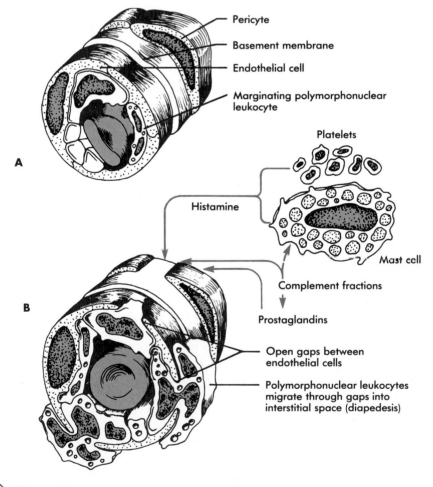

◇ Figure 4-1

Early vascular responses to injury. Initial transient vasoconstriction **(A)** is soon followed by vasodilation **(B).** Vasodilation is caused by action of histamine, prostaglandins, and other vasodilatory substances. Dilation causes intercellular gaps to occur, which allows egress of plasma and emigration of leukocytes. *(From Bryant WM:* CIBA-GEIGY, Clin Symp, *1977.)*

vascular tone. The vasoconstriction slows blood flow into the area of injury, promoting blood coagulation. Within minutes, histamine and prostaglandins E_1 and E_2, elaborated by white blood cells, cause vasodilation and open small spaces between endothelial cells, which allows plasma to leak and leukocytes to migrate into interstitial tissues. Fibrin from the transudated plasma causes lymphatic obstruction, and the transudated plasma—aided by obstructed lymphatics—accumulates in the area of injury, functioning to dilute contaminants. This fluid collection is called *edema* (Figure 4-1).

The cardinal signs of inflammation are redness (erythema) and swelling (edema), with warmth and pain—*rubor et tumour cum calore et dolore* (Celsius, [30 B.C.-A.D. 38]) and loss of function—*functio laesa* (Virchow, 1821-1902). Warmth and erythema are caused by vasodilation; swelling is caused by transudation of fluid; and pain and loss of function are caused by histamine, kinins, and prostaglandins released by leukocytes, as well as by pressure from edema.

The cellular phase of inflammation is triggered by the activation of serum complement by tissue trauma. Complement-split products, particularly C3a and C5a, act as chemotactic factors and cause polymorphonuclear leukocytes (neutrophils) to stick to the side of blood vessels (margination) and then migrate through the vessel walls (diapedesis). Once in contact with foreign materials (such as bacteria), the neutrophils release the contents of their lysosomes (degranulation). The lysosomal enzymes (consisting primarily of proteases) work to destroy bacteria and other foreign materials and to digest necrotic tissue. Clearance of debris is

also aided by monocytes, such as macrophages, which phagocytize foreign and necrotic materials. With time, lymphocytes accumulate at the site of tissue injury. The lymphocytes are in the B or T groups. B lymphocytes are able to recognize antigenic material, produce antibodies that assist the remainder of the immune system in identifying foreign materials, and interact with complement to lyse foreign cells. T lymphocytes are divided into the following three principal subgroups: helper T cells, which stimulate B cell proliferation and differentiation; suppressor T cells, which work to regulate the function of helper T cells; and cytotoxic (killer) T cells, which lyse cells bearing foreign antigens.

The inflammatory stage is sometimes referred to as the *lag phase,* because this is the period during which no significant gain in wound strength occurs (because little collagen deposition is taking place). The principal material holding a wound together during the inflammatory stage is fibrin, which possesses little tensile strength (Figure 4-2).

FIBROPLASTIC STAGE. The strands of fibrin, which are derived from the coagulation of blood, crisscross wounds to form a latticework on which fibroblasts can begin laying down ground substance and tropocollagen. This is the fibroplastic stage of wound repair. The ground substance consists of several mucopolysaccharides, which act to cement collagen fibers together. The fibroblasts transform local and circulating pluripotential mesenchymal cells that begin tropocollagen production on the third or fourth day after tissue injury. Fibroblasts also secrete fibronectin, a protein that performs

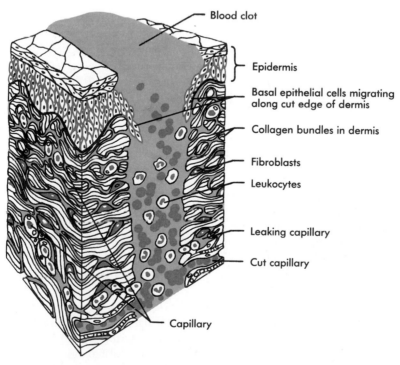

- Blood clot
- Epidermis
- Basal epithelial cells migrating along cut edge of dermis
- Collagen bundles in dermis
- Fibroblasts
- Leukocytes
- Leaking capillary
- Cut capillary
- Capillary

◇ Figure 4-2

Inflammatory stage of wound repair. Wound fills with clotted blood, inflammatory cells, and plasma. Adjacent epithelium begins to migrate into wound, and undifferentiated mesenchymal cells begin to transform into fibroblasts. *(From Bryant WM: CIBA-GEIGY, Clin Symp, 1977.)*

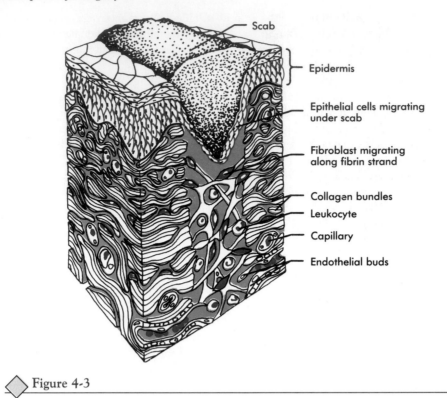

Scab
Epidermis
Epithelial cells migrating under scab
Fibroblast migrating along fibrin strand
Collagen bundles
Leukocyte
Capillary
Endothelial buds

◇ **Figure 4-3**

Migratory phase of fibroplastic stage of wound repair. Continued epithelial migration occurs, leukocytes dispose of foreign and necrotic materials, capillary ingrowth begins, and fibroblasts migrate into wound along fibrin strands. *(From Bryant WM:* CIBA-GEIGY, Clin Symp, *1977.)*

several functions. Fibronectin helps stabilize fibrin, assists in recognizing foreign material that should be removed by the immune system, acts as a chemotactic factor for fibroblasts, and helps to guide macrophages along fibrin strands for eventual phagocytosis of fibrin by the macrophages.

The fibrin network is also used by new capillaries, which bud from existing vessels along the margins of the wound and run along fibrin strands to cross the wound. As fibroplasia continues, with increasing ingrowth of new cells, fibrinolysis occurs, which is caused by plasmin brought in by the new capillaries to remove the fibrin strands that have become unnecessary (Figure 4-3).

Fibroblasts deposit tropocollagen, which undergoes cross-linking to produce collagen. Initially, collagen is produced in excessive amounts and is laid down in a haphazard manner. The poor orientation of fibers decreases the effectiveness of a given amount of collagen to produce wound strength, so an overabundance of collagen is necessary to strengthen the healing wound initially. Despite the poor organization of collagen, wound strength rapidly increases during the fibroplastic stage, which normally lasts 2 to 3 weeks. If a wound is placed under tension at the beginning of fibroplasia, it tends to pull apart along the initial line of injury. However, if the wound were to be placed under tension near the end of fibroplasia, it would open along the junction between old collagen previously on the edges of the wound and newly deposited collagen. Clinically, the wound at the end of the fibroplastic stage will be stiff because of the excessive amount of collagen, erythematous because of the high degree of vascularization, and able to withstand 70% to 80% as much tension as uninjured tissue (Figure 4-4).

REMODELING STAGE. The final stage of wound repair, which continues indefinitely, is known as the *remodeling stage,* although some use the term *wound maturation.* During this stage, many of the previous randomly laid collagen fibers are destroyed as they are replaced by new collagen fibers, which are oriented to better resist tensile forces on the wound. During this stage, wound strength increases slowly but not with the same magnitude of increase seen during the fibroplastic stage. Wound strength never reaches more than 80% to 85% of the strength of uninjured tissue. Because of the collagen fibers' more efficient orientation, fewer of them are necessary, and the excess is removed, which softens the scar. As wound metabolism lessens, vascularity is decreased, which diminishes wound erythema. Elastin found in normal skin and ligaments is not replaced during wound healing, so injuries in those tissues cause a loss of flexibility along the scarred area (Figure 4-5).

A final process, which begins near the end of fibroplasia and continues during the early portion of remodeling, is wound contraction. In most cases, wound contraction plays a beneficial role in wound repair, although the exact mechanism

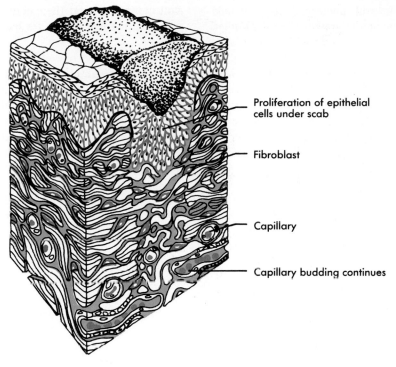

Proliferation of epithelial cells under scab

Fibroblast

Capillary

Capillary budding continues

◇ Figure 4-4

Proliferative phase of fibroplastic stage of wound repair. Proliferation increases epithelial thickness, collagen fibers are haphazardly laid down by fibroblasts, and budding capillaries begin to establish contact with their counterparts from other sites in wound. *(From Bryant WM:* CIBA-GEIGY, Clin Symp, *1977.)*

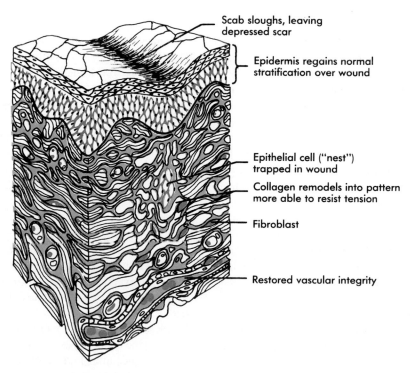

Scab sloughs, leaving depressed scar

Epidermis regains normal stratification over wound

Epithelial cell ("nest") trapped in wound

Collagen remodels into pattern more able to resist tension

Fibroblast

Restored vascular integrity

◇ Figure 4-5

Remodeling stage of wound repair. Epithelial stratification is restored, collagen is remodeled into more efficiently organized patterns, fibroblasts slowly disappear, and vascular integrity is reestablished. *(From Bryant WM:* CIBA-GEIGY, Clin Symp, *1977.)*

that contracts a wound is still unclear. During wound contraction the edges of a wound migrate toward each other. In a wound in which the edges are not or will not be placed in apposition, wound contraction diminishes the size of the wound. However, contraction can cause problems, such as those seen in victims of third-degree (full-thickness) burns of skin, who develop deforming and debilitating contractures if not given skin grafts. Another example of detrimental contraction is seen in individuals suffering sharply curved lacerations, who frequently are left with a mound of tissue on the concave side of the scar because of wound contraction, even when the edges are well readapted. Contraction can be lessened by placement of a layer of epithelium between the free edges of a wound. Surgeons use this phenomenon when they place skin grafts on the bared periosteum during a vestibuloplasty or on full-thickness burn wounds.

SURGICAL SIGNIFICANCE OF WOUND HEALING CONCEPTS

The surgeon can create conditions that either augment or impede the natural wound repair process. Adherence to surgical principles facilitates optimal wound healing, with reestablishment of tissue continuity, minimization of scar size, and restoration of function. It should be remembered that no wound in skin, oral mucosa, or muscle heals without scar formation. The surgeon's goal with respect to scar formation is not to prevent a scar, but rather to produce a scar that minimizes loss of function and looks as inconspicuous as possible.

FACTORS THAT IMPAIR WOUND HEALING

Four factors that can impair wound healing in an otherwise healthy individual are foreign material, necrotic tissue, ischemia, and wound tension.

FOREIGN MATERIAL. Foreign material is everything the host organism's immune system views as "nonself," including bacteria, dirt, suture material, and so on. Foreign materials cause three basic problems. First, bacteria can proliferate and cause an infection in which bacterial proteins that destroy host tissue are released. Second, nonbacterial foreign materials act as havens for bacteria by sheltering them from host defenses and thus promoting infection. Third, foreign material is often antigenic and can stimulate a chronic inflammatory reaction that decreases fibroplasia.

NECROTIC TISSUE. Necrotic tissue in a wound causes two problems. The first is that its presence serves as a barrier to the ingrowth of reparative cells. The inflammatory stage is then prolonged to allow white blood cells to remove the necrotic debris through the processes of enzymatic lysis and phagocytosis. The second problem is that, similar to foreign material, necrotic tissue serves as a protected niche for bacteria. Necrotic tissue frequently includes blood that

collects in a wound (hematoma), where it can serve as an excellent nutrient source for bacteria.

ISCHEMIA. Decreased blood supply to a wound interferes with wound repair in several ways. It can lead to further tissue necrosis and also lessen the conveyance to a wound of necessary antibodies, white blood cells, and antibiotics, which increases the chances of a wound infection. Wound ischemia decreases the delivery of oxygen and the nutrients necessary for wound healing. Ischemia can be caused by several things, including tight or incorrectly located sutures, improperly designed flaps, excessive external pressure on a wound, internal pressure on a wound (seen, for example, with hematomas), systemic hypotension, peripheral vascular disease, and anemia.

TENSION. Tension on a wound is the final factor that can impede wound healing. If sutures are used to overcome excessive wound tension, the tissue encompassed by the sutures will be strangulated, producing ischemia. If sutures are removed too early in the healing process, the wound under tension will probably reopen and then heal with excessive scar formation and wound contraction. If sutures are left in too long in an attempt to overcome wound tension, the wound will still tend to spread open during the remodeling stage of healing, and the tract into the epithelium through which the sutures ran will epithelialize and leave a permanent disfiguring mark.

HEALING BY PRIMARY AND SECONDARY INTENTION

Clinicians use the terms *primary intention* and *secondary intention* to describe the two basic methods of wound healing. In healing by primary intention, the edges of a wound in which there is no tissue loss are placed in essentially the same anatomic position they held before injury and are allowed to heal. Wound repair then occurs with minimal scar formation, because the tissues would not "perceive" that an injury had occurred. Strictly speaking, healing by primary intention is only a theoretic ideal, impossible to attain clinically; however, the term is generally used to designate wounds in which the edges are closely reapproximated. This method of wound repair lessens the amount of reepithelialization, collagen deposition, contraction, and remodeling necessary during healing. Therefore healing occurs more rapidly, with a lower risk of infection and with less scar formation than in wounds allowed to heal by secondary intention. Examples of wounds that heal by primary intention include well-repaired lacerations or incisions, well-reduced bone fractures, and anatomic nerve reanastomoses of recently severed nerves. In contrast, healing by secondary intention implies that a gap is left between the edges of an incision or laceration or between bone or nerve ends after repair or that tissue loss has occurred in a wound that prevents close approximation of wound edges. These situations require a large amount of epithelial migration, collagen deposition, contraction, and remodeling during healing. Healing is slower and produces more scar tissue than is the case with healing by primary intention. Examples of wounds allowed to heal by secondary intention include extraction sockets, poorly reduced fractures, deep ulcers, and large avulsive injuries of any soft tissue.

Some surgeons use the term *tertiary intention* to refer to the healing of wounds through the use of tissue grafts over large wounds healing by secondary intention.

HEALING OF EXTRACTION SOCKETS

The removal of a tooth initiates the same sequence of inflammation, epithelialization, fibroplasia, and remodeling seen in prototypic skin or mucosal wounds. As previously mentioned, sockets heal by secondary intention, and many months must pass before a socket heals to the degree to which it becomes difficult to distinguish from the surrounding bone when viewed radiographically.

When a tooth is removed, the remaining empty socket consists of cortical bone (the radiographic lamina dura) covered by torn periodontal ligaments, with a rim of oral epithelium (gingiva) left at the coronal portion. The socket fills with blood, which coagulates and seals the socket from the oral environment.

The inflammatory stage occurs during the first week of healing. White blood cells enter the socket to remove contaminating bacteria from the area and begin to break down any debris, such as bone fragments, that are left in the socket. Fibroplasia also begins during the first week, with the ingrowth of fibroblasts and capillaries. The epithelium migrates down the socket wall until it either reaches a level at which it contacts epithelium from the other side of the socket or it encounters the bed of granulation tissue (tissue filled with numerous immature capillaries and fibroblasts) under the blood clot over which it can migrate. Finally, during the first week of healing, osteoclasts accumulate along the crestal bone.

The second week is marked by the large amount of granulation tissue that fills the socket. Osteoid deposition has begun along the alveolar bone lining the socket. In smaller sockets the epithelium may have become fully intact by this point.

The processes begun during the second week continue during the third and fourth weeks of healing, with epithelialization of most sockets complete at this time. The cortical bone continues to be resorbed from the crest and walls of the socket, and new trabecular bone is laid down across the socket. It is not until 4 to 6 months after extraction that the cortical bone lining a socket is fully resorbed; this is recognized radiographically when there is loss of a distinct lamina dura. As bone fills the socket, the epithelium moves toward the crest and eventually becomes level with adjacent crestal gingiva. The only visible remnant of the socket after 1 year is the rim of poorly vascularized fibrous (scar) tissue that remains on the edentulous alveolar ridge.

BONE HEALING

The events that occur during normal wound healing of soft-tissue injuries (inflammation, fibroplasia, and remodeling) also take place during the repair of an injured bone. But in contrast to soft tissues, osteoblasts and osteoclasts are also involved, to reconstitute and remodel the damaged ossified tissue.

Osteogenic cells (osteoblasts) important to bone healing are derived from the following three sources: periosteum, endosteum, and circulating pluripotential mesenchymal cells. Osteoclasts, derived from monocyte precursor cells, function to resorb necrotic bone and bone that needs to be remodeled. Osteoblasts then lay down osteoid, which, if completely immobile during healing, goes on to calcify.

The terms *primary intention* and *secondary intention* are appropriate for descriptions of bone repair.* If a bone is fractured and the free ends of the bone are more than a millimeter or so apart, the bone heals by secondary intention; that is, during the fibroplastic stage of healing a large amount of collagen must be laid down to bridge the bony gap (Figure 4-6). The fibroblasts and osteoblasts actually produce so much fibrous matrix that the healing tissue extends circumferentially beyond the free ends of the bone and forms what is called a *callus* (Figure 4-7). Under normal conditions the fibrous tissue, including the callus, ossifies. During the remodeling stage, bone that was haphazardly produced is resorbed by osteoclasts, and osteoblasts lay down new bone directed to resist low-grade tensions placed on the bone (Figure 4-8).

Healing of bone by primary intention occurs when the bone is either incompletely fractured, so that the fractured ends do not become separated from each other (greenstick fracture), or when a surgeon closely reapproximates and rigidly stabilizes the fractured ends of a bone (anatomic reduction of the fracture). In both of these situations, little fibrous tissue is produced, and reossification of the tissue within the fracture area occurs quickly, with minimal callus formation. The surgical technique that comes closest to allowing bone to heal by primary intention is anatomic reduction of the fracture (put the ends of fractured bones back into their normal relationship), with the application of bone plates that rigidly hold the ends of the bone together. This minimizes the distance between the ends of a fractured bone, so that ossification across the fracture gap can occur with little intervening fibrous tissue formation.

Two factors of importance to proper bone healing are vascularity and immobility. The fibrous connective tissue that forms in a bony fracture site requires a high degree of vascularity (which carries blood with a normal oxygen content) for eventual ossification. If vascularity or oxygen supply are sufficiently compromised, cartilage forms instead of bone. Furthermore, if vascularity or oxygen supply are poor, the fibrous tissue does not chondrify or ossify.

Bone must be placed under some tension to stimulate continued osteoblastic bone formation. Bone is formed perpendicular to lines of tension, to help withstand the forces placed on it. This is the basis of the functional matrix concept

---

*The term *fracture* used with respect to bone repair includes not only traumatically injured bone but also bone cuts purposely made by a surgeon during reconstructive surgery.

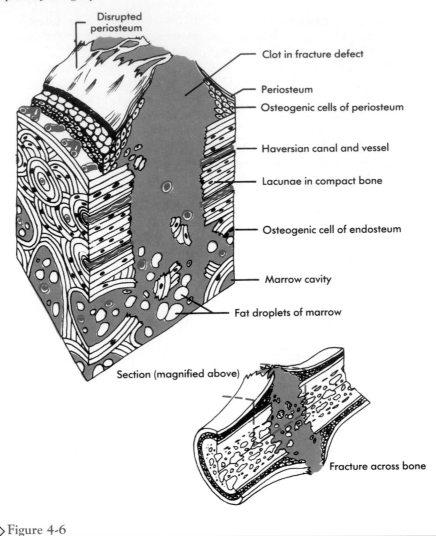

Disrupted periosteum

Clot in fracture defect

Periosteum

Osteogenic cells of periosteum

Haversian canal and vessel

Lacunae in compact bone

Osteogenic cell of endosteum

Marrow cavity

Fat droplets of marrow

Section (magnified above)

Fracture across bone

◇ Figure 4-6

Early phase of fibroplastic stage of bone repair. Osteogenic cells from periosteum and marrow proliferate and differentiate into osteoblasts, osteoclasts, and chondroblasts, and capillary budding begins. *(From Bryant WM:* CIBA-GEIGY, Clin Symp, *1977.)*

of bone remodeling. However, excessive tension or torque placed on a healing fracture site produces mobility there. This mobility compromises vascularity of the wound and favors the formation of cartilage or fibrous tissue rather than bone along the fracture line, and in a contaminated fracture it promotes wound infection (Figure 4-8).

IMPLANT OSSEOINTEGRATION

The discovery of osseointegration by Branemark and his research team in the 1960s forced a reexamination of traditional concepts of wound healing. Before acceptance of his findings it was thought than any foreign material placed through an epithelial surface would eventually be expelled by the body. This would occur as the epithelium bordering the foreign material migrated down along the interface with the foreign material, finally fully surrounding the portion of the foreign body protruding into the body, causing the material to be completely external to the epithelial barrier. For a

dental implant, this meant eventual loosening of the implant.

The innate tendency of epithelium to surround and externalize foreign material was thought to be the result of the principle of contact inhibition, discussed previously, whereby any epithelial surface disrupted by any force or object triggers epithelial growth and migration. The epithelium continues to spread until it contacts other epithelial cells and is inhibited from further lateral growth. Branemark found that if an inert foreign material was placed through an epithelial barrier and allowed to develop intimate contact with underlying bone, epithelial migration down into the bone along the implant surface would not occur. However, if, instead, the implant had an intervening layer of connective tissue between itself and the bone, epithelium would migrate down the implant, externalizing it. Thus, when an implant integrated with bone (osseointegration), lateral growth of epithelium stopped, without contact inhibition as it was classically conceived to function (Figure 4-9).

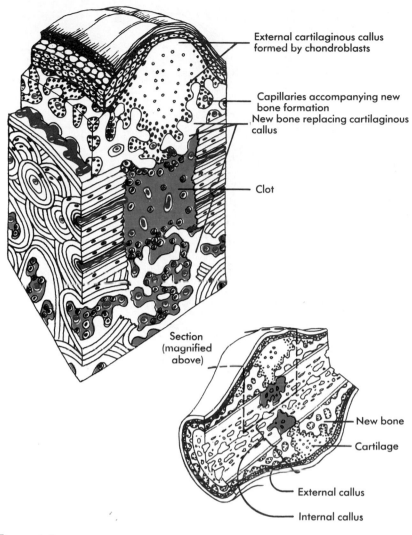

External cartilaginous callus formed by chondroblasts

Capillaries accompanying new bone formation

New bone replacing cartilaginous callus

Clot

Section (magnified above)

New bone

Cartilage

External callus

Internal callus

◇ Figure 4-7

Late phase of fibroplastic stage of bone repair. Osteoclasts resorb necrotic bone. In areas of sufficient oxygen tension, osteoblasts lay down new bone; in areas of low oxygen tension, chondroblasts lay down cartilage. Also capillary ingrowth continues, and internal and external calluses form. *(From Bryant WM: CIBA-GEIGY, Clin Symp, 1977.)*

The reasons why epithelium does not continue to migrate when it meets a bone-implant interface are not known. Nonetheless, dentistry has used this aberration in normal wound healing principles to provide integrated metal posts (implants) that are extremely useful to stabilize dental prostheses. Surgeons use similar techniques to place implants through skin in other body sites to stabilize prosthetic ears, eyes, noses, and so on.

Wound healing around dental implants involves the two basic factors of healing of bone to the implant and healing of alveolar soft tissue to the implant. Dental implants made of pure titanium will be used in the discussion of healing around dental implants; similar healing occurs around properly placed implants made of other inert materials.

Bone healing onto the surface of an implant must occur before any soft tissue forms between the bone and implant surfaces. Maximizing the likelihood of bone winning this race with soft tissue to cover the implant requires the following: (1) a short distance between the bone and implant, (2) viable bone at or very near the surface of the bone along the implant, (3) no movement of the implant while bone is attaching to its surface, and (4) an implant surface free of contamination by organic or inorganic materials.

A short distance between the bone and implant depends on preparing a bony site into which the implant fits precisely. Minimizing bone damage during site preparation preserves the viability of bone near the implant surface. Much of the damage caused by preparing an implant site is the result of heat from friction during the cutting process. Limiting heat production and rapidly dissipating the heat created at the site help protect the viability of bone along the cut surface. This is accomplished by using sharp bone-cutting instruments and

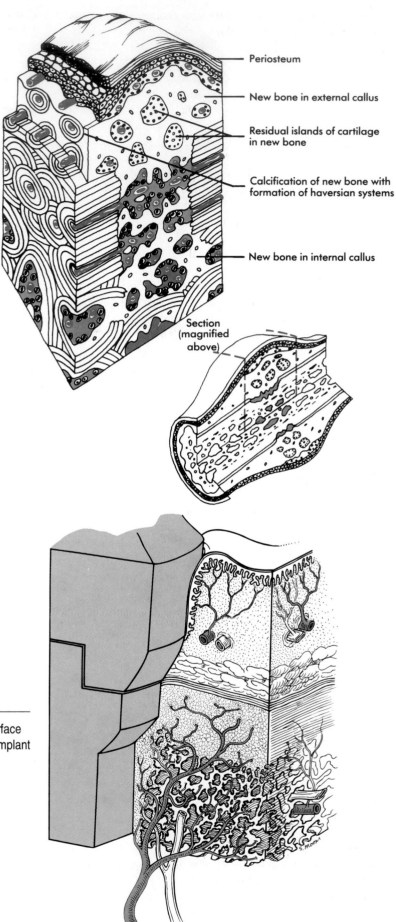

Periosteum

New bone in external callus

Residual islands of cartilage in new bone

Calcification of new bone with formation of haversian systems

New bone in internal callus

Section (magnified above)

◇ Figure 4-8

Remodeling stage of bone repair. Osteoclasts remove unnecessary bone, and osteoblasts lay new bone tissue in response to stresses placed on bone. New haversian systems develop as concentric layers of cortical bone are deposited along blood vessels. Calluses gradually decrease in size. *(From Bryant WM:* CIBA-GEIGY, Clin Symp, *1977.)*

◇ Figure 4-9

Osseointegrated implant with direct bone-implant contact. Surface epithelium migration along implant halted by the direct bone-implant integration.

limited cutting speeds to limit frictional heat and by keeping the bone cool with irrigation during site preparation. Additional damage to the cut surface of bone may occur if the site becomes infected. This is minimized by using systemic and/or topical antibiotics and aseptic surgical techniques.

Movement along the healing bone-implant interface is prevented by keeping forces off of the implant during the critical portion of the healing period. Countersinking implants and using low-profile healing screws decrease the ability of any forces to be delivered to the implant. Covering the top of the implant with gingiva during healing further protects it. Implants that are threaded or otherwise fit tightly into the prepared site are better protected from movement than nonthreaded or loose implants. Eventually, once initial integration has occurred, some limited daily pressure on the implant (1000 μm of strain) will actually hasten cortical bone deposition on the implant surface.

Finally, the surface to which bone is intended to attach must be free of surface contaminants. Such contaminants include bacteria, oil, glove powder, foreign metals, and foreign proteins. The surface of an implant intended to osseointegrate must not be handled with bare or gloved fingers, a forceps made of a metal different than the implant, machine oil, or any soap used to try to clean a contaminated implant.

The surface of pure titanium implants is completely covered by a 2000-Å-thick layer of titanium oxide. This stabilizes the surface, and it is to this oxidized surface that bone must attach for osseointegration to occur.

Regardless of how much care is taken to minimize damage to bone during implant site preparation, a superficial layer of bone along the surface of a prepared implant site becomes nonviable as a result of thermal and vascular trauma. Although the living cells in the bone die, the inorganic bone structure remains. Under the influence of local growth factors, bone cells directly underlying this bone structure and blood-borne undifferentiated mesenchymal cells repopulate and remodel the bony scaffold with osteoblasts, osteoclasts, and osteocytes. The nonviable bone is slowly replaced with new, viable cortical bone through the process of creeping substitution. Cutting cones move through the bone at a rate of 40 μm/day, removing dead bone and leaving new osteoid.

At the implant surface, glycosaminoglycans secreted by osteocytes coat the oxide layer. Soon osteoblasts begin to secrete a layer of osteoid over the proteoglycan layer. Bone then goes on to form if proper conditions, such as no implant movement and good oxygen supply, continue during the months required for healing. The greater the amount of available implant surface, the greater the amount of implant osseointegration. Thus longer or wider-diameter implants and those with sandblasted rather than polished surfaces have more surface available for osseointegration.

The initial deposition of bone must occur before epithelium migrates onto or fibrous connective tissue forms on the implant surface. If soft tissue arrives first at any part of the implant surface, bone will never replace the soft tissue at that site. If too much of the implant surface becomes covered with soft tissue rather than bone, and the implant will not become sufficiently osseointegrated to use for a dental prosthesis.

Clinicians have found that in some circumstances they can selectively aid the bone-forming process in its race to cover a surface before soft tissue fills the site. An example of this is the use of woven membranes that have a pore size adequate to allow oxygen and other nutrients to reach the bone grown beneath the membrane, while keeping fibroblasts and other tissue elements outside the membrane. By selectively excluding soft tissues, bone is "guided" into a desired position, thus the term used to describe this process, *guided-tissue regeneration.*

The component of an implant that extends through the oral mucosa also has the ability to alter the contact-inhibition process that normally controls closure of openings through epithelium. In this case, once oral epithelium reaches the surface of a titanium abutment, it seems to stop migrating and secretes a ground substance that attaches the soft tissue to the metal. A hemidesmosomal, basal lamina system forms, further strengthening soft tissue attaching to the implant abutment.

Nerve Injury and Repair

Peripheral nerve injuries represent a unique situation with respect to wound healing. Although the tissue around an injured nerve goes through the stages of inflammation, fibroplasia, and remodeling, the nerve itself goes through other changes.

A brief review of a peripheral nerve's anatomy is necessary before discussing its healing. Peripheral nerves consist of cell bodies that are located in or near the spinal cord or brainstem, with axons that travel to peripheral nerve endings. Both myelinated and unmyelinated axons travel together, grouped in fascicles that are surrounded by the nerve sheath (epineurium).

When a nerve is crushed or severed, the axon distal to the site of injury undergoes Wallerian degeneration and eventually leaves only an empty nerve sheath.* The axon proximal to the area of damage degenerates in a proximal direction for a portion of or for the entire distance back to the cell body.* If the sheath has not been severed, this process is called *axonotmesis.* With axonotmesis the proximal end of the axon begins to bud within 2 days and regenerates down the nerve sheath, with the axon growing about 1 to 1.5 mm per day. If no obstruction exists, nerve function generally returns after a period that depends on the distance from the cell body to the target end-organ.

If the nerve sheath is severed, *neurotmesis* has occurred. In this situation, axonal degeneration occurs in the same manner as with axonotmesis. However, while the axon is regenerating, fibroplasia of tissue surrounding the severed nerve tends to obstruct the proximal end of the nerve, frequently preventing the axon from reaching the end-organ. When the regenerating axon reaches such an obstruction, it may begin randomly branching, in an attempt to find the distal portion of the nerve sheath or to find a path around the obstruction, thus creating

---

*The terms *axial* and *proximal* used in the description of nerves and bones refer to positions farthest away from (distal) or nearest to (proximal) the central nervous system.

a new nerve sheath as it grows. If the axon is unable to circumvent the obstruction, it may simply form a haphazard bundle of nerve tissue, called a *neuroma,* which may cause a dysesthesia (unpleasant sensation) in the case of a sensory nerve injury.

Nerves that are damaged near the periphery, that is, within 2 cm of the end-organ, do not require close approximation of severed ends, because the axons can frequently find the proper end-organ by random branching. (Chapter 29 contains an expanded discussion of nerve injury and repair.)

BIBLIOGRAPHY

Peacock EE Jr: *Wound repair,* ed 3, Philadelphia, 1984, WB Saunders.

Shafer WG, Hine MK, Levy BM: *A textbook of oral pathology,* ed 4, Philadelphia, 1983, WB Saunders.

Wong EKM, The biology of alveolar healing following the removal of impacted teeth. In Alling C, Helfrick J, Alling R, editors: *Impacted teeth,* Philadelphia, 1993, WB Saunders.

PRINCIPLES OF ASEPSIS

JAMES R. HUPP

CHAPTER OUTLINE

I t would be difficult for a person living in an industrialized society during the twentieth century not to have been exposed to concepts of personal and public hygiene. Personal cleanliness and public sanitation have been ingrained in the culture of modern civilized societies through parental and public education and have been reinforced by government regulations and media advertising. This awareness contrasts starkly with earlier centuries, when the importance of hygienic measures for the control of infectious diseases was not widely appreciated. The monumental work of Semmelweis, Koch, and Lister led to enlightenment about asepsis, so that today the use of aseptic techniques seems almost instinctive.

Despite continued advancements in the area of infection control, health professionals must still learn and practice techniques that limit the spread of contagions. There are two reasons that this is especially true for dentists performing surgery. First, to perform surgery the dentist must violate an epithelial surface, the most important barrier against infection. Second, during most oral surgical procedures the dentist, assistants, and equipment become contaminated with the patient's blood and saliva.

COMMUNICABLE PATHOGENIC ORGANISMS

Two of the most important pieces of knowledge in any conflict are the identity of the enemy and the enemy's strengths and weaknesses. In the case of oral surgery, the opposition includes virulent bacteria, mycobacteria, viruses, and fungi. The opposition's strengths are the various means that organisms use to survive destruction, and the weakness is their susceptibility to chemical and physical agents. With an understanding of the "enemy" the dentist can make rational decisions about infection control.

BACTERIA

UPPER RESPIRATORY TRACT FLORA. Normal oral flora contains the microorganisms usually present in the saliva and on the surfaces of oral tissues in healthy, immunocompetent individuals who have not been exposed to agents that alter the composition of oral organisms. A complete description of this flora can be found in Chapter 16. In brief, normal oral flora consists of aerobic gram-positive cocci (primarily streptococci), actinomycetes, anaerobic bacteria, and candidal species (Table 5-1). The total number of oral organisms is held in check by the following four main processes: (1) rapid epithelial turnover with desquamation; (2) host immunologic factors, such as salivary IgA; (3) dilution by salivary flow; and (4) competition between oral organisms for available nutrients and attachment sites. Any agent—physical, biologic, or chemical—that alters any of the forces that keep oral microbes under control will permit potentially pathologic organisms to overgrow and set the stage for a wound infection.

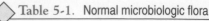

Table 5-1. Normal microbiologic flora

Region	Bacteria
Oral cavity	Aerobic, gram-positive organisms—primarily *Streptococcus* spp.
	Actinomyces spp.
	Anaerobic bacteria, including *Bacteroides melaninogenicus*
	Candida spp.
Nasal cavity	Aerobic gram-positive organisms—primarily *Streptococcus* spp.
	In children: *Haemophilus influenzae* frequently present
	In adults: *Staphylococcus aureus* frequently present
Facial skin	*Staphylococcus* spp., primarily *S. epidermidis*, occasionally *S. aureus*
	Corynebacterium diphtheriae
	Propionibacterium acnes
All areas below clavicles, including hands	*Staphylococcus epidermidis*
	Corynebacterium diphtheriae
	Gram-negative aerobes, such as *Escherichia coli*, *Klebsiella* spp., and *Proteus* spp.
	Anaerobic enteric organisms, including *Bacteroides fragilis*

The flora of the nose and paranasal sinuses consists primarily of gram-positive aerobic streptococci and anaerobes. In addition, many children harbor *Haemophilus influenzae* bacteria in these areas, and many adults have *Staphylococcus aureus* as a part of their transient or resident nasal and paranasal sinus flora. The normal flora in this region of the body is limited by the presence of ciliated, respiratory epithelium, secretory immunoglobulins, and epithelial desquamation. The epithelial cilia move organisms trapped in mucus into the alimentary tract.

MAXILLOFACIAL SKIN FLORA. The skin of the maxillofacial region has surprisingly few resident organisms in its normal flora. The bacteria *Staphylococcus epidermidis* and *Corynebacterium diphtheriae* are the predominant species present. *Propionibacterium acnes* is found in pores and hair follicles, and many individuals carry *S. aureus,* spread from the nose, on their facial skin (Table 5-1).

The skin has several means of preventing surface organisms from entering. The most superficial layer of skin is comprised of keratinized epithelial cells that resist mild trauma. In addition, epithelial cells are joined by tight bonds that resist bacterial entrance. The skin undergoes a process of continued desquamation, which removes bacteria before they are able to form large colonies. Skin is subjected to desiccation, which slows bacterial multiplication, and the sebum produced by glands found in hair follicles is bacteriostatic. Finally, organisms must compete for limited amounts of nutrients.

Skin flora can be altered by processes such as occlusive dressings (which prevent skin desiccation and desquamation), by dirt or dried blood (which provide increased nutrients for organisms), or by antimicrobial agents (which alter the fine balance between various organisms).

NONMAXILLOFACIAL FLORA. The flora below the region of the clavicles, especially the pelvic region and unwashed fingertips, comprises an ever-increasing number of aerobic gram-negative and anaerobic enteric organisms. Knowledge of these bacteria is important for dental surgeons when they are preparing for surgery or when patients require venipuncture or catheterization.

VIRAL ORGANISMS

Viruses are ubiquitous in the environment, but fortunately only a few pose a threat to the patient and the surgical team. The two viral organisms that cause the most difficulty are the hepatitis B virus and the human immunodeficiency virus (HIV). These two viruses have differences in their susceptibility to inactivation that are important to understand when attempting to prevent their spread. Each virus is described here with respect to hardiness and usual mode of transmission. In addition, there is a brief description of the circumstances in which the clinician might suspect that an individual is carrying one of these viruses, which may allow the surgical team to take necessary precautions.

HEPATITIS VIRUSES. Hepatitis A, B, C, and D viruses are responsible for most infectious hepatic diseases. Hepatitis A is spread primarily by contact with the feces of infected individuals; hepatitis C may spread either through contaminated feces or by contaminated blood. Hepatitis B and D are spread by contact with any human secretion. The hepatitis B virus therefore has the most serious risk of transmission for the dentist, staff, and patients. It is usually transmitted by the introduction of infected blood into the bloodstream of a susceptible person, but infected individuals may also secrete large amounts of the virus in their saliva, which can enter an individual through any moist mucosal surface or epithelial (skin or mucosal) wound. Minute quantities of the virus have been found capable of transmitting disease (only 10^5 to 10^7 virions/mL of blood). Unlike most viruses, the hepatitis virus is exceptionally resistant to desiccation and chemical disinfectants, including alcohols, phenols, and quaternary ammonium compounds. Therefore the hepatitis B virus is difficult to contain, particularly when oral surgery is being performed.

Fortunately, there are means of inactivating the virus, including halogen-containing disinfectants (such as iodophor and hypochlorite), formaldehyde, ethylene oxide gas, all types of properly performed heat sterilization, and irradiation. These methods can be used to minimize the spread of hepatitis B from one patient to another.

However, in addition to preventing patient-to-patient spread, the dentist and staff also need to take precautions to protect themselves from contamination, because several instances have occurred in which dentists have been the primary source of a hepatitis B epidemic. Dentists who

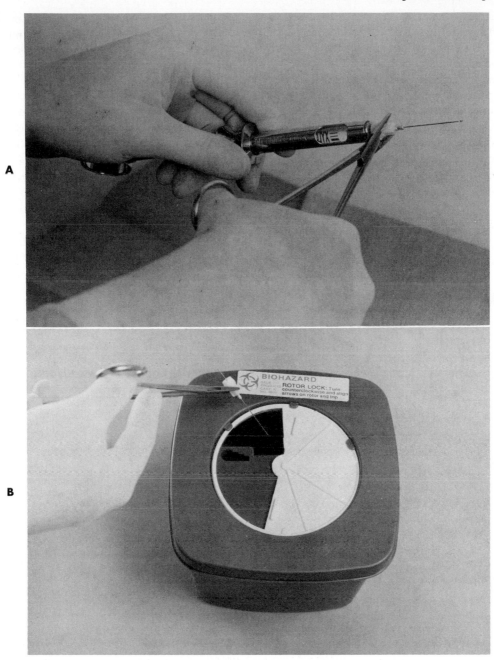

◇ Figure 5-1

A, Technique of removing needle from syringe, using needle holder to grasp it, thereby preventing possibility of pricking. **B,** Proper disposal of sharp, disposable supplies into well-marked, rigid container to prevent accidental inoculation of office staff or cleaning workers with contaminated debris.

perform oral surgical procedures are exposed to blood and saliva; therefore the dental surgery team should wear barriers to protect against contaminating any open wounds on the hands and any exposed mucosal surfaces. This includes wearing gloves, a face mask, and eyeglasses or goggles during surgery. The dental staff should continue to wear these protective devices when cleaning instruments and when handling impressions, casts, or specimens from patients. A common means of hepatitis inoculation is injury with a needle or blade that is contaminated with blood or saliva. Such an injury can be prevented by holding the sheath with an instrument during the resheathing of needles or using the needle to scoop on the sheath after use, taking care never to apply or remove a blade from a scalpel handle or a needle from a syringe without an instrument (Figure 5-1, *A*), and disposing of used blades, needles,and other sharp disposable items into rigid, well-marked receptacles specially designed for contaminated sharp objects (Figure 5-1, *B*). Also, members of the dental staff should receive hepatitis B vaccinations, which have been shown to reduce an individual's susceptibility to hepatitis B infection effectively, although the longevity of protection has not been definitively determined (Figure 5-2). Finally, office-cleaning personnel and commercial laboratory technicians can be protected by proper labeling of contaminated objects and proper disposal of sharp objects (Table 5-2).

Recognition of all individuals known to be carriers of hepatitis B would aid in knowing when special precautions were necessary. However, only about half of the people infected with hepatitis B ever have clinical signs and symptoms of the infection, and some individuals who have completely recovered from the disease still shed intact virus particles in their secretions.

The concept of universal precautions was developed to address the inability of health care providers to specifically identify all patients with communicable diseases. The theory on which the universal precautions concept is based is that protection of self, staff, and patients from contamination by using barrier techniques when treating all patients, as if they all had a communicable disease, ensures that everyone is protected from those who do have an infectious process.

Universal precautions typically include having all doctors and staff who come in contact with patient blood or secretions, whether directly or in aerosol form, wear barrier devices, including a face mask, eye protection, and gloves. Universal precaution procedures go on to include decontaminating or disposing of all surfaces that are exposed to patient blood, tissue, and secretions. Finally, universal precautions mandate avoidance of touching, and thereby contaminating, surfaces (for example, the dental record, telephone, and so on) with contaminated gloves or instruments.

HUMAN IMMUNODEFICIENCY VIRUS.   The human immunodeficiency virus (HIV), which causes acquired immunodeficiency virus (AIDS), acts in a fashion similar to other sexually transmitted infectious disease agents because of its relative inability to survive outside the host organism. That is, transfer of the virions from one individual to another requires direct contact between virus-laden blood or secretions from the infected host organism and a mucosal surface or epithelial wound of the potential host. Evidence has shown that the HIV loses its infectivity once desiccated. In addition, extremely few people carrying the HIV secrete the virus in their saliva, and those who do tend to secrete extremely small amounts. There is no epidemiologic evidence to support HIV infection by saliva alone. Even the blood of patients who are HIV-positive has low concentrations of infectious particles (10^6 particles/mL as compared with 10^{13} particles/mL in hepatitis patients). This probably explains why professionals who are not in any of the known high-risk groups for HIV positivity have an extremely low probability of contracting it, even when exposed to the blood and secretions of large numbers of patients who are HIV-positive during the performance of surgery or when accidentally autoinoculated with infected blood or secretions. Nevertheless, until the transmis-

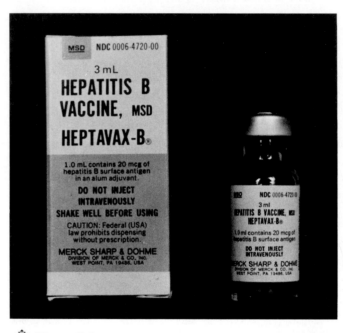

 Figure 5-2

Vaccine used to help prevent transmission of hepatitis B to vaccinated individuals.

◇ Table 5-2. Methods designed to limit the spread of hepatitis viruses

From infected patient to other patients	From infected patient to dental staff
Use of disposable materials	Learning to recognize individuals likely to be carriers
Disinfecting surfaces	Use of barrier technique (gloves, face mask, eye protection) during surgery, when handling contaminated
A. With halogen compounds	objects, and during cleanup
1. Iodophors	Prompt disposal of sharp objects into well-labeled protective containers
2. Hypochlorite (bleach)	Disposal of needles immediately after use or resheathing in-use instruments
B. With aldehydes	Use of an instrument to place a scalpel blade on or take one off a blade handle
1. Formaldehyde	Hepatitis B vaccine
2. Glutaraldehyde	
Sterilize reusable instruments	
A. With heat	
B. With ethylene oxide gas	

sion of HIV becomes fully understood, prudent surgeons will take steps to prevent the spread of infection from the HIV-carrying patient to themselves and their assistants through the use of universal precautions, including barrier techniques.

The universal precaution techniques of preventing the spread of the hepatitis B virus from patient to patient are entirely adequate for prevention of HIV spread. In fact, the patient who is HIV-positive and has AIDS is actually at more risk from the dentist than vice versa, because the immunodeficiency predisposes these patients to infections with unusual pathogens.

In general, the precautions used for bacterial, mycotic, and other viral processes will protect the dentist, office staff, and other patients from the spread of the virus that causes AIDS (Table 5-2).

It is also important that patients with depressed immune function be afforded extra care, to prevent the spread of contagions to them. Thus all patients infected with HIV who have CD4+ T-lymphocyte counts of less than 200/μL or category B or C HIV infection should be treated by doctors and staff free of clinically evident infectious diseases. These patients should not be put in a circumstance in which they are forced to sit close to other patients with clinically apparent disease or symptoms of communicable diseases.

Mycobacterial Organisms

The only mycobacterial organism of significance to most dentists is *Mycobacterium tuberculosis.* Although tuberculosis is an uncommon disease in the United States and Canada, the immigration of individuals from Southeast Asia, where tuberculosis is common, brought a new reservoir of *M. tuberculosis* organisms. Patients who are infected with HIV are another group of individuals who may harbor TB organisms. In addition, some newer strains of TB have become resistant to the drugs commonly used to treat TB. Therefore it is still important that measures be followed to prevent the spread of tuberculosis from patients to the dental staff.

Tuberculosis is transmitted primarily through exhaled aerosols that carry *M. tuberculosis* bacilli (Mtb) from the infected lungs of one individual to the lungs of another individual. Droplets are produced by those with untreated TB during breathing, coughing, sneezing, speaking, and forced expiration. Mtb is not a highly contagious microorganism. However, transmission can also occur via inadequately sterilized instruments, because although Mtb organisms do not form spores, they are highly resistant to desiccation and to most chemical disinfectants. To prevent transmission of tuberculosis from an infected individual to the dental staff, the staff should wear face masks whenever treating or in close contact with these patients. The organisms are sensitive to heat, ethylene oxide, and irradiation; therefore, to prevent their spread from patient to patient, all reusable instruments and supplies should be sterilized with heat or ethylene oxide gas.

When safe to do so, patients with untreated TB should have their surgery postponed until they can receive treatment for their TB.

Aseptic Technique and Universal Precautions ⎯⎯⎯⎯⎯◇

Terminology

Different terms are used to describe various means of preventing infection. However, despite their differing definitions, terms such as *disinfection* and *sterilization* are often used interchangeably. This can lead to the misconception that a certain technique or chemical has sterilized an object when it has merely reduced the level of contamination. Therefore the dental surgeon must be aware of the precise definition of words used for the various techniques of asepsis.

Sepsis is the breakdown of living tissue by the action of microorganisms and is usually accompanied by inflammation. Thus the mere presence of microorganisms, such as in bacteremia, does not constitute a septic state. *Asepsis* refers to the avoidance of sepsis. *Medical asepsis* is the attempt to keep patients, health care staff, and objects as free as possible of agents that cause infection. *Surgical asepsis* is the attempt to prevent microbes from gaining access to surgically created wounds.

Antiseptic and *disinfectant* are terms that are often misused. Both refer to substances that can prevent the multiplication of organisms capable of producing sepsis. The difference is that antiseptics are applied to living tissue, whereas disinfectants are used on inanimate objects.

Sterility is the freedom from viable forms of microorganisms. It represents an absolute state; there are no degrees of sterility.

Sanitization is the reduction of the number of viable microorganisms to levels judged safe by public health standards. It should not be confused with sterilization.

Decontamination is similar to sanitization, except it is not connected to public health standards.

Concepts

Chemical and physical agents are the two principal means of reducing the number of microbes on a surface. Antiseptics, disinfectants, and ethylene oxide gas are the major chemical means of killing microorganisms on surfaces. Heat, irradiation, and mechanical dislodgment are the primary physical means of eliminating viable organisms (Box 5-1).

The microbes that cause human disease include bacteria, viruses, mycobacteria, parasites, and fungi. The microbes within these groups have variable ability to resist chemical or physical agents. The microorganisms most resistant to elimination are bacterial endospores. Therefore, in general, any method of sterilization or disinfection that kills endospores is also capable of eliminating bacteria, viruses, mycobacteria, fungi, mold, and parasites. This concept is used in monitoring the success of disinfection and sterilization techniques.

TECHNIQUES OF INSTRUMENT STERILIZATION

Any means of instrument sterilization to be used in office-based oral and maxillofacial surgery must be reliable, practical, and safe for the instruments. The three methods generally available for instrument sterilization are dry heat, moist heat, and ethylene oxide gas.

STERILIZATION WITH HEAT.

Heat is one of the oldest means of destroying microorganisms. Pasteur used heat to reduce the number of pathogens in liquids for preservation. Koch was the first to use heat for sterilization. He found that 1½ hours of dry heat at 100° C would destroy all vegetative

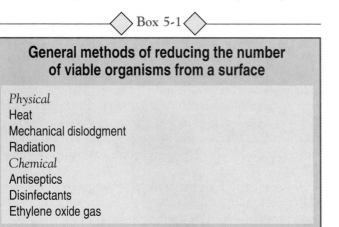

───── ◇ Box 5-1 ◇ ─────

General methods of reducing the number of viable organisms from a surface

Physical
Heat
Mechanical dislodgment
Radiation
Chemical
Antiseptics
Disinfectants
Ethylene oxide gas

bacteria, but that 3 hours of dry heat at 140° C was necessary to eliminate the spores of anthrax bacilli. Koch then tested moist heat and found it a more efficient means of heat sterilization, because it reduces the temperature and time necessary to kill spores. Moist heat is probably more effective, because dry heat oxidizes cell proteins, a process requiring extremely high temperatures, whereas moist heat causes destructive protein coagulation quickly at relatively low temperatures.

Because spores are the most resistant forms of microbial life, they can be used to monitor sterilization techniques. The spore of the bacteria *Bacillus stearothermophilus* is extremely resistant to heat and is therefore used to test the reliability of heat sterilization. These bacilli can be purchased by hospitals and private offices and run through the sterilizer with the equipment being sterilized. A laboratory then places the heat-treated spores into culture. If no growth occurs, the sterilization procedure was successful (Figure 5-3).

It has been shown that 6 months after sterilization the possibility of organisms entering the sterilization bag increases; therefore all sterilized items should be labeled with an expiration date that is 6 months in the future.

Dry heat. Dry heat is a method of sterilization that can be provided in most dental offices, because the necessary equipment is no more complicated than a thermostatically controlled oven and a timer. Dry heat is most commonly used to sterilize glassware and bulky items that can withstand heat

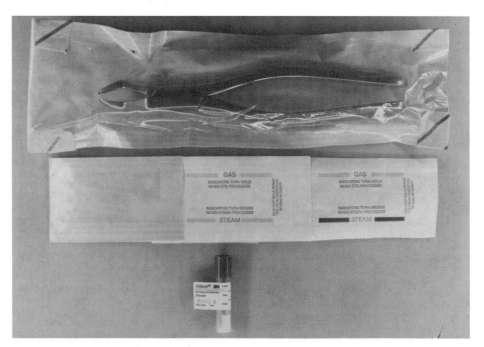

◇ Figure 5-3 ─────────────────────

Tests of sterilization equipment. Color-coded packaging is made of paper and cellophane; test areas on package change color on exposure to sterilizing temperatures *(top)* or to ethylene oxide gas *(center)*. *Bottom*, vial contains spores of *B. stearothermophilus*, which is used for testing efficiency of heat-sterilization equipment.

but are susceptible to rust. The success of sterilization depends not only on attaining a certain temperature but also on maintaining the temperature for a sufficient amount of time. The following factors therefore must be considered when using dry heat: (1) warm-up time for the oven and the materials to be sterilized, (2) the heat conductivity of the materials, and (3) airflow throughout the oven and through the objects being sterilized. In addition, time for the sterilized equipment to cool after heating must be taken into consideration. The time necessary for dry-heat sterilization limits its practicality in the ambulatory setting, because it lengthens the turnover time and forces the dentist to have many duplicate instruments.

The advantages of dry heat are the relative ease of use and the unlikelihood of damaging heat-resistant instruments. The disadvantages are the time necessary and the potential damage to heat-sensitive equipment. Guidelines for the use of dry-heat sterilization are provided in Table 5-3.

Moist heat. Moist heat is more efficient than dry heat for sterilization, because it is effective at much lower temperatures and requires less time. The reason for this is based on several physical principles. First, water boiling at 100° C takes less time to kill organisms than does dry heat at the same temperature, because water is better than air at transferring heat. Second, it takes approximately 7 times as much heat to convert boiling water to steam as it takes to cause the same amount of room-temperature water to boil. When steam comes into contact with an object, the steam condenses and almost instantly releases that stored heat energy, which quickly denatures vital cell proteins. Saturated steam placed under pressure (autoclaving) is even more efficient than nonpressurized steam. This is because increasing pressure in a container of steam increases the boiling point of water so that the new steam entering a closed container gradually becomes hotter. Temperatures attainable by steam under pressure include 109° C at 5 psi (pounds per square inch), 115° C at 10 psi, 121° C at 15 psi, and 126° C at 20 psi (Table 5-3).

The container usually used for providing steam under pressure is known as an *autoclave* (Figure 5-4). It works by creating steam and then, through a series of valves, increasing the steam pressure so that the steam becomes superheated. Equipment placed into an autoclave should be packaged to allow the free flow of steam to the equipment, such as by placing instruments in paper bags or wrapping them in cotton cloth.

Simply placing instruments in boiling water or free-flowing steam results in disinfection rather than sterilization, because at the temperature of 100° C, many spores and certain viruses survive.

The advantages of sterilization with moist heat are its effectiveness, speed, and the relative availability of office-proportioned autoclaving equipment. Disadvantages include the tendency of moist heat to dull and rust instruments and the cost of autoclaves (Table 5-4).

GASEOUS STERILIZATION. Certain gases exert a lethal action on bacteria by destroying enzymes and other biochemical structures essential for viability. Of the several gases available for sterilization, ethylene oxide is the most commonly used. It is a highly flammable gas and is mixed with Freon, CO_2, or nitrogen to make it safer to use. Because ethylene oxide gas is at room temperature, it can readily diffuse through porous materials, such as plastic and rubber. At 50° C it is effective for killing all organisms, including spores, within 3 hours. However, because it is highly toxic to animal tissue, equipment exposed to ethylene oxide must be aerated for 8 to 12 hours at 50° to 60° C or at ambient temperatures for 4 to 7 days.

The advantages of ethylene oxide for sterilization are its effectiveness for sterilizing porous materials, large equipment, and materials sensitive to heat or moisture. The disadvantages are the need for special equipment and the length of sterilization and aeration time necessary to reduce tissue toxicity. This technique is rarely practical for dental use, unless the dentist has easy access to a large facility willing to gas sterilize dental equipment.

TECHNIQUES OF INSTRUMENT DISINFECTION

CHEMICAL DISINFECTANTS. Many dental instruments cannot withstand the temperatures required for heat sterilization. Therefore, if gaseous sterilization is not available and absolute sterility is not required, chemical disinfection can be performed. Chemical agents with potential disinfectant capabilities have been classified as being high, intermediate, or low in biocidal activity. The classification is based on the agent's ability to inactivate vegetative bacteria, tubercle bacilli, bacterial spores, nonlipid viruses, and/or lipid viruses. Agents with low biocidal activity are effective only against vegetative bacteria and lipid viruses, immediate disinfectants are effective against all microbes except bacterial spores, and agents

◇ Table 5-3. Guidelines for dry-heat and steam sterilization

Temperature	Duration of treatment or exposure*
Dry heat	
121° C (250° F)	6-12 hr
140° C (285° F)	3 hr
150° C (300° F)	2½ hr
160° C (320° F)	2 hr
170° C (340° F)	1 hr
Steam	
116° C (240° F)	60 min
118° C (245° F)	36 min
121° C (250° F)	24 min
125° C (257° F)	16 min
132° C (270° F)	4 min
138° C (280° F)	1.5 min

*Times for dry heat treatments do not begin until temperature of oven reaches goal. Use spore tests weekly to judge effectiveness of sterilization technique and equipment. Use temperature-sensitive monitors each time equipment is used, to indicate that sterilization cycle was initiated.

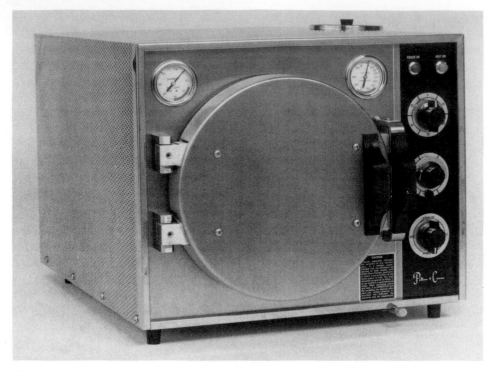

◇ Figure 5-4

Office-proportioned autoclave that can be used as both steam and dry-heat sterilizer. *(Courtesy Pelton and Crane, Inc, Charlotte, NC.)*

◇ Table 5-4. Comparison of dry-heat versus moist-heat sterilization techniques

	Dry heat	Moist heat
Principal antimicrobial effect	Oxidizes cell proteins	Denatures cell proteins
Time necessary to achieve sterilization	Long	Short
Equipment complexity and cost	Low	High
Tendency to dull or rust instruments	Low	High
Availability of equipment sized for office use	Good	Good

◇ Table 5-5. Classification system for the biocidal effects of chemical disinfectants

Level of biocidal activity*	Vegetative bacteria	Lipid viruses	Nonlipid viruses	Tubercle bacilli	Bacterial spores
Low	+	+	−	−	−
Intermediate	+	+	+	+	−
High	+	+	+	+	+

*In absence of gross organic materials on surfaces being disinfected.

with high activity are biocidal for all microbes. The classification depends not only on innate properties of the chemical but also, and just as important, on how the chemical is used (Table 5-5).

Substances acceptable for disinfecting dental instruments for surgery include glutaraldehyde, iodophors, chlorine compounds, and formaldehyde, with the glutaraldehyde-containing compounds being the most commonly used. Table 5-6 summarizes the biocidal activity of most of the acceptable disinfecting agents when used properly. Alcohols are not suitable for general dental disinfection, because they evaporate too rapidly, but they can be used to disinfect local anesthetic cartridges. Quaternary ammonium compounds are not recommended for dentistry, because they are not effective against the hepatitis B virus and become inactivated by soap and anionic agents.

Certain procedures must be followed to ensure maximal disinfection, regardless of which disinfectant solution is used. The agent must be properly reformulated or discarded periodically, as specified by the manufacturer. Instruments must remain in contact with the solution for the designated period, and, during that time, no new contaminated instruments should be added to the solution. All instruments must be washed free of blood or other gross contaminating proteins before being placed in the solution. Finally, after disinfection, the instruments should be rinsed free of chemicals and used immediately.

An outline of the preferred method of sterilization for selected dental instruments is presented in Table 5-7.

◇ Table 5-6. Biocidal activity of various chemical disinfectants

Generic	Brand names	Exposure time	Activity level*	
			Intermediate	High
Formaldehyde 3%				
8% or		≥30 min	+	
8% in 70% alcohol		10 hr		+
Glutaraldehyde 2% with nonionic ethoxylates of linear alcohols	Wavicide, Sterall			
Room temperature		≥10 min	+	
40°-45° C		4 hr		+
60° C		1 hr		+
Glutaraldehyde 2% alkaline with phenolic buffer	Sporcidin			
Diluted 1:16		≥10 min	+	
Full strength		7 hr		+
Glutaraldehyde 2% alkaline	Cidex, Procide, Glutarex, Omnicide	≥10 min	+	
		10 hr		+
1% Chlorine compound	Clorox			
Diluted 1:5		≥30 min	I	
O-phenylphenol 9% plus O-benzyl-p-chlorophenol 1%	Omni II			
Diluted 1:32		≥10 min	+	
Iodophors 1% iodine	Betadine, Isodine	≥30 min	+	

*Grossly visible contamination, such as blood, must be removed before chemical disinfection to maximize biocidal activity.

◇ Table 5-7. Methods of sterilization or disinfection of selected dental instruments

Items	Steam autoclave	Dry heat oven	Chemical disinfection sterilization
	15-30 min required per cycle	1-1½ hr required per cycle	*
Stainless instruments (loose), restorative burs	++	++	−
Instruments in packs	++	+ (small packs)	−
Instrument tray setups, surgical or restorative	+ (size limit)	++	−
Rustable instruments	(only when coated with chemical protectant)	++	−
Handpiece (autoclave)	++	−	−
Handpiece (non + autoclavable)	−	−	± (iodophor disinfectant)
Angle attachments†	+	+	−
Rubber items	++	−	−
Rag wheels	++	+	−
Removable prosthetics	−	−	+‡
Heat-resistant plastic evacuators	++	+	−

*Chemical disinfecting/sterilizing solutions are not the method of choice for sterilization of any items used in the mouth. In some circumstances they may be used when other, more suitable procedures have been precluded.

†Confirm with manufacturer that attachment is capable of withstanding heat sterilization.

‡Rinse well, immerse in 1:10 household bleach solution (5% to 6% sodium hypochlorite) for 5 minutes. Rinse. Repeat disinfection before returning to patient.

MAINTENANCE OF STERILITY

DISPOSABLE MATERIALS. Materials and drugs used during oral and maxillofacial surgery, such as sutures, local anesthetics, scalpel blades, and syringes with needles, are sterilized by the manufacturer with a variety of techniques, including gases, autoclaving, filtration, and irradiation. The dentist must only remove the material or drug from its container properly to maintain sterility. Most surgical supplies are double-wrapped; the only common exception is scalpel blades. The outer wrapper is designed to be handled in a nonsterile fashion and usually is sealed in a manner that allows an unsterile individual to unwrap it and to pass in a sterile manner the surgical material contained in the sterile inner wrapper. The unsterile individual can either allow the surgical

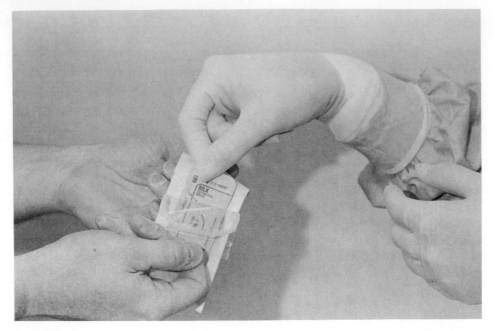

◇ Figure 5-5

Method of sterilely transferring double-wrapped sterile supplies from clean individual *(ungloved hands)* to sterilely gowned individual *(gloved hands)*. Package is designed to be peeled open from one end, without touching sterile interior of package. Sterile contents are then prominently presented to recipient.

material in the inner wrapper to drop onto a sterile part of the surgical field or allow another individual to remove the wrapped material in a sterile manner (Figure 5-5). Scalpel blades are handled in a similar fashion; the unwrapped blade can be dropped onto the field or grasped in a sterile manner by another individual.

SURGICAL FIELD MAINTENANCE. An absolutely sterile surgical field is impossible to attain. For oral and maxillofacial procedures, even a relatively clean field is difficult to maintain because of oral and upper respiratory tract contamination. Therefore during oral and maxillofacial surgery the goal is to prevent any organisms from the surgical staff or other patients from entering the patient's wound.

Once instruments are sterilized or disinfected, they should be set up for use during surgery in a manner that limits the likelihood of contamination by organisms foreign to the patient's maxillofacial flora. Use a flat platform, such as a Mayo stand, and place two layers of sterile towels or waterproof paper on it. Then lay the instrument pack on the platform and open out the edges in a sterile fashion (Figure 5-6). Anything placed on the platform should be either sterile or disinfected. Care should be taken not to allow excessive moisture to get on the towels or paper, because if they become saturated, they can allow bacteria from the unsterile under-surface to seep up to the sterile instruments.

OPERATORY DISINFECTION

The various surfaces present in the dental operatory have different requirements concerning disinfection that depend on the potential for contamination and the degree of patient contact with the surface. The most serious disease, possessing the greatest potential for patient-to-patient spread from surface transfer, is serum hepatitis. Any surface that a patient contacts is a potential carrier of infectious organisms. The dental chair itself comes in direct contact with every patient and therefore requires frequent disinfection, because there is no practical means of differentiating patients who carry hepatitis from patients who do not. Fortunately, many chemical disinfectants, including chlorine compounds and glutaraldehyde, can prevent transfer of the hepatitis viruses when used on surfaces in certain concentrations (0.2% for chlorine, 2% for glutaraldehyde). Most headrests can easily be covered with single-use, disposable headrest covers; the rest of the dental chair can be quickly sprayed with a disinfectant. Countertops usually come into contact with patients only indirectly, through objects that have touched patients being placed there. Although it may not be feasible to wipe counters clean after every patient, counters should be periodically disinfected, especially before surgical procedures. Limiting the number of objects left on counters in operatories will make periodic cleaning easier and more effective.

Soap dispensers and sink faucets are another source of contamination. Unless they can be activated without using the

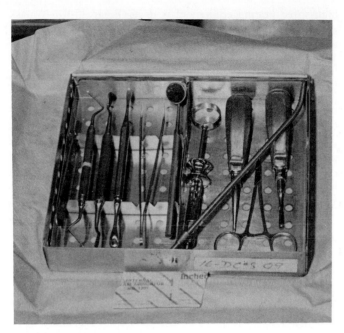

 Figure 5-6

Instruments to be used for extraction of erupted tooth, seen here after two layers of wrapping used during sterilization have been opened. Only the corners of package are grasped, preserving sterility of both interior of wrapping material and instruments. Notice color-coded sterility indicator included when package was wrapped.

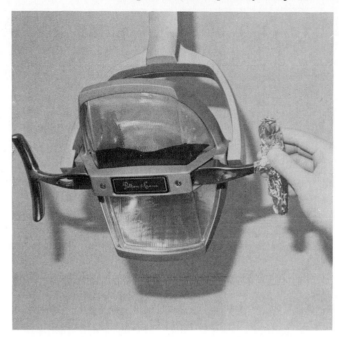

Figure 5-7

Rectangle of sterilized aluminum foil used on light handle to help prevent introduction of contamination from handle to patient.

hands, they should be frequently disinfected, because many bacteria survive—even thrive—in a soapy environment (discussed later in this section). This is one reason soap is not the ideal agent when preparing hands for surgery.

Most oral surgery requires frequent redirection of the light source. A simple way to do this is by sterilizing large squares of aluminum foil that can then be placed over the light handle to allow light manipulation without cross-contamination of patients (Figure 5-7).

Anesthetic equipment used to deliver gases, such as oxygen or nitrous oxide, may also spread patient-to-patient infection. Plastic nasal cannulas are designed to be discarded after one use. Nasal masks and the tubing leading to the mask from the source of the gases are available in disposable form.

SURGICAL STAFF PREPARATION

The preparation of the operating team for oral and maxillofacial surgery differs according to the nature of the procedure being performed and the location of the surgery. The two basic types of personnel asepsis to be discussed are the *clean* technique and the *sterile* technique. Antiseptics are used during each of the techniques, so they are discussed first.

ANTISEPTICS. Antiseptics are used to prepare the surgical team's hands and arms before gloves are donned and to disinfect the surgical site. Because antiseptics are used on living tissue, they are designed to have low tissue toxicity while maintaining disinfecting properties. The three antiseptics most commonly used in dentistry are iodophors, chlorhexidine, and hexachlorophene.

Iodophors, such as polyvinylpyrrolidone-iodine (povidone-iodine) solution, have the broadest spectrum of antiseptic action, being effective for both gram-positive and gram-negative bacteria, most viruses, *M. tuberculosis* organisms, spores, and fungi. Iodophors are usually formulated in a 1% iodine solution. The scrub form has an added anionic detergent. Iodophors are preferred over noncompounded solutions of iodine, because they are much less toxic to tissue than free iodine and more water-soluble. However, iodophors are contraindicated for use on individuals sensitive to iodinated materials, those with untreated hypothyroidism, and pregnant women. Iodophors exert their effect over a period of several minutes, so the solution should remain in contact with the surface for at least a few minutes for maximal effect.

Chlorhexidine and hexachlorophene are other useful antiseptics. Chlorhexidine is used extensively worldwide and is available in the United States both as a skin-preparation solution and for internal use. The potential for systemic toxicity with repeated use of hexachlorophene has limited its use. Both agents are more effective against gram-positive than gram-negative bacteria, which makes them useful for maxillofacial prepping. Chlorhexidine and hexachlorophene are more effective when used repeatedly during the day, because they accumulate on the skin and leave a residual

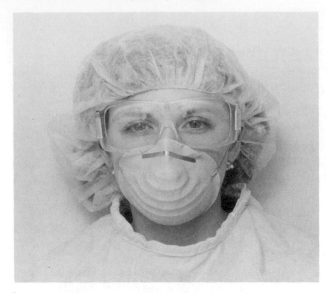

◇ **Figure 5-8**

Surgeon ready for office oral surgery, wearing clean gown over street clothes, mask over nose and mouth, cap covering scalp hair, clean gloves, and shatter-resistant eye protection. Nondangling earrings are acceptable in clean technique.

antibacterial effect after each wash. However, their ineffectiveness against tubercle bacilli, spores, and many viruses makes them less effective than iodophors.

CLEAN TECHNIQUE.   The clean technique is generally used for office-based surgery that does not specifically require a sterile technique. Office oral surgical procedures that call for a sterile technique include any surgery in which skin is incised or any procedure such as the placement of certain maxillofacial implants. The clean technique is designed as much to protect the dental staff and other patients from a particular patient as it is to protect the patient from pathogens that the dental staff may harbor.

When using a clean technique, the dental staff can wear clean street clothing but should be covered by long-sleeved laboratory coats (Figure 5-8). Preferably, a dental uniform can be worn instead of street clothes, with no further covering or covered by a long-sleeved surgical gown.

Gloves should be worn by dentists whenever they are providing dental care, because they have no practical means of identifying which patients are carrying pathogenic microorganisms, such as the hepatitis B virus. When the clean technique is used, the hands should be washed with antiseptic soap and dried on a disposable towel before gloving. Gloves should be sterile and put on using an appropriate technique to maintain sterility of the external surfaces. The technique of sterile self-gloving is illustrated in Figure 5-9.

The need for wearing masks and eye protection is also based on the inability to identify patients carrying infectious microorganisms. In general, eye protection should be worn when blood or saliva are dispersed, such as when high-speed cutting equipment is used (Figure 5-8). A mask should be used whenever aerosols are created or a surgical wound is to be made.

There is usually no absolute need to prepare the operative site when using the clean technique. But when surgery in the oral cavity is performed, the perioral skin may be decontaminated with the same solutions used to scrub the hands, and the oral cavity prepared by brushing or rinsing with chlorhexidine gluconate (0.12%) or an alcohol-based mouthwash. These procedures will reduce the amount of skin or oral mucosal contamination of the wound and decrease the microbial load of any aerosols made while using high-speed drills in the mouth. The dentist may desire to drape the patient loosely, to protect the patient's clothes and to keep objects from accidentally entering the patient's eyes.

During an oral surgical procedure, only sterile water or sterile saline solution should be used to irrigate open wounds. Irrigation can be delivered by a disposable injection syringe, a reusable bulb syringe, or an irrigation pump connected to a bag of intravenous solution.

STERILE TECHNIQUE.   The sterile technique is used for office-based surgery when clean wounds are created, when implants are placed, or when surgery is performed in an operating room.* Its purpose is to minimize the number of organisms that enter wounds created by the surgeon. It requires a strict attention to detail and cooperation among the members of the surgical team.

The surgical hand and arm scrub is another means of lessening the chance of contaminating a patient's wound. Although sterile gloves are worn, gloves can be torn (especially during oral-maxillofacial surgical procedures), thereby exposing the patient to the surgeon's hands. By proper scrubbing with antiseptic solutions, the surface bacterial level of the hands and arms is reduced.

There are several acceptable methods of performing a surgical hand and arm scrub. Most hospitals have a surgical scrub protocol that should be followed when performing surgery in that institution. Standard to most techniques is the use of an antiseptic soap solution, a moderately stiff brush, and a fingernail cleaner. The hands and forearms are wetted in a scrub sink, and the hands are kept above the level of the elbows after wetting, until the hands and arms are dried. A copious amount of antiseptic soap is applied to the hands and arms from either wall dispensers or antiseptic-impregnated scrub brushes. The antiseptic soap is allowed to remain on the arms while any dirt is removed from underneath each fingernail tip using a sharp-tipped fingernail cleaner. Then more antiseptic soap is applied and scrubbing is begun, with repeated firm strokes of the scrub brush on every surface of the hands and arms up to approximately 5 cm below the elbow. Scrub techniques based on the number of strokes to each surface are more reliable than a set time for scrubbing. An individual's scrub

---

*A clean wound is a wound made through intact skin that has been treated with an antiseptic.

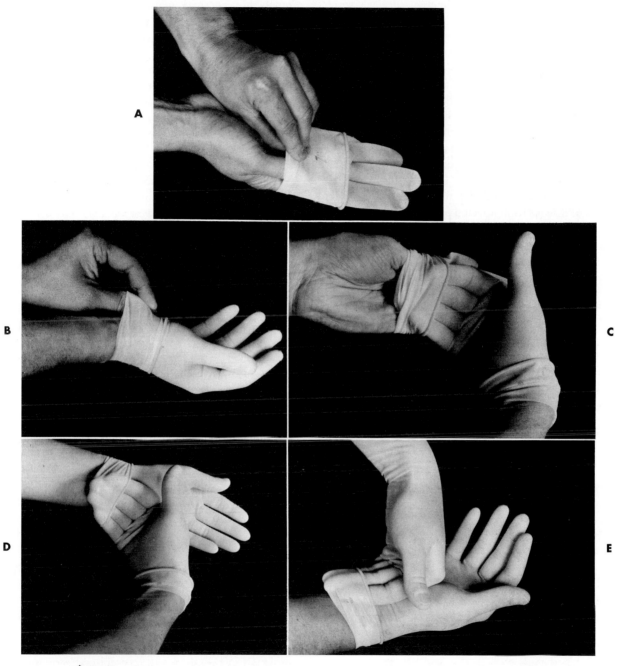

◇ Figure 5-9

Technique of sterile self-gloving. **A,** Fingers of right hand are placed into right glove; fingers of left hand hold interior edge of cuff. **B,** Right hand slowly pushes into glove, while left hand pulls glove on. Cuff of right glove is left unturned at this stage. **C,** Right hand is placed inside cuff of left glove, and left hand is then placed into opening of left glove. Care is taken not to allow right hand to touch interior of left glove. Right hand remains only on exterior surface of left glove. **D,** Left hand slowly pushes into left glove, while right hand helps to push glove on. After fingers of left hand are completely in place, right hand turns cuff down onto forearm, taking care not to let right glove touch any nonsterile surface. **E,** Fingers of left gloved hand are inserted into cuff of right glove and are used to turn that cuff down, which completes self-gloving procedure.

technique should follow a routine that has been designed to ensure that no forearm or hand surface is left improperly prepared. An example of an acceptable surgical scrub technique is shown in Chapter 31.

POSTSURGICAL ASEPSIS.   A few principles of postsurgical care are useful to prevent the spread of pathogens. Wounds should be inspected or dressed by hands that have been cleaned and covered with clean gloves. When there are several patients waiting, those without infectious problems should be seen first, and those with problems such as a draining abscess should be seen afterwards.

Finally, after any surgery the contaminated materials should be disposed of in such a way that the staff and other patients will not be infected. The most common risk for transmission of disease from infected patients to the staff is by accidental needle sticks or scalpel lacerations, which are best prevented by immediately disposing of all sharp, disposable supplies into rigid, well-marked containers designed for that use. For environmental protection, contaminated supplies should be discarded in properly labeled bags and given to a reputable waste-management company.

BIBLIOGRAPHY

ADA Councils on Dental Materials, Instruments, and Equipment; Dental Practice; and Dental Therapeutics: Infection control recommendations of the dental office and the dental laboratory, *J Am Dent Assoc* 118(suppl):1, 1992.

Cottone JA, Terezhalmy GT, Molinari JA: *Practical infection control in dentistry,* ed 2, Baltimore, 1996, Williams & Wilkins.

Finkbeiner BL, Johnson CS: *Mosby's comprehensive dental assisting,* St Louis, 1995, Mosby.

Miller CH, Palenik CJ: *Infection control and management of hazardous materials for the dental team,* St Louis, 1998, Mosby.

Torres HO, Ehrlich A: *Modern dental assisting,* ed 5, Philadelphia, 1995, WB Saunders.

PRINCIPLES OF EXODONTIA

For most people, dentists and lay people alike, the term *oral surgery* usually implies removal of a tooth. The atraumatic extraction of a tooth is a procedure that requires finesse, knowledge, and skill on the part of the surgeon. The purpose of this section is to present the principles of exodontia and the instrumentation, techniques, and management of patients who are undergoing extraction surgery.

Chapter 6 presents the armamentarium commonly employed for office oral surgery procedures. The basic instrumentation and the fundamental application to its surgical purpose are discussed. Many variations of the instruments presented here are available.

Chapter 7 presents the basic aspects of how to remove an erupted tooth atraumatically. The preoperative assessment and preparation of the patient is discussed briefly. The position of the patient in the chair and the position of the surgeon, the surgeon's hands, and the dental assistant for removal of each tooth are discussed. The armamentarium and movements necessary to extract each tooth are discussed in detail.

Chapter 8 presents the basic aspects of managing complicated extractions. Complicated extractions refers primarily to retrieving tooth roots and teeth that are likely to fracture or for some other reason have an obstacle to extraction. In these situations, surgical removal of bone or surgical sectioning of the tooth is required.

Chapter 9 presents the fundamental aspects of management of impacted teeth. The rationale for timely removal of impacted teeth is presented in the initial portion of the chapter. This is followed by a discussion of classification and determination of degree of difficulty of the impaction. Finally, a brief description is given of the basic surgical techniques required to remove impacted third molars.

Chapter 10 presents the techniques for managing the patient in the postoperative period. This chapter discusses postoperative instructions that should be given to the patient, as well as postoperative medications.

Chapter 11 presents the common surgical complications that are encountered in the removal of teeth. Emphasis is placed on anticipating the complication and taking measures to prevent or minimize the complication.

Finally, Chapter 12 discusses the medical and legal considerations involved in basic exodontia. An important portion of this chapter discusses the concept of informed consent for the patient.

CHAPTER

6

ARMAMENTARIUM FOR BASIC ORAL SURGERY

LARRY J. PETERSON

CHAPTER OUTLINE

The purpose of this chapter is to introduce the instrumentation required to perform routine oral surgical procedures. These instruments are used for a wide variety of purposes, including both soft tissue and hard tissue procedures. This chapter deals primarily with a description of the instruments; subsequent chapters discuss the actual use of the instruments in the variety of ways for which they are intended.

INSTRUMENTS TO INCISE TISSUE

Most surgical procedures begin with an incision. The instrument for making an incision is the scalpel, which is composed of a handle and a disposable, sterile sharp blade. The most commonly used handle is the no. 3 handle, but occasionally the longer, more slender no. 7 handle will be used (Figure 6-1). The tip of the scalpel handle is prepared to receive a variety of differently shaped scalpel blades that can be inserted onto a slotted receiver.

The most commonly used scalpel blade for intraoral surgery is the no. 15 blade (Figure 6-2). It is relatively small and can be used to make incisions around teeth and through mucoperiosteum. It is similar in shape to the larger no. 10 blade, which is used for large skin incisions. Other commonly used blades for intraoral surgery are the no. 11 blade and the no. 12 blade. The no. 11 blade is a sharp-pointed blade that is used primarily for making small stab incisions, such as for incising an abscess. The hooked no. 12 blade is useful for mucogingival procedures in which incisions must be made on the posterior aspect of teeth or in the maxillary tuberosity area.

The scalpel blade is carefully loaded onto the handle with a needle holder to avoid lacerating the operator's fingers. The blade is held on the superior edge, where it is reinforced with

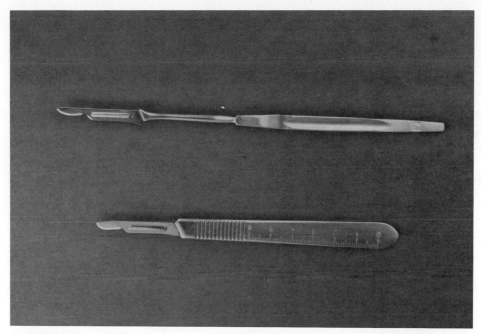

◇ **Figure 6-1**

Scalpels are composed of handle and sharp, disposable blade. *Top scalpel,* No. 7 handle with no. 15 blade. *Bottom scalpel,* More commonly used no. 3 handle.

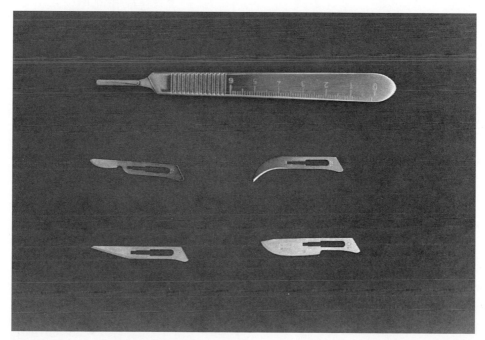

◇ **Figure 6-2**

Scalpel blades used in oral surgery include no. 15 *(upper left),* no. 12 *(upper right),* no. 11 *(lower left),* and no. 10 *(lower right).* No. 3 scalpel handle is above.

a small rib, and the handle is held so that the male portion of the fitting is pointing upward (Figure 6-3, *A*). The knife blade is then slid onto the handle until it clicks into position (Figure 6-3, *B*). The knife is unloaded in a similar fashion. The needle holder grasps the most proximal end of the blade (Figure 6-3,

C) and lifts it to disengage it from the male fitting. It is then slid off the knife handle in the opposite direction (Figure 6-3, *D*). The used blade is discarded into a proper rigid-sided "sharps" container.

When using the scalpel to make an incision, the surgeon

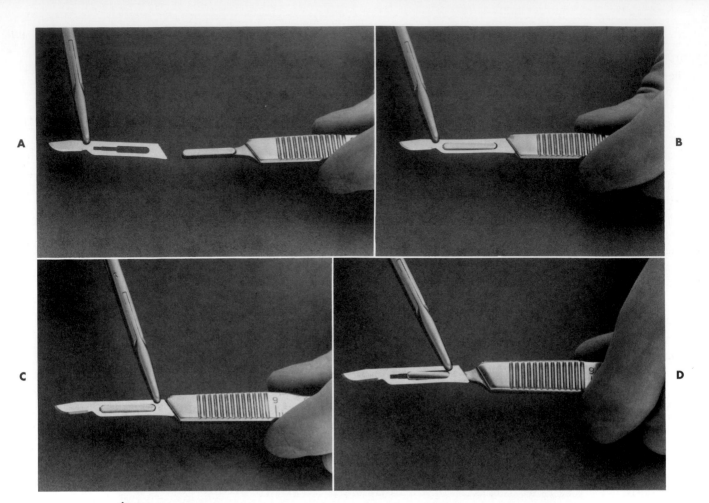

◇ Figure 6-3

A, When loading scalpel blade, surgeon holds blade in needle holder and handle, with male portion of fitting pointing upward. **B,** Blade is then slid into handle until it clicks into place. **C,** To remove blade, the surgeon uses needle holder to grasp proximal end of blade and lifts it to disengage it from fitting. **D,** Blade is then slid off handle.

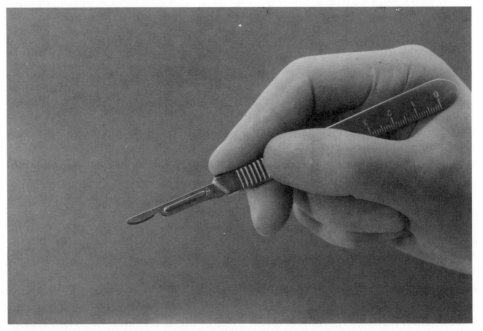

◇ Figure 6-4

Scalpel is held in pen grasp to allow maximal control.

holds it in the pen grasp (Figure 6-4) to allow maximal control of the blade as the incision is made. Mobile tissue should be held firmly to stabilize it so that as the incision is made, the blade will incise, not displace, the mucosa. When a mucoperiosteal incision is made, the knife should be pressed down firmly so that the incision penetrates the mucosa and periosteum with the same stroke.

Scalpel blades are designed for single-patient use. They are dulled very easily when they come into contact with hard tissue such as bone and teeth. If several incisions through mucoperiosteum to bone are required, it may be necessary to use a second blade during a single operation. It is important to remember that dull blades do not make clean, sharp incisions in soft tissue and therefore should be replaced when they become dull.

INSTRUMENTS FOR ELEVATING MUCOPERIOSTEUM

After an incision through mucoperiosteum has been made, the mucosa and periosteum should be reflected from the underlying bone in a single layer with a periosteal elevator. The instrument that is most commonly used is the no. 9 Molt periosteal elevator (Figure 6-5, *A*). This instrument has a sharp, pointed end and a broader flat end. The pointed end is used to reflect dental papillae from between teeth, and the broad end is used for elevating the tissue from the bone.

Some surgeons prefer to use round-ended Molt periosteal elevators. This type of periosteal elevator can be single-ended (Figure 6-5, *B*) or double-ended (Figure 6-5, *C* and *D*). The cutting edge of the Molt periosteal elevator is thin and sharp, resulting in a clean separation of the periosteum from the bone.

The periosteal elevator can be used to reflect soft tissue by three methods. First, the pointed end can be used in a prying motion to elevate soft tissue. This is most commonly used when elevating a dental papilla from between teeth. The second method is the push stroke, in which the broad end of the instrument is slid underneath the flap, separating the periosteum from the underlying bone. This is the most efficient stroke and results in the cleanest reflection of the periosteum. The third method is a pull, or scrape, stroke. This is occasionally useful in some areas but tends to shred or tear the periosteum unless it is done carefully.

The periosteal elevator can also be used as a retractor. Once the periosteum has been elevated, the broad blade of the periosteal elevator is pressed against the bone, with the mucoperiosteal flap elevated into its reflected position.

When teeth are to be extracted, the soft tissue attachment around the tooth must be released from the tooth. The instrument most commonly used for this is the no. 1 Woodson periosteal elevator (Figure 6-6). This instrument is relatively small and delicate and can be used to loosen the soft tissue via the gingival sulcus. The pointed end of the no. 9 periosteal elevator can also be used for this purpose.

INSTRUMENTS FOR CONTROLLING HEMORRHAGE

When incisions are made through tissue, small arteries and veins are incised, causing bleeding that may require more than simple pressure to control. When this is necessary, an instrument called a *hemostat* is used (Figure 6-7, *A*). Hemostats come in a variety of shapes, may be relatively small and delicate or larger, and are either straight or curved. The hemostat most commonly used in oral surgery is a curved hemostat (Figure 6-7, *B*).

The hemostat has a relatively long, delicate beak, used to grasp tissue, and a locking handle. The locking mechanism allows the surgeon to clamp the hemostat onto a vessel, and then let go of the instrument, which will remain clamped onto the tissue.

In addition to its use as an instrument for controlling bleeding, the hemostat is especially useful in oral surgery to remove granulation tissue from tooth sockets and to pick up small root tips, pieces of calculus, fragments of amalgam restorations, and any other small particles that have dropped into the mouth or wound area.

INSTRUMENTS TO GRASP TISSUE

In performing soft tissue surgery it is frequently necessary to stabilize soft tissue flaps in order to pass a suture needle. Tissue forceps most commonly used for this purpose are the Adson forceps (Figure 6-8). These are delicate forceps with small teeth, which can be used to gently hold tissue and thereby stabilize it. When this instrument is used, care should be taken not to grasp the tissue too tightly, thereby crushing it. Adson forceps are also available without teeth.

When working in the posterior part of the mouth, the Adson forceps may be too short. A longer forceps that has similar shape is the Stillies forceps. This forceps is usually 7 to 9 inches long and can easily grasp tissue in the posterior part of the mouth and still leave enough of the instrument protruding beyond the lips for the surgeon to control it (Figure 6-8, *B*).

Occasionally, it is more convenient to have an angled forceps. Such a forceps is the college, or cotton, forceps (Figure 6-8, *C*). Although this forceps is not especially useful for handling tissue, it is an excellent instrument for picking up small fragments of tooth, amalgam, or other foreign material, and for placing or removing gauze packs. This instrument is commonly used in tray systems.

In some types of surgery, especially when removing larger amounts of fibrous tissue, such as in an epulis fissuratum, forceps with locking handles and teeth that will grip the tissue firmly are necessary. In this situation the Allis tissue forceps are used (Figure 6-9, *A* and *B*). The locking handle allows the forceps to be placed in the proper position and then to be held

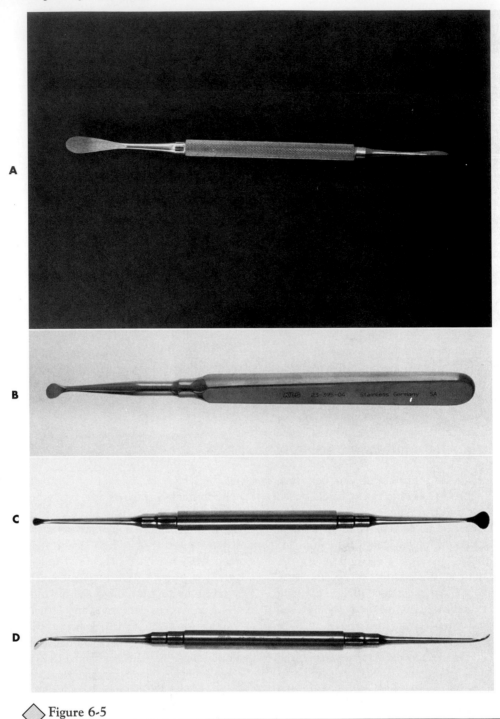

◇ Figure 6-5

A, No. 9 Molt periosteal elevator is most commonly used in oral surgery. **B,** A single-ended Molt periosteal elevator with a sharp round end may be used to elevate the mucoperiosteum. **C** and **D,** The double-ended Molt periosteal elevator has a large and small end to provide the surgeon the appropriate-size end for the specific task.

by an assistant to provide the necessary tension for proper dissection of the tissue. The Allis forceps should never be used on tissue that is to be left in the mouth, because they cause a relatively large amount of tissue destruction as a result of crushing injury (Figure 6-9, *C*).

Russian tissue forceps are large, round-ended tissue forceps (Figure 6-10, *A*) that are most useful in oral surgery to pick up teeth that have been elevated from their sockets (Figure 6-10, *B*). The round end allows a positive grip on a tooth or tooth fragment, so that it is not likely to slip out of the instrument's

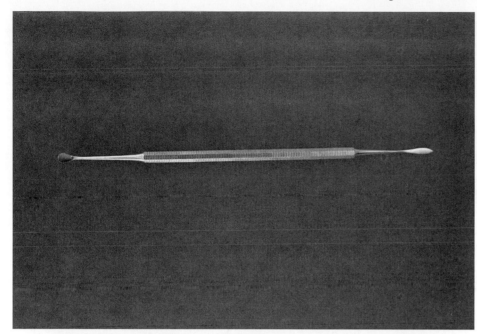

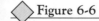

Figure 6-6

No. 1 Woodson periosteal elevator is used to loosen soft tissue from teeth before extraction.

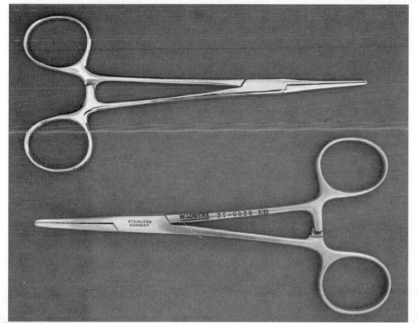

A

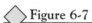

Figure 6-7

A, Hemostats used in oral surgery are usually small, curved mosquito type *(top)*. **B,** Curved hemostat *(side)*.

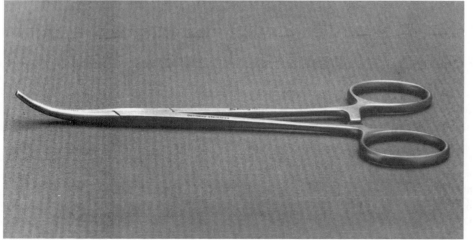

B

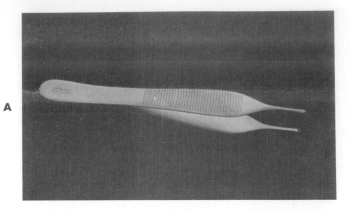

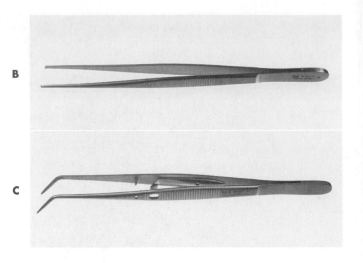

◇ Figure 6-8

A, Small, delicate Adson tissue forceps are used to gently stabilize soft tissue for suturing or dissection. **B,** The Stillies pickup is longer than the Adson pickup and is used to handle tissue in the more posterior aspect of the mouth. **C,** The college pliers is an angled forceps that is used for picking up small objects in the mouth or from the Mayo stand.

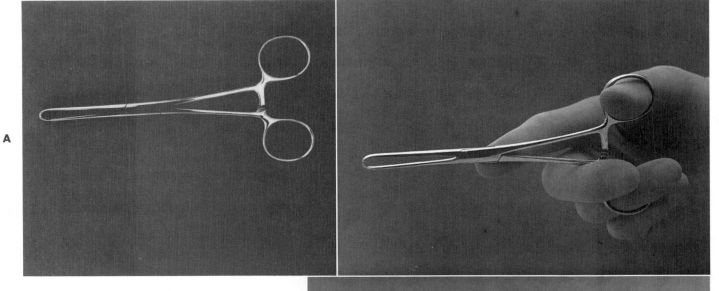

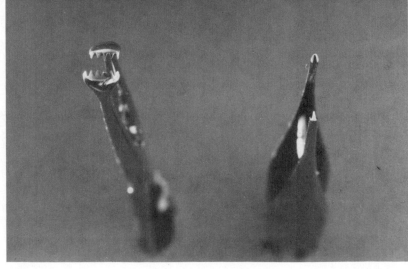

◇ Figure 6-9

A, Allis tissue forceps are useful for grasping and holding tissue that will be excised. **B,** Allis forceps are held in same fashion as needle holder. **C,** Comparison of Adson beaks with Allis beaks shows difference in their usage.

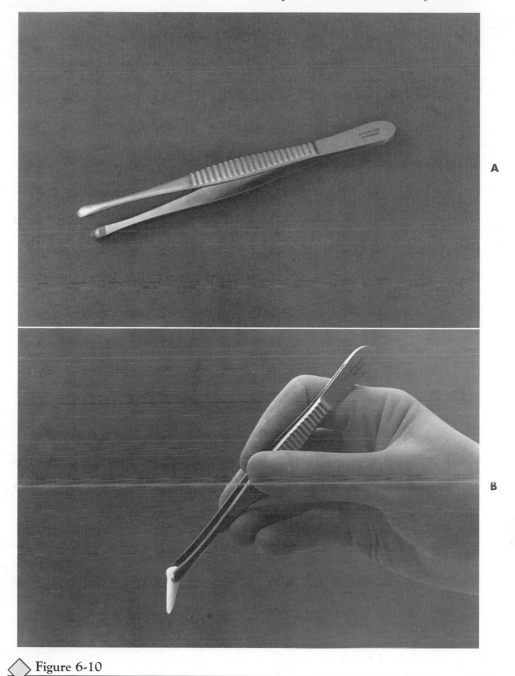

◇ **Figure 6-10**

A, Russian tissue forceps are round-ended pickups. **B,** Russian forceps are especially useful for grasping teeth that are loose in mouth.

grip, as commonly occurs with the hemostat. The Russian forceps are also useful for placing gauze in the mouth when the surgeon is isolating a particular area for surgery.

INSTRUMENTS FOR REMOVING BONE

RONGEUR FORCEPS

The instrument most commonly used for removing bone is the rongeur forceps. This instrument has sharp blades that are squeezed together by the handles, cutting or pinching through the bone. Rongeur forceps have a leaf spring between the handle, so that when hand pressure is released, the instrument will open. This allows the surgeon to make repeated cuts of bone without reopening the instrument (Figure 6-11, *A*). The two major designs for rongeur forceps are a side-cutting forceps and the side-cutting/end-cutting forceps (Figure 6-11, *B*).

The side-cutting/end-cutting forceps (Blumenthal rongeurs) are more practical for most dentoalveolar surgical procedures that require bone removal. Because they are end-cutting, these forceps can be inserted into sockets for removal of interradicular bone, but they can also be used to remove sharp edges of bone. Rongeurs can be used to remove large amounts of bone efficiently and quickly. Because

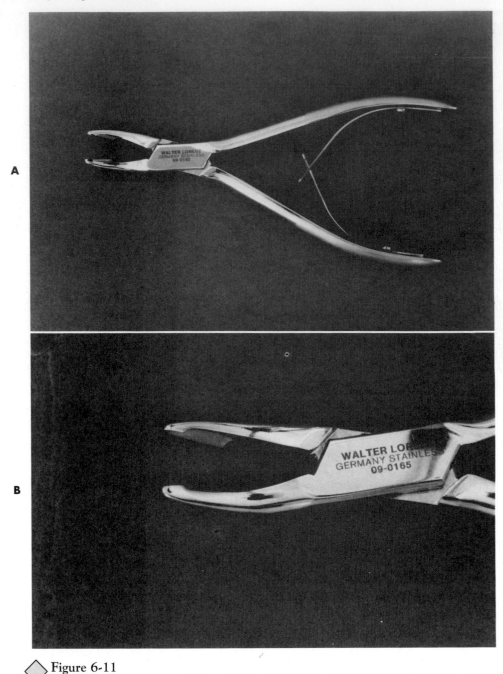

Figure 6-11

A, Rongeurs are bone-cutting forceps that have spring-loaded handles. **B,** Blumenthal rongeurs are combination end-cutting and side-cutting blades. They are preferred for oral surgery procedures.

rongeurs are relatively delicate instruments, the surgeon should not use the forceps to remove large amounts of bone in single bites. Rather, smaller amounts of bone should be removed in each of multiple bites. Likewise, the rongeurs should not be used to remove teeth, because this practice will quickly dull and destroy the instrument. Rongeurs are usually quite expensive, so care should be taken to keep them in working order.

CHISEL AND MALLET

One of the obvious methods of bone removal is to use a surgical chisel and mallet (Figure 6-12, *A, B,* and *C*). Bone is

usually removed with a monobevel chisel, and teeth are usually sectioned with a bibevel chisel. The success of chisel use depends on the sharpness of the instrument. Therefore it is necessary to sharpen the chisel before it is sterilized for the next patient. Some chisels have carbide tips and can be used more than once between sharpenings. A mallet with a nylon facing imparts less shock to the patient, is less noisy, and is therefore recommended.

BONE FILE

Final smoothing of bone before suturing the mucoperiosteal flap back into position is usually performed with a small bone

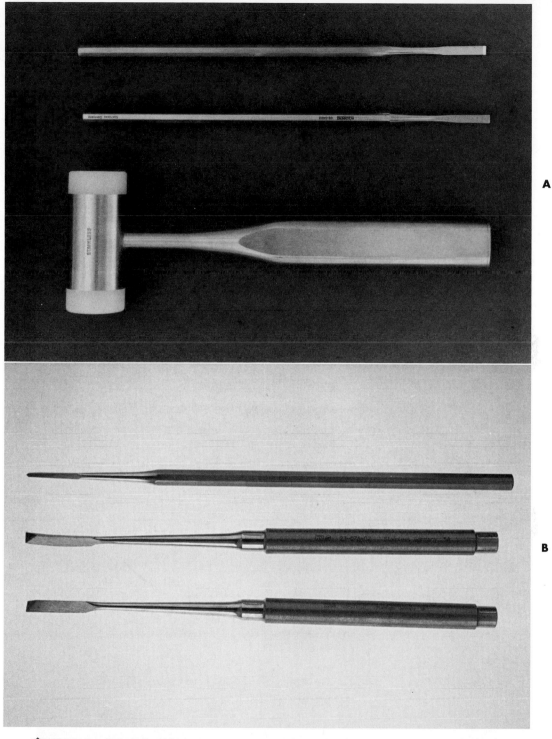

⬦ **Figure 6-12**

A, Surgical chisel and mallet can be used for removing bone and sectioning teeth. **B,** Additional chisels are straight unibevel chisel, curved unibevel chisel, or straight bibevel chisel. *Continued*

file (Figure 6-13, *A*). The bone file is usually a double-ended instrument with a small and large end. It cannot be used efficiently for removal of large amounts of bone, and it is used only for final smoothing. The teeth of the bone file are arranged in such a fashion that they remove bone only on a *pull* stroke (Figure 6-13, *B*). Pushing the bone file results only in burnishing and crushing the bone and should be avoided.

BUR AND HANDPIECE

A final method for removing bone is with a bur and handpiece. This is the technique that most surgeons use when removing

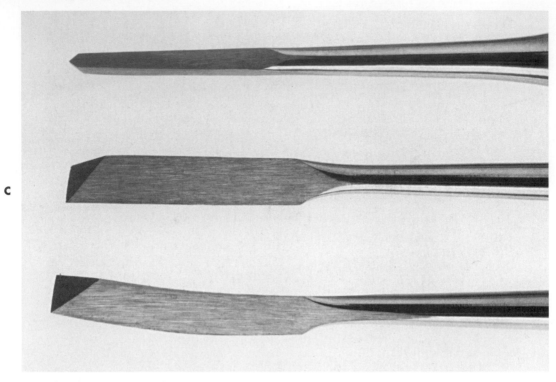

C

◇ **Figure 6-12, cont'd**

C, A close-up view of the chisel working end shows the bibevel end, the straight unibevel end, and the curved unibevel end.

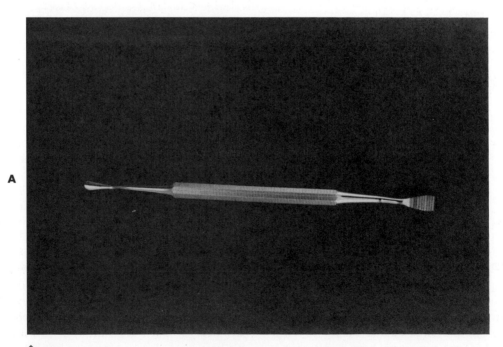

A

◇ **Figure 6-13**

A, Double-ended bone file is used for smoothing small, sharp edges or spicules of bone.   *Continued*

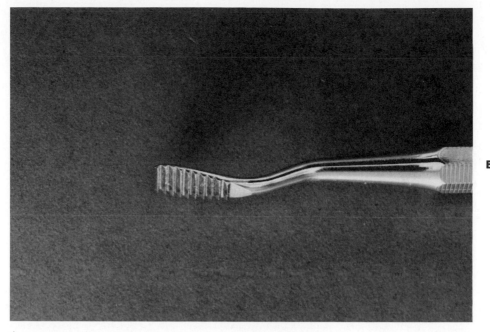

◆ Figure 6-13, cont'd

B, Teeth of bone file are effective only in pull stroke.

bone for surgical removal of teeth. Relatively high-speed handpieces with sharp carbide burs remove cortical bone efficiently. Burs such as a no. 557 or no. 703 fissure bur or a no. 8 round bur are used. When large amounts of bone must be removed, such as in torus reduction, a large bone bur that resembles an acrylic bur is used.

The handpiece that is used must be completely sterilizable in a steam autoclave. When a handpiece is purchased, the manufacturer's specifications must be checked carefully to ensure that this is possible. The handpiece should have relatively high speed and torque (Figure 6-14). This allows the bone removal to be done rapidly and allows efficient sectioning of teeth. The handpiece must not exhaust air into the operative field as dental drills do. Most high-speed turbine drills used for routine restorative dentistry must not be used. The reason is that the air exhausted into the wound may be forced into deeper tissue planes and produce tissue emphysema, a potentially dangerous occurrence.

INSTRUMENTS TO REMOVE SOFT TISSUE FROM BONY DEFECTS ◇

The periapical curette is an angled, double-ended instrument used to remove soft tissue from bony defects (Figure 6-15). The principal use is to remove granulomas or small cysts from periapical lesions, but it is also used to remove small amounts of granulation tissue debris from the tooth socket.

The periapical curette is distinctly different from the periodontal curette in design and function.

INSTRUMENTS FOR SUTURING MUCOSA ◇

Once a surgical procedure has been completed, the mucoperiosteal flap is returned to its original position and held in place by sutures. The needle holder is the instrument used to place the sutures.

NEEDLE HOLDER

The needle holder is an instrument with a locking handle and a short, stout beak. For intraoral placement of sutures, a 6-inch (15-cm) needle holder is usually recommended (Figure 6-16). The beak of the needle holder is shorter and stronger than the beak of the hemostat (Figure 6-17, *A*). The face of the beak of the needle holder is crosshatched to permit a positive grasp of the suture needle and suture. The hemostat has parallel grooves on the face of the beaks, thereby decreasing the control over needle and suture. Therefore the hemostat should not be used for suturing (Figure 6-17, *B*).

To properly control the locking handles and to direct the relatively long needle holder, the surgeon must hold the instrument in the proper fashion (Figure 6-18). The thumb and ring finger are inserted through the rings. The index finger is held along the length of the needle holder to steady and direct it. The second finger aids in controlling the locking mechanism. The index finger should not be put through

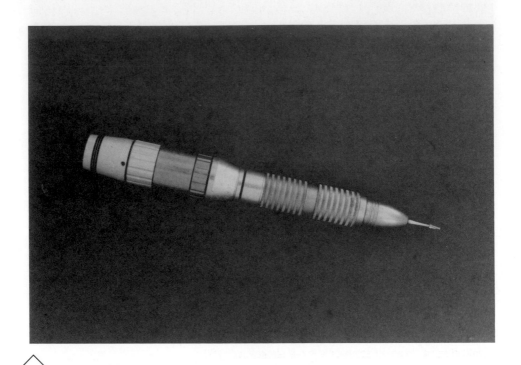

Typical moderate speed, high-torque, sterilizable handpiece with 703 bur.

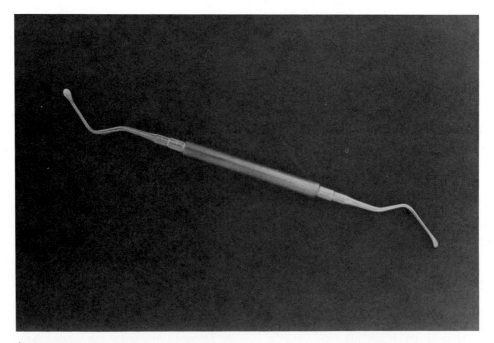

◇ **Figure 6-15**

Periapical curette is a double-ended, spoon-shaped instrument used to remove soft tissue from bony defects.

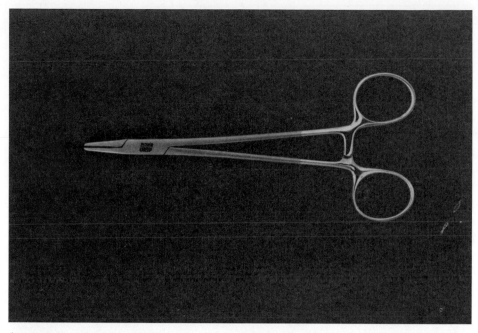

◇ Figure 6-16

Needle holder has locking handle and short, stout beak.

the finger ring, because this will result in dramatic decrease in control.

NEEDLE

The needle used in closing mucosal incisions is usually a small half-circle or three eighths-circle suture needle. It is curved to allow the needle to pass through a limited space, where a straight needle could not reach. Suture needles come in a large variety of shapes, from very small to very large (Figure 6-19, *A*). The tips of suture needles are either tapered, such as a sewing needle, or have triangular tips that allow them to be cutting needles (Figure 6-19, *B*). A cutting needle will pass through mucoperiosteum more easily than the tapered needle. The cutting portion of the needle extends about one-third the length of the needle, and the remaining portion of the needle is round. The suture can be threaded through the eye of the needle or can be purchased already swaged on by the manufacturer (Figure 6-19, *C*). If the dentist chooses to load his own needles for the sake of economy, he must use needles that have eyes, as has a typical sewing needle. If the dentist chooses to use the disposable needles, then the suture will be swaged onto the needle. Needles that have eyes are larger at the tip and may cause slightly increased tissue injury compared with the swaged-on needles.

The curved needle is held approximately two thirds of the distance between the tip and the end of the needle (Figure 6-20). This allows enough of the needle to be exposed to pass through the tissue, while allowing the needle holder to grasp the needle in its strong portion to prevent bending of the needle. Techniques for placing sutures are discussed in Chapter 8.

SUTURE MATERIAL

Many types of suture materials are available. The materials are classified by size, resorbability, and whether or not they are monofilament or polyfilament.

The size of suture is designated by a series of zeros. The size most commonly used in the suturing of oral mucosa is 3-0 (000). A larger size suture would be 2-0, or 0. Smaller sizes would be 4-0, 5-0, and 6-0 sutures. Sutures of very fine size such as 6-0 are usually used in conspicuous places on the skin, such as the face, because smaller sutures usually cause less scarring. Sutures of size 3-0 are large enough to prevent tearing through mucosa, are strong enough to withstand the tension placed on them intraorally, and are strong enough for easy knot-tying with a needle holder.

Sutures may be resorbable or nonresorbable. Non-resorbable suture materials include such types as silk, nylon, and stainless steel. The most commonly used nonresorbable suture in the oral cavity is silk. Nylon and stainless steel are rarely used in the mouth. Resorbable sutures are primarily made of gut. Although the term *catgut* is often used to designate this type of suture, gut actually is derived from the serosal surface of sheep intestines. Plain catgut resorbs relatively quickly in the oral cavity, rarely lasting longer than 5 days. Gut that has been treated by tanning solutions (chromic acid) and is therefore called *chromic gut* lasts longer, up to 10 to 12 days. Several synthetic resorbable sutures are also available. These are materials that are long chains of polymers braided into suture material. Examples are polyglycolic acid and polylactic acid. These materials are slowly resorbed, taking up to 4 weeks before they are resorbed. Such long-lasting resorbable sutures are rarely indicated in the oral cavity.

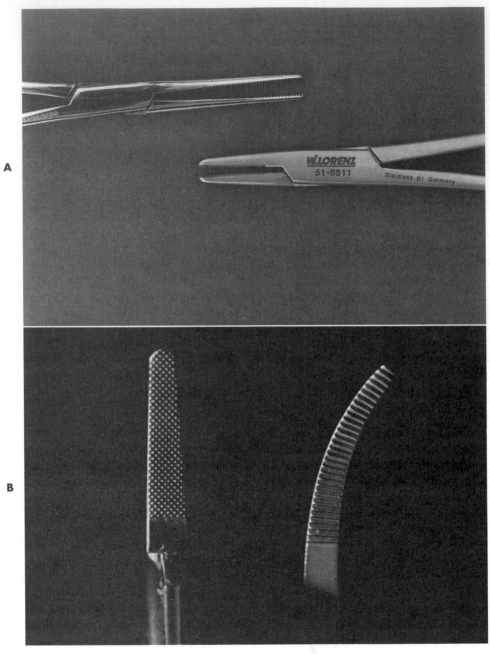

◇ **Figure 6-17**

A, Hemostat *(top)* has longer, thinner beak compared with needle holder *(bottom)* and therefore should not be used for suturing. **B,** Face of shorter beak of needle holder is crosshatched to ensure positive grip on needle *(left).* Face of hemostat has parallel grooves that do not allow firm grip on needle *(right).*

Finally, sutures are classified based on whether or not they are monofilament or polyfilament. Monofilament sutures are sutures such as both plain and chromic gut, nylon, and stainless steel. Polyfilament sutures are silk, polyglycolic acid, and polylactic acid. Sutures that are made of braided material are easy to handle and tie and rarely come untied. The cut ends are usually soft and nonirritating to the tongue and surrounding soft tissues. However, because of the multiple filaments, they tend to "wick" oral fluids along the suture to the underlying tissues. This wicking action may carry bacteria along with the saliva. Monofilament sutures do not cause this wicking action but may be more difficult to tie, tend to come untied, and are stiffer and therefore more irritating to the tongue and soft tissues.

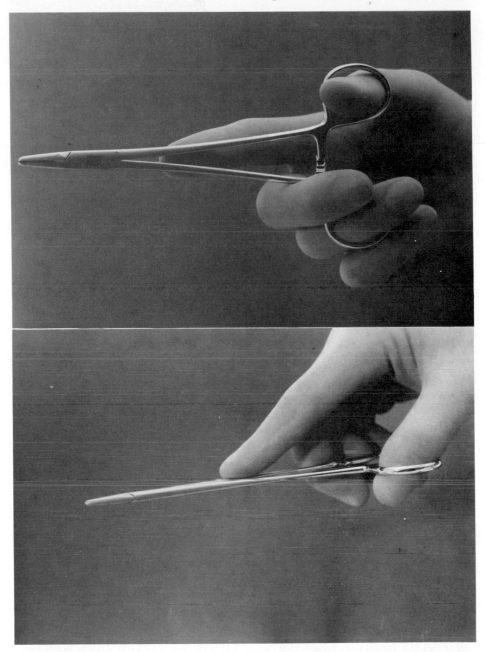

◇ **Figure 6-18**

Needle holder is held by using thumb and ring finger in rings and first and second finger to control instrument.

The most commonly used suture for the oral cavity is 3-0 black silk. The size 3-0 has the appropriate amount of strength; the polyfilament nature of the silk makes it easy to tie and easily tolerated by the patient's soft tissues. The black color makes the suture easy to see when the patient returns for suture removal. Sutures that are holding mucosa together usually stay no longer than 5 to 7 days, so the wicking action is of little clinical importance.

Techniques for suturing and knot-tying are presented in Chapter 7.

SCISSORS

The final instruments necessary for placing sutures are suture scissors (Figure 6-21). Suture scissors usually have relatively long handles and thumb and finger rings. They are held in the same way as the needle holder. The suture scissors usually have short cutting edges, because their sole purpose is to cut sutures (Figure 6-22). The most commonly used suture scissors are the Dean scissors. These have slightly curved handles and serrated blades that make cutting sutures easier.

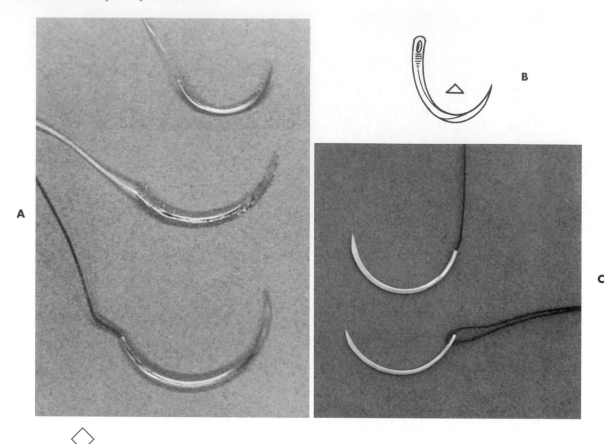

◇ ──

A, Comparison of needles used in oral surgery. Top is P-3 needle, which is usually 4-0 size suture. Middle is FS-2 needle, and bottom is X-1. All are cutting needles. **B,** Tip of needle used to suture mucoperiosteum is triangular in cross-section to make it a cutting needle. **C,** Suture may be threaded through needle eye or can be purchased already swaged onto needle.

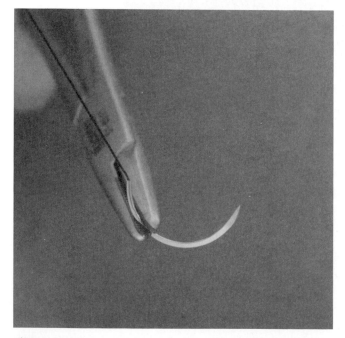

◇ **Figure 6-20**
──
Needle holder grasps curved needle two thirds of the distance from tip of needle.

An additional type of scissors is designed for soft tissue. The two major types of tissue scissors are the Iris scissors and the Metzenbaum scissors (Figure 6-23). The Iris scissors are small, sharp-pointed delicate tools used for fine work. The Metzenbaum scissors are blunt-nosed scissors used for undermining soft tissue, as well as for cutting. Tissue scissors such as the Iris or Metzenbaum scissors should not be used to cut sutures, because the suture material will dull the edges of the blades and make them less effective for cutting tissue.

INSTRUMENTS FOR RETRACTING SOFT TISSUE ────────◇

It is critical to have good vision and good access to perform good surgery. To this end there are a variety of retractors that have been designed to retract the cheeks, tongue, and muco-periosteal flaps.

The two most popular cheek retractors are the right-angle Austin retractor (Figure 6-24) and the offset broad Minnesota retractor (Figure 6-25). Both of these retractors can retract the cheek and a mucoperiosteal flap simultaneously. Before the

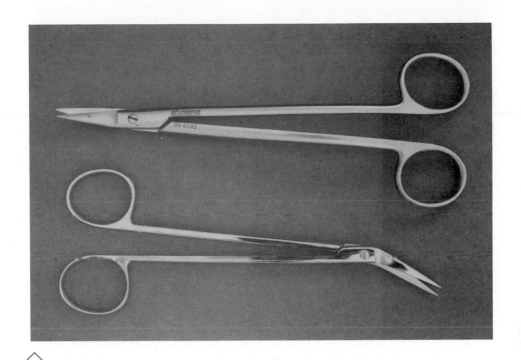

Suture scissors have long handles and short blades. Blades may be angled slightly in either of two directions.

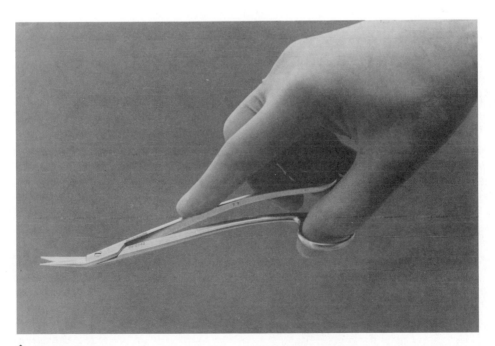

◇ **Figure 6-22**

Suture scissors should be held in same fashion as needle holder.

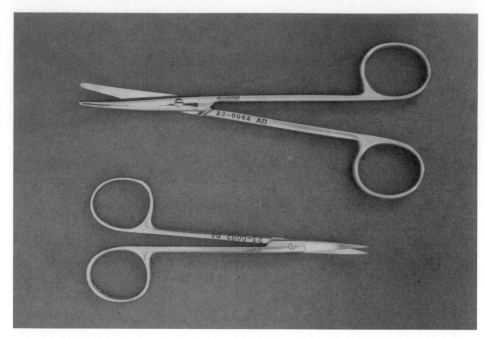

◇ **Figure 6-23**

Soft tissue scissors are of two designs. Iris scissors are small, sharp-pointed scissors. Metzenbaum scissors *(top)* are longer, delicate, blunt-nosed scissors.

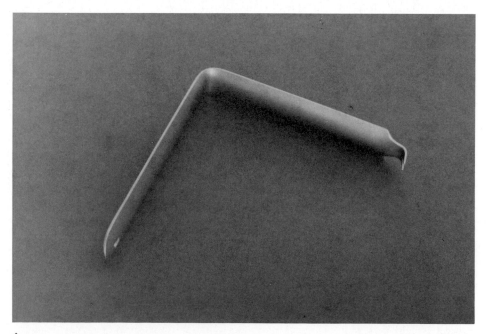

◇ **Figure 6-24**

Austin retractor is a right-angle retractor that can be used to retract cheek, tongue, or flaps.

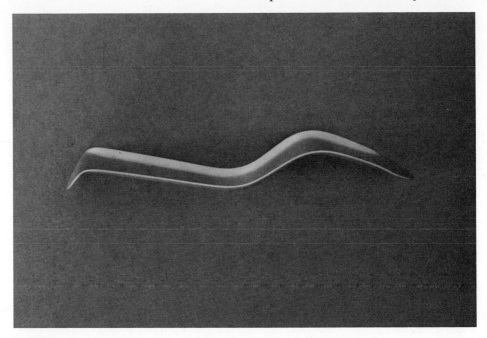

◆ Figure 6-25

Minnesota retractor is an offset retractor used for retraction of cheeks and flaps.

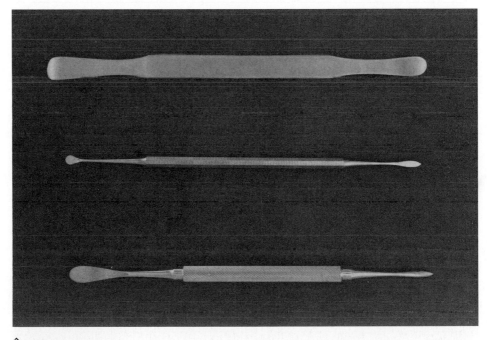

◆ Figure 6-26

Periosteal elevators such as Woodson and no. 9 Molt are useful to retract flaps. Seldin retractor *(top)* is broader instrument that provides broader retraction and increased visualization.

flap is created, the retractor is held loosely in the cheek, and once the flap is reflected the retractor is placed on the bone and is then used to retract the flap.

In addition to the Austin and Minnesota retractors, there are other retractors designed more specifically to reflect soft tissue flaps. The Seldin retractor is typical of this kind (Figure 6-26).

Although this retractor may look similar to a periosteal elevator, the leading edge is not sharp but rather is dull and should not be used to reflect mucoperiosteum. The periosteal elevator is often used as the primary instrument to retract soft tissue. Once the flap has been reflected, the periosteal elevator is positioned on bone and held there to reflect the tissue.

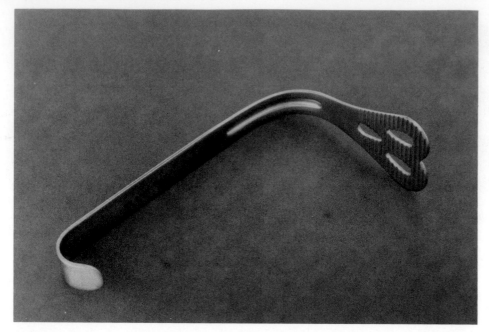

◇ Figure 6-27

Weider retractor is a large retractor designed to retract tongue. Serrated surface helps to engage tongue, so that it can be held securely.

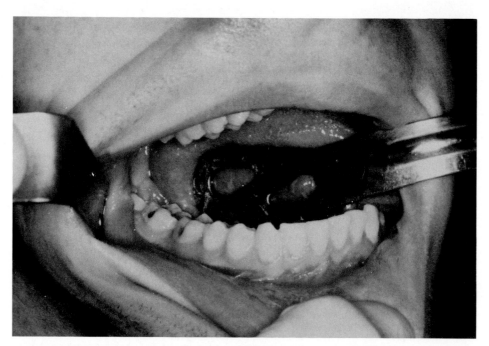

◇ Figure 6-28

Weider retractor is used to hold tongue away from surgical field. Austin retractor is used to retract cheek.

The instrument most commonly used to retract the tongue is the mouth mirror. This is usually part of every basic setup, because it has both the usual use and use as a tongue retractor. The Weider tongue retractor is a broad, heart-shaped retractor that is serrated on one side, so that it can more firmly engage the tongue and retract it medially and anteriorly (Figure 6-27). When this retractor is used, care must be taken not to position it so far posteriorly that it causes gagging (Figure 6-28).

The towel clip can be used to hold the tongue. When a biopsy procedure is to be performed on the posterior aspect of the tongue, the most positive way to control the tongue is by holding the anterior tongue with a towel clip. Local anesthesia must be profound where the clip is placed.

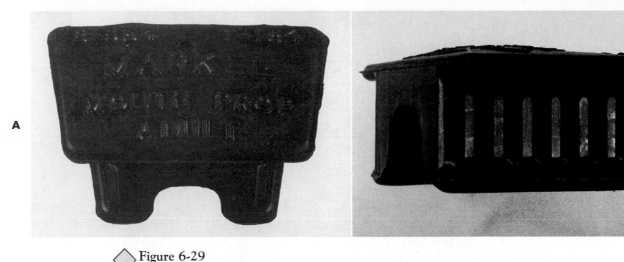

◇ Figure 6-29

A, Rubber bite block is used to hold mouth open in position chosen by patient. **B,** The sides of the bite block are corrugated to provide a surface for the teeth to engage.

INSTRUMENTS TO HOLD THE MOUTH OPEN ◇

When performing extractions of mandibular teeth, it is necessary to support the mandible to prevent stress on the temporomandibular joints. By having the patient's jaw supported on a bite block, the joints will be protected. The bite block is just what the name implies (Figure 6-29, *A* and *B*). It is a rubber block on which the patient can rest the teeth. The patient opens his or her mouth to a comfortably wide position, and the rubber bite block is inserted, which holds the mouth in the desired position. Should the surgeon need the mouth to open wider, the patient must open wide and the bite block must be positioned more to the posterior of the mouth.

The side-action mouth prop, or Molt mouth prop, (Figure 6-30) can be used by the operator to open the mouth wider if necessary. This mouth prop has a ratchet-type action, opening the mouth wider as the handle is closed. This type of mouth prop should be used with caution, because great pressure can be applied to the teeth and temporomandibular joint, and injury may occur with injudicious use. This type of mouth prop is useful in patients who are deeply sedated.

INSTRUMENTS FOR PROVIDING SUCTION ◇

To provide adequate visualization, blood, saliva, and irrigating solutions must be suctioned from the operative site. The surgical suction is one that has a smaller orifice than the type used in general dentistry, so that the tooth sockets can be suctioned in case a root tip is fractured and adequate visualization is necessary. Many of these suctions are designed with several orifices, so that the soft tissue will not become aspirated into the suction hole and cause tissue injury (Figure 6-31, *A*).

The Fraser suction has a hole in the handle portion that can be covered as the requirement dictates. When hard tissue is being cut under copious irrigation, the hole is covered so that the solution is removed rapidly. When soft tissue is being suctioned, the hole is uncovered to prevent tissue injury (Figure 6-31, *B*).

INSTRUMENTS TO TRANSFER STERILE INSTRUMENTS ◇

The transfer forceps are heavy forceps used to move instruments from one sterile area to another (Figure 6-32, *A*). These forceps are usually right-angled forceps with heavy jaws, so that instruments such as extraction forceps can be moved from one area to another and small items can be handled without dropping them (Figure 6-32, *B* and *C*). The transfer forceps are stored in a container that is usually filled with a bactericidal solution, such as glutaraldehyde. The container must be emptied and new solution placed at least every other day. The container should be thoroughly washed and autoclaved at least once per week.

INSTRUMENT TO HOLD TOWELS AND DRAPES IN POSITION ◇

When drapes are placed around a patient, they must be held together with a towel clip (Figure 6-33). This instrument has a locking handle and finger and thumb rings. The action ends of the towel clip are sharp, curved points that penetrate the towels and drapes. When this instrument is used, the operator must take extreme caution not to pinch the patient's underlying skin.

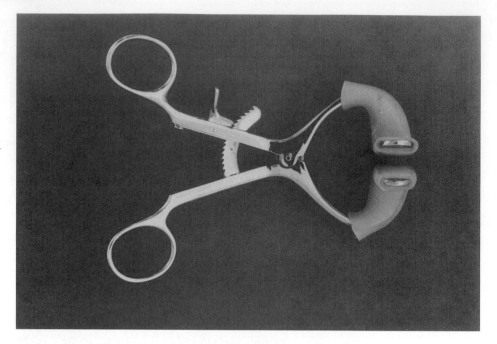

◇ Figure 6-30

Side-action, or Molt, mouth prop can be used to open patient's mouth when patient is unable to cooperate, such as during sedation.

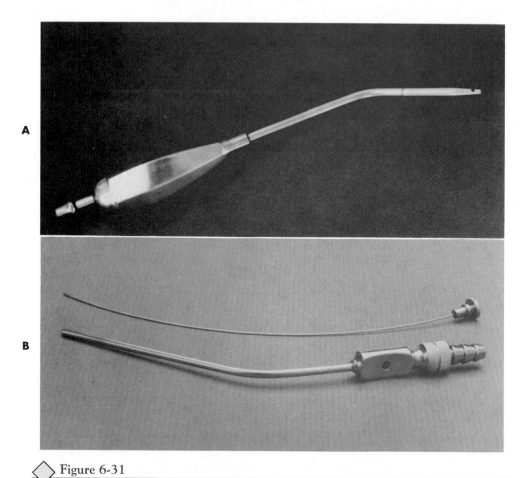

A

B

◇ Figure 6-31

A, Typical surgical suction has small-diameter tip. Suction tip has hole in side to prevent tissue injury because of excess suction pressure. **B,** Fraser suction tip has blade in handle, to allow operator more control over amount of suction power. Wire stylet is used to clean tip when bone or tooth particles plug suction.

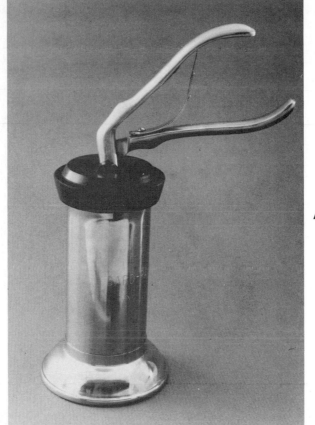

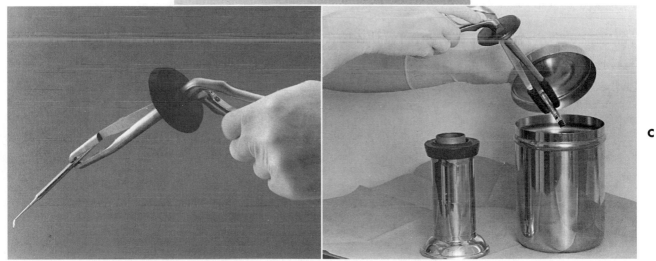

⬦ Figure 6-32

A, Transfer forceps are used to move sterile instruments from one sterile area to another. **B,** These forceps are sturdy enough to move instruments without fear of loosing grip on them. **C,** Transfer forceps can also be used to handle small items, such as anesthetic cartridges.

INSTRUMENTS FOR
IRRIGATION ⬦

When a handpiece and bur are used to remove bone, it is essential that the area be irrigated with a steady stream of irrigating solution, usually sterile saline. The irrigation cools the bur and prevents bone-damaging heat buildup. The irri-

gation also increases the efficiency of the bur by washing away bone chips from the flutes of the bur and by providing a certain amount of lubrication. Additionally, once a surgical procedure is completed and before the mucoperiosteal flap is sutured back into position, the surgical field should be irrigated thoroughly with saline. A large plastic syringe with a blunt 18-gauge needle is used for irrigation purposes. Although the syringe is disposable, it can be sterilized multiple times before

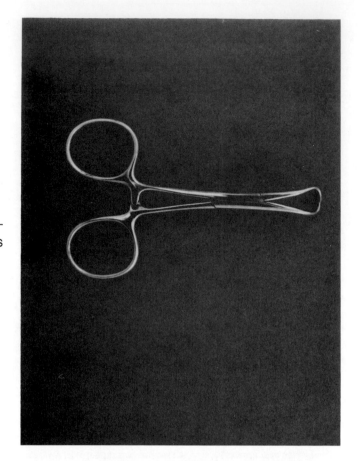

Figure 6-33

Towel clip is used to hold drapes in position. Sharp points penetrate towels and locking handles maintain drape in position.

A

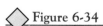
Figure 6-34

A, Bulb or regular syringes may be used to carry irrigation solution to operative site. **B,** The self-loaded syringe is spring-loaded to allow filling simply by releasing the plunger.

B

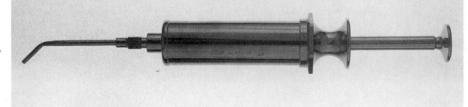

it must be discarded. The needle should be blunt and smooth so that it does not damage soft tissue, and it should be angled for more efficient direction of the irrigating stream (Figure 6-34, *A* and *B*).

DENTAL ELEVATORS

One of the most important instruments used in the extraction procedure is the dental elevator. These instruments are used to luxate teeth (loosen them) from the surrounding bone. Loosening teeth before the application of the dental forceps can frequently make a difficult extraction easier. By luxating the teeth before the application of the forceps, the clinician can minimize the incidence of broken roots and teeth. Finally, luxation of teeth before forceps application facilitates the removal of a broken root should it occur, because the root will be loose in the dental socket. In addition to their role in loosening teeth from the surrounding bone, dental elevators are also used to expand alveolar bone. By expanding the buccocortical plate of bone, the surgeon facilitates the removal of a tooth that has a limited and somewhat obstructed path for removal. Finally, elevators are used to remove broken or surgically sectioned roots from their sockets. Elevators are designed with specific shapes, to facilitate their removal of roots from sockets.

COMPONENTS

The three major components of the elevator are the handle, the shank, and the blade (Figure 6-35). The handle of the elevator is usually of generous size, so that it can be held comfortably in the hand to apply substantial but controlled force. The application of specifically applied force is critical in the proper use of dental elevators. In some situations, crossbar or T-bar handles are used. These instruments must be used with caution, because they can generate a very large amount of force (Figure 6-36).

The shank of the elevator simply connects the handle to the working end, or blade, of the elevator. The shank is generally of substantial size and is strong enough to transmit the force from the handle to the blade.

The blade of the elevator is the working tip of the elevator and is used to transmit the force to the tooth, bone, or both.

TYPES

The biggest variation in the type of elevator is in the shape and size of the blade. The three basic types of elevators are the straight, or gouge, type; the triangle, or pennant-shape, type; and the pick type. The straight, or gouge, type elevator is the most commonly used elevator to luxate teeth (Figure 6-37, *A*). The blade of the straight elevator has a concave surface on one side, so that it can be used in the same fashion as a shoehorn (Figure 6-37, *B* and *C*). The small straight elevator, no. 301, is frequently used for beginning the luxation of an erupted tooth, before application of the forceps (Figure 6-38). The larger straight elevator is used to displace roots from their sockets and is also used to luxate teeth that are more widely spaced. The most com-

monly used large straight elevator is the no. 34S, but the no. 46 and no. 77R are also occasionally used. The shape of the blade of the straight elevator can be angled from the shank, allowing this instrument to be used in the more posterior aspects of the mouth. Two examples of the angled-shank elevator with a blade similar to the straight elevator are the Miller elevator and the Potts elevator.

The second most commonly used elevator is the triangular, or pennant-shaped, elevator (Figure 6-39). These elevators are provided in pairs, a left and a right. The triangle-shaped elevator is most useful when a broken root remains in the tooth socket, and the adjacent socket is empty. A typical example would be when a mandibular first molar is fractured, leaving the distal root in the socket but the mesial root removed with the crown. The tip of the triangle shaped elevator is placed into the socket, with the shank of the elevator resting on the buccal plate of bone. It is then turned in a wheel-and-axle type of rotation, with the sharp tip of the elevator engaging the cementum of the remaining distal root; the elevator is then turned and the root delivered. There are many variations in the types and angulation of the triangle-shaped elevators, but the Cryer is the most common type.

The third type of elevator that is used with some frequency is the pick type elevator. This type of elevator is used to remove roots. The heavy version of the pick is the Crane pick (Figure 6-40). This instrument is used as a lever to elevate a broken root from the tooth socket. It is usually necessary to drill a hole with a bur, approximately 3 mm deep into the root. The tip of the pick is then inserted into the hole, and, with the buccal plate of bone as a fulcrum, the root is elevated from the tooth socket. Occasionally, the sharp point can be used without preparing a purchase point by engaging the cementum of the tooth.

The second type of pick is the root tip pick, or apex elevator (Figure 6-41). The root tip pick is a delicate instrument that is used to tease small root tips from their sockets. It must be emphasized that this instrument is a thin instrument and cannot be used as a wheel-and-axle or lever type of elevator as is the Cryer elevator or the Crane pick. The root tip pick is used to tease the very small root end of a tooth.

EXTRACTION FORCEPS

The instruments that come to mind when thinking of the removal of a tooth are the extraction forceps. These instruments are used for removing the tooth from the alveolar bone. They are designed in many styles and configurations, to adapt to the variety of teeth for which they are used. There are several basic designs that each have a multiplicity of variations for individual operator preferences. This section deals with the basic fundamental designs and mentions only in passing several of the variations.

COMPONENTS

The basic components of dental extraction forceps are the handle, hinge, and beaks (Figure 6-42). The handles are usually of adequate size to be handled comfortably and deliver sufficient pressure and leverage to remove the required tooth.

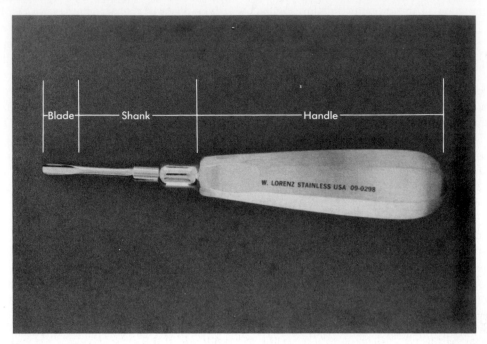

◈ Figure 6-35

Three major components of an elevator are handle, shank, and blade.

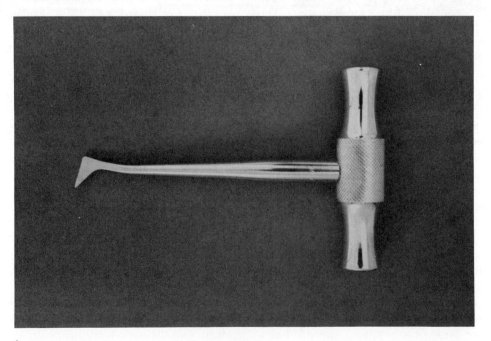

◈ Figure 6-36

Crossbar handle is used on certain elevators. This type of handle can generate large amounts of force and therefore must be used with caution.

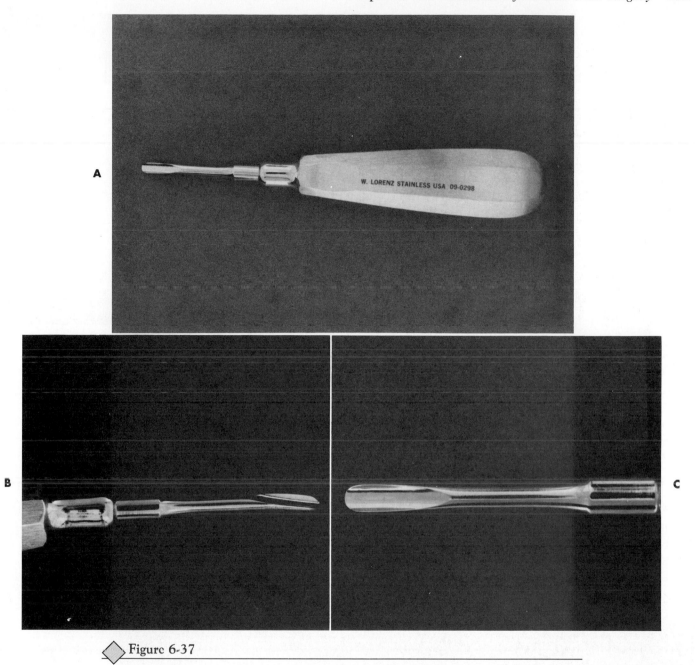

◇ Figure 6-37

A, Straight elevator is most commonly used elevator. **B** and **C,** Blade of straight elevator is concave on its working side.

The handles have a serrated surface, to allow a positive grip and prevent slippage.

The handles of the forceps are held differently, depending on the position of the tooth to be removed. Maxillary forceps are held with the palm underneath the forceps, so that the beak is directed in a superior direction (Figure 6-43). The forceps used for removal of mandibular teeth are held with the palm on top of the forceps, so that the beak is pointed down toward the teeth (Figure 6-44). The handles of the forceps are usually straight but may be curved. This provides the operator with a sense of "better fit" (Figure 6-45).

The hinge of the forceps, like the shank of the elevator, is merely a mechanism for connecting the handle to the beak. The hinge transfers and concentrates the force applied to the handles to the beak. One distinct difference in styles does exist. The usual American type of forceps has a hinge in a horizontal direction and is used as has been described (Figure 6-42 and 6-43). The English preference is for a vertical hinge and corresponding vertically positioned handle (Figure 6-46, *A*). Thus the English style handle and hinge are used with the hand held in a vertical direction as opposed to a horizontal direction (Figure 6-46, *B*).

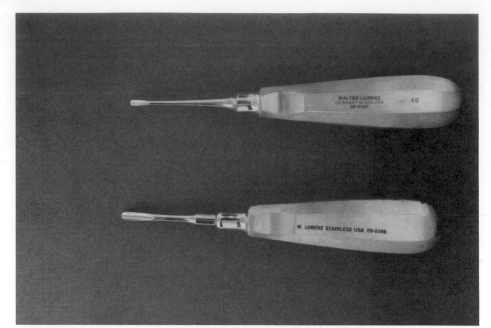

◇ **Figure 6-38**

Blade of small straight elevator is about half the width of a large straight elevator.

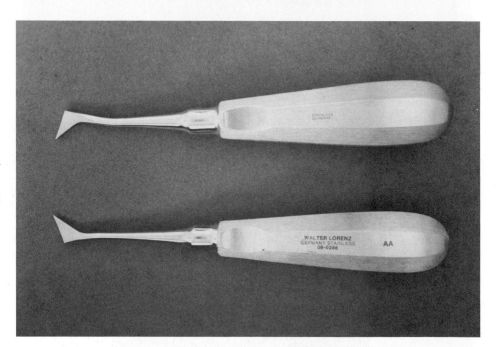

◇ **Figure 6-39**

Triangular-shaped elevators (Cryer) are pairs of instruments and are therefore used for specific roots.

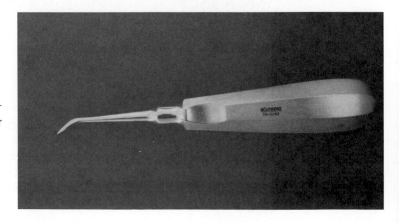

◇ **Figure 6-40**

Crane pick is a heavy instrument used to elevate whole roots or even teeth after purchase point has been prepared with bur.

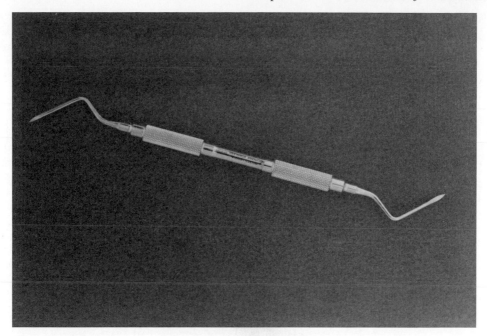

◇ Figure 6-41

Delicate root tip pick is used to tease small root tip fragments from socket.

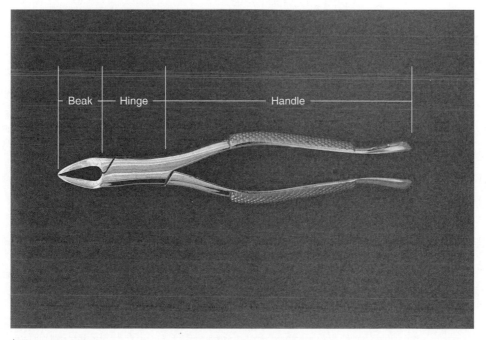

◇ Figure 6-42

Basic components of extraction forceps are handle, hinge, and beaks.

The beaks of the extraction forceps are the source of the greatest variation among forceps. The beak is designed to adapt to the tooth root at the junction of the crown and root. It is important to remember that the beaks of the forceps are designed to be adapted to the *root structure* of the tooth and not to the crown of the tooth. In a sense then, there are beaks designed for single-rooted teeth, two-rooted teeth, and three-rooted teeth. The design variation is such that the tips of the beaks will adapt closely to the various root formations, decreasing the chance for root fracture. The more closely the beak of the forceps adapts to the tooth roots, the more efficient will be the extraction and the less chance for untoward complications.

A final design variation is in the width of the beak. Some

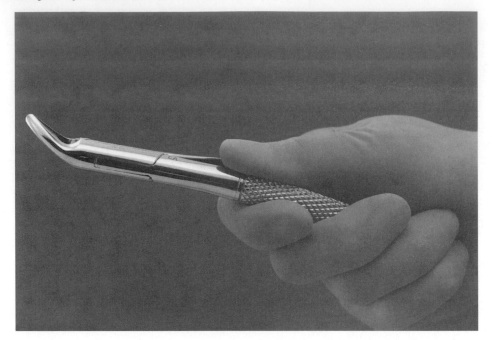

◇ **Figure 6-43**

Forceps used to remove maxillary teeth are held with palm under handle.

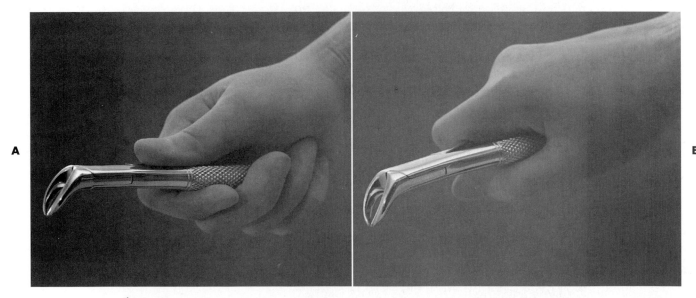

A ◇ **Figure 6-44** B

A, Forceps used to remove mandibular teeth are held with palm on top of forceps. **B,** Firmer grip for delivering greater amounts of rotational force can be achieved by moving thumb around and under handle.

forceps are narrow, because their primary use is to remove narrow teeth, such as incisor teeth. Other forceps are somewhat broader, because the teeth they are designed to remove are substantially wider, such as lower molar teeth. Forceps designed to remove a lower incisor can be used to remove a lower molar, but the beaks are so narrow that they

will be inefficient for that application. Similarly, the broader molar forceps would not adapt to the narrow space allowed by the narrow lower incisor and therefore could not be used in that situation.

The beaks of the forceps are angled so that they can be placed parallel to the long axis of the tooth, with the

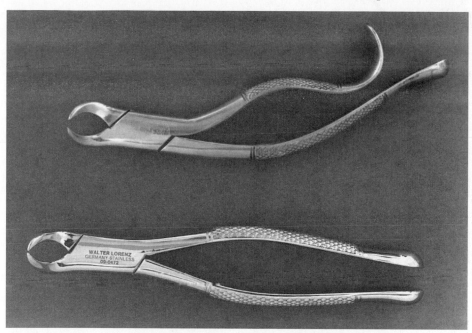

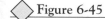

◇ **Figure 6-45**

Straight handles are usually preferred, but curved handles are preferred by some surgeons.

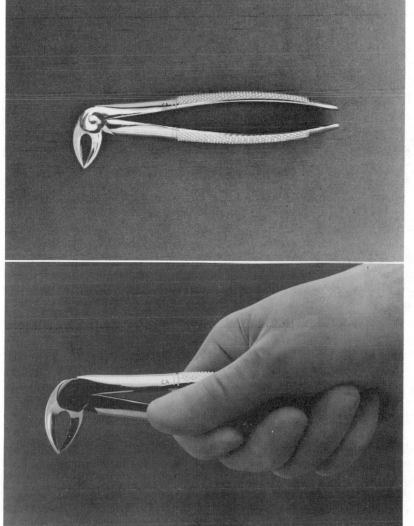

A

B

◇ **Figure 6-46**

A, English style of forceps have hinge in vertical direction.
B, English style of forceps are held in vertical direction.

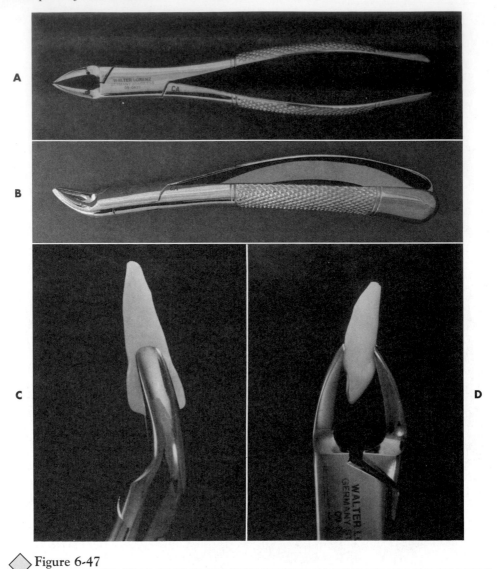

◇ Figure 6-47

A, Superior view of no. 150 forceps. **B,** Side view of no. 150 forceps. **C** and **D,** No. 150 forceps adapted to maxillary central incisor.

handle in a comfortable position. Therefore the beaks of maxillary forceps are usually parallel to the handles. Maxillary molar forceps are offset in a bayonet fashion to allow the operator to comfortably reach the posterior aspect of the mouth and yet keep the beaks parallel to the long axis of the tooth. The beak of mandibular forceps is usually set perpendicular to the handles, which allows the surgeon to reach the lower teeth and maintain a comfortable, controlled position.

MAXILLARY FORCEPS

The removal of maxillary teeth requires the use of instruments designed for single-rooted teeth, as well as for teeth with three roots. The maxillary incisors, canine teeth, and premolar teeth are all considered to be single-rooted teeth. The maxillary first premolar frequently has a bifurcated root, but because this occurs in the apical one third, it has no influence on the design

of the forceps. The maxillary molars are usually trifurcated and therefore require extraction forceps, which will adapt to that configuration.

The single-rooted maxillary teeth are usually removed with maxillary universal forceps, usually number 150 (Figure 6-47). The no. 150 forceps are slightly curved when viewed from the side and are essentially straight when viewed from above. The beaks of the forceps curve to meet only at the tip. The slight curve of the no. 150 allows the operator to reach not only the incisors, but also the bicuspids in a comfortable fashion. The beak of the no. 150 forceps has been modified slightly to form the no. 150A forceps (Figure 6-48). The no. 150A is useful for the maxillary premolar teeth and should not be used for the incisors, because their adaptation to the roots of the incisors is poor.

In addition to the no. 150 forceps, there are also straight forceps. The no. 1 (Figure 6-49), which can be used for

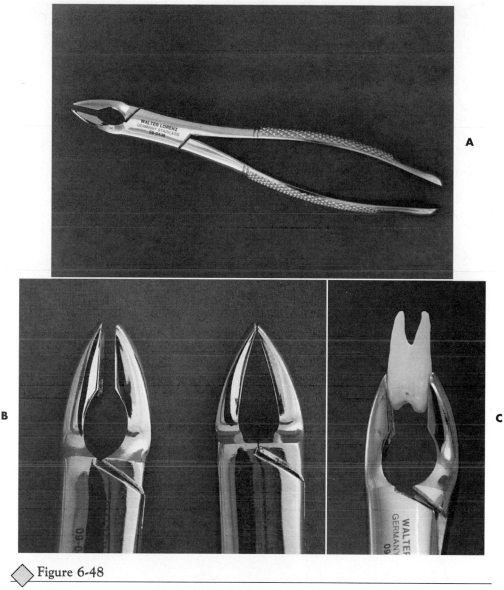

◇ **Figure 6-48**

A, Superior view of no. 150A forceps. **B,** No. 150A forceps have parallel beaks that do not touch. **C,** Adaptation of no. 150A forceps to maxillary premolar.

maxillary incisors and canines are slightly easier to use than the no. 150 for incisors.

The maxillary molar teeth are three-rooted teeth with a single palatal root and a buccal bifurcation. Therefore forceps that are adapted to fit the maxillary molars must have a smooth, concave surface for the palatal root and a beak with a pointed design that will fit into the buccal bifurcation on the buccal beak. This requires that the molar forceps come in pairs, a left and a right. Additionally, the molar forceps should be offset so that the operator can reach the posterior aspect of the mouth and remain in the correct position. The most commonly used molar forceps are the no. 53 right and left (Figure 6-50). These forceps are designed to fit anatomically around the palatal beak, and the pointed buccal beak fits into the buccal bifurcation. The beak is offset to allow for good positioning.

A design variation is shown in the no. 88 right and left forceps, which have a longer, more accentuated, pointed beak formation (Figure 6-51). These forceps are known as upper cowhorn forceps. They are particularly useful for maxillary molars whose crowns are severely decayed. The sharply pointed beaks may reach deeper into the trifurcation to sound dentin. The major disadvantage is that they crush alveolar bone, and when used on intact teeth without due caution, fracture of large amounts of buccal alveolar bone may occur.

Occasionally, maxillary second molars and erupted third molars have a single conically shaped root. In this situation, forceps with broad, smooth beaks that are offset from the handle can be useful. The no. 210S forceps exemplify this design (Figure 6-52). Another design variation is shown in the offset molar forceps with very narrow beaks. These are used

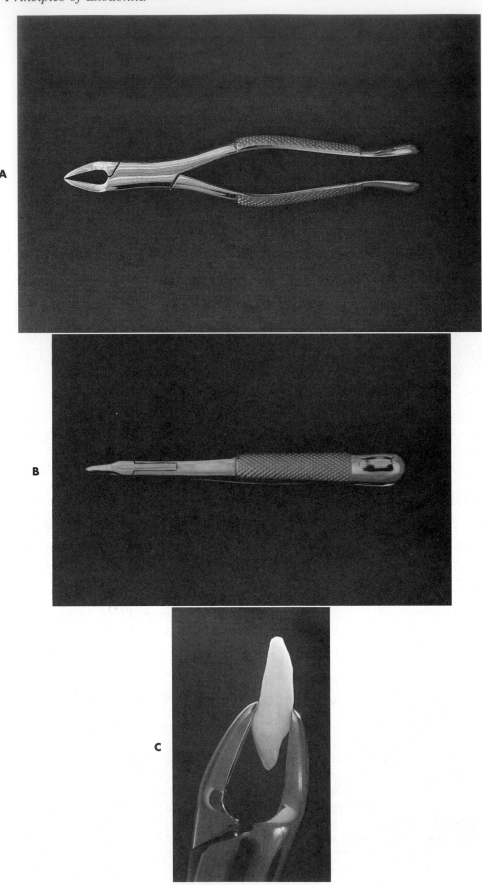

◇ **Figure 6-49**

A, Superior view of the no. 1 forceps. **B,** Side view of the no. 1 forceps. **C,** No. 1 forceps adapted to incisor.

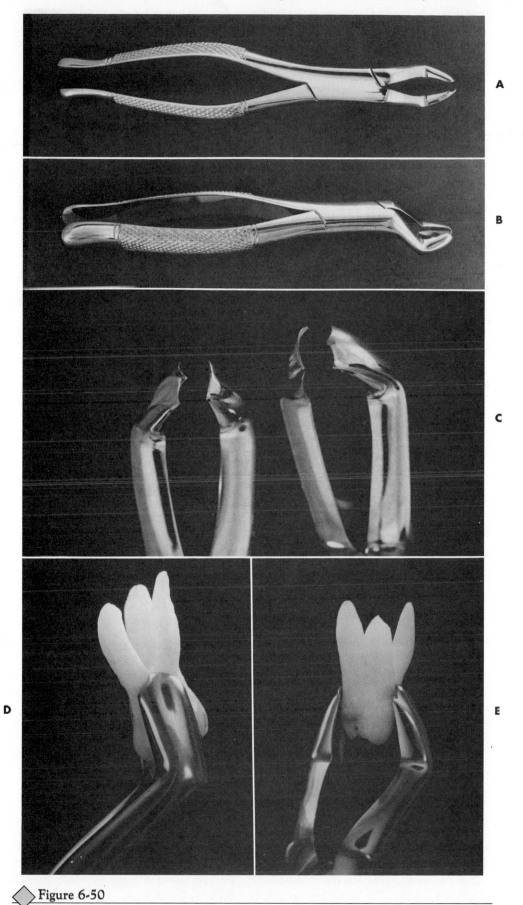

◇ **Figure 6-50**

A, Superior view of the no. 53L forceps. **B,** Side view of no. 53L forceps. **C,** *Right,* No. 53L; *left,* no. 53R.
D and **E,** No. 53L adapted to maxillary molar.

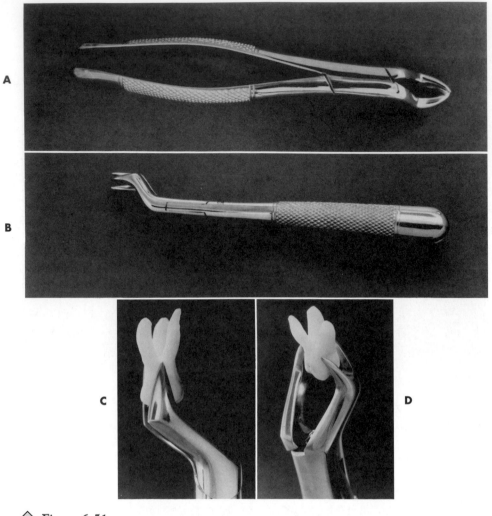

◇ **Figure 6-51**

A, Superior view of no. 88L forceps. **B,** Side view of no. 88L forceps. **C** and **D,** No. 88R adapted to maxillary molar.

primarily to remove broken maxillary molar roots but can be used for removal of narrow premolars and for lower incisors. These forceps, the no. 286, are also known as root tip forceps (Figure 6-53).

A smaller version of the no. 150, the no. 150S, is useful for removing primary teeth (Figure 6-54). These adapt well to all maxillary primary teeth and can be used as universal primary tooth forceps.

MANDIBULAR FORCEPS

Extraction of mandibular teeth requires forceps that can be used for single-rooted teeth for the incisors, canines, and premolars and for two-rooted teeth for the molars. The forceps most commonly used for the single-rooted teeth are the lower universal forceps, or the no. 151 (Figure 6-55). These have handles similar in shape to the no. 150, but the beaks are pointed inferiorly for the lower teeth. The beaks are smooth and relatively narrow and meet only at the tip. This allows the

beaks to fit at the cervical line of the tooth and grasp the root.

The no. 151A forceps have been modified slightly for mandibular premolar teeth (Figure 6-56). They should not be used for other lower teeth, because their form prevents adaptation to the roots of the teeth.

The English style of vertical-hinge forceps are used occasionally for the single-rooted teeth in the mandible (Figure 6-57). Great force can be generated with these forceps, and, unless care is used, the incidence of root fracture is high with this instrument. Therefore it is rarely used by the beginning surgeon.

The mandibular molars are bifurcated, two-rooted teeth that allow the use of forceps that anatomically adapt to the tooth. Because the bifurcation is on both the buccal and the lingual sides, only single molar forceps are necessary for the left and right in contradistinction to the maxilla, with which a right- and left-paired molar forceps set is required.

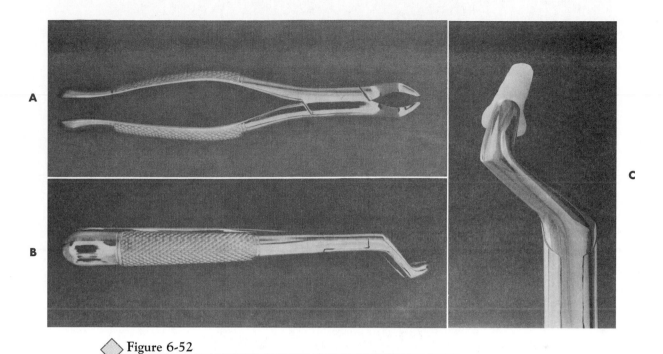

◇ **Figure 6-52**

A, Superior view of no. 210S forceps. **B,** Side view of no. 210S forceps. **C,** No. 210S adapted to maxillary molar.

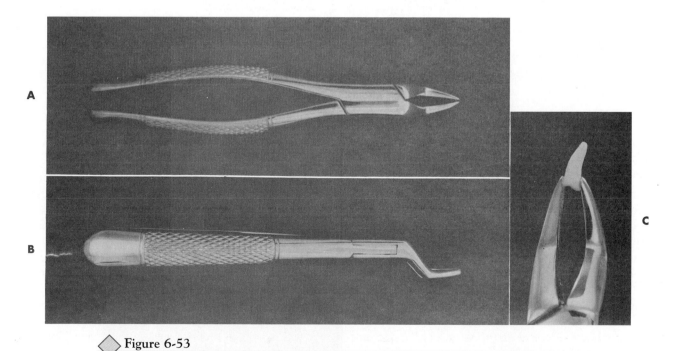

◇ **Figure 6-53**

A, Superior view of no. 286 forceps. **B,** Side view of no. 286 forceps. **C,** No. 286 adapted to broken root.

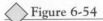 **Figure 6-54**

No. 150S *(bottom)* is smaller version of no. 150 forceps and is used for primary teeth.

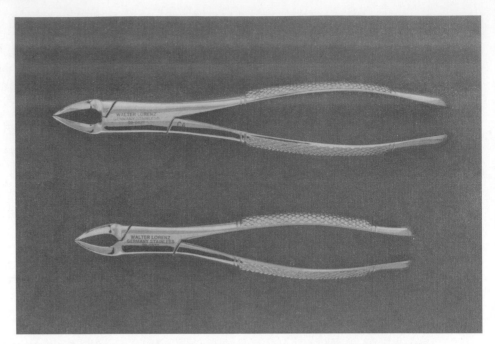

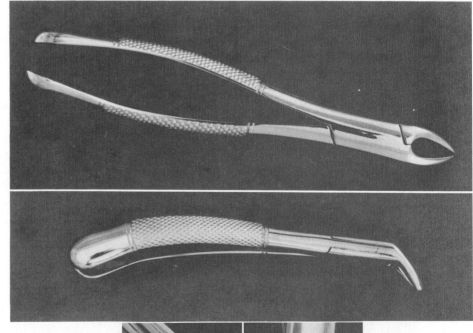

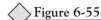 **Figure 6-55**

A, Superior view of no. 151 forceps. **B,** Side view of no. 151 forceps. **C** and **D,** No. 151 forceps adapted to mandibular incisor.

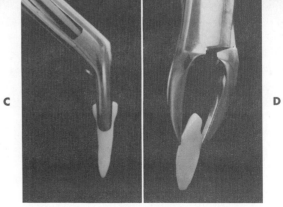

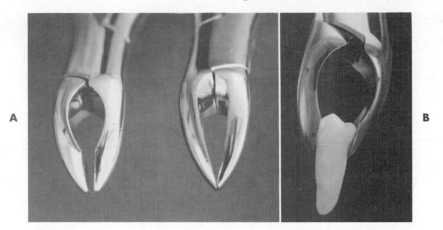

◇ **Figure 6-56**

A, No. 151A forceps have beaks that are parallel and do not adapt well to roots of most teeth. **B,** No. 151A forceps adapted to a lower premolar tooth. Note lack of close adaptation of tips of beak to root of tooth.

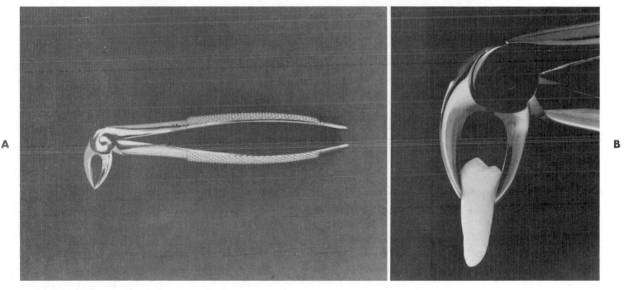

◇ **Figure 6-57**

A, Side view of English style of forceps. **B,** Forceps adapted to lower premolar.

The most useful lower molar forceps are the no. 17 (Figure 6-58). These forceps are usually straight-handled, and the beaks are set obliquely downward. The beaks have bilateral pointed tips in the center to adapt into the bifurcation of the molar teeth. The remainder of the beak adapts well to the bifurcation. Because of the pointed tips, the no. 17 forceps cannot be used for molar teeth, which have fused, conically shaped roots. For this purpose the no. 222 forceps are useful (Figure 6-59). They are similar in design to the no. 17, but the beaks are shorter and do not have pointed tips to prevent them from being used. The most common tooth for which the no. 222 is useful is the erupted mandibular third molar.

The major design variation in lower molar forceps is the no. 23, the so-called cowhorn forceps (Figure 6-60). These instruments are designed with two pointed heavy beaks that enter into the bifurcation of the lower molar. After the forceps are seated into the correct position, the tooth is elevated by squeezing the handles of the forceps together tightly. The beaks are squeezed into the bifurcation, using the buccal and lingual cortical plates as fulcrums, and the tooth is literally squeezed out of the socket. As with the English style of forceps, improper use of cowhorn forceps can result in an increase in the incidence of untoward effects, such as fractures of the alveolar bone. The beginning surgeon should use cowhorn forceps with caution.

The no. 151 is also adapted for primary teeth. The no. 151S

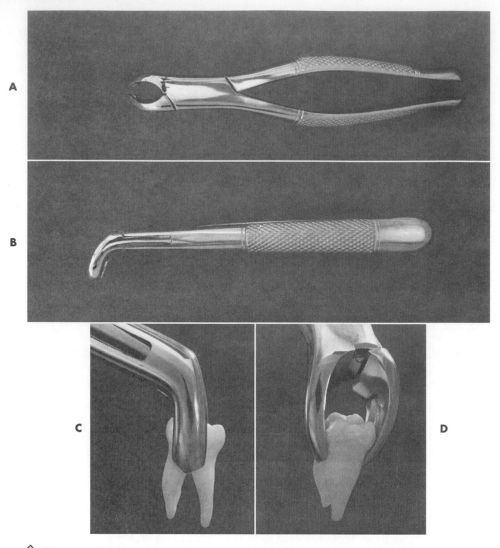

◇ **Figure 6-58**

A, Superior view of no. 17 molar forceps. **B,** Side view of no. 17 molar forceps. **C** and **D,** No. 17 forceps adapted to lower molar.

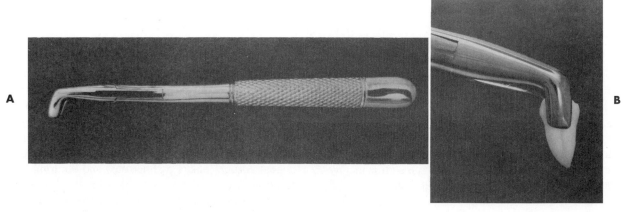

◇ **Figure 6-59**

A, Side view of no. 222 forceps. **B,** No. 222 forceps adapted to lower third molar.

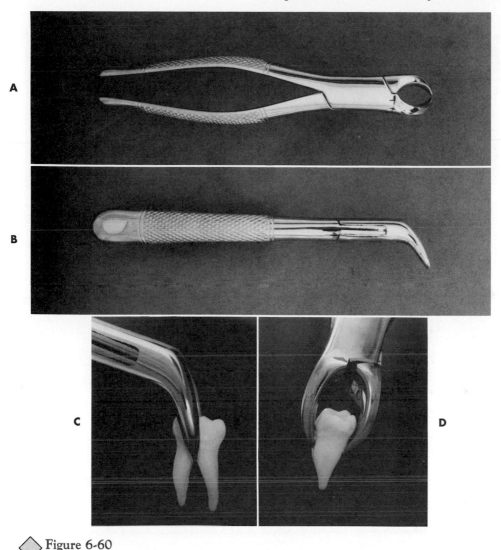

◇ Figure 6-60

A, Superior view of cowhorn forceps. **B,** Side view of cowhorn forceps. **C** and **D,** Cowhorn forceps adapted to lower molar tooth.

is the same general design as the no. 151 but is scaled down to adapt to the primary teeth. A single pair of forceps is adequate for removal of all primary mandibular teeth (Figure 6-61).

INSTRUMENT TRAY SYSTEMS ◇

Many surgeons find it practical to use the "tray" method to assemble instruments. Standard sets of instruments are packaged together, sterilized, and unwrapped at surgery. The typical basic extraction pack includes a local anesthesia syringe, a needle, a local anesthesia cartridge, a Woodson elevator, a periapical curette, a small and large straight elevator, a pair of college pliers, a curved hemostat, a towel

clip, an Austin retractor, a suction, and gauze (Figure 6-62). The required forceps would be added to this tray.

A tray used for surgical extractions would include the items from the basic extraction tray plus a needle holder and suture, a pair of suture scissors, a periosteal elevator, a blade handle and blade, Adson tissue forceps, a bone file, a tongue retractor, a root tip pick, Russian tissue forceps, a pair of Cryer elevators, a rongeur, and a handpiece and bur (Figure 6-63). These instruments permit incision and reflection of soft tissue, removal of bone, sectioning of teeth, retrieval of roots, debridement of the wound, and suturing of the soft tissue.

The biopsy tray includes the basic tray, plus a blade handle and blade, needle holder and suture, suture scissors, Metzenbaum scissors, Allis tissue forceps, Adson tissue forceps, and curved hemostat (Figure 6-64). These instru-

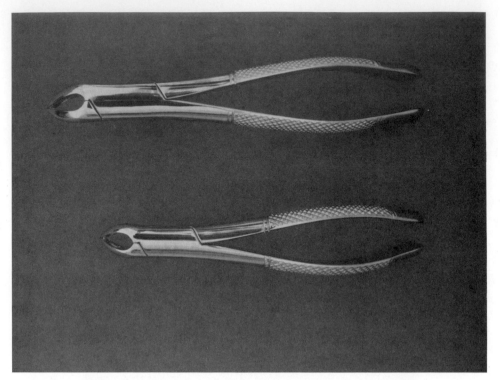

Figure 6-61

No. 151S *(bottom)* is smaller version of no. 151 and is used to extract primary teeth.

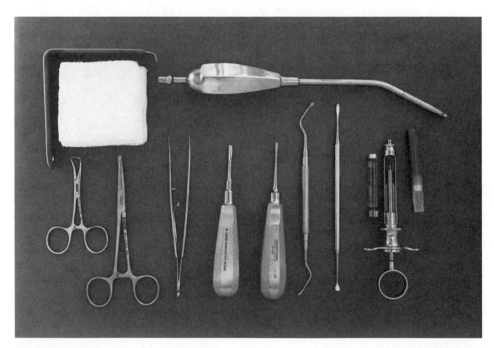

Figure 6-62

Typical basic extraction tray.

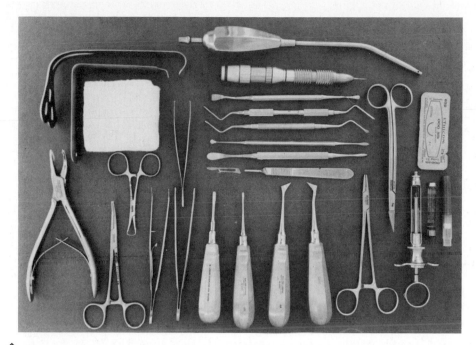

◈ **Figure 6-63**

Surgical extraction tray adds necessary instrumentation to reflect soft tissue flaps, remove bone, section teeth, retrieve roots, and suture flaps back into position.

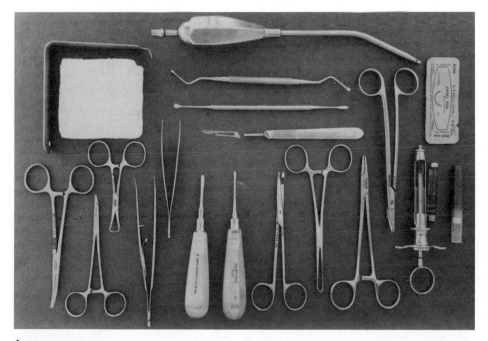

◈ **Figure 6-64**

Biopsy tray adds equipment necessary to remove soft tissue specimen and suture wound closed.

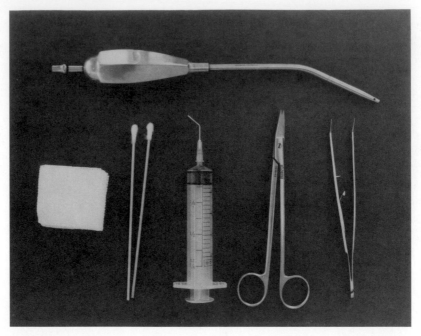

◇ **Figure 6-65**

Postoperative tray includes instruments necessary to remove sutures and irrigate mouth.

ments permit incision and dissection of a soft tissue specimen and closure of the wound with sutures.

The postoperative tray has the necessary instruments to irrigate the surgical site and remove sutures (Figure 6-65). It usually includes scissors, college pliers, irrigation syringe, applicator sticks, gauze, and suction.

The appendix includes prices for the instruments listed for these trays. A casual review of the cost of the surgical instruments will reflect why the surgeon and staff should make every effort to take good care of instruments.

BIBLIOGRAPHY

Findlay IA: The classification of dental elevators, *Br Dent J* 109:219, 1960.

Kandler HJ: The design and construction of dental elevators, *J Dent* 10:317, 1982.

Lilly GE et al: Reaction of oral tissues to suture materials, *Oral Surg* 28:432, 1969.

Macht SD, Krizek TJ: Sutures and suturing: current concepts, *J Oral Surg* 36:710, 1978.

CHAPTER

7

PRINCIPLES OF
UNCOMPLICATED EXODONTIA

LARRY J. PETERSON

CHAPTER OUTLINE ⸺◇

Extraction of teeth is a procedure that incorporates the principles of surgery and many principles from physics and mechanics. When these principles are applied correctly, a tooth can probably be removed intact from the alveolar process without untoward sequelae. This chapter presents the principles of surgery and mechanics for uncomplicated tooth extraction. In addition to a discussion of the fundamental underlying principles, there also is a detailed description of techniques for removal of specific teeth with specific instruments.

At the outset it is important to remember that removal of a tooth does not require a large amount of brute force but rather can be accomplished with finesse and controlled force in such a manner that the tooth is not pulled from the bone but instead is gently lifted from the alveolar process. During the preoperative period the degree of difficulty that is anticipated for removing a particular tooth is assessed. If the preoperative assessment leads the surgeon to believe that the degree of difficulty will be high and the initial attempts at tooth removal confirm this, a deliberate surgical approach—not an application of excessive force—should be taken. Excessive force may injure local tissues and destroy surrounding bone and teeth. Moreover, excessive force heightens the intraoperative discomfort and anxiety of the patient.

PAIN AND ANXIETY CONTROL

The removal of a tooth is a challenge to the dentist, because profound local anesthesia is required to prevent pain during the extraction, and control of the patient's anxiety is necessary to prevent psychologic distress. Local anesthesia must be absolutely profound to eliminate sensation from the pulp, periodontal ligament, and buccolingual soft tissues.

It is equally important for the dentist to recognize the anxiety that invariably exists in patients about to undergo tooth extraction. Few patients face this procedure with tran-

quility, and even patients with no overt signs of anxiety are likely to have internal feelings of distress.

LOCAL ANESTHESIA

Profound anesthesia is needed if the tooth is to be removed without pain for the patient; therefore it is essential that the surgeon remember the precise innervations of all teeth and surrounding soft tissue and the kinds of injection necessary to anesthetize those nerves totally. Tables 7-1 and 7-2 summarize the sensory innervation of the teeth and surrounding tissue and the recommended injections for extraction. It is important to remember that in areas of nerve transition there is almost always some overlap. For example, in the region of the mandibular second premolar, the buccal soft tissues are innervated primarily by the mental branch of the inferior alveolar nerve but also by terminal branches of the long buccal nerve. Therefore it may be necessary to supplement the inferior alveolar nerve block with a long buccal nerve block to achieve adequate anesthesia of the buccal soft tissue when extracting this particular tooth.

 Table 7-1. Sensory innervation of jaws

Nerve	Teeth	Soft tissue
Inferior alveolar nerve	All mandibular teeth	Buccal soft tissue of premolars, canine, and incisors
Lingual nerve	None	Lingual soft tissue of all teeth
Long buccal nerve	None	Buccal soft tissue of molars
Anterior superior alveolar nerve	Maxillary incisors and canine tooth	Buccal soft tissue of incisors and canine
Middle superior alveolar nerve	Maxillary premolars and portion of first molar tooth	Buccal soft tissue of premolars
Posterior superior alveolar nerve	Maxillary molars except for portion of first molar tooth	Buccal soft tissue of molars
Anterior palatine nerve	None	Lingual soft tissue of molars and premolars
Nasopalatine nerve	None	Lingual soft tissue of incisors and canine

Table 7-2. Recommended injections for extraction of specific teeth*

Tooth	Pulpal anesthetic	Buccal soft tissue	Lingual soft tissue
Maxilla			
Central incisor	Infiltration at apex	Infiltration	Nasopalatine nerve block
Lateral incisor	Infiltration at apex	Infiltration	Nasopalatine nerve block
Canine	Infiltration at apex	Infiltration	Nasopalatine nerve block
First premolar	Infiltration at apex	Infiltration	Anterior palatine nerve block
Second premolar	Infiltration at apex	Infiltration	Anterior palatine nerve block
First molar	Infiltration over mesial root *and* infiltration over second molar apex	Infiltration over mesial root *and* infiltration over second molar apex	Anterior palatine nerve block
Second molar	Infiltration at apex	Infiltration	Anterior palatine nerve block
Third molar	Infiltration at apex	Infiltration	Anterior palatine nerve block
Mandible			
Central incisor	Inferior alveolar nerve block	Inferior alveolar nerve block	Lingual nerve block
Lateral incisor	Inferior alveolar nerve block	Inferior alveolar nerve block	Lingual nerve block
Canine	Inferior alveolar nerve block	Inferior alveolar nerve block	Lingual nerve block
First premolar	Inferior alveolar nerve block	Inferior alveolar nerve block	Lingual nerve block
Second premolar	Inferior alveolar nerve block	Inferior alveolar nerve block	Lingual nerve block
First molar	Inferior alveolar nerve block	Long buccal nerve block	Lingual nerve block
Second molar	Inferior alveolar nerve block	Long buccal nerve block	Lingual nerve block
Third molar	Inferior alveolar nerve block	Long buccal nerve block	Lingual nerve block

*For teeth that border transitional areas innervated by two different nerves, additional infiltration injections may be required.

When anesthetizing a maxillary tooth for extraction, the surgeon should anesthetize the adjacent teeth, as well. During the extraction process the adjacent teeth are usually subjected to certain amounts of pressure, which may be sufficient to cause the patient pain. This is also true for mandibular extractions, but the mandibular-block anesthetic usually produces sufficient anesthesia.

Profound local anesthesia results in the loss of all pain, temperature, and touch sensations but does not anesthetize the proprioceptive fibers of the involved nerves. Thus the patient feels a sensation of pressure, especially when the force is intense. The surgeon must therefore remember that the patient will need to distinguish between sharp pain and the dull, albeit intense, feeling of pressure.

In spite of profound soft tissue anesthesia and apparent pulpal anesthesia, the patient may continue to have sharp pain as the tooth is luxated. This is especially likely when the teeth have a pulpitis or the surrounding soft and hard tissues are inflamed or infected. A technique that should be employed in these situations is the periodontal ligament injection. When this injection is delivered properly and the local anesthetic solution injected under pressure, there is immediate profound local anesthesia in almost all situations. The anesthesia is relatively short-lived, so the surgical procedure should be one that can be accomplished within 15 or 20 minutes.

It is important to keep in mind the pharmacology of the various local anesthetic solutions that are used, so that they can be employed properly. Table 7-3 summarizes the commonly used local anesthetics and the amount of time they can

be expected to provide profound anesthesia. The dentist must remember that pulpal anesthesia of maxillary teeth after local infiltration lasts a much shorter time than does pulpal anesthesia of mandibular teeth after block anesthesia. Also, pulpal anesthesia disappears 60 to 90 minutes before soft tissue anesthesia does. Therefore it is quite possible that a patient may still have lip anesthesia after having lost pulpal anesthesia and may be experiencing pain.

There are limits to how much local anesthetic can be safely used in a given patient. To provide profound anesthesia for multiple tooth extractions, it may be necessary to inject multiple cartridges of local anesthetic. Thus it is important to know how many cartridges of a given local anesthetic solution can be administered safely. Table 7-4 summarizes in two different ways the maximal amounts of local anesthetic that can be used. First, each local anesthetic has a recommended maximal dosage based on milligrams per kilogram. The second column in Table 7-4 is the number of cartridges that can safely be used on a healthy 70-kg adult. It is rarely necessary to exceed this dosage, even in patients larger than 70 kg. Patients who are smaller, especially children, should be given proportionally less local anesthetic. The most likely victim of overdose is the small child to whom 3% mepivacaine (Carbocaine) is administered. For a patient who weighs 20 kg, the recommended maximal amount of mepivacaine is 100 mg. If the child is given two cartridges of 1.8 mL each, the dose amounts to 108 mg. Therefore a third cartridge of 3% mepivacaine should be avoided. It is wise to remember that the smallest amount of local anesthetic solution sufficient to provide profound anesthesia is the proper amount.

SEDATION

Management of patient anxiety must be a major consideration in oral surgical procedures. Anxiety is a more important factor in oral surgical procedures than in other areas of dentistry. Patients are frequently already in pain and may be agitated and fatigued, both of which lower the patient's ability to deal with pain or pain-producing situations. Patients who are to have extractions may have predetermined concepts of how painful such a procedure will be; they have seen other patients, including family members, who have reported how painful it is to have a tooth extraction. They are thus convinced that the procedure they are about to undergo will be uncomfortable. There are also potential psychologic complications when surgical procedures are being performed. The removal of teeth

◇ **Table 7-3.** Duration of anesthesia

Local anesthetic	Maxillary teeth	Mandibular teeth	Soft tissue
Group 1*	10-20 min	40-60 min	2-3 hr
Group 2†	50-60 min	90-100 min	3-4 hr
Group 3‡	1½ hr	3 hr	4-9 hr

*Group 1: Local anesthetics without vasoconstrictors
   Mepivacaine 3%
   Prilocaine 4%
†Group 2: Local anesthetics with vasoconstrictors
   Lidocaine   2% with 1:50,000 or 1:100,000 epinephrine
   Mepivacaine 2% with 1:20,000 levonordephrine
   Prilocaine   4% with 1:400,000 epinephrine
†Group 3: Long-acting local anesthetics
   Bupivacaine   0.5% with 1:200,000 epinephrine
   Etidocaine   1.5% with 1:200,000 epinephrine

◇ **Table 7-4.** Recommended maximal local anesthetic doses

Drug/solution	Maximal number of mg/kg	Number of cartridges for 70 kg (154 lb)—adult	Number of cartridges for 20 kg (44 lb)—child
Lidocaine 2% with 1:100,000 epinephrine	5	10	3
Mepivacaine 2% with 1:20,000 levonordephrine	5	10	3
Mepivacaine 3% (no vasoconstrictor)	5	6	2
Prilocaine 4% with 1:200,000 epinephrine	5	6	2
Bupivacaine 0.5% with 1:200,000 epinephrine	1.5	10	3
Etidocaine 1.5% with 1:200,000 epinephrine	8	15	5

causes a variety of reactions; a patient may mourn for lost body parts or perceive the extraction as a confirmation that youth has passed. In such situations, patients would like to avoid the extraction, and, because they cannot, they become doubly agitated.

Finally, anxiety is likely to be higher because the procedure is truly uncomfortable. As noted before, although the sharp pain is eliminated by local anesthetic, there is still a considerable amount of pressure sensation. Other noxious stimuli are present during an extraction procedure, such as the cracking of bone and clicking of instruments. For these reasons, prudent dentists use a prospective planned method of anxiety control to prepare themselves and their patients for the anxiety associated with tooth extraction.

Anxiety control may sometimes consist of a proper explanation of the planned procedure, including assurance that there will be no sharp pain and an expression of concern, caring, and empathy from the dentist. For the mildly anxious patient with a caring dentist, no pharmacologic assistance is necessary.

As patient anxiety increases, it becomes necessary to employ pharmacologic assistance. Fundamental to all anxiety-control techniques is a thorough explanation of the procedure and an expression of concern. These are augmented with drugs given in a variety of ways. Preoperative orally administered drugs, such as diazepam, may provide a patient with rest the night before the surgery and some relief of anxiety in the morning. However, orally administered drugs are usually not profound enough to control moderate-to-severe anxiety once the patient enters the operative suite.

Sedation by inhalation of nitrous oxide and oxygen is frequently the technique of choice and may be the sole technique required for many patients who have mild-to-moderate anxiety. If the dentist is skilled in the use of nitrous oxide and the patient requires a routine, uncomplicated surgical procedure, nitrous oxide sedation is frequently sufficient.

An extremely anxious patient who is to have several uncomplicated extractions may require parenteral sedation, usually by the intravenous route. Intravenous sedation with anxiolytic drugs, such as diazepam or midazolam with or without a narcotic, allows patients with moderate anxiety to undergo surgical procedures with minimal psychologic stress. If the dentist is not skilled at using this modality, the patient should be referred to a dentist or oral surgeon who can provide it.

Further discussion of the techniques of oral, inhalation, or intravenous sedation is beyond the scope of this text.

Presurgical Medical Assessment ⬦

When evaluating a patient preoperatively, it is critical that the surgeon examine the patient's medical status. Patients may have a variety of maladies that require treatment modification before the required surgery can be performed safely. Special measures may be needed to control bleeding, prevent infection, and prevent worsening of the patient's preexisting disease state. This information is discussed in detail in Chapter 1. The reader should refer to that chapter for information regarding the specifics of altering treatment for medical management reasons.

Indications for Removal of Teeth ⬦

Teeth are removed from the mouth for a variety of reasons. Although the position of modern dentistry is that all possible measures should be taken to preserve and maintain teeth in the oral cavity, it is still necessary to remove some of them. This section discusses a variety of general indications for removing teeth. It must be remembered that these indications are recommendations and not absolute rules.

Severe Caries

Perhaps the most common and widely accepted reason to remove a tooth is that it is so severely carious that it cannot be restored. The extent to which the tooth is carious and is judged to be nonrestorable is a judgment call to be made between the dentist and the patient.

Pulpal Necrosis

A second, closely aligned rationale for removing a tooth is the presence of pulp necrosis or irreversible pulpitis that is not amenable to endodontics. This may be the result of a patient declining endodontic treatment or of a root canal that is tortuous, calcified, and untreatable by standard endodontic techniques. Also included in this general indication category is the endodontic failure. In this situation, endodontic treatment has been done but has failed to relieve pain or provide drainage.

Severe Periodontal Disease

A common reason for tooth removal is severe and extensive periodontal disease. If severe adult periodontitis has existed for some time, there is excessive bone loss and irreversible tooth mobility. In these situations the hypermobile teeth should be extracted.

Orthodontic Reasons

Patients who are about to undergo orthodontic correction of crowded dentition frequently require the extraction of teeth to provide space for tooth alignment. The most commonly extracted teeth are the maxillary and mandibular first premolars, but second premolars or a mandibular incisor may occasionally require extraction for this same reason.

Malopposed Teeth

Teeth that are malopposed or malpositioned may be indicated for removal in several situations. If they traumatize soft tissue and cannot be repositioned by orthodontic treatment, they should be extracted. A common example of this is the maxillary third molar, which erupts in severe buccal version and causes ulceration and soft tissue trauma in the cheek. Another example is malopposed teeth that are hypererupted because of the loss of teeth in the opposing arch. If prosthetic rehabilitation is to be carried out in the opposing arch, the hypererupted teeth may interfere with construction of an adequate prosthesis. In this situation the malopposed teeth should be considered for extraction.

CRACKED TEETH

A clear but uncommon indication for extraction of teeth is a tooth that is cracked or has a fractured root. The cracked tooth can be painful and is unmanageable by a more conservative technique. Even endodontic and complex restorative procedures cannot relieve the pain of a cracked tooth.

PREPROSTHETIC EXTRACTIONS

Teeth occasionally interfere with the design and proper placement of prosthetic appliances, that is, full dentures, partial dentures, or fixed partial dentures. When this happens, preprosthetic extractions are necessary.

IMPACTED TEETH

Impacted teeth should be considered for removal. If it is clear that a partially impacted tooth is unable to erupt into a functional occlusion because of inadequate space, interference from adjacent teeth, or some other reason, it should be scheduled for surgical removal. If there are contraindications for removing the impacted tooth, such as medical compromise, full bony impaction in a patient who is over the age of 35, or advanced age, then the tooth may be retained. See Chapter 9 for a more thorough discussion of this topic.

SUPERNUMERARY TEETH

Supernumerary teeth are usually impacted and should be removed. A supernumerary tooth may interfere with eruption of succedaneous teeth and has the potential for causing their resorption and displacement.

TEETH ASSOCIATED WITH PATHOLOGIC LESIONS

Teeth that are involved in pathologic lesions may require removal. In some situations the teeth can be retained and endodontic therapy performed. However, if maintaining the tooth compromises the complete surgical removal of the lesion, the tooth should be removed.

PRERADIATION THERAPY

Patients who are to receive radiation therapy for a variety of oral tumors should have serious consideration given to removing teeth in the line of radiation therapy. See Chapter 19 for a more thorough discussion of the effects of radiation therapy on the teeth and jaws.

TEETH INVOLVED IN JAW FRACTURES

Patients who sustain fractures of the mandible or the alveolar process occasionally must have teeth removed. In a majority of situations the tooth involved in the line of fracture can be maintained, but if the tooth is injured or severely luxated from the surrounding bony tissue, its removal may be necessary to prevent infection.

ESTHETICS

Occasionally a patient requires removal of teeth for esthetic reasons. In these situations teeth may be severely stained, as with tetracycline staining or fluorosis, or they may be severely malopposed and usually protruding. Although other techniques, such as bonding, can be employed to relieve the staining problem, and orthodontic or osteotomy procedures can be used to correct severe protrusion, the patient may choose to have extraction and prosthetic reconstruction.

ECONOMICS

A final indication for removal of teeth is economic. All of the indications for extraction already mentioned may become stronger if the patient is unwilling or unable financially to support the decision to maintain the tooth. The inability of the patient either to pay for the procedure or to take enough time from work to allow it to be performed may require that the tooth be removed.

CONTRAINDICATIONS FOR THE REMOVAL OF TEETH

Even if a given tooth meets one of the requirements for removal, in some situations the tooth should not be removed because of other factors or contraindications to extraction. These factors, like the indications, are relative in their strength. In some situations the contraindication can be modified by the use of additional care or treatment, and the indicated extraction can be performed. In other situations, however, the contraindication may be so significant that the tooth should not be removed until the severity of the problem has been resolved. Generally, the contraindications are divided into the two groups of systemic contraindications and local contraindications.

SYSTEMIC CONTRAINDICATIONS

Systemic contraindications preclude extraction because the patient's systemic health is such that the ability to withstand the surgical insult may be compromised (see Chapter 1). One systemic contraindication is a group of diseases called *severe uncontrolled metabolic disease*. Brittle diabetes and end-stage renal disease with severe uremia are part of this group. Patients with mild diabetes or well-controlled severe diabetes can be treated as reasonably normal patients. It is only when the disease process becomes uncontrolled that the patient should not have a tooth removed.

Patients who have uncontrolled leukemias and lymphomas should not have teeth removed until the leukemias can be brought under control. The potential complications are infection as a result of nonfunctioning white cells and excessive bleeding as a result of an inadequate number of platelets. Patients with any of a variety of severe uncontrolled cardiac diseases should also have their extractions deferred until the disease can be brought under control. Patients with severe myocardial ischemia, such as unstable angina pectoris, and patients who have had a recent myocardial infarction should not have a tooth extracted. Patients who have severe uncontrolled hypertension should also have extractions deferred, because persistent bleeding, acute myocardial insufficiency, and cerebrovascular accidents are more likely to occur as a result of stress caused by the extraction. Patients who have severe, uncontrolled cardiac dysrhythmias should have their extraction procedures deferred as well.

Pregnancy is a relative contraindication; patients who are in the first or last trimester should have their extractions deferred if possible. The latter part of the first trimester and the first month of the last trimester may be as safe as the middle trimester for a simple uncomplicated extraction, but more extensive surgical procedures should be deferred until after the child has been delivered.

Patients who have a severe bleeding diathesis, such as hemophilia, or severe platelet disorders should not have teeth extracted until the coagulopathy has been corrected. Most severe bleeding disorders can be controlled by the administration of coagulation factors or platelet transfusions. Close coordination with the patient's hematologist can result in an uncomplicated recovery from the extraction procedure in most situations. Similarly, patients who take anticoagulants can have routine extractions performed when care is taken to manage the patient appropriately.

Finally, patients who take or have taken a variety of medications should have surgery performed with caution. Drugs to watch for include corticosteroids, immunosuppressives, and cancer chemotherapeutic agents.

Local Contraindications

There are several local contraindications to extractions of indicated teeth. The most important and most critical is a history of therapeutic radiation for cancer. Extractions performed in an area of radiation may result in osteoradionecrosis and therefore must be done with extreme caution. Chapter 19 discusses this in detail.

Teeth that are located within an area of tumor, especially a malignant tumor, should not be extracted. The surgical procedure for extraction could disseminate cells and thereby hasten the metastatic process.

Patients who have severe pericoronitis around an impacted mandibular third molar should not have the tooth extracted until the pericoronitis has been treated. Nonsurgical treatment should include irrigations, antibiotics, and removal of the maxillary third molar to relieve impingement on the edematous soft tissue overlying the mandibular impaction. If the mandibular third molar is removed in the face of severe pericoronitis, the incidence of postoperative infection, which is potentially life threatening, increases. If the pericoronitis is mild and the tooth can be removed without a surgical flap or

bone removal, then immediate extraction may be performed. However, if flap reflection and bone surgery are required, the infection should be controlled first.

Finally, the acute dentoalveolar abscess must be mentioned. It is abundantly clear from many prospective studies that the most rapid resolution of an infection secondary to pulpal necrosis is obtained when the tooth is removed as early as possible. Therefore acute infection is not a contraindication to extraction. However, it may be difficult to extract such a tooth because the patient may not be able to open his or her mouth sufficiently wide, or it may be difficult to reach a state of adequate local anesthesia. If access and anesthesia considerations can be met, the tooth should be removed as early as possible.

Clinical Evaluation of Teeth for Removal ⟶◇

In the preoperative assessment period the tooth to be extracted should be examined carefully to assess the difficulty of the extraction. A variety of factors must be specifically examined to make the appropriate assessment.

Access to Tooth

The first factor to be exaimined in preoperative assessment is the extent to which the patient can open his or her mouth. Any limitation of opening may compromise the ability of the surgeon to do a routine uncomplicated extraction. If the patient's opening is substantially compromised, the surgeon should plan for a surgical approach to the tooth instead of a forceps extraction. Additionally, the surgeon should look for the cause of the reduction of opening. The most likely causes are trismus associated with infection, temporomandibular joint dysfunction (especially internal joint derangement with displacement of the disk without reduction), and muscle fibrosis.

The location and position of the tooth to be extracted within a dental arch should be examined. A properly aligned tooth has a normal access for placement of elevators and forceps. However, crowded or otherwise malopposed teeth may present difficulty in positioning the proper forceps onto the tooth for extraction. When access is a problem, a compromise forceps must be chosen, or a surgical approach may be indicated.

Mobility of Tooth

The mobility of the tooth to be extracted should be assessed preoperatively. Greater-than-normal mobility is frequently seen with severe periodontal disease. If the teeth are excessively mobile, an uncomplicated tooth removal should be expected, and there should be more involved and complicated soft tissue management after the extraction (Figure 7-1, *A*).

Teeth that have less-than-normal mobility should be carefully assessed for the presence of hypercementosis or ankylosis of the roots. Ankylosis is often seen with primary

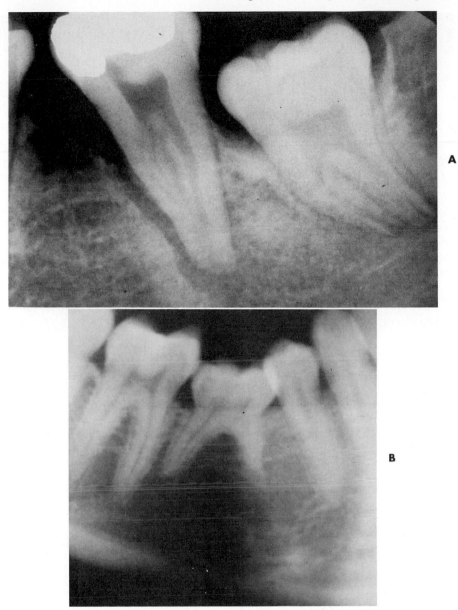

◇ Figure 7-1

A, Tooth with severe periodontal disease with bone loss and wide periodontal ligament space. This kind of tooth is easy to remove. **B,** Retained mandibular second primary molar with an absent succedaneous tooth. It is submerged, and likelihood for ankylosed roots is high.

molars that are retained and have become submerged (Figure 7-1, *B*) and is also seen occasionally in nonvital teeth that have had endodontic therapy many years before the extraction. If the tooth is thought to be ankylosed, it is wise to plan for a surgical removal of the tooth as opposed to a forceps extraction.

CONDITION OF THE CROWN

The assessment of the crown of the tooth before the extraction should be related to the presence of large caries or restorations in the crown. If large portions of the crown have been destroyed by caries, there is increased likelihood of crushing the crown during the extraction and thus more difficulty in removing the tooth (Figure 7-2). Similarly, the presence of large amalgam restorations will produce a weakness in the crown, and the restoration will probably fracture during the extraction process (Figure 7-3). In these two situations it is critical that the forceps be applied as far apically as possible so as to grasp the root portion of the tooth instead of the crown.

If the tooth to be extracted has a large accumulation of calculus, the gross accumulation should be removed with a scaler or ultrasonic cleaner before extraction. The reasons for this are that calculus interferes with the placement of the forceps in the appropriate fashion, and fractured calculus

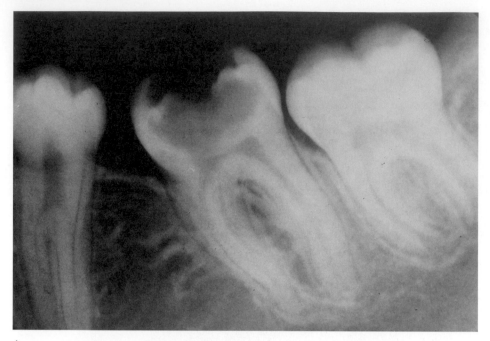

◇ **Figure 7-2**

Teeth with large carious lesions are likely to fracture during extraction, which makes extraction more difficult.

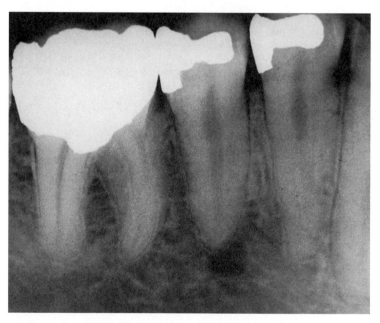

◇ **Figure 7-3**

Teeth with large amalgam restorations. These are likely to be fragile and to fracture when extraction forces are applied.

may contaminate the empty tooth socket once the tooth is extracted.

The surgeon should also assess the condition of the adjacent teeth. If the adjacent teeth have large amalgams or crowns or have had root canal therapy, it is important to keep this in mind when elevators and forceps are used to mobilize and remove the indicated tooth. If the adjacent teeth have large restorations, the surgeon should use elevators with extreme caution, because fracture of the restorations may occur (Figure 7-4). The patient should be informed before the surgical procedure about possible damage to these restorations.

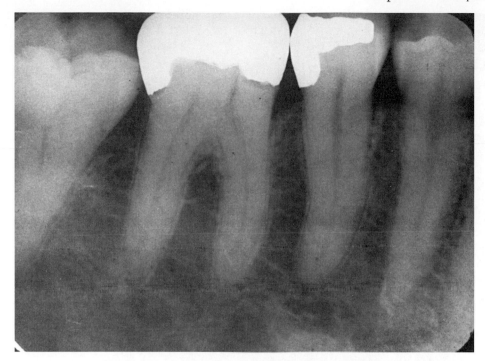

◇ **Figure 7-4**

Mandibular first molar. If it is to be removed, surgeon must take care not to fracture amalgam in second premolar with elevators or forceps.

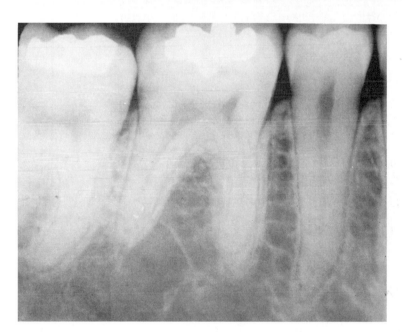

◇ **Figure 7-5**

Properly exposed radiographs for extraction of mandibular first molar.

RADIOGRAPHIC EXAMINATION OF TOOTH FOR REMOVAL ◇

It is essential that proper radiographs be taken of the tooth to be removed. In general, periapical radiographs provide the most accurate and detailed information concerning the tooth, its roots, and the surrounding tissue. Panoramic radiographs are used frequently, but their greatest usefulness is for impacted teeth as opposed to erupted teeth.

For radiographs to have their maximal value they must meet certain criteria. First of all, they must be properly exposed, with adequate penetration and good contrast. The radiographic film should have been properly positioned, so that it shows all portions of the crown and roots of the tooth under consideration without distortion (Figure 7-5). The radiograph must be properly processed, with good fixation, drying, and mounting. The mounting should be labeled with the patient's name and the date on which the film was exposed. The radiograph should be mounted in the American Dental Association standardized method, which is to view the radiograph as if you are looking at the patient; the raised dot on the film faces the observer. Finally, the radiograph must be

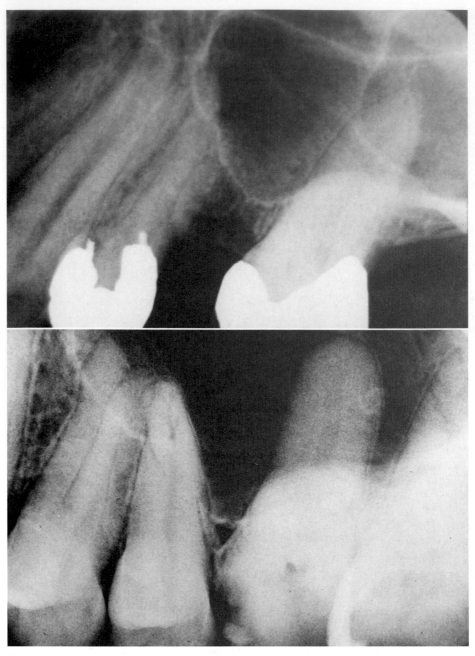

◇ **Figure 7-6**

Maxillary molar teeth immediately adjacent to sinus present increased danger of sinus exposure.

mounted on a view box that is visible to the surgeon during the operation. Radiographs that are taken but not available during surgery are of no value.

The relationship of the tooth to be extracted to adjacent erupted and unerupted teeth should be noted. If it is a primary tooth, the relationship of its roots to the underlying succedaneous tooth should be carefully noted. It is possible that the extraction of the primary teeth can injure or dislodge the underlying tooth. If surgical removal of a root or part of a root is necessary, the relationship of the root structures of adjacent teeth must be known. Bone removal should be

performed judiciously whenever it is necessary, but it is particularly important to be careful if adjacent roots are close to the root being removed.

Relationship of Associated Vital Structures

When performing extractions of the maxillary molars, it is essential to be aware of the proximity of the molar's roots to the floor of the maxillary sinus. If there is only a thin layer of bone between the sinus and the roots of the molar teeth, there is increased potential for perforation of the maxillary sinus

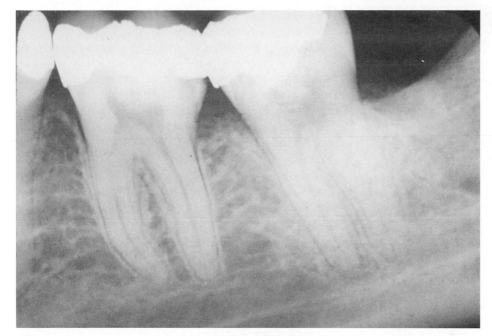

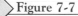 Figure 7-7

Mandibular molar teeth that are close to inferior alveolar canal. Third molar removal is procedure most likely to result in injury to nerve.

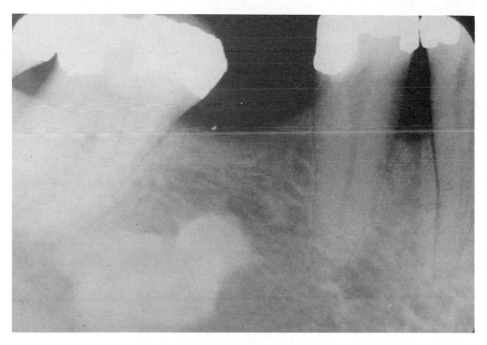

Figure 7-8

Before premolar extractions that require a surgical flap are performed, it is essential to know relationship of mental foramen to root apices. Note radiolucent area at apex of second premolar, which represents mental foramen.

during the extraction. Thus the surgical treatment plan may be altered to an open surgical technique, with division of the maxillary molar roots into individual roots before the extraction proceeds (Figure 7-6).

The inferior alveolar canal may approximate the roots of the mandibular molars. Although the removal of an erupted tooth rarely impinges on the inferior alveolar canal, if an impacted tooth is to be removed, it is important that the relationship between the molar roots and the canal be assessed. Such an extraction may lead to injury to the canal and cause consequent anesthesia of the inferior alveolar nerve (Figure 7-7).

A periapical radiograph taken before the removal of mandibular premolar teeth should include the mental foramen.

Should a surgical flap be required to retrieve a premolar root, it is essential that the surgeon know where the mental foramen is to avoid injuring the mental nerve during flap development (Figures 7-3 and 7-8).

CONFIGURATION OF ROOTS

Radiographic assessment of the tooth to be extracted probably contributes most to the determination of difficulty of the extraction. The first factor to evaluate is the number of roots on the tooth to be extracted. Most teeth have the typical number of roots, in which case the surgical plan can be carried out in the usual fashion, but many teeth do have an abnormal number of roots. If the number of roots is known before the

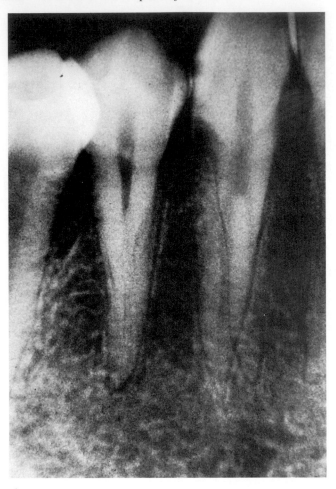

◇ **Figure 7-9**

Mandibular canine tooth with two roots. Knowledge of this fact preoperatively may result in less traumatic extraction.

tooth is extracted, an alteration in the plan can be made to prevent fracture of the additional roots (Figure 7-9).

The surgeon must know both the curvature of the roots and the degree of root divergence to plan the extraction procedure. Roots of the usual number and of average size may still diverge substantially and thus make the total root width so wide that it prevents extraction with normal forceps. In situations of excess curvature with wide divergence, surgical extraction may be required (Figure 7-10).

The shape of the individual root must be taken into consideration. Roots may have short, conical shapes that make them very easy to remove. However, long roots with severe and abrupt curves or hooks at their apical end are more difficult to remove. The surgeon must have knowledge of the roots' shapes before surgery to allow an adequate plan to be made (Figure 7-11).

The size of the root must be assessed. Teeth with short roots are easier to remove than teeth with long roots. A long root that is bulbous as a result of hypercementosis is even more difficult to remove. The periapical radiographs of older patients should be examined carefully for evidence of hypercementosis, because this process seems to be a result of aging (Figure 7-12).

The surgeon should look for evidence of caries extending into the roots. Root caries may substantially weaken the root and make it more liable to fracture when the force of the forceps is applied (Figure 7-13).

Root resorption, either internal or external, should be assessed on examination of the radiograph. Like root caries, root resorption weakens the root structure and renders it more likely to be fractured. Surgical extraction may be considered in situations of extensive root resorption (Figure 7-14).

The tooth should be evaluated for previous endodontic

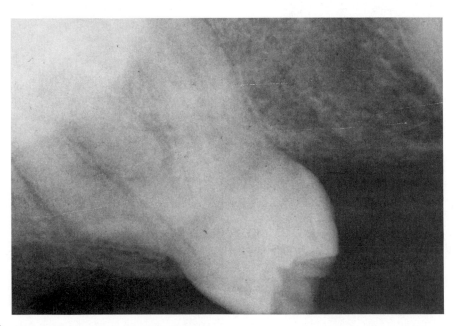

◇ **Figure 7-10**

Widely divergent roots of this maxillary first molar make extraction more difficult.

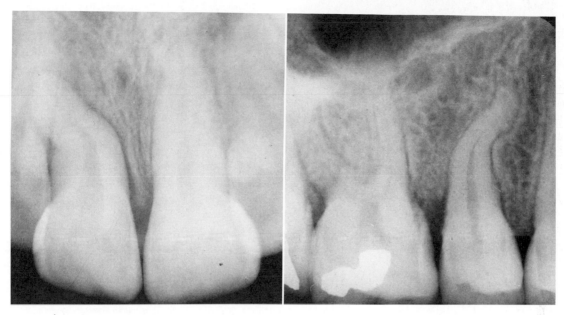

◇ Figure 7-11

Curvature of roots of these two teeth is unexpected. Preoperative radiographs allow surgeon to plan extraction more carefully.

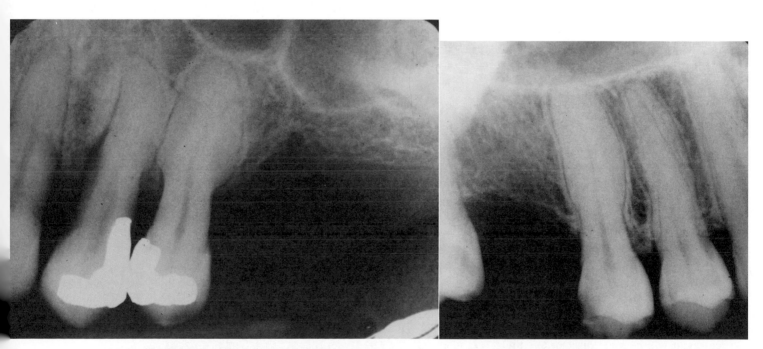

◇ Figure 7-12

Hypercementosis increases difficulty of these extractions, because roots are larger at apical end than at cervical end. Surgical extraction will probably be required.

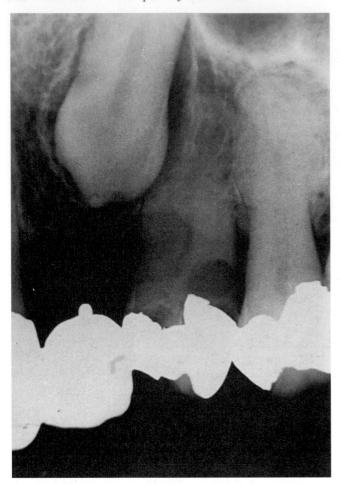

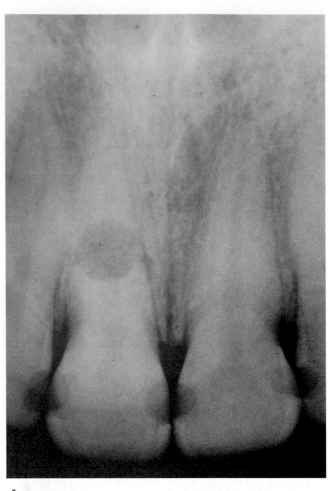

◇ **Figure 7-13**

Root caries in first premolar tooth make extraction more difficult, because fracture of tooth is likely. Note hypercementosis of second premolar.

◇ **Figure 7-14**

Internal resorption of root makes closed extraction almost impossible, because fracture of root will almost surely occur.

therapy. If there was endodontic therapy many years before the extraction process, there may be ankylosis or the tooth root may be more brittle. In both of these situations, surgical extraction may be indicated (Figure 7-15).

CONDITION OF SURROUNDING BONE

Careful examination of the periapical radiograph indicates the density of the bone surrounding the tooth to be extracted. Bone that is more radiolucent is likely to be less dense, which makes the extraction easier. On the other hand, if the bone appears to be radiographically opaque (indicating increased density) with evidence of condensing osteitis or other sclerosis-like processes, it will be more difficult to extract.

The surrounding bone should also be examined carefully for evidence of apical pathology. Teeth that have nonvital pulps may have periapical radiolucencies that represent granulomas or cysts. It is important to be aware of the presence of such lesions, because they should be removed at the time of surgery (Figure 7-16).

SUMMARY

Presurgical assessment of the patient includes evaluation of the level of anxiety, determination of health status and any necessary modifications of routine procedures, evaluation of the clinical presentation of the tooth to be removed, and radiographic evaluation of the tooth root and bone. All four of these major factors must be weighed when estimating the difficulty of the extraction. If any factor or combination of factors presents a level of difficulty that seems too great, the dentist should refer the patient to an oral and maxillofacial surgeon.

PATIENT AND SURGEON PREPARATION ◇

Surgeons must prevent inadvertent injury or transmission of infection to their patients or to themselves. The concept of universal precautions states that all patients must be viewed as

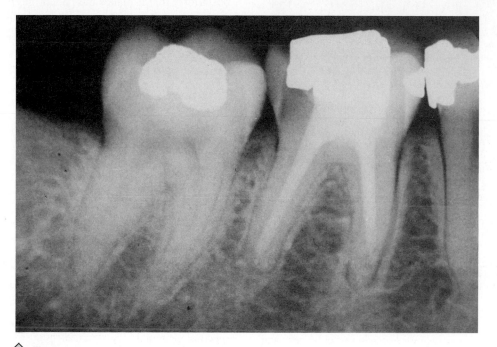

◇ Figure 7-15

Tooth made brittle by previous endodontic therapy. It is thus more difficult to remove.

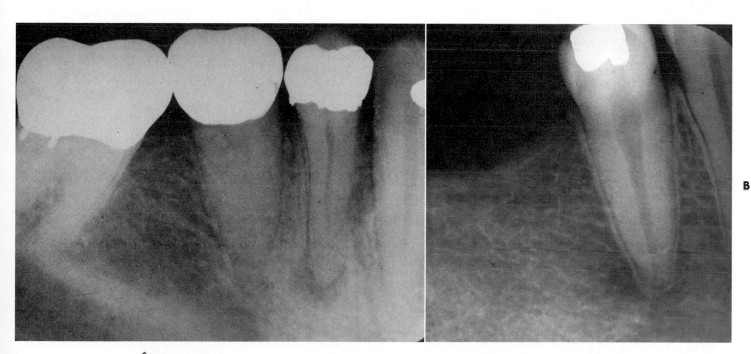

◇ Figure 7-16

A, Periapical radiolucency. Surgeon must be aware of this before extraction so that proper management can be delivered. **B,** Periapical radiolucency around mandibular premolar represents mental foramen. Surgeon must be aware that this is not pathologic condition. Note intact lamina dura is in **B** but not in **A.**

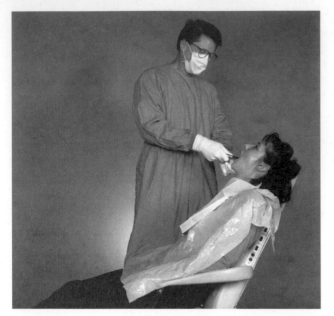

◇ **Figure 7-17**

Surgeon, prepared by wearing protective eyeglasses, mask, and gloves. Surgeons should have short or pinned-back hair and should wear long-sleeved smocks that are changed daily or sooner if they become soiled. Patient should have full, waterproof drape.

having blood-borne diseases that can be transmitted to the surgical team. To prevent this transmission, surgical gloves, surgical mask, and eyewear with side shields are required. (See Chapter 5 for a detailed discussion of this topic.) Additionally, most authorities recommend that the surgical team wear long-sleeve gowns that can be changed when they become visible soiled (Figure 7-17).

If the surgeon has long hair, it is essential that the hair be held in position with barrettes or other holding devices or be covered with a surgical cap. It is a major breach in aseptic technique to allow the surgeon's hair to hang over the patient's face and mouth (Figure 7-18).

Before the patient undergoes the surgical procedure, a minimal amount of draping is necessary. A sterile drape should be put across the patient's chest to decrease the risk of contamination (Figure 7-17). A head drape with either a hair-covering cap or a towel is also recommended.

Before the extraction, patients should vigorously rinse their mouths with an antiseptic mouth rinse, such as chlorhexidine. This reduces the gross bacterial contamination in the patient's mouth, which helps to reduce the incidence of postoperative infection.

To prevent teeth or fragments of teeth from falling into the mouth and potentially being swallowed or aspirated into the lungs, many surgeons prefer to place a 4 × 4-inch gauze loosely into the back of the mouth (Figure 7-19). This oral partition serves as a barrier so that should a tooth slip from the forceps or shatter under the pressure of the forceps, it will be caught in the gauze rather than be swallowed or aspirated. The surgeon must take care that the gauze is not positioned so far

posteriorly that it makes the patient gag. The surgeon should explain the purpose of the partition, to gain the patient's acceptance and cooperation for allowing the gauze to be placed.

CHAIR POSITION FOR FORCEPS EXTRACTION ────────────◇

The position of the patient, chair, and operator is critical for successful completion of the extraction. The best position is one that is comfortable for both the patient and surgeon and allows the surgeon to have maximal control of the force that is being delivered to the patient's tooth through the forceps. The correct position allows the surgeon to keep the arms close to the body and provides stability and support; it also allows the surgeon to keep the wrists straight enough to deliver the force with the arm and shoulder and not with the hand. The force delivered can thus be controlled in the face of sudden loss of resistance from a root or bone fracture.

Dentists usually stand during extractions, so the positions for a standing surgeon will be described first. Modifications that are necessary to operate in a seated position will be presented later.

For a maxillary extraction the chair should be tipped backward so that the maxillary occlusal plane is at an angle of about 60 degrees to the floor. The height of the chair should be such that the height of the patient's mouth is at or slightly below the operator's elbow level (Figure 7-20). During an operation on the maxillary right quadrant, the patient's head should be turned substantially toward the operator, so that adequate access and visualization can be achieved (Figure 7-21). For extraction of teeth in the maxillary anterior portion of the arch, the patient should be looking straight ahead (Figure 7-22). The position for the maxillary left portion of the arch is similar, except that the patient's head is turned slightly toward the operator (Figure 7-23).

For the extraction of mandibular teeth the patient should be positioned in a more upright position, so that when the mouth is opened widely, the occlusal plane is parallel to the floor. A bite block should be used to stabilize the mandible when the extraction forceps is used. Even though the surgeon will support the jaw, the additional support provided by the bite block will result in less stress being transmitted to the jaws. The chair should be lower than for extraction of maxillary teeth, and the surgeon's arm is inclined downward to approximately a 120-degree angle at the elbow (Figure 7-24), which provides a comfortable, stable position that is more controllable than the higher position. During removal of the mandibular right posterior teeth the patient's head should be turned severely toward the surgeon to allow adequate access to the jaw, and the surgeon should maintain the proper arm and hand position (Figure 7-25). When removing teeth in the anterior region of the mandible, the surgeon should rotate around to the side of the patient (Figures 7-26 and 7-27). When operating on the left posterior mandibular region, the surgeon should stand in front of the patient, but the patient's head should not turn quite so severely toward the surgeon (Figure 7-28).

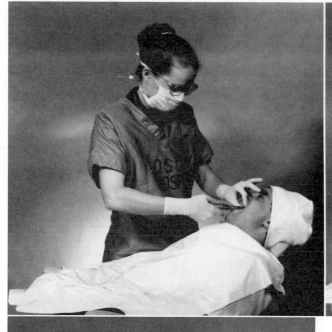

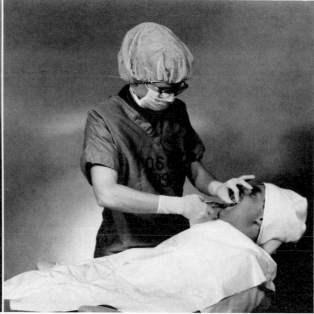

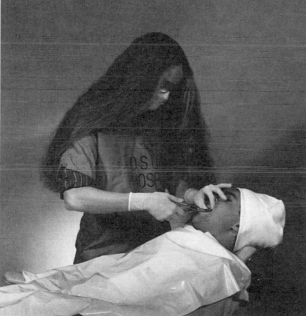

◇ Figure 7-18

A, If dentist's hair is long, it should be tied so that it stays in place and does not drape into surgical field. **B**, As alternative, dentist's hair can be placed under surgical cap. **C**, Long and uncontrolled hair that drapes into surgical field is unacceptable.

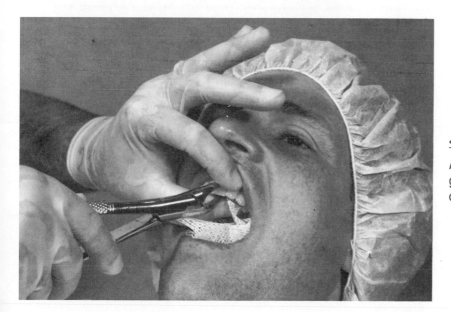

◇ Figure 7-19

A gauze partition can be placed in the mouth to help guard against loss of tooth or tooth fragments into the oral pharynx.

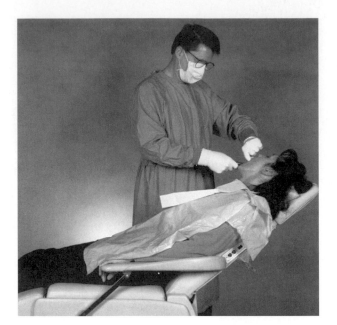

Figure 7-20

Patient positioned for maxillary extraction: tilted back so that maxillary occlusal plane is at about 60-degree angle to floor. Height of chair should put patient's mouth slightly below surgeon's elbow.

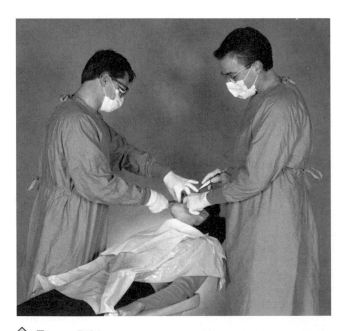

Figure 7-21

Extraction of teeth in maxillary right quadrant. Note that surgeon turns patient's head toward self.

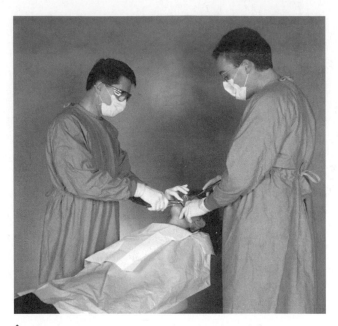

Figure 7-22

Extraction of anterior maxillary teeth. Patient looks straight ahead.

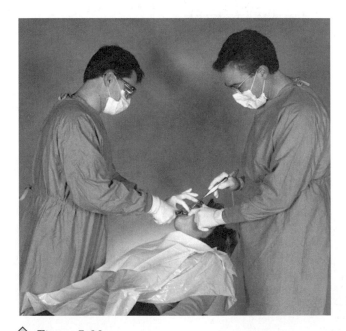

Figure 7-23

Patient with head turned slightly toward surgeon for extraction of maxillary left posterior teeth.

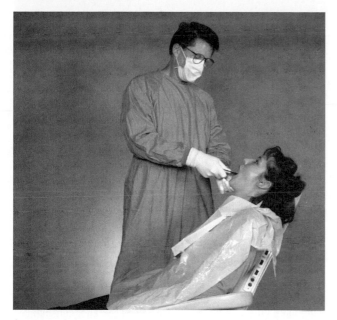

Figure 7-24

For mandibular extractions, patient is more upright, so that mandibular occlusal plane of opened mouth is parallel to floor. Height of chair is also lower to allow operator's arm to be straighter.

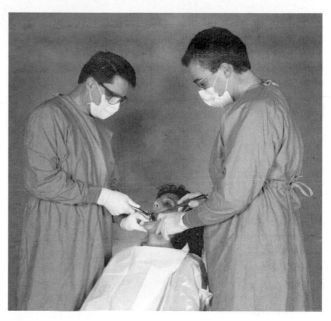

Figure 7-26

For extraction of mandibular anterior teeth, surgeon stands at side of patient, who looks straight ahead.

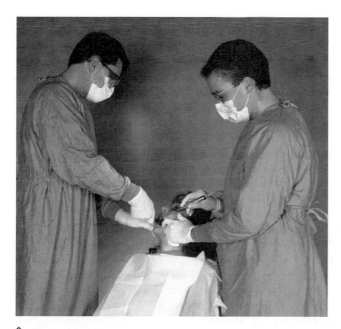

Figure 7-25

Patient with head turned toward surgeon for removal of mandibular right teeth.

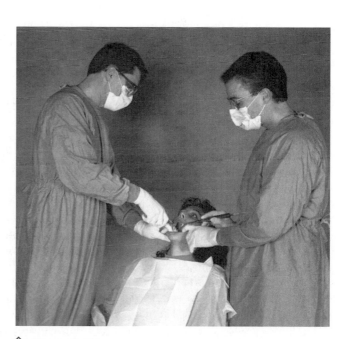

Figure 7-27

When English style of forceps are used for anterior mandibular teeth, patient's head is positioned straight.

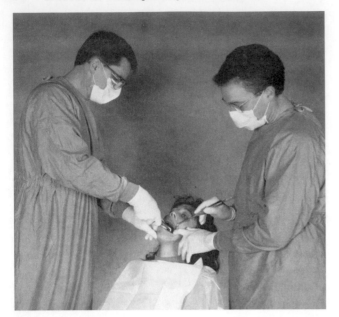

◇ **Figure 7-28**

For extraction of mandibular posterior teeth, patient turns slightly toward surgeon.

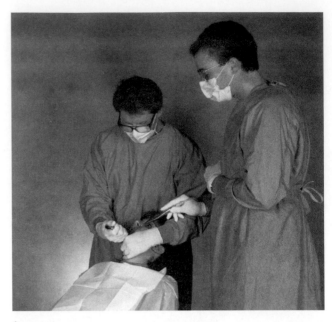

◇ **Figure 7-29**

Behind-the-patient approach for extraction of posterior right mandibular teeth. This allows surgeon to be in comfortable, stable position.

Some surgeons prefer to approach the mandibular teeth from a posterior position. This allows the left hand of the surgeon to support the jaw better, but it requires that the forceps be held opposite the usual method and that the surgeon view the field with a more upside-down perspective. The left hand of the surgeon goes around the patient's head and supports the jaw. The usual behind-the-patient approach is seen in Figures 7-29 and 7-30.

If the surgeon chooses to sit while performing extractions, there are several modifications. For maxillary extractions the patient is positioned in a reclining position similar to that used when the surgeon is standing. However, the patient is not reclined quite as much, and therefore the maxillary occlusal plane is not perpendicular to the floor as it is when the surgeon is standing. The patient should be lowered as far as possible, so that the level of the patient's mouth is as near as possible to the surgeon's elbow (Figure 7-31). The arm and hand position for extraction of the maxillary anterior and posterior teeth is similar to the position used for the same extractions performed while standing (Figure 7-32).

As when the surgeon is standing, for extraction of teeth in the lower arch the patient is a bit more upright than for extraction of maxillary teeth. The surgeon can work from the front of the patient (Figures 7-33 and 7-34) or from behind the patient (Figures 7-35 and 7-36). When English style of forceps are used, the surgeon's position is usually behind the patient (Figure 7-37). It should be noted that the surgeon and the assistant have hand and arm positions similar to those used when the surgeon is in the standing position.

MECHANICAL PRINCIPLES INVOLVED IN TOOTH EXTRACTIONS ◇

The removal of teeth from the alveolar process employs the use of the following mechanical principles and simple machines: the lever, wedge, and wheel and axle.

Elevators are used primarily as levers. A lever is a mechanism for transmitting a modest force—with the mechanical advantages of a long lever arm and a short effector arm—into a small movement against great resistance (Figure 7-38). When an elevator is used for tooth extraction, a purchase point can be made and a crane pick can be used to elevate the tooth or a tooth root from the socket (Figure 7-39). The small, straight elevator is frequently used to help mobilize teeth in a similar fashion, without the preparation of a purchase point.

The second machine that is useful is the wedge (Figure 7-40). It is useful in several different ways for the extraction of teeth. First the beaks of the extraction forceps are usually narrow at their tips; they broaden as they go superiorly. When the forceps are used, there should be a conscious effort made to force the tips of the forceps into the periodontal ligament space to expand the bone and force the tooth out of the socket (Figure 7-41). The wedge principle is also useful when a straight elevator is used to luxate a tooth from its socket. A small elevator is forced into the periodontal ligament space, which displaces the root toward the occlusion and therefore out of the socket (Figure 7-42).

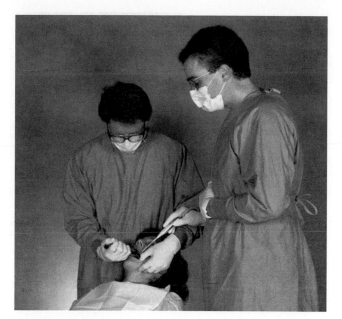

◇ Figure 7-30

Behind-the-patient approach for extraction of posterior left mandibular teeth. Hand is positioned under forceps.

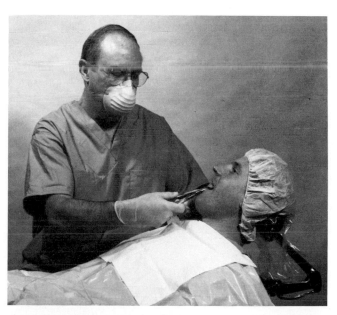

◇ Figure 7-31

In seated position, patient is positioned as low as possible so that mouth is level with surgeon's elbow.

The third machine used in tooth extraction is the wheel and axle, which is most closely identified with the triangular, or pennant-shaped, elevator. When one root of a multiple-rooted tooth is left in the alveolar process, the pennant-shaped elevator is positioned into the socket and turned. The handle then serves as the axle, and the tip of the triangular elevator

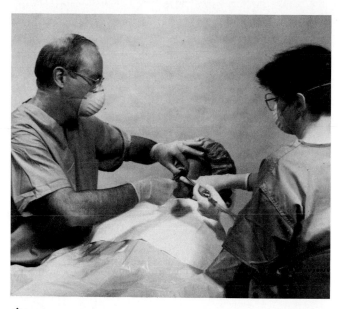

◇ Figure 7-32

For extraction of maxillary teeth, patient is reclined back approximately 60 degrees. Hand and forceps positions are same as for standing position.

acts as a wheel and engages and elevates the tooth root from the socket (Figure 7-43).

PRINCIPLES OF FORCEPS USE ◇

The primary instrument used to remove a tooth from the alveolar process is the extraction forceps. Although elevators may help in the luxation of a tooth, the instrument that does most of the work is the forceps. The goal of forceps use is twofold: (1) expansion of the bony socket by use of the wedge-shaped beaks of the forceps and the movements of the tooth itself with the forceps, and (2) removal of the tooth from the socket.

There are five major motions that the forceps can apply to luxate the teeth and expand the bony socket. The first is apical pressure, which accomplishes two goals. Although there is minimal movement of the tooth in an apical direction, there is expansion of the tooth socket by the insertion of the beaks down into the periodontal ligament space (Figure 7-44). Thus apical pressure of the forceps on the tooth causes bony expansion. A second accomplishment of apical pressure is that the center of the tooth's rotation is displaced apically. Because the tooth is moving in response to the force placed on it by the forceps, the forceps becomes the instrument of expansion. If the fulcrum is high (Figure 7-45), a larger amount of force is placed on the apical region of the tooth, which increases the chance of fracturing the root end. If the beaks of the forceps are forced into the periodontal ligament space, the center of

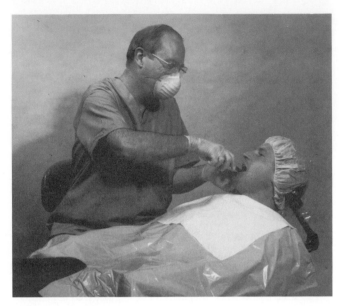

◈ **Figure 7-33**

For extraction of mandibular teeth, operator's hand and arm position is similar to that used for standing position. Patient is placed more upright so mandibular occlusal plane of open mouth is nearly parallel to floor. Surgeon's opposite hand helps support mandible.

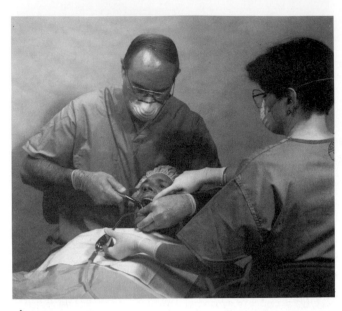

◈ **Figure 7-35**

For removal of anterior teeth, surgeon moves to position behind patient, so that mandible and alveolar process can be supported by surgeon's opposite hand.

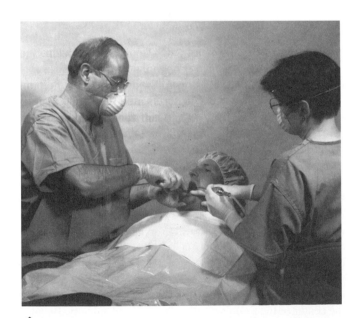

◈ **Figure 7-34**

For removal of mandibular posterior teeth, patient's head is turned toward surgeon.

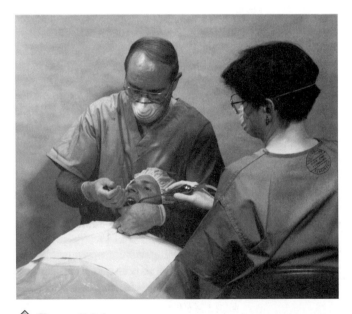

◈ **Figure 7-36**

The behind-the-patient position can be used for removal of mandibular posterior teeth. Hand is positioned under forceps for maximum control.

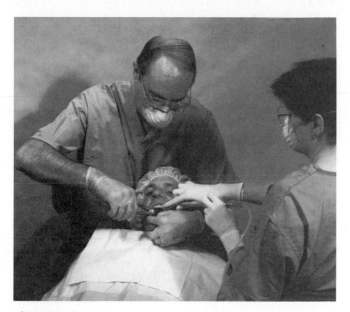

Figure 7-37

When English style of forceps is used, a behind-the-patient position is preferred.

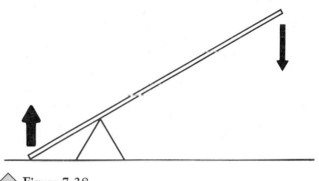

Figure 7-38

First-class lever transforms small force and large movement to small movement and large force.

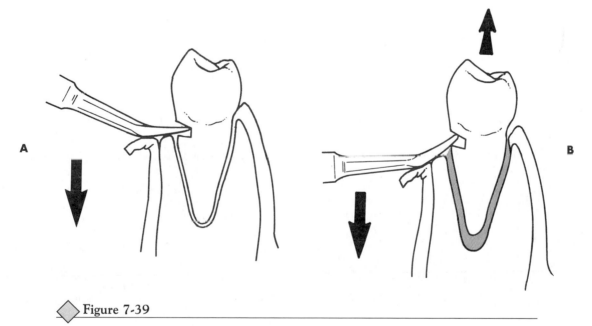

Figure 7-39

In removal of this mandibular premolar tooth, purchase point has been placed in tooth, which creates first-class lever situation. When Crane pick is inserted into purchase point and handle forces apically **(A),** tooth is elevated occlusally out of socket with buccoalveolar bone used as fulcrum **(B).**

rotation is moved apically, which results in greater movement of the expansion forces at the crest of the ridge and less force moving the apex of the tooth lingually (Figure 7-46). This process decreases the chance for apical root fracture.

The second major pressure or movement applied by forceps is the buccal force. Buccal pressures result in expansion of the buccal plate, particularly at the crest of the ridge (Figure 7-47). It is important to remember that although buccal pressure causes expansion forces at the crest of the ridge, it also causes lingual apical pressure.

Third, lingual pressure is similar to the concept of buccal pressure but is aimed at expanding the linguocrestal bone and, at the same time, avoiding excessive pressures on the buccal apical bone (Figure 7-48).

Fourth, rotational pressure, as the name implies, rotates the tooth, which causes some internal expansion of the tooth socket. Teeth with single, conical roots, such as the maxillary incisors, and mandibular premolars, whose roots are not curved, are most amenable to luxation by this technique (Figure 7-49). Teeth that have other than conical roots or that have multiple roots—especially if those roots are curved—are more likely to fracture under this type of pressure.

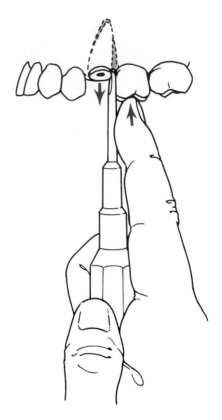

◇ Figure 7-40

Wedge can be used to expand, split, and displace portions of substance that receives it.

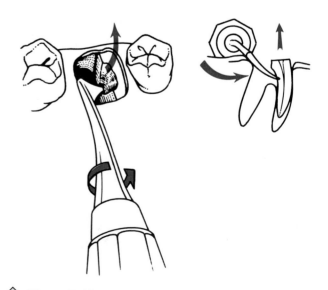

◇ Figure 7-42

Small, straight elevator, used as wedge to displace tooth root from its socket. Its use in this fashion gives this elevator the nickname *shoehorn*.

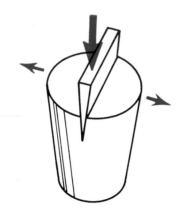

◇ Figure 7-41

Beaks of forceps act as wedge to expand alveolar bone and displace tooth in occlusal direction.

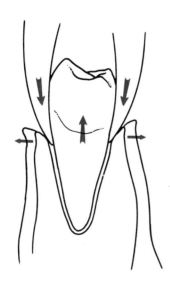

◇ Figure 7-43

Triangular elevator in role of wheel-and-axle machine, used to retrieve root from socket.

Finally, tractional forces are useful for delivering the tooth from the socket once adequate bony expansion is achieved. Tractional forces should be limited to the final portion of the extraction process and should be gentle (Figure 7-50).

In summary, there are a variety of forces that can be used

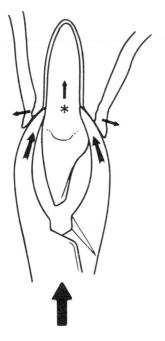

◇ **Figure 7-44**

Extraction forceps should be seated with strong apical pressure to expand crestal bone and to displace center of rotation(*) as far apically as possible.

to remove teeth. A strong apical force is always useful and should be applied whenever forceps are adapted to the tooth. Most teeth are removed by a combination of buccal and lingual forces. Because maxillary buccal bone is usually thinner and the palatal bone is a thicker cortical bone, maxillary teeth are usually removed by strong buccal forces and less vigorous palatal forces. In the mandible the buccal bone is thinner from the midline posteriorly to the area of the molars. Therefore the incisors, canines, and premolars are removed primarily as a result of strong buccal force and less vigorous lingual pressures. The mandibular molar teeth have stronger buccal bone and usually require a stronger lingual pressure than the other teeth in the mouth. As mentioned earlier, rotational forces are useful for single-rooted teeth that have conical roots and no severe curvatures at the root end. The maxillary incisors, particularly the central incisor and mandibular premolars (especially the second premolar), are most amenable to rotational forces.

PROCEDURE FOR CLOSED EXTRACTION ◇

An erupted root can be extracted in one of the following two major ways: closed or open. The closed technique is also known as the *simple*, or *forceps* technique. The open technique is also known as the *surgical*, or *flap*, technique. This section discusses the closed, or forceps, extraction technique; the open technique is discussed in Chapter 8.

The closed technique is the most frequently used technique and is given primary consideration for almost every extrac-

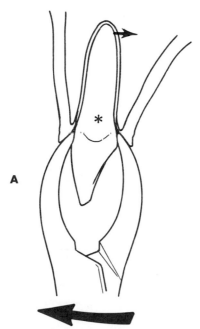

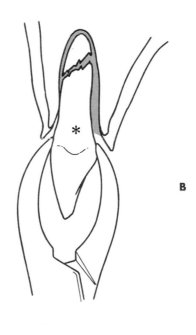

A **B**

◇ Figure 7-45

If center of rotation is not far enough apically, it is too far occlusally, which results in excess movement of tooth apex **(A). B,** Excess motion of root apex caused by high center of rotation results in fracture of root apex.

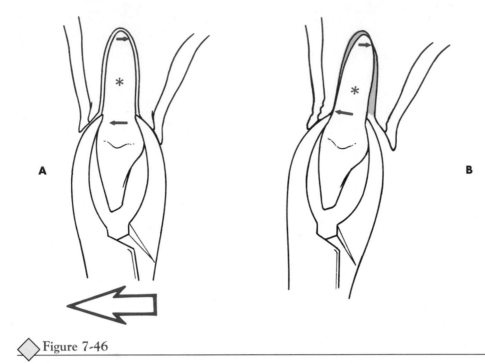

Figure 7-46

If forceps is seated apically, center of rotation is displaced apically, and there are less apical pressures generated **(A).** This results in greater expansion of buccal cortex, less movement of apex of tooth, and therefore less chance of fracture of root **(B).**

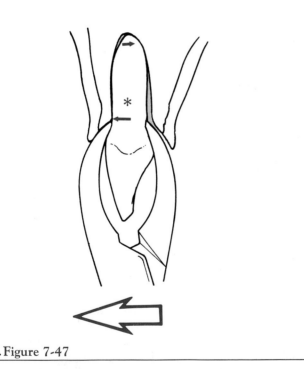

Figure 7-47

Buccal pressure applied to tooth will expand buccocortical plate toward crestal bone, with some lingual expansion at apical end of root.

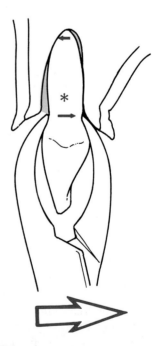

Figure 7-48

Lingual pressure will expand linguocortical plate at crestal area and slightly expand buccal bone at apical area.

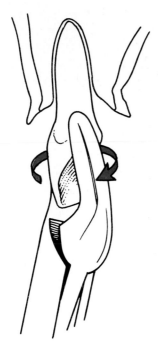

Figure 7-49

Rotational forces, useful for teeth with conical roots, such as maxillary incisors and mandibular premolars.

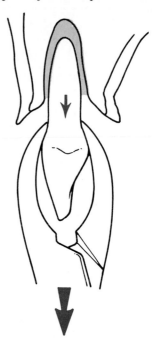

Figure 7-50

Tractional forces, useful for final removal of tooth from socket. They should always be small forces, because teeth are not "pulled."

tion. The open technique is used when there is reason to believe that excessive force is necessary to remove the tooth or when a substantial amount of the crown is missing and access to the root of the tooth is difficult. The correct technique for any situation should lead to an atraumatic extraction; the wrong technique may result in an excessively traumatic extraction.

Whatever technique is chosen, the fundamental requirements for a good extraction remain the same. These requirements are the following: (1) adequate access and visualization of the field of surgery, (2) an unimpeded pathway for the removal of the tooth, and (3) the use of controlled force to luxate and remove the tooth.

For the tooth to be removed from the bony socket, it is necessary to expand the alveolar bony walls to allow the tooth root an unimpeded pathway, and it is necessary to tear the periodontal ligament fibers that hold the tooth in the bony socket. The use of elevators and forceps as levers and wedges with steadily increasing force can accomplish these two objectives.

There are five general steps in the closed-extraction procedure.

Step 1: Loosening of soft tissue attachment from the tooth. The first step in removing a tooth by the closed-extraction technique is to loosen the soft tissue from around the tooth with a sharp instrument, such as the Woodson elevator or the sharp end of the no. 9 periosteal elevator (Figure 7-51). The purpose of loosening the soft tissue from the tooth is twofold. First, it allows the surgeon to ensure that profound anesthesia has been achieved. When this step has been performed the

dentist informs the patient that the surgery is about to begin, and that the first step will be to push the soft tissue away from the tooth. A small amount of pressure is felt at this step, but there is no sensation of sharpness or discomfort. The surgeon then begins the soft tissue–loosening procedure, gently at first and then with increasing force.

The second reason that the soft tissue is loosened is to allow the tooth-extraction forceps to be positioned more apically, without interference from or impingement on the soft tissue of the gingiva. As the soft tissue is loosened away from the tooth, it is slightly reflected, which thereby increases the width of the gingival sulcus and allows easy entrance of the beveled wedge tip of the forceps beaks.

If a straight elevator is to be used to luxate the tooth, the Woodson elevator is also used to reflect the tooth's adjacent gingival papilla where the straight elevator will be inserted (Figure 7-52). This allows the elevator to be placed directly onto alveolar bone, without crushing or injuring the gingival papilla.

Step 2: Luxation of the tooth with a dental elevator. The next step is to begin the luxation of the tooth with a dental elevator, usually the straight elevator. Expansion and dilation of the alveolar bone and tearing of the periodontal ligament require that the tooth be luxated in several ways. The straight elevator is inserted perpendicular to the tooth into the interdental space, after reflection of the interdental papilla (Figure 7-53). The elevator is then turned in such a way that the inferior portion of the blade rests on the alveolar bone and the superior, or occlusal, portion of the blade is turned toward the tooth being extracted (Figure 7-54). Strong, slow, forceful

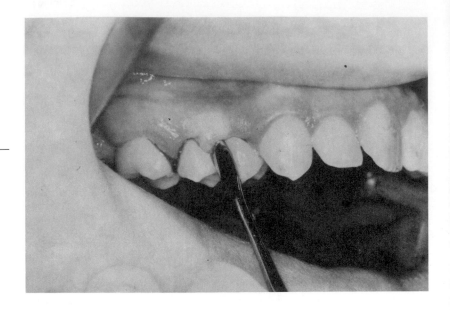

◇ **Figure 7-51**

Woodson elevator, used to loosen gingival attachment from tooth.

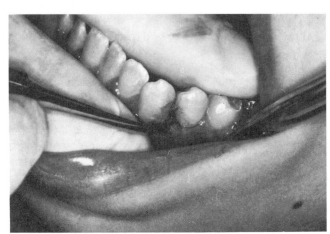

◇ **Figure 7-52**

Reflection of gingival papilla to allow straight elevator to be used to luxate tooth without injury to papilla.

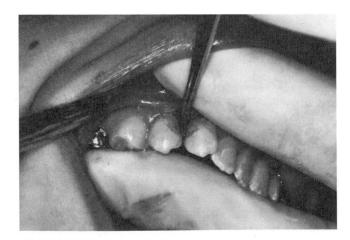

◇ **Figure 7-53**

Small, straight elevator, inserted perpendicular to tooth after papilla has been reflected.

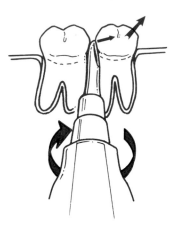

◇ **Figure 7-54**

Handle of small straight elevator, turned so that occlusal side of elevator blade is turned toward tooth.

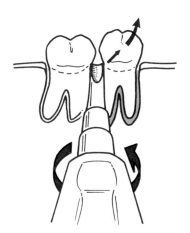

◇ **Figure 7-55**

Handle of elevator, which may be turned in opposite direction to displace tooth further from socket. This can be accomplished only if there is no tooth adjacent posteriorly.

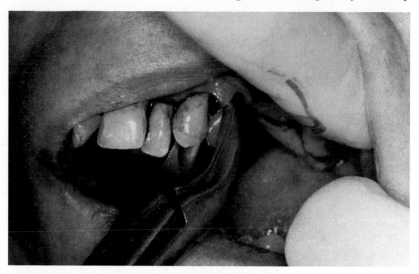

Tips of forceps beak, forced apically under soft tissue.

turning of the handle moves the tooth in a posterior direction, which results in some expansion of the alveolar bone and tearing of the periodontal ligament. If the tooth is intact and in contact with stable teeth anterior and posterior to it, the amount of movement achieved with the straight elevator will be minimal. The usefulness of this step is greater if there is no tooth posterior to the tooth being extracted or if it is broken down to an extent that the crowns do not inhibit movement of the tooth.

In certain situations the elevator can be turned in the opposite direction and more vertical displacement of the tooth will be achieved, which can possibly result in complete removal of the tooth (Figure 7-55).

Luxation of teeth with a straight elevator should be performed with caution. Excessive forces can damage and even displace the teeth adjacent to those being extracted. This is especially true if the adjacent tooth has a large restoration or carious lesion. It must be kept in mind that this is only the initial step, and that the forceps are the major instrument for tooth luxation in most situations.

Step 3: Adaptation of the forceps to the tooth. The proper forceps are then chosen for the tooth to be extracted. The beaks of the forceps should be shaped to adapt anatomically to the tooth, apical to the cervical line, that is, to the root surface. The forceps are then seated onto the tooth so that the tips of the forceps beaks grasp the root underneath the loosened soft tissue (Figure 7-56). The lingual beak is usually seated first and then the buccal beak. Care must be taken to confirm that the tips of the forceps beaks are beneath the soft tissue and not engaging an adjacent tooth. Once the forceps have been positioned on the tooth, the surgeon grasps the handles of the forceps at the very ends to maximize mechanical advantage and control (Figure 7-57).

If the tooth is malopposed in such a fashion that the usual forceps cannot grasp the tooth without injury to adjacent teeth, another forceps should be employed. The maxillary root forceps can often be useful for crowded lower anterior teeth (Figure 7-58).

The beaks of the forceps must be held parallel to the long axis of the tooth, so that the forces generated by the application of pressure to the forceps handle can be delivered along the long axis of the tooth for maximal effectiveness in dilating and expanding the alveolar bone. If the beaks are not parallel to the long axis of the tooth, there is increased likelihood of fracturing the tooth root.

The forceps are then forced apically as far as possible to grasp the root of the tooth as apically as possible. This accomplishes two things. First, the beaks of the forceps act as wedges to dilate the crestal bone on the buccal and lingual aspects. Second, by forcing the beaks apically the center of rotation (or fulcrum) of the forces applied to the tooth is displaced toward the apex of the tooth, which results in greater effectiveness of bone expansion and less likelihood of fracturing the apical end of the tooth.

At this point the surgeon's hand should be grasping the forceps firmly, with the wrist locked and the arm held against the body; the surgeon should be prepared to apply force with the shoulder and upper arm without any wrist pressure. The surgeon should be standing straight, with the feet comfortably apart.

Step 4: Luxation of the tooth with the forceps. The surgeon begins to luxate the tooth by using the motions discussed earlier. The major portion of the force is directed toward the thinnest and therefore weakest bone. Thus in the maxilla and all but the molar teeth in the mandible the major movement is labial and buccal, that is, toward the thinner layer of bone. The surgeon uses slow, steady force to displace the tooth buccally. The motion is deliberate and slow and gradually increases in force. The tooth is then moved again toward the opposite direction with slow, deliberate, strong pressure. As

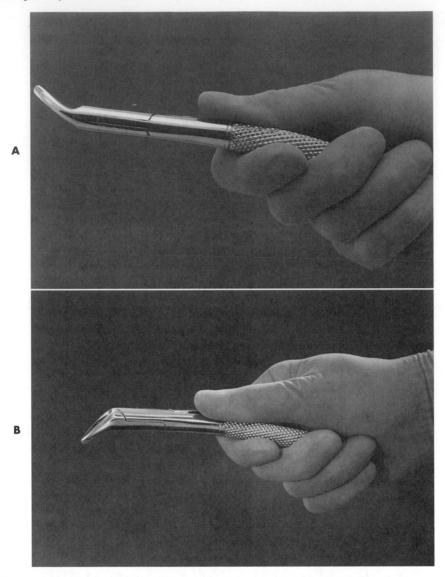

◆ **Figure 7-57**

Forceps handles, held at very ends to maximize mechanical advantage and control. **A,** Maxillary universal forceps. **B,** Mandibular universal forceps.

the alveolar bone begins to expand, the forceps are reseated apically with a strong, deliberate motion, which causes additional expansion of the alveolar bone and further displaces the center of the rotation apically. Buccal and lingual pressures continue to expand the alveolar socket. For some teeth, rotational motions are then used to help expand the tooth socket and tear the periodontal ligament attachment.

Beginning surgeons have a tendency to apply inadequate pressure for insufficient amounts of time. The following three factors must be reemphasized: (1) the forceps must be seated apically as far as possible and reseated periodically during the extraction; (2) the forces applied in the buccal and lingual directions should be slow, deliberate pressures and not jerky wiggles; and (3) the force should be held for several seconds, to allow the bone time to expand. It must be remembered that

teeth are not pulled but rather gently lifted from the socket once the alveolar process has been sufficiently expanded.

Step 5: Removal of the tooth from the socket. Once the alveolar bone has expanded sufficiently and the tooth has been luxated, a slight tractional force, usually directed buccally, can be used. Tractional forces should be minimized, because this is the last motion that is used once the alveolar process is sufficiently expanded and the periodontal ligament completely severed.

It is useful to remember that luxation of the tooth with the forceps and removal of the tooth from the bone are separate steps in the extraction. Luxation is directed toward expansion of the bone and disruption of the periodontal ligament. The tooth is not removed from the bone until these two goals are accomplished. The novice surgeon should realize that the

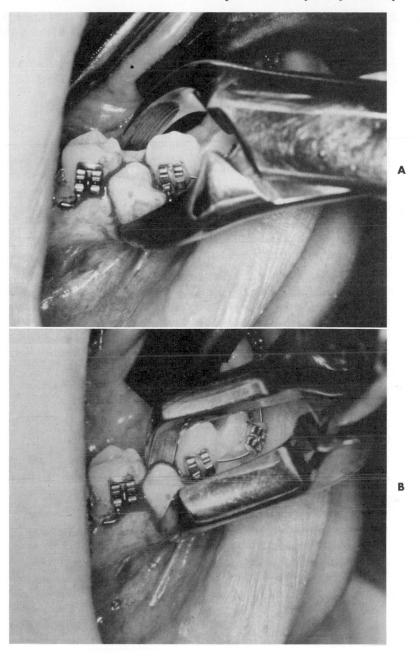

◇ **Figure 7-58**

A, No. 151 forceps, too wide to grasp premolar to be extracted without luxating adjacent teeth. **B,** Maxillary root forceps, which can be adapted easily to tooth for extraction.

major role of the forceps is not to remove the tooth but rather to expand the bone so that the tooth can be removed.

For teeth that are malopposed or have unusual positions in the alveolar process the luxation with the forceps and removal from the alveolar process will be in unusual directions. The surgeon must develop a sense for the direction the tooth wants to move and then be able to move it in that direction. Careful preoperative assessment and planning help to make this determination during the extraction.

ROLE OF THE OPPOSITE HAND

When using the forceps and elevators to luxate and remove teeth, it is important that the surgeon's opposite hand play an active role in the procedure. For the right-handed operator, the left hand has a variety of functions. It is responsible for reflecting the soft tissues of the cheeks, lips, and tongue to provide adequate visualization of the area of surgery. It helps to protect other teeth from the forceps, should they release suddenly from the tooth socket. It helps to stabilize the patient's head during the extraction process. In some situations, large amounts of force are required to expand heavy alveolar bone, and therefore the patient's head requires active assistance to be held steady. The opposite hand plays an important role in supporting and stabilizing the lower jaw when mandibular teeth are being extracted. It is often necessary to apply considerable pressure to expand heavy mandibular bone, and such forces can cause discomfort and even injury to the temporomandibular joint unless they are counteracted by a steady hand. A bite block placed on the contralateral side is also used to help support the jaw in this situation. Finally, the opposite hand supports the alveolar process and provides tactile information to the operator concerning the expansion of the alveolar process during the luxation period. In some situations it is impossible for the opposite hand to perform all of these functions at the same time, so the surgeon requires an assistant to help with some of them.

ROLE OF ASSISTANT DURING EXTRACTION

For a successful outcome in any surgical procedure, it is essential to have a competent assistant. During the extraction the assistant plays a variety of important roles that contribute to making the surgical experience atraumatic.

The assistant helps the surgeon to visualize and gain access to the operative area. The assistant reflects the soft tissue of the cheeks and tongue so that the surgeon can have an unobstructed view of the surgical field. Even during a closed extraction the assistant can reflect the soft tissue so that the surgeon can apply the instruments to loosen the soft tissue attachment and adapt the forceps to the tooth and tooth root in the most effective manner.

Another major activity of the assistant is to suction away blood, saliva, and the irrigating solutions used during the surgical procedure. This prevents fluids from accumulating and makes proper visualization of the surgical field possible. Suctioning is also important for patient comfort, because most patients are unable to tolerate an accumulation of blood or other fluids in their mouths. During a surgical procedure it is almost impossible for the assistant to suction too much.

During the extraction the assistant should also help to protect the teeth of the opposite arch, which is especially important when removing lower posterior teeth. If traction forces are necessary to remove a lower tooth, occasionally the tooth releases suddenly and the forceps strike the maxillary teeth and sometimes fracture a tooth cusp. The assistant should hold either a suction tip or a finger against the maxillary teeth to protect them from an unexpected blow.

During the extraction of mandibular teeth the assistant may play an important role by supporting the mandible during the application of the extraction forces. A surgeon who uses his or her own hand to reflect the soft tissue may not be able to support the mandible. If this is the case, the assistant plays an important role in stabilizing the mandible to prevent temporomandibular joint discomfort. Most often the surgeon stabilizes the mandible, which makes this role less important for the assistant.

The assistant also provides psychologic and emotional support for the patient by helping to alleviate patient anxiety during the surgery. The assistant is important in gaining the patient's confidence and cooperation by using positive language and physical contact with the patient during the preparation and performance of the surgery. The assistant should avoid making casual, offhand comments that may increase the patients' anxiety and lessen their cooperation.

SPECIFIC TECHNIQUES FOR REMOVAL OF EACH TOOTH

This section describes specific techniques for the removal of each tooth in the mouth. In some situations, several teeth are grouped together (for example, the maxillary anterior teeth) because the technique for their removal is essentially the same.

MAXILLARY TEETH

In the correct position for extraction of maxillary left or anterior teeth, the left index finger of the surgeon should reflect the lip and cheek tissue, and the thumb should rest on the palatal alveolar process (Figure 7-59). In this way the left hand is able to reflect the soft tissue of the cheek, stabilize the patient's head, support the alveolar process, and provide tactile information to the surgeon regarding the progress of the extraction. When such a position is used during the extraction of a maxillary molar, the surgeon can frequently feel with the left hand the palatal root of the molar becoming free in the alveolar process before realizing it with the forceps or extracting hand. For the right side, the index finger is positioned on the palate and the thumb on the buccal aspect.

MAXILLARY INCISOR TEETH.
The maxillary incisor teeth are extracted with the upper universal forceps (no. 150), although other forceps can be used. The maxillary incisors generally have conical roots, with the lateral ones being slightly longer and more slender. The lateral incisor is more likely also to have a distal curvature on the apical one third of the root, so this must be checked radiographically before the tooth is extracted. The alveolar bone is thin on the labial side and heavier on the palatal side, which indicates that the major expansion of the alveolar process will be in the buccal direction. The initial movement is slow, steady, and firm in the labial direction, which expands the crestal buccal bone. A less vigorous palatal force is then used, followed by a slow, firm, rotational force. Rotational movement should be minimized for the lateral incisor, especially if a curvature exists on the

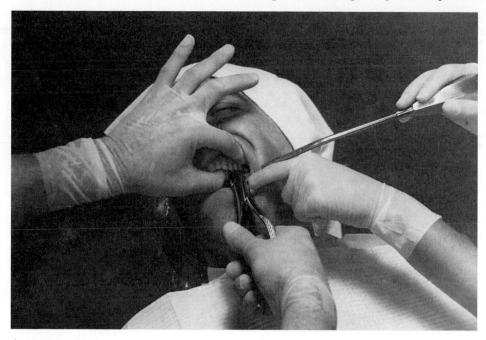

◇ **Figure 7-59**

Extraction of maxillary left posterior teeth. Left index finger reflects lip and cheek and supports alveolar process on buccal aspect. Thumb is positioned on palatal aspect of alveolar process and supports alveolar process. Head is steadied by this grip, and tactile information is gained regarding tooth and bone movement.

tooth. The tooth is delivered in the labial-incisal direction with a small amount of tractional force (Figure 7-60).

MAXILLARY CANINE.   The maxillary canine is usually the longest tooth in the mouth. The root is oblong in cross section and usually produces a bulge called the canine eminence on the anterior surface of the maxilla. The result is that the bone over the labial aspect of the maxillary canine is usually quite thin. In spite of the thin labial bone, this tooth can be difficult to extract simply because of its long root. Additionally, it is not uncommon for a segment of labial alveolar bone to fracture from the labial plate and be removed with the tooth.

The preferred forceps for removing the maxillary canine is the upper universal (no. 150) forceps. As with all extractions, the initial placement of the beaks of the forceps on the canine tooth should be as far apically as possible. The initial movement is to the buccal aspect, with return pressure to the palatal. As the bone is expanded and the tooth mobilized, the forceps should be repositioned apically. A small amount of rotational force may be useful in expanding the tooth socket, especially if the adjacent teeth are missing or have just been extracted. After the tooth has been well luxated, it is delivered from the socket in a labial-incisal direction with labial tractional forces (Figure 7-61).

If, during the luxation process with the forceps, the surgeon feels a portion of the labial bone fracture, a decision must be made concerning the next step. If the palpating finger indicates that a relatively small amount of bone has fractured free and is attached to the canine tooth, the extraction should continue in the usual manner, with caution taken not to tear the soft tissue. However, if the palpating finger indicates that a relatively large portion of labial alveolar plate has fractured, the surgeon should stop the surgical procedure at this point. Usually the fractured portion of bone is attached to periosteum and therefore is viable. The surgeon should use a thin periosteal elevator to raise a small amount of mucosa from around the tooth, down to the level of the fractured bone. The canine tooth should then be stabilized with the extraction forceps, and the surgeon should attempt to free the fractured bone from the tooth, with the periosteal elevator as a lever to separate the bone from the tooth root. If this can be accomplished, the tooth can be removed and the bone left in place attached to the periosteum. Normal healing should occur. If the bone becomes detached from the periosteum during these attempts, it should be removed, because it is probably nonvital and may actually prolong wound healing. This procedure can be used whenever alveolar bone is fractured during extraction.

Prevention of fractured labial plate is important. If during the luxation process with the forceps a normal amount of pressure has not resulted in any movement of the tooth, the surgeon should seriously consider doing an open extraction. By reflecting a soft tissue flap and removing a small amount of bone, the surgeon may be able to remove the stubborn canine tooth without fracturing a larger amount of labial bone.

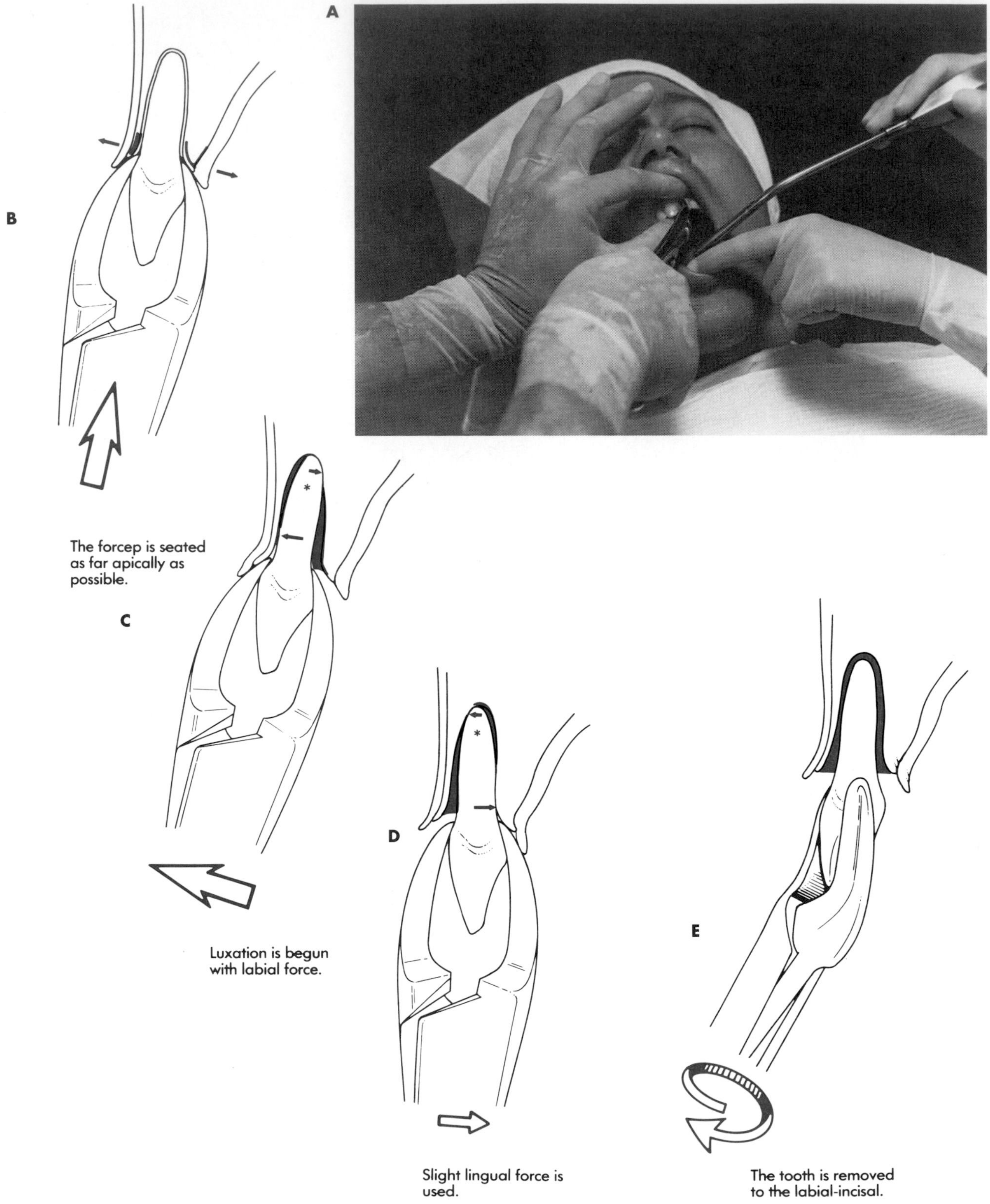

The forcep is seated as far apically as possible.

Luxation is begun with labial force.

Slight lingual force is used.

The tooth is removed to the labial-incisal.

◇ Figure 7-60

A, Maxillary incisors are extracted with no. 150 forceps. Left hand grasps alveolar process. Assistant helps reflect and protect soft tissue. **B,** Forceps are seated as far apically as possible. **C,** Luxation is begun with labial force. **D,** Slight lingual force is used. **E,** Tooth is delivered to labial incisor with rotational, tractional movement.

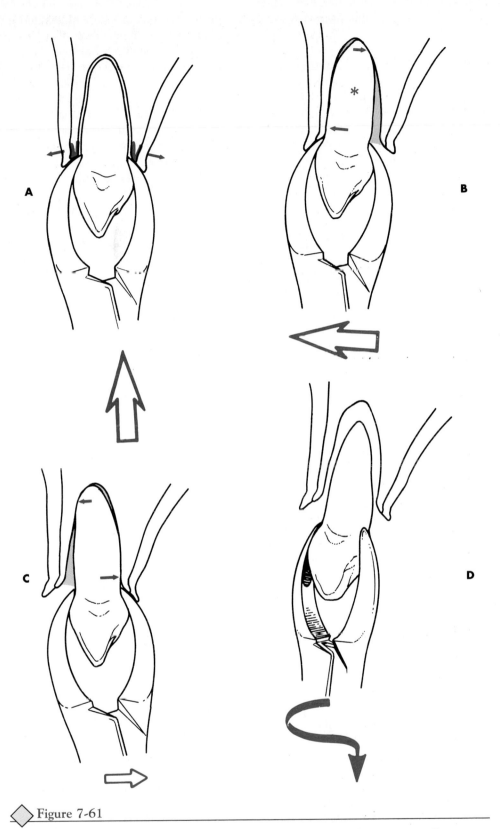

◇ Figure 7-61

A, Hand and forceps position for removal of maxillary canine is similar to that for incisors. Forceps are seated as far apically as possible. **B,** Initial movement is buccally. **C,** Small amounts of lingual force are applied. **D,** Tooth is delivered in labial-incisal direction with slight rotational force.

By using the open technique, there will be an overall reduction in the amount of bone loss and a reduction in postoperative healing time.

MAXILLARY FIRST PREMOLAR. The maxillary first premolar is a single-rooted tooth in its first two thirds, with a bifurcation into a buccolingual root usually occurring in the apical one third to one half. These roots may be extremely thin and are subject to fracture, especially in older patients in whom bone density is great and bone elasticity is small (Figure 7-62). Perhaps the most common root fracture when extracting teeth in adults occurs with this tooth. As with other maxillary teeth, the buccal bone is relatively thin compared with the palatal bone.

The forceps of choice once again is the upper universal (no. 150) forceps. Alternatively, the no. 150A forceps can be used for removal of the maxillary first premolar.

Because of the high likelihood of root fracture, the tooth should be luxated as much as possible with the straight elevator. If root fracture does occur, a mobile root tip can be removed more easily than one which has not been well luxated.

Because of the bifurcation of the tooth into two relatively thin root tips, extraction forces should be carefully controlled during removal of the maxillary first premolar. Initial movements should be buccal. Palatal movements are made with relatively small amounts of force to prevent fracture of the palatal root tip, which is harder to retrieve. When the tooth is luxated buccally, the most likely tooth root to break is the labial. When the tooth is luxated in the palatal direction, the most likely root to break is the palatal root. Of the two root tips, the labial is easier to retrieve because of the thin, overlying bone. Therefore buccal pressures should be greater than palatal pressures. Any rotational force should be avoided. Final delivery of the tooth from the tooth socket is with tractional force in the occlusal direction and slightly buccal (Figure 7-62).

MAXILLARY SECOND PREMOLAR. The maxillary second premolar is a single-rooted tooth for the root's entire length. The root is thick and has a blunt end. Consequently, the root of the second premolar fractures only rarely. The overlying alveolar bone is similar to that of other maxillary teeth in that it is relatively thin toward the bucca, with a heavy palatal alveolar palate.

The recommended forceps is the maxillary universal forceps, or no. 150; the no. 150A is preferred by some surgeons. The forceps are forced as far apically as possible so as to gain maximal mechanical advantage in removing this tooth. Because the tooth root is relatively strong and blunt, the extraction requires relatively strong movements to the bucca, back to the palate, and then in the bucco-occlusal direction with a rotational, tractional force (Figure 7-63).

MAXILLARY MOLAR. The maxillary first molar has three large and relatively strong roots. The buccal roots are usually relatively close together, and the palatal root diverges widely toward the palate. If the two buccal roots are also widely divergent, it becomes difficult to remove this tooth by closed, or forceps, extraction. Once again the overlying alveolar bone is similar to that of other teeth in the maxilla; the buccal plate is thin and the palatal cortical plate is thick and heavy. When evaluating this tooth radiographically, the dentist should note the size, curvature, and apparent divergence of the three roots. Additionally, the dentist should look carefully at the relationship of the tooth roots to the maxillary sinus. If the sinus is in close proximity to the roots and the roots are widely divergent, there is increased likelihood of sinus perforation caused by removal of a portion of the sinus floor during tooth removal. If this appears to be likely after preoperative evaluation, the surgeon should strongly consider a surgical extraction.

The forceps usually used for extraction of the maxillary molars are the paired forceps no. 53R and no. 53L. These forceps have tip projections on the buccal beaks to fit into the buccal bifurcation. Some surgeons prefer to use the no. 89 and no. 90 forceps, which are sometimes called the *upper cowhorn forceps*. These forceps are especially useful if the crown of the molar tooth has large caries or large restorations.

The upper molar forceps are adapted to the tooth and seated apically as far as possible in the usual fashion (Figure 7-64). The basic extraction movement is to use strong buccal and palatal pressures, with stronger forces toward the bucca than toward the palate. Rotational forces are not useful for extraction of this tooth because of its three roots. As was mentioned in the discussion of the extraction of the maxillary first premolar, it is preferable to fracture a buccal root than a palatal root, because it is easier to retrieve the buccal roots. Therefore if the tooth has widely divergent roots and the dentist suspects that one root may be fractured, the tooth should be luxated in such a way as to prevent fracturing the palatal root. The dentist must minimize palatal force, because this is the force that fractures the palatal root. Strong, slow, steady, buccal pressure expands the buccocortical plate and tears the periodontal ligament fibers that hold the palatal root in its position. Palatal forces should be used but kept to a minimum.

The maxillary second molar's anatomy is similar to that of the maxillary first molar except that the roots tend to be shorter and less divergent, with the buccal roots more commonly fused into a single root. This means that the tooth is more easily extracted by the same technique described for the first molar.

The erupted maxillary third molar frequently has conical roots and is usually extracted with the no. 210S forceps, which are universal forceps used for both the left and right sides. The tooth is usually easily removed, because the buccal bone is thin and the roots are usually fused and conical. The erupted third molar is also frequently extracted by the use of elevators alone. It is important to visualize the maxillary third molar clearly on the preoperative radiograph, because the root anatomy of this tooth is quite variable and often small, dilacerated, hooked roots exist in this area. Retrieval of fractured roots in this area can be very difficult.

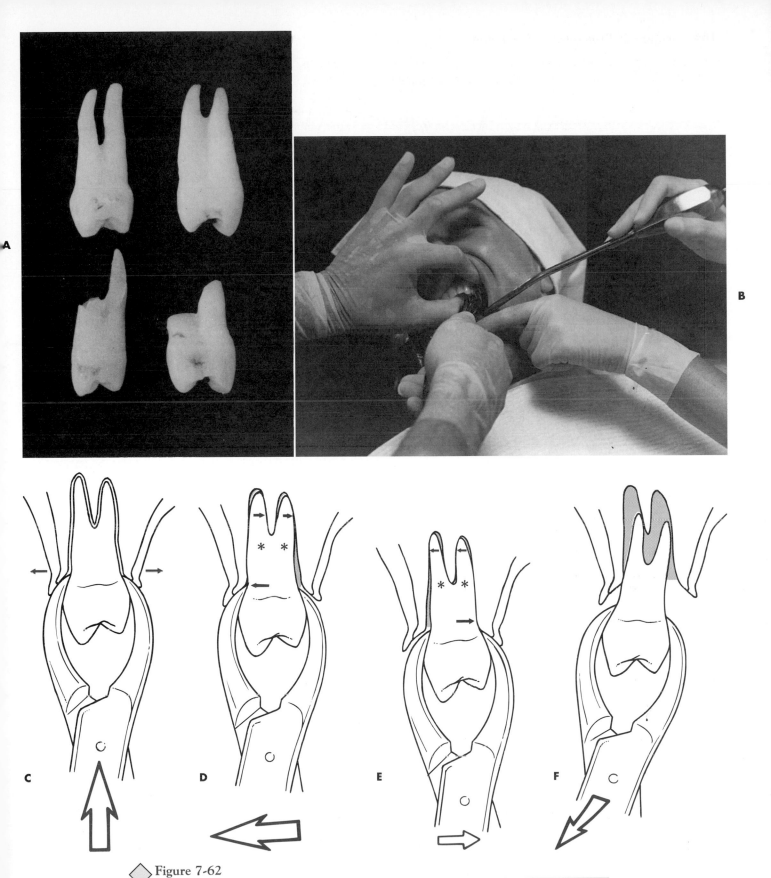

A, Maxillary first premolar has two thin roots that are quite subject to fracture during extraction. **B,** Maxillary premolars are removed with no. 150 forceps. Hand position is similar to that used for anterior teeth. **C,** Firm apical pressure is applied first to lower center of rotation as far as possible and to expand crestal bone. **D,** Buccal pressure is applied initially to expand buccocortical plate. Note that apices of roots are pushed lingually and are therefore subject to fracture. **E,** Palatal pressure is applied but less vigorously than buccal pressure. **F,** Tooth is delivered in bucco-occlusal direction with combination of buccal and tractional forces.

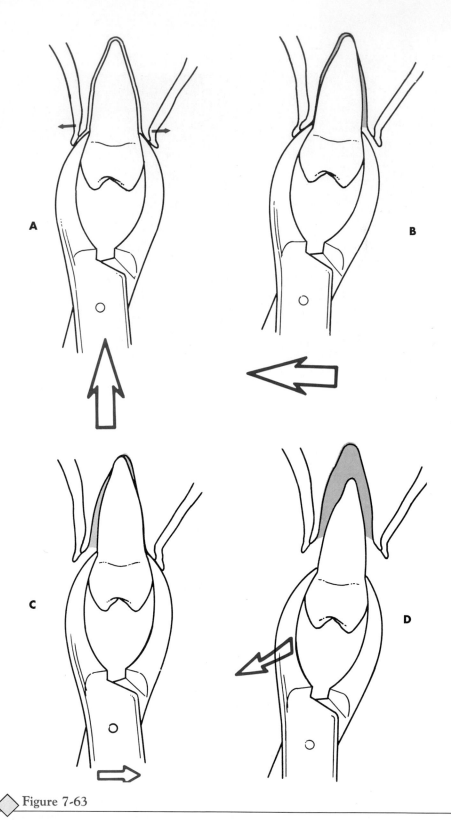

◇ Figure 7-63

A, When extracting maxillary second premolar, forceps is seated as far apically as possible. **B,** Luxation is begun with buccal pressure. **C,** Very slight lingual pressure is used. **D,** Tooth is delivered in bucco-occlusal direction.

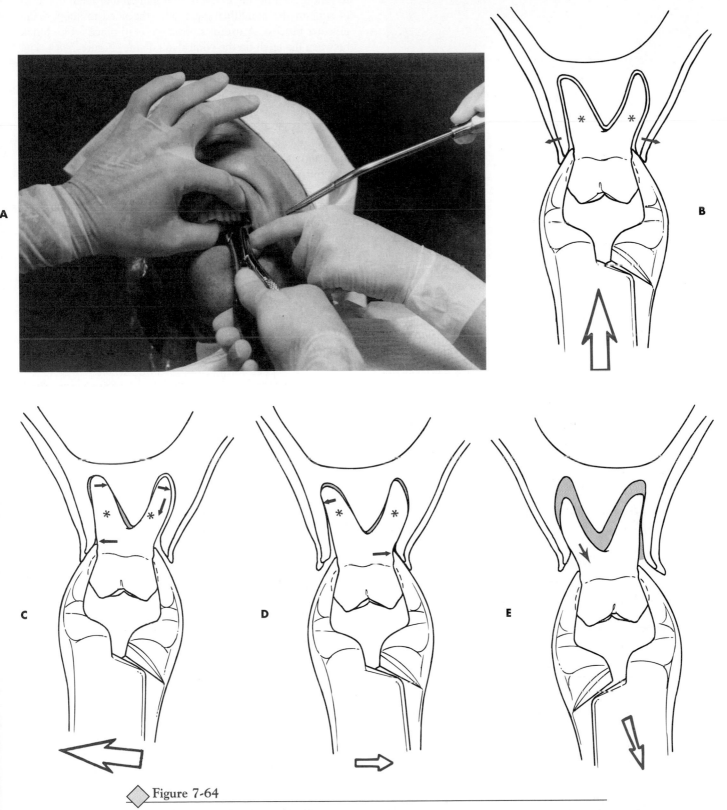

Figure 7-64

A, Extraction of maxillary molars. Soft tissue of lips and cheek is reflected, and alveolar process is grasped with opposite hand. **B,** Forceps beaks are seated apically as far as possible. **C,** Luxation is begun with strong buccal force. **D,** Lingual pressures are used only moderately. **E,** Tooth is delivered in bucco-occlusal direction.

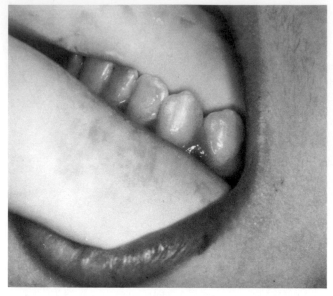

Figure 7-65

Extraction of mandibular left posterior teeth. Surgeon's left index finger is positioned in buccal vestibule, reflecting cheek, and second finger is positioned in lingual vestibule, reflecting tongue. Thumb is positioned under chin. Jaw is grasped between fingers and thumb to provide support during extraction.

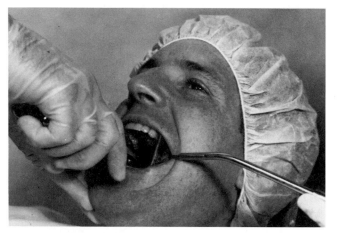

Figure 7-66

To provide support for the mandible to prevent excessive temporomandibular joint pressures, a rubber bite block can be placed between the teeth on the contralateral side.

MANDIBULAR TEETH

When removing lower molar teeth the index finger of the left hand is in the buccal vestibule and the second finger is in the lingual vestibule, reflecting the lip, cheek, and tongue (Figure 7-65). The thumb of the left hand is placed below the chin so that the jaw is held between the fingers and thumb, which support the mandible and minimize temporomandibular joint pressures. There is less tactile information provided by this technique, but during extraction of mandibular teeth the need to support the mandible supersedes the need to support the alveolar process. A useful alternative is to place a bite block between the teeth on the contralateral side (Figure 7-66). The bite block allows the patient to help provide stabilizing forces to limit the pressure on the temporomandibular joints. The surgeon's hand should continue to provide additional support to the jaw.

MANDIBULAR ANTERIOR TEETH. The mandibular incisors and canines are similar in shape, with the incisors being shorter and slightly thinner and the canine roots being longer and somewhat heavier. The incisor roots are more likely to be fractured, because they are somewhat thin and therefore should be removed only after adequate preextraction luxation. The alveolar bone that overlies the incisors and canines is quite thin on the labial and lingual sides. The bone over the canine may be somewhat thicker, especially on the lingual side.

The usual forceps employed to remove these teeth is the lower universal (no. 151) forceps. Alternative choices are the no. 151A or the English style of Ashe forceps. The forceps beaks are positioned on the teeth and seated apically with strong force. The extraction movements are generally in the labial and lingual directions, with equal pressures both ways. Once the tooth has become luxated and mobile, rotational movement may be used to expand the alveolar bone further. The tooth is removed from the socket with tractional forces in a labial-incisal direction (Figure 7-67).

MANDIBULAR PREMOLARS. The mandibular premolars are among the easiest teeth to remove. The roots tend to be straight and conical, albeit sometimes slender. The overlying alveolar bone is thin on the buccal aspect and somewhat heavier on the lingual side.

The forceps usually chosen for extraction of the mandibular premolars are the lower universal (no. 151) forceps. The no. 151A forceps and the English style of forceps are both popular alternatives for extraction of these teeth.

The forceps are forced apically as far as possible, with the basic movements being toward the buccal aspect, returning to the lingual aspect, and, finally, rotating. Rotational movement is used more when extracting these teeth than any others, except perhaps the maxillary central incisor. The tooth is then delivered in the occlusobuccal direction (Figure 7-68). Careful preoperative radiographic assessment must be performed to assure the operator that no root curvature exists in the apical third of the tooth. If such a curvature does exist, the rotational movements should be reduced or eliminated from the extraction procedure (Figure 7-69).

MANDIBULAR MOLARS. The mandibular molars are usually two-rooted, with roots of the first molar more widely divergent than those of the second molar. Additionally, the roots may converge at the apical one third, which increases the difficulty of extraction. The roots are generally heavy and strong. The overlying alveolar bone is heavier than the bone

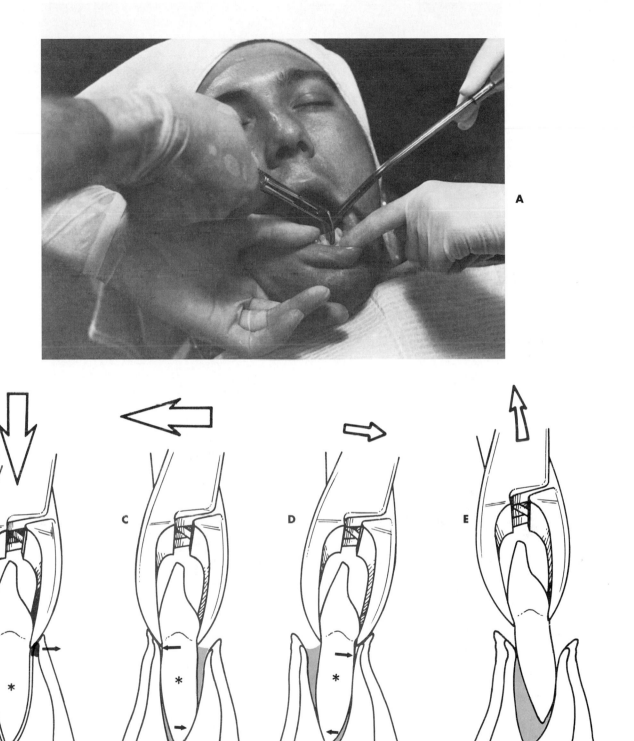

◇ Figure 7-67

A, When extracting mandibular anterior teeth, no. 151 forceps are used. Assistant reflects lip, and surgeon stabilizes jaw with left hand. **B,** Forceps are seated apically as far as possible. **C,** Moderate labial pressure is used to initiate luxation process. **D,** Lingual force is used to continue expansion of bone. **E,** Tooth is delivered in labial-incisal direction.

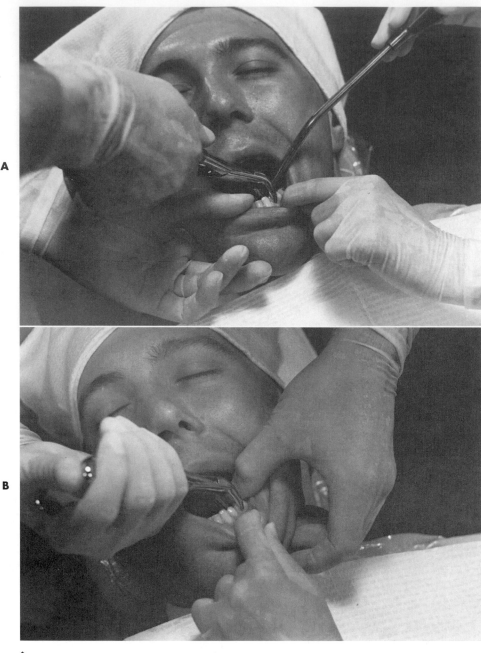

◇ Figure 7-68

A, Extraction of mandibular premolar. Jaw is stabilized, soft tissue is reflected, and no. 151 forceps is positioned. **B,** Hand position is modified slightly for behind-the-patient technique.

Continued

on any other teeth in the mouth. The combination of relatively long, strong, divergent roots with heavy overlying buccolingual bone makes the mandibular first molar the most difficult of all teeth to extract.

The forceps usually used for extraction of the mandibular molars are the no. 17 forceps, which have small tip projections on both beaks to fit into the bifurcation of the tooth roots. The forceps are adapted to the root of the tooth in the usual fashion, and strong apical pressure is applied to set the beaks of the forceps apically as far as possible.

Strong buccolingual motion is then used to expand the tooth socket and allow the tooth to be delivered in the bucco-occlusal direction. The linguoalveolar bone around the second molar is thinner than the buccal plate, so the second molar can be more easily removed with stronger lingual than buccal pressures (Figure 7-70).

If the tooth roots are clearly bifurcated, the no. 23, or cowhorn, forceps can be used. These forceps are designed to be closed forcefully with the handles, thereby squeezing the beaks of the forceps into the bifurcation. This creates force

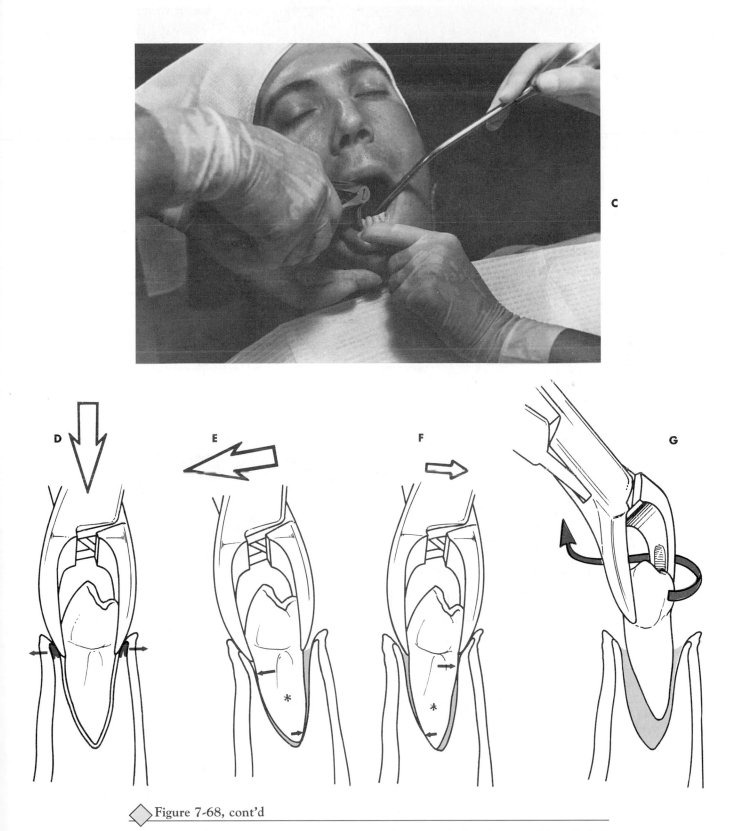

◇ Figure 7-68, cont'd

C, English style of forceps can also be used. **D,** Forceps is seated apically as far as possible to displace center of rotation and to begin expansion of crestal bone. **E,** Buccal forceps is applied to begin luxation process. **F,** Slight lingual pressure is used. **G,** Tooth is delivered with rotational, tractional force.

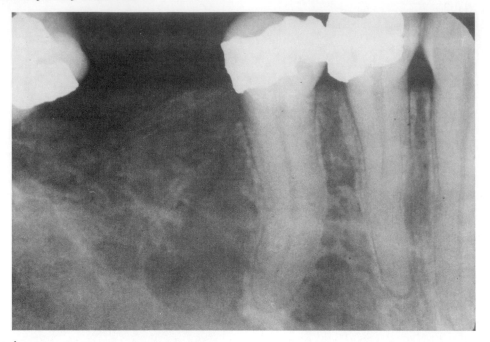

◇ **Figure 7-69**

If curvature of premolar root exists, rotational extraction forces will result in fracture of curved portion of root, and therefore such forces should be minimized.

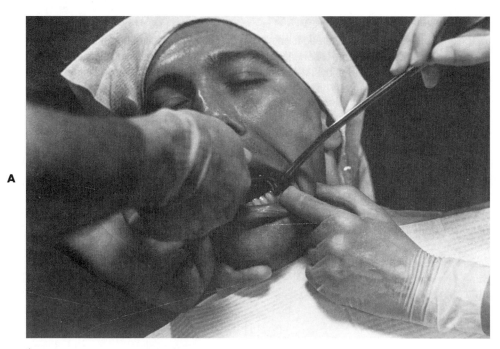

◇ **Figure 7-70**

A, Mandibular molars are extracted with no. 17 or no. 23 forceps. Hand positions of surgeon and assistant are same for both forceps.

Continued

against the crest of the alveolar ridge on the buccolingual aspects and literally forces the tooth superiorly directly out of the tooth socket (Figure 7-71). If initially this is not successful, the forceps are given buccolingual movements to expand the alveolar bone, and more squeezing of the handles is performed. Care must be taken with these forceps to prevent

damaging the maxillary teeth, because the lower molar may actually pop out of the socket and thus release the forceps to strike the upper teeth (Figure 7-71).

Erupted mandibular third molars usually have fused conical roots. Because there is not usually a bifurcation, the no. 222 forceps—a short-beaked, right-angled forceps—is

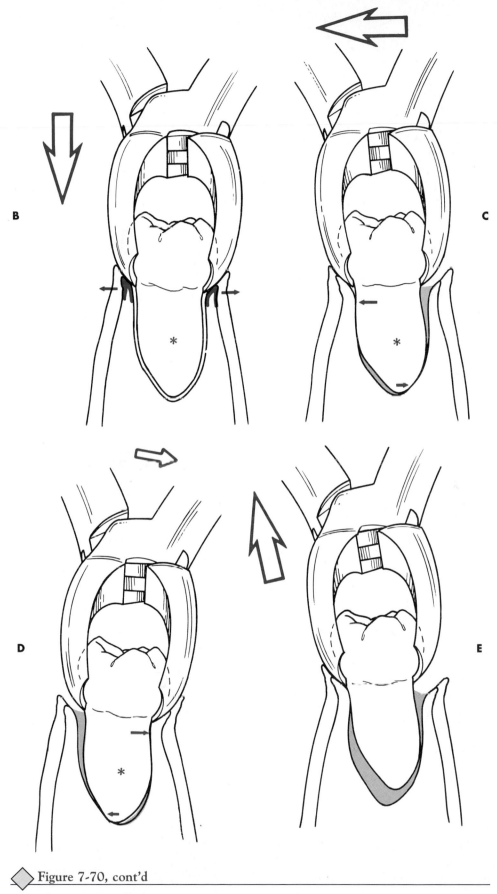

◈ Figure 7-70, cont'd

B, No. 17 forceps is seated as far apically as possible. **C,** Luxation of molar is begun with strong buccal movement. **D,** Strong lingual pressure is used to continue luxation. **E,** Tooth is delivered in bucco-occlusal direction.

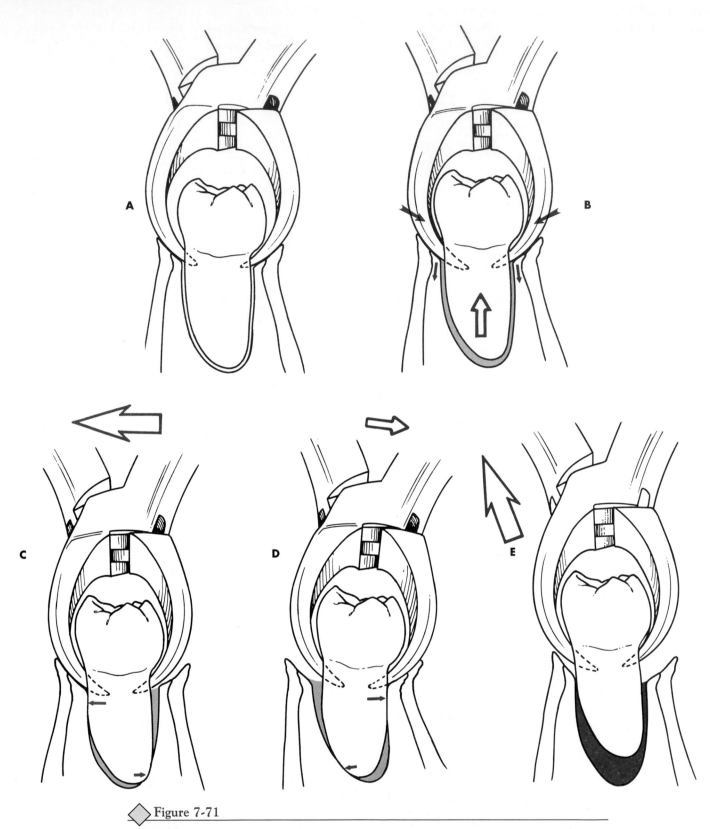

◈ Figure 7-71

A, No. 23 forceps is carefully positioned to engage bifurcation area of lower molar. **B,** Handles of forceps are squeezed forcibly together, which causes beaks of forceps to be forced into bifurcation and exerts tractional forces on tooth. **C,** Strong buccal forces are then used to expand socket. **D,** Strong lingual forces are used to luxate tooth further. **E,** Tooth is delivered in bucco-occlusal direction with buccal and tractional forces.

used to extract this tooth. The lingual plate of bone is definitely thinner than the buccocortical plate, so most of the extraction forces should be delivered to the lingual aspect. The third molar is delivered in the linguo-occlusal direction. The erupted mandibular third molar that is in function can be a deceptively difficult tooth to extract. The dentist should give serious consideration to using the straight elevator to achieve a moderate degree of luxation before applying the forceps. Pressure should be gradually increased, and attempts to mobilize the tooth should be made before final strong pressures are delivered.

MODIFICATIONS FOR EXTRACTION OF PRIMARY TEETH

It is rarely necessary to remove primary teeth before substantial root resorption has occurred. However, when removal is required, it must be done with a great deal of care, because the roots of the primary teeth are very long and delicate and subject to fracture. This is especially true because the succedaneous tooth causes resorption of coronal portions of the root structure and thereby weakens it. The forceps usually used are adaptations of the upper and lower universal forceps, the no. 150S and the no. 151S. They are adapted and forced apically in the usual fashion, with slow, steady pressures toward the buccal aspect and return movements toward the lingual aspect. Rotational motions may be employed but should be minimal and used judiciously with multirooted teeth. The dentist should pay careful attention to the direction of least resistance and deliver the tooth into that path. If the roots of the primary molar tooth embrace the crown of the permanent premolar, the surgeon should consider sectioning the tooth. Occasionally, the roots hold the crown of the premolar firmly enough in their grasp to cause it to be extracted also.

POSTEXTRACTION CARE OF THE TOOTH SOCKET ——◇

Once the tooth has been removed from the socket, it is necessary to provide proper care. The socket should be débrided only if necessary. If there is a periapical lesion visible on the preoperative radiograph, and there was no granuloma attached to the tooth when it was removed, the periapical region should be carefully curetted to remove the granuloma or cyst. If there is any obvious debris, such as calculus, amalgam, or tooth fragment, remaining in the socket, it should be gently removed with a curette or suction tip (Figure 7-72). However, if neither periapical lesion nor debris is present, the socket *should not* be curetted. The remnants of the periodontal ligament and the bleeding bony walls are in the best condition to provide for rapid healing. Vigorous curettage of the socket wall merely produces additional injury and may delay healing.

The expanded buccolingual plates should be compressed back to their original configuration. Finger pressure should be applied to the buccolingual cortical plate to gently but firmly compress the plates to their original position or ap-

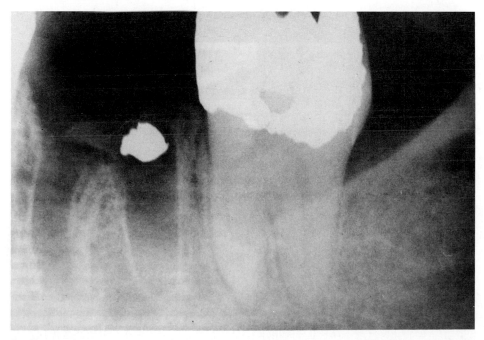

◇ Figure 7-72

Amalgam fragment left in this tooth socket after extraction, because surgeon failed to inspect and debride surgical field.

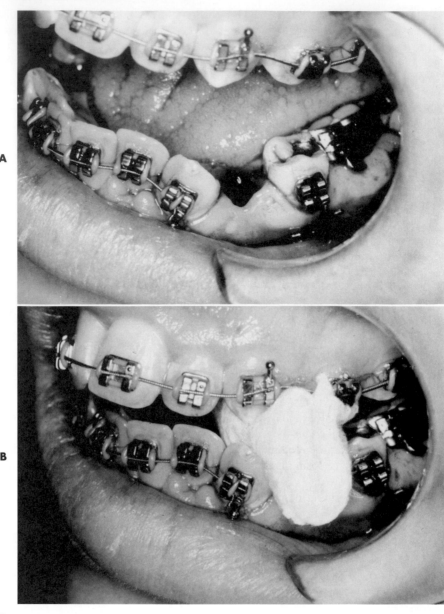

◇ **Figure 7-73**

A, After extraction of single tooth, small space exists where crown of tooth was. **B,** Gauze pad (2 × 2-inch) is folded in half twice and placed into space. When patient bites on gauze, pressure is transmitted to gingiva and socket.

Continued

proximate them even more closely, if possible. This helps to prevent bony undercuts that may have been caused by excessive expansion of the buccocortical plate, especially after first molar extraction.

If the teeth were removed because of periodontal disease, there may be an accumulation of excess granulation tissue around the gingival cuff. If this is the case, special attention should be given to removing this granulation tissue with a curette or hemostat. The arterioles of granulation tissue have little or no capacity to retract and constrict, which leads to bothersome bleeding if excessive granulation tissue is left.

Finally, the bone should be palpated through the overlying mucosa to check for any sharp, bony projections. If any exist, the mucosa should be reflected and the sharp edges smoothed judiciously with a bone file.

To gain initial control of hemorrhage, a moistened 2 × 2-inch gauze is placed over the extraction socket. The gauze should be positioned so that when the patient closes the teeth together, it fits into the space previously occupied by the crown of the tooth. The pressure of biting the teeth together is placed on the gauze and is transmitted to the socket. This pressure results in hemostasis. If the gauze is simply placed

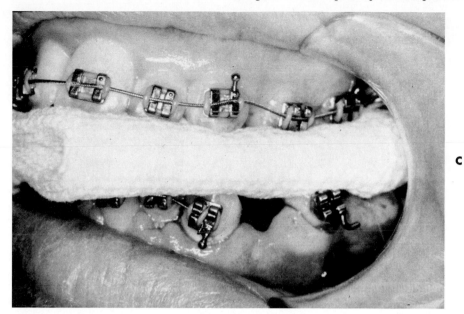

⬦ Figure 7-73, cont'd

C, If large gauze is used, pressure goes on teeth, not on gingiva and socket.

on the occlusal table, the pressure applied to the bleeding socket is insufficient to achieve adequate hemostasis (Figure 7-73). A larger gauze sponge (4 × 4-inch) may be required if multiple teeth have been extracted or if the opposing arch is edentulous.

The extraction of multiple teeth at one sitting is a more involved and complex procedure. It is discussed in Chapter 8.

BIBLIOGRAPHY

Berman SA: Basic principles of dentoalveolar surgery. In Peterson LJ, editor: *Principles of oral and maxillofacial surgery,* Philadelphia, 1992, JB Lippincott.

Byrd DL: Exodontia: modern concepts, *Dent Clin North Am* 15:273, 1971.

PRINCIPLES OF COMPLICATED EXODONTIA

LARRY J. PETERSON

The removal of most erupted teeth can be achieved by closed, or forceps, delivery, but occasionally this technique does not suffice. The surgical, or open, extraction technique is the method used for recovering roots that were fractured during routine extraction or teeth that cannot be extracted by the routine closed methods for a variety of reasons. Also, removal of multiple teeth during one surgical session requires more than the simple removal of teeth as described in Chapter 7. Small flaps are usually required for recontouring and smoothing bone.

This chapter discusses techniques for surgical tooth extraction. The principles of flap design, development, management, and suturing are explained, as are the principles of surgical extraction of single-rooted and multirooted teeth.

Also discussed are the principles involved in multiple extractions and concomitant alveoloplasty.

PRINCIPLES OF FLAP DESIGN, DEVELOPMENT, AND MANAGEMENT ———————◇

The term *flap* indicates a section of soft tissue that (1) is outlined by a surgical incision, (2) carries its own blood supply, (3) allows surgical access to underlying tissues, (4) can be replaced in the original position, and (5) can be maintained with sutures and is expected to heal. Soft tissue flaps are frequently used in oral surgical, periodontal, and endodontal procedures to gain access to underlying tooth and bone structures. To perform a tooth extraction properly, the dentist must have a clear understanding of the principles of design, development, and management of soft tissue flaps.

DESIGN PARAMETERS FOR SOFT TISSUE FLAPS

To provide adequate exposure and promote rapid healing, the surgeon must design the flap correctly. He must keep in mind several parameters when designing a flap for a specific situation.

When the flap is outlined, the base of the flap must be broader than the free margin to preserve an adequate blood supply. This means that all areas of the flap must have a source of uninterrupted vasculature to prevent ischemic necrosis of the entire flap or portions of it (Figure 8-1).

The flap must be of adequate size for several reasons. Sufficient soft tissue reflection is required to provide necessary visualization of the area. Adequate access also must exist for the insertion of all instruments required to perform the

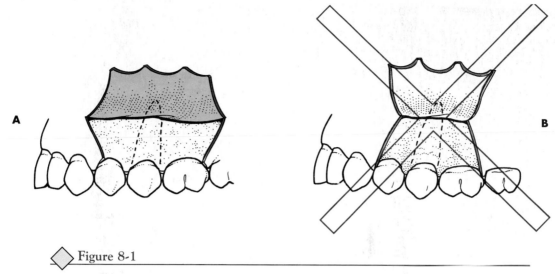

◇ Figure 8-1

A, Flap must have base that is broader than free gingival margin. **B,** If flap is too narrow at base, blood supply may be inadequate, which may lead to flap necrosis.

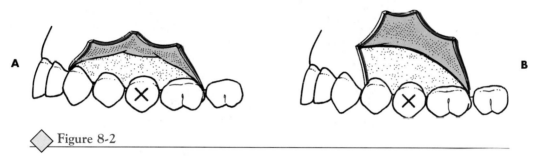

◇ Figure 8-2

A, To have sufficient access to root of second premolar, envelope flap should extend anteriorly, mesial to canine, and posteriorly, distal to first molar. **B,** If releasing incision (three-cornered flap) is used, flap extends mesial to first premolar.

surgery. In addition, the flap must be held out of the operative field by a retractor that must rest on intact bone. There must be enough flap reflection to permit the retractor to hold the flap without tension. Furthermore, soft tissue heals across the incision, not along the length of the incision, and sharp incisions heal more rapidly than torn tissue. Therefore a long, straight incision with adequate flap reflection heals more rapidly than a short, torn incision, which heals slowly by secondary intention. For an envelope flap to be of adequate size, the length of the flap in the anteroposterior dimension usually extends two teeth anterior and one tooth posterior to the area of surgery (Figure 8-2, *A*). If a relaxing incision is made, the incision should extend one tooth anterior and one tooth posterior to the area of surgery (Figure 8-2, *B*).

The flap should be a full-thickness mucoperiosteal flap. This means that the flap includes the surface mucosa, the submucosa, and the periosteum. Because the goal of the surgery is to remove or reshape the bone, all overlying tissue must be reflected from it. In addition, full-thickness flaps are necessary because the periosteum is the primary tissue

responsible for bone healing, and replacement of the periosteum in its original position hastens that healing process. Also, torn, split, and macerated tissue heals more slowly than a cleanly reflected, full-thickness flap.

The incisions that outline the flap must be made over intact bone that will be present after the surgical procedure is complete. If the pathologic condition has eroded the buccocortical plate, the incision must be at least 6 or 8 mm away from it. In addition, if bone is to be removed over a particular tooth, the incision must be sufficiently distant from it so that after the bone is removed, the incision is 6 to 8 mm away from the bony defect created by surgery. If the incision line is unsupported by sound bone, it tends to collapse into the bony defect, which results in wound dehiscence and delayed healing (Figure 8-3).

The flap should be designed to avoid injury to local vital structures in the area of the surgery. The two most important structures that can be damaged are both located in the mandible; these are the lingual nerve and the mental nerve. When making incisions in the posterior mandible, especially

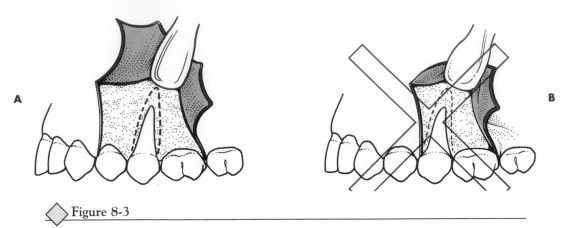

◇ Figure 8-3

A, When designing flap, it is necessary to anticipate how much bone will be removed so that after surgery is complete, incision rests over sound bone. In this situation, vertical release was one tooth anterior to bone removal and left an adequate margin of sound bone. **B,** When releasing incision is made too close to bone removal, delayed healing results.

in the region of the third molar, incisions should be well away from the lingual aspect of the mandible. In this area the lingual nerve may be closely adherent to the lingual aspect of the mandible, and incisions in this area may result in the severing of that nerve, with consequent prolonged temporary or permanent anesthesia of the tongue. In the same way, surgery in the apical area of the mandibular premolar teeth should be carefully planned and executed to avoid injury to the mental nerve. Envelope incisions should be used if at all possible, and releasing incisions should be well anterior or posterior to the area of the mental nerve.

Flaps in the maxilla rarely endanger any vital structures. On the facial aspect of the maxillary alveolar process, no nerves or arteries exist that are likely to be damaged. When reflecting a palatal flap, the dentist must remember that the major blood supply to the palate comes through the greater palatine artery, which emerges from the greater palatine foramen at the posterior lateral aspect of the hard palate. This artery courses forward and has an anastomosis with the nasopalatine artery. The nasopalatine nerves and arteries exit the incisive foramen to supply the anterior palatal gingiva. If the anterior palatal tissue must be reflected, both the artery and the nerve can be incised at the level of the foramen without much risk. There is little likelihood of bothersome bleeding, and the nerve regenerates quickly. The temporary numbness usually does not bother the patient. However, vertical releasing incisions in the posterior aspect of the palate should be avoided, because they usually sever the greater palatine artery within the tissue, which results in bleeding that may be difficult to control and that can lead to ischemic necrosis of the tissue.

Releasing incisions should be used only when necessary and not routinely. Envelope incisions usually provide the adequate visualization required for tooth extraction in most areas. When vertical releasing incisions are necessary, only a single vertical incision should be used, which is usually at the anterior end of the envelope component. The vertical releasing incision is not a straight vertical incision but is oblique, to allow the base of the flap to be broader than the free gingival margin. A vertical releasing incision should be made so that it does not cross bony prominences, such as the canine eminence. To do so would increase the likelihood of tension in the suture line, which would result in wound dehiscence.

Vertical releasing incisions should cross the free gingival margin at the line angle of a tooth and should not be directly on the facial aspect of the tooth nor directly in the papilla (Figure 8-4). Incisions that cross the free margin of the gingiva directly over the facial aspect of the tooth do not heal properly because of tension; the result is a defect in the attached gingiva. Because the facial bone is frequently quite thin, such incisions will also result in vertical clefting of the bone. Incisions that cross the gingival papilla damage the papilla unnecessarily and increase the chances for localized periodontal problems; such incisions should be avoided.

TYPES OF MUCOPERIOSTEAL FLAPS

A variety of intraoral tissue flaps can be used. The most common incision is the envelope, or sulcular, incision, which produces the envelope flap. In the dentulous patient the incision is made in the gingival sulcus to the crestal bone, through the periosteum, and the full-thickness mucoperiosteal flap is reflected apically (Figure 8-2, *A*). This usually provides sufficient access to perform the necessary surgery.

If the patient is edentulous, the envelope incision is made along the scar at the crest of the ridge. There are no vital structures in this area, and the envelope incision can be as long as is required to provide adequate access. The tissue can be reflected buccally or lingually as necessary for the removal of a mandibular torus.

If the envelope incision has a vertical releasing incision, it is a three-cornered flap, with corners at the posterior end of the envelope incision, at the inferior aspect of the vertical incision, and at the superior aspect of the vertical releasing incision

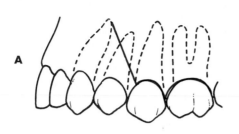
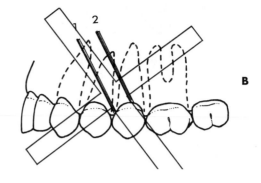

◆ Figure 8-4

A, Correct position for end of vertical releasing incision is at line angle (mesiobuccal angle in this figure) of tooth. Likewise, incision does not cross canine eminence. Crossing such bony prominences results in increased chance for wound dehiscence. **B,** These two incisions are made incorrectly. *(1)* Incision crosses prominence over canine tooth, which increases risk of delayed healing. Incision through papilla results in unnecessary damage. *(2)* Incision crosses attached gingiva directly over facial aspect of tooth, which is likely to result in soft tissue defect and periodontal deformity.

(Figure 8-5). This incision provides for greater access with a shorter envelope incision. When greater access is necessary in an apical direction, especially in the posterior aspect of the mouth, this incision is frequently necessary. The vertical component is more difficult to close and may cause some mildly prolonged healing, but if care is taken when suturing, the healing period is not noticeably lengthened.

The four-cornered flap is an envelope incision with two releasing incisions. Two corners are at the superior aspect of the releasing incision, and two corners are at either end of the envelope component of the incision (Figure 8-6). Although this flap provides substantial access in areas that have limited antero-posterior dimension, it is rarely indicated. When releasing incisions are necessary, a three-cornered flap usually suffices.

An incision that is used occasionally to approach the root apex is a semilunar incision (Figure 8-7). This incision avoids trauma to the papillae and gingival margin but provides limited access, because the entire root of the tooth is not visible. This incision is most useful for periapical surgery of a limited extent. The horizontal component of the semilunar incision should not cross major prominences, such as the canine eminence.

Two incisions are useful on the palate. The first is the Y incision, which is named for its shape. This incision is useful for surgical access to the bony palate for removal of a maxillary palatal torus. The tissue overlying the torus is usually quite thin and must be reflected carefully. The anterolateral extensions of the midline incision are anterior to the region of the canine tooth. They are anterior enough in this position that they do not sever major branches of the greater palatine artery; therefore bleeding is not usually a problem (Figure 8-8).

Another flap that is used occasionally on the palate is the pedicle flap. This flap is designed to be mobilized from one area and then rotated to fill a soft tissue defect in another area. The pedicled palatal flap is used primarily for closure of oroantral communications (see Chapter 20).

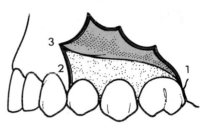

◆ Figure 8-5

Vertical releasing incision converts envelope incision into three-cornered flap.

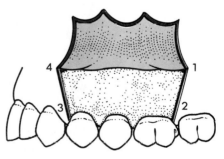

◆ Figure 8-6

Vertical releasing incisions at either end of envelope incision convert envelope incision into four-cornered flap.

TECHNIQUE FOR DEVELOPING A MUCOPERIOSTEAL FLAP

There are several specific considerations for developing flaps for surgical tooth extraction. The first step is to incise the soft tissue to allow reflection of the flap. The no. 15 blade is used in a no. 3 scalpel handle and is held in the pen grasp (Figure 8-9). The blade is held at a slight angle to the teeth, and the

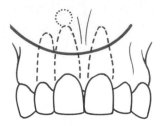

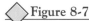Figure 8-7

Semilunar incision, designed to avoid marginal attached gingiva when working on root apex. It is most useful when only small amount of access is necessary.

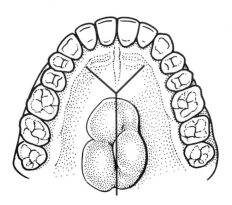

Figure 8-8

Y incision is useful on palate for adequate access to remove palatal torus. Two anterior limbs serve as releasing incisions to provide for greater access.

incision is made posteriorly to anteriorly in the gingival sulcus by drawing the knife toward the operator. One smooth continuous stroke is used while keeping the knife blade in contact with bone throughout the entire incision (Figures 8-10 and 8-11).

The scalpel blade is an extremely sharp instrument, but it dulls rapidly when it is pressed against bone, such as when making a mucoperiosteal incision. If more than one flap is to be reflected, the surgeon should change blades between incisions.

If a vertical releasing incision is made, the tissue is reflected apically, with the opposite hand tensing the alveolar mucosa so that the incision can be made cleanly through it. If the alveolar mucosa is not tensed, the knife will not incise cleanly through the mucosa, and a jagged incision will result.

Reflection of the flap begins at the papilla. The sharp end of the Woodson elevator or the no. 9 periosteal elevator begins a reflection (Figure 8-12). The sharp end is slipped underneath the papilla in the area of the incision and turned laterally to pry the papilla away from the underlying bone. This technique is used along the entire extent of the free gingival incision. If it is difficult to elevate the tissue at any one spot, the incision is probably incomplete, and that area should be reincised. Once the entire free edge of the flap has been reflected with the sharp end of the elevator, the broad end is used to reflect the mucoperiosteal flap to the extent desired.

If a three-cornered flap is used, the initial reflection is accomplished with the sharp end of the Woodson elevator on the first papilla only. Once the flap reflection is started, the broad end of the periosteal elevator is inserted at the middle corner of the flap, and the dissection is carried out with a pushing stroke, posteriorly and apically. This facili-

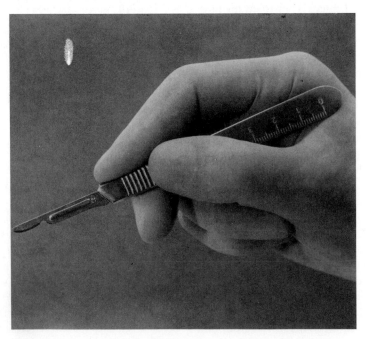

Figure 8-9

Scalpel handle is held in pen grasp for maximal control and tactile sensitivity.

tates the rapid and atraumatic reflection of the soft tissue flap (Figure 8-13).

Once the flap has been reflected the desired amount, the periosteal elevator is used as a retractor to hold the flap in its proper reflected position. To accomplish this effectively the retractor is held perpendicular to the bone tissue while resting on sound bone and not trapping soft tissue between the

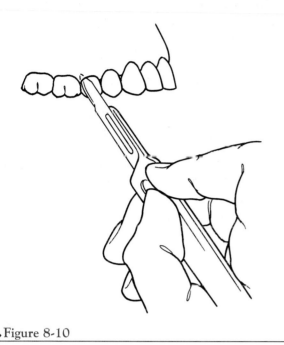

◇Figure 8-10

No. 15 blade is used to incise gingival sulcus.

retractor and bone. The periosteal elevator therefore is maintained in its proper position, and the soft tissue flap is held without tension (Figure 8-14). The Seldin elevator or the Minnesota or Austin retractors can be used in a similar fashion when broader exposure is necessary. The retractor should not be forced against the soft tissue in an attempt to pull the tissue out of the field. Instead, the retractor is positioned in the proper place and held firmly against the bone. By retracting in this fashion the surgeon can focus primarily on the surgical field and not on the retractor, and there is less chance of an inadvertent flap tear.

PRINCIPLES OF SUTURING

Once the surgical procedure is completed and the wound properly irrigated and debrided, the flap must be repositioned in its original position or in a new position if necessary and held in place with sutures. Sutures perform multiple functions. The most obvious and important function that sutures perform is to coapt wound margins; that is, to hold the flap in position and approximate the two wound edges. The sharper the incision and the less trauma inflicted on the wound margin, the more probable is healing by primary intention. If the space between the two wound edges is minimal, wound healing will be rapid and complete. If tears or excessive trauma to the wound edges occur, wound healing will be by secondary intention.

Sutures also aid in hemostasis. If the underlying tissue is bleeding, the surface mucosa or skin should not be closed, because the bleeding in the underlying tissues may continue and result in the formation of a hematoma. Surface sutures aid

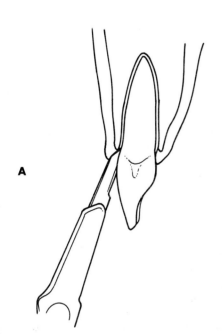

A

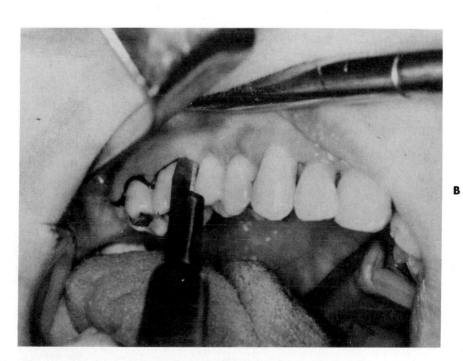

B

◇Figure 8-11

A, Knife is angled slightly away from tooth and incises soft tissue, including periosteum, at crestal bone.
B, Incision is started posteriorly and is carried anteriorly, with care taken to incise completely through interdental papilla.

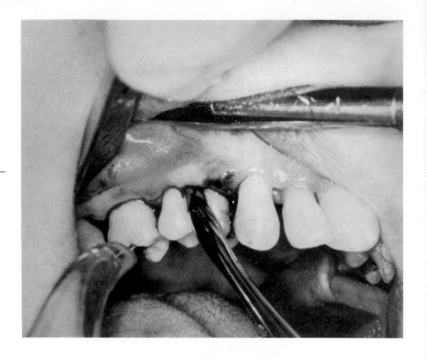

◆ **Figure 8-12**

Reflection of flap is begun by using sharp end of periosteal elevator to pry away interdental papilla.

◆ **Figure 8-13**

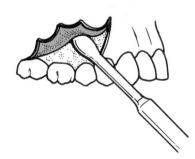

When three-cornered flap is used, only anterior papilla is reflected with sharp end of elevator. Broad end is then used with push stroke to elevate posterosuperiorly.

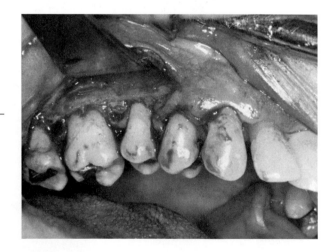

◆ **Figure 8-14**

Periosteal elevator (Seldin elevator) is used to reflect mucoperiosteal flap. Elevator placed perpendicular to bone and held in place by pushing firmly against bone, not by pushing it apically against soft tissue.

◆ **Figure 8-15**

A, Figure-eight stitch, occasionally placed over top of socket to aid in hemostasis. **B,** This is usually performed to help maintain piece of oxidized cellulose in tooth socket.

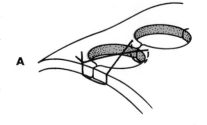

A

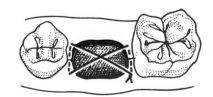

B

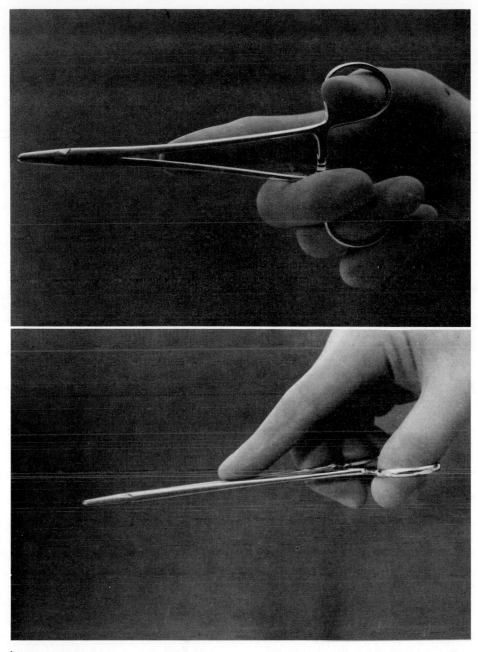

◈ Figure 8-16

Needle holder is held with thumb and ring finger. Index finger extends along instrument for stability and control.

in hemostasis but only as a tamponade in a generally oozing area, such as a tooth socket. Overlying tissue should never be sutured tightly in an attempt to gain hemostasis in a bleeding tooth socket.

Sutures help hold a soft tissue flap over bone. This is an extremely important function, because bone that is not covered with soft tissue becomes nonvital and requires an excessively long time to heal. When mucoperiosteal flaps are reflected from alveolar bone, it is important that the extent of the bone be recovered with the soft tissue flaps. Unless appropriate suture techniques are employed, the flap may retract away from the bone, which exposes it and results in delayed healing.

Sutures may aid in maintaining a blood clot in the alveolar socket. A special stitch, such as a figure-eight stitch, can provide a barrier to clot displacement (Figure 8-15). However, it should be emphasized that suturing across an open wound socket plays a minor role in maintaining the blood clot in the tooth socket.

The armamentarium includes a needle holder, a suture needle, and suture material. The needle holder of choice is 15 cm in length and has a locking handle. It is held with the thumb and ring finger through the rings and with the index finger along the length of the needle holder to provide stability and control (Figure 8-16).

The suture needle usually used in the mouth is a small ⅜

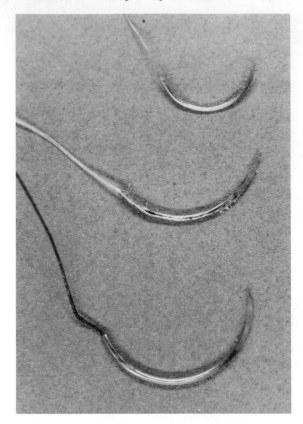

Figure 8-17

Needle used in oral surgery is ⅜ circle cutting needle. Middle needle is F5-2, and lower needle is X-1.

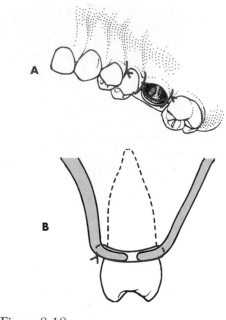

Figure 8-18

A, Flap held in place with sutures in papillae. **B,** Cross-sectional view of suture.

to ½ circle with a reverse cutting edge. The cutting edge helps the needle pass through the relatively tough mucoperiosteal flap. Needle sizes and shapes have been assigned numbers. The most common needle shapes used in oral surgery are the FS-2 and X-1 (Figure 8-17).

The suture material most commonly used in the mouth is black silk. This is a nonresorbable, multifilament, dyed material that is easy to see, is well tolerated by the soft tissue and tongue, is easy to tie, and does not come untied easily. Alternative materials are plain and chromic catgut. These are both resorbable and do not require removal by the surgeon. The usual suture size used in the mouth is 3-0. Some surgeons prefer 4-0 suture.

The technique used for suturing is deceptively difficult. The use of the needle holder and the technique that is necessary to pass the curved needle through the tissue are difficult to learn. The following discussion presents the technique employed in suturing; practice is necessary before suturing can be performed with skill and finesse.

When the envelope flap is repositioned into its correct location, it is held in place with sutures that are placed through the papillae only. Sutures are not placed across the empty tooth socket, because the edges of the wound would not be supported over sound bone (Figure 8-18). When reapproximating the flap, the suture is passed first through

the mobile (usually facial) tissue; the needle is regrasped with the needle holder and passed through the attached tissue of the lingual papilla. If the two margins of the wound are close together, the experienced surgeon may be able to insert the needle through both sides of the wound in a single pass. However, it is best to use two passes in most situations (Figure 8-19).

When passing the needle through the tissue, the needle should enter the surface of the mucosa at a right angle, to make the smallest possible hole in the mucosal flap (Figure 8-20). If the needle passes through the tissue obliquely, the suture will tear through the surface layers of the flap when the suture knot is tied, which results in greater injury to the soft tissue.

When passing the needle through the flap, the surgeon must ensure that an adequate bite of tissue is taken, to prevent the suture from pulling through the soft tissue flap. Because the flap that is being sutured is a mucoperiosteal flap and should not be tied tightly, a relatively small amount of tissue is necessary. The minimal amount of tissue between the suture and the edge of the flap should be 3 mm. Once the sutures are passed through both the mobile flap and the immobile lingual tissue, they are tied with an instrument tie (Figure 8-21).

The surgeon must remember that the purpose of the stitch is merely to reapproximate the tissue, and therefore the suture should not be tied too tightly. Sutures that are too tight cause ischemia of the flap margin and result in tissue necrosis, with tearing of the suture through the tissue. Thus sutures that are too tightly tied result in wound dehiscence more frequently than sutures that are loosely tied. As a clinical guideline, there should be no blanching or obvious ischemia of the wound edges. If this occurs, the suture should be removed and replaced. The knot should be positioned so that it does not fall

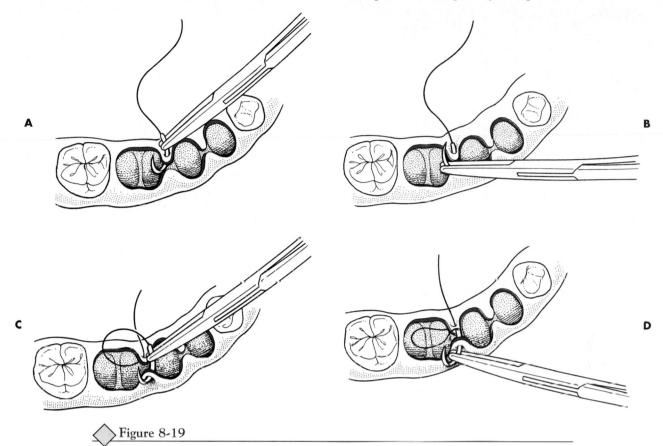

Figure 8-19

When mucosal flap is back in position, suture is passed through two sides of socket in separate passes of needle. **A,** Needle is held by needle holder and passed through papilla, usually of mobile tissue first. **B,** Needle holder is then released from needle; it regrasps needle on underside of tissue and is turned through flap. **C,** Needle is then passed through opposite side of soft tissue papilla in similar fashion. **D,** Finally, needle holder grasps needle on opposite side to complete passing of suture through both sides of mucosa.

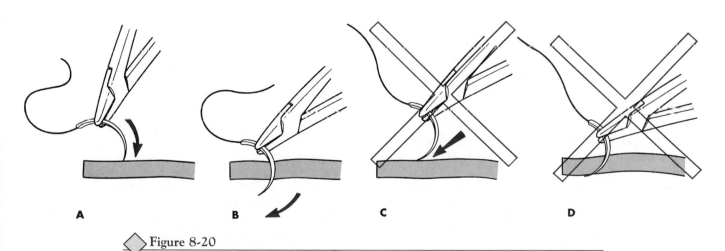

Figure 8-20

When passing through soft tissue of mucosa, needle should enter surface of tissue at right angle **(A). B,** Needle holder should be turned so that needle passes easily through tissue at right angles. **C,** If needle enters soft tissue at acute angle and is pushed rather than turned through tissue, tearing of mucosa with needle or with suture is likely to occur **(D).**

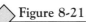

◇ Figure 8-21

Most intraoral sutures are tied with instrument tie. **A,** Suture is pulled through tissue until short tail of suture (approximately 1½ to 2 inches long) remains. Needle holder is held horizontally by right hand in preparation for knot-tying procedure. **B,** Left hand then wraps long end of suture around needle holder twice in clockwise direction to make two loops of suture around needle holder. **C,** Surgeon then opens needle holder and grasps short end of suture near its end. **D,** Ends of suture are then pulled to tighten knot. Needle holder should not pull at all until knot is nearly tied, to avoid lengthening that portion of suture.

Continued

over the incision line, because this causes additional pressure on the incision. Therefore the knot should be positioned to the side of the incision.

If a three-cornered flap is used, the vertical end of the incision must be closed separately. Two sutures usually are required to close the vertical end properly. Before the sutures are inserted, the Woodson periosteal elevator should be used to elevate slightly the nonflap side of the incision, freeing the margin to facilitate passage of the needle through the tissue (Figure 8-22). The first suture is placed across the papilla, where the vertical release incision was made. This is a known, easily identifiable landmark that is most important when repositioning a three-cornered flap. The remainder of the envelope portion of the incision is then closed, followed by closure of the vertical component. The slight reflection of the nonflap side of the incision greatly eases the placing of sutures.

The sutures are left in place for approximately 5 to 7 days. After this time they play no useful role and, in fact, probably increase the contamination of the underlying submucosa. When sutures are removed, the surface debris that has collected on them should be cleaned off with a cotton-tipped applicator stick soaked in peroxide, chlorhexidine, iodophor, or other antiseptic solution. The suture is cut with sharp,

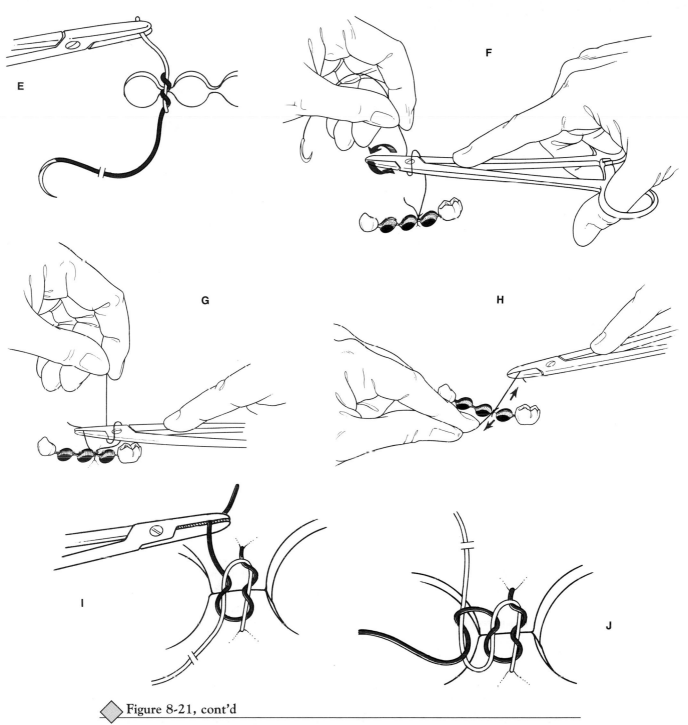

⬦ Figure 8-21, cont'd

E, End of first step of surgeon's knot. Note that double wrap has resulted in double overhand knot. This increases friction in knot and will keep wound edges together until second portion of knot is tied. **F,** Needle holder is then released from short end of suture and held in same position as when knot-tying procedure began. Left hand then makes single wrap in counterclockwise direction. **G,** Needle holder then grasps short end of suture at its end. **H,** This portion of knot is completed by pulling this loop firmly down against previous portion of knot. **I,** This completes surgeon's knot. Double loop of first pass holds tissue together until second portion of square knot can be tied. **J,** Most surgeons add third throw to their instrument tie. Needle holder is repositioned in original position, and one wrap is placed around needle holder in original clockwise direction. Short end of suture is grasped and tightened down firmly to form second square knot. Final throw of three knots is tightened firmly.

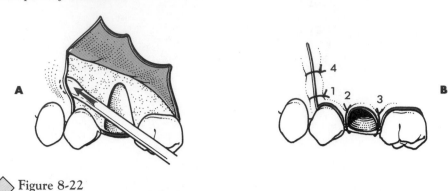

◇ Figure 8-22
_____

A, To make the suturing of three-cornered flap easier, Woodson elevator is used to elevate small amount of fixed tissue so that suture can be passed through entire thickness of mucoperiosteum. **B,** When three-cornered flap is repositioned, first suture is placed at occlusal end of vertical releasing incision. Papillae are then sutured sequentially, and finally, if necessary, superior aspect of releasing incision is sutured.

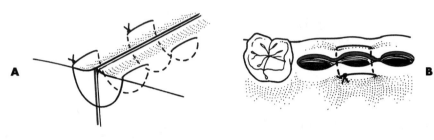

◇ Figure 8-23
_____

A, Horizontal mattress suture is sometimes used to close soft tissue wounds. Use of this suture decreases number of individual sutures that have to be placed but, more important, compresses wound together slightly and everts wound edges. **B,** Single horizontal mattress suture can be placed across both papillae of tooth socket and serves as two individual sutures.

pointed suture scissors and removed by pulling it toward the incision line (not away from the suture line).

There are many configurations of sutures. The simple interrupted suture is the one most commonly used in the oral cavity. This suture simply goes through one side of the wound, comes up through the other side of the wound, and is tied in a knot at the top. These sutures can be placed relatively quickly, and the tension on each suture can be adjusted individually. If one suture is lost, the remaining sutures stay in position.

A suture technique that is useful for suturing two papillae with a single stitch is the horizontal mattress suture (Figure 8-23). A slight variation of that suture is the figure-eight suture, which holds the two papilla in position and puts a cross over the top of the socket so that may help hold the blood clot in position (see Figure 8-15).

If the incision is long, continuous sutures can be used efficiently. When using this technique, a knot does not have to be made for each stitch, which makes it quicker to suture a long-span incision. The continuous simple suture can be either locking or nonlocking (Figure 8-24). The horizontal mattress suture also can be used in a running fashion. A disadvantage of the continuous suture is that if one suture pulls through, the entire suture line becomes loose.

PRINCIPLES AND TECHNIQUES FOR SURGICAL EXTRACTION ───────────◇

Surgical extraction of an erupted tooth is a technique that should not be reserved for the extreme situation. A prudently employed open extraction technique may be more conservative and cause less operative morbidity than a closed extraction. Forceps extraction techniques that require great force may result not only in removal of the tooth but also of large amounts of associated bone and occasionally the floor of the maxillary sinus (Figure 8-25). If a soft tissue flap is reflected and a proper amount of bone removed or if the tooth is sectioned, the bone loss may be less. The morbidity of fragments of bone that are literally torn from the jaw by the

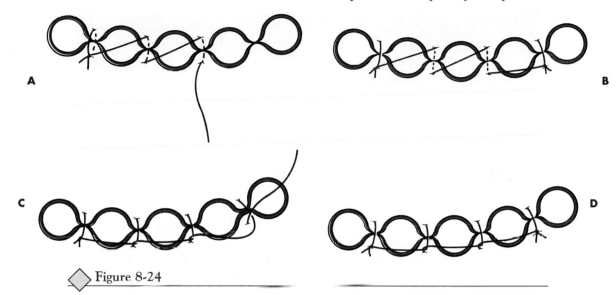

A

B

C

D

◆ Figure 8-24

When multiple sutures are to be placed, incision can be closed with running or continuous suture. **A,** First papilla is closed and knot tied in usual way. Long end of suture is held, and adjacent papilla is sutured, without knot being tied but just with suture being pulled firmly through tissue. **B,** Succeeding papillae are then sutured until final one is sutured and final knot is tied. Final appearance is with suture going across each empty socket. **C,** Continuous locking stitch can be made by passing long end of suture underneath loop before it is pulled through tissue. **D,** This puts suture on both deep periosteal and mucosal surfaces directly across papilla and may aid in more direct apposition of tissues.

conservative closed technique exceeds by far the morbidity of controlled surgical extraction.

INDICATIONS FOR SURGICAL EXTRACTION

It is prudent for the surgeon to evaluate carefully each patient and each tooth to be removed for the possibility of an open extraction. Although the vast majority of decisions will be to perform a closed extraction, the surgeon must be aware continually that open extraction may be the less morbid of the two.

As a general guideline, surgeons should consider performing an elective surgical extraction when they perceive a possible need for excessive force to extract a tooth. The term *excessive* means that the force will probably result in a fracture of bone, a tooth root, or both. In any case the excessive bone loss, the need for additional surgery to retrieve the root, or both can cause undue morbidity. The following are examples of situations in which closed extraction may require excessive force.

The dentist should strongly consider performing an open extraction after initial attempts at forceps extraction have failed. Instead of applying unnecessarily great amounts of force that may not be controlled, the surgeon should simply reflect a soft tissue flap, section the tooth, remove some bone, and extract the tooth in sections. In these situations the philosophy of "divide and conquer" results in the most efficient extraction.

If the preoperative assessment reveals that the patient has heavy or especially dense bone, particularly on the bucco-cortical plate, surgical extraction should be considered (Figure 8-26). The extraction of most teeth depends on the expansion

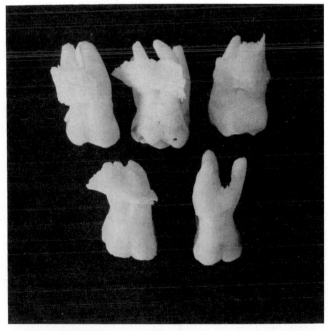

◆ Figure 8-25

Forceps extraction of these teeth resulted in removal of bone and tooth instead of just tooth.

of the buccocortical plate. If this bone is especially heavy, adequate expansion is less likely to occur, and fracture of the root is more likely. Dense bone in the older patient warrants even more caution. Whereas young patients have bone that is more elastic and more likely to expand with controlled force,

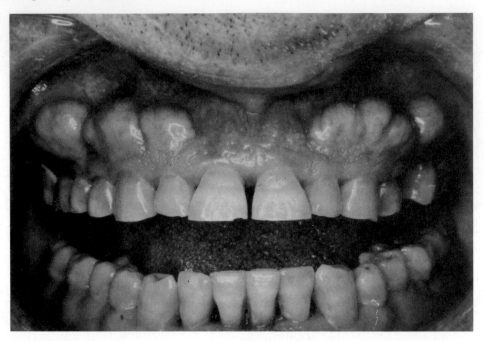

◇ **Figure 8-26**

Heavy buccal plate suggests difficult forceps extraction. This may be easier if performed by open technique.

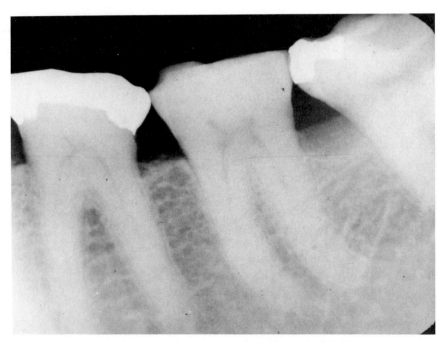

◇ **Figure 8-27**

Teeth that exhibit evidence of bruxism may have denser bone and stronger periodontal ligame attachment, which make them more difficult to extract.

older patients usually have denser, more highly calcified bone that is less likely to provide adequate expansion during luxation of the tooth.

Occasionally, the dentist treats a patient who has very short clinical crowns with evidence of severe attrition. If such attrition is the result of bruxism, or a grinding habit, it is likely that the teeth are surrounded by dense, heavy bone with strong periodontal ligament attachment (Figure 8-27). The surgeon should exercise extreme caution if removal of such teeth is attempted with a closed technique. An open technique usually results in a quicker, easier extraction.

Careful review of the preoperative radiographs may reveal

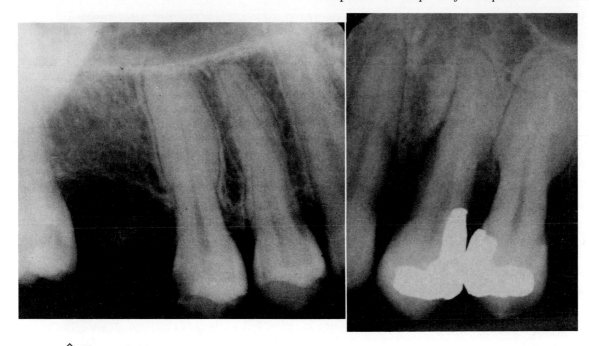

◇ Figure 8-28

Hypercementosis of root makes forceps delivery difficult.

tooth roots that are likely to cause difficulty if the tooth is extracted by the standard forceps technique. One condition commonly seen among older patients is hypercementosis. In this situation, cementum has continued to be deposited on the tooth and has formed a large bulbous root that is difficult to remove through the available tooth socket opening. Great force used to expand the bone may result in fracture of the root or buccocortical bone and in a more difficult extraction procedure (Figure 8-28).

Roots that are widely divergent, especially the maxillary first molar roots (Figure 8-29) or roots that have severe dilaceration or hooks, also are difficult to remove without fracturing one or more of the roots (Figure 8-30). By reflecting a soft tissue flap and dividing the roots prospectively with a bur, a more controlled and planned extraction can be performed and will result in less morbidity overall.

If the maxillary sinus has expanded to include the roots of the maxillary molars, extraction may result in removal of a portion of the sinus floor along with the tooth. If the roots are divergent, such a situation is even more likely to occur (Figure 8-31).

Teeth that have crowns with extensive caries, especially root caries, or that have large amalgam restorations are candidates for open extraction (Figure 8-32). Although the tooth is grasped primarily by the root, a portion of the force is applied to the crown. Such pressures can crush and shatter the crowns of teeth with extensive caries or large restorations. Open extraction can circumvent the need for extensive force and result in a quicker, easier extraction. Teeth with crowns that have already been lost to caries and that present as retained roots should also be considered for open extraction.

If there is extensive periodontal disease around such teeth, it may be possible to deliver them easily with straight elevators or Cryer elevators. However, if the bone is firm around the tooth and there is no periodontal disease, the surgeon should consider an open extraction.

Technique for Open Extraction of Single-Rooted Tooth

The technique for open extraction of a single-rooted tooth is relatively straightforward but requires attention to detail, because several decisions must be made during the operation. Single-rooted teeth are those that have resisted attempts at closed extraction or that have fractured at the cervical line and therefore exist only as a root. The technique is essentially the same for both.

The first step is to provide adequate visualization and access by reflecting a sufficiently large mucoperiosteal flap. In most situations an envelope flap that is extended two teeth anterior and one tooth posterior to the tooth to be removed is sufficient. If a releasing incision is necessary, it should be placed at least one tooth anterior to the extraction site (see Figure 8-2).

Once an adequate flap has been reflected and is held in its proper position by a periosteal elevator, the surgeon must determine the need for bone removal. There are several options at this point. First, the surgeon may attempt to reseat the extraction forceps under direct visualization and therefore achieve a better mechanical advantage and remove the tooth with no bone removal at all (Figure 8-33).

The second option is to grasp a bit of buccal bone under the buccal beak of the forceps to obtain a better mechanical

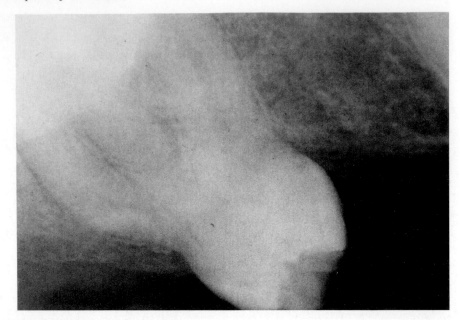

◇ Figure 8-29

Widely divergent roots increase likelihood of fracture of bone, tooth root, or both.

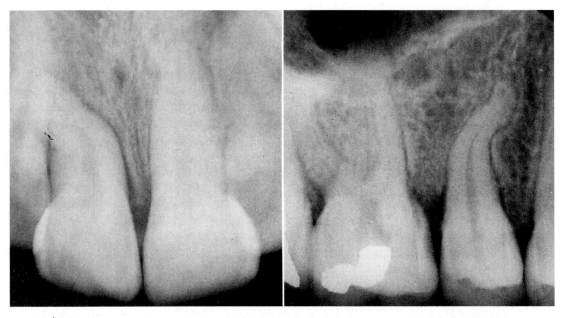

◇ Figure 8-30

Severe dilaceration of roots may result in fracture of root unless surgical extraction is performed.

advantage and grasp of the tooth root. This may allow the surgeon to luxate the tooth sufficiently to remove it without any additional bone removal (Figure 8-34). A small amount of buccal bone is pinched off and removed with the tooth.

The third option is to use the straight elevator as a shoehorn elevator by forcing it down the periodontal ligament space of the tooth. (Figure 8-35). The index finger of the surgeon's

hand must support the force of the elevator so that the total movement is controlled and no slippage of the elevator occurs. A small wiggling motion should be used to help expand the periodontal ligament space, which allows the small straight elevator to enter the space and act as a wedge to displace the root occlusally.

The final option is to proceed with bone removal over the

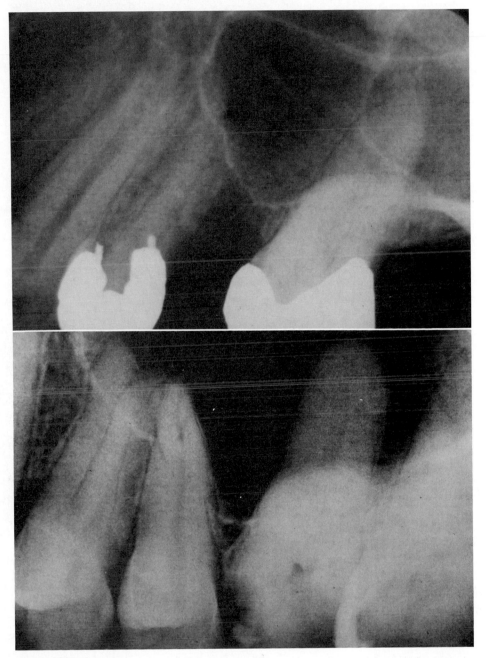

◇ Figure 8-31

Maxillary molar teeth "in" floor of maxillary sinus increase chance of fracture of sinus floor, with resulting sinus perforation.

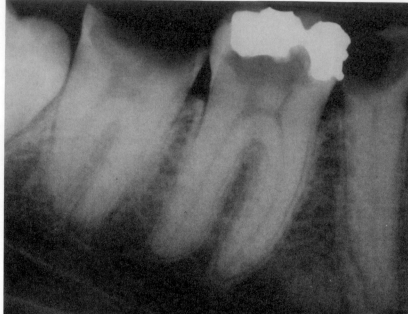

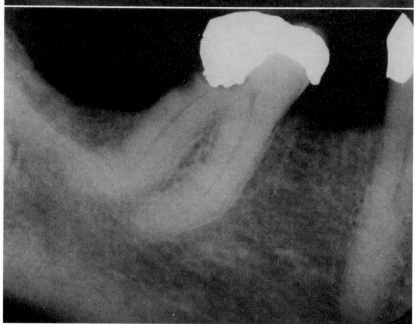

 Figure 8-32

Large caries or large restorations may lead to fracture of crown of tooth and therefore to more difficult extraction.

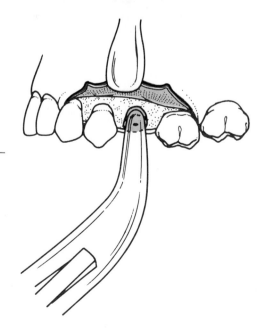

 Figure 8-33

Small envelope flap can be reflected to expose fractured root. Under direct visualization, forceps can be seated more apically into periodontal ligament space, which eliminates need for bone removal.

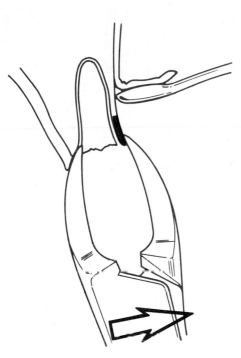

◇ **Figure 8-34**

If root is fractured at level of bone, buccal beak of forceps can be used to remove small portion of bone at same time that it grasps root.

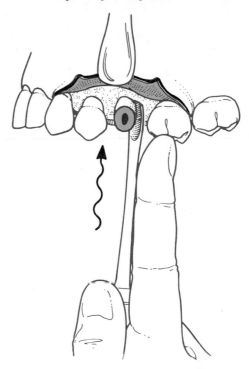

◇ **Figure 8-35**

Small straight elevator can be used as shoehorn to luxate broken root. When straight elevator is used in this position, hand must be securely supported on adjacent teeth to prevent inadvertent slippage of instrument from tooth and subsequent injury to adjacent tissue.

area of the tooth. The surgeon who makes the decision to remove some buccal bone from the tooth may use either the bur or the chisel. If the bone is thin, a chisel is convenient and frequently requires hand pressure only. However, most surgeons currently prefer a bur to remove the bone. The width of buccal bone that is removed is essentially the same width as the tooth in a mesiodistal direction (Figure 8-36). In a vertical dimension, bone should be removed approximately one-half to two-thirds the length of the tooth root (Figure 8-37). This amount of bone removal sufficiently reduces the amount of force necessary to displace the tooth and makes removal relatively easy. Either a small straight elevator (Figure 8-38) or a forceps can be used to remove the tooth (Figure 8-39).

If the tooth is still difficult to extract after removal of bone, a purchase point can be made in the root with the bur at the most apical portion of the area of bone removal (Figure 8-40). This hole should be about 3 mm in diameter and depth to allow the insertion of an instrument. A heavy elevator, such as a Crane pick, can be used to elevate or lever the tooth from its socket (Figure 8-41).

The bone edges should be checked; if sharp, they should be smoothed with a bone file. Edge sharpness is checked by replacing the soft tissue flap and gently palpating it with a finger. Removal of bone with a rongeur is rarely indicated, because it tends to remove too much bone.

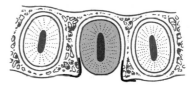

◇ **Figure 8-36**

When removing bone from buccal surface of tooth or tooth root to facilitate removal of that root, mesiodistal width of bone removal should be approximately same as mesiodistal dimension of tooth root itself. This allows unimpeded path for removal of root in buccal direction.

Once the tooth is delivered, the entire surgical field should be thoroughly irrigated with copious amounts of saline. Special attention should be directed toward the most inferior portion of the flap (where it joins the bone), because this is a common place for debris to settle, especially in mandibular extractions. If the debris is not removed carefully by curettage or irrigation, it can cause delayed healing or even a small subperiosteal abscess in the ensuing 3 to 4 weeks. The flap is then set in its original position and sutured into place with 3-0 black silk sutures.

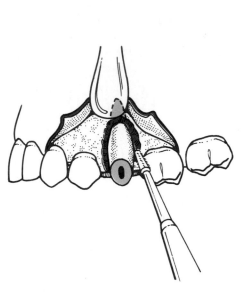

◆ **Figure 8-37**

Bone is removed with bone-cutting bur after reflection of standard envelope flap. Bone should be removed approximately one half to two thirds length of tooth root.

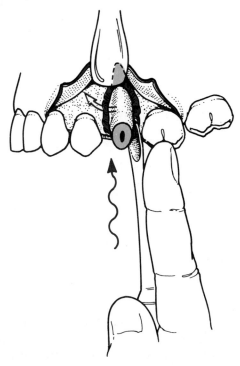

◆ **Figure 8-38**

Once appropriate amount of buccal bone has been removed, shoe-horn elevator can be used down palatal aspect of tooth to displace tooth root in buccal direction. It is important to remember that when elevator is used in this direction, surgeon's hand must be firmly supported on adjacent teeth to prevent slippage of instrument and injury to adjacent soft tissues.

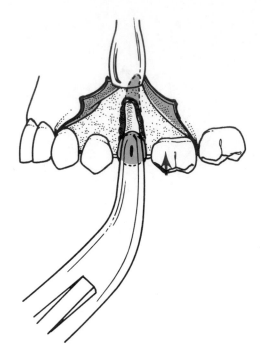

◆ **Figure 8-39**

After bone has been removed and tooth root luxated with straight elevator, forceps can be used to remove root.

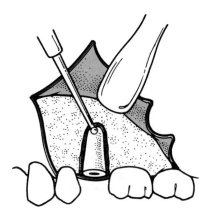

◆ **Figure 8-40**

If tooth root is quite solid in bone, buccal bone can be removed and purchase point made for insertion of elevator.

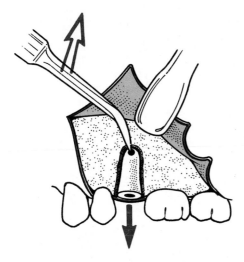

◇ Figure 8-41

Stout elevator, such as Crane pick, is then inserted into purchase point, and tooth is elevated from its socket.

TECHNIQUE FOR SURGICAL REMOVAL OF MULTIROOTED TEETH

If the decision is made to perform an open extraction of a multirooted tooth, such as a mandibular or maxillary molar, the same surgical technique employed for the single-rooted tooth is generally used. The major difference is that the tooth may be divided with a bur to convert a multirooted tooth into several single-rooted teeth. If the crown of the tooth remains intact, the crown portion is sectioned in such a way as to facilitate removal of roots. However, if the crown portion of the tooth is missing and only the roots remain, the goal is to separate the roots to make them easier to remove with elevators.

Removal of the lower first molar with an intact crown is usually done by sectioning the tooth buccolingually and thereby dividing the tooth into a mesial half (with mesial root and half of the crown) and a distal half. An envelope incision is also made, and a small amount of crestal bone is removed. Once the tooth is sectioned, it is luxated with straight elevators to begin the mobilization process. The sectioned tooth is treated as a lower premolar tooth and is removed with a lower universal forceps. The flap is repositioned and sutured (Figure 8-42).

The surgical technique begins with the reflection of an adequate flap (Figure 8-43, A and B). The surgeon selects either an envelope or three-cornered flap as the requirement for access and personal preference dictate. Evaluation of the need for sectioning roots and removing bone is made at this stage, as it was with the single-rooted tooth. Occasionally forceps, elevators, or both are positioned with direct visualization to achieve better mechanical advantage and to remove the tooth without removing the bone.

However, in most situations a small amount of crestal bone should be removed, and the tooth should be divided. Tooth sectioning is usually accomplished with a straight handpiece with a straight bur, such as the no. 8 round bur, or with a fissure bur, such as the no. 557 or no. 703 bur (Figure 8-43, C).

Once the tooth is sectioned, the small straight elevator is used to luxate and mobilize the sectioned roots (Figure 8-43, D). The straight elevator may be used to actually deliver the mobilized sectioned tooth (Figure 8-43, E). If the crown of the tooth is sectioned, upper or lower universal forceps are used to remove the individual portions of the sectioned tooth (Figure 8-43, F). If the crown is missing, then straight and triangular elevators are employed to elevate the tooth roots from the sockets. Sometimes a remaining root may be difficult to remove, and additional bone removal (as is described for a single-rooted tooth) may be necessary. Occasionally it is necessary to prepare a purchase point with the bur and to use an elevator, such as the Crane pick, to elevate the remaining root.

After the tooth and all the root fragments have been removed, the flap is repositioned and the surgical area palpated for sharp bony edges. If any are present, they are smoothed with a bone file. The wound is thoroughly irrigated and debrided of loose fragments of tooth, bone, calculus, and other debris. The flap is repositioned again and sutured in the usual fashion (Figure 8-43, G).

An alternative method for removing the lower first molar is to reflect the soft tissue flap and remove sufficient buccal bone to expose the bifurcation. Then the bur is used to section the mesial root from the tooth and convert the molar into a single-rooted tooth (Figure 8-44). The crown with the mesial root intact is extracted with no. 17 lower molar forceps. The remaining mesial root is elevated from the socket with a Cryer elevator. The elevator is inserted into the empty tooth socket and rotated, using the wheel-and-axle principle. The sharp tip of the elevator engages the cementum of the remaining root, which is elevated occlusally from the socket. If the interradicular bone is heavy, the first rotation or two of the Cryer elevator removes the bone, which allows the elevator to engage the cementum of the tooth on the second or third rotation.

If the crown of the mandibular molar has been lost, the procedure again begins with the reflection of an envelope flap and removal of a small amount of crestal bone. The bur is used to section the two roots into mesial and distal components (Figure 8-45, A). The small straight elevator is used to mobilize and luxate the mesial root, which is delivered from its socket by insertion of the Cryer elevator into the slot prepared by the dental bur (Figure 8-45, B). The Cryer elevator is rotated in the wheel-and-axle manner, and the mesial root is delivered occlusally from the tooth socket. The opposite member of the paired Cryer instruments is inserted into the empty root socket and rotated through the interradicular bone to engage and deliver the remaining root (Figure 8-45, C).

Extraction of maxillary molars with widely divergent buccal and palatal roots that require excessive force to extract can be removed more prudently by dividing the root into several sections. This three-rooted tooth must be divided in a pattern different from that of the two-rooted mandibular

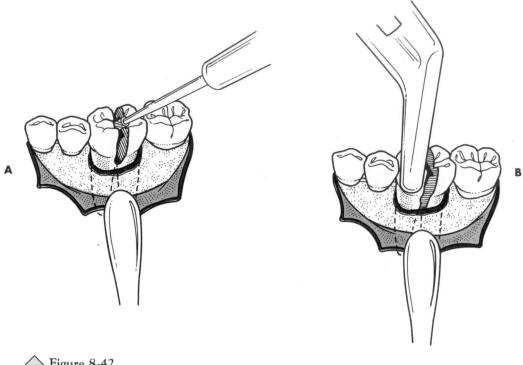

◇ **Figure 8-42**

If lower molar is difficult to extract, it can be sectioned into single-rooted teeth. **A,** Envelope incision is reflected, and small amount of crestal bone is removed to expose bifurcation. Drill is then used to section the tooth into mesial and distal halves. **B,** Lower universal forceps is used to remove two crown-root portions separately.

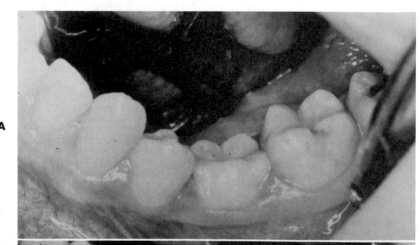

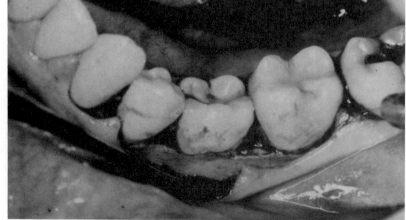

◇ **Figure 8-43**

A, This primary second molar cannot be removed by closed technique because of tipping of adjacent teeth into occlusal path of withdrawal and of high likelihood of ankylosis. **B,** Envelope incision is made, extending two teeth anteriorly and one tooth posteriorly.

Continued

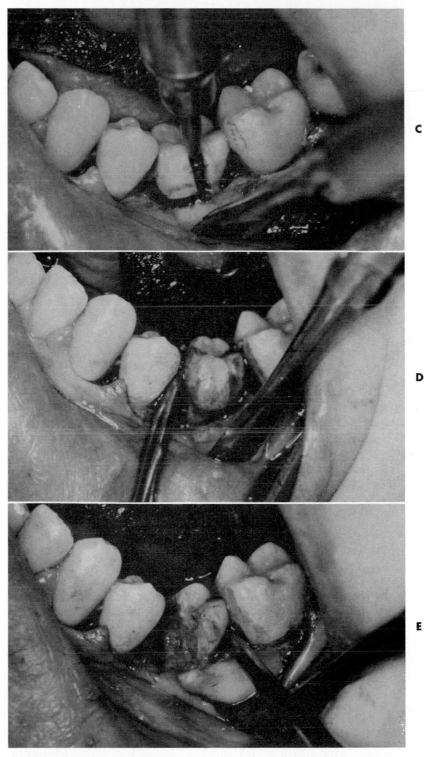

◇ Figure 8-43, cont'd

C, Small amount of crestal bone is removed, and tooth is sectioned into two portions with bur. **D,** Small straight elevator is used to luxate and deliver mesial portion of crown and mesial root. **E,** Distal portion is luxated with small straight elevator. *Continued*

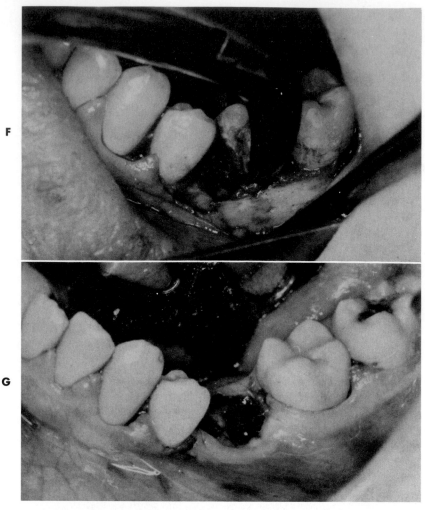

◆ Figure 8-43, cont'd

F, No. 151 forceps is used to deliver remaining portion of tooth. **G,** Wound is irrigated and flap approximated with gut sutures in papillae.

molar. If the crown of the tooth is intact, the two buccal roots are sectioned from the tooth, and the crown is removed along with the palatal root.

The standard envelope flap is reflected, and a small portion of crestal bone is removed to expose the trifurcation area. The bur is used to section off the mesiobuccal and distobuccal roots (Figure 8-46, *A*). With gentle but firm bucco-occlusal pressure, the upper molar forceps delivers the crown and palatal root along the long axis of the root (Figure 8-46, *B*). No palatal force should be delivered with the forceps to the crown portion, because this results in fracture of the palatal root. The entire delivery force should be in the buccal direction. A small straight elevator is then used to luxate the buccal roots (Figure 8-46, *C*), which can then be delivered either with a Cryer elevator used in the usual fashion (Figure 8-46, *D*) or with a straight elevator. If straight elevators are used, the surgeon should remember that the maxillary sinus may be very close to these roots, so apically directed forces must be kept to a minimum and carefully controlled. The

entire force of the straight elevator should be in a mesiodistal direction, and slight pressure should be applied apically.

If the crown of the maxillary molar is missing or fractured, the roots should be divided into two buccal roots and a palatal root. The same general approach as before is used. An envelope flap is reflected and retracted with a periosteal elevator. A moderate amount of buccal bone is removed to expose the tooth for sectioning (Figure 8-47, *A*). The roots are sectioned into the two buccal roots and a single palatal root. Next the roots are luxated with a straight elevator and delivered with Cryer elevators, according to the preference of the surgeon (Figure 8-47, *B* and *C*). Occasionally, there is enough access to the roots so that a maxillary root forceps or upper universal forceps can be used to deliver the roots independently (Figure 8-47, *D*). Finally, the palatal root is delivered after the two buccal roots have been removed. The small straight elevator can be used efficiently for this, because there is usually much loss of interradicular bone by this time. The elevator is forced down the periodontal ligament space on

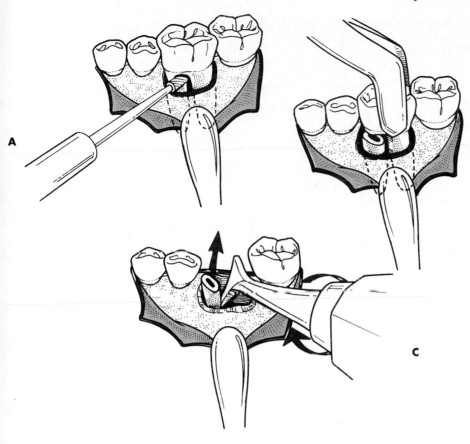

◇ **Figure 8-44**

A, Alternative method of sectioning is to use bur to remove mesial root from first molar. **B,** No. 17 forceps is then used to grasp crown of tooth and remove the crown and distal root. **C,** Cryer elevator is then used to remove mesial root. Its point is inserted into empty socket of distal root and turned in wheel-and-axle fashion, with sharp point engaging interseptal bone and root and elevating mesial root from its socket.

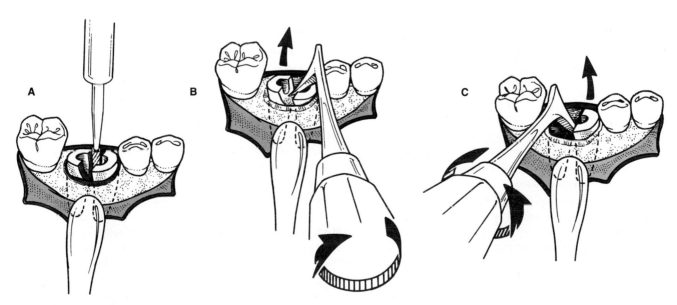

◇ **Figure 8-45**

A, When crown of lower molar is lost because of fracture or caries, small envelope flap is reflected, and small amount of crestal bone is removed. Bur is then used to section tooth into two individual roots. **B,** After small straight elevator has been used to mobilize roots, Cryer elevator is used to elevate distal root. Tip of elevator is placed into slot prepared by bur, and elevator is turned to deliver the root. **C,** Opposite member of paired Cryer elevators is then used to deliver remaining tooth root with same type of rotational movement.

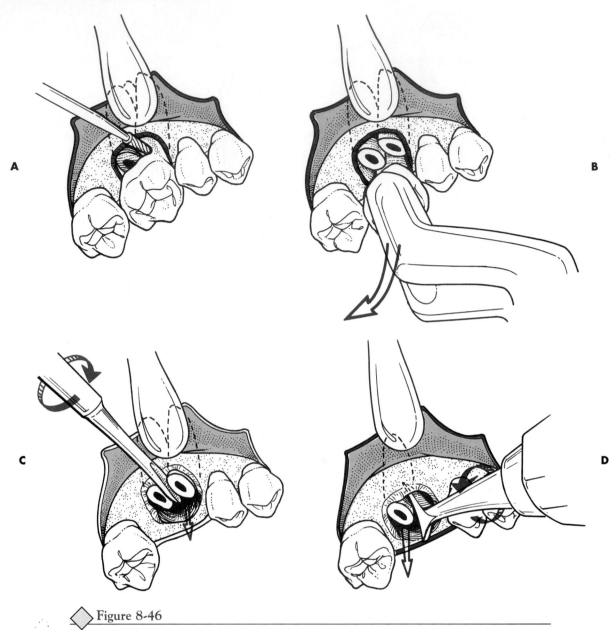

◇ Figure 8-46

A, When intact maxillary molar must be divided for judicious removal (as when there is extreme divergence of roots), small envelope incision is made, and small amount of crestal bone is removed. This allows bur to be used to section buccal roots from crown portion of tooth. **B,** Upper molar forceps is then used to remove crown portion of tooth along with palatal root. Tooth is delivered in bucco-occlusal direction, and no palatal pressure is used, because it would probably cause fracture of palatal root from crown portion. **C,** Straight elevator is then used to mobilize buccal roots and can occasionally be used to deliver these roots. **D,** Cryer elevator can be used in usual fashion by placing tip of elevator into empty socket and rotating it to deliver remaining root.

the palatal aspect with gentle, controlled wiggling motions, which causes displacement of the tooth in the bucco-occlusal direction (Figure 8-47, *E*).

REMOVAL OF SMALL ROOT FRAGMENTS AND ROOT TIPS

If fracture of the apical one third (3 to 4 mm) of the root occurs during a closed extraction, an orderly procedure should be used to remove the root tip from the socket. Initial attempts

should be made to extract the root fragment by a closed technique, but the surgeon should begin a surgical technique if the closed technique is not immediately successful. Whichever technique is chosen, the following two requirements for extraction are of critical importance: excellent light and excellent suction, preferably with a suction tip of small diameter. It is impossible to remove a small root tip fragment unless the surgeon can clearly visualize it. It is also important that an irrigation syringe be available to irrigate blood and

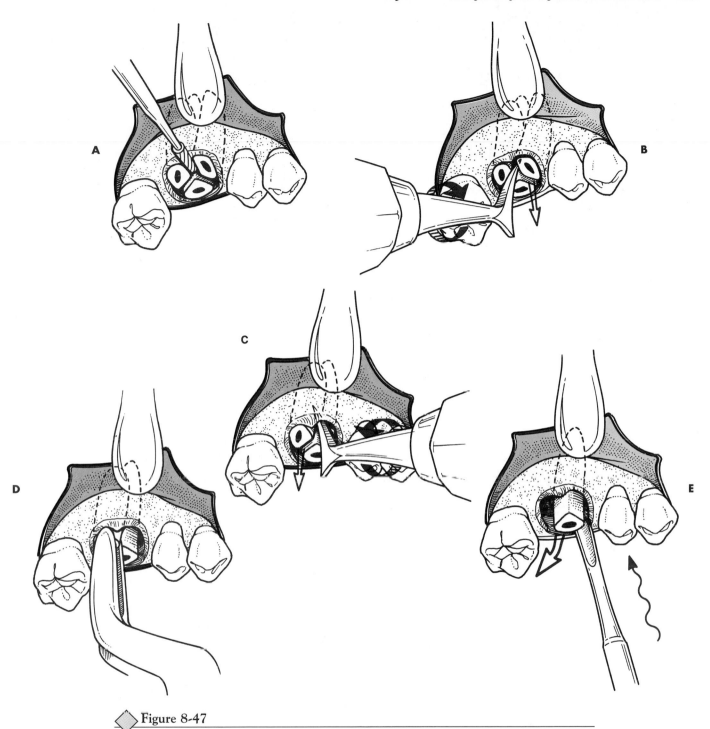

⬧ Figure 8-47

A, If crown of upper molar has been lost to caries or has been fractured from roots, small envelope incision is reflected, and small amount of crestal bone is removed. Bur is then used to section three roots into independent portions. **B,** After roots have been luxated with small straight elevator, mesiobuccal root is delivered with Cryer elevator placed into slot prepared by bur. **C,** Once mesiobuccal root has been removed, Cryer elevator is again used to deliver distal buccal root. Tip of Cryer elevator is placed into empty socket of mesiobuccal root and turned in usual fashion to deliver tooth root. **D,** Maxillary root forceps can occasionally be used to grasp and deliver remaining root. Palatal root can then be delivered either with straight elevator or with Cryer elevator. If straight elevator is used, it is placed between root and palatal bone and gently wiggled in effort to displace palatal root in bucco-occlusal direction. **E,** Small straight elevator can be used to elevate and displace remaining root of maxillary third molar in bucco-occlusal direction with gentle wiggling pressures.

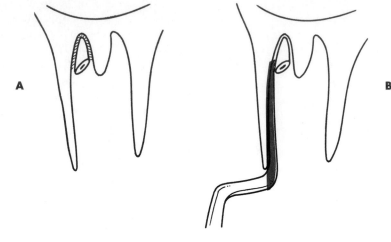

◇ **Figure 8-48**

A, When small (2 to 4 mm) portion of root apex is fractured from tooth, root tip pick can be used to retrieve it. **B,** Root tip pick is teased into periodontal ligament space and used to luxate root tip gently from its socket.

debris from around the root tip so that it can be clearly seen.

The closed technique for root tip retrieval is defined as *any technique that does not require reflection of soft tissue flaps and removal of bone.* Closed techniques are most useful when the tooth was well luxated and mobile before the root tip fractured. If sufficient luxation occurred before the fracture, the root tip often is mobile and can be removed with the closed technique. However, if the tooth was not well mobilized before the fracture, the closed technique is less likely to be successful. The closed technique is also less likely to be successful if there is a bulbous hypercementosed root with bony interferences that prevent extraction of the root tip fragment. Also, severe dilaceration of the root end may prevent the use of the closed technique.

Once the fracture has occurred, the patient should be repositioned so that adequate visualization (with proper lighting), irrigation, and suction are achieved. The tooth socket should be irrigated vigorously and suctioned with a small suction tip, because the loose tooth fragment occasionally can be irrigated from the socket. Once irrigation and suction are completed, the surgeon should inspect the tooth socket carefully to assess whether the root has been removed from the socket.

If the irrigation-suction technique is unsuccessful, the next step is to tease the loose root apex from the socket with a root tip pick. A root tip pick is a delicate instrument and cannot be used as the Cryer elevator can to remove bone and elevate entire roots. The root tip pick is inserted into the periodontal ligament space, and the root is teased out of the socket (Figure 8-48). Neither excessive apical nor lateral force should be applied to the root tip pick. Excessive apical force could result in displacement of the root tip into other anatomic locations, such as the maxillary sinus. Excessive lateral force could result in the bending or fracture of the end of the root tip pick.

Endodontic files can remove root tips in certain situations.

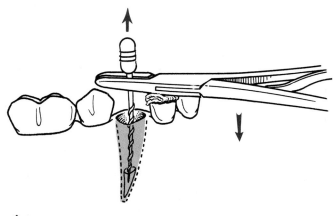

◇ **Figure 8-49**

Endodontic file can be inserted into pulp canal to engage tooth. Needle holder grasps file, and with adjacent tooth used as fulcrum (gauze pad protects tooth), root can be elevated from socket.

After proper visualization of the root canal is achieved, an endodontic file of a size appropriate to fit the canal is selected and screwed into the root canal of the fragment until it firmly engages the root tip. The shank of the file is gripped with a needle holder, which is used as a lever to lift the root fragment from the socket (Figure 8-49). The tooth that is used as the fulcrum should be protected with a gauze or cotton roll. If the file pulls out of the root canal, a larger file should be screwed into the canal and the technique attempted again. Endodontic files are not useful for removing root tips with nonvisible canals, hypercementosed root fragments, bony interferences, or teeth with severe curvatures or dilacerations that prevent access to the root canal. If a firm grasp can be obtained in the root canal, this technique can be successful even for root tips that were not well mobilized before the fracture occurred.

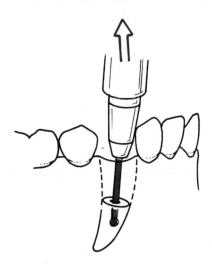

Figure 8-50

When large portion of root (approximately half) remains in socket, no. 4 round bur can be drilled into tooth and dental engine stopped. Handpiece is then removed from socket, and friction between bur and tooth sometimes allows tooth to be elevated when handpiece is removed.

A technique that is similar in concept to the endodontic file technique involves the use of a dental drill with a small, round (no. 4) bur to drill into the tooth root. The drill is stopped, but the bur remains in the tooth. There may be sufficient friction between the bur and the tooth to permit the root to be removed when the drill is removed from the socket. This technique is more useful for larger root fragments than for small root tips, such as those of the maxillary first premolar (Figure 8-50).

The root tip also can be removed with the small straight elevator used as a shoehorn. This technique is indicated more often for the removal of larger root fragments than for small root tips. The technique is similar to that of the root tip pick, because the small straight elevator is forced into the periodontal ligament space, where it acts like a wedge to deliver the tooth fragment toward the occlusal plane (Figure 8-51). Strong apical pressure should be avoided, because it may force the root into the underlying tissues. This is more likely to occur in the maxillary premolar and molar areas, where tooth roots can be displaced into the maxillary sinus. When the straight elevator is used in this fashion, the surgeon's hand must always be supported on an adjacent tooth or a solid bony prominence. This support allows the surgeon to deliver carefully controlled force and to decrease the possibility of displacing tooth fragments or the instrument. The surgeon must be able to visualize clearly the top of the fractured root to see the periodontal ligament space. The straight elevator must be inserted into this space and not merely pushed down into the socket.

If the closed technique is unsuccessful, the surgeon should switch without delay to the open technique. It is important for the surgeon to recognize that a smooth, efficient, properly performed open retrieval of a root fragment is less traumatic than a prolonged, time-consuming, frustrating attempt at closed retrieval.

There are two main open techniques for removing root tips. The first is simply an extension of the technique described for surgical removal of single-rooted teeth. A soft tissue flap is reflected and retracted with a periosteal elevator. Bone is removed with a chisel or bur to expose the buccal surface of the tooth root. The root is buccally delivered with a small straight elevator. The flap is repositioned and sutured (Figure 8-52).

A modification of the open technique just described can be performed to deliver the root fragment without removal of the entire buccal plate overlying the tooth. This technique is known as the *open-window* technique. A soft tissue flap is reflected in the usual fashion, and the apex area of the tooth fragment is located. A dental bur is used to remove the bone overlying the apex of the tooth and expose the root fragment. An instrument is then inserted into the window, and the tooth is displaced out of the socket (Figure 8-53). The preferred flap technique is the three-cornered flap, because there is a need for more extensive exposure of the apical areas. This approach is especially indicated when the buccocrestal bone must be left intact. An important and common example is the removal of maxillary premolars for orthodontic purposes especially in adults.

POLICY FOR LEAVING ROOT FRAGMENTS

When a root tip has fractured, when closed approaches of removal have been unsuccessful, and when the open approach may be excessively traumatic, the surgeon may consider leaving the root in place. As with any surgical approach, the surgeon must balance the benefits of surgery against the risks of surgery. In some situations the risks of removing a small root tip may outweigh the benefits.

Three conditions must exist for a tooth root to be left in the alveolar process. First, the root fragment must be small, usually no more than 4 to 5 mm in length. Second, the root must be deeply embedded in bone and not superficial, to prevent subsequent bone resorption from exposing the tooth root and interfering with the prosthesis that will be constructed over the edentulous area. Third, the tooth involved must not be infected, and there must be no radiolucency around the root apex. This lessens the likelihood that subsequent infections will result from leaving the root in position. If these three conditions exist, then consideration can be given to leaving the root.

For the surgeon to leave a small, deeply embedded, noninfected root tip in place, the risk of surgery must be greater than the benefit. This risk is considered to be greater if one of the following three conditions exists. First, the risk is too great if removal of the root will cause excessive destruction of surrounding tissue; that is, if excessive amounts of bony tissue must be removed to retrieve the root. For example, reaching a small palatal root tip of a maxillary first molar may require the removal of large amounts of bone.

Second, the risk is too great if removal of the root endangers vital structures, most commonly the inferior alveolar nerve, either at the mental foramen area or along the course of the canal. If surgical retrieval of a root may result

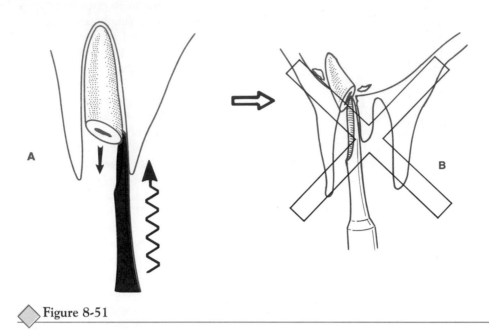

◆ **Figure 8-51**

A, When larger portion of tooth root is left behind after extraction of tooth, small straight elevator can sometimes be used as wedge, or shoehorn, to displace tooth in occlusal direction. It is important to remember that pressure applied in such fashion should be in gentle wiggling motions; excessive pressure should not be applied. **B,** Excessive pressure in apical direction results in displacement of tooth root into undesirable places, such as maxillary sinus.

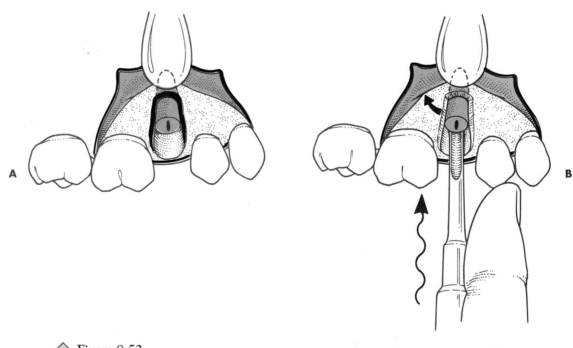

◆ **Figure 8-52**

A, If root cannot be retrieved by closed techniques, soft tissue flap is reflected, and bone overlying root is removed with bur. **B,** Small straight elevator is then used to luxate root buccally by wedging straight elevator into palatal periodontal ligament space.

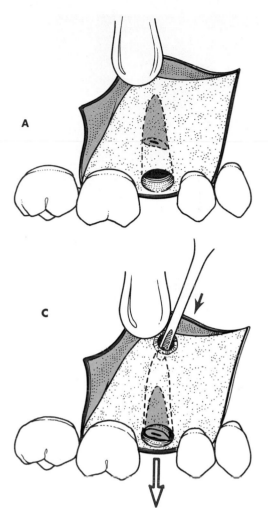

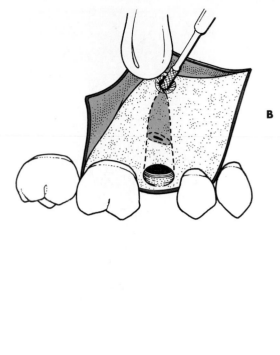

◇ Figure 8-53

A, Open-window approach for retrieving root is indicated when bucco-crestal bone must be maintained. Three-cornered flap is reflected to expose area overlying apex of root fragment being recovered. **B,** Bur is used to uncover apex of root and allow sufficient access for insertion of straight elevator. **C,** Small straight elevator is then used to displace tooth out of tooth socket.

in a permanent or even a prolonged temporary anesthesia of the inferior alveolar nerve, the surgeon should seriously consider leaving the root tip in place.

Finally, the risks outweigh the benefits if attempts at recovering the root tip can displace the root into tissue spaces or into the maxillary sinus. The roots most often displaced into the maxillary sinus are those of the maxillary molars. If the preoperative radiograph shows that the bone is thin over the roots of the teeth and that the separation between the teeth and maxillary sinus is small, the prudent surgeon will choose to leave a small root fragment rather than risk displacing it into the maxillary sinus. Likewise, roots of the mandibular second and third molars can be displaced into the submandibular space during attempts to remove them. During retrieval of any root tip, apical pressure may displace teeth into tissue spaces or into the sinus.

If the surgeon elects to leave a root tip in place, a strict protocol must be observed. The patient must be informed that, in the surgeon's judgment, leaving the root in its position will do less harm than surgery. In addition, radiographic documentation of the root tip's presence and position must be obtained and retained in the patient's record. The fact that the patient was informed of the decision to leave the root tip in position must be recorded in the patient's chart. Also, the patient must be recalled for several routine periodic follow-ups over the ensuing year to track the fate of this root. The patient should be instructed to contact the surgeon immediately should any problems develop in the area of the retained root.

MULTIPLE EXTRACTIONS ─◇

If multiple adjacent teeth are to be extracted at a single sitting, slight modifications of the routine extraction procedure must be made to facilitate a smooth transition from a dentulous to an edentulous state that allows for proper rehabilitation with a fixed or removable prosthesis. This section discusses those modifications.

The order in which multiple teeth are extracted deserves some discussion. Maxillary teeth usually should be removed first for several reasons. First of all, an infiltration anesthetic has a more rapid onset and also disappears more rapidly, which means that the surgeon can begin the surgical procedure sooner after the injections have been given but also that surgery should not be delayed, because profound anesthesia is lost more quickly in the maxilla. In addition, maxillary teeth should be removed first, because during the extraction process debris such as portions of amalgams, fractured crowns, and

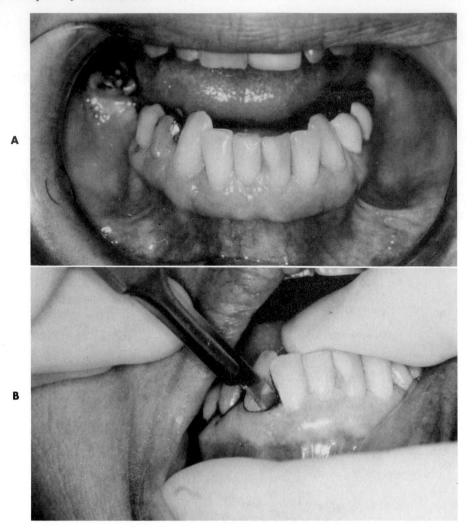

◇ Figure 8-54

A, This patient's remaining teeth are to be extracted. Note broad zone of attached gingiva in adequate vestibular depth. **B,** After adequate anesthesia is achieved, soft tissue attachment to teeth is incised with no. 15 blade. Incision is carried around necks of teeth and through interdental papilla.

Continued

bone chips may fall into the empty sockets of the lower teeth if the lower surgery is performed first. Also maxillary teeth are removed with a major component of buccal force. There is little or no vertical traction force used in removal of these teeth, as is commonly required with mandibular teeth. Therefore mandibular extractions that follow maxillary extractions are usually easier to perform. A single minor disadvantage for extracting maxillary teeth first is that if hemorrhage is not controlled in the maxilla before mandibular teeth are extracted, the hemorrhage may interfere with visualization during mandibular surgery. Hemorrhage is usually not a major problem, because hemostasis should be achieved in one area before the surgeon turns his attention to another area of surgery, and the surgical assistant should be able to keep the surgical field free from blood with adequate suction.

Extraction usually begins with extraction of the most posterior teeth first. This allows for the more effective use of dental elevators to luxate and mobilize teeth before the forceps are used to extract the tooth. The two teeth that are the most difficult to remove, the molar and canine, should be extracted last. Removal of the teeth on either side weakens the bony socket on the mesial and distal side of these teeth, and their subsequent extraction is made easier.

In summary, if a maxillary and mandibular left quadrant are to be extracted, the following order is recommended: (1) maxillary posterior teeth, leaving the first molar; (2) maxillary anterior teeth, leaving the canine; (3) maxillary molar; (4) maxillary canine; (5) mandibular posterior teeth, leaving the first molar; (6) mandibular anterior teeth, leaving the canine; (7) mandibular molar; and (8) mandibular canine.

The surgical procedure for removing multiple adjacent teeth is modified slightly. The first step in removing a single tooth is to loosen the soft tissue attachment from around the tooth (Figure 8-54, *A* and *B*). When performing multiple extractions, the soft tissue reflection is extended slightly to form a small envelope flap to expose the crestal bone only (Figure 8-54, *C*).

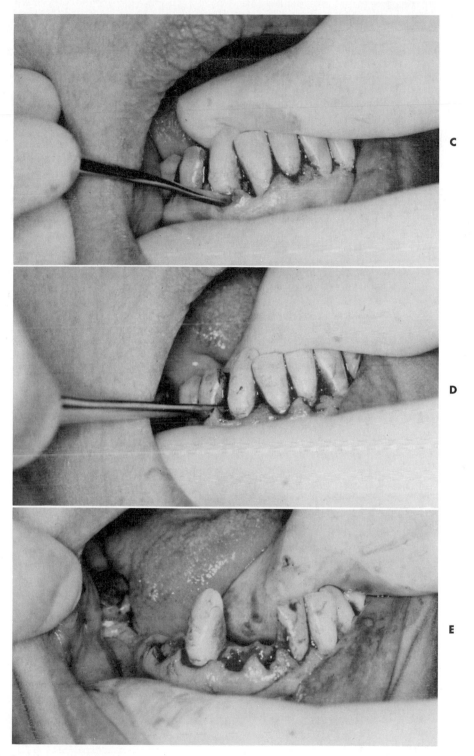

◇ **Figure 8-54, cont'd**

C, Woodson elevator is used to reflect labial soft tissue just to crest of labioalveolar bone. **D,** Small straight elevator is used to luxate teeth before forceps are used. Note that surgeon's opposite hand is reflecting soft tissue and stabilizing mandible. **E,** Teeth adjacent to mandibular canine are extracted first, which makes extraction of remaining canine tooth easier to accomplish.   *Continued*

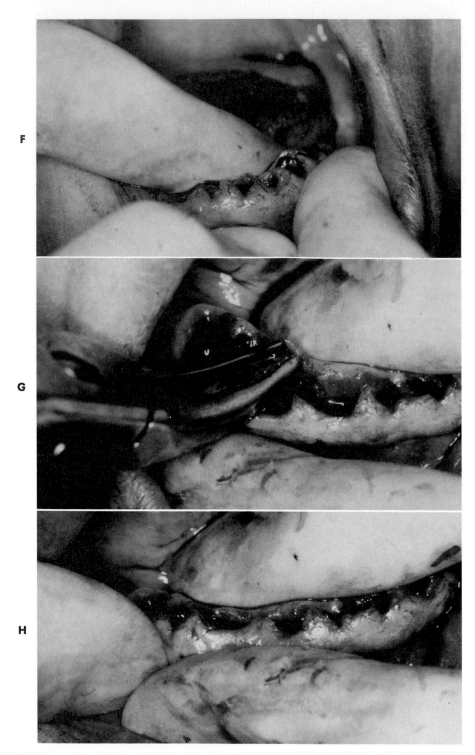

◇ Figure 8-54, cont'd

F, Alveolar plates are compressed firmly together to reestablish presurgical buccolingual width of alveolar process. Because of mild periodontal disease, there is excess soft tissue, which will be trimmed to prevent excess flabby tissue on crest of ridge. **G,** Rongeur forceps are used to remove only bone that is sharp and protrudes above reapproximated soft tissue. **H,** After soft tissue has been trimmed and sharp bony projections removed, tissue is checked one final time for completeness of soft tissue surgery.

Continued

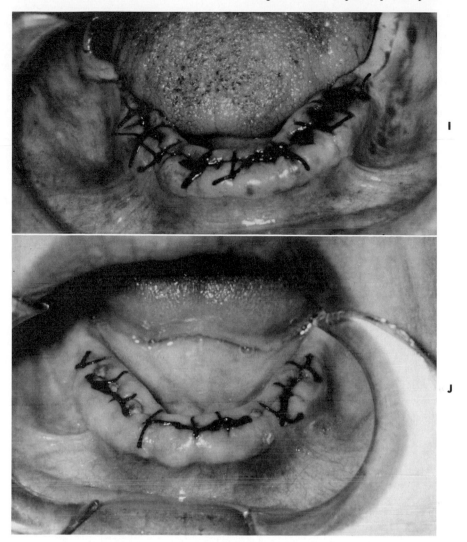

Figure 8-54, cont'd

I, Tissue is closed with interrupted black silk sutures across papilla. This approximates soft tissue at papilla but leaves tooth socket open. Soft tissue is not mobilized to achieve primary closure, because this would tend to reduce vestibular height. **J,** Patient returns for suture removal 1 week later. Normal healing has occurred, and sutures are ready for removal. Note that broad band of attached tissue remains on ridge, similar to what existed in preoperative situation (see **A**).

The teeth are luxated with the straight elevator (Figure 8-54, *D*) and delivered with forceps in the usual fashion (Figure 8-54, *E*). If removing any of the teeth is likely to require excessive force, the surgeon should remove a small amount of buccal bone to prevent fracture and bone loss.

After the extractions are completed, the buccolingual plates are pressed together with firm pressure (Figure 8-54, *F*). The soft tissue is repositioned, and the surgeon palpates the ridge to determine if there are any areas of sharp bony spicules or obvious undercuts. If any exist, the bone rongeur is used to remove the larger areas of interference, and the bone file is used to smooth any sharp spicules (Figure 8-54, *G*). The area is irri-

gated thoroughly with sterile saline. The soft tissue is inspected for the presence of excess granulation tissue. If any is present, it should be removed, because it may prolong postoperative hemorrhage. The soft tissue is then reapproximated and inspected for excess gingiva. If the teeth are being removed because of severe periodontitis with bone loss, it is not uncommon for the soft tissue flaps to overlap and cause redundant tissue. If this is the situation, the gingiva should be trimmed so that no overlap occurs when the soft tissue is apposed (Figure 8-54, *H*). However, if there is no redundant tissue, the surgeon must not try to gain primary closure over the extraction sockets. If this is done, the depth of the vestibule decreases, which may interfere with denture construction and wear. Finally, the papilla are sutured into position (Figure 8-54, *I* and *J*). Interrupted or continuous sutures are used, depending on the preference of the surgeon.

In some patients a more extensive alveoloplasty following multiple extractions is necessary. Chapter 12 has an in-depth discussion of this technique.

BIBLIOGRAPHY

Berman SA: Basic principles of dentoalveolar surgery. In LJ Petersen, editor: *Principles of oral and maxillofacial surgery,* Philadelphia, 1992, JB Lippincott.

Cerny R: Removing broken roots: a simple method, *Aust Dent J* 23:351, 1978.

PRINCIPLES OF MANAGEMENT OF IMPACTED TEETH

LARRY J. PETERSON

An impacted tooth is one that fails to erupt into the dental arch within the expected time. The tooth becomes impacted because eruption is prevented by adjacent teeth, dense overlying bone, or excessive soft tissue. Because impacted teeth do not erupt, they are retained for the patient's lifetime unless removed surgically.

The term *unerupted* includes both impacted teeth and teeth that are in the process of erupting. The term *embedded* occasionally is used interchangeably with the term *impacted*.

Teeth most often become impacted because of inadequate dental arch length and space in which to erupt; that is, the total alveolar bone arch length is smaller than the total tooth arch length. The most common impacted teeth are the maxillary and mandibular third molars, followed by the maxillary canines and mandibular premolars. The third molars are the most frequently impacted, because they are the last teeth to erupt and therefore are the most likely to have inadequate space into which to erupt.

In the anterior maxilla, the canine tooth also is commonly prevented from erupting by crowding from other teeth. The canine tooth usually erupts after the maxillary lateral incisor and maxillary first premolar. If space is inadequate to allow eruption, the canine tooth becomes impacted. In the anterior mandible a similar situation affects the mandibular premolars, because they erupt after the mandibular first molar and mandibular canine. Therefore, if there is inadequate room for eruption, one of the premolars, usually the second premolar, remains unerupted and becomes impacted.

As a general rule, all impacted teeth should be removed unless removal is contraindicated. Extraction should be performed as soon as the dentist determines that the tooth is impacted. Removal of impacted teeth becomes more difficult with advancing age. The dentist should *not* recommend that impacted teeth be left in place until they cause difficulty. If the tooth is left in place until problems arise, there is an increased incidence of local tissue morbidity, loss of adjacent teeth and bone, and potential injury to adjacent vital structures. Additionally, if removal of impacted teeth is deferred until they cause problems later in life, surgery is more likely to be complicated and hazardous, because the patient may have compromising systemic diseases. A fundamental precept of the philosophy of dentistry is that problems should be prevented. Preventive dentistry dictates that impacted teeth be removed before complications arise.

This chapter discusses the management of impacted teeth. It is not a thorough nor in-depth discussion of the technical aspects of surgical impaction removal. Rather, its goal is to provide both the information necessary for proper management and a basis for determining the difficulty of surgery.

INDICATIONS FOR REMOVAL OF IMPACTED TEETH ⎯⎯⎯◇

All impacted teeth should be considered for removal as soon as the diagnosis is made. The average age for the eruption of the third molar is age 20, although eruption may continue in some patients until age 25. During normal development the lower third molar begins its development in a horizontal angulation, and as the tooth develops and the jaw grows, the angulation changes from horizontal to mesioangular to vertical. Failure of rotation from the mesioangular to the vertical direction is the most common cause of the tooth remaining impacted. The second major factor is that the mesiodistal dimension of the teeth versus the length of the jaw is such that there is inadequate room in the alveolar process anterior to the anterior border of the ramus to allow the tooth to erupt into position.

As noted earlier, some third molars will continue to erupt after age 20, coming into final position by age 25. Multiple factors are associated with continued eruption. When late eruption occurs, the unerupted tooth is usually covered only with soft tissue or very slightly with bone. These teeth are almost always in a vertical position and are relatively superficially positioned with respect to the occlusal plane of the adjacent second molar. Finally and perhaps most importantly, there is sufficient space between the anterior border of the ramus and the second molar tooth to allow eruption.[14,15] Likewise, if the tooth does not erupt after age 20, it is most likely covered with bone, is a mesioangular impaction, is located lower in the alveolar process near the cervical level of the adjacent second molar, and there is inadequate space to allow eruption. Therefore the dentist and surgeon can use these parameters to predict whether or not a tooth will erupt into the arch or remain impacted.

Early removal reduces the postoperative morbidity and allows for the best healing.[1,7,8,10] Younger patients tolerate the procedure better and recover more quickly and with less interference to their daily lives. Periodontal healing is better in the younger patient, because there is better and more complete regeneration of bone and better reattachment of gingival tissue to the adjacent tooth. Moreover, the procedure is easier to perform in younger patients. The ideal time for removal of impacted third molars is after the roots of the teeth are one-third formed and before they are two-thirds formed, usually during the late teenage years, between ages 16 and 18.

If impacted teeth are left in the alveolar process, it is highly probable that one or more of several problems will result.[6,9] To prevent this, impacted teeth should be removed.

PREVENTION OF PERIODONTAL DISEASE

Erupted teeth adjacent to impacted teeth are predisposed to periodontal disease (Figures 9-1 and 9-2). The mere presence of an impacted mandibular third molar decreases the amount of bone on the distal aspect of an adjacent second molar (Figure 9-1). Because the most difficult tooth surface to keep clean is the distal aspect of the last tooth in the arch, the patient may have gingival inflammation with apical migration of the gingival attachment on the distal aspect of the second molar. With even minor gingivitis the causative bacteria have access to a large portion of the root surface, which results in the early formation of severe periodontitis (Figure 9-2). Patients with impacted mandibular third molars often have deep periodontal pockets on the distal aspect of the second molars but have normal sulcular depth in the remainder of the mouth.

The accelerated periodontal problem resulting from an impacted third molar is especially serious in the maxilla. As a periodontal pocket expands apically, it becomes involved with the distal furcation of the maxillary second molar relatively early, which makes advancement of the periodontal disease more rapid and severe. In addition, treatment of the localized periodontal disease around the maxillary second molar is more difficult because of the distal furcation involvement.

By removing the impacted third molars early, periodontal disease can be prevented, and there is a greater likelihood of bony healing and bone fill into the area previously occupied by the crown of the third molar.[7,8,10]

PREVENTION OF DENTAL CARIES

When a third molar is impacted or partially impacted, the bacteria that cause dental caries can be exposed to the distal aspect of the second molar, as well as to the third molar. Even in situations in which no obvious communication between the mouth and the impacted third molar exists, there may be enough communication to allow for caries production (Figures 9-3 to 9-5).

PREVENTION OF PERICORONITIS

When a tooth is partially impacted with a large amount of soft tissue over the axial and occlusal surfaces, the patient frequently has one or more episodes of pericoronitis.[5] Pericoronitis is an infection of the soft tissue around the crown of a partially impacted tooth and is caused by the normal oral

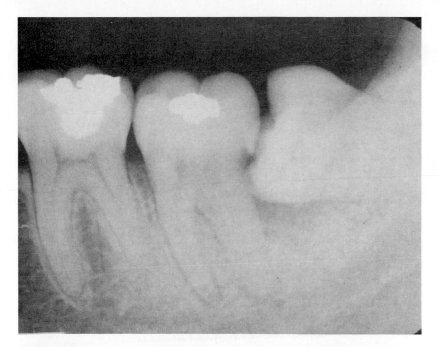

Figure 9-1

Radiograph of mandibular third molar impacted against second molar, with bone loss resulting from presence of third molar.

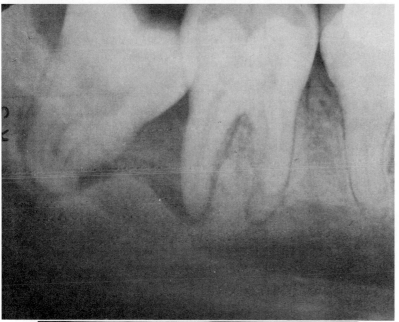

Figure 9-2

Radiographs showing variations of mandibular third molar impacted against second molar, with severe bone loss secondary to periodontal disease and third molar.

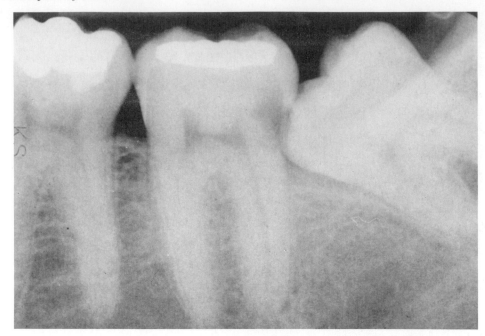

◆ **Figure 9-3**

Radiograph of caries in mandibular second molar secondary to presence of impacted third molar.

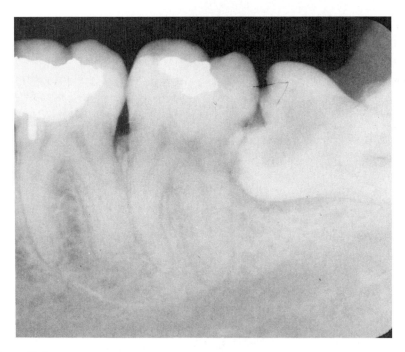

◆ **Figure 9-4**

Radiograph of caries in mandibular impacted molar.

flora. For most patients, the bacteria and host defenses maintain a delicate balance, but host defenses cannot eliminate the bacteria. If the host defenses are compromised (for example, during minor illnesses, such as the flu or an upper respiratory infection, or from severe fatigue), infection can occur. Thus, although the impacted tooth has been present for some time without infection, if the patient experiences a mild, transient decrease in host defenses, pericoronitis may result.

Pericoronitis also can arise secondary to minor trauma from a maxillary third molar. The soft tissue that covers the occlusal surface of the partially erupted mandibular third molar (known as the *operculum*) can be traumatized and become swollen.

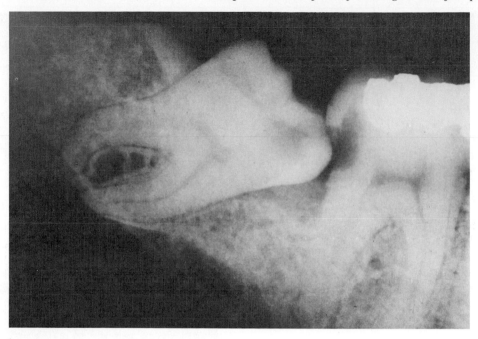

◈ **Figure 9-5**

Radiograph of caries in both impacted third molar and second molar.

Often the maxillary third molar further traumatizes the already swollen operculum, which causes increased swelling that again can be traumatized more easily. This spiraling cycle of trauma and swelling is often interrupted only by removal of the maxillary third molar.

Another common cause of pericoronitis is entrapment of food under the operculum. During eating, a small amount of food may be packed into the pocket between the operculum and the impacted tooth. Because this pocket cannot be cleaned, it is invaded by bacteria, and pericoronitis begins.

Pericoronitis is caused by streptococci and a large variety of anaerobic bacteria, the usual bacteria that inhabit the gingival sulcus. Pericoronitis can be treated initially by mechanically débriding the large periodontal pocket that exists under the operculum by using hydrogen peroxide as an irrigating solution. Hydrogen peroxide not only mechanically removes bacteria with its foaming action, it also reduces the number of anaerobic bacteria by releasing oxygen into the usually anaerobic environment of the oral cavity. Other irrigates, such as chlorhexidine or iodophors, can reduce the bacterial population of the pocket.

Pericoronitis can present as a very mild infection or as a severe infection that requires hospitalization of the patient. Just as the severity of the infection varies, the treatment and management of this problem vary from very mild to aggressive.

In its mildest form, pericoronitis is a localized tissue swelling and soreness. For patients with a mild infection, irrigation and curettage by the dentist, followed by home irrigations by the patient, usually suffice.

If the infection is slightly more severe, with a large amount of local soft tissue swelling that is traumatized by a maxillary third molar, the dentist should consider extracting the maxillary third molar in addition to local irrigation.

For patients who have, in addition to local swelling and pain, mild facial swelling, mild trismus secondary to inflammation extending into the muscles of mastication, and a low-grade fever, the dentist should consider administering an antibiotic along with irrigation and extraction. The antibiotic of choice is penicillin.

Pericoronitis can lead to serious fascial space infections. Because the infection begins in the posterior mouth, it can spread rapidly into the fascial spaces of the mandibular ramus and the lateral neck. If a patient develops trismus (with an inability to open the mouth more than 20 mm), a temperature of greater than 101° F, facial swelling, pain, and malaise, the patient should be referred to an oral and maxillofacial surgeon, who may admit the patient to the hospital.

Patients who have had one episode of pericoronitis, although managed successfully by these methods, will continue to have episodes of pericoronitis, unless the offending mandibular third molar is removed. The patient should be informed that the tooth should be removed at the earliest possible time, to prevent recurrent infections. The mandibular third molar should not be removed until the signs and symptoms of pericoronitis have been completely resolved. The incidence of postoperative complications, specifically dry socket and postoperative infection, increases if the tooth is removed during the time of active infection.

Prevention of pericoronitis can be achieved by removing the impacted third molars before they penetrate the oral mucosa and are visible. Although excision of the surrounding

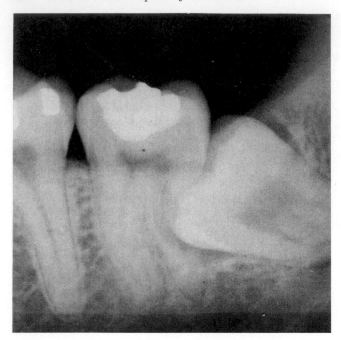

◆ **Figure 9-6**

Root resorption of second molar as result of impacted third molar.

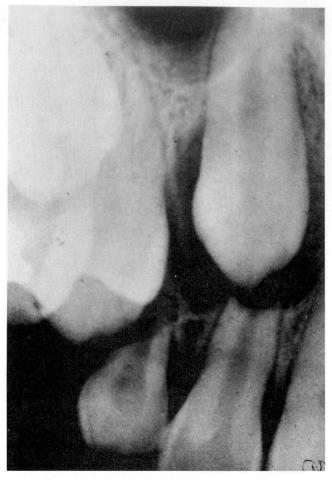

◆ **Figure 9-7**

Root resorption of maxillary lateral incisors as result of impacted canine.

soft tissue, or operculectomy, has been advocated as a method for preventing pericoronitis without removal of the impacted tooth, it is very painful and usually does not work. The soft tissue excess tends to recur, because it drapes over the impacted tooth and causes regrowth of the operculum. The overwhelming majority of cases of pericoronitis can be prevented only by extraction of the tooth.

Prevention of Root Resorption

Occasionally, an impacted tooth causes sufficient pressure on the root of an adjacent tooth to cause root resorption (Figures 9-6 and 9-7). Although the process by which root resorption occurs is not well defined, it appears to be similar to the resorption process primary teeth undergo in the presence of the succedaneous teeth. Removal of the impacted tooth may result in salvage of the adjacent tooth by cemental repair. Endodontic therapy may be required to save these teeth.

Impacted Teeth under a Dental Prosthesis

When a patient has an edentulous area restored, impacted teeth in the area should be removed before the prosthetic appliance is constructed. There are several reasons for this. After teeth are extracted, the alveolar process slowly undergoes resorption. Thus the impacted tooth becomes closer to the surface of the bone, giving the appearance of erupting. The denture may compress the soft tissue on the impacted tooth, which is no longer covered with bone; the result is ulceration of the overlying soft tissue and initiation of an odontogenic infection (Figure 9-8).

Impacted teeth should be removed before a prosthesis is constructed because, if the impacted tooth must be removed after construction, the alveolar ridge may be so altered by the extraction that the prosthesis becomes unattractive and less functional (Figure 9-9). In addition, if removal of impacted teeth in edentulous areas is achieved before the prosthesis is made, the patient is probably in good physical condition. Waiting until the overlying bone has resorbed and an ulceration with infection occurs does not produce a favorable situation for extraction. If extraction is postponed, the patient will be older and more likely to be in poorer health. Furthermore, the mandible may have become atrophic, which increases the likelihood of fracture during tooth removal (Figure 9-10).

Prevention of Odontogenic Cysts and Tumors

When impacted teeth are retained within the alveolar process, the associated follicular sac also is retained. Although in most patients the dental follicle maintains its original size, it may undergo cystic degeneration and become a dentigerous cyst or keratocyst. If the patient is closely followed, the cyst can be

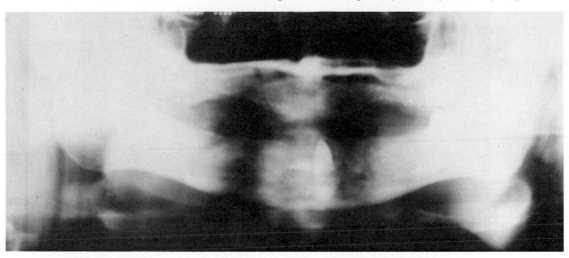

◇ Figure 9-8

Impacted tooth retained under denture. Tooth is now at surface and is causing infection.

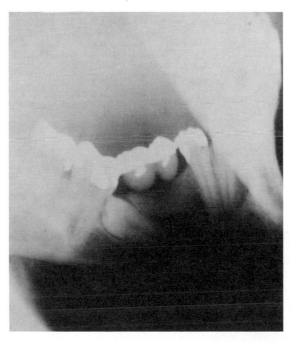

◇ Figure 9-9

Impacted tooth under fixed bridge. Tooth must be removed and may jeopardize bridge.

diagnosed by the dentist before it reaches large proportions (Figure 9-11). However, unmonitored cysts can reach enormous sizes (Figure 9-12). As a general guideline, if the follicular space around the crown of the tooth is greater than 3 mm, the diagnosis of a dentigerous cyst is a reasonable one.

In the same way that odontogenic cysts can occur around impacted teeth, odontogenic tumors can arise from the epithelium contained within the dental follicle. The most

common odontogenic tumor to occur in this region is the ameloblastoma. Ameloblastomas in this area usually must be treated aggressively by excision of the overlying soft tissue and of at least a portion of the mandible. Occasionally, other odontogenic tumors may occur in conjunction with impacted teeth (Figure 9-13).

Although the overall incidence of odontogenic cysts and tumors around impacted teeth is not high,[13] the overwhelming majority of pathologic conditions of the mandibular third molar are associated with unerupted teeth. It is therefore recommended that impacted teeth be removed to prevent the occurrence of cysts and tumors.

TREATMENT OF PAIN OF UNEXPLAINED ORIGIN

Occasionally, patients come to the dentist complaining of pain in the retromolar region of the mandible for no obvious reasons. If conditions such as myofascial pain dysfunction syndrome and temporomandibular joint disorder are excluded and if the patient has an unerupted tooth, removal of the tooth sometimes results in resolution of the pain.

PREVENTION OF FRACTURE OF THE JAW

An impacted third molar in the mandible occupies space that is usually filled with bone. This may weaken the mandible and render the jaw more susceptible to fracture (Figure 9-14).

If the jaw fractures through the area of an impacted third molar, the impacted third molar frequently is removed before the fracture is reduced and intermaxillary fixation is applied.

FACILITATION OF ORTHODONTIC TREATMENT

In patients who require retraction of second and first molars by orthodontic techniques, the presence of impacted third molars may interfere with the treatment. It is therefore rec-

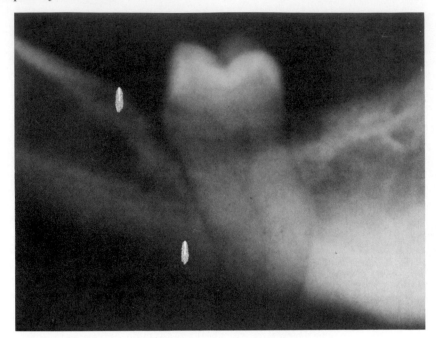

◇ Figure 9-10

Impaction in atrophic mandible, which may result in jaw fracture during extraction.

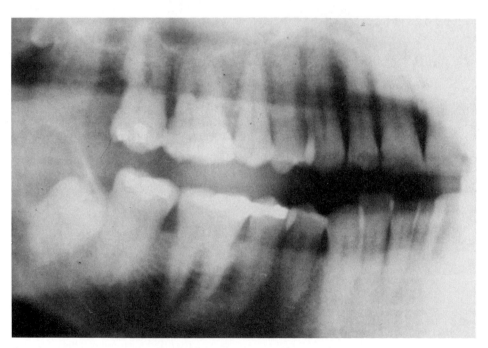

◇ Figure 9-11

Small dentigerous cyst arising around impacted tooth.

ommended that impacted third molars be removed before orthodontic therapy is begun.

Another consideration is that, after orthodontic treatment has been concluded, there may be crowding of the mandibular incisor teeth. This has been attributed to the mesial force transmitted to the molar and premolar teeth by impacted third molars, especially mesially inclined impactions.[11,12] Several other factors influence crowding. Growth of the maxilla stops before growth of the mandible. If the upper and lower incisors are in a proper overbite and overjet relationship, and the mandible continues to grow after the maxilla stops growing, then the mandibular incisors become crowded to accommo-

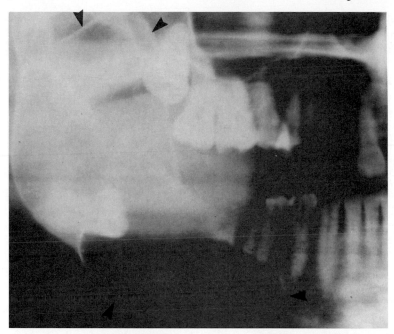

◇ **Figure 9-12**

Large dentigerous cyst that extends from coronoid process to mental foramen. Cyst has displaced impacted third molar to inferior border of mandible.

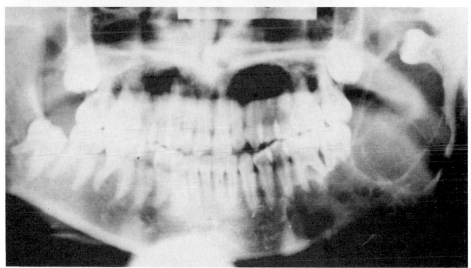

◇ **Figure 9-13**

Large ameloblastoma in mandible as result of impacted third molar.

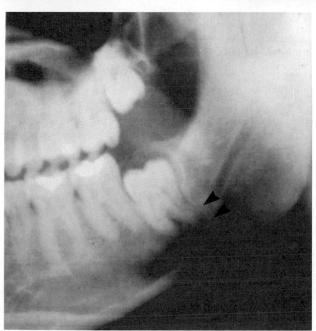

◇ **Figure 9-14**

Fracture of mandible that occurred through location of impacted third molar.

date the constriction imposed on them by the maxillary incisors. This explanation appears sound, because crowding occurs after the age at which the maxilla stops growing and the mandible continues forward growth.

Many orthodontists still refer their patients to surgeons for removal of impacted third molars after orthodontic treatment is complete. Although the surgeon should explain that there are other reasons for surgery, he should support the decision to remove impacted teeth to help prevent crowding.

OPTIMAL PERIODONTAL HEALING

As noted earlier, one of the most important indications for removal of impacted third molars is to preserve the periodontal health. A great deal of attention has been given to the two primary parameters of periodontal health following third molar surgery; that is, bone height on the distal aspect of the second molar and attachment level on the distal aspect of the second molar.

Recent studies have provided information on which to base the likelihood of optimum periodontal tissue healing.[2-4] The two most important factors have been shown to be the extent of the preoperative intrabony defect on the distal aspect of the second molar and the patient's age at the time of surgery. If there is a large amount of distal bone missing because of the presence of the impacted tooth and the associated follicle, there is a lower likelihood of decreasing the intrabony pocket. Likewise, if the patient is older, then the likelihood of optimum bony healing is likewise decreased. Patients whose third molars are removed before age 25 are more likely to have better bone healing than those whose impacted teeth are removed after age 25.[3] In the younger patient, not only is the initial periodontal healing better but the long-term continued regeneration of the periodonteum is clearly better.[3]

As mentioned previously, unerupted teeth may continue to erupt until age 25. Because the terminal portion of the eruption process occurs relatively slowly, there is increased chance for development of pericoronitis and larger amounts of contact between the third molar and second molar. Both of these factors decrease the possibility for optimum periodontal healing. However, it should be noted that the completely bony impacted third molar in a patient older than age 30 should probably be left in place unless some specific pathology develops. Removal of such asymptomatic completely impacted third molars in older patients will clearly result in pocket depths and alveolar bone loss, which will be greater than if the tooth were left in place.

CONTRAINDICATIONS FOR REMOVAL OF IMPACTED TEETH

All impacted teeth should be removed unless specific contraindications justify leaving them in position. When the potential benefits outweigh the potential complications and risks, the procedure should be performed. Similarly, when the risks are greater than the potential benefits, the procedure

should be deferred. Contraindications for the removal of impacted teeth primarily involve the patient's physical status.

EXTREMES OF AGE

The third molar tooth bud can be seen radiographically by age 6. Some surgeons think that removal of the tooth bud at age 7 to 9 can be accomplished with minimal surgical morbidity and therefore should be performed at this age. However, most surgeons believe that it is not possible to predict accurately if the forming third molar will be impacted. The consensus is that very early removal of third molars should be deferred until an accurate diagnosis of impaction can be made.

The most common contraindication for the removal of impacted teeth is advanced age. As a patient ages, the bone becomes highly calcified and therefore less flexible and less likely to bend under the forces of tooth extraction. The result is that more bone must be surgically removed to displace the tooth from its socket.

Similarly, as patients age, they respond less favorably and with more postoperative sequelae. An 18-year-old patient may have 1 or 2 days of discomfort and swelling after the removal of an impacted tooth, whereas a similar procedure may result in a 4- or 5-day recovery period for a 50-year-old patient.

Finally, if a tooth has been retained in the alveolar process for many years without periodontal disease, caries, or cystic degeneration, it is unlikely that these unfavorable sequelae will occur. Therefore in an older patient (usually over age 40) with an impacted tooth that shows no signs of disease and that has a layer of overlying bone (usually at least 4 mm) the tooth should not be removed (Figure 9-15). The dentist caring for the patient should check the impacted tooth radiographically every 1 or 2 years to ensure that no adverse sequela occurs.

If the impacted tooth shows signs of cystic formation or periodontal disease involving either the adjacent tooth or the impacted tooth, if it is a single impacted tooth underneath a prosthesis with thin overlying bone, or if it becomes symptomatic as the result of infection, the tooth must be removed.

COMPROMISED MEDICAL STATUS

Similar to extremes of age, compromised medical status contraindicates the removal of an impacted tooth. Frequently, compromised medical status and advancing age go hand-in-hand. If the impacted tooth is asymptomatic, its surgical removal must be viewed as elective. If the patient's cardiovascular or respiratory function or host defenses for combating infection are compromised or if the patient has a serious acquired or congenital coagulopathy, the surgeon must consider leaving the tooth in the alveolar process. On the other hand, if the tooth becomes symptomatic, the surgeon must work carefully with the patient's physician to remove the tooth with the least operative and postoperative medical sequelae.

PROBABLE EXCESSIVE DAMAGE TO ADJACENT STRUCTURES

If the impacted tooth lies in an area in which its removal may seriously jeopardize adjacent nerves, teeth, or previously constructed bridges, it may be prudent to leave the tooth in

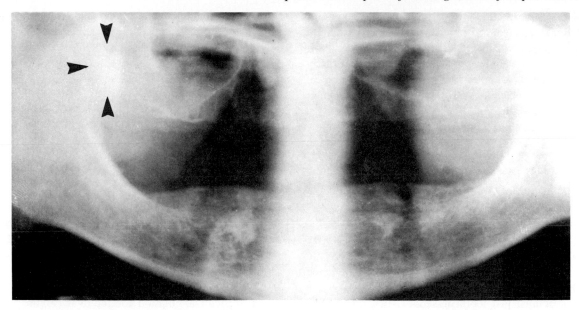

◇ Figure 9-15

Impacted maxillary right third molar in 63-year-old patient. It should not be extracted, because it is deeply embedded and there are no signs of disease.

place. When the dentist makes the decision not to remove a tooth, the reasons must be weighed against potential future complications. For younger patients who may suffer the sequelae of impacted teeth, it may be wise to remove the tooth while taking special measures to prevent damage to adjacent structures. However, for the older patient with no signs of impending complications and for whom the probability of such complications is low, the impacted tooth should not be removed. A classic example of such a case is the elderly patient with a potentially severe periodontal defect on the distal aspect of the second molar but in whom removal of the third molar would almost surely result in the loss of the second molar. In this situation the impacted tooth should not be removed.

Summary

The preceding discussion of indications and contraindications for the removal of impacted third molars has been designed to point out that there are risks and benefits for removing impacted teeth in each individual patient. Patients who present with one or more pathologic symptoms or problems should have their impacted teeth removed. Most of the symptomatic, pathologic problems that result from impacted third molars occur because of partially erupted teeth and occur less commonly with a complete bony impaction.

It is less clear what should be done with impacted teeth before they cause symptoms or problems. In making a decision as to whether or not an impacted third molar should be removed, a variety of factors must be considered. First, the available room in the arch into which the tooth can erupt must be considered. If adequate room exists, then the clinician may choose to defer removal of the tooth until eruption is complete.

A second consideration is the status of the impacted tooth and the age of the patient. It is critical to remember that the average age of complete eruption is 20, but that eruption may continue to occur up to age 25. A tooth that appears to be a mesioangular impaction at age 17 may eventually become more vertical and erupt into the mouth. If insufficient room exists to accommodate the tooth and a soft tissue operculum exists over the posterior aspect, then pathologic sequelae are likely to occur.

Although there have been some attempts at making very early predictions of whether or not a tooth was going to be impacted, these efforts have not yet resulted in a reliable predictive model. However, by the time the patient reaches age 18, the dentist and surgeon can reasonably predict whether there will be adequate room into which the tooth can erupt with sufficient clearance of the anterior ramus to prevent soft tissue operculum formation. At this time, if surgical removal is chosen, soft tissue and bone tissue healing will occur at its maximal level. At age 18 or 19, if the diagnosis for inadequate room for functional eruption can be made, then the asymptomatic third molar can be removed, and the long-term periodontal health of the second molar will be maximized.

Classification Systems of Impacted Teeth ◇

Removal of impacted teeth can be either extremely difficult or relatively straightforward and easy. To determine the degree of difficulty preoperatively, the surgeon should examine the patient methodically. The primary factor determining the difficulty of the removal is accessibility. Accessibility is determined by the ease of exposing the tooth, of preparing a pathway for its delivery, and of preparing a purchase point (or taking advantage of a natural purchase point). With careful classification of the impacted teeth using a variety of systems, the surgeon can approach the proposed surgery in an orderly fashion and predict whether any extraordinary surgical approaches will be necessary or if the patient will encounter any postoperative problems.

The majority of the classifying results from analysis of the radiograph. For most situations the periapical radiograph provides adequate detail and should be the radiograph most commonly employed. The panoramic radiograph shows a more accurate picture of the total anatomy of the region and can be used as an adequate substitute.

For each patient the dentist should carefully analyze the factors discussed in this section. By combining these factors, the dentist can assess the difficulty of the surgery and elect to extract the impacted teeth that are within his skill level. However, for the patient's sake the dentist should refer the patient to a specialist if a tooth presents a difficult surgical problem.

ANGULATION

The first classification system employs a description of the angulation of the long axis of the impacted third molar with respect to the long axis of the second molar. Because teeth at certain inclinations have ready-made pathways for withdrawal, whereas pathways for teeth of other inclinations require the removal of substantial amounts of bone, this classification system provides an initial evaluation of the difficulty of extractions.

The mesioangular impaction is generally acknowledged as the least difficult impaction to remove (Figure 9-16). The mesioangular impacted tooth is tilted toward the second molar in a mesial direction. This type of impaction is also the most commonly seen and comprises approximately 43% of all impacted teeth.

In a severe mesial inclination the impacted tooth is horizontal (Figure 9-17). This type of impaction usually is considered more difficult to remove than the mesioangular impaction. Horizontal impactions occur less frequently and are seen only in approximately 3% of all mandibular impactions.

In the vertical impaction the long axis of the impacted tooth runs in the same direction as the long axis of the second molar. This impaction occurs with the second greatest frequency, accounts for approximately 38% of all impactions, and is third in difficulty of removal (Figure 9-18).

Finally, the distoangular impaction is the tooth with the most difficult angulation for removal (Figure 9-19). In the distoangular impaction the long axis of the third molar is angled distally or posteriorly away from the second molar. This impaction is the most difficult to remove because the tooth has a withdrawal pathway that runs into the mandibular ramus, and its removal requires greater surgical intervention. Distoangular impactions occur uncommonly and account for approximately only 6% of all impacted third molars. Erupted third molars may be in a distoangular position. When this occurs, they routinely are extremely difficult to remove compared with the removal of other erupted teeth.

In addition to the relationship between the angulation of the

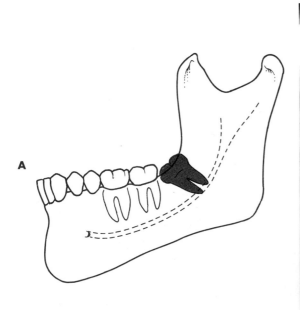
A
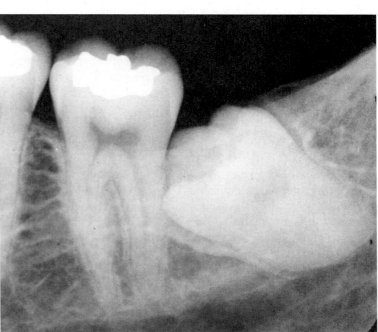
B

◆ **Figure 9-16**

A, Mesioangular impaction—most common and easiest impaction to remove. **B,** Mesioangular impaction is usually in close proximity to second molar.

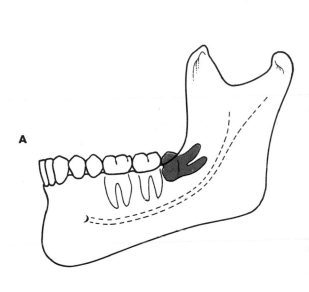
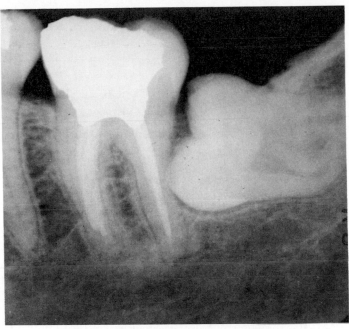

◇ Figure 9-17

A, Horizontal impaction—uncommon and more difficult to remove than mesioangular impaction. **B,** Occlusal surface of horizontal impacted third molar is usually immediately adjacent to root of second molar, which often produces early severe periodontal disease.

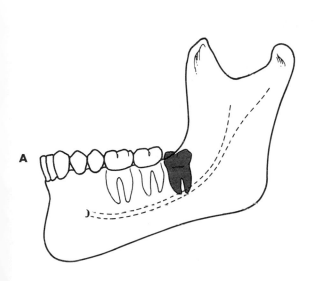
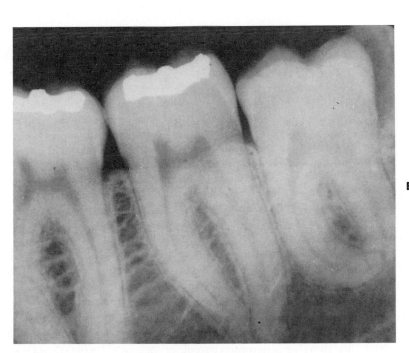

◇ Figure 9-18

A, Vertical impaction—second most common impaction and second most difficult to remove. **B,** Vertical impaction is frequently covered on its posterior aspect with bone of anterior ramus of mandible.

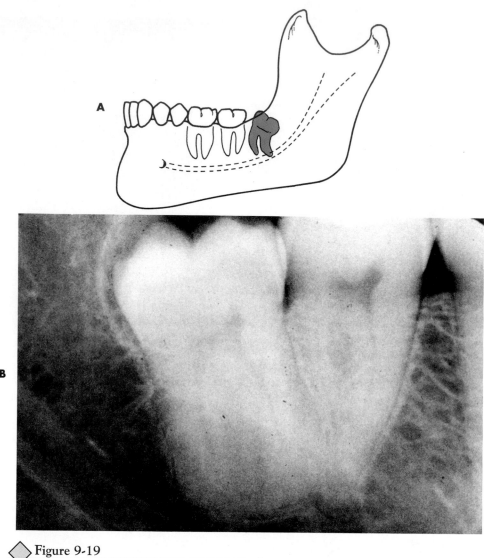

◇ Figure 9-19

A, Distoangular impaction—uncommon and most difficult of the four types to remove. **B,** Occlusal surface of distoangular impaction is usually embedded in ramus of mandible and requires significant bone removal for extraction.

long axes of the second and third molars, the teeth also can be angled in a buccal or lingual direction. As was noted earlier, the linguocortical plate of the mandible becomes thinner as it progresses posteriorly. Therefore most mandibular third molars are angled toward the lingual direction or in lingual version. Occasionally, a tooth is angled toward the buccal aspect of the mandible or in buccal version.

Rarely, a tooth is a transverse impaction, that is, in an absolutely horizontal position in a buccolingual direction. The occlusal surface of the tooth can face either the buccal or lingual direction. To determine buccal or lingual version accurately, the dentist must take a perpendicular occlusal film. However, this determination usually is not necessary, because the surgeon can make this identification early in the operation, and the buccal or lingual position of the tooth does not greatly influence the difficulty of the surgery.

RELATIONSHIP TO ANTERIOR BORDER OF RAMUS

Another method for classifying impacted mandibular third molars is based on the amount of impacted tooth that is covered with the bone of the mandibular ramus. This classification is known as the *Pell and Gregory classification* and is sometimes referred to as the *Pell and Gregory classes 1, 2, and 3.* For this classification it is important that the surgeon carefully examine the relationship between the tooth and the anterior part of the ramus. If the mesiodistal diameter of the crown is completely anterior to the anterior border of the mandibular ramus, it is in a class 1 relationship. If the tooth is angled in a vertical direction, the chances for the tooth to erupt into a normal position are good (Figure 9-20).

If the tooth is positioned posteriorly so that approximately one half is covered by the ramus, the tooth's relationship with

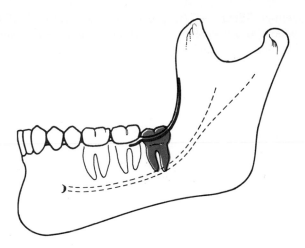

Figure 9-20

Pell and Gregory class 1 impaction. Mandibular third molar has sufficient anteroposterior room (anterior-to-anterior border of ramus) to erupt.

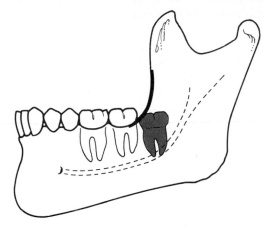

Figure 9-22

Pell and Gregory class 3 impaction. Impacted third molar is completely embedded in bone of ramus of mandible.

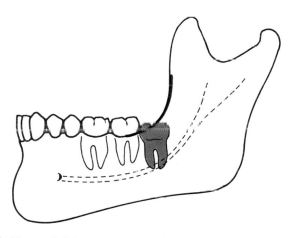

Figure 9-21

Pell and Gregory class 2 impaction. Approximately half is covered by anterior portion of ramus of mandible.

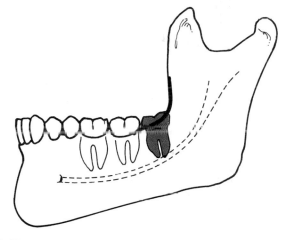

Figure 9-23

Pell and Gregory class A impaction. Occlusal plane of impacted tooth is at same level as occlusal plane of second molar.

the ramus is class 2. In the class 2 situation the tooth cannot become completely free from bone, because a small shelf of bone overlies the distal portion of the tooth (Figure 9-21). A class 3 relationship between the tooth and ramus occurs when the tooth is located completely within the mandibular ramus (Figure 9-22). It should be obvious that the class 1 relationship will provide the greatest accessibility to the impacted tooth and therefore will be easiest to remove. The class 3 relationship provides the least accessibility and therefore presents the greatest difficulty.

RELATIONSHIP TO OCCLUSAL PLANE

The depth of the impacted tooth compared with the height of the adjacent second molar provides the next classification system for determining the difficulty of impaction removal.

This classification system also was suggested by Pell and Gregory and is called *Pell and Gregory A, B, and C* classification. In this classification the degree of difficulty is measured by the thickness of the overlying bone; that is, the degree of difficulty increases as the depth of the impacted tooth increases. As the tooth becomes less accessible and it becomes more difficult to section the tooth and to prepare purchase points, the overall difficulty of the operation increases substantially.

A class A impaction is one in which the occlusal surface of the impacted tooth is level or nearly level with the occlusal plane of the second molar (Figure 9-23). A class B impaction is an impacted tooth with an occlusal surface between the occlusal plane and the cervical line of the second molar (Figure 9-24). Finally, the class C impaction is one in which the occlusal surface of the impacted tooth is below the cervical line of the second molar (Figure 9-25).

SUMMARY

The three classification systems discussed so far are used in conjunction to determine the difficulty of an extraction. For example, a mesioangular impaction with a class 1 ramus and a class A depth is easy to remove and is essentially the extraction of an erupted tooth (Figure 9-26). However, as the ramus relationship changes to a class 2 and the depth of the impaction increases to a class B, the degree of difficulty becomes greater. A horizontal impaction with a class 2 ramus relationship and a class B depth is a moderately difficult extraction and one that most general practitioners do not want

to attempt (Figure 9-27). Finally, the most difficult of all impactions is a distoangular impaction with a class 3 ramus relationship at a class C depth. Even specialists view removing this tooth as a surgical challenge (Figure 9-28).

ROOT MORPHOLOGY

Just as the root morphology of the erupted tooth has a major influence on the degree of difficulty of a closed extraction, root morphology plays a major role in determining the degree of difficulty of the impacted tooth's removal. Several factors must be considered when assessing the morphologic structure of the root.

The first consideration is the length of the root. As

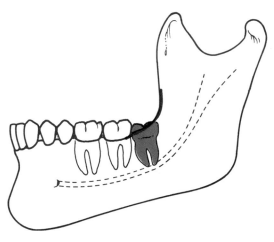

Figure 9-24

Pell and Gregory class B impaction. Occlusal plane of impacted tooth is between occlusal plane and cervical line of second molar.

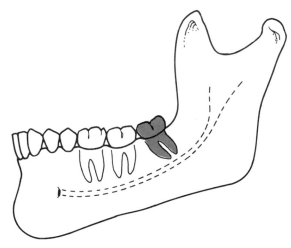

Figure 9-26

Mesioangular impaction with class 1 ramus relationship and class A depth. All three classifications make it easiest type of impaction to remove.

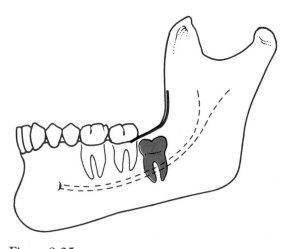

Figure 9-25

Pell and Gregory class C impaction. Impacted tooth is below cervical line of second molar.

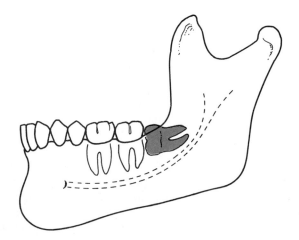

Figure 9-27

Horizontal impaction with class 2 ramus relationship and class B depth make it moderately difficult to extract.

discussed earlier, the optimal time for removal of an impacted tooth is when the root is one-third to two-thirds formed. When this is the case, the ends of the roots are blunt and almost never fracture (Figure 9-29). If the tooth is not removed during the formative stage and the entire length of the root develops, the possibility increases for abnormal root morphology and for fracture of the root tips during extraction. If the root development is insufficient (that is, less than one-third complete), the tooth is more difficult to remove, because it tends to roll in its crypt like a ball in a socket, which prevents easy elevation (Figure 9-30). The next factor to be assessed is

whether the roots are fused into a single, conical root (Figure 9-31) or if they are separate and distinct roots. The fused, conical roots are easier to remove than widely separate roots (Figure 9-32).

The curvature of the tooth roots also plays a role in the difficulty of the extraction. Severely curved or dilacerated roots are more difficult to remove than straight or slightly curved roots (Figure 9-32). The surgeon should examine the apex area of the radiograph carefully to assess the presence of small, abnormal, and sharply hooked roots that probably fracture if the surgeon does not give them special consideration.

The direction of the tooth root curvature is also important to examine preoperatively. During removal of a mesioangular impaction, roots that are curved gently in the distal direction (following along the pathway of extraction) can be removed without the force that can cause fracture of the roots. However, if the roots of a mesioangular impaction are curved mesially, the roots almost always fracture or must be sectioned before the tooth can be delivered.

The total width of the roots in the mesiodistal direction should be compared with the width of the tooth at the cervical line. If the tooth root width is greater, the extraction will be more difficult. More bone must be removed or the tooth must be sectioned before extraction.

Finally, the surgeon should assess the periodontal ligament space. Although in most patients the periodontal ligament space is of normal dimensions, it sometimes is wider or narrower. The wider the periodontal ligament space, the easier the tooth is to remove (Figure 9-33). A third molar that is in the proper stage of development for removal has a relatively broad periodontal ligament space, which eases extraction. However, older patients, especially those above age 40, tend

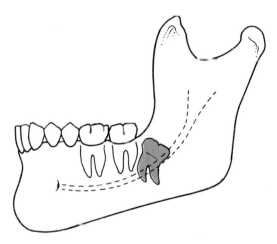

◇ Figure 9-28

Impaction with distoangular, class 3 ramus relationship and class C depth make it extremely difficult to remove.

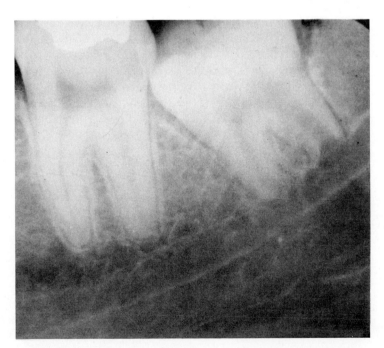

◇ Figure 9-29

Roots that are two-thirds formed, which are less difficult to remove.

to have a much narrower periodontal ligament space, which thereby increases the difficulty of the extraction.

SIZE OF FOLLICULAR SAC

The size of the follicle around the impacted tooth can help determine the difficulty of the extraction. If the follicular sac

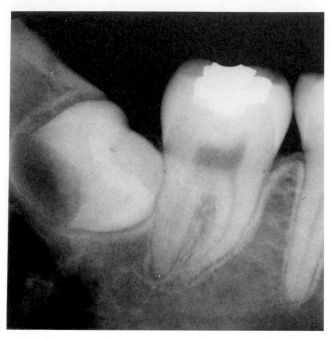

◇ **Figure 9-30**

Lack of root development. If extraction is attempted, crown will roll around in crypt, which makes it difficult to remove.

is wide (almost cystic in size), much less bone must be removed, which makes the tooth easier to extract (Figure 9-34). (Young patients are more likely to have large follicles, which is another factor that makes extractions easier in younger patients.) However, if the follicular space around the crown of the tooth is narrow or nonexistent, the surgeon must create space around the entire crown, which increases both the difficulty of the procedure and the time required to remove the tooth. The surgeon must carefully examine the follicle size when determining the difficulty of an extraction.

DENSITY OF SURROUNDING BONE

The density of the bone surrounding the tooth plays a role in determining the difficulty of the extraction. Although some clues can be seen on the radiographs, variations in radiograph density and angulation render interpretations based on radiographs unreliable. Bone density is best determined by the patient's age. Patients who are age 18 or younger have bone densities favorable for tooth removal. The bone is less dense, is more likely to be pliable, and expands and bends somewhat, which allows the socket to be expanded by elevators or by luxation forces applied to the tooth itself. Additionally, the bone is easier to cut with a dental drill and can be removed more rapidly than denser bone.

Conversely, patients who are older than age 35 have denser bone and thus decreased flexibility and ability to expand. In these patients the surgeon must remove all interfering bone, because it is not possible to expand the bony socket. In addition, as the bone increases in density, it becomes more difficult to remove with a dental drill, and the bone removal process takes longer.

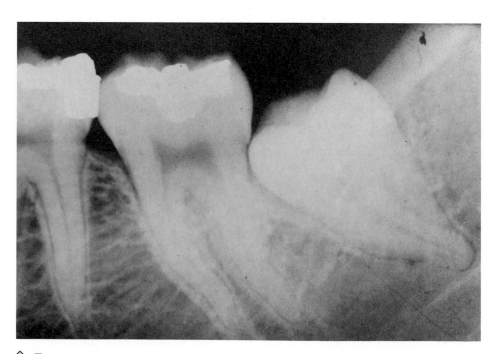

◇ **Figure 9-31**

Fused roots with conical shape.

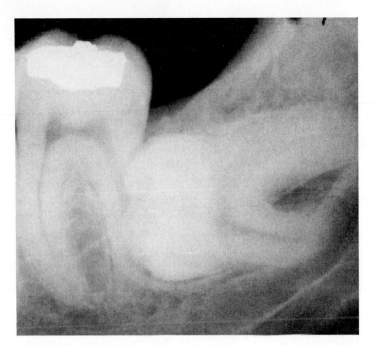

◆ Figure 9-32

Divergent roots with severe curvature. Such roots are more difficult to remove.

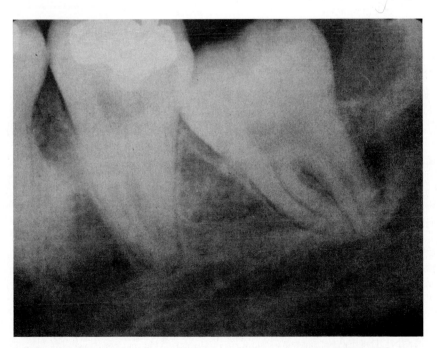

◆ Figure 9-33

Wide periodontal ligament space. Such space makes extraction process less difficult.

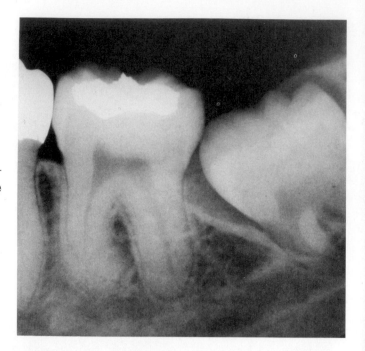

 Figure 9-34

Large follicular sac. When space of sac is large, amount of required bone removal is decreased.

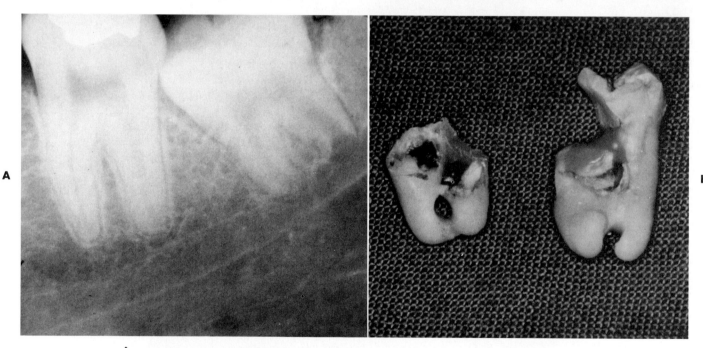

A   **B**

◇ **Figure 9-35**

A, Radiographic view of mandibular third molar suggests that it is surrounding or adjacent to inferior alveolar neurovascular canal. **B,** Hole and indentation in two roots of mandibular third molar indicate position of roots of this tooth to inferior alveolar canal. When this tooth was removed, inferior alveolar neurovascular bundle was severed. This is not same tooth as shown in **A.**

CONTACT WITH MANDIBULAR SECOND MOLAR

If there is space between the second molar and the impacted third molar, the extraction will be easier. However, if the tooth is a mesioangular or horizontal impaction, it is frequently in direct contact with the adjacent second molar. To remove the third molar safely without injuring the second molar the surgeon must be cautious with pressure from elevators or with the bur when removing bone. If the second molar has caries or a large restoration or root canal, the surgeon must take special care not to fracture the restoration or a portion of the carious crown (Figure 9-17, *B*).

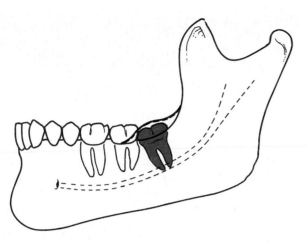

◇ **Figure 9-36**

Soft tissue impaction in which crown of tooth is covered by soft tissue only and can be removed without bone removal.

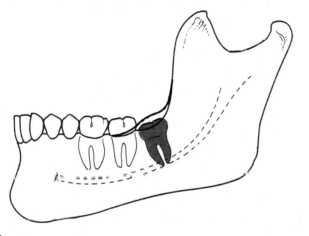

◇ **Figure 9-37**

Partial bone impaction in which part of tooth, usually posterior aspect, is covered with bone and requires either bone removal or tooth sectioning for extraction.

RELATIONSHIP TO INFERIOR ALVEOLAR NERVE

Impacted mandibular third molars frequently have roots that are superimposed on the inferior alveolar canal on radiographs. Although the canal is usually on the buccal aspect of the tooth, it is in close proximity to the tooth. Therefore one of the potential sequelae of impacted third molar removal is damage to or bruising of the inferior alveolar nerve. This usually results in some altered sensation (paresthesia or anesthesia) of the lower lip on the injured side. Although this altered sensation is usually brief (lasting only a few days), it may extend for weeks or months; on rare occasions it can be permanent. If the root ends of the tooth appear to be close to the inferior alveolar nerve, the surgeon must take special care to avoid injuring the nerve (Figure 9-35), which makes the procedure more difficult.

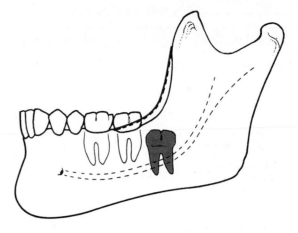

◇ **Figure 9-38**

Complete bone impaction in which tooth is completely covered with bone and requires extensive removal of bone for extraction.

NATURE OF OVERLYING TISSUE

The preceding systems all classify factors that make third molar extraction easier or more difficult. The classification system discussed in this section does not fit into this category. However, it is the system used by most dental insurance companies and the one by which the surgeon charges for his services.

According to this scheme, the three types of impactions are soft tissue impaction, partial bony impaction, and full bony impaction. An impaction is defined as a *soft tissue impaction* when the height of the tooth's contour is above the level of the alveolar bone, and the superficial portion of the tooth is covered by soft tissue only (Figure 9-36). To remove the soft tissue impaction, the surgeon must incise the soft tissue and reflect a small soft tissue flap to obtain access to the tooth to elevate it from its socket. The soft tissue impaction is usually the easiest of the three extractions.

The partial bone impaction occurs when the superficial portion of the tooth is covered by soft tissue, but the height of the tooth's contour is below the level of the surrounding alveolar bone (Figure 9-37). To remove the tooth, the surgeon must incise the soft tissue, reflect a soft tissue flap, and remove the bone above the height of the contour. The surgeon may need to divide the tooth in addition to removing bone.

The complete bone impaction is an impacted tooth that is completely encased in bone so that, when the surgeon reflects the soft tissue flap, no tooth is visible (Figure 9-38). To remove the tooth, extensive amounts of bone must be removed, and the tooth almost always must be sectioned. The complete bony impaction is often the most difficult to remove.

Although this classification is used extensively, it frequently has no relationship to the difficulty of the extraction. The parameters of angulation, ramus relationship, root morphology, and patient age are more important than this system. The surgeon should use all of the information available to determine the difficulty of the proposed surgery. See Boxes 9-1 and 9-2.

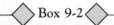

◇ Box 9-1 ◇

Factors that make impaction surgery less difficult

1. Mesioangular position
2. Class 1 ramus
3. Class A depth
4. Roots one-third to two-thirds formed*
5. Fused conical roots
6. Wide periodontal ligament*
7. Large follicle*
8. Elastic bone*
9. Separated from second molar
10. Separated from inferior alveolar nerve*
11. Soft tissue impaction

*Present in the young patient.

◇ Box 9-2 ◇

Factors that make impaction surgery more difficult

1. Distoangular
2. Class 3 ramus
3. Class C depth
4. Long, thin roots*
5. Divergent curved roots
6. Narrow periodontal ligament*
7. Thin follicle*
8. Dense, inelastic bone*
9. Contact with second molar
10. Close to inferior alveolar canal
11. Complete bone impaction

*Present in older patients.

MODIFICATION OF CLASSIFICATION SYSTEMS FOR MAXILLARY IMPACTED TEETH

The classification systems for the maxillary impacted third molar are essentially the same as for the impacted mandibular third molar. However, several distinctions and additions must be made to assess more accurately the difficulty of removal during the treatment-planning phase of the procedure.

In regard to angulation, the three types of maxillary third molars are the vertical impaction (Figure 9-39, *A*), the distoangular impaction (Figure 9-39, *B*), and the mesioangular impaction (Figure 9-39, *C*). The vertical impaction occurs approximately 63% of the time, the distoangular approximately 25%, and the mesioangular position approximately 12% of the time. Rarely, other positions, such as a transverse, inverted, or horizontal position, are encountered; these unusual positions account for less than 1% of impacted maxillary third molars.

The same angulations in mandibular third molar extractions cause opposite degrees of difficulty for maxillary third molar extractions. Vertical and distoangular impactions are the easiest to remove, whereas mesioangular impactions are the most difficult (exactly the opposite of impacted mandibular third molars). Mesioangular impactions are more difficult to remove because the bone that overlies the impaction and that must be removed or expanded is on the posterior aspect of the tooth and is much heavier than in the vertical or distoangular impaction. In addition, access to the mesioangularly positioned tooth is more difficult.

The position of the maxillary third molar in a buccopalatal direction is also important for determining the difficulty of the removal. Most maxillary third molars are angled toward the buccal aspect of the alveolar process, which makes the overlying bone in that area thin and therefore easy to remove

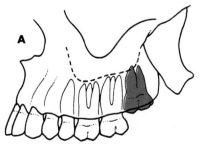
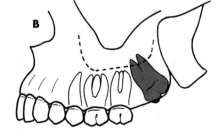
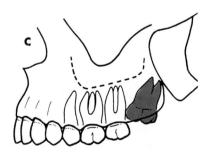

◇ Figure 9-39

A, Vertical impaction of maxillary third molar. This angle accounts for 63% of impactions. **B,** Distoangular impaction of maxillary third molar. This angle accounts for 25% of impactions. **C,** Mesioangular impaction of maxillary third molar. This angle accounts for 12% of impactions.

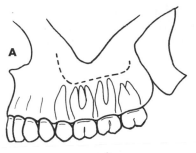 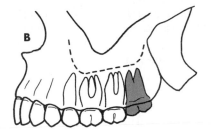 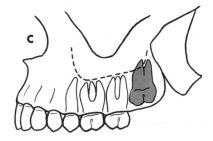

Figure 9-40

A, Pell and Gregory class A occlusal surface of third molar is at same level as that of second molar. **B,** Pell and Gregory class B occlusal surface of third molar is located between occlusal plane and cervical line of second molar. **C,** Pell and Gregory class C impacted maxillary third molar is deep to cervical line of second molar.

or to expand. Occasionally, the impacted maxillary third molar is positioned toward the palatal aspect of the alveolar process. This makes the tooth much more difficult to extract, because greater amounts of bone must be removed to gain access to the underlying tooth. A combination of radiographic assessment and clinical digital palpation of the tuberosity area can determine if the maxillary third molar is in the buccopalatal position. If the tooth is positioned toward the bucca, there is a definite palpable bulge in the area, whereas if the tooth is positioned palatally, there is a bony deficit in that region. When either is determined by clinical examination, the surgeon must anticipate a longer, more difficult procedure.

The Pell and Gregory A, B, and C classification used to diagnose the depth of impaction in the mandible also is used in the maxilla (Figure 9-40). Preoperative assessment of the remaining classifications are the same. The factors that influence the difficulty of mandibular impacted third molar removal are the same for maxillary third molar removal. For example, the individual impacted tooth root morphology plays a substantial role in determining the degree of extraction difficulty. The most common factor that causes difficulty with maxillary third molar removal is a thin, nonfused root with erratic curvature (Figure 9-41). The majority of maxillary third molars have fused roots that are conical. However, the surgeon should examine the preoperative radiograph carefully to ensure that this is the situation with each individual impaction. The surgeon also should check the periodontal ligament, because the wider the ligament space the less difficult the tooth is to remove. Also, similar to mandibular third molars, the periodontal ligament space tends to decrease as the patient increases in age.

The follicle surrounding the crown of the impacted tooth also has an influence on the difficulty of the extraction. If the follicular space is broad, the tooth will be easier to remove than if the follicular space is thin or nonexistent.

Bone density is also an important factor in maxillary impaction removal and is related closely to the age of the patient. The younger the patient, the less dense and more elastic—and therefore more expandable—is the bone surrounding the impacted third molar. As the patient ages, the

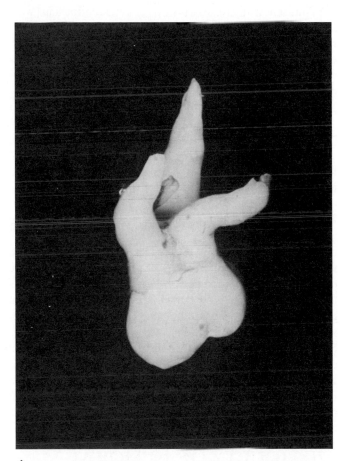

Figure 9-41

Maxillary third molar has most erratic and bizarre root formation of all teeth.

bone becomes more dense and less elastic, and the tooth becomes more difficult to remove.

The relationship to the adjacent second molar tooth also influences the difficulty of the extraction. It may require that additional bone be removed to displace the tooth from underneath the second molar. Also, because the use of elevators is common in the removal of maxillary third molars, the surgeon must be aware of the existence of large restorations or caries in the adjacent second molar. Injudicious use of elevators can result in the fracture of restorations or carious teeth.

The type of impaction, with respect to overlying tissue, also must be considered for maxillary third molars. The classification system used for mandibular teeth is the same as the system that is used for maxillary teeth: soft tissue impaction, partial bone impaction, and complete bone impaction. The definitions of these types of impactions are precisely the same as those used for the mandibular third molars.

Two additional factors influence the difficulty of maxillary third molar removal but do not exist for the mandibular third molars. Both are related to the structure and position of the maxillary sinus. First, the maxillary sinus is in intimate contact with the roots of the molar teeth, and, frequently, the maxillary third molar actually forms a portion of the posterior sinus wall. If this is the case, removal of the maxillary third molar may result in maxillary sinus complications, such as sinusitis or an oroantral fistula. The presence of the maxillary sinus does not necessarily make the removal of the impacted tooth more difficult, but it increases the likelihood of postoperative complications and morbidity.

Finally, in maxillary third molar removal the tuberosity of the posterior maxilla can be fractured. Such fractures are possible when several factors exist. Bone that is denser and less elastic, such as in older patients, is easily fractured. Also a large maxillary sinus makes the surrounding alveolar bone thin and more susceptible to fracture when excessive force is applied. A root morphology that is not fused but has divergent roots requires greater force to remove and can make fracture more likely. In addition, mesioangular impactions increase the possibility of fractures (Figure 9-39, *C*). In these situations the overlying tuberosity is heavier, but the surrounding bone is usually thinner. When the surgeon prepares a purchase point at the mesiocervical line, if the bone is nonelastic (as in older patients), if the tooth is multirooted with large bulbous roots (as in older patients), if the maxillary sinus is large and expanded to include the roots of the impacted third molar, or if the surgeon must use excessive force to elevate the tooth, fracture of the tuberosity becomes a greater risk. Management of the fractured tuberosity is discussed in Chapter 11.

DIFFICULTY OF REMOVAL OF OTHER IMPACTED TEETH

After the mandibular and maxillary third molars the next most commonly impacted tooth is the maxillary canine. If the patient seeks orthodontic care, the orthodontist will frequently request that the maxillary canine simply have the overlying soft and hard tissue removed so that the tooth can be manipulated into its proper position by orthodontic appliances. If the tooth is located superiorly in a class B or C position and is angled toward the labial aspect, the surgeon should uncover the tooth using an apically repositioned flap. This technique is used because, if the overlying soft tissue is simply removed and the tooth brought into position with orthodontic appliances, the surrounding soft tissue is likely to be alveolar mucosa instead of attached keratinized gingiva. The tooth is exposed by making an incision anterior, inferior, and posterior to the tooth; a small flap is elevated and retracted; the overlying bone is removed with a hand chisel or a bur; and the soft tissue flap is repositioned apically and sutured. Usually, a temporary periodontal pack is used until adequate healing has occurred. After 7 to 10 days the orthodontist can cement a bracket to the tooth and begin to manipulate it into position, or the surgeon can bond the bracket to the tooth at the time of surgery. Although this prolongs the surgery, the postoperative recovery is usually more rapid, and the orthodontist can begin mechanics earlier (Fig 9-42).

If the tooth is positioned toward the palatal aspect, the tooth may be either repositioned or removed. If the tooth is repositioned, it is surgically exposed and moved into position orthodontically. In this procedure the overlying soft tissue is excised; flaps are not needed to gain attached tissue. Because the bone in the palate is thicker, a bur is usually necessary to remove the overlying bone. The exposed tooth then is managed in the same manner as is the labially positioned tooth.

If the dentist decides the tooth should be removed, he must determine if the tooth is positioned labially, toward the palate, or in the middle of the alveolar process. If the tooth is on the labial aspect, it is easy to reflect a soft tissue flap and to remove the underlying bone and the tooth. However, if the tooth is on the palatal aspect or in the intermediate buccolingual position, it is much more difficult to remove. Therefore when assessing the impacted maxillary canine for removal the surgeon's most important assessment is of the buccolingual position of the tooth.

Similar considerations are necessary for other impactions, such as mandibular premolars and supernumerary teeth. The supernumerary tooth in the midline of the maxilla, called a *mesiodens,* is almost always found on the palate and should be approached from a palatal direction when it is removed.

SURGICAL PROCEDURE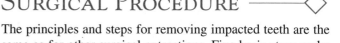

The principles and steps for removing impacted teeth are the same as for other surgical extractions. Five basic steps make up the technique. The first step is to have adequate exposure of the area of the impacted tooth. This means that the reflected soft tissue flap must be of an adequate dimension to allow the surgeon to retract the soft tissue and perform the necessary surgery. The second step is to assess the need for bone removal and to remove a sufficient amount of bone to expose the tooth for sectioning and delivery. The third step is to divide the tooth with a bur or chisel to allow the tooth to be extracted without removing excessive amounts of bone. In the fourth step the sectioned tooth is delivered from the alveolar process with the appropriate elevators. Finally, the wound is thoroughly

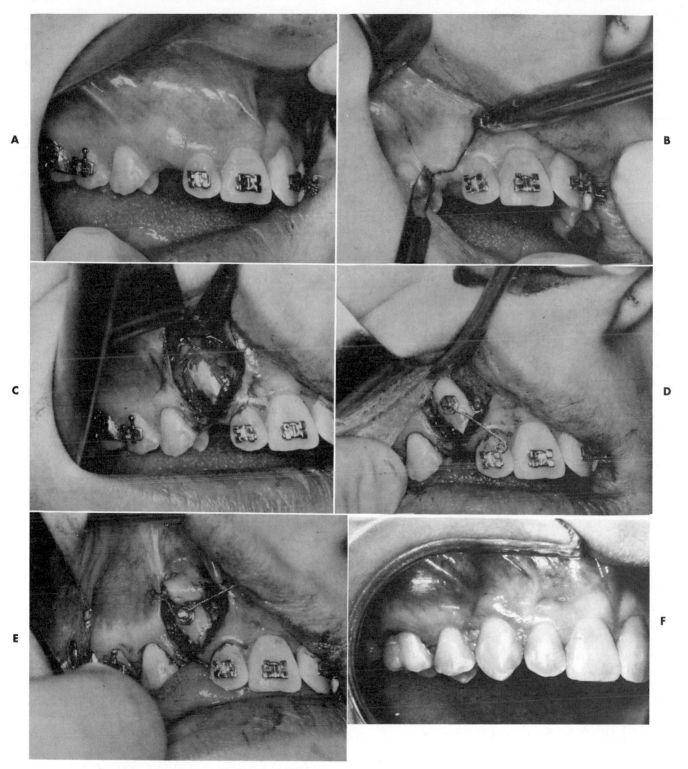

◇ Figure 9-42

A, Labially positioned impacted maxillary canine. Tooth should be uncovered with apically positioned flap procedure to preserve attached gingiva. **B,** Mucoperiosteal flap is outlined, allowing for repositioning of keratinized mucosa over exposed tooth. **C,** When flap is reflected, thin overlying bone is removed. **D,** Tissue is retracted and bracket bonded to teeth. **E,** Flap is sutured apically to tooth. **F,** After 6 months, exposed tooth is in desired position, with broad zone of attached gingiva.

cleansed with irrigation and mechanical débridement with a curette and is closed with simple interrupted sutures. The following discussion elaborates on these steps for the removal of impacted third molars.

Although the surgical approach to the removal of impacted teeth is similar to other surgical tooth extractions, it is important to keep in mind several distinct differences. For instance, the typical surgical extraction of a tooth or tooth root requires the removal of a relatively small amount of bone. However, when an impacted tooth (especially a mandibular third molar) is extracted, the amount of bone that must be removed to deliver the tooth is substantially greater. This bone also is much denser than it is for typical surgical extractions, and its removal requires better instrumentation and a higher degree of surgical skill.

Impacted teeth also frequently require sectioning, whereas other types of tooth extractions do not. Although erupted maxillary and mandibular molars occasionally are divided for removal, it is not a routine step in the extraction of these teeth. However, with impacted mandibular third molars, the surgeon is required to divide the tooth in a substantial majority of patients. The surgeon must therefore have the necessary equipment for such sectioning and the necessary skills and experience for dividing the tooth along the proper planes.

Unlike most other types of surgical tooth extractions, for an impacted tooth removal the surgeon must be able to balance the degree of bone removal and sectioning. Essentially, all impacted teeth can be removed without sectioning if a large amount of bone is removed. But the removal of excessive amounts of bone unnecessarily prolongs the healing period and may result in a weakened jaw. Therefore the surgeon should remove most mandibular third molars only after sectioning them. On the other hand, removal of a small amount of bone with multiple divisions of the tooth may cause the tooth sectioning process to take an excessively long time and thus prolong the operation unnecessarily. The surgeon must remove an adequate amount of bone and section the tooth into a reasonable number of pieces both to hasten healing and to minimize the time of the surgical procedure.

Step 1. Reflecting adequate flaps for accessibility. The difficulty of removing an impacted tooth depends on its accessibility. To gain access to the area and to visualize the overlying bone that must be removed, the surgeon must reflect an adequate mucoperiosteal flap. The reflection must be of a dimension adequate to allow the placement and stabilization of retractors and instruments for the removal of bone.

In most situations the envelope flap is the preferred technique. The envelope flap is easier to close and heals better than the three-cornered flap. However, if the surgeon requires greater access to the more apical areas of the tooth, which might stretch and tear the envelope flap, the surgeon should consider using a three-cornered flap.

The preferred incision for the removal of an impacted mandibular third molar is an envelope incision that extends from the mesial papilla of the mandibular first molar, around the necks of the teeth to the distobuccal line angle of the second molar, and then posteriorly to and laterally up the anterior border of the mandible (Figure 9-43, *A*). The incision must not continue posteriorly in a straight line, because the mandible diverges laterally, as well as posteriorly. An incision that extends straight posteriorly falls off the bone and into the sublingual space and may damage the lingual nerve, which is in close proximity to the mandible in the area of the third molar. If this nerve is traumatized, the patient probably will have a lingual nerve anesthesia, which may be distracting to the patient. The incision must always be on bone; therefore the surgeon should palpate the retromolar area carefully before beginning the incision.

The flap is reflected laterally to approximately the external oblique ridge with a periosteal elevator (Figure 9-43, *B*). The surgeon should not reflect beyond the external oblique ridge, because this results in increased morbidity and an increased number of complications following surgery. The retractor is placed on the buccal shelf, just at the external oblique ridge and is stabilized by applying pressure toward the bone, which results in a retractor that is stable and does not continually traumatize the soft tissue. The Austin and the Minnesota retractors are the most commonly used for flap reflection when removing mandibular third molars.

If the impacted third molar is deeply embedded in bone and requires more extensive bone removal, a releasing incision may be useful (Figure 9-43, *C* and *D*). The flap created by this incision can be reflected farther apically, without risk of tearing the tissue.

The recommended incision for the maxillary third molar is also an envelope incision. It extends posteriorly from the distobuccal line angle of the second molar and anteriorly to the mesial aspect of the first molar (Figure 9-44, *A* and *B*). In situations in which much access is required (for example, in a deeply embedded impaction), a release incision extending from the mesial aspect of the second molar can be used (Figure 9-44, *C* and *D*).

In the removal of third molars it is vital that the flap be large enough for adequate access and visibility of the surgical site. The flap must have a broad base if the release incision is used. The incision must be made with a smooth stroke of the scalpel, which is kept in contact with bone throughout the entire incision so that the mucosa and periosteum are completely incised. This allows a full-thickness mucoperiosteal flap to be reflected. The incision should be designed so that it can be closed over solid bone (rather than over a bony defect). This is achieved by extending the incision at least one tooth anterior to the surgical site when a vertical releasing incision is used. The incision should avoid vital anatomic structures. Only a single releasing incision should be used.

Step 2. Removal of overlying bone. Once the soft tissue is elevated and retracted so that the surgical field can be visualized, the surgeon must make a judgment concerning the amount of bone to be removed. In some situations the tooth can be sectioned with a chisel and delivered without bone removal. In most cases, however, some bone removal is required.

Although chisels can be used to remove bone overlying impacted teeth, most surgeons and patients prefer that bone be

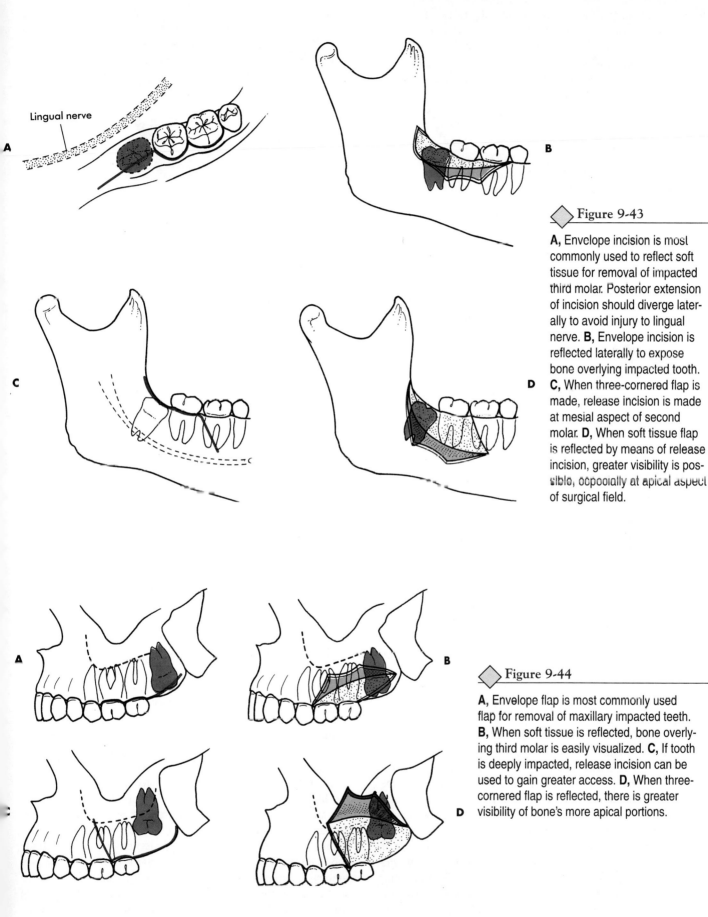

◇ Figure 9-43

A, Envelope incision is most commonly used to reflect soft tissue for removal of impacted third molar. Posterior extension of incision should diverge laterally to avoid injury to lingual nerve. **B,** Envelope incision is reflected laterally to expose bone overlying impacted tooth. **C,** When three-cornered flap is made, release incision is made at mesial aspect of second molar. **D,** When soft tissue flap is reflected by means of release incision, greater visibility is possible, especially at apical aspect of surgical field.

◇ Figure 9-44

A, Envelope flap is most commonly used flap for removal of maxillary impacted teeth. **B,** When soft tissue is reflected, bone overlying third molar is easily visualized. **C,** If tooth is deeply impacted, release incision can be used to gain greater access. **D,** When three-cornered flap is reflected, there is greater visibility of bone's more apical portions.

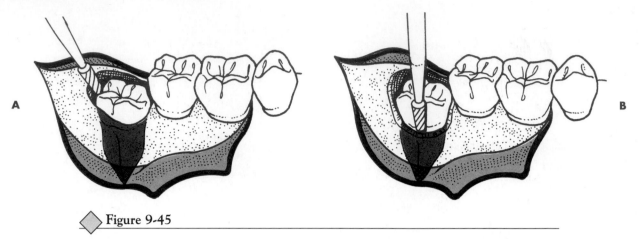

◇ **Figure 9-45**

A, After soft tissue has been reflected, bone overlying occlusal surface of tooth is removed with Fisher bur. **B,** Bone on buccodistal aspect of impacted tooth is then removed with bur.

removed with a drill. The preferred instrument is a handpiece with adequate speed, high torque, and the ability to be sterilized completely, usually in a steam autoclave.

The bone on the occlusal aspect and on the buccal and distal aspects down to the cervical line of the impacted tooth should be removed initially. The amount of bone that must be removed varies with the depth of the impaction, the morphology of the roots, and the angulation of the tooth. Rarely, if ever, is bone removed on the lingual aspect of the mandible because of the likelihood of damaging the lingual nerve.

The burs that are used to remove the bone overlying the impacted tooth vary with surgeons' preferences. A large round bur, such as a no. 8, is desirable, because it is an end-cutting bur and can be used effectively for drilling with a pushing motion. The tip of a fissure bur, such as a no. 703 bur, does not cut well, but the edge removes bone rapidly and sections teeth quickly when used in a lateral direction.

The typical bone removal for the extraction of an impacted mandibular tooth is illustrated in Figure 9-45. The bone on the occlusal aspect of the tooth is removed first to expose the crown of the tooth. Then the cortical bone on the buccal aspect of the tooth is removed down to the cervical line. Next, the bur can be used to remove bone between the tooth and the cortical bone in the cancellous area of the bone with a maneuver called *ditching*. This provides access for elevators to gain purchase points.

For maxillary teeth, bone is removed primarily on the buccal aspect of the tooth, down to the cervical line to expose the entire clinical crown. Additional bone must be removed on the mesial aspect of the tooth to allow an elevator an adequate purchase point to deliver the tooth. Because the bone overlying maxillary teeth is usually thin, it can be removed easily with a unibevel chisel with only hand pressure.

Step 3. Sectioning the tooth. Once sufficient amounts of bone have been removed from around the impacted tooth, the surgeon should assess the need to section the tooth. Sectioning allows portions of the tooth to be removed separately with elevators through the opening provided by bone removal.

The direction in which the impacted tooth should be divided depends primarily on the angulation of the impacted tooth. Although minor modifications are necessary for teeth with divergent roots or for teeth that are more deeply or less deeply impacted, the most important determinant is the tooth's angulation.

Tooth sectioning can be performed with either a bur or chisel; however, the bur is used by most surgeons. If a chisel is used, it must be extremely sharp, and the blows delivered to it by the mallet must be sharp and forceful enough to split the tooth. For the conscious patient the sound of the chisel striking the tooth may be bothersome.

When the bur is used, the tooth is sectioned three-fourths of the way toward the lingual aspect. A straight elevator is inserted into the slot made by the bur and rotated to split the tooth. The bur should not be used to section the tooth completely through in the lingual direction, because this is more likely to injure the lingual nerve.

The mesioangular impaction is usually the least difficult to remove of the four basic angulation types. After sufficient bone has been removed, the distal half of the crown is sectioned off at the buccal groove to just below the cervical line on the distal aspect. This portion is delivered. The remainder of the tooth is removed with a no. 301 elevator placed at the mesial aspect of the cervical line. A mesioangular impaction also can be removed by preparing a purchase point in the tooth with the drill and using a Crane pick elevator to elevate the tooth from the socket (Figure 9-46).

The next most difficult impaction to remove is the horizontal impaction. After sufficient bone has been removed down to the cervical line to expose the superior aspect of the distal root and the majority of the buccal surface of the crown, the tooth is sectioned by dividing the crown of the tooth from the roots at the cervical line. The crown of the tooth is removed, and the roots are displaced with a Cryer elevator into the space previously occupied by the crown. If the roots of an impacted third molar are divergent, they may require sectioning into two separate portions to be delivered individually (Figure 9-47).

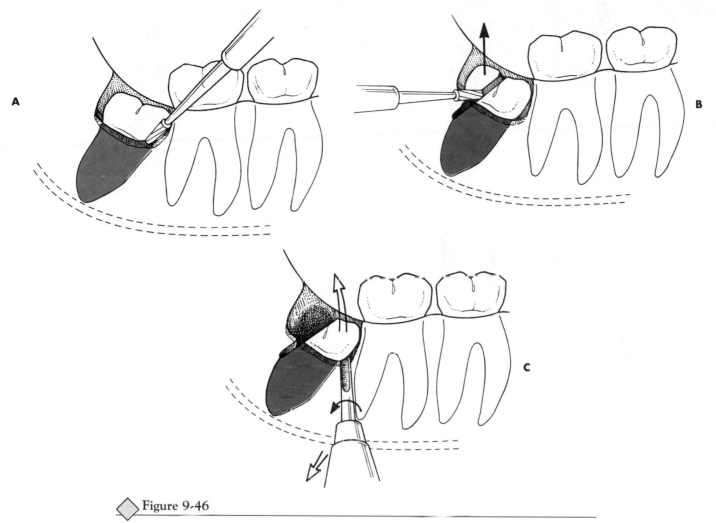

◇ Figure 9-46

A, When removing mesioangular impaction, buccodistal bone are removed to expose crown of tooth to cervical line. **B,** Distal aspect of crown is then sectioned from tooth. Occasionally it is necessary to section entire tooth into two portions rather than to section distal portion of crown only. **C,** After distal portion of crown has been delivered, small straight elevator is inserted into purchase point on mesial aspect of third molar, and tooth is delivered with rotational and lever motion of elevator.

The vertical impaction is one of the two most difficult impactions to remove. The procedure of bone removal and sectioning is similar to the mesioangular impaction; that is, the occlusal buccal and distal bone is removed. The distal half of the crown is sectioned and removed, and the tooth is elevated by applying an elevator at the mesial aspect of the cervical line of the tooth. This is more difficult than a mesioangular removal, because access around the mandibular second molar is difficult to obtain and requires the removal of substantially more bone on the buccal and distal sides (Figure 9-48).

The most difficult tooth to remove is the distoangular impaction. After sufficient bone is removed from the bucco-occlusal and the distal sides of the tooth, the crown is sectioned from the roots just above the cervical line. The entire crown is usually removed, because it interferes with visibility and access to the root structure of the tooth. If the roots are fused, a Cryer or straight elevator can be used to elevate the tooth into the space previously occupied by the crown. If the roots are divergent, they usually are sectioned into two pieces and delivered individually. Extracting this impaction is difficult, because much distal bone must be removed, and the tooth tends to be elevated distally and into the ramus portion of the mandible (Figure 9-49).

Impacted maxillary teeth rarely are sectioned, because the overlying bone is usually thin and relatively elastic. In situations in which the bone is thicker or the patient is older (and therefore the bone not so elastic), tooth extraction is usually accomplished by bone removal rather than tooth sectioning. Under no circumstances should a chisel be used to section maxillary teeth, because displacement of the tooth into the maxillary sinus is highly likely.

In general, impacted teeth elsewhere in the mouth are usually sectioned only at the cervical line. This permits removal of the crown portion of the tooth, displacement of the

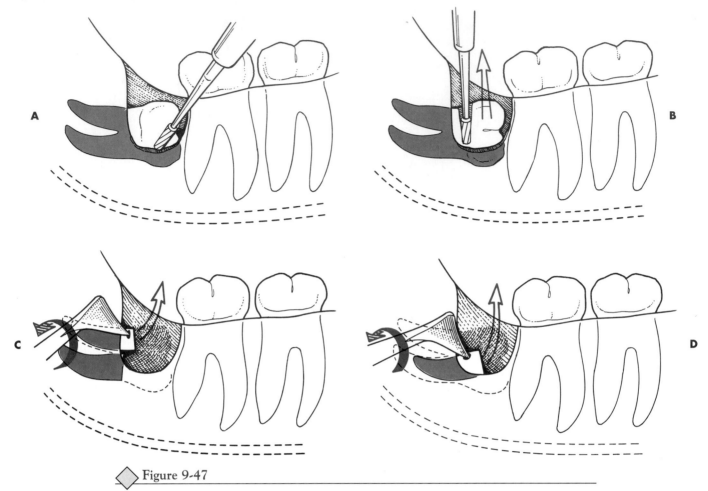

◇ Figure 9-47

A, During removal of horizontal impaction, bone overlying tooth (that is, bone on distal and buccal aspect of tooth) is removed with bur. **B,** Crown is then sectioned from roots of tooth and delivered from socket. **C,** Roots are then delivered together or independently by Cryer elevator used with rotational motion. Roots may require separation into two parts; occasionally, purchase point is made in root to allow Cryer elevator to engage it. **D,** Mesial root of tooth is elevated in similar fashion.

root portion into the space previously occupied by the crown, and removal of the root portion.

Step 4. Delivery of the sectioned tooth with elevator. Once adequate bone has been removed to expose the tooth and the tooth has been sectioned in the appropriate fashion, the tooth is delivered from the alveolar process with dental elevators. In the mandible the most frequently used elevators are the straight elevator, the paired Cryer elevator, and the Crane pick.

An important difference between the removal of an impacted mandibular third molar and of a tooth elsewhere in the mouth is that there is almost no luxation of the tooth for the purpose of expansion of the buccal or linguocortical plate. Instead, bone is removed and teeth are sectioned to prepare an unimpeded pathway for delivery of the tooth. Application of excessive force may result in unfavorable fracturing of the tooth, of excessive buccal bone, of the adjacent second molar, or possibly of the entire mandible. Elevators are designed not to deliver excessive force but to engage the tooth or tooth root

and to apply force in the proper direction. Some highly skilled surgeons use the periapical curette to remove sectioned roots from their sockets. Because the impacted tooth has never sustained occlusal forces, the periodontal ligament is weak and permits the easy displacement of the tooth root if appropriate bone is removed and force is delivered in the proper direction.

Delivery of maxillary third molars is accomplished with small straight elevators such as the no. 301 elevator, which luxates the tooth distobuccally. Some surgeons prefer angled elevators, such as the Potts or Miller elevators, which aid in gaining access to the impacted tooth. The elevator tip is inserted into the area at the mesial cervical line, and force is applied to displace the tooth in the distobuccal direction (Figure 9-50). The surgeon should be cautious about applying excessive pressure anteriorly to avoid damage to the root of the maxillary second molar. In addition, as pressure is applied to displace the tooth posteriorly, the surgeon should have a

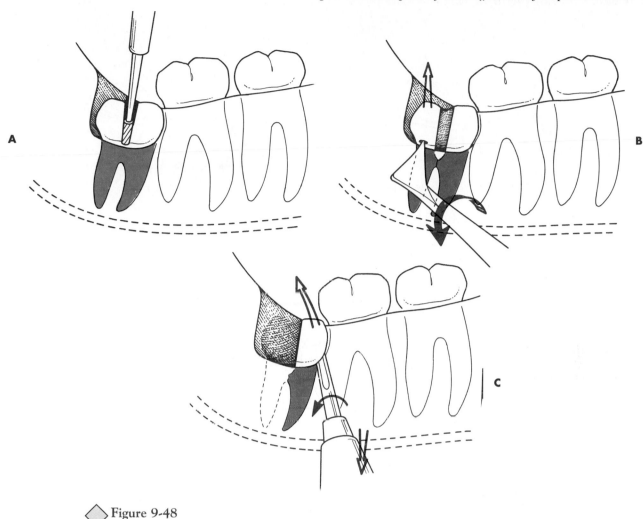

◇ **Figure 9-48**

A, When removing vertical impaction, bone on occlusal, buccal, and distal aspects of crown is removed, and tooth is sectioned into mesial and distal sections. If tooth has fused single root, distal portion of crown is sectioned off in manner similar to that depicted for mesioangular impaction. **B,** Posterior aspect of crown is elevated first with Cryer elevator inserted into small purchase point in distal portion of tooth. **C,** Small straight elevator no. 301 is then used to elevate mesial aspect of tooth by rotary and lever type of motion.

finger on the tuberosity of the maxilla (especially if the impaction is mesioangular) so that if a fracture does occur, steps can be taken to salvage the tuberosity of the maxilla.

Step 5. Débridement of wound and wound closure. Once the impacted tooth is removed from the alveolar process, the surgeon must direct attention to débriding the wound of all particulate bone chips and debris. The surgeon should irrigate the wound with sterile saline and take special care to irrigate thoroughly under the reflected soft tissue flap. The periapical curette should be used to mechanically débride both the superior aspect of the socket and the inferior edge of the reflected soft tissue to remove any particulate material that might have accumulated during surgery. The bone file should be used to smooth any sharp, rough edges of bone. A mosquito hemostat can be employed to remove any remnants of the

dental follicle. Once the follicle is grasped, it is lifted with a slow, steady pressure and will pull free from the surrounding hard and soft tissue. A final irrigation and a thorough inspection should be performed before the wound is closed.

The closure of the incision usually should be a primary closure. If the flap was well designed and not traumatized during the surgical procedure, it will fit closely back into its original position. The initial suture should be made through the attached tissue on the posterior aspect of the second molar. Additional sutures are placed posteriorly from that position and anteriorly through the papilla on the mesial side of the second molar. Usually three or four sutures are necessary to close an envelope incision. If a release incision was used, attention must be directed to closing that portion of the incision, as well.

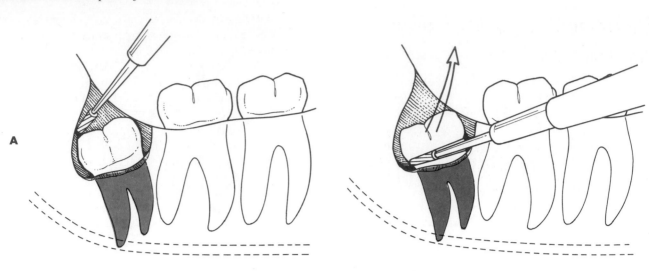

A

B

◇ **Figure 9-49**

A, For distoangular impaction, occlusal, buccal, and distal bone is removed with bur. It is important to remember that more distal bone must be taken off than for vertical or mesioangular impaction. **B,** Crown of tooth is sectioned off with bur, and crown is delivered with straight elevator. **C,** Purchase point is put into remaining root portion of tooth, and roots are delivered by Cryer elevator with wheel-and-axle type of motion. If roots diverge, it may be necessary in some cases to split them into independent portions.

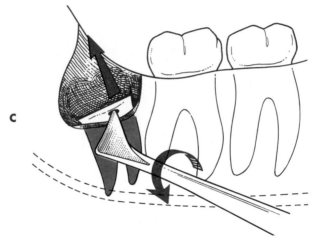

C

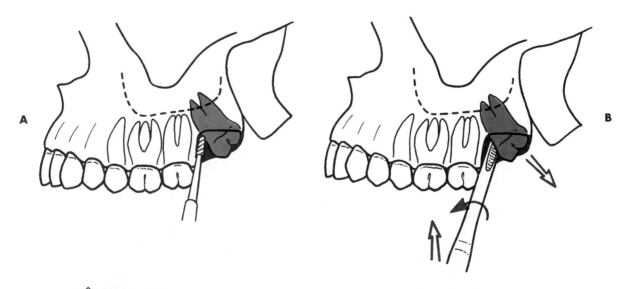

A

B

◇ **Figure 9-50**

Delivery of impacted maxillary third molar. **A,** Once soft tissue has been reflected, small amount of buccal bone is removed with bur or hand chisel. **B,** Tooth is then delivered by small straight elevator, with rotational and lever types of motion. Tooth is delivered in distobuccal and occlusal direction.

PERIOPERATIVE PATIENT MANAGEMENT ◇

The removal of impacted third molars is a surgical procedure that is associated with a large amount of patient anxiety. In addition, this surgical procedure can involve unpleasant noises and sensations. As a result, surgeons who routinely perform surgical removal of impacted third molars commonly recommend to their patients some type of profound anxiety control such as a general anesthetic or deep intravenous sedation.

The choice of technique is based on the surgeon's preference. However, the goals are to achieve a level of patient comfort that allows the surgeon to work rapidly and efficiently and that limits the patient's experience to the minimal number of unpleasant effects. Whether a deep intravenous sedative or a light general anesthetic is used, most surgeons intend their patients to have a profound amnesia of the procedure. Thus the patient has little if any unpleasant memory of the surgical experience.

In addition to the increased need for pain and anxiety control, a variety of medications are required to control the sequelae of third molar extraction surgery. The surgeon should consider writing a prescription for a potent oral analgesic for every patient who undergoes surgical removal of an impacted third molar. Enough tablets should be prescribed to last for 3 or 4 days. Combinations of codeine, or codeine congeners, with aspirin or acetaminophen commonly are used. Nonsteroidal antiinflammatory analgesics may be of some value for certain patients.

To minimize the swelling common after the surgical removal of impacted third molars, some surgeons prefer to give parenteral steroids. Intravenous administration of a modest amount of a glucocorticoid steroid provides sufficient antiinflammatory activity to give relief to swelling. Although many different regimens and protocols for steroids exist, a relatively common one is the single administration of 8 mg of dexamethasone before surgery. This is a relatively long-acting steroid, and its efficacy in controlling third molar postsurgical swelling is documented. Although steroids given in this manner have few side effects or contraindications, the general philosophy of weighing the risks and benefits of drug administration must be followed carefully before the decision is made to give these drugs routinely.

Another medication that sometimes is used is an antibiotic. If a patient has had a preexisting pericoronitis, it is common to prescribe antibiotics for a few days after surgery. However, if the patient is healthy and there is no systemic indication for antibiotics nor a preexisting local infection, antibiotics usually are not prescribed.

The normal postoperative experience of a patient after surgical removal of an impacted third molar is more involved than after a routine extraction. The patient can expect a modest amount of swelling in the area of the surgery for 3 to 4 days, with the swelling completely dissipating by about 10 days. A modest amount of discomfort usually follows the procedure. This discomfort can be effectively controlled with potent oral analgesics. Patients usually require analgesics for 2 or 3 days

on a routine basis and intermittently for several more days. The patient may have some mild soreness in the region for 2 to 3 weeks after the surgery.

Patients who have had mandibular third molars surgically removed frequently have mild-to-moderate trismus. This inability to open the mouth interferes with the patient's normal oral hygiene and eating habits. Patients should be warned that they will be unable to open their mouths normally following surgery. The trismus gradually resolves, and the ability to open the mouth should return to normal by 10 to 14 days after surgery.

All of the sequelae of the surgical removal of impacted teeth are of less intensity in the young, healthy patient and of far greater intensity in the older, more debilitated patient. Even healthy adult patients between the ages of 35 to 40 years have a significantly more difficult time following the extraction of impacted third molars than do healthy 17-year-old patients.

REFERENCES

1. Bruce RA, Frederickson GC, Small GS: Age of patients and morbidity associated with mandibular third molar surgery, *J Am Dent Assoc* 101:240, 1980.
2. Kugelberg CF: Periodontal healing two and four years after impacted lower third molar surgery, *Int J Oral Maxillofac Surg* 19:341, 1990.
3. Kugelberg CF, Ahlstrom U, Ericson S et al: The influence of anatomical, pathophysiological and other factors on periodontal healing after impacted lower third molar surgery, *J Clin Periodontol* 18:37, 1991.
4. Kugelberg CF, Ahlstrom U, Ericson S et al: Periodontal healing after impacted lower third molar surgery in adolescents and adults, *Int J Oral Maxillofac Surg* 20:18, 1991.
5. Leone SA, Edenfield MJ, Coehn ME: Correlation of acute pericoronitis and the position of the mandibular third molar, *Oral Surg Oral Med Oral Pathol* 62:245, 1986.
6. Lysell L, Rohlin M: A study of indications used for removal of the mandibular third molar, *Int J Oral Maxillofac Surg* 17:161, 1988.
7. Marmary J et al: Alveolar bone repair following extraction of impacted mandibular third molars, *Oral Surg Oral Med Oral Pathol* 61:324, 1986.
8. Meister F Jr et al: Periodontal assessment following surgical removal of mandibular third molars, *Gen Dentistry* 14:120, 1986.
9. Nordenram A, Hultin M, Kjellman O et al: Indications for surgical removal of the mandibular third molar, *Swed Dent J* 11:23-29, 1987.
10. Osborne WH, Snyder AJ, Tempel TR: Attachment levels and crevicular depths at the distal aspect of mandibular second molars following removal of adjacent third molars, *J Periodontol* 53:93, 1982.
11. Richardson JE, Dent M: The effect of mandibular first premolar extraction on third molar space, *Angle Orthod* 59:291, 1986.
12. Richardson ME: The role of the third molar in the cause of late lower arch crowding: a review, *Am J Orthod Dentofac Orthop* 95:79, 1989.
13. Stanley HR, Alattar M, Collett WK et al: Pathological sequelae of "neglected" impacted third molars, *J Oral Pathol* 17:113, 1988.

14. Venta I, Murtomaa H, Turtola L et al: Assessing the eruption of lower third molars on the basis of radiographic features, *Br J Oral Maxillofac Surg* 29:259, 1991.

15. Venta I, Murtomaa H, Turtola L et al: Clinical follow-up study of third molar eruption from ages 20 to 26 years, *Oral Surg Oral Med Oral Pathol* 72:150, 1991.

16. von Wowern N, Nielsen HO: The fate of impacted lower third molars after the age of 20, *Int J Oral Maxillofac Surg* 18:277, 1989.

BIBLIOGRAPHY

Bean LR, King DR: Periocoronitis: its nature and etiology, *J Am Dent Assoc* 83:1074, 1971.

ChinQuee TA et al: Surgical removal of the fully impacted mandibular third molar: the influence of flap design and alveolar bone height on the periodontal status of the second molar, *J Periodontol* 56:625, 1985.

Laskin DM: Indications and contraindications for removal of impacted third molars, *Dent Clin North Am* 13:919, 1969.

Lytle JJ: Indications and contraindications for removal of the impacted tooth, *Dent Clin North Am* 23:333, 1979.

Pell GJ, Gregory GT: Report on a ten-year study of a tooth division technique for the removal of impacted teeth, *Am J Orthod* 28:660, 1942.

Peterson LJ: Principles of management of impacted teeth. In Peterson LJ, editor: *Principles of oral and maxillofacial surgery,* Philadelphia, 1992, JB Lippincott.

CHAPTER 10

POSTOPERATIVE PATIENT MANAGEMENT

LARRY J. PETERSON

CHAPTER OUTLINE ◇

O nce the surgical procedure has been completed, patients should be given proper instructions on how to care for themselves for the remainder of the day of surgery and for a few days afterward. If the patient is to receive intravenous sedation, the postoperative management instructions must be discussed *before* the sedation is given. These instructions should also be repeated to the patient's escort before discharge from the office.

Postoperative instructions should predict what the patient is likely to experience, explain why these phenomena occur, and tell the patient how to manage and control the typical postoperative sequelae. The instructions must be given to the patient orally and on a written sheet. The instruction sheet should describe the typical problems and their management. It should also include a phone number at which the surgeon can be reached in an emergency. The language must be clear and simple enough to be followed by all patients. A typical postoperative instruction sheet is found in Appendix VII.

This chapter discusses common postoperative problems and methods of controlling them.

CONTROL OF POSTOPERATIVE BLEEDING ◇

Once an extraction has been completed, the initial maneuver to control postoperative bleeding is the placement of a small, damp gauze pack directly over the empty socket. Large packs that cover the occlusal surfaces of the teeth do not apply pressure to the bleeding socket and should not be used (Figure 10-1). The gauze should be moistened so that the oozing blood does not coagulate in the gauze and then dislodge the clot when the gauze is removed. The patient should be instructed to bite firmly on this gauze for at least 30 minutes and not to chew on the gauze but rather to hold it without opening or closing the mouth. Talking should be kept to a minimum for 3 or 4 hours.

Patients should be informed that it is normal for a tooth socket to ooze slightly for 24 hours after the extraction procedure. They should be warned that a small amount of blood and a large amount of saliva will appear to be a large amount of blood. If the bleeding is more than a slight ooze, the patient should be instructed on how to reapply a small, damp gauze pack directly over the area of the extraction. The patient should be instructed to hold this second gauze pack in place for as long as 1 hour to gain control of bleeding.

Patients should be cautioned about things that may aggravate the bleeding and that should therefore be avoided. Patients who smoke should be encouraged to avoid smoking for the first 12 hours or, more commonly, if they must smoke, to draw on the cigarette very lightly. The negative pressure created by this suction in the mouth may promote bleeding and should be discouraged. The patient should be told not to suck on a straw when drinking; this also creates negative pressure. The patient should be advised not to spit during the first 12 hours after surgery. The process of spitting involves negative pressure and mechanical agitation of the extraction, which

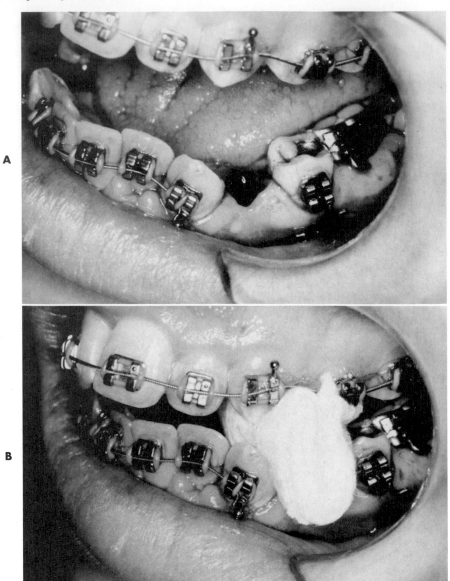

A

B

◇ Figure 10-1

A, Fresh extraction site will bleed excessively unless a properly positioned gauze pack is placed. **B,** Small gauze pack is placed to fit only in area of extraction. This permits pressure to be applied directly to socket.   *Continued*

may prolong bleeding. Patients who object to having blood in the mouth should be encouraged to bite firmly on a piece of gauze to control the hemorrhage and to swallow their saliva instead of spitting it out. Finally, no strenuous exercise should be performed for the first 12 to 24 hours after extraction, because the increased circulation may result in bleeding.

Patients should be warned that there may be some oozing during the night and that they will probably have some blood on their pillows. This will prevent many frantic telephone calls to the surgeon in the middle of the night.

Patients should also be instructed that if they are worried about their bleeding, they should call to get additional advice. Prolonged bleeding, bright red bleeding, or large clots in the patient's mouth are all indications for a return visit. The dentist should then examine the area closely and apply appropriate measures to control the bleeding (see Chapter 11).

ECCHYMOSIS

Some patients have blood that oozes submucosally and subcutaneously, which appears as a bruise in the oral tissues on the face (Figure 10-2). Blood in the subcutaneous tissues is known as *ecchymosis*. This is usually seen in older patients because of their decreased tissue tone and weaker intercellular attachment. Ecchymosis is not dangerous and does not increase pain or infection. The patient, however, should be

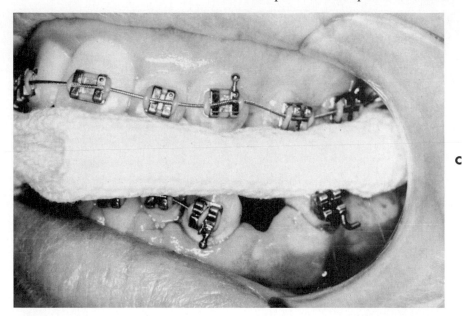

c

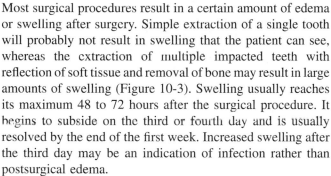

◇ Figure 10-1, cont'd

C, Large or mispositioned gauze pack is not effective in controlling bleeding. Pressure of biting is not directed to socket.

warned that ecchymosis may occur, because if they awaken on the second postoperative day and see bruising in the cheek or submandibular area, they may become very apprehensive about their progress. This is easily preventable by postoperative instructions.

EDEMA

Most surgical procedures result in a certain amount of edema or swelling after surgery. Simple extraction of a single tooth will probably not result in swelling that the patient can see, whereas the extraction of multiple impacted teeth with reflection of soft tissue and removal of bone may result in large amounts of swelling (Figure 10-3). Swelling usually reaches its maximum 48 to 72 hours after the surgical procedure. It begins to subside on the third or fourth day and is usually resolved by the end of the first week. Increased swelling after the third day may be an indication of infection rather than postsurgical edema.

Once the surgery is completed and the patient is ready to be discharged, application of ice packs to the area may help minimize the swelling and make the patient feel more comfortable; it also provides the patient with some active involvement in their own care. Ice should not be placed directly on the skin, but rather a layer of dry cloth should be placed between the ice container and the tissue to prevent superficial tissue damage. The ice bag should be kept on the local area for 20 minutes and then left off for 20 minutes. Ice-pack application should be maintained for no more than 24 hours, because longer application does not help. Ice packs are only minimally effective in controlling edema.

On the second postoperative day, neither ice nor heat should be applied to the face. On the third and subsequent postoperative days, application of heat may help to resolve the swelling more quickly. Heat sources such as hot water bottles and heating pads are recommended. Patients should be warned to avoid high-level heat for long periods to keep from burning or injuring the skin.

It is most important that patients anticipate some amount of swelling. They should also be warned that the swelling may tend to wax and wane, occurring more in the morning and less in the evening because of postural variation. Patients should be informed that a moderate amount of swelling is a normal and healthy reaction of the tissue to the trauma of surgery. They should not be concerned or frightened by it, because it will resolve within a few days.

TRISMUS

Extraction of teeth may result in trismus, or limitation in opening the mouth. This is the result of inflammation involving the muscles of mastication. The trismus may be a result of multiple injections of local anesthetic, especially if the injections have penetrated muscles. The muscle most likely to be involved is the medial pterygoid muscle, which may be inadvertently penetrated by the local anesthetic needle during the inferior alveolar nerve block.

Surgical extraction of impacted mandibular third molars frequently results in trismus, because the inflammatory response to the surgical procedure is sufficiently widespread to involve several muscles of mastication. Trismus usually is not severe and does not hamper the patient's activity. However, to prevent alarm, patients should be warned that this phenomenon may occur.

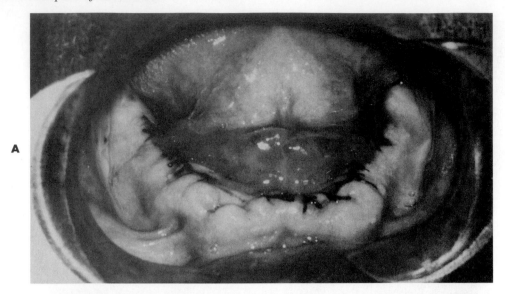

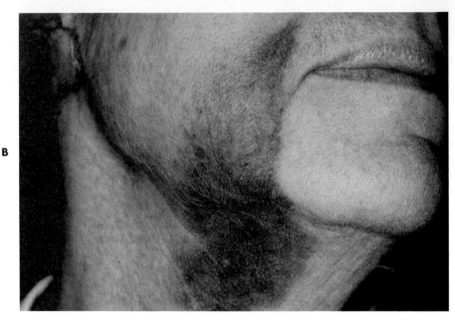

◇ Figure 10-2

A, Moderate ecchymosis of floor of mouth, which was evident at time of suture removal on sixth day after multiple extractions. **B,** Moderate widespread ecchymosis of right side of face and neck in elderly patient after extraction of several mandibular teeth.

DIET ◇

Patients who have had extractions may avoid eating because of local pain or fear of pain when eating. Therefore they should be given very specific instructions regarding their postoperative diet. A high-calorie, high-volume liquid diet is best for the first 12 to 24 hours.

The patient must have an adequate intake of fluids, usually at least 2 quarts, during the first 24 hours. The fluids should be juices, milk, or water.

Food in the first 12 hours should be soft and cool. Cool and cold foods help keep the local area comfortable. Ice cream and milkshakes, unlike solid foods, tend not to cause local trauma nor initiate rebleeding episodes.

If the patient had multiple extractions in all areas of the mouth, a soft diet is recommended for several days after the surgical procedure. In most situations, patients have surgery only in an isolated quadrant or half of the mouth, which leaves the opposite side free to chew. The patient should be advised to return to a normal diet as soon as possible.

Patients who are diabetic should be encouraged to return to their normal insulin and diet routine as soon as possible. For

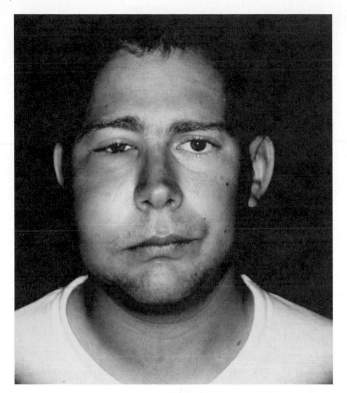

◇ Figure 10-3

Extraction of impacted right maxillary and mandibular third molars 2 days before photograph was taken. Patient exhibits moderate amount of facial edema, which will resolve within 1 week of surgery.

such patients the surgeon should plan surgery in only one side of the mouth at each surgical sitting, thereby not interfering with the normal dietary intake.

ORAL HYGIENE ◇

Patients should be advised that keeping the teeth and mouth reasonably clean results in a more rapid healing of their surgical wounds. On the day of surgery the patient can gently brush the teeth that are away from the area of surgery in the usual fashion. They should avoid brushing the teeth immediately adjacent to the extraction site to prevent a new bleeding episode and to avoid pain.

On the following day the patient should begin gentle rinses with warm salt water. A saline solution can be prepared by dissolving one-half teaspoon of salt in an 8-ounce glass of warm water. The water should be warm but not hot enough to burn the tissue. Most patients can resume their preoperative oral hygienic methods by the third or fourth day after surgery. Dental floss should be used in the usual fashion on teeth anterior and posterior to the extraction sites as soon as the patient is comfortable enough to do so.

If oral hygiene is likely to be compromised following extractions in multiple areas of the mouth, local antibiotic mouth rinses with agents such as chlorhexidine may be used. Twice-daily rinses for approximately 1 week after surgery may result in more rapid healing.

CONTROL OF POSTOPERATIVE PAIN AND DISCOMFORT ◇

All patients expect a certain amount of pain after a surgical procedure, so it is important for the dentist to discuss this issue carefully with each patient before discharge from the office. The surgeon must help the patient have a realistic expectation of what type of pain may occur. The surgeon must therefore pay attention to the patient's concerns and preconceived ideas of how much pain is likely to occur. Patients who tell the surgeon that they expect a great deal of pain after surgery should not be ignored and told to take an aspirin if it hurts, because these are the patients most likely to return for pain medication. It is important for the surgeon to assure patients, especially the latter group, that their postoperative pain can be effectively managed.

The pain a patient may experience after a surgical procedure such as tooth extraction is highly variable and depends a great deal on the patient's preoperative frame of mind. The surgeon who spends several minutes discussing these issues with the patient before surgery will be able to recommend the most appropriate medication.

All patients should be given advice concerning analgesics before they are discharged. Even the surgeon who believes that no analgesics are necessary should recommend that the patient take aspirin or acetaminophen postoperatively to prevent initial discomfort when the effect of the local anesthetic disappears. Patients who are expected to have a higher level of pain should be given prescriptions for analgesics that will control the pain. The surgeon should also take care to advise the patient that the goal of analgesic medication is management of pain and not elimination of all soreness.

The surgeon must understand the three characteristics of the pain that occurs after tooth extraction. First, it is usually not severe and can be managed in most patients with mild analgesics. Second, the peak pain experience occurs about 12 hours after the extraction and diminishes rapidly after that. Finally, the pain from extraction rarely persists longer than 2 days after surgery. With these factors kept in mind, the patients can best be advised regarding the effective use of analgesics.

The first dose of analgesic medication should be taken before the effect of the local anesthetic subsides. If this is done, the patient will not experience the intense, sharp pain that follows the loss of the local anesthesia. By preventing the sudden onset of surgical pain, the subsequent control of it is more easily and predictably achieved with mild analgesics. Postoperative pain is much more difficult to overcome if administration of analgesic medication is delayed.

For some patients who are scheduled to undergo more extensive surgical procedures, preoperative dosing with nonsteroidal analgesics may be useful. Not only is the analgesic effect of the drug active at the time of the cessation of the local anesthetic effect, but there also may be some antiinflammatory effect that may actually reduce the pain sensations. If local anesthetic is used and there are no

◇ Table 10-1. Normal dosages for nonsteroidal antiinflammatory drugs (NSAIDs)

Brand name	Generic name	Adult dosage	Maximum daily dose
p-Aminophenol			
Tylenol	Acetaminophen	500-1000 mg q4h	4000 mg
Salicylates			
Aspirin	Aspirin	500-1000 mg q4h	4000 mg
Dolobid	Diflunisal	500 mg q8h	1500 mg
Propionic Acids			
Advil, Motrin, etc.	Ibuprofen	200-800 mg q4-6h	3200 mg
Naprosyn	Naproxen	275-500 mg bid	1000 mg
Anaprox	Naproxen sodium	275-550 mg bid	1475 mg
Orudis	Ketoprofen	50-75 mg q8h	300 mg
Ansaid	Flurbiprofen	50-100 mg bid	300 mg
Indol			
Clinoril	Sulindac	150-200 mg bid	400 mg
Lodine	Etodolac	200-400 mg tid	1200 mg
Phenylacetic Acids			
Voltaren	Diclofenac sodium	25-75 mg bid-tid	200 mg
Oxicams			
Feldene	Piroxicam	10-20 mg qd	20 mg
Fenamates			
Meclomen	Meclofenamate sodium	100 mg 8h	400 mg
Ketoralac Tromethamine			
Toradol oral	Ketoralac	10 mg q6h	40 mg
Toradol IV/IM	Ketoralac	15-30 mg q6h	150 mg

restrictions for preoperative oral intake, the surgeon may wish to consider routine use of a preoperative dose of a drug, such as 600 mg of ibuprofen.

The strength of the analgesic is also of importance. Potent analgesics are not required in most extraction situations; instead, analgesics with a lower potency per dose are effective. The patient can then be told to take one, two, or three tablets as necessary to control their pain. By allowing the patient to assume an active role in determining the amount of medication to take, a more precise and realistic control can be achieved. Patients should be warned that taking too much of the medication will result in drowsiness and an increased chance of an upset stomach. In most situations, patients should take their medication with some type of food to decrease its irritating effect on the stomach.

Aspirin has been amply demonstrated to be an effective medication to control the pain and discomfort of a tooth extraction. This drug works primarily peripherally, interfering with prostaglandin synthesis. The surgeon should prescribe a combination aspirin-narcotic medication that delivers 500 to 1000 mg of aspirin per dose. If the patient cannot tolerate aspirin, acetaminophen in a similar dosage is a good alternative drug. Aspirin has the disadvantage of causing a decrease in platelet aggregation. Acetaminophen does not have this characteristic, so some surgeons prefer its use to decrease the incidence of postoperative bleeding episodes. However, aspirin remains the drug of choice for control of mild-to-moderate pain after tooth extraction. Nonsteroidal antiinflammatory analgesics (NSAIDs), such as ibuprofen, are

also useful for patients who have had a tooth extraction. Well-controlled studies have documented their effectiveness. Normal useful dosages of several commonly used drugs are listed in Table 10-1.

Centrally acting analgesics are also frequently used to control pain after tooth extraction. The most commonly used drugs are codeine and the codeine congeners such as oxycodone, hydrocodone, and dihydrocodeine. These narcotics are well absorbed from the gut, and when used in equipotent dosages, produce similar pain relief, drowsiness, and gastrointestinal upset (Table 10-2). They are rarely used alone; instead, they are formulated with other analgesics, primarily aspirin or acetaminophen. When codeine is used, the amount of codeine is frequently designated by a numbering system. Compounds labeled no. 1 have 7.5 mg of codeine, no. 2 has 15 mg, no. 3 has 30 mg, and no. 4 has 60 mg.

When a combination of analgesic drugs is used, the dentist must keep in mind that it is necessary to provide 500 to 1000 mg of aspirin or acetaminophen every 6 hours to achieve maximal effectiveness from the nonnarcotic. Many of the compound drugs have only 300 mg of aspirin or acetaminophen added to the narcotic. An example of a rational approach would be to prescribe a compound containing 300 mg of aspirin and 15 mg of codeine (no. 2). The usual adult dose would be two tablets of this compound every 4 hours. This two-tablet (30 mg of codeine and 600 mg of aspirin) dose provides a nearly ideal analgesia. Should the patient require stronger analgesic action, three tablets can be taken with increased effectiveness of both aspirin and codeine. Doses that

...

 Table 10-2. Normal dosages of narcotic analgesics

Oral narcotic	Usual dosage
Codeine	30 mg q4h
Oxycodone	5 mg q4h
Hydrocodone	5 mg q4h
Dihydrocodine	30 mg q4h
Pentazocine	50 mg q4h
Meperidine	100 mg q4h

 Table 10-3. Commonly used combination analgesics

Brand name	Amount (mg)	Amount (mg)
Codeine-aspirin	**Codeine**	**Aspirin**
Empirin		
No. 3	30	325
No. 4	60	325
Fiorinal*	30	325
Codeine-acetaminophen	**Codeine**	**Acetaminophen**
Fioricet*	30	325
Phenopehn		
No. 3	30	325
No. 4	60	325
Tylenol		
No. 2	15	300
No. 3	30	300
No. 4	60	300
Oxycodone-aspirin	**Oxycodone**	**Aspirin**
Percodan	5	325
Percdodan-Demi	2.5	325
Oxycodone-acetaminophen	**Oxycodone**	**Acetaminophen**
Percocet	5	325
Tylox	5	500
Hydrocodone-aspirin	**Hydrocodone**	**Aspirin**
Lortab ASA	5	500
Hydrocodone-acetaminophen	**Hydrocodone**	**Acetaminophen**
Vicodin	5	500
Vicodine ES	7.5	750
Lorcet HD	5	500
Lorcet Plus	7.5	650
Lorcet 10/650	10	650
Lortab 2.5/500	2.5	500
Lortab 5/500	5	500
Dihydrocodeine-aspirin	**Dihydrocodeine**	**Aspirin**
Synalgos-DC†	16	350
Propoxyphene-acetaminophen	**Propoxphene**	**Acetaminophen**
Darvocet N-1000	100	650

*Also contains butalbital.
†Also contains caffeine.

supply 30 or 60 mg of codeine but only 300 mg of aspirin fail to take advantage of aspirin's analgesic effect (Table 10-3).

Other drugs that can be used as analgesics that produce their effects centrally are pentazocine, meperidine, and hydromorphone. Pentazocine and meperidine are useful but definitely second-choice drugs compared with the aspirin-codeine combination.

Narcotic analgesics are controlled by the Drug Enforcement Administration (DEA). To write prescriptions for these drugs the dentist must have a DEA permit and number. The drugs are categorized into four basic schedules based on their liability for abuse. Several important differences exist between Schedule II and Schedule III drugs in regard to writing prescriptions (see Appendix V).

It is important to emphasize that the most effective method of controlling pain is to build a close relationship between surgeon and patient. Specific time must be spent discussing the issue of postoperative discomfort, with concern clearly expressed by the surgeon. Prescriptions should be given with clear instructions about when to begin the medication and how to take it at each interval. If these procedures are followed, mild analgesics given for a short time (usually no longer than 2 to 3 days) will be all that is required.

Control of Infection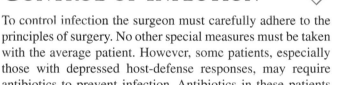

To control infection the surgeon must carefully adhere to the principles of surgery. No other special measures must be taken with the average patient. However, some patients, especially those with depressed host-defense responses, may require antibiotics to prevent infection. Antibiotics in these patients should be administered before the surgical procedure is begun (see Chapter 16). Additional antibiotics after the surgery are usually not necessary. A surgeon who decides to give additional antibiotics must carefully discuss the timing of administration with the patient so that a clear understanding is reached.

Postoperative Follow-Up Visit

All patients should be given a return appointment so that the surgeon can check the patient's progress after the surgery. In routine, uncomplicated procedures a follow-up visit at 1 week is usually adequate. If sutures are to be removed, that can be done at the 1-week postoperative appointment.

Moreover, patients should be informed that should any question or problem arise, they should call their dentist and request an earlier follow-up visit. The most likely reasons for an earlier visit are prolonged and bothersome bleeding, pain that is not responsive to the prescribed medication, and infection.

If a patient who has had surgery begins to develop swelling with surface redness and pain on the third postoperative day or later, the patient can be assumed to have developed an infection until this is proven otherwise. The patient should be instructed to call for an appointment at the dentist's office as soon as possible. The surgeon must then inspect the patient carefully to confirm or rule out the diagnosis of infection. If an infection is diagnosed, appropriate therapeutic measures should be taken.

Postsurgical pain that decreases at first but on the third or fourth day begins to increase, yet is accompanied by no swelling or other signs of infection, is probably a sign of "dry socket." This annoying problem is simple to manage but requires that the patient return to the office several times (see Chapter 11).

It is important that the patient know that the dentist is available to answer any postoperative questions or to treat any postoperative problems that arise. Even if a postoperative follow-up visit does not appear to be necessary, one should be made to give the patient an opportunity to discuss any postoperative sequelae.

OPERATIVE NOTE FOR THE RECORDS

The surgeon must enter into the records a note of what transpired during each visit. Some critical factors must be entered into the chart. The first is the date of the operation and a brief identification of the patient. This is followed by a statement of the diagnosis and reason for the extraction (for example, nonrestorable caries or severe periodontal disease).

Comments regarding the patient's pertinent medical history, medications, and vital signs should be mentioned next in the chart. This information should be noted in the chart before the surgery is performed, to confirm that the dentist has reviewed these issues with the patient and that the patient's current status is satisfactory for the surgical procedure.

A brief mention should be made of the oral examination. During any routine long-term care of a patient, the dentist should examine the soft tissues of the face, mouth, and upper neck periodically. If this is done at the time of surgery, it should be noted in the chart.

The surgeon should enter into the chart the type and amount of anesthetic used and the technique that was chosen for injection. For example, if the drug was lidocaine with a vasoconstrictor, the dentist would write down the number of milligrams of lidocaine and of epinephrine. If the inferior alveolar nerve block technique was used, that would be indicated in this portion of the note, as would any use of nitrous oxide or intravenous sedation.

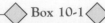

◇ Box 10-1 ◇

Operative note

1. Date
2. Patient name and identification
3. Diagnosis
4. Review of medical history, medications, and vital signs
5. Oral examination
6. Anesthesia: amount and type of block technique that was used
7. Procedure, including description of progress or complications
8. Discharge instructions
9. Medications prescribed and their amounts
10. Return appointment: date and time
11. Signature (legible or printed underneath)

The surgeon should then write a brief note concerning the procedure that was performed, which should include a description of progress and any complications. A description of the patient's tolerance of the procedure should also be included.

A comment concerning the discharge instructions, including mention of the postoperative instruction list that was given to the patient, is recorded.

The prescribed medications are listed, including the name of the drug, its dosage, and the total number of tablets. Finally, the date of the return appointment is recorded in the chart (see Box 10-1 and Appendix IV).

BIBLIOGRAPHY

Forsgren H et al: Effect of cold dressings in the postoperative course in oral surgery, *Int J Oral Surg* 14:223, 1985.

Seymour RA, Walton JG: Pain control after third molar surgery, *Int J Oral Surg* 13:457, 1984.

Seymour RA, Meechan JG, Blair GS: An investigation into postoperative pain after third molar surgery under local analgesia, *Br J Oral Maxillofac Surg* 23:410, 1985.

PREVENTION AND MANAGEMENT OF SURGICAL COMPLICATIONS

LARRY J. PETERSON

CHAPTER OUTLINE ◇

This chapter discusses the variety of complications of oral surgical procedures. It is divided into two sections, intraoperative and postoperative complications. These are surgical, not medical, complications; the latter are discussed in Chapter 4.

PREVENTION OF COMPLICATIONS ◇

It is axiomatic that the best and easiest way to manage a complication is to prevent it from happening. Prevention of surgical complications is best accomplished by a thorough preoperative assessment and comprehensive treatment plan. Only when these are routinely performed can the surgeon expect to have minimal complications. It is important to realize that even with such planning, complications occasionally occur. In situations in which the dentist has planned carefully, the complication is often expected and can be managed in a routine manner. For example, when extracting a maxillary first premolar, which has long thin roots, it is far easier to remove the buccal root than the palatal root. Therefore the surgeon uses more force toward the buccal root than toward the palatal root. If a root does fracture, it is then the buccal root rather than the palatal root, and the subsequent retrieval is easier.

Surgeons must perform surgery that is within their own ability. Surgeons must therefore carefully evaluate their training and ability before deciding to perform a specific surgical task. It is inappropriate for a dentist with limited experience in the management of impacted third molars to undertake the surgical extraction of a deeply embedded tooth. The incidence of operative and postoperative complications is unacceptably high in this situation. Surgeons must be cautious of unwarranted optimism, which clouds their judgment and prevents them from delivering the best possible care to the patient. The dentist must keep in mind that referral to a specialist is an option that should always be exercised if there is any suspicion that the planned surgery is beyond the dentist's own skill level. In some situations this is not only a moral obligation but a medicolegal responsibility.

In planning a surgical procedure the first step is always a thorough review of the patient's medical history. Several of the complications to be discussed in this chapter are caused by inadequate attention to medical histories that would have revealed the presence of a complicating factor. Patients with compromised physical status will have local surgical complications that could have been prevented had the surgeon taken a more thorough medical history.

One of the primary ways to prevent complications is by taking adequate radiographs and reviewing them carefully (see Chapter 7). The radiograph must include the entire area of surgery, including the apices of the roots of the teeth to be extracted and the local and regional anatomic structures, such as the maxillary sinus and the inferior alveolar canal. The surgeon must look for the presence of abnormal tooth root morphology. After careful examination of the radiographs, the surgeon occasionally must alter the treatment plan to prevent the complications that might be anticipated with a routine forceps (closed) extraction. Instead, the surgeon should consider surgical approaches to removing teeth in such cases.

After an adequate medical history has been taken and the radiographs have been analyzed, the surgeon must do the preoperative planning. This is not simply a preparation of a detailed surgical plan but is also a plan for managing patient anxiety and pain and postoperative recovery (instructions and modifications of normal activity for the patient). Thorough preoperative instructions and explanations for the patient are essential in preventing the majority of complications that occur in the postoperative period. If the instructions are not thoroughly explained nor their importance made clear, the patient is less likely to follow them.

Finally, to keep complications at a minimum, the surgeon must always follow the basic surgical principles. There should always be clear visualization and access to the operative field, which requires adequate light, adequate soft tissue reflection (including lips, cheeks, tongue, and soft tissue flaps), and adequate suction. The teeth to be removed must have an unimpeded pathway for removal. Occasionally, bone must be removed and teeth must be sectioned to achieve this goal. Controlled force is of paramount importance; this means "finesse," not "force." The surgeon must follow the prin-

ciples of asepsis, atraumatic handling of tissues, hemostasis, and thorough débridement of the wound after the surgical procedure. Violation of these principles leads to an increased incidence and severity of surgical complications.

COMPLICATIONS OCCURRING DURING THE OPERATIVE PROCEDURE

Complications that occur during the operation fall into several categories. The following discussion divides complications into groups primarily characterized by the tissue involved, although clearly several complications involve both soft and hard tissues.

SOFT TISSUE INJURIES

Injuries to the soft tissue of the oral cavity are almost always the result of the surgeon's lack of adequate attention to the delicate nature of the mucosa and the use of excessive and uncontrolled force. The surgeon must continue to pay careful attention to the soft tissue while working primarily on the bone and tooth structure.

The most common soft tissue injury is the tearing of the mucosal flap during surgical extraction of a tooth. This is usually the result of an inadequately sized envelope flap, which is retracted beyond the tissue's ability to stretch (Figure 11-1). This results in a tearing, usually at one end of the incision. Prevention of this complication is twofold: (1) create adequately sized flaps to prevent excess tension on the flap and

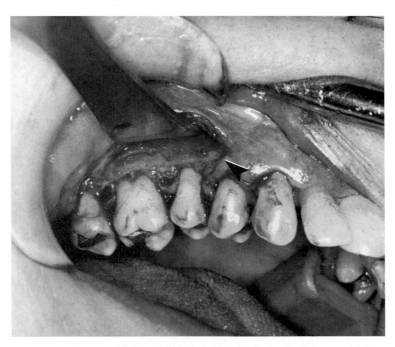

◇ **Figure 11-1**

Torn envelope incision resulting from inadequately sized envelope flap.

(2) use small amounts of retraction force on the flap. If a tear does occur in the flap, the flap should be carefully repositioned once the surgery is complete. In most patients, careful suturing of the tear results in adequate but delayed healing. If the tear is especially jagged, the surgeon may consider excising the edges of the torn flap to create a smooth flap margin for closure. This latter step should be performed with caution, because excision of excessive amounts of tissue leads to closure of the wound under tension and probable wound dehiscence.

If the area of surgery is near the apex of a tooth, there is an increased incidence of envelope-flap tearing as a result of excessive retractional forces. In this situation a release incision to create a three-cornered flap should be used to gain access to the bone.

The second soft tissue injury that occurs with some frequency is inadvertent puncturing of the soft tissue. Instruments, such as a straight elevator or periosteal elevator, may slip from the surgical field and puncture or tear into adjacent soft tissue. Once again, this injury is the result of using uncontrolled force instead of finesse and is best prevented by the use of controlled force, with special attention given to the supporting fingers or support from the opposite hand in anticipation of slippage. If the instrument slips from the tooth or bone, the fingers thus catch the hand before injury occurs (Figure 11-2). When a puncture wound does occur, the treatment is aimed primarily at preventing infection and allowing healing to occur, usually by secondary intention. If

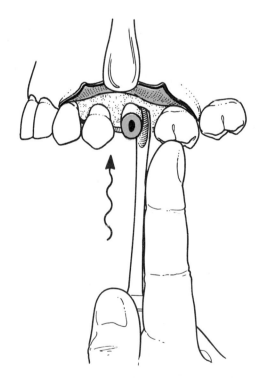

◇ Figure 11-2

Method of holding instruments that may slip. Instruments must be used in a fashion that provides adequate support for surgeon's hand if instruments slip.

the wound bleeds excessively, it should be controlled by direct pressure on the soft tissue. Once hemostasis is achieved, the wound is usually left open and not sutured, so that if a small infection were to occur, there would be an adequate pathway for drainage.

Abrasions or burns of the lips and corners of the mouth are usually the result of the rotating shank of the bur rubbing on the soft tissue (Figure 11-3). When the surgeon is intent on the cutting end of the bur, the assistant should be aware of the location of the shank of the bur in relation to the cheeks and lips. If such an abrasion does develop, the dentist should advise the patient to keep it covered with Vaseline or an antibiotic ointment. It is important that the patient keep the ointment only on the abraded area and not spread onto intact skin, because it is quite likely to result in a rash. These abrasions usually take 5 to 10 days to heal. The patient should keep the area moist with the ointment during the entire healing period to prevent eschar formation, scarring, and delayed healing and to keep the area reasonably comfortable.

INJURIES TO OSSEOUS STRUCTURES

The extraction of a tooth requires that the surrounding alveolar bone be expanded to allow an unimpeded pathway for tooth removal. However, in some situations the bone fractures and is removed with the tooth instead of expanding. The most likely cause of fracture of the alveolar process is the use of excessive force with a forceps, which fractures large portions of cortical plate. If the surgeon realizes that excessive force is necessary to remove a tooth, a soft tissue flap should be elevated and controlled amounts of bone removed so that the tooth can be delivered easily. If this principle is not adhered to and the dentist continues to use excessive or uncontrolled force, fracture of the bone will probably occur.

The most likely places for bony fracture are the buccocortical plate over the maxillary canine, the buccocortical plate over the maxillary molars (especially the first molar), portions of the floor of the maxillary sinus associated with maxillary molars, the maxillary tuberosity, and the labial bone on mandibular incisors (Figure 11-4). All of these bony injuries are caused by excessive force from the forceps.

The primary method of preventing these fractures is to perform a careful preoperative examination of the alveolar process both clinically and radiographically. Surgeons should inspect the root form of the tooth to be removed and assess the proximity of the roots to the maxillary sinus (Figure 11-5). They should also check the thickness of the buccocortical plate overlying the tooth to be extracted (Figure 11-6). If the roots diverge widely or lie close to the sinus, or if there is heavy buccocortical bone, surgeons must take special measures to prevent fracturing excessive portions of bone. Age is a factor to be considered, because the bones of elderly patients are likely to be less elastic and therefore more likely to fracture rather than expand.

The surgeon who determines preoperatively that a high probability exists for bone fracture should consider performing the extraction by the surgical technique. Using this method the surgeon can remove a smaller, more controlled amount of

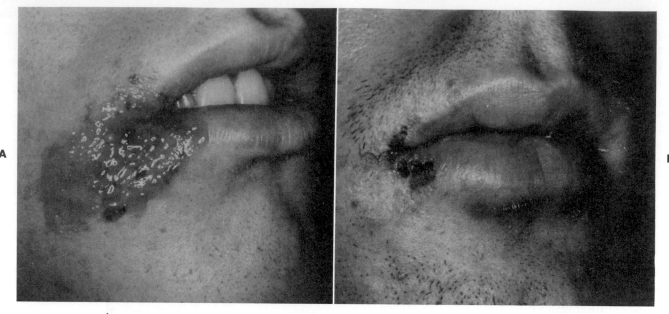

Figure 11-3

A, Abrasion of lip as result of shank of bur rotating on soft tissue. Wound should be kept covered with antibiotic ointment. **B,** Healing should occur rapidly, as seen in this photo taken 5 days later.

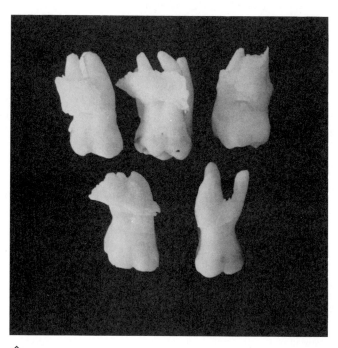

Figure 11-4

Teeth that were removed by forceps extraction. Bone was removed with teeth.

bone, which results in more rapid healing and a more ideal ridge form for prosthetic reconstruction. When the maxillary molar lies close to the maxillary sinus, surgical exposure of the tooth, with sectioning of the tooth roots into two or three portions, will prevent the removal of a portion of the maxillary

sinus floor. This prevents the formation of a chronic oroantral fistula, which requires secondary procedures to close.

In summary, prevention of fractures of large portions of the cortical plate depends on preoperative radiographic and clinical assessment, avoidance of the use of excessive amounts of uncontrolled force, and the early decision to perform an open extraction with removal of controlled amounts of bone and sectioning of multirooted teeth. During a forceps extraction, if the appropriate amount of tooth mobilization does not occur early, then the wise and prudent dentist will alter the treatment plan to the surgical technique instead of pursuing the closed method.

Management of fractures of the alveolar bone takes several different routes, depending on the type and severity of the fracture. If the bone has been completely removed from the tooth socket along with the tooth, it should *not* be replaced. The surgeon should simply make sure that the soft tissue has been replaced and repositioned over the remaining bone to prevent delayed healing. The surgeon must also smooth any sharp edges that may have been caused by the fracture. If such sharp edges of bone exist, the surgeon should reflect a small amount of soft tissue and use a bone file to round off the sharp edges.

The surgeon who has been supporting the alveolar process with the fingers during the extraction will feel the fracture of the buccocortical plate when it occurs. At this time the bone remains attached to the periosteum and will heal if it can be separated from the tooth and left attached to the overlying soft tissue. The surgeon must carefully dissect the bone with its associated soft tissue away from the tooth. For this procedure the tooth must be stabilized with the forceps, and a small sharp instrument, such as a Woodson periosteal elevator, should be

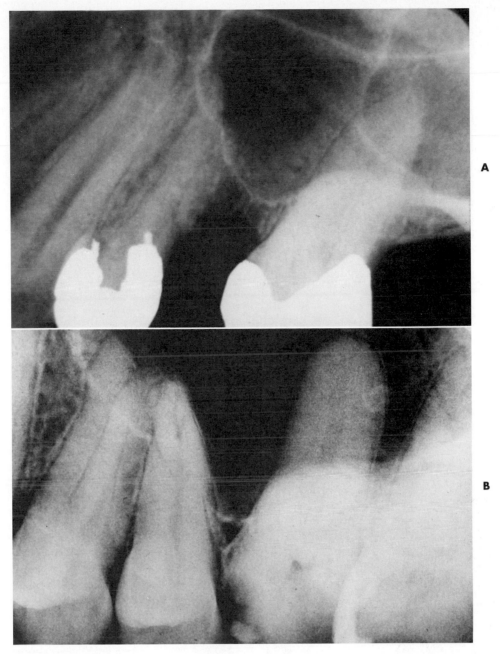

A

B

◇ Figure 11-5

Floor of sinus associated with roots of teeth. If extraction is required, tooth should be removed surgically.

used to elevate the buccal bone from the tooth root. It is important to realize that if the soft tissue flap is reflected from the bone, the blood supply to the overlying bone will be severed and the bone will then undergo necrosis. Once the bone and soft tissue have been elevated from the tooth, the tooth is removed and the bone and soft tissue flap are reapproximated and secured with sutures. When treated in this fashion, there is a high probability that the bone will heal in a more favorable ridge form for prosthetic reconstruction than if the bone had been removed along with the tooth. Therefore it is worth the special effort to dissect the bone from the tooth.

Fracture of a large section of bone in the maxillary tuberosity area is a situation of special concern. The maxillary tuberosity is especially important for the construction of a stable retentive maxillary denture. If a large portion of this tuberosity is removed along with the maxillary tooth, denture stability may be compromised. The fracture of the maxillary tuberosity most commonly results from extraction of an erupted maxillary third molar or from a second molar if it happens to be the last tooth in the arch (Figure 11-7).

If this type of fracture occurs during an extraction, treatment is similar to that just discussed for other bony

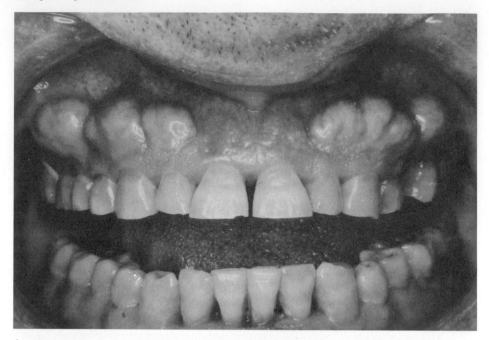

◇ Figure 11-6

Patient with heavy buccocortical plate who requires open extraction.

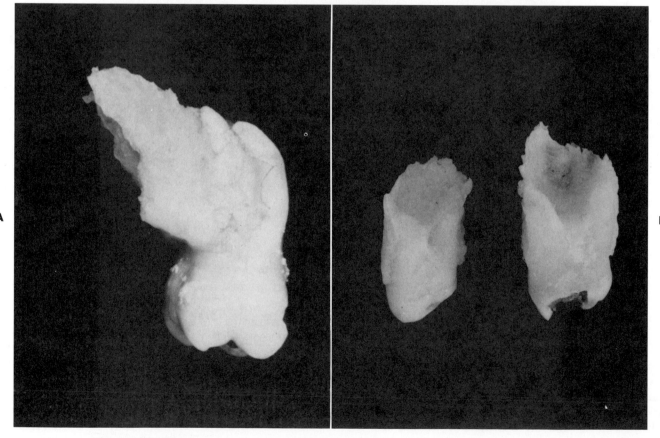

◇ Figure 11-7

Tuberosity removed with maxillary second molar, which eliminates important prosthetic retention area and exposes maxillary sinus. **A,** Buccal view of bone removed with tooth. **B,** Superior view, looking onto sinus floor, which was removed with tooth.

fractures. The surgeon using finger support for the alveolar process during the fracture (if the bone remains attached to the periosteum) should take extreme measures to ensure the survival of that bony segment. If at all possible, the bony segment should be dissected away from the tooth and the tooth removed in the usual fashion. The tuberosity is then stabilized with sutures as indicated earlier.

However, if the tuberosity is excessively mobile and cannot be dissected from the tooth, the surgeon has several options. The first option is to splint the tooth being extracted to adjacent teeth and defer the extraction for 6 to 8 weeks, during which time the bone will heal; the tooth is then extracted with an open surgical technique. The second option is to section the crown of the tooth from the roots and allow the tuberosity and tooth root section to heal. After 6 to 8 weeks the surgeon can reenter the area and remove the tooth roots in the usual fashion. If the maxillary molar tooth is infected, these two techniques should be used with caution.

If the maxillary tuberosity is completely separated from the soft tissue, the usual steps are to smooth the sharp edges of the remaining bone and to replace and suture the remaining soft tissue. The surgeon must check carefully for an oroantral communication and treat as necessary.

Fractures of the maxillary tuberosity should be viewed as a grave complication. The major therapeutic goal of management is to maintain the fractured bone in place and to provide the best possible environment for healing.

OROANTRAL COMMUNICATIONS

Removal of maxillary molars occasionally results in communication between the oral cavity and the maxillary sinus. If the maxillary sinus is large, if there is no bone between the roots of the teeth and the maxillary sinus, and if the roots of the tooth are widely divergent, then there is an increased probability that a portion of the bony floor of the sinus will be removed with the tooth. If this complication occurs, appropriate measures are necessary to prevent a variety of sequelae. The two sequelae of most concern are postoperative maxillary sinusitis and formation of a chronic oroantral fistula. The probability that either of these two sequelae will occur is related to the size of the oroantral communication and the management of the exposure.

As with all complications, prevention is the easiest and most efficient method of managing the situation. Preoperative radiographs must be carefully evaluated for the tooth-sinus relationship whenever maxillary molars are to be extracted. If the sinus floor seems to be very close to the tooth roots and the tooth roots are widely divergent, the surgeon should avoid a closed forceps extraction and perform a surgical removal with sectioning of tooth roots (Figure 11-5). Large amounts of force should be avoided in the removal of such maxillary molars.

Diagnosis of the oroantral communication can be made in several ways. The first is to examine the tooth once it is removed. If there is a section of bone adhering to the root ends of the tooth, the surgeon can be relatively certain that a communication between the sinus and mouth exists. If a small

amount of bone or no bone adheres to the molars, a communication may exist anyway. To confirm the presence of a communication, the best technique is to use the nose-blowing test. The patient's nose is occluded by pinching the nostrils together, and the patient is asked to blow gently through the nose while the surgeon observes the area of the tooth extraction. If a communication exists, there will be passage of air through the tooth socket and bubbling of blood in the socket area.

After the diagnosis of oroantral communication has been established, the surgeon must determine the approximate size of the communication, because the treatment will depend on the size of the opening. If the communication is small (2 mm in diameter or less), no additional surgical treatment is necessary. The surgeon should take measures to ensure the formation of a high-quality blood clot in the socket and then advise the patient to take sinus precautions to prevent dislodgement of the blood clot.

Sinus precautions are aimed at preventing increases or decreases in the maxillary sinus air pressure that would dislodge the clot. Patients should be advised to avoid blowing the nose, violent sneezing, sucking on straws, and smoking. Patients who smoke and who cannot stop even temporarily should be advised to smoke in small puffs, not in deep drags, to avoid pressure changes.

The surgeon must not probe through the socket into the sinus with a periapical curette or a root tip pick. It is possible that the bone of the sinus has been removed without perforation of the sinus lining. To probe the socket with an instrument might unnecessarily lacerate the membrane. Probing of the communication may also introduce foreign material, including bacteria, into the sinus and thereby further complicate the situation. Probing of the communication is therefore absolutely contraindicated.

If the opening between the mouth and sinus is of moderate size (2 to 6 mm) additional measures should be taken. To help ensure the maintenance of the blood clot in the area, a figure-eight suture should be placed over the tooth socket (Figure 11-8). The patient should also be told to follow sinus precautions. Finally, the patient should be prescribed several medications to help lessen the possibility that maxillary sinusitis will occur. Antibiotics, usually penicillin or erythromycin, should be prescribed for 7 days. In addition, a decongestant nasal spray should be prescribed to shrink the

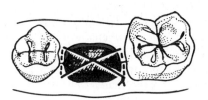

◇ Figure 11-8

Figure-eight stitch over socket of tooth. This stitch helps secure blood clot.

nasal mucosa to keep the ostium of the sinus patent. As long as the ostium is patent and normal sinus drainage can occur, there is a decreased possibility of sinusitis and sinus infection. An oral decongestant is sometimes recommended.

If the sinus opening is large (7 mm or larger) the dentist should consider closing the sinus communication with a flap procedure. This usually requires that the patient be referred to an oral and maxillofacial surgeon, because flap development and closure of a sinus opening are somewhat complex procedures that require skill and experience. The most commonly used flap is a buccal flap. This technique mobilizes buccal soft tissue to cover the opening and provide for a primary closure. It may also require that some of the alveolar process be reduced in height to allow the communication to be closed. This technique should be performed as soon as possible, preferably on the same day in which the opening occurred. The same sinus precautions and medications are usually required (see Chapter 20).

The recommendations just described hold true for patients who have no preexisting sinus disease. If a communication does occur, it is important that the dentist inquire specifically about a history of sinusitis and sinus infections. If the patient has a history of chronic sinus disease, even small oroantral communications will heal poorly and may result in permanent oroantral communication. Therefore creation of an oroantral communication in patients with chronic sinusitis is cause for referral to an oral and maxillofacial surgeon for definitive care (see Chapter 20).

The majority of oroantral communications treated in the methods just recommended will heal uneventfully. Patients should be followed up carefully for several weeks to ensure that this has occurred. Even patients who return within a few days with a small communication usually heal spontaneously if there is no maxillary sinusitis. These patients should be followed up closely and referred to an oral and maxillofacial surgeon if the communication persists for longer than 2 weeks. Closure of oroantral fistulae is important because air, water, food, and bacteria go from the oral cavity into the sinus, often causing a chronic sinusitis condition. Additionally, if the patient is wearing a full maxillary denture, there is loss of good suction and therefore retention of the denture is compromised.

FRACTURES OF THE MANDIBLE

Fracture of the mandible during extraction is a rare complication; it is associated almost exclusively with the surgical removal of impacted third molars. A mandibular fracture is usually the result of the application of a force exceeding that needed to remove a tooth and often occurs during the use of dental elevators. However, when lower third molars are deeply impacted, even small amounts of force may cause a fracture. Fractures may also occur during removal of impacted teeth from a severely atrophic mandible. Should such a fracture occur, it must be treated by the usual methods used for jaw fractures. The fracture must be adequately reduced and stabilized with intermaxillary fixation. Usually this means that the patient should be referred to an oral and maxillofacial surgeon for definitive care.

INJURIES TO ADJACENT TEETH

When the dentist extracts a tooth, the focus of attention is on that particular tooth and the application of forces to luxate and deliver it. When the surgeon's total attention is thus focused, likelihood of injury to the adjacent teeth increases. The surgeon should mentally step back from time to time to survey the entire surgical field to prevent injury to adjacent teeth.

The most common injury to adjacent teeth is the inadvertent fracture of either a restoration or a severely carious tooth while the surgeon is attempting to luxate the tooth to be removed with an elevator (Figure 11-9). If a large restoration exists or if the adjacent tooth is severely carious, the surgeon should warn the patient preoperatively that there is a possibility of fracturing it during the extraction. Prevention of such a fracture is primarily achieved by avoiding application of instrumentation and force on the restoration or carious tooth. This means that the straight elevator should be used with great caution or not used at all to luxate the tooth before extraction. If a restoration is dislodged or fractured, the surgeon should make sure that the displaced restoration is removed from the mouth and does not fall into the empty tooth socket. Once the surgical procedure has been completed, the injured tooth should be treated by placement of a temporary restoration. The patient should be informed that the fracture has occurred and that a permanent restoration must be placed (see Chapter 12).

Inappropriate use of the extraction instruments may luxate the adjacent tooth. This is prevented by judicious use of force with elevators and forceps. If the tooth to be extracted is crowded and has overlapping adjacent teeth, such as is commonly seen in the mandibular incisor region, thin, narrow forceps such as the no. 286 forceps, may be useful for the extraction (Figure 11-10). Forceps with broader beaks should be avoided, because they will cause injury and luxation of the adjacent teeth.

If an adjacent tooth is luxated or partially avulsed, the treatment goal is to reposition the tooth into its appropriate position and stabilize it so that adequate healing occurs. This usually requires that the tooth simply be repositioned in the tooth socket and left alone. The occlusion should be checked to ensure that the tooth has not been displaced into a hypererupted and traumatic occlusion. Occasionally, the luxated tooth is very mobile. If this is the case, the tooth should be stabilized with the least possible rigid fixation to maintain the tooth in its position. A simple silk suture that crosses the occlusal table and is sutured to the adjacent gingiva is usually sufficient. Rigid fixation with circumdental wires and arch bars results in increased chances for external root resorption and ankylosis of the tooth and therefore should usually be avoided (see Chapter 24).

Teeth in the opposite arch may also be injured as a result of uncontrolled tractional forces. This usually occurs when a tooth is inadequately mobilized by buccolingual forces and excessive tractional forces are used. The tooth suddenly releases from the socket, and the forceps strikes against the teeth of the opposite arch and chips or fractures a cusp. This is more likely to occur with extraction of lower teeth, because

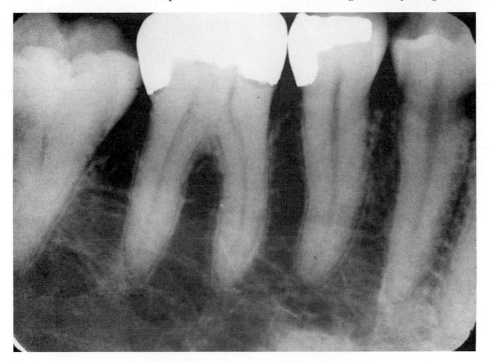

◇ Figure 11-9

Large restoration in tooth adjacent to tooth to be extracted. Use of straight elevator to luxate tooth before use of forceps should be performed with great caution, if at all.

these teeth may require more vertical tractional forces for their delivery, especially when using the no. 23 (cowhorn) forceps. Prevention of this type of injury can be accomplished by several methods. First and primary, the surgeon should avoid the use of excessive tractional forces. The tooth should be adequately luxated with apical, buccolingual, and rotational forces to minimize the need for tractional forces.

Even when this is done, however, occasionally a tooth releases unexpectedly. The surgeon or assistant should protect the teeth of the opposite arch by simply holding a finger or suction tip against them to absorb the blow should the forceps be released in that direction. If such an injury occurs, the tooth should be smoothed or restored as necessary to keep the patient comfortable until a permanent restoration can be constructed.

A complication that every dentist believes can never happen—but happens surprisingly often—is extraction of the wrong tooth. This should never occur if appropriate attention is given to the planning and execution of the surgical procedure. This problem may be the result of inadequate attention to the preoperative assessment. If the tooth to be extracted is grossly carious, it is less likely that the wrong tooth will be removed. The wrong tooth is most commonly extracted when the dentist is asked to remove teeth for orthodontic purposes, especially from patients who are in mixed dentition stages and whose orthodontists have asked for unusual extractions. Careful preoperative planning and clinical assessment of which

tooth is to be removed before the forceps are applied is the main method of preventing this complication.

If the wrong tooth is extracted and the dentist realizes this error immediately, the tooth should be gently rinsed with normal saline and replaced immediately into the tooth socket. If the extraction is for orthodontic purposes, the dentist should contact the orthodontist immediately and discuss whether or not the tooth that was removed can substitute for the tooth that should have been removed. If the orthodontist believes the original tooth must be removed, the extraction should be deferred for 3 or 4 weeks, until the fate of the replanted tooth can be assessed. If the wrongfully extracted tooth has regained its attachment to the alveolar process, then the originally planned extraction can proceed. The surgeon should not extract the contralateral tooth until a definite alternative treatment plan is made.

If the surgeon does not recognize that the wrong tooth was extracted until the patient returns for a postoperative visit, little can be done to correct the problem. Replantation of the extracted tooth after it has dried cannot be accomplished successfully.

When the wrong tooth is extracted, it is important to inform the patient, the patient's parents (if the patient is a minor), and any other dentist involved with the patient's care, such as the orthodontist. In some situations the orthodontist may be able to adjust the treatment plan so that extraction of the wrong tooth necessitates only a minor adjustment.

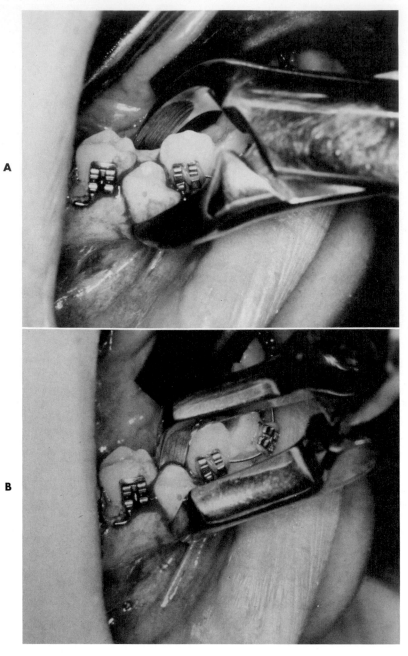

◇ **Figure 11-10**

A, Crowded teeth that prevent adaptation of usual forceps. **B,** Surgeon should use thin-beaked forceps, such as maxillary root tip forceps.

COMPLICATIONS WITH THE TOOTH BEING EXTRACTED

ROOT FRACTURE. The most common complication associated with the tooth being extracted is fracture of its roots. Long, curved, divergent roots that lie in dense bone are most likely to be fractured. The main method of preventing fracture of roots is to perform an open extraction technique and to remove bone to decrease the amount of force necessary to remove the tooth. Recovery of the fractured root with a surgical approach has been discussed in Chapter 8.

ROOT DISPLACEMENT. The tooth root that is most commonly displaced into unfavorable anatomic spaces is the maxillary molar root, which is forced into the maxillary sinus. If a root of a maxillary molar is being removed, with a straight elevator being used with excess apical pressure as a wedge in the periodontal ligament space, the tooth root can be displaced into the maxillary sinus. If this occurs, the surgeon must make several assessments to prescribe the appropriate treatment. First, the surgeon must identify the size of the root lost into the sinus. It may be a root tip of several millimeters, an entire tooth root, or the entire tooth. The surgeon must next assess if there has been any infection of the tooth or periapical tissues. If the tooth is not infected, management is easier than if the tooth has been acutely infected. Finally, the surgeon must assess the preoperative condition of the maxillary sinus. For the patient who has a healthy maxillary sinus, it is easier to manage a displaced root than if the sinus has been chronically infected.

If the displaced tooth fragment is a small (2 or 3 mm) root tip and the tooth and sinus have no preexisting infection, the surgeon should make a minimal attempt at removing the root. First, a radiograph of the fractured tooth root should be taken to document its position and size. Once that has been accomplished, the surgeon should irrigate through the small opening in the socket apex and then suction the irrigating solution from the sinus via the socket. This occasionally flushes the root apex from the sinus through the socket. The surgeon should check the suction solution and confirm radiographically that the root has been removed. If this technique is not successful, no additional surgical procedure should be performed through the socket, and the root tip should be left in the sinus. The small, noninfected root tip can be left in place, because it is quite unlikely that it will cause any troublesome sequelae. Additional surgery in this situation will cause more patient morbidity than leaving the root tip in situ. If the root tip is left in the sinus, measures should be taken similar to those taken when leaving any root tip in place. The patient must be informed of the decision and given proper follow-up instructions.

The oroantral communication should be managed as already discussed, with a figure-eight suture over the socket, sinus precautions, antibiotics, and a nasal spray to prevent infection and keep the ostium open. The most likely occurrence is that the root apex will fibrose onto the sinus membrane with no subsequent problems. If the tooth root is infected or the patient has chronic sinusitis, the patient should be referred to an oral and maxillofacial surgeon for removal of the root tip.

If a large root fragment or the entire tooth is displaced into the maxillary sinus, it should be removed (Figure 11-11). The usual method is a Caldwell-Luc approach into the maxillary sinus in the canine fossa region and then removal of the tooth. This procedure is performed by the oral and maxillofacial surgeon to whom the patient should be referred (see Chapter 20).

Impacted maxillary third molars are occasionally displaced into the maxillary sinus (from which they are removed via a Caldwell-Luc approach) or posteriorly into the infratemporal space. During elevation of the tooth the elevator may force the tooth posteriorly through the periosteum into the infratemporal fossa. The tooth is usually lateral to the lateral pterygoid plate and inferior to the lateral pterygoid muscle.

If there is good access and light, the surgeon should make a single cautious effort to retrieve the tooth with a hemostat. The tooth is usually not visible, and blind probing will result in further displacement. If the tooth is not retrieved after a single effort, the incision should be closed and the operation stopped.

The patient should be informed that the tooth has been displaced and will be removed later. Antibiotics should be given to help decrease the possibility of an infection, and routine postoperative care should be provided.

During the initial healing time, fibrosis occurs and stabilizes the tooth in a rather firm position. The tooth is removed 4 to 6 weeks later. Preoperative lateral and posteroanterior radiographs are taken to locate the tooth in all three planes of space. After the area is anesthetized, a long needle (usually a spinal needle) is used to locate the tooth. The surgeon then dissects along the needle until the tooth is located. Because this surgical procedure is complex, it is usually performed by an oral and maxillofacial surgeon.

The displaced tooth lies medial to the ramus of the mandible and may interfere with wide opening of the mouth. There is also the small likelihood of a late infection occurring. Although possible, it is very unlikely that the tooth will migrate after initial fibrosis has occurred. If no mandibular restriction exists, the patient may elect not to have the tooth removed. If this decision is made, the surgeon must document that the patient understands the situation and the potential complications.

Fractured mandibular molar roots that are being removed with apical pressures may be displaced through the linguocortical plate and into the submandibular fascial space. The linguocortical bone over the roots of the molars becomes thinner as it progresses posteriorly. Mandibular third molars, for example, frequently have dehiscence in the overlying lingual bone and may be actually sitting in the submandibular space preoperatively. Even small amounts of apical pressure result in displacement of the root into that space. Prevention of displacement into the submandibular space is primarily achieved by avoiding all apical pressures when removing the mandibular roots.

Pennant-shaped elevators, such as the Cryer, are used to elevate the broken tooth root. If the root disappears during the root removal, the dentist should make a single effort to remove it. The index finger of the left hand is inserted onto the lingual aspect of the floor of the mouth in an attempt to place pressure against the lingual aspect of the mandible and force the root back into the socket. If this works, the surgeon may be able to tease the root out of the socket with a root tip pick. If this effort is not successful on the initial attempt, the dentist should abandon the procedure and refer the patient to an oral and maxillofacial surgeon. The usual, definitive procedure of removing such a root tip is to reflect a soft tissue flap on the lingual aspect of the mandible and gently dissect the overlying mucoperiosteum until the root tip can be found. As with teeth that are displaced into the maxillary sinus, if the root fragment is small and was not infected preoperatively, the oral and maxillofacial surgeon may elect to leave the root in its position, because surgical retrieval of the root may be an extensive procedure.

Occasionally, the crown of a tooth or an entire tooth might be lost down the oropharynx. If this occurs, the patient should

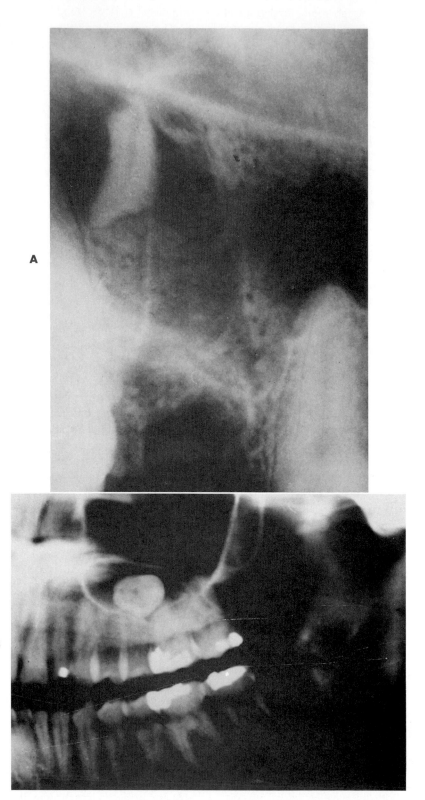

◇ Figure 11-11

A, Large root fragment displaced into maxillary sinus. Fragment should be removed with Caldwell-Luc approach. **B,** Tooth in maxillary sinus is maxillary third molar that was displaced into sinus during elevation of tooth. This tooth must be removed from sinus, probably with Caldwell-Luc approach.

be turned toward the dentist, into a mouth-down position, as much as possible. The suction device can then be used to help remove the tooth. The patient should be encouraged to cough and spit the tooth out onto the floor.

In spite of these efforts, the tooth may be swallowed or aspirated. If the patient has no coughing or respiratory distress, it is most likely that the tooth was swallowed and has traveled down the esophagus into the stomach. However, if the patient has a violent episode of coughing that continues, the tooth may have been aspirated beyond the larynx into the trachea.

If aspiration is suspected, the patient should be transported to an emergency room and a chest radiograph taken to determine the specific location of the tooth. Consultation should be requested from the emergency room physician regarding the possibility of removing the tooth with a bronchoscope. The urgent management of aspiration is to maintain the patient's airway and breathing. Supplemental oxygen may be appropriate if respiratory distress appears to be occurring.

If the tooth has been swallowed, there is high probability that it will pass through the GI tract within 2 to 4 days. Because teeth are usually not jagged or sharp, unimpeded passage occurs in almost all situations. However, it may be prudent to have the patient go to an emergency room and have a radiograph of the abdomen taken to confirm the tooth's presence in the GI tract instead of in the respiratory tract. Follow-up radiographs are probably not necessary, because the usual fate of swallowed teeth is passage.

INJURIES TO ADJACENT STRUCTURES

During the process of tooth extraction it is possible to injure adjacent tissues. The prudent surgeon evaluates all adjacent anatomic areas preoperatively and designs a surgical procedure to prevent injury to these tissues. The structures most likely to be injured during extraction are the branches of the fifth cranial nerve, which provide innervation to the mucosa and skin. The most frequently involved specific branches are the mental nerve, the lingual nerve, the buccal nerve, and the nasopalatine nerve. The nasopalatine and buccal nerves are frequently sectioned during the creation of flaps for removal of impacted teeth. The area of sensory innervation of these two nerves is relatively small, and reinnervation of the affected area usually occurs rapidly. Therefore the nasopalatine and long buccal nerves can be surgically sectioned without sequelae or complications.

Surgical removal of mandibular premolar roots or impacted mandibular premolars and periapical surgery in the area of the mental nerve and mental foramen must be performed with great care. If the mental nerve is injured, the patient will have an anesthesia or paresthesia of the lip and chin. If the injury is the result of flap reflection or simple manipulation, the altered sensation usually disappears in a few weeks to a few months. If the mental nerve is sectioned at its exit from the mental foramen or torn along its course, it is likely that mental nerve function will not return, and the patient will have a permanent state of anesthesia. If surgery is to be performed

in the area of the mental nerve or the mental foramen, it is imperative that surgeons have a keen awareness of the potential morbidity from injury to this nerve. If surgeons have any question concerning their ability to perform the indicated surgical procedure, they should refer the patient to an oral and maxillofacial surgeon. If a three-corner flap is to be used in the area of the mental nerve, the vertical releasing incision must be placed far enough anterior to avoid severing any portion of the mental nerve. Rarely is it advisable to make the vertical releasing incision at the interdental papilla between the canine and first premolar.

The lingual nerve rarely regenerates if it is severely traumatized. Incisions made in the retromolar pad region of the mandible should be placed to avoid severing this nerve. The lingual nerve is anatomically located directly against the lingual aspect of the mandible in the retromolar pad region. Therefore incisions made for surgical exposure of impacted third molars or of bony areas in the posterior molar region should be made well to the buccal aspect of the mandible. Prevention of injury to the lingual nerve is of paramount importance for controlling this difficult complication.

Finally, the inferior alveolar nerve may be traumatized along the course of its intrabony canal. The most common place of injury is the area of the mandibular third molar. Removal of impacted third molars may crush or sharply injure the nerve in its canal. This complication is common enough during the extraction of third molars that it is important to inform patients on a routine basis that it is a possibility. The surgeon must then take every precaution possible to avoid injuring the nerve during the extraction.

Another major structure that can be traumatized during an extraction procedure in the mandible is the temporo-mandibular joint. Removal of mandibular molar teeth frequently requires the application of a substantial amount of force. If the jaw is inadequately supported during the extraction, the patient may experience pain in this region. Controlled force and adequate support of the jaw prevents this. The use of a bite block on the contralateral side may provide adequate balance of forces so that injury and pain do not occur. The surgeon must also support the jaw as described earlier. If the patient complains of pain in the temporomandibular joint immediately after the extraction procedure, the surgeon should recommend the use of moist heat, rest for the jaw, a soft diet, and 1000 mg of aspirin every 4 hours for several days. Patients who cannot tolerate aspirin should be given an aspirin substitute, such as acetaminophen.

SUMMARY

Prevention of complications should be a major goal of the surgeon. Skillful management of complications when they do occur is the *sine qua non* of the wise and mature surgeon.

The surgeon who anticipates a high probability of an unusual specific complication should inform the patient and explain the anticipated management and sequelae. Notation of this should be made in the informed consent that the patient signs.

COMPLICATIONS OCCURRING DURING THE POSTOPERATIVE PERIOD ◇

Unexpected and undesirable sequelae may be postoperative complications of the surgical procedure. The postoperative complications can be grouped into the two major categories of those related to bleeding and those related to delayed wound healing and infection. This section discusses these two general groups of problems.

BLEEDING

Extraction of teeth is a surgical procedure that presents a severe challenge to the body's hemostatic mechanism. There are several reasons for this challenge. First, the tissues of the mouth and jaws are highly vascular. Second, the extraction of a tooth leaves an open wound, with both soft tissue and bone open, which allows additional oozing and bleeding. Third, it is almost impossible to apply dressing material with enough pressure and sealing to prevent additional bleeding during surgery. Fourth, patients tend to play with the area of surgery with their tongues and occasionally dislodge blood clots, which initiates secondary bleeding. The tongue also may cause secondary bleeding by creating small negative pressures that suction the blood clot from the socket. Finally, salivary enzymes may lyse the blood clot before it has organized and before the ingrowth of granulation tissue.

As with all complications, prevention of bleeding is the best way to manage this problem. One of the prime factors in preventing bleeding is the taking of a thorough history from the patient regarding this specific potential problem. Several questions should be asked of the patient concerning any history of bleeding. If there are affirmative answers to any of these questions, the surgeon should take special efforts to control bleeding.

The first question that patients should be asked is if they have ever had a problem with bleeding in the past. The surgeon should inquire about bleeding after previous tooth extractions or previous surgery (such as a tonsillectomy) and persistent bleeding after accidental lacerations. The surgeon must listen carefully to the patient's answers to these questions, because the patient's idea of "persistent" may actually be normal. For example, it is quite normal for a socket to ooze small amounts of blood for the first 12 to 24 hours after extraction. However, if a patient relates a history of bleeding that persisted for more than 1 day or that required special attention from the dentist, then the surgeon's degree of suspicion should be elevated substantially.

The surgeon should inquire about any family history of bleeding. If anyone in the patient's family has or had a history of prolonged bleeding, further inquiry about its cause should be pursued. Most congenital bleeding disorders are familial, inherited characteristics. These congenital disorders vary from very mild to very profound, the latter requiring substantial efforts to control.

The patient should next be asked about any medications currently being taken that may interfere with coagulation. Five drug groups can potentiate the patient's bleeding. The first is aspirin. Aspirin taken before the extraction interferes with platelet function, which may prolong bleeding as a result of decreased platelet aggregation and platelet plug formation in small arterioles. If the patient admits to aspirin intake in the immediate preoperative period, the surgeon may wish to take special measures to control bleeding.

The second drug group is the anticoagulants. Patients are often given anticoagulants to "thin" their blood to prevent intravascular coagulation. Patients who have had a myocardial infarction or pulmonary embolism or those who have prosthetic heart valves or venous thrombosis may be taking anticoagulants to prevent additional intravascular coagulation. The method of management for these patients is discussed later.

The third drug group is broad-spectrum antibiotics. These drugs may cause a change in intestinal flora, which may decrease vitamin K production. Vitamin K is necessary for the liver to produce adequate quantities of coagulation factors II, VII, IX, and X. If a patient has a history of prolonged broad-spectrum antibiotic therapy, the surgeon should be suspicious of decreased hemostasis.

The next drug that can interfere with hemostasis is alcohol. Patients who have taken large amounts of alcohol for long periods of time may have sufficient cirrhosis of the liver to decrease production of the liver-dependent coagulation factors. Patients who are known alcoholics should be handled with special care, because they will have a decreased ability to coagulate after surgery.

The fifth group of drugs are the anticancer, or cancer chemotherapeutic, drugs. These drugs interfere with the hematopoietic system and reduce the number of circulating platelets; in other words, patients receiving chemotherapy may have increased bleeding as a result of a decreased number of circulating platelets.

These five groups of drugs—aspirin, anticoagulants, antibiotics, alcohol, and anticancer drugs—can be easily remembered, because they all start with the letter *A*. The dentist who is about to perform an extraction should know that the patient is taking none of these five "letter *A* drugs." If the patient *is* taking one of them, the dentist should be prepared to take special measures to control the bleeding.

The final question that the surgeon should ask the patient when determining the likelihood of prolonged bleeding is about several specific systemic diseases. These include nonalcoholic liver disease, primarily hepatitis, and hypertension. Patients who have elevated blood pressures (180 to 200 systolic) may have prolonged bleeding following surgery, even in the face of adequate local measures.

The patient who has a known or suspected coagulopathy should be evaluated by laboratory testing before surgery is performed, to determine the severity of the disorder. The best screening test for acquired coagulopathies is the prothrombin time (PT). The PT is reported as two numbers. The first is a control time, which is usually approximately 12 seconds. The

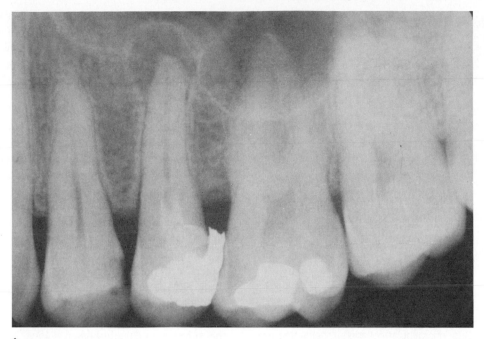

◇ **Figure 11-12**

Granuloma of second premolar. Surgeon should not curette periapically around this second premolar to remove granuloma, because risk for sinus perforation is high.

second is a patient test time. To have a reasonably good chance of achieving hemostasis by local measures, the patient's PT should be within 1.5 times the control time; that is, 18 seconds or less if the control is 12 seconds. If the PT is longer than 18 seconds, the dentist should consult with the patient's physician before performing surgical procedures. If the PT is less than 18 seconds, the bleeding should be controllable by the usual local measures.

A more contemporary means to measure the status of anticoagulation is to use the International Normalized Ratio (INR). This value takes into account both the patient's PT and the control. Normal anticoagulated status for most medical indications will have an INR of 2.0 to 3.0. This roughly corresponds to a PT ratio of 1.3 to 2.0. Therefore it is reasonable to perform extractions on patients who have an INR of 2.5 or below. With special precautions, it is reasonably safe to do minor amounts of surgery in patients with an INR of up to 3.0, if special local hemostatic measures are taken.

Primary control of bleeding during surgery depends on gaining control of all factors that may prolong bleeding. Surgery should be as atraumatic as possible, with clean incisions and gentle management of the soft tissue. Care should be taken not to crush the soft tissue, because crushed tissue tends to ooze for long periods. Sharp bony spicules should be smoothed or removed. All granulation tissue should be curetted from the periapical region of the socket and from around the necks of adjacent teeth and soft tissue flaps. This should be deferred when anatomic restrictions, such as the sinus or inferior alveolar canal, are present (see Figure 11-12). The wound should be inspected carefully for the presence of any specific bleeding arteries. If such arteries exist in the soft tissue, they should be controlled with direct pressure or, if pressure fails, by clamping the artery with a hemostat and ligating it with a resorbable suture. For most oral surgical procedures, direct pressure over the soft tissue bleeding area for 5 minutes results in complete control.

The surgeon should also check for bleeding from the bone. Occasionally a small, isolated vessel bleeds from a bony foramen. If this occurs, the foramen can be crushed with the closed ends of the hemostat, thereby occluding the bleeding vessel. Once these measures have been accomplished, the bleeding socket is covered with a damp 2- × 2-inch sponge that has been folded to fit directly into the area from which the tooth was extracted. The patient bites down firmly on this gauze for at least 30 minutes. The surgeon should not dismiss the patient from the office until hemostasis has been achieved. This requires that the surgeon check the patient's extraction socket about 15 minutes after the completion of surgery. The patient should open the mouth widely, the gauze should be removed, and the area should be inspected carefully for any persistent oozing. Initial control should have been achieved. New damp gauze is then folded and placed into position, and the patient is told to leave it in place for an additional 30 minutes.

If bleeding persists, and careful inspection of the socket reveals that no arterial bleeding exists, the surgeon should take additional measures to achieve hemostasis. Several different materials can be placed in the socket to help gain hemostasis (Figure 11-13). The most commonly used and the least expensive is the absorbable gelatin sponge (for example, Gelfoam). This material is placed in the extraction socket and held in place with a figure-eight suture placed over the socket.

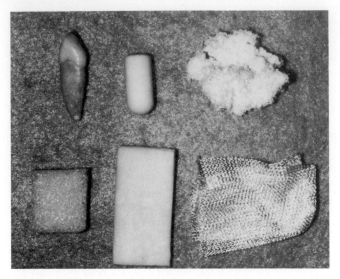

◇ **Figure 11-13**

Material that can be used in a bleeding socket. Clockwise from the canine tooth: collagen plug, microfibular collagen, regenerated oxidized cellulose, collagen tape, and absorbable gelatin sponge.

The absorbable gelatin sponge forms a scaffold for the formation of a blood clot, and the suture helps maintain the sponge in position during the coagulation process. A gauze pack is then placed over the top of the socket and is held with pressure.

A second material that can be used to control bleeding is oxidized regenerated cellulose (for example, Surgicel). This material promotes coagulation better than the absorbable gelatin sponge, and it can be packed into the socket under pressure. The gelatin sponge becomes very friable when wet and cannot be packed into a bleeding socket. When the cellulose is packed into the socket, it almost always causes delayed healing of the socket. Therefore packing the socket with cellulose is reserved for more persistent bleeding.

If the surgeon has special concerns about the patient's ability to clot, a liquid preparation of topical thrombin (prepared from bovine thrombin) can be saturated onto a gelatin sponge and inserted into the tooth socket. The thrombin bypasses all steps in the coagulation cascade and helps to convert fibrinogen to fibrin enzymatically, which forms a clot. The sponge with the topical thrombin is secured in place with a figure-eight suture. A gauze pack is placed over the extraction site in the usual fashion.

A final material that can be used to help control a bleeding socket is collagen. Collagen promotes platelet aggregation and thereby helps accelerate blood coagulation. Collagen is currently available in several different forms. Microfibular collagen (for example, Avitene) is available as a fibular material that is loose and fluffy but can be packed into a tooth socket and held in by suturing and gauze packs, as with the other materials. A more highly cross-linked collagen is supplied as a plug (for, example, Collaplug) or as a tape (for example, Collatape). These materials are more readily packed

into a socket (Figure 11-14) and are easier to use. They are also more expensive.

Even after primary hemostasis has been achieved, patients occasionally return to the dentist with bleeding from the extraction site, referred to as *secondary bleeding*. The surgeon must have an orderly, planned regimen to control this secondary bleeding. The patient should be positioned in the dental chair, and all blood, saliva, and fluids should be suctioned from the mouth. The surgeon should visualize the bleeding site carefully with good light to determine the precise source of bleeding. If it is clearly seen to be a generalized oozing, the bleeding site is covered with a folded, damp 2- × 2-inch sponge held in place with firm pressure by the surgeon's finger for at least 5 minutes. This measure is sufficient to control most bleeding. The reason for the bleeding is usually some secondary trauma that is potentiated by the patient's continuing to suck on the area or to spit blood from the mouth instead of continuing to apply pressure with a gauze sponge.

If 5 minutes of this treatment does not control the bleeding, the surgeon must administer a local anesthetic so that the socket can be treated more aggressively. Block techniques are to be encouraged instead of local infiltration techniques. Infiltration with solutions containing epinephrine cause vasoconstriction and may control the bleeding temporarily. However, when the effects of the epinephrine dissipate, rebound hemorrhage with recurrent bothersome bleeding may occur.

Once local anesthesia has been achieved, the surgeon should gently curette out the tooth extraction socket and suction all areas of old blood clot. The specific area of bleeding should be identified as clearly as possible. As with primary bleeding, the soft tissue should be checked for diffuse oozing versus specific artery bleeding. The bone tissue should be checked for small nutrient artery bleeding or general oozing. The same measures described for control of primary bleeding should be used. The surgeon must then decide if a hemostatic agent should be inserted into the bony socket. The use of an absorbable gelatin sponge with topical thrombin held in position with a figure-eight stitch and reinforced with application of firm pressure from a small, damp gauze pack is standard for local control of secondary bleeding. This technique works well in almost every bleeding socket. In many situations an absorbable gelatin sponge and gauze pressure are adequate. The patient should be given specific instructions on how to apply the gauze packs directly to the bleeding site should additional bleeding occur. Before the patient with secondary bleeding is discharged from the office, the surgeon should monitor the patient for at least 30 minutes to ensure that adequate hemostatic control has been achieved.

If hemostasis is not achieved by any of the local measures just discussed, the surgeon should consider performing additional laboratory screening tests to determine if the patient has a profound hemostatic defect. The dentist usually requests a consultation from a hematologist, who orders the typical screening tests. These tests are for the PT, partial thromboplastin time (PTT), platelet count, and template

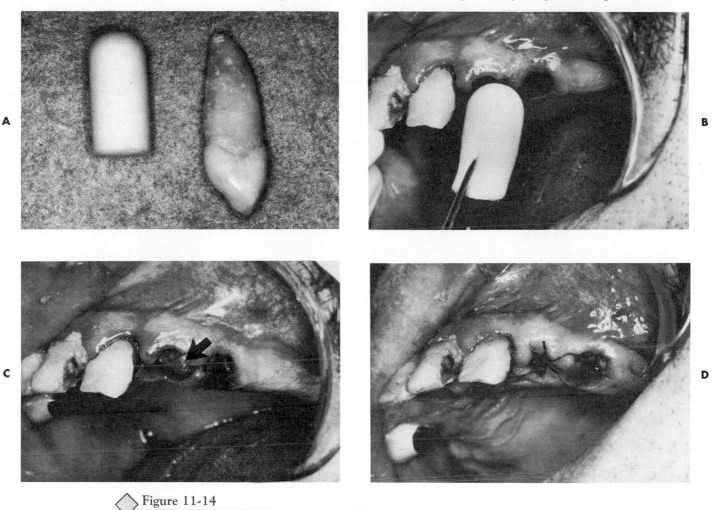

◇ **Figure 11-14**

A, Collagen shaped into the form of a plug is similar in size to the root of a maxillary canine. **B** and **C,** The collagen plug is placed into the socket with a cotton pliers *(arrow)*. **D,** A figure-eight suture is placed over the socket to maintain the collagen in the socket.

bleeding time. The PT is used to find defects in the extrinsic coagulation cascade, which is affected primarily by acquired deficiencies. The PTT is used primarily for discovering deficiencies in the intrinsic system, or congenital deficiencies. The platelet count is an assessment of the quantitative status of the platelets, and the template bleeding time is a measure of platelet function in conjunction with small vessel function. Abnormalities in these tests should prompt the hematologist to investigate the patient's hemostatic system further.

Patients with known bleeding disorders, such as hemophilia A (factor VIII deficiency), hemophilia B (factor IX deficiency), von Willebrand's disease, or platelet disorders (quantitative or qualitative), require special measures for extractions to be performed safely. Extractions in the patient with a diagnosed coagulopathy usually should be performed by an oral and maxillofacial surgeon, who often works in conjunction with a hematologist. The usual technique employed for control of bleeding in the factor-deficiency patient is to administer a transfusion with enough factor replacement to achieve initial hemostasis. The patient is then

given an antifibrinolytic agent, such as aminocaproic acid (Amicar), for 10 days following the extraction. With this technique the amount of coagulation factor to be transfused can be kept to a minimum, and hospitalization is usually not required.

A final hemostatic complication relates to intraoperative and postoperative bleeding into the adjacent soft tissues. Blood that escapes into tissue spaces, especially subcutaneous tissue spaces, appears as bruising of the overlying soft tissue 2 to 5 days after the surgery. This bruising is termed *ecchymosis*. Ecchymosis is seen when many extensive soft tissue flaps have been reflected and occurs more frequently and to a greater extent in elderly patients than in younger patients (Figure 11-15). Patients who undergo procedures more complicated than a simple tooth extraction and who are older than age 50 should be warned that they may have some ecchymosis of the submandibular region and that ecchymosis may extend into the neck and upper anterior chest. Ecchymosis does not increase the potential for infection or other sequelae, but it can be distressing for the patient who

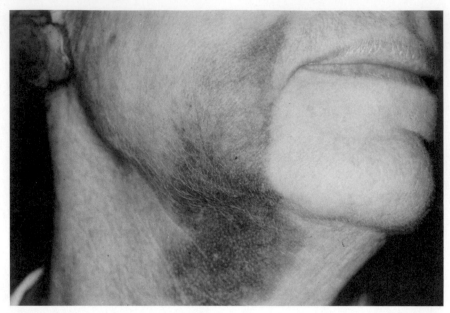

◇ **Figure 11-15**

Ecchymosis in elderly patient who underwent routine extraction of multiple mandibular teeth. Resultant widespread ecchymosis is not uncommon after this type of procedure.

does not expect it. There is probably no way to prevent ecchymosis, but it can be minimized by performing the most atraumatic surgery possible. The patient should be told that the application of moist heat may hasten the resolution of ecchymosis.

DELAYED HEALING AND INFECTION

The most common cause of delayed wound healing is infection. Infection is a rare complication following routine dental extraction and is seen primarily after oral surgery that involves the reflection of soft tissue flaps and bone removal. Prevention of infection following surgical flap procedures can best be achieved by careful asepsis and thorough wound débridement after surgery. This means that the area of bone removal under the flap must be irrigated copiously with saline and that all foreign debris must be removed with a curette. Some patients are predisposed to postoperative wound infections and should be given perioperative prophylactic antibiotics (see Chapter 16).

Another problem of delayed healing is wound dehiscence. If a soft tissue flap is replaced and sutured without an adequate bony foundation, the unsupported soft tissue flap often sags and separates along the line of incision. A second cause of dehiscence is suturing the wound under tension. If the soft tissue flap is sutured under tension, the sutures cause ischemia of the flap margin with subsequent tissue necrosis, which allows the suture to pull through the flap margin and results in wound dehiscence. Therefore sutures should always be placed in tissue without tension and tied loosely enough to prevent blanching of the tissue.

Dry socket, or alveolar osteitis, causes delayed healing but is not associated with an infection. This postoperative complication causes moderate-to-severe pain but is without the usual signs and symptoms of infection, such as fever, swelling, and erythema. The term *dry socket* describes the appearance of the tooth extraction socket when the pain begins. In the usual clinical course, pain develops on the third or fourth day after removal of the tooth. On examination the tooth socket appears to be empty, with a partially or completely lost blood clot, and the bone surfaces of the socket are exposed. The exposed bone is extremely sensitive and is the source of the pain. The dull, aching pain is moderate to severe, usually throbs, and frequently radiates to the patient's ear. The area of the socket has a bad odor, and the patient frequently complains of a bad taste.

The etiology of alveolar osteitis is not absolutely clear, but it appears to be the result of high levels of fibrinolytic activity in and around the tooth extraction socket. This fibrinolytic activity results in lysis of the blood clot and subsequent exposure of the bone. The fibrinolytic activity may be the result of subclinical infections, inflammation of the marrow space of the bone, or other factors. The occurrence of a dry socket after a routine tooth extraction is relatively rare (2% of extractions), but it is quite frequent after the removal of impacted mandibular third molars (20% of extractions).

Prevention of the dry socket syndrome requires that the surgeon minimize trauma and bacterial contamination in the area of surgery. The surgeon should perform atraumatic surgery with clean incisions and soft tissue reflection. Following the surgical procedure, the wound should be thoroughly débrided and irrigated with large quantities of saline. Small amounts of antibiotics, such as tetracycline, placed in the socket alone or on a gelatin sponge may help to decrease the incidence of dry socket in mandibular third molars. The incidence of dry socket can also be decreased by preoperative and postoperative rinses with antimicrobial mouthrinses, such as chlorhexidine. Well-controlled studies indicate that the incidence of dry socket after impacted mandibular third molar surgery can be reduced by up to 50%.

The treatment of alveolar osteitis is dictated by the single therapeutic goal of relieving the patient's pain during the period of healing. If the patient receives no treatment, there is no sequela other than continued pain (treatment does not hasten healing). Treatment is straightforward and consists of gentle irrigation and insertion of a medicated dressing. First, the tooth socket is gently irrigated with saline. The socket should not be curetted down to bare bone, because this increases both the amount of exposed bone and the pain. Usually the entire blood clot is not lysed, and the part that is intact should be retained. The socket is carefully suctioned of all excess saline, and a small strip of iodoform gauze soaked with the medication is inserted into the socket. The medication contains the following principle ingredients: eugenol, which obtunds the pain from the bone tissue; a topical anesthetic, such as benzocaine; and a carrying vehicle, such as balsam of Peru. The medication can be made by the surgeon's pharmacist or can be obtained as a commercial preparation from dental supply houses.

The medicated gauze is gently inserted into the socket, and the patient usually experiences profound relief from pain within 5 minutes. The dressing is changed every day or every other day for the following 3 to 6 days, depending on the severity of the pain. The socket is gently irrigated with saline at each dressing change. Once the patient's pain decreases, the dressing should not be replaced, because it acts as a foreign body and further prolongs wound healing.

BIBLIOGRAPHY

Birn H: Etiology and pathogenesis of fibrinolytic alveolitis, *Int J Oral Surg* 2:211, 1973.

Hall HD, Bildman BS, Hand CD: Prevention of dry socket with local application of tetracycline, *J Oral Surg* 29:35, 1971.

Kohn MW, Chase DC, Marciani RD: Surgical misadventures, *Dent Clin North Am* 17:533, 1973.

Larsen PE: The effect of chlorhexidine rinse on the incidence of alveolar osteitis following the surgical removal of impacted mandibular third molars, *J Oral Maxillofac Surg* 49:932, 1991.

Moake JL: Common bleeding problems, *Ciba Found Symp* 35(3):1, 1983.

Osbon DB: Postoperative complications following dentoalveolar surgery, *Dent Clin North Am* 17:483, 1973.

Redding SW, Stiegler KE: Dental management of the classic hemophiliac with inhibitors, *Oral Surg* 56:145, 1983.

Steinberg MJ, Moores JF: Use of INR to assess degree of anticoagulation in patients who have dental procedures, *Oral Surg Oral Med Oral Pathol Oral Radiol Endod* 80:175, 1995.

Sweet JB, Butter DP, Drager JL: Effects of lavage techniques with third molar surgery, *Oral Surg* 41:152, 1976.

Troulis MJ, Head TW, Lederc JC: What is the INR? *J Canadian Dent Assoc* 62(suppl):428, 1996.

Waite DE: Maxillary sinus, *Dent Clin North Am* 15:349, 1971.

MEDICOLEGAL CONSIDERATIONS

RICHARD L. SMALL AND MYRON R. TUCKER

CHAPTER OUTLINE ———◇

I n recent years there has been an increase in the number of malpractice claims brought against dentists. This trend has had a profound impact on several aspects of dentistry. Some of the most common lawsuits are related to extraction of the wrong tooth, failure to diagnose a problem, and lack of proper informed consent. The stress associated with the increased possibility of litigation influences the entire office. Malpractice insurance premiums are high, contributing to increased patient costs. Dentists feel pressured into practicing "defensive dentistry," second-guessing sound clinical decisions based on concerns about potential litigation.

The influence of litigation on dentistry has resulted in an effort by the profession to reduce the risk of legal liability by more closely examining treatment decisions, improved documentation, and better dentist-patient relationships. Reviewing all aspects of dental practice to provide the best possible patient care and to reduce unnecessary legal liability is termed *risk management.*

Although there is no substitute for sound clinical practice, many lawsuits are prompted by nontreatment issues. These often include miscommunication and misunderstanding between the dentist and patient and poor record-keeping, which in turn present opportunities for patient's lawyers to criticize. This chapter reviews concepts of liability, risk management, methods of risk reduction and actions that should be taken if a malpractice suit is filed.

LEGAL CONCEPTS INFLUENCING LIABILITY ———◇

To understand the responsibility of the dentist in risk management, it is important to review several legal concepts pertaining to the practice of dentistry.

Malpractice is generally defined as professional negligence. Professional negligence occurs when treatment provided by the dentist fails to comply with "standards of care" exercised by other dentists in similar situations. In other words, professional negligence occurs when professionals fail to have or exercise the degree of skill ordinarily possessed and demonstrated by members of their profession practicing under similar circumstances.

In most states the standard of care is defined by that which an ordinarily skilled, educated, and experienced dentist would do under similar circumstances. Many states adhere to a national standard for dental specialists. Malpractice occurs when the patient proves that the dentist failed to comply with this minimal level of care, which resulted in injury.

In most malpractice cases the patient must prove all of the following four elements of a malpractice claim: (1) the applicable standard of care (legal duty), (2) breach of standard of care, (3) injury, and (4) the breach caused the injury. The burden of proving malpractice lies with the plaintiff/patient. The patient must prove by a preponderance of the evidence all four elements of the claim.

First, there must be a professional relationship between the dentist and patient before a legal duty or obligation is owed to exercise appropriate care. This relationship can be established if the dentist accepts the patient or otherwise begins treatment. Second, a breach or failure to provide treatment that satisfies the standard of care must be demonstrated. This standard of care does not obligate the dentist to provide the highest level of treatment exercised by the most skilled dentist or that which is taught in dental school. The standard of care is intended to be a "common denominator" defined by what average practitioners would ordinarily do under similar circumstances. Third, it must be shown that the failure to provide this standard of care was the cause of the patient's injury. Finally, there must have been some form of damage demonstrated.

Dentists are not liable for inherent risks of treatment that occur in the absence of negligence. For example, a dentist is not liable if a patient experiences a numb lip following a properly performed third molar extraction. This is a recognized complication. A dentist can be legally liable for a numb lip if the patient proves it was caused by negligence (the numbness was caused by a careless incision, careless use of a bur or other instrument, and so on).

Recently, several suits have charged the dentist with *breach of contract*. This charge has traditionally been applied to business transactions and has not normally been used in disputes between patients and dentists. However, some courts have recently ruled that a patient and dentist may actually have a contractual agreement to produce a specific result and that failure to achieve this objective may result in a breach of contract. In many states an alleged promise or guarantee as to the result is not enforceable unless it is in writing. Overly aggressive marketing can lead to contractual liability.

Marketing pressures sometimes lead to written advertisements or promotions that can be interpreted as guaranteed results. Patients who have difficulty chewing after delivery of new dentures, if originally promised that they would be able to eat any type of food without difficulty, might consider such promises breach of contract. Dissatisfaction with esthetics or function is often linked to unreasonable expectations, sometimes fueled by ineffective communication or excessive salesmanship.

The *statute of limitations* generally provides a time limit for filing a malpractice suit against a dentist. This limit, however, varies widely from state to state. In some states the statute of limitations begins when an incident occurs. In other states the statute of limitations is extended for a short period after the alleged malpractice is discovered (or when a "reasonable" person would have discovered it).

Several other factors can extend the statute of limitations in many states. These include children under 18 or the age of majority, fraudulent concealment of negligent treatment by the dentist or leaving a nontherapeutic foreign object in the body (for example, broken bur or file).

RISK REDUCTION ◇

The foundation for all dental practice should be sound clinical procedures. However, properly addressing other aspects of patient care and office policy may considerably reduce potential legal liability. These aspects include dentist-patient and staff-patient communication, patient information, informed consent, proper documentation, and appropriate management of complications. Additionally, note that patients with reasonable expectations and a favorable relationship with their dentist are less likely to sue and more likely to tolerate complications.

PATIENT INFORMATION AND OFFICE COMMUNICATION

A solid dentist-patient relationship is key to any risk-management program. Well-informed patients generally have a much better understanding of potential complications and more realistic expectations about treatment outcomes. This can be accomplished by providing patients with as much information as possible on proposed treatment, alternatives and risks, and benefits and limitations of each. If done properly, the informed consent process can improve rapport. Patients are given this information to help them better understand their care so they can make informed decisions. The information should be communicated in a positive manner, and not presented in a defensive way.

Patients value and expect a discussion with their dentist about their care. Brochures and other types of informational packages help provide patients with both general and specific information about general dental and oral surgical care. Patients requiring oral surgical procedures will benefit from information on the nature of their problem, recommended treatment and alternatives, expectations, and possible complications. This information should have a well-organized format that is easily understood and is written in layman's language. Informed consent is discussed in detail in the following section.

When a dentist has a specific discussion with a patient or gives a patient an informational package, it should be documented in the patient's chart. Complications discussed earlier can be reviewed if they occur later. In general, patients with reasonable expectations create fewer problems. This theme will be repeated throughout this chapter.

INFORMED CONSENT

In addition to providing quality care, effective communication and good rapport should become a standard part of office management objectives. Dentists can be sued not only for negligent treatment but also for failing to properly inform patients about the treatment to be rendered, reasonable alternatives, and the reasonable benefits, risks, and complications of each. In fact, in some states, treatment without a proper informed consent is considered battery.

The concept of informed consent is that the patient has a right to consider known risks and complications inherent to treatment. This enables the patient to make a knowlegeable, voluntary decision whether to proceed with recommended treatment or elect another option. If a patient is properly advised of inherent risks and a complication occurs in the absence of negligence, the dentist is not legally liable. However, a dentist can be held liable when an inherent risk occurs after the dentist fails to obtain the patient's *informed* consent. The rationale for liability is that the patient was denied the opportunity to refuse treatment after being properly advised of risks associated with the treatment and reasonable options.

Current concepts of informed consent are based as much on providing the patient the necessary information as on actually obtaining a consent or signature for a procedure. In addition to fulfilling the legal obligations, there are several benefits of obtaining the proper informed consent from patients. First, well-informed patients who understand the nature of the problem and have realistic expectations are less likely to sue. Second, a properly presented and documented informed consent often prevents frivolous claims based on misunderstanding or unrealistic expectations. Finally, obtaining an informed consent offers the dentist the opportunity to develop better rapport with the patient by demonstrating a greater personal interest in the patient's well-being.

The requirements of an informed consent vary from state to state. Initially, informed consent was to inform patients that bodily harm or death may result from a procedure. It did not require discussion of minor, unlikely complications that seldom occur and infrequently result in ill effects. However, some states have currently adopted the concept of "material risk," which requires dentists to discuss *all* aspects material to the patient's decision to undergo treatment, even if it is not customary in the profession to provide such information. A risk is material when a reasonable person is likely to attach significance to it in assessing whether to have the proposed therapy.

In many states, dentists have a nondeligable duty to obtain the patient's consent. Although staff can present the consent form, the dentist should review treatment recommendations, options, and the risks and benefits of each option and be available to answer questions. Although not required by the standard of care in many states, it is adviseable to get the patient's written consent for invasive dental procedures. Parents or guardians must sign for minors. Legal guardians must sign for individuals with mental or similar incapacities. In certain regions of the country, it is helpful to have consent forms written in other languages or have multilingual staff members available.

Informed consent consists of the following three phases: (1) discussion, (2) written consent, and (3) documentation in the patient's chart. The informed consent should include frank discussions and information about the following items: (1) the specific problem, (2) proposed treatment, (3) anticipated or common side effects, (4) possible complications and approximate frequency of occurrence, (5) anesthesia, (6) treatment alternatives, and (7) uncertainties about final outcome, including a statement that the treatment has no absolute guarantees.

This information must be presented so that the patient has no difficulty understanding it. A variety of video presentations are available describing dental and surgical procedures and the associated risks and benefits. These can be used as part of the informed consent process but should not replace direct discussions between the dentist and patient. At the conclusion of the presentation the patient should be given an opportunity to ask any additional questions.

After these presentations or discussions a written informed consent should be signed by the patient. The written consent should summarize in easily understandable terms the items presented. Some states presume that if the information is not on the form, it was not discussed. It should also be documented that the patient can read and speak English; if not, the presentation and written consent should be given in the patient's language.

To ensure that the patient understands each specific paragraph of the consent form, the dentist should consider having the patient initial each paragraph on the consent form. An example of an informed consent document appears in Appendix VIII. At the conclusion of the discussion, the informed consent document should be signed by the patient, the dentist, and at least one witness. In the case of a minor the informed consent should be signed by both the patient and parent or legal guardian. In some states, minors may sign the informed consent for their own treatment if they are married or pregnant. Before assuming this to be the case, local regulations should be verified.

The third and final phase of the informed consent procedure is to document in the patient's chart that an informed consent was obtained after the dentist discussed treatment options, risks, and benefits. The dentist should record the fact that consent discussions took place and should also record other events, such as videos shown, brochures given, and so on. The written consent form should be included.

There are three special situations in which an informed consent may deviate from these guidelines. First, a patient may specifically ask not to be informed of all aspects of the treatment and complications (this must be specifically documented in the chart). Second, it may be harmful in some cases to provide all of the appropriate information to the patient. This is termed *the therapeutic privilege* for not obtaining a complete informed consent. It is somewhat controversial and would rarely apply to routine oral surgical and dental procedures. Third, a complete informed consent may not be necessary in an emergency, when the need to proceed with treatment is so urgent that unnecessary delays to obtain an informed consent may result in further harm to the patient. This also applies to management of complications during a surgical procedure. It is assumed that if failure to manage a condition immediately would result in further patient harm, then treatment should proceed without a specific informed consent.

Patients have the right to know if there are any risks

associated with their decision to reject certain forms of treatment. This *informed refusal* should be clearly documented in the chart, along with specific information given to the patient informing them of the risk and consequence of refusing treatment. Patients who do not appear for needed treatment should be sent a letter warning them of potential problems that may arise if they do not seek treatment. Copies of these letters should be kept in the patient's chart.

RECORDS AND DOCUMENTATION

Poor record-keeping is one of the most common problems encountered in the defense of a malpractice suit. When the quality of patient care is questioned, the records supposedly reflect what was done and why. Poor records provide plaintiff attorneys with an opportunity to claim that patient care also must have been substandard. Even though a perfect record is neither possible nor required, records should reasonably reflect the diagnosis, treatment, consent, complications, and other key events.

Adequate documentation of the diagnosis and treatment is one of the most important aspects of patient care. Well-documented charts are the cornerstone of any risk-managment program. If dentists do not document fundamental clinical findings supporting the diagnosis and treatment, attorneys may question the need for treatment in the first place. Some argue that if an item is not charted, it did not happen. The following items are helpful when recorded in the chart:

1. Chief complaint
2. Dental history
3. Past medical history
4. Current medication
5. Allergies
6. Clinical and radiographic findings and interpretations
7. Recommended treatment and other alternatives
8. Informed consent
9. Therapy actually instituted
10. Recommended follow-up treatment
11. Referrals to other general dentists, specialists, or other medical practitioners

Frequently overlooked information that should be recorded in the chart includes the following:

1. Prescriptions and refills dispensed to the patient
2. Messages or other discussions related specifically to patient care (including phone calls)
3. Consultations obtained
4. Results of laboratory tests
5. Clinical observations of progress or outcome of treatment
6. Recommended adjunct follow-up care
7. Appointments made or recommended
8. Postoperative instructions and orders given
9. Warnings to the patient, including issues related to lack of compliance, failure to appear for appointments, failure to obtain or take medication, instructions to see other dentists or physicians, or instructions on participation in any activity that might jeopardize the patient's health
10. Missed appointments

Corrections should be made by drawing a single line through any information to be deleted. Correct information can be inserted above, or added below, along with a contemporaneous date. The single-line deletion should be initialed and dated. No portion of the chart should be discarded, obliterated, erased, or altered in any fashion. In some states it is a felony to alter records with the intent to deceive.

REFERRAL TO ANOTHER GENERAL DENTIST OR SPECIALIST

In many cases, dentists may think that the recommended treatment is beyond their level of training or experience and may choose to refer a patient to another general dentist or specialist. A referral slip or letter should clearly indicate the basis for referral and what the specialist is being asked to do. The referral should be recorded in the chart. A written referral to a specialist may ask the specialist to provide a written report detailing the diagnosis and treatment plan.

A patient's refusal to pursue a referral should be clearly noted in the chart. If a patient refuses to seek treatment from a specialist, the dentist must decide whether the recommended treatment is within his or her expertise. If not, the dentist should not provide this particular treatment, even if the patient insists. A patient's refusal to seek care from a specialist does not relieve the dentist of liablity for injuries or complications resulting from care outside the dentist's level of training and expertise.

Dental specialists should carefully evaluate all referred patients. For example, extracting or treating the wrong tooth is a common allegation in court. When in doubt the specialist should contact the referring dentist and discuss the case. Any change in the treatment plan provided by the specialist should be documented in both the referring dentist's and specialist's charts. Any revised plan or recommendation must be approved by the patient to avoid informed consent problems.

COMPLICATIONS

Less-than-desirable results can occur despite the dentist's best efforts in diagnosis, treatment planning, and surgical technique. A poor result does not necessarily suggest that a practitioner is guilty of negligence or other wrongdoing. However, when complications occur, it is mandatory that the dentist immediately begin to address the problem in an appropriate fashion.

In most instances the dentist should advise the patient of the complication. Examples of such situations are loss of or failure to recover a root tip; breaking a dental instrument, such as an endodontic file, in a tooth; perforation of the maxillary sinus; damage to adjacent teeth; or inadvertent fracture of surrounding bone. In these instances the dentist should clearly outline proposed management of the problem, including specific instructions to the patient, further treatment that may be necessary, and referral to an oral and maxillofacial surgeon when appropriate.

It is advisable to consider and discuss reasonable treatment options that may still produce reasonable results. For example, when teeth are extracted for orthodontic purposes, the first premolar may accidently be extracted when the orthodontist preferred extraction of the second premolar. Before removing any other teeth or alarming the patient and parents, the dentist should call the orthodontist to discuss the affect on treatment outcome and available treatment modifications. The patient and parents should be notified that the wrong tooth was extracted but that the orthodontist indicated that the treatment can proceed without significantly compromising the result.

The lack of reasonable modifications of the original treatment plan is more challenging. The dentist may have to consider a more expensive plan, such as implants, and should also consider funding additional treatment.

Another common complication is altered sensation following third molar removal. The chart should reflect the existence and extent of the problem. It may be useful to use a diagram to document the area involved. The density and severity of the deficit should be noted after testing, if possible. The chart should reflect the progress of the condition each time the patient returns for follow up. Ultimately, the patient may require a referral to an oral and maxillofacial surgeon with experience in diagnosing and treating nerve injuries. In most cases the referral should occur within approximately 3 months following the injury if there is no significant improvement. Excessive delays may limit the effectiveness of future treatment. Documentation of the patient's progress helps justify the decision to delay the referral.

PATIENT MANAGEMENT PROBLEMS

NONCOMPLIANT PATIENT

Dentists and staff should routinely chart lack of compliance, including missed appointments and cancellations and failure to follow advice to take medications, seek consultations, wear appliances, or return for routine visits. Efforts to advise patients of risks associated with failing to follow instructions should also be recorded.

When the patient's health may be jeopardized by continued noncompliance, consider writing a letter to the patient identifying the potential harm. Advise the patient that the office will not be responsible if these and other problems develop as a result of the patient's noncompliance. If the patient's care is eventually terminated, the accumulation of detailed chart entries documenting the noncompliance should justify why the dentist is unwilling to continue care.

PATIENT ABANDONMENT

A legal duty is owed to the patient once a doctor-patient relationship is established. This occurs when a patient has been accepted by the office, the initial evaluation has been completed, and treatment has begun. The dentist is usually obligated to provide care until the treatment is completed. There may be instances, however, when it is impossible or unreasonable for a dentist to complete a treatment plan because of several problems. Such problems include the

patient's failure to return for necessary appointments, follow explicit instructions, take medication, seek recommended consultations, and stop activities that may inhibit the treatment plan or otherwise jeopardize the dentist's ability to achieve acceptable results. This may include a total breakdown of communication and loss of rapport between the dentist and patient.

In these cases it is usually necessary for the dentist to follow certain steps before discontinuing treatment, to avoid being accused of patient abandonment. First, the chart must document the activities leading to the patient's termination. The patient should be adequately warned (if possible) that termination will result if the undesired activity does not stop. The patient should be warned of the potential harm that may result if such activity continues and the reason why the harm may occur. After being told why the office is no longer willing to provide treatment, the patient should be given a reasonable opportunity to find a new dentist (30 to 45 days is common). The office should continue treatment during this period if the patient is in need of emergency care or care is required to avoid harm to the patient's health or to treatment progress.

When it has been decided that the dentist-patient relationship cannot continue, the dentist must take the following steps to terminate the relationship:

A letter should be sent to the patient, indicating the intent to withdraw from the case and the unwillingness to provide further treatment. It should include the following information:

1. The reasons supporting the decision to discontinue treatment.
2. If applicable, the potential harm caused by the patient (or parent's) undesired activity.
3. Past warnings by the office that did not alter the patient's actions and continued to put the patient at risk (or jeopardized the dentist's ability to achieve an acceptable result).
4. A warning that the patient's treatment is not completed, and the patient should immediately seek another dentist, or, alternatively, go to a hospital or teaching clinic in the area for immediate examination or consultation. Include a warning that if the patient fails to follow this advice, the patient's dental health may continue to be jeopardized and any treatment progress may be lost or worse.
5. An offer to continue treating the patient for a reasonable period and for emergencies until the patient locates another dentist.

This letter should be sent by certified mail to ensure and document that the patient did in fact receive it. If other dentists are treating the patient, consider advising them of this decision. Consult local counsel if there are any concerns of confidentiality or if there is a particularly sensitive reason behind this decision.

The dentist must continue to remain available for treatment of emergency problems until the patient has had adequate time to seek treatment from another dentist. This must be communicated in the letter outlined above.

The dentist must offer to forward copies of all pertinent records that affect patient care. Nothing must be done to inhibit efforts of subsequent treatment to complete patient care.

Patients who are HIV-positive or who have similar diseases cannot be terminated because of their disease, because this action may violate the Handicapped Civil Rights Act and other federal or state laws. These patients cannot be refused treatment based on their disease. Patients who are HIV-positive or have AIDS are considered handicapped under these laws.[2] Legal counsel should be consulted if there is another valid reason to terminate such a patient.

Exceptions do exist to these suggested guidelines. Dentists must evaluate each situation carefully. Occasions may occur when the dentist does not wish to lose contact with a patient or lose the ability to observe and follow a complication. Terminating treatment will often anger a patient, who may in turn seek legal advice if experiencing a complication. The office may elect to complete treatment in such cases.

If treatment continues, the chart should carefully reflect all warnings to the patient about potential harm and the increased chance that acceptable results may not be achieved. In certain cases the patient may be asked to sign a revised consent form that includes the following information:

1. The patient realizes that he or she has been noncompliant or has otherwise not followed advice.
2. The above activities either jeopardized the patient's health or the dentist's ability to achieve acceptable results or has unreasonably increased the chances of complication.
3. The dentist will continue treatment, but there are no assurances that the results will be acceptable. Complications may occur requiring additional care, and the patient (or the patient's legal guardian) will accept full responsibility if any of the above events occur and will not hold the dentist responsible.

COMMON AREAS OF DENTAL LITIGATION

Litigation has involved all aspects of dental practice and nearly every specific type of treatment. There are a few areas with a high incidence of legal action.

Removal of the wrong tooth usually results from a communication breakdown between the general dentist and oral surgeon or the patient and dentist. When in doubt the dentist must confirm the tooth to be extracted by radiograph, clinical examination, or discussion with the referring dentist. If there is a difference of opinion regarding the proposed treatment, the patient and the referring dentist should be notified and the outcome of any subsequent conversation documented. A short follow-up letter confirming the final decision may also be helpful in documenting this decision. If the wrong tooth is in fact extracted, this should be handled in the manner described earlier in this chapter.

Nerve injuries are often grounds for suits, with attorneys claiming that the nerve injuries resulted from extractions, implants, endodontic treatment, or other procedures. These allegations are usually coupled with allegations of insufficient informed consent. Because nerve injuries are a known complication of mandibular extractions or mandibular implants posterior to the mental foramen, patient advocates claim the patient had a right to accept these risks as part of treatment. If the dentist can visualize conditions that increase this risk, the patient should be advised and the condition documented. An example would be to specifically note the relationship of the inferior alveolar nerve to the third molar tooth to be extracted, when these appear to be in very close proximity.

Failure to diagnose can be related to several areas of dentistry. One of the most common problems is a lesion that is seen on examination but is not adequately documented and no treatment or follow up is instituted. If the lesion causes further problems or a subsequent biopsy documents long-standing pathology or a malignancy, this may be viewed as negligence. This problem can be avoided by following up on any potentially abnormal finding. Chart an initial diagnosis or seek a consultation from a specialist. If the lesion has resolved by the next visit, record that fact so the issue is closed. If the patient is referred to another doctor, follow up to document the patient's progress, including whether or not the patient's condition was successfully treated.

Failure to diagnose periodontal disease is often the area of criticism and legal action. A periodontal examination should be a part of routine dental evaluations and therefore becomes the primary responsibility of the general dentist. The status of the problem, suggestions for treatment, referrals, and progress or resolution of the problem must be clearly documented.

Implant complications or failure is another common area of litigation. As with any procedure the patient should be informed of the complication's associated reconstruction and long-term outcome. The need for careful long-term hygiene and follow up should be explained. The potential detrimental effect of patient habits such as smoking should be explained and documented. Dentists placing implants should consider using a customized consent form, summarizing common complications and stressing the importance of patient follow-up care and oral hygiene.

Failure to provide appropriate referral to another dentist or specialist can be a source of legal problems. Dentists usually determine the appropriate time to refer a patient to a specialist for initial care or management of a complication. Failure to refer patients for complicated treatment not routinely performed by the dentist or delayed referral for management of a complication frequently becomes the basis for litigation. Referrals to specialists can greatly reduce liability risks. Specialists are accustomed to treating more difficult cases and complications. Specialists with whom the dentist has a good relationship can also diffuse patient-management problems by being objective and caring and reassuring angry patients. The general dentist and specialist may discuss ways of relieving the expense of addressing a complication and completing treatment.

Temporomandibular joint disorders sometimes become more apparent after dental procedures requiring prolonged opening or manipulation, such as tooth extraction or endodontic treatment. It is important to document any preexisting condition in the pretreatment assessment. The risk of temporomandibular joint pain or other dysfunction as a result of a procedure should be included in the informed consent when indicated. If the patient is in dire need of care that may aggravate or cause a temporomandibular joint condition, a customized consent form should be drafted and signed. It should clearly define the problem, giving the patient options, and ultimately confirm the patient's authorization to proceed.

WHEN A PATIENT THREATENS TO SUE

Whenever a patient, the patient's attorney, or any other representative of the patient informs the dentist that a malpractice suit is being considered, several precautions should be taken.

First, all such threats should be documented and reported immediately to the malpractice insurance carrier. The dentist should follow the advice of the malpractice carrier, institutional risk-management team, or the attorney assigned to the case. These individuals will usually respond to the threat. Because the first indication of a potential claim is usually a request for records, the office should comply with state law regarding what must be provided (usually copies of care and treatment records, not the originals). Patients sometimes request the original chart and radiographs for a variety of reasons. The law in many states indicates that the records are owned by the dental office and that the dental office has a legal obligation to maintain original records for a specified period. Patients are entitled to a legible copy, and dental offices are entitled to a reasonable reimbursement for the same. Patients do not own the records merely because they paid for care and treatment.

Second, the dentist and staff should not discuss the case with the patient (or representative of the patient) once a law suit is threatened or made. All requests for information or other contact should be forwarded to the carrier or attorney representing the dentist. All arguments with the patient or representative should be avoided. The dentist must not admit liability or fault or agree to waive fees. Any such statement or admission made to the patient or patient's representative may be used against the dentist later as an "admission against the dentist's interest."

Finally, it is imperative that no additions, deletions, or changes of any sort be made in the patient's dental record. Records must not be misplaced or destroyed. Seek legal advice before attempting to clarify an entry.

During the process of malpractice litigation, dentists may be called to give a deposition. This may be as the defendant in a case or as an expert witness. Although this is quite routine for attorneys, the procedure is often unnerving and emotional for dentists, particularly when testifying in their own defense.

The following are some suggestions that should be considered when giving a deposition related to a malpractice case:

1. Be prepared. Know your records well. Review all chart entries, test results, and any other relevant information. In complex cases, consider reviewing textbook knowledge of the subject but consult with your attorney before reviewing anything other than your record.
2. Never answer a question unless you are sure you understand it. Listen carefully to the question and provide a succinct answer to the question. Stop talking after you answer the question. A lawsuit cannot be won but can be lost at deposition.
3. Do not speculate. If you need to review records, radiographs, or other information, do so before answering a question, rather than guessing.
4. Be careful when agreeing that any particular expert author or text is "authoritative." Once you make such a statement you may be placed in a situation in which you did something or disagreed with something the "expert" has written. In most states, you can be impeached by anything the author states, once you agree that he is "authoritative."
5. Do not argue unnecessarily with the other attorney. Do not show your temper. This will only educate your adversary as to what is necessary to upset you in front of the jury at trial. They expect dentists to act professionally.
6. Follow the advice of your lawyer. The attorney is there to represent your interests. Even if the attorney is retained by the insurance company, he or she is required to represent your interests, not that of the insurance company or anyone else.

Most anxiety related to litigation comes from the fear of the unknown. Most dental practitioners have limited or no exposure to litigation. It must be kept in mind that dentists prevail in most cases. Only about 10% of cases go to trial, and dentists win well over 80% of these cases.

Unfortunately, a malpractice trial requires a tremendous investment of time, energy, and emotion, all of which detracts from patient care. Most dentists have no choice; they must defend themselves. Dentists who are prepared and who possess reasonable expectations of each step of the litigation process usually experience less anxiety.

MANAGED CARE ISSUES

The influence of managed health care has greatly changed many aspects of dentistry. This includes the doctor-patient relationship and the way decisions are made regarding which treatment alternatives are most appropriate. Dentists are often placed in the middle of a conflict between a desire to provide optimal treatment and a health care plan's willingness to approve appropriate, needed care.

Traditionally, the patient chose whether to elect a compromised treatment plan or even no treatment. Under managed care, however, some patients are being forced to accept compromised treatment or no treatment, based on administrative decisions that may be driven more by cost-containment pressures than sound dental judgment.

In some cases a "gag provision" is included in a dentist's contract with a mangaged care organization. This prevents the dentist from criticizing managed care organizations and sometimes prevents a dentist from presenting an alternative for care not covered by the third party provider. This obviously creates a conflict between a contractual agreement with the company and the ethical and professional responsibility of the dentist to the patient. In some states this provision is illegal and unenforceable.

In 1995 the ADA Council on Ethics, Bylaws, and Judicial Affairs issued the following statement underscoring dentists' obligation to provide appropriate care:

> Dentists who enter into managed care agreements may be called upon to reconcile the demands placed on them to contain costs with the needs of their patients. Dentists must not allow these demands to interfere with the patient's right to select a treatment option based on informed consent. Nor should dentists allow anything to interfere with the free exercise of their professional judgement or their duty to make appropriate referrals if indicated. Dentists are reminded that contract obligations do not excuse them from their ethical duty to put the patient's welfare first.[1]

Dentists may have a responsibility to advise patients that a "compromised" treatment plan has been approved by the managed care organization. The dentist should seek the patient's consent to provide such treatment after the pertinent risks, complications, and limitations have been reviewed, along with an explanation of more optimal treatment options. Dentists should consider advising in written form both patients and third party payers of reasonably expected outcomes when the appropriate treatment is not available because of improper decisions by third providers.

SUMMARY ◇

In addition to providing sound technical care, the dentist must address several other aspects of patient care to minimize unnecessary legal liability. The dentist should develop the best possible rapport with patients, through improved communication and by providing any information that may enhance patient understanding of treatment. Adequate documentation of all aspects of patient care is also necessary. Clinicians face a constant struggle to document quality care and advice to the patient. The law only requires that such efforts be reasonable, not perfect.

This chapter is intended to provide suggestions to be considered by individual dentists. It is not intended to in any way establish, influence, or modify the standard of care. Medical and dental malpractice laws vary from state to state. When confronted with medicolegal issues, all health care providers should consult local counsel familiar with the laws and regulations that apply in their jurisdiction.

REFERENCES

1. ADA Counsel on Ethics, Bylaws and Judicial Affairs: How to reconcile participation in managed care plans with their ethical obligations, *ADA News,* p 12, Feb 6, 1995.
2. Americans with Disabilities Act of 1990, 42 USC, section 12101.

BIBLIOGRAPHY

Informed consent package for dentists, Physicians Insurance Company of Michigan, 1994.

Nora RL: Dental malpractice: its causes and cures, *Quintessence Int* 17:121, 1986.

Risk Retention Group: The informed consent process, Rosemont, Ill, 1994, AAOMS Mutual Insurance Company.

Small RL: How to avoid being sued for malpractice, *J Mich Dent Assoc* 75:45, 1993.

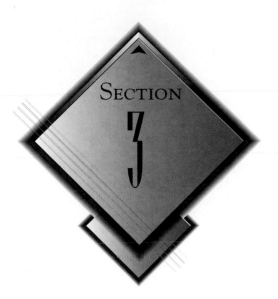

SECTION

3

PREPROSTHETIC SURGERY

In spite of dentistry's improved ability to maintain dentition a large portion of the population continues to require replacement of some or all of their teeth. Surgical improvement of the denture-bearing area and surrounding tissue (preprosthetic surgery) offers an exciting and demanding challenge in the area of dental practice.

Many minor modifications of the alveolar ridge and vestibular areas can greatly improve denture stability and retention. Several surgical techniques frequently employed for this purpose are described and illustrated in Chapter 13. In some cases, patients have severe bone changes or soft tissue abnormalities that require more extensive surgical preparation before implant placement or before the prosthetic appliance can be properly constructed and worn. Procedures that improve prosthesis retention and stability are discussed and illustrated in Chapter 14.

One of the most exciting frontiers in dentistry is the area of implantology. Proper placement of implants and subsequent prosthetic reconstruction can provide patients with a more natural and efficient substitution for their lost dentition. Depending on the circumstances, several types of implant systems may be used. Chapter 15 discusses the various types of implant systems currently in use and their advantages, disadvantages, and indications for use.

CHAPTER 13

BASIC PREPROSTHETIC SURGERY

MYRON R. TUCKER

OBJECTIVES OF PREPROSTHETIC SURGERY ⎯⎯⎯◇

Despite the enormous progress in the technology available to preserve the dentition, there is still a need for prosthetic restoration and rehabilitation of the masticatory system in patients who are edentulous or partially edentulous. Nearly 10% of the American population, including 35% of those over age 65, are currently totally edentulous, and millions of people have experienced a partial loss of their dentition.[10]

The prosthetic replacement of lost or congenitally absent teeth frequently involves surgical preparation of the remaining oral tissues to support the best possible prosthetic replacement. Often oral structures, such as frenal attachments and exostosis, have no significance when teeth are present but become obstacles to proper prosthetic appliance construction after tooth loss. The challenge of prosthetic rehabilitation of the patient includes restoration of the best masticatory function possible combined with restoration or improvement of dental and facial esthetics. Maximal preservation of hard and soft tissue during preprosthetic surgical preparation is also mandatory. The oral tissues are difficult to replace once they are lost.

The objective of preprosthetic surgery is to create proper supporting structures for subsequent placement of prosthetic appliances. The best denture support has the following characteristics:[9]
1. No evidence of intraoral or extraoral pathologic conditions.
2. Proper jaw relationship in the anteroposterior, transverse, and vertical dimensions.
3. Alveolar processes that are as large as possible and of the proper configuration. (The ideal shape of the alveolar

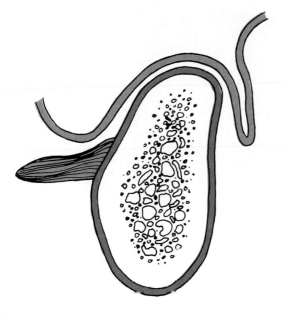

◇ Figure 13-1

Ideal shape of alveolar process in denture-bearing area.

process is a broad U-shaped ridge, with the vertical components as parallel as possible [Figure 13-1].)
4. No bony or soft tissue protuberances or undercuts.
5. Adequate attached keratinized mucosa in the primary denture-bearing area.
6. Adequate vestibular depth.
7. Adequate form and tissue coverage for possible implant placement.

PRINCIPLES OF PATIENT EVALUATION AND TREATMENT PLANNING ——◇

Before any surgical or prosthetic treatment, a thorough evaluation outlining the problems to be solved and a detailed treatment plan should be developed for each patient. It is imperative that no preparatory surgical procedure be undertaken without a clear understanding of the desired design of the final prosthesis.

Preprosthetic surgical treatment must begin with a thorough history and physical examination of the patient. An extremely important aspect of the history is to obtain a clear idea of the patient's chief complaint and expectations of surgical and prosthetic treatment. Esthetic and functional goals of the patient must be assessed carefully and a determination made of whether these expectations can be met. Psychologic factors and the adaptability of patients are important determinants of their ability to function adequately with full or partial dentures. Information on success or failure with previous prosthetic appliances may be helpful in determining the patient's attitude toward and adaptability to

prosthetic treatment. The history should include important information such as the patient's risk status for surgery, with particular emphasis on systemic diseases that may affect bone or soft tissue healing.

An intraoral and extraoral examination of the patient should include an assessment of the existing tooth relationships if any remain, amount and contour of remaining bone, quality of soft tissue overlying the primary denture-bearing area, vestibular depth, location of muscle attachments, jaw relationships, and presence of soft tissue or bony pathologic conditions.

EVALUATION OF SUPPORTING BONY TISSUE

Examination of the supporting bone should include visual inspection, palpation, radiographic examination, and in some cases evaluation of models. Abnormalities of the remaining bone can often be assessed during the visual inspection; however, because of bony resorption and location of muscle or soft tissue attachments, many bony abnormalities may be obscured. Palpation of all areas of the maxilla and mandible, including both the primary denture-bearing area and vestibular area, is necessary.

Evaluation of the denture-bearing area of the maxilla includes an overall evaluation of the bony ridge form. No bony undercuts or gross bony protuberances that block the path of denture insertion should be allowed to remain in the area of the alveolar ridge, buccal vestibule, or palatal vault. Palatal tori that require modification should be noted. Adequate posttuberosity notching must exist for posterior denture stability and peripheral seal.

The remaining mandibular ridge should be evaluated visually for overall ridge form and contour, gross ridge irregularities, tori, and buccal exostosis. In cases of moderate-to-severe resorption of alveolar bone, ridge contour cannot be adequately assessed by visual inspection alone. Muscular and mucosal attachments near the crest of the ridge may obscure underlying bony anatomy, particularly in the area of the posterior mandible, where a depression can frequently be palpated between the external oblique line and mylohyoid ridge areas. The location of the mental foramen and mental neurovascular bundle can be palpated in relation to the superior aspect of the mandible, and neurosensory disturbances can be noted.

Evaluation of the interarch relationship of the maxilla and the mandible is extremely important and includes an examination of the anteroposterior and vertical relationships, as well as any possible skeletal asymmetries that may exist between the maxilla and mandible. The anteroposterior relationship must be evaluated with the patient in the proper vertical dimension. Overclosure of the mandible may result in a class III skeletal relationship but may appear normal if evaluated with the mandible in the proper postural position. Lateral and posteroanterior cephalometric radiographs with the jaws in proper postural position may be helpful in confirming a skeletal discrepancy. Careful attention must be paid to the interarch distance, particularly in the posterior areas, where

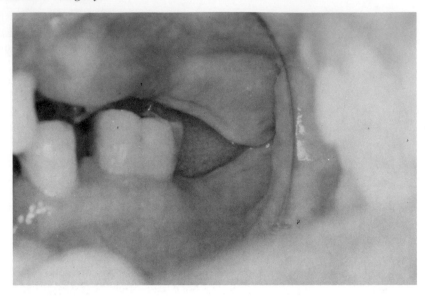

◇ Figure 13-2

Examination of interarch relationships in proper vertical dimension often reveals lack of adequate space for prosthetic reconstruction. In this case, bony and fibrous tissue excess in tuberosity area must be reduced to provide adequate space for partial denture construction.

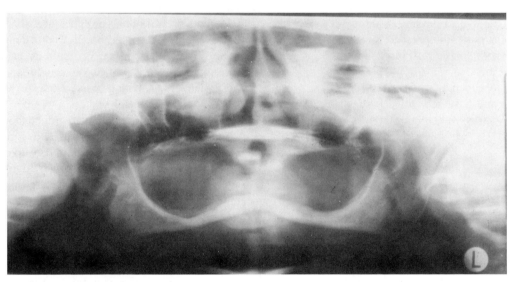

◇ Figure 13-3

Radiograph demonstrating atrophic mandibular and maxillary alveolar ridges. Note pneumatization of maxillary sinus.

vertical excess of the tuberosity, either bony tissue or soft tissue, may impinge on space necessary for placement of a prosthesis that is properly constructed (Figure 13-2).

Proper radiographs are an important part of the initial diagnosis and treatment plan. Panoramic radiographic techniques provide an excellent overview assessment of underlying bony structure and pathologic conditions.[2] Radiographs should disclose bony pathologic lesions, impacted teeth or portions of remaining roots, the bony pattern of the alveolar ridge, and the size and pneumatization of the maxillary sinus (Figure 13-3).

EVALUATION OF SUPPORTING SOFT TISSUE

Assessment of the quality of tissue of the primary denture-bearing area overlying the alveolar ridge is of utmost importance. The amount of keratinized tissue firmly attached to the underlying bone in the denture-bearing area should be

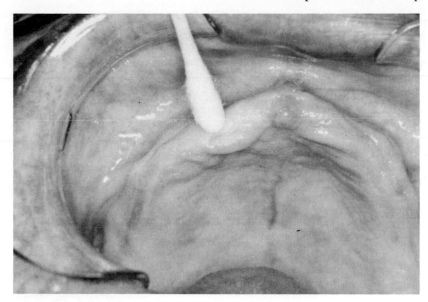

◇ Figure 13-4

Palpation reveals hypermobile tissue that will not provide adequate base in denture-bearing area.

distinguished from poorly keratinized or freely movable tissue. Palpation discloses hypermobile fibrous tissue inadequate for a stable denture base (Figure 13-4).

The vestibular areas should be free of inflammatory changes, such as scarred or ulcerated areas caused by denture pressure or hyperplastic tissue resulting from an ill-fitting denture. Tissue at the depth of the vestibule should be supple and without irregularities, for maximal peripheral seal of the denture. Assessment of vestibular depth should include manual manipulation of the adjacent muscle attachments. By tensing the soft tissue adjacent to the area of the alveolar ridge, the dentist can note muscle or soft tissue attachments (including frena) that approximate the crest of the alveolar ridge and are often responsible for the loss of peripheral seal of the denture during speech and mastication.

The lingual aspect of the mandible should be inspected with a mouth mirror in the linguovestibular area to determine the level of attachment of the mylohyoid muscle in relation to the crest of the mandibular ridge and the attachment of the genioglossus muscle in the anterior mandible. The linguovestibular depth should be evaluated with the tongue in several positions, because movement of the tongue accompanied by elevation of the mylohyoid and genioglossus muscles is a common cause of movement and displacement of the lower denture.

TREATMENT PLANNING

Before any surgical intervention, a treatment plan addressing the patient's identified oral problems should be formulated. The dentist responsible for prosthesis construction should assume responsibility for seeking surgical consultation when necessary. Long-term maintenance of the underlying bone and soft tissue, as well as of the prosthetic appliances, should be kept in mind at all times. Hasty treatment planning, without

consideration for long-term results, can often result in unnecessary loss of bone or soft tissue and improper functioning of the prosthetic appliance. For example, when there appears to be a soft tissue excess over the alveolar ridge area, the most appropriate long-term treatment plan may involve grafting bone or an alloplastic material, such as hydroxyapatite (HA), to improve the contour of the alveolar ridge. Maintenance of the redundant soft tissue may be found necessary to improve the results of the grafting procedure. If this tissue were removed without any consideration of the possible long-term benefits of a grafting procedure, both the opportunity for improved immediate function and the opportunity for long-term maintenance of bony tissue and soft tissue would be lost.

Preprosthetic surgical preparation of the denture-supporting areas begins early in the treatment sequence. It may be desirable to delay definitive soft tissue procedures until underlying bony problems have been adequately resolved. However, when bone or alloplastic grafting or other, more complex treatment of bony abnormalities is not required, both bony and soft tissue preparation can be completed simultaneously.

RECONTOURING OF THE ALVEOLAR RIDGES ────◇

Irregularities of the alveolar bone found either at the time of tooth extraction or after a period of initial healing require recontouring before final prosthetic construction. The objectives of this recontouring should be to provide the best possible tissue contour for prosthesis support while maintaining as much bone and soft tissue as possible.

SIMPLE ALVEOLOPLASTY ASSOCIATED WITH REMOVAL OF MULTIPLE TEETH

The simplest form of alveoloplasty consists of the compression of the lateral walls of the extraction socket after simple tooth removal. In many cases of single tooth extraction, digital compression of the extraction site adequately contours the underlying bone, provided that there are no gross irregularities of bone contour in the area after extraction. However, when multiple irregularities exist, more extensive recontouring often is necessary.

A conservative alveoloplasty in combination with multiple extractions is carried out after all of the teeth in the arch have been removed as described in Chapter 8. The specific areas requiring alveolar recontouring are obvious if this sequence is followed. Whether alveolar ridge recontouring is performed at the time of tooth extraction or after a period of healing, the technique is essentially the same. Bony areas requiring recontouring should be exposed using an envelope type of flap. A mucoperiosteal incision along the crest of the ridge, with adequate extension anteroposterior to the area to be exposed, and flap reflection allow adequate visualization and access to the alveolar ridge. Where adequate exposure is not possible, small vertical releasing incisions may be necessary. The primary objectives of mucoperiosteal flap reflection are to allow for adequate visualization and access to the bony structures that require recontouring and to protect soft tissue adjacent to this area during the procedure. Although releasing incisions often create more discomfort during the healing period, this technique is certainly preferred to the possibility

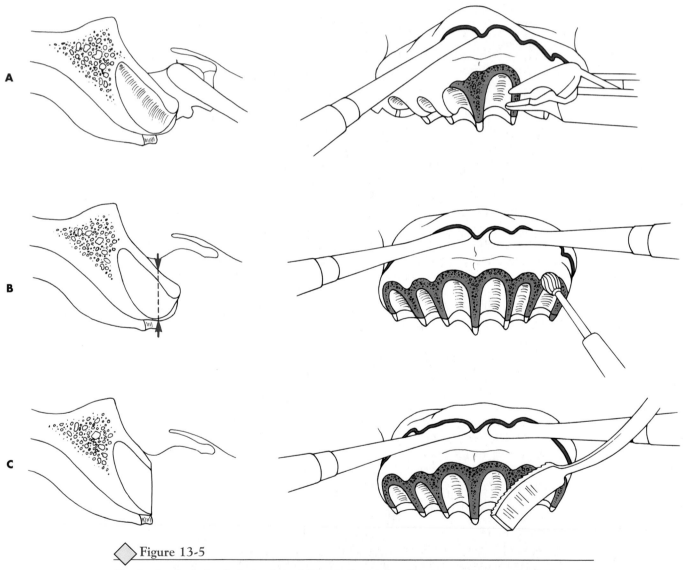

◇ Figure 13-5

Simple alveoloplasty eliminates buccal irregularities and undercut areas by removing labiocortical bone. **A,** Elevation of mucoperiosteal flap, exposure of irregularities of alveolar ridge, and removal of gross irregularity with rongeur. **B,** Bone bur in rotating handpiece can also be used to remove bone and smooth labiocortical surface. **C,** Use of bone file to smooth irregularities and achieve final desired contour.

of an unanticipated tear in the edges of a flap when inadequate exposure could not be achieved with an envelope flap. Regardless of flap design, the mucoperiosteum should be reflected only to the extent that adequate exposure to the area of bony irregularity can be achieved. Excessive flap reflection may result in devitalized areas of bone, which will resorb more rapidly after surgery, and a diminished soft tissue adaptation to the alveolar ridge area.

Depending on the degree of irregularity of the alveolar ridge area, recontouring can be accomplished with a rongeur, a bone file, or a bone bur in a handpiece, alone or in combination (Figure 13-5). In any case, copious saline irrigation should be used throughout the recontouring procedure. After recontouring, the flap should be reapproximated by digital pressure and the ridge palpated to ensure that all irregularities have been removed (Figure 13-6). After copious

irrigation, the edges of the flaps can be trimmed to remove excess tissue and sutured with interrupted or continuous sutures. If an extensive incision has been made, continuous suturing tends to be less annoying to the patient and provides for easier postoperative hygiene because of the elimination of knots and loose suture ends along the incision line.

When a sharp knife-edge ridge exists in the mandible the sharp superior portion of the alveolus can be removed in a manner similar to that described for simple alveoloplasty. After local anesthesia is obtained, a crestal incision is made, extending along the alveolar ridge, approximately 1 cm beyond either end of the area requiring recontouring (Figure 13-7). After minimal reflection of the mucoperiosteum, a rongeur can be used to remove the major portion of the sharp area of the superior aspect of the mandible. A bone file is used to smooth the superior aspect of the mandible. After copious

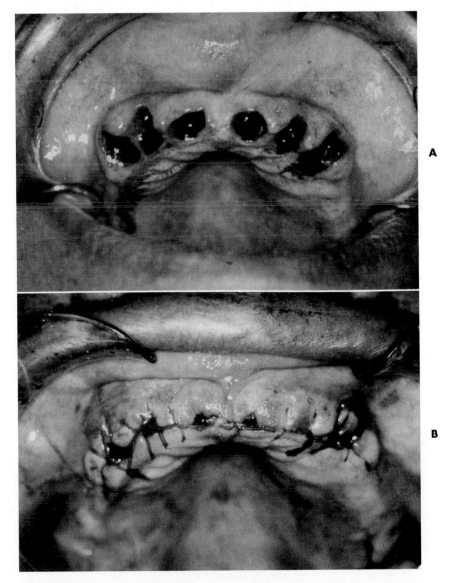

A

B

◇ Figure 13-6

A, Clinical appearance of maxillary ridge after removal of teeth and before bony recontouring.
B, Properly contoured alveolar ridge free of irregularities and bony undercuts.

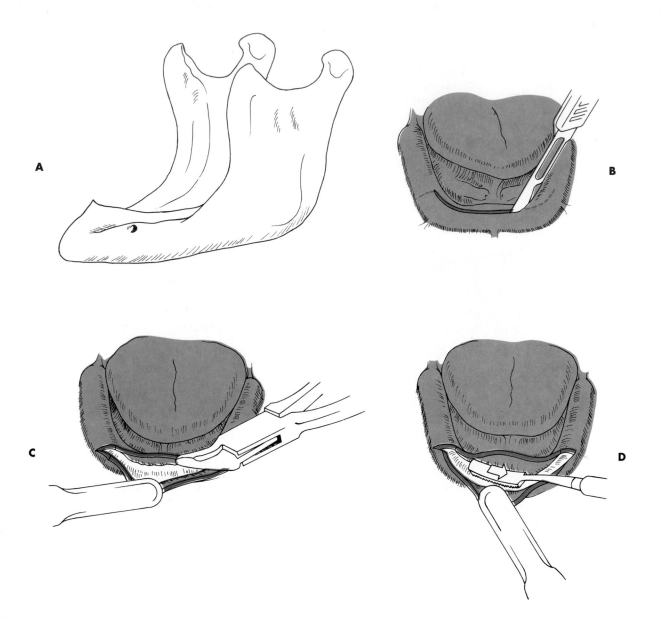

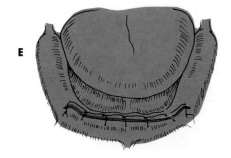

◇ Figure 13-7

Recontouring of a knife-edge ridge. **A,** Lateral view of mandible, with resorption resulting in knife-edge alveolar ridge. **B,** Crestal incision extends 1 cm beyond each end of area to be recontoured. (Vertical releasing incisions are occasionally necessary at posterior ends of initial incision.) **C,** Rongeur used to eliminate bulk of sharp bony projection. **D,** Bone file used to eliminate any minor irregularities. (Bone bur and handpiece can also be used for this purpose.) **E,** Continuous suture technique for mucosal closure.

irrigation, this area is closed with continuous or interrupted sutures. Before removal of any bone, strong consideration should be given to reconstruction of proper ridge form using alloplastic materials, which is discussed later in this chapter and in Chapter 14.

INTRASEPTAL ALVEOLOPLASTY

An alternative to the removal of alveolar ridge irregularities by the simple alveoloplasty technique is the use of an intraseptal alveoloplasty, or Dean's technique, involving the removal of intraseptal bone and the repositioning of the labial cortical bone, rather than removal of excessive or irregular areas of the labial cortex.[3] This technique is best used in an area where the ridge is of relatively regular contour and adequate height but presents an undercut to the depth of the labial vestibule because of the configuration of the alveolar ridge. It can be accomplished at the time of tooth removal or in the early initial postoperative healing period.

After exposure of the crest of the alveolar ridge by reflection of the mucoperiosteum, a small rongeur can be used to remove the intraseptal portion of the alveolar bone (Figure 13-8). After adequate bone removal has been accomplished, digital pressure should be sufficient to fracture the labiocortical plate of the alveolar ridge inward to approximate the palatal plate area more closely. Occasionally, small vertical cuts at either end of the labiocortical plate will facilitate repositioning of the fractured segment. By using a bur or osteotome inserted through the distal extraction area, the labial cortex is scored without perforation of the labial mucosa. Digital pressure on the labial aspect of the ridge is necessary to determine when the bony cut is complete and to ensure that the mucosa is not damaged. After positioning of the labiocortical plate, any slight areas of bony irregularity can be contoured with a bone file, and the alveolar mucosa can be reapproximated with interrupted or continuous suture techniques. A splint or an immediate denture lined with a soft lining material can then be inserted to maintain the bony position until initial healing has taken place.

There are several advantages to this type of technique. The labial prominence of the alveolar ridge can be reduced without significantly reducing the height of the ridge in this area. The periosteal attachment to the underlying bone can also be maintained, thereby reducing postoperative bone resorption and remodeling. Finally, the muscle attachments to the area of the alveolar ridge can be left undisturbed in this type of procedure. Michael and Barsaun[7] reported the results of a study comparing the effects of postoperative bone resorption following three alveoloplasty techniques. In their study, nonsurgical extraction, labial alveoloplasty, and an intraseptal alveoloplasty technique were compared to evaluate postoperative bony resorption. The initial postoperative results were similar, but the best long-term maintenance of alveolar ridge height was achieved with nonsurgical extractions, and the intraseptal alveoloplasty technique resulted in less resorption than did removal of labiocortical bone for reduction of ridge irregularities.

The main disadvantage of this technique is the decrease in ridge thickness that obviously occurs with this procedure. If the ridge form remaining after this type of alveoplasty is excessively thin, this may preclude placement of implants at some point in the future. For this reason the intraseptal alveoplasty should reduce the thickness of the ridge in an amount sufficient only to reduce or eliminate undercuts.

MAXILLARY TUBEROSITY REDUCTION

Horizontal and/or vertical excess of the maxillary tuberosity area may be a result of excess bone, an increase in the thickness of soft tissue overlying the bone, or both. A preoperative radiograph is often useful to determine the extent to which bone and soft tissue contribute to this excess and to locate the floor of the maxillary sinus. Recontouring of the maxillary tuberosity area may be necessary to remove bony ridge irregularities or to create adequate interarch space, which will allow proper construction of prosthetic appliances in the posterior areas. Surgery can be accomplished using local anesthetic infiltration or posterosuperior alveolar and greater palatine blocks. Access to the tuberosity for bone removal is accomplished by making a crestal incision that extends up the posterior aspect of the tuberosity area. The most posterior aspect of this incision is often best made with a no. 12 scalpel blade. Reflection of a full-thickness mucoperiosteal flap is completed in both the buccal and palatal directions to allow adequate access to the entire tuberosity area (Figure 13-9). Bone can be removed using either a side-cutting rongeur or rotary instruments, with care taken to avoid perforation of the floor of the maxillary sinus. If the maxillary sinus is inadvertently perforated, no specific treatment is required, provided that the sinus membrane has not been violated. After the appropriate amount of bone has been removed, the area should be smoothed with a bone file and copiously irrigated with saline. The mucoperiosteal flaps can then be readapted. Excess, overlapping soft tissue resulting from the bone removal is excised in an elliptic fashion. A tension-free closure over this area is important, particularly if the floor of the sinus has been perforated. Sutures should remain in place for approximately 7 days. Initial denture impressions can be completed approximately 4 weeks after surgery.

In the event of a gross sinus perforation involving an opening in the sinus membrane, the use of postoperative antibiotics and sinus decongestants is recommended. Penicillin or a penicillin derivative is usually the antibiotic of choice, unless contraindicated by allergy. Sinus decongestants, such as pseudoephedrine with or without an antihistamine, are adequate. Both the antibiotic and decongestant should be given for 7 to 10 days postoperatively. The patient is informed of the potential complications and cautioned against creating excessive sinus pressure, such as nose blowing, for 10 to 14 days.

BUCCAL EXOSTOSIS AND EXCESSIVE UNDERCUTS

Excessive bony protuberances and resulting undercut areas are more common in the maxilla than the mandible. A local anesthetic should be infiltrated around the area requiring bony

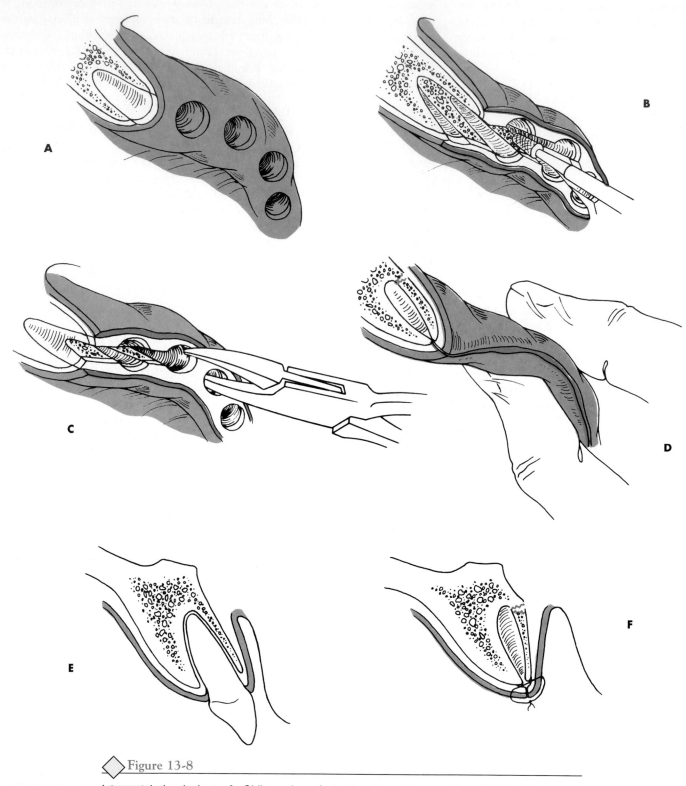

◇ Figure 13-8

Intraseptal alveoloplasty. **A,** Oblique view of alveolar ridge, demonstrating slight facial undercut. **B,** Minimal elevation of mucoperiosteal flap, followed by removal of intraseptal bone using fissure bur and handpiece. **C,** Rongeur used to remove intraseptal bone. **D,** Digital pressure used to fracture labiocortex in palatal direction. **E,** Cross- sectional view of alveolar process. **F,** Cross-sectional view of alveolar process after tooth removal and intraseptal alveoloplasty. By fracturing labiocortex of alveolar process in palatal direction, labial undercut can be eliminated without reducing vertical height of alveolar ridge.

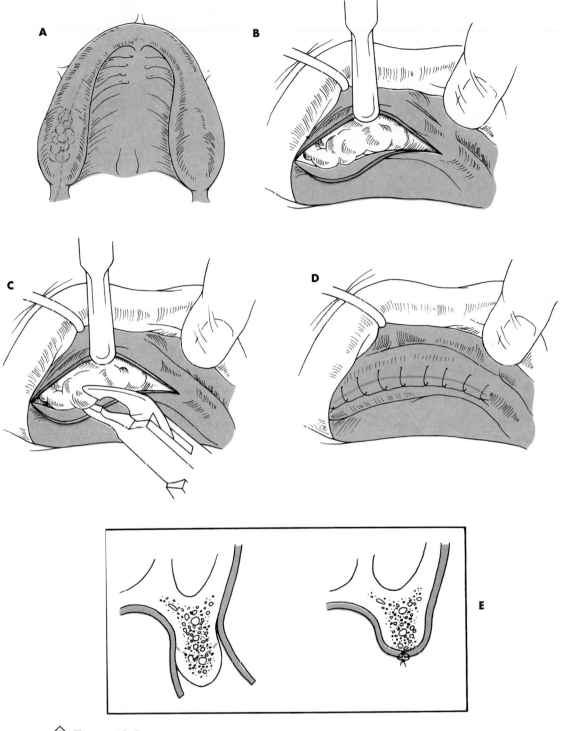

◇ Figure 13-9

Bony tuberosity reduction. **A,** Incision extended along crest of alveolar ridge distally to superior extent of tuberosity area. **B,** Elevated mucoperiosteal flap provides adequate exposure to all areas of bony excess. **C,** Rongeur used to eliminate bony excess. **D,** Tissue reapproximated with continuous suture technique. **E,** Cross-sectional view of posterior tuberosity area, showing vertical reduction of bone and reapposition of mucoperiosteal flap. (In some cases, removal of large amounts of bone produces excessive soft tissue, which can be excised before closure to prevent overlapping.)

reduction. For mandibular buccal exostosis, inferior alveolar blocks may also be required to anesthetize bony areas. A crestal incision extends 1 to 1.5 cm beyond each end of the area requiring contour, and a full-thickness mucoperiosteal flap is reflected to expose the areas of bony exostosis. If adequate exposure cannot be obtained, vertical releasing incisions are necessary to provide access and prevent trauma to the soft tissue flap. If the areas of irregularity are small, recontouring with a bone file may be all that is required; larger areas may necessitate use of a rongeur or rotary instrument (Figure 13-10). After completion of the bone recontouring, soft tissue is readapted, and visual inspection and palpation ensure that no irregularities or bony undercuts exist. Interrupted or continuous suturing techniques are used to close the soft tissue incision, and the sutures are removed in approximately 7 days. Denture impressions can be made 4 weeks postoperatively.

Although extremely large areas of bony exostosis generally require removal, small undercut areas are often best treated by being filled with either autogenous or allogeneic bone material or with an alloplastic material such as hydroxyapatite (HA). Such a situation might occur in the anterior maxilla or mandible, where removal of the bony buccal protuberance results in a narrowed crest in the alveolar ridge area and a less desirable area of support for the denture, as well as an area that may resorb more rapidly.

Local anesthetic infiltration is generally sufficient when filling in buccal undercut areas. After a vertical incision is made in the anterior maxillary or mandibular areas, a small periosteal elevator is used to create a subperiosteal tunnel extending the length of the area to be filled in with bone or HA (Figure 13-11). HA is placed with syringes provided by the manufacturer, and digital pressure is used to contour the material to its proper configuration. The incision is closed with interrupted or continuous sutures. When small undercuts are obliterated, splints are usually unnecessary. However, in larger defects a splint can often be used to help contain and contour the HA material and mold it to its proper configuration during the healing phase. If a splint is used, it should remain for 5 to 7 days. Sutures are removed at 7 days postoperatively, and denture impressions can be taken 3 to 4 weeks after surgery.

Another technique that may be employed to correct contour defects involves open exposure of the area to be grafted, placement of graft material, and the use of a membrane covering over the grafted tissue to facilitate guided bone regeneration. This type of bone grafting is discussed in Chapters 14 and 15.

LATERAL PALATAL EXOSTOSIS

The lateral aspect of the palatal vault may be somewhat irregular because of the presence of lateral palatal exostosis. This presents problems in denture construction because of the undercut created by the exostosis and the narrowing of the palatal vault. Occasionally, these exostoses are large enough that the mucosa covering the area becomes ulcerated.

Local anesthetic in the area of the greater palatine foramen and infiltration in the area of the incision are necessary. A crestal incision is made from the posterior aspect of the tuberosity, extending slightly beyond the anterior area of the exostosis, which requires recontouring (Figure 13-12). Reflection of the mucoperiosteum in the palatal direction should be accomplished with careful attention to the area of the palatine foramen to avoid damage to the blood vessels as they leave the foramen and extend forward. After adequate exposure, a rotary instrument or bone file can be used to remove the excess bony projection in this area. The area is irrigated with sterile saline and closed with continuous or interrupted sutures. No surgical splint or packing is generally required after this procedure.

MYLOHYOID RIDGE REDUCTION

One of the more common areas interfering with proper denture construction in the mandible is the mylohyoid ridge area. In addition to the actual bony ridge, with its easily damaged thin covering of mucosa, the muscular attachment to this area often is responsible for dislodging the denture. When this ridge is extremely sharp, denture pressure may produce significant pain in this area. Relocation of the mylohyoid muscle to improve this condition is discussed in Chapter 14. In cases of severe resorption the external oblique line and the mylohyoid ridge area may actually form the most prominent areas of the posterior mandible, with the midportion of the mandibular ridge existing as a concave structure. In such cases, augmentation of the posterior aspect of the mandible rather than removal of the mylohyoid ridge may be found beneficial (see Chapter 14). There are, however, some cases that can be improved by reduction of the mylohyoid ridge area.

Inferior alveolar, buccal, and lingual nerve blocks are required for mylohyoid ridge reduction. A linear incision is made over the crest of the ridge in the posterior aspect of the mandible. Extension of the incision too far to the lingual aspect should be avoided, because this may cause potential trauma to the lingual nerve. A full-thickness mucoperiosteal flap is reflected, which exposes the mylohyoid ridge area and mylohyoid muscle attachments (Figure 13-13). The mylohyoid muscle fibers are removed from the ridge by sharply incising the muscle attachment at the area of bony origin. When the muscle is released, the underlying fat is visible in the surgical field. After reflection of the muscle, a rotary instrument or bone file can be used to remove the sharp prominence of the mylohyoid ridge. Immediate replacement of the denture is desirable, because it may help facilitate a more inferior relocation of the muscular attachment; however, this is somewhat unpredictable and may actually be best managed by a procedure to lower the floor of the mouth (see Chapter 14).

GENIAL TUBERCLE REDUCTION

As the mandible begins to undergo resorption, the area of the attachment of the genioglossus muscle in the anterior portion of the mandible may become increasingly prominent. In some cases the tubercle may actually function as a shelf against which the denture can be constructed, but it usually requires reduction to construct the prosthesis properly. Before a

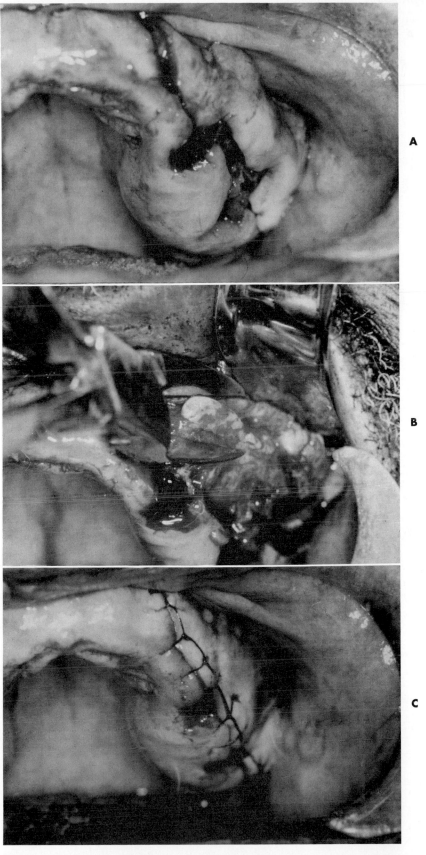

◇ Figure 13-10

Removal of buccal exostosis. **A,** Gross irregularities of buccal aspect of alveolar ridge. Following tooth removal, incision is completed over crest of alveolar ridge. (Note vertical releasing incision in cuspid area.) **B,** Exposure and removal of buccal exostosis with rongeur. **C,** Soft tissue closure using continuous suture technique.

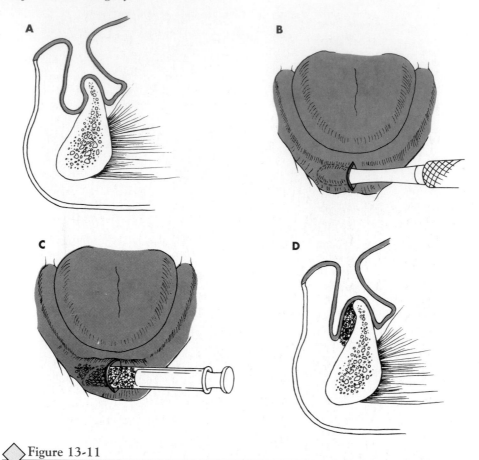

⬦ Figure 13-11

Removal of mandibular buccal undercut. **A,** Cross-sectional view of anterior portion of mandible, which, if corrected by removal of labiocortical bone, would result in knife-edge ridge. **B,** Vertical incision is made and subperiosteal tunnel developed in depth of undercut area. **C,** Syringe containing hydroxyapatite (HA) is placed in subperiosteal tunnel. **D,** Cross-sectional view after filling defect with HA.

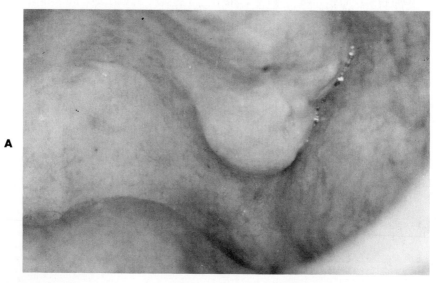

⬦ Figure 13-12

Removal of palatal bony exostosis. **A,** Small palatal exostosis that interferes with proper denture construction in this sarea.

Continued

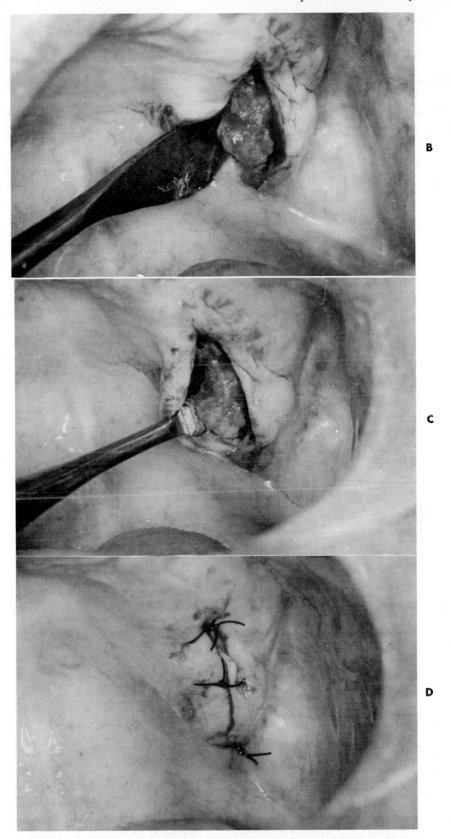

◇ Figure 13-12, cont'd

B, Crestal incision and mucoperiosteal flap reflection to expose palatal exostosis. **C,** Use of bone file to remove bony excess. **D,** Soft tissue closure.

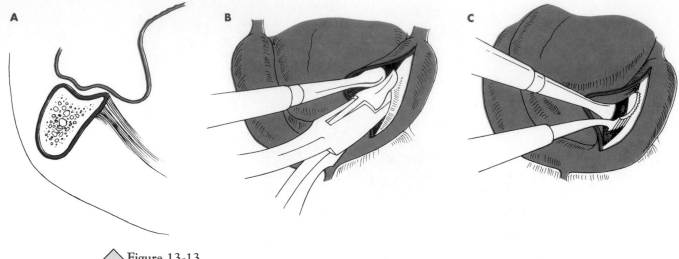

◆ Figure 13-13

Mylohyoid ridge reduction. **A,** Cross-sectional view of posterior aspect of mandible, showing concave contour of the superior aspect of ridge from resorption. Mylohyoid ridge and external oblique lines form highest portions of ridge. (This can generally best be treated by alloplastic augmentation of mandible but in rare cases may also require mylohyoid ridge reduction.) **B,** Crestal incision and exposure of lingual aspect of mandible for removal of sharp bone in mylohyoid ridge area. Rongeur or bur in rotating handpiece can be used to remove bone. **C,** Bone file used to complete recontouring of mylohyoid ridge.

decision to remove this prominence is made, consideration should be given to possible augmentation of the anterior portion of the mandible rather than reduction of the genial tubercle. If augmentation is the preferred treatment, the tubercle should be left to add support to the graft in this area. Local anesthetic infiltration and bilateral lingual nerve blocks should provide adequate anesthesia. A crestal incision is made from each premolar area to the midline of the mandible. A full-thickness mucoperiosteal flap is dissected lingually to expose the genial tubercle. The genioglossus muscle attachment can be removed by a sharp incision. Smoothing with a bur or a rongeur followed by a bone file removes the genial tubercle. The genioglossus muscle is left to reattach in a random fashion. As with the mylohyoid muscle and mylohyoid ridge reduction, a procedure to lower the floor of the mouth may also benefit the anterior mandible.

TORI REMOVAL ◇
MAXILLARY TORI

Maxillary tori consist of bony exostosis formation in the area of the palate. The origin of maxillary tori is unclear. They are found in 20% of the female population, approximately twice the prevalence in males.[6] Tori may have multiple shapes and configurations, ranging from a single smooth elevation to a multiloculated pedunculated bony mass. Tori present few problems when the maxillary dentition is present and only occasionally interfere with speech or become ulcerated from frequent trauma to the palate. However, when the loss of teeth necessitates full or partial denture construction, tori often interfere with proper design and function of the prosthesis.

Nearly all large maxillary tori should be removed before full or partial denture construction. Smaller tori may often be left, because they do not interfere with prosthetic construction or function. Even small tori necessitate removal when they are irregular, extremely undercut, or in the area where a posterior palatal seal would be expected.

Bilateral greater palatine and incisive blocks and local infiltration provide the necessary anesthesia for tori removal. A linear incision in the midline of the torus with oblique vertical releasing incisions at one or both ends is generally necessary (Figure 13-14). Because the mucosa over this area is extremely thin, care must be taken in reflecting the tissue from the underlying bone, a particularly difficult task when the tori are multiloculated. When tori with a small pedunculated base are present, an osteotome and mallet may be used to remove the bony mass. For larger tori it is usually best to section the tori into multiple fragments with a bur in a rotary handpiece. Careful attention must be paid to the depth of the cuts, to avoid perforation of the floor of the nose. After sectioning, individual portions of the tori can be removed with a mallet and osteotome or a rongeur, and the area can be smoothed with a large bone bur. The entire bony projection does not necessarily require removal, but a smooth regular area without undercuts should be created, without extension into the area where a posterior palatal seal would be placed. Tissue is readapted by finger pressure and inspected to determine the amount of excess mucosa that may require removal. It is important to retain enough tissue to allow a tension-free closure over the entire area of exposed bone. The mucosa is reapproximated and sutured; an interrupted suture technique is often required, because the thin mucosa may not

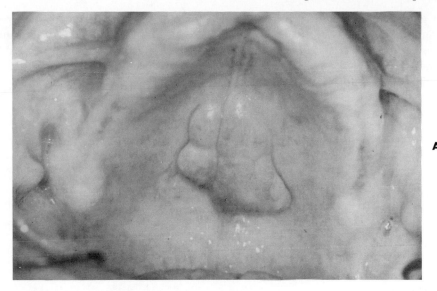

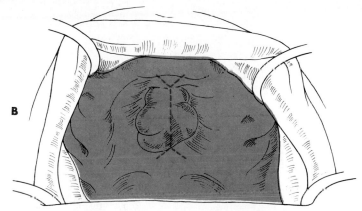

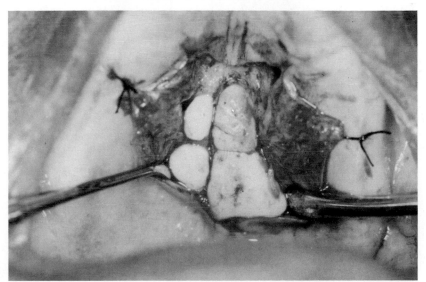

◇ Figure 13-14

Removal of palatal torus. **A,** Typical appearance of maxillary torus. **B,** Midline incision with anteroposterior oblique releasing incisions. **C,** Mucoperiosteal flaps retracted with silk sutures to improve access to all areas of torus.   *Continued*

retain sutures well. To prevent hematoma formation, some form of pressure dressing must be placed over the area of the palatal vault. Vaseline gauze formed into a pack and adapted to the palate can be sutured in place with 2-0 silk sutures tied to the lateral aspects of the palatal vault, which suspends the Vaseline pack in place under pressure against the palatal bone. A temporary denture or prefabricated splint relieved with a soft liner and placed in the center of the palate to prevent pressure necrosis can also be used to support the thin mucosa and prevent hematoma formation.

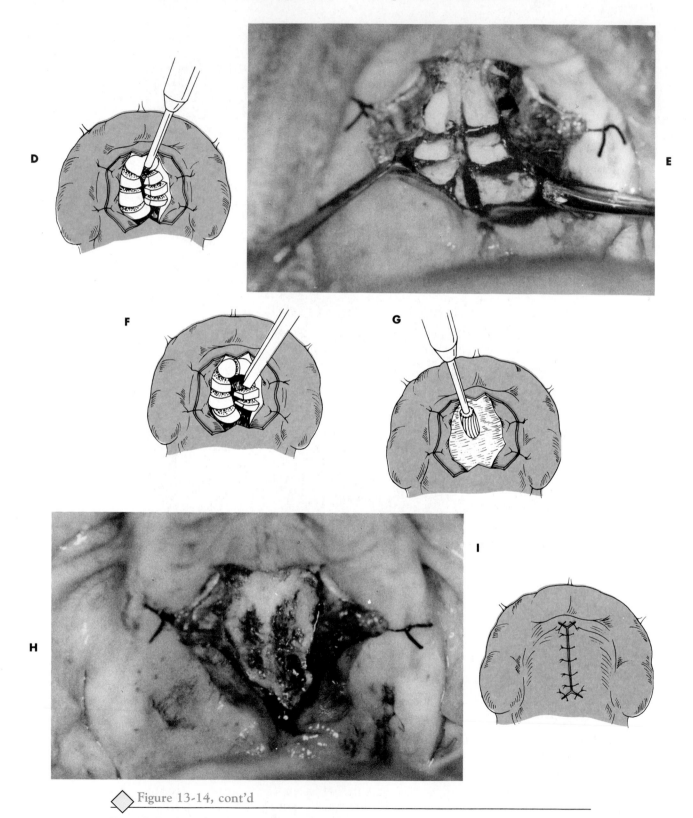

◇ Figure 13-14, cont'd

D and **E,** Sectioning of torus using fissure bur. **F,** Small osteotome used to remove sections of torus. **G** and **H,** Large bone bur used to produce the final desired contour. **I,** Soft tissue closure.

The major complications of maxillary tori removal include postoperative hematoma formation, fracture or perforation of the floor of the nose, and necrosis of the flap. Local care, including vigorous irrigation and good hygiene, and support with soft tissue conditioners in the splint or denture usually provide adequate treatment.

MANDIBULAR TORI

Mandibular tori are bony protuberances on the lingual aspect of the mandible that usually occur in the premolar area. The origins of this bony exostosis are uncertain, and the lesions may slowly increase in size. Occasionally, extremely large tori interfere with normal speech or tongue function during eating, but these tori rarely require removal when teeth are present. After the removal of lower teeth and before the construction of partial or complete dentures, it may be necessary to remove mandibular tori to facilitate denture construction.

Bilateral lingual and inferior alveolar injections provide adequate anesthesia for tori removal. A crest of the ridge incision should be made, extending 1 to 1.5 cm beyond each end of the tori to be reduced. When bilateral tori are to be removed simultaneously, it is best to leave a small band of tissue attached at the midline between the anterior extent of the two incisions. Leaving this tissue attached helps eliminate potential hematoma formation in the anterior floor of the mouth and will maintain as much of the lingual vestibule as possible in the anterior mandibular area. As with maxillary tori, the mucosa over the lingual tori is generally very thin and should be reflected carefully to expose the entire area of bone to be recontoured (Figure 13-15). When the torus has a small pedunculated base, a mallet and osteotome may be used to cleave the tori from the medial aspect of the mandible. The line of cleavage can be directed by creating a small trough with a bur and a handpiece before using an osteotome. It is extremely important to ensure that the direction of the initial bur trough (or the osteotome if it is used alone) is parallel with the medial aspect of the mandible to avoid an unfavorable fracture of the lingual or inferior cortex. The bur can also be

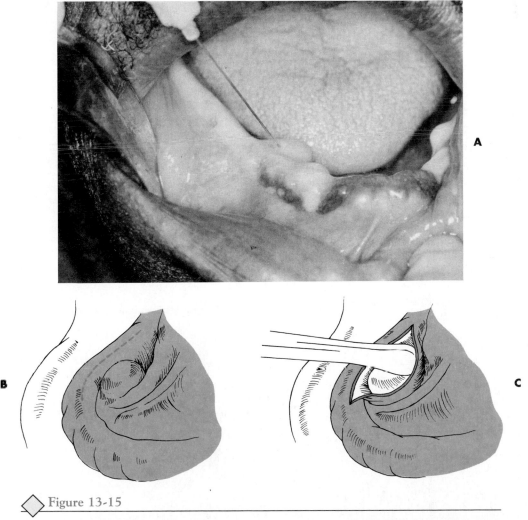

Figure 13-15

Removal of mandibular tori. **A,** After block local anesthetic is administered, ballooning of thin mucoperiosteum over area of tori can be accomplished by placing bevel of local anesthetic needle against torus and injecting local anesthetic subperiosteally. (This greatly facilitates reflection of mucoperiosteal flap.) **B,** Outline of crestal incision. **C,** Exposure of torus. *Continued*

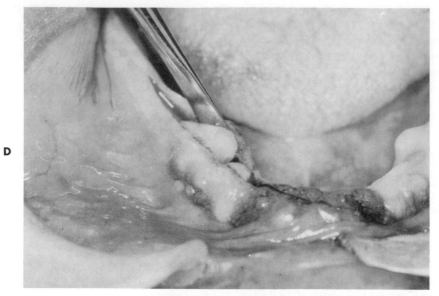

D

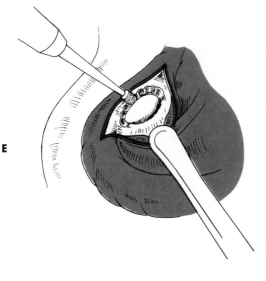

E

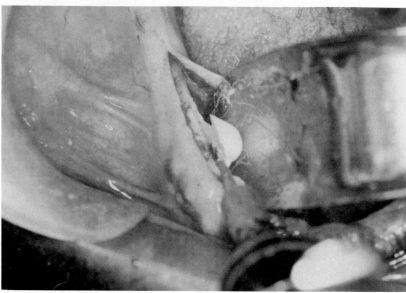

F

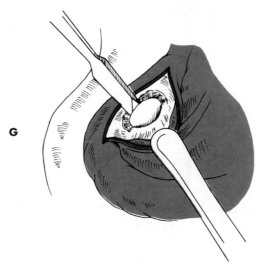

G

◇ **Figure 13-15, cont'd**

D, Exposure of torus. **E** and **F,** Fissure bur and handpiece used to create small trough between mandibular ridge and torus. **G,** Use of small osteotome to complete removal of torus from the mandible.

Continued

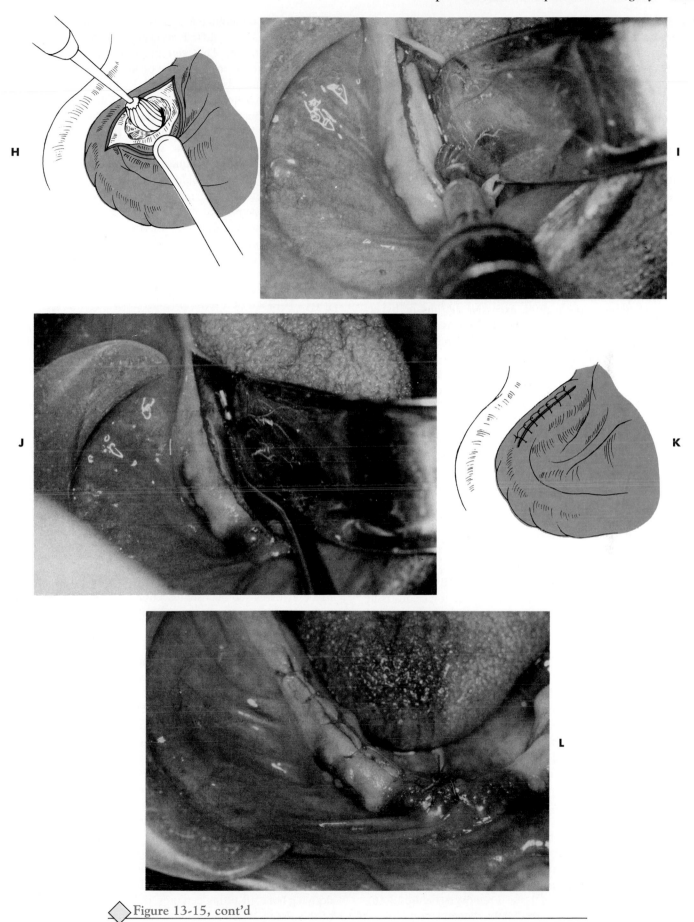

◆ Figure 13-15, cont'd

H to **J,** Use of bone bur and bone file to eliminate minor irregularities. **K** and **L,** Tissue closure.

used to deepen the trough so that a small instrument can be levered against the mandible to fracture the lingual tori to allow its removal. A bone bur or file can then be used to smooth the lingual cortex. The tissue should be readapted and palpated to evaluate contour and elimination of undercuts. An interrupted or continuous suture technique is used to close the incisions. Gauze packs placed in the floor of the mouth and retained for 12 hours are generally helpful in reducing postoperative edema and hematoma formation. In the event of wound dehiscence or exposed bone in the area of a mucosal perforation, treatment with local care, including frequent vigorous saline irrigation, is usually sufficient.

Soft Tissue Abnormalities

Abnormalities of the soft tissue in the denture-bearing and peripheral tissue areas include excessive fibrous or hyper-mobile tissue; inflammatory lesions, such as inflammatory fibrous hyperplasia of the vestibule and inflammatory papillary hyperplasia of the palate; and abnormal muscular and frenal attachments. With the exception of pathologic and inflammatory lesions, many of the other conditions do not present problems when the patient has a full dentition. However, when loss of teeth necessitates prosthetic reconstruction, alteration of the soft tissue is often necessary. Immediately after tooth removal, muscular and frenal attachments initially do not present problems but may eventually interfere with proper denture construction as bony resorption takes place.

Long-term treatment planning before any soft tissue surgery is mandatory. Soft tissue that initially appears to be flabby and excessive may be quite useful if future ridge augmentation procedures are necessary. Oral mucosa is difficult to replace once it is removed. The only exception to this usefulness of excess tissue is when pathologic soft tissue lesions require removal.

Maxillary Tuberosity Reduction (Soft Tissue)

The primary objective of soft tissue maxillary tuberosity reduction is to provide adequate interarch space for proper denture construction in the posterior area and a firm mucosal base of consistent thickness over the alveolar ridge denture-bearing area. Maxillary tuberosity reduction may require the removal of soft tissue and bone to achieve the desired result. The amount of soft tissue available for reduction can often be determined by evaluating a presurgical panoramic radiograph. If a radiograph is not of the quality necessary to determine soft tissue thickness, this depth can be measured with a sharp probe after local anesthesia is obtained at the time of surgery.

Local anesthetic infiltration in the posterior maxillary area is sufficient for a tuberosity reduction. An initial elliptic incision is made over the tuberosity in the area requiring reduction, and this section of tissue is removed (Figure 13-16).

After tissue removal, the medial and lateral margins of the excision must be thinned to remove excess soft tissue, which allows further soft tissue reduction and provides a tension-free soft tissue closure. This can be accomplished by digital pressure on the mucosal surface of the adjacent tissue while sharply excising tissue tangential to the mucosal surface (Figure 13-17). After the flaps are thinned, digital pressure can be used to approximate the tissue to evaluate the vertical reduction that has been accomplished. If adequate tissue has been removed, the area is sutured with interrupted or continuous suturing techniques. If too much tissue has been removed, no attempt should be made to close the wound primarily. A tension-free approximation of the tissue to bone should be accomplished, which allows the open wound area to heal by secondary intention. Sutures are removed in 5 to 7 days, and impressions can generally be taken 3 to 4 weeks postoperatively.

Mandibular Retromolar Pad Reduction

The need for removal of mandibular retromolar hypertrophic tissue is rare. Local anesthetic infiltration in the area requiring excision is sufficient. An elliptic incision is made to excise the greatest area of tissue thickness in the posterior mandibular area. Slight thinning of the adjacent areas is carried out with the majority of the tissue reduction on the labial aspect. Excess removal of tissue in the submucosal area of the lingual flap may result in damage to the lingual nerve and artery. The tissue is approximated with continuous or interrupted sutures.

Lateral Palatal Soft Tissue Excess

Soft tissue excess on the lateral aspect of the palatal vault often interferes with proper construction of the denture. As with bony abnormalities of this area, soft tissue hypertrophy often narrows the palatal vault and creates slight undercuts, which interfere with denture construction and insertion.

One technique suggested for removal of lateral palatal soft tissue involves submucosal resection of the excess tissue in a manner similar to the previously described soft tissue tuberosity reduction. However, the amount and extension of soft tissue removal under the mucosa is much more extensive and creates the risk of damage to the greater palatine vessels, with possible sloughing of the lateral palatal soft tissue area.

The preferred technique requires superficial excision of the soft tissue excess. Local anesthetic infiltrated in the greater palatine area and anterior to the soft tissue mass is sufficient. With a sharp scalpel blade in the tangential fashion, the superficial layers of mucosa and underlying fibrous tissue can be removed to the extent necessary to eliminate undercuts in soft tissue bulk (Figure 13-18). Following removal of this tissue, a surgical splint lined with a tissue conditioner can be inserted for 5 to 7 days to aid in healing.

Unsupported Hypermobile Tissue

Excessive hypermobile tissue without inflammation on the alveolar ridge is generally the result of resorption of the underlying bone, ill-fitting dentures, or both. Before the excision of this tissue, a determination must be made of whether the

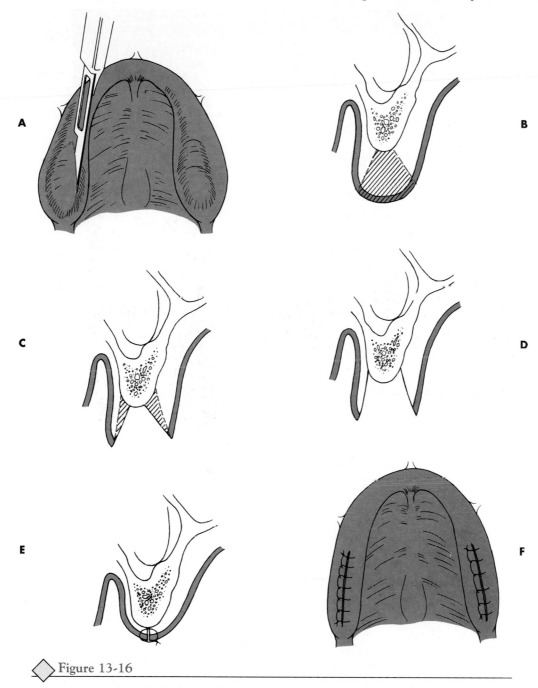

⬥ Figure 13-16

Maxillary soft tissue tuberosity reduction. **A,** Elliptic incision around soft tissue to be excised in tuberosity area. **B,** Soft tissue area excised with initial incision. **C,** Undermining of buccal and palatal flaps to provide adequate soft tissue contour and tension-free closure. **D,** View of final tissue removal. **E** and **F,** Soft tissue closure.

underlying bone should be augmented with a graft. If a bony deficiency is the primary cause of soft tissue excess, then augmentation of the underlying bone is the treatment of choice. Augmentation is discussed in detail in Chapter 14. If adequate alveolar height remains after reduction of the hypermobile soft tissue, then excision may be indicated.

A local anesthetic is injected adjacent to the area requiring tissue excision. Removal of hypermobile tissue in the alveolar ridge area consists of two parallel full-thickness incisions on the buccal and lingual aspects of the tissue to be excised (Figure 13-19). A periosteal elevator is used to remove the excess soft tissue from the underlying bone. A tangential excision of small amounts of tissue in the adjacent areas may be necessary to allow for adequate soft tissue adaptation during closure. These additional excisions should be kept to a minimum whenever possible to avoid removing too much soft tissue and to prevent detachment of periosteum from underlying bone. Continuous or interrupted sutures are used to

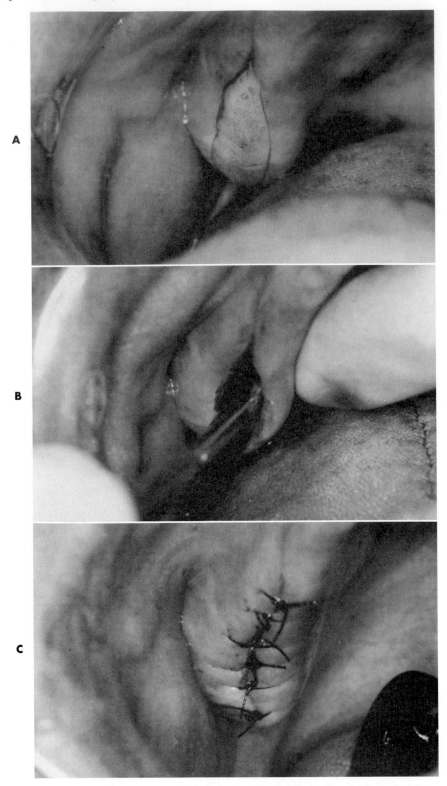

◇ Figure 13-17

Maxillary soft tissue tuberosity reduction. **A,** Elliptic incision. **B,** Thinning of mucosal flaps by removal of underlying soft tissue. Digital pressure used to stabilize the tissue flaps during submucosal excision. **C,** Tension-free readaptation of flaps.

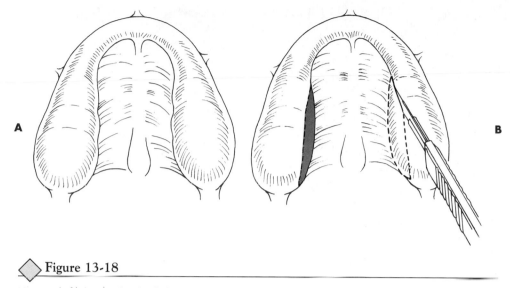

◆ **Figure 13-18**

Removal of lateral palatal soft tissue. **A,** View of excessive palatal tissue creating narrow palatal vault and undercut areas. **B,** Tangential excision of excess soft tissue.

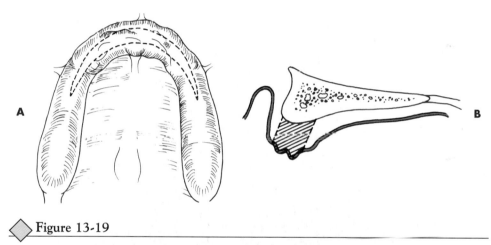

◆ **Figure 13-19**

Removal of hypermobile unsupported tissue. **A,** Outline of incisions for removal of crestal area of hypermobile tissue. **B,** Cross-sectional area demonstrating amount of tissue to be excised. (This type of tissue excision should be considered only if adequate ridge height will remain after removal of tissue. If excision of this tissue will result in inadequate ridge height and obliteration of vestibular depth, some type of augmentation procedure should be considered.)

approximate the remaining tissue and are removed 7 days after surgery. Denture impressions can usually be taken 3 to 4 weeks after surgery. One possible complication of this type of procedure is the obliteration of the buccal vestibule as a result of tissue undermining necessary to obtain tissue closure.

Hypermobile tissue in the crestal area of the mandibular alveolar ridge frequently consists of a small cordlike band of tissue. If no underlying sharp bony projection is present, this tissue can best be removed by a supraperiosteal soft tissue excision. Local anesthetic is injected adjacent to the area requiring tissue removal. The cordlike band of fibrous connective tissue can be elevated by using pickups and scissors, and the scissors can be used to excise the fibrous

tissue at the attachment to the alveolar ridge (Figure 13-20). No suturing is generally necessary for this technique, and a denture with a soft liner can be reinserted immediately.

INFLAMMATORY FIBROUS HYPERPLASIA

Inflammatory fibrous hyperplasia, also called *epulis fissuratum* or *denture fibrosis,* is a generalized hyperplastic enlargement of mucosa and fibrous tissue in the alveolar ridge and vestibular area, which most often results from ill-fitting dentures. In the early stages of fibrous hyperplasia, when fibrosis is minimal, nonsurgical treatment with a denture in combination with a soft liner is frequently sufficient for reduction or elimination of this tissue. When the condition has

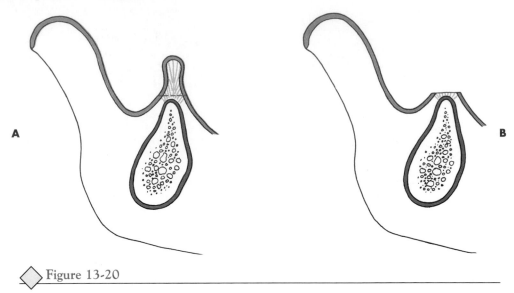

⬦ Figure 13-20

Supraperiosteal removal of hypermobile tissue on mandibular alveolar ridge. **A,** Hypermobile tissue on superior aspect of ridge. **B,** Pickups and scissors are used to excise the cordlike mobile fibrous tissue without perforating periosteum.

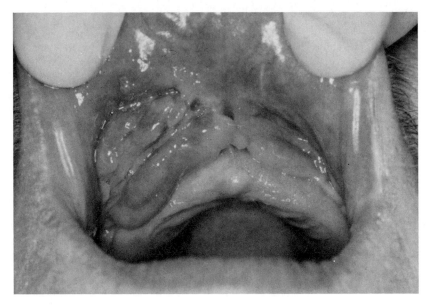

⬦ Figure 13-21

Inflammatory fibrous hyperplasia of labiovestibular area.

been present for some time, significant fibrosis exists within the hyperplastic tissue. This will not respond to nonsurgical treatment (Figure 13-21); excision of the hyperplastic tissue is the treatment of choice.

Three techniques can be used for successful treatment of inflammatory fibrous hyperplasia. Local anesthetic infiltration in the area of the redundant tissue is sufficient for anesthesia. When the area to be excised is minimally enlarged, electrosurgical techniques provide good results for tissue excision. If the tissue mass is extensive, large areas of excision using electrosurgical techniques may result in excessive

vestibular scarring. Simple excision and reapproximation of the remaining tissue is preferred. The redundant areas of tissue are grasped with tissue pickups, a sharp incision is made at the base of the excessive fibrous tissue down to the periosteum, and the hyperplastic tissue is removed (Figure 13-22). The adjacent tissue is gently undermined and reapproximated using interrupted or continuous sutures.

When there are areas of gross tissue redundancy, excision frequently results in total elimination of the vestibule. In such cases, excision of the epulae, with peripheral mucosal repositioning and secondary epithelialization is preferable

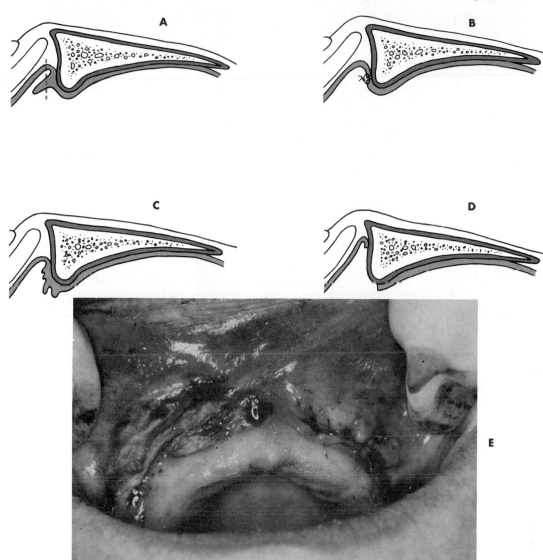

◇ Figure 13-22

A, Small, well-localized area of fibrous hyperplasia. This area can be removed with simple excision. **B,** Closure of wound margins. **C,** Large area of inflammatory fibrous hyperplasia. Removal and primary closure would result in elimination of labial vestibule. **D,** After supraperiosteal removal of excess tissue, mucosal edge is sutured to periosteum at depth of vestibule. **E,** Postoperative view of Figure 13-21. The smaller well-localized area on patient's left has been removed and closed primarily. The larger area of excessive tissue on right has been removed and wound margin sutured to periosteum at depth of vestibule, which leaves exposed periosteum.

(see Figure 13-22). In this procedure the hyperplastic soft tissue is excised superficial to the periosteum from the alveolar ridge area. A clean supraperiosteal bed is created over the alveolar ridge area, and the unaffected margin of the tissue excision is sutured to the most superior aspect of the vestibular periosteum with an interrupted suture technique. A surgical splint or denture lined with soft tissue conditioner is inserted and worn continuously for the first 5 to 7 days, with removal only for oral saline rinses. Secondary epithelialization usually takes place, and denture impressions can be made within 4 weeks.

The hyperplastic tissue usually represents only the result of an inflammatory process; however, other pathologic conditions may exist. It is therefore imperative that representative tissue samples *always* be submitted for pathologic examination after removal.

INFLAMMATORY PAPILLARY HYPERPLASIA OF THE PALATE

Inflammatory papillary hyperplastic tissue formation in the palate is frequently a result of mechanical irritation and is seen most often in patients who wear prosthetic appliances. Other

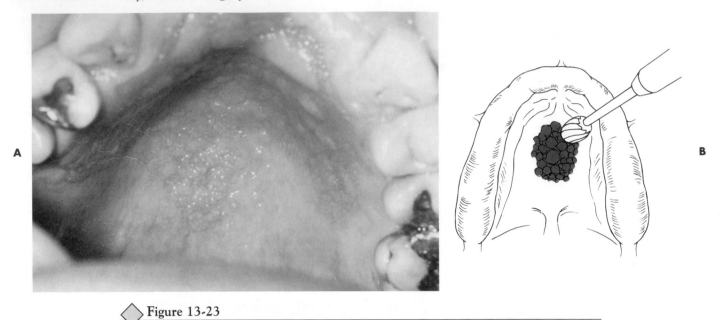

Figure 13-23

Inflammatory papillary hyperplasia of palate. **A,** Clinical appearance. **B,** Diagram of removal of papillary hyperplasia of palate using bur for abrasion of mucosa.

potential contributing factors to this process include poor hygiene, fungal infections, and the associated inflammation. This condition usually appears as multiple nodular projections in the palatal tissue. Although it was once thought to represent a precancerous condition, this has not been substantiated.[1] Because the process appears to be primarily inflammatory rather than neoplastic, total full-thickness incision is not necessary. In fact, in the very early stages, nonsurgical treatment, such as proper denture adjustment combined with a tissue conditioner, may eliminate or reduce this problem.

If removal is required, a mucosal excision superficial to the periosteum is recommended and can generally be performed with local anesthetic infiltration in the palatal area. Regardless of the technique used for removal of this tissue, a specimen should be obtained and submitted for histopathologic examination. Guernsey[4] described a technique using electrosurgical loops for excision of the palatal mucosa. When electrosurgical techniques are used, it is important to maintain a split-thickness excision, so that palatal bone is not cauterized. An alternative technique that eliminates this possibility is split-thickness excision done sharply with a scalpel.[8] However, palatal form and access to the area of excision may limit the use of this scalpel technique in certain situations. Techniques to abrade the superficial layer of palatal mucosa are also effective for treatment. A coarsely fluted acrylic or bone bur or dermabrasion brush in a rotating handpiece can be used for this purpose (Figure 13-23). Other techniques that can be considered for superficial tissue removal include cryosurgery and the use of lasers. Following tissue incision, insertion of a splint or denture containing soft tissue liner provides improved patient comfort during the healing period. Second-

ary epithelialization usually takes place in approximately 4 weeks.

LABIAL FRENECTOMY

Labial frenal attachments consist of thin bands of fibrous tissue covered with mucosa, extending from the lip and cheek to the alveolar periosteum. The level of frenal attachments may vary from the height of the vestibule to the crest of the alveolar ridge and even to the incisal papilla area in the anterior maxilla. With the exception of the midline labial frenum in association with a diastema, frenal attachments generally do not present problems when the dentition is intact. However, the construction of a denture may be complicated when it is necessary to accommodate a frenal attachment. Movement of the soft tissue adjacent to the frenum may create discomfort and ulceration and may interfere with the peripheral seal and dislodge the denture.

Three surgical techniques are effective in removal of frenal attachments. The simple excision and the Z-plasty techniques are effective when the mucosal and fibrous tissue band is relatively narrow. A localized vestibuloplasty with secondary epithelialization is often preferred when the frenal attachment has a wide base.

Local anesthetic infiltration is sufficient for surgical treatment of frenal attachments. Care must be taken to avoid excessive anesthetic infiltration directly in the frenum area, because it may obscure the anatomy that must be visualized at the time of excision. In all cases it is helpful to have the surgical assistant elevate and evert the lip during this procedure. For the simple excision technique a narrow elliptic incision around the frenal area down to the periosteum is completed (Figure 13-24). The fibrous frenum is then sharply dissected from the underlying periosteum and soft tissue, and the margins of the wound are gently undermined and reapproximated. Placement of the first suture should be at the maximal depth of the vestibule and should include both edges of mucosa and underlying periosteum at the height of the vestibule beneath the anterior nasal spine (see Figure 13-24). This will reduce hematoma formation and allow for adaptation of the tissue to the maximal height of the vestibule. The remainder of the incision should then be closed with interrupted sutures. Occasionally, it is not possible to approximate the portion of the excision closest to the alveolar ridge crest; this will undergo secondary epithelialization without difficulty.

In the Z-plasty technique an excision of the fibrous connective tissue is done, similar to that in the simple excision procedure just described. After excision of the fibrous tissue, two oblique incisions are made in a Z fashion, one at each end of the previous area of excision (Figure 13-25). The two pointed flaps are then gently undermined and rotated to close the initial vertical incision horizontally. The two small oblique extensions also require closure. This technique may decrease the amount of vestibular ablation sometimes seen after linear excision of a frenum.

A third technique for removal of the frenum involves a localized vestibuloplasty with secondary epithelialization. This procedure is especially advantageous when the base of the frenal attachment is extremely wide, as in many mandibular anterior frenal attachments. Local anesthetic is infiltrated primarily in the supraperiosteal areas along the margins of the frenal attachments. An incision is made through mucosal tissue and underlying submucosal tissue, without perforating the periosteum. A supraperiosteal dissection is completed by undermining the mucosal and submucosal tissue with scissors or by digital pressure on a sponge placed against the periosteum. After a clean periosteal layer is identified, the edge of the mucosal flap is sutured to the periosteum at the maximal depth of the vestibule, and the exposed periosteum is allowed to heal by secondary epithelialization (Figure 13-26). A surgical splint or denture containing soft tissue liner is often useful in the initial healing period. This technique is also useful in localized broad-based muscle attachments, such as those frequently seen in the lateral maxillary areas.

LINGUAL FRENECTOMY

An abnormal lingual frenal attachment usually consists of mucosa, dense fibrous connective tissue, and, occasionally, superior fibers of the genioglossus muscle. This attachment binds the tip of the tongue to the posterior surface of the mandibular alveolar ridge. Even when no prosthesis is required, such attachments can affect speech. After loss of teeth, this frenal attachment interferes with denture stability, because each time the tongue is moved, the frenal attachment is tensed, and the denture is dislodged.

Bilateral lingual blocks and local infiltration in the anterior area provide adequate anesthesia for a lingual frenectomy. The tip of the tongue is best controlled with a traction suture. Surgical release of the lingual frenum requires incising the attachment of the fibrous connective tissue at the base of the tongue in a transverse fashion, followed by closure in a linear direction, which completely releases the anterior portion of the tongue (Figure 13-27). A hemostat can be placed across the frenal attachment at the base of the tongue for approximately 3 minutes, which provides vasoconstriction and a nearly bloodless field during the surgical procedure. After removal of the hemostat, an incision is created through the area previously closed in the hemostat. Careful attention must be given to blood vessels at the inferior aspect of the tongue and floor of the mouth region and to the submandibular duct openings, which must be protected during the incision and suturing. The tongue is retracted superiorly, and the margins of the wound are carefully undermined and closed parallel to the midline of the tongue. Occasionally, a lingual frenum release must also be accompanied by a small soft tissue-releasing procedure performed between the opening of the submandibular duct and the lingual aspect of the mandible. If access is available, this can be done in a fashion similar to the release above the submandibular ducts. However, if only a short tissue band exists in this area, a localized supraperiosteal dissection removing the fibrous attachment from the lingual aspect of the alveolar ridge is sufficient.

IMMEDIATE DENTURES ———◇

The decision may be made to insert dentures at the time of tooth removal and bony recontouring. Hartwell[5] cites several advantages of an immediate denture technique. The insertion of a denture after extraction offers immediate psychologic and esthetic benefits to patients, whereas alternatively they may be edentulous for some time. The immediate insertion of a denture after surgery also functions to splint the surgical site, which results in the reduction of postoperative bleeding and edema and improved tissue adaptation to the alveolar ridge. Another advantage is that the vertical dimension can be most easily reproduced with an immediate denture technique. Disadvantages include the need for frequent alteration of the denture postoperatively and the construction of a new denture after initial healing has taken place.

Surgical treatment for immediate denture insertion can be accomplished in stages, with extraction of the posterior dentition in the maxilla and the mandible done before anterior extraction. This allows for initial healing of the posterior areas and facilitates the denture construction. Following the initial healing period of the posterior segments, new records are taken, and models are mounted on a semiadjustable articulator. After replacement of the model teeth with prosthetic teeth, the cast of the alveolar ridge area is then carefully recontoured (Figure 13-28).

Immediate denture surgery generally involves the most conservative technique possible in removal of the remaining teeth. An intraseptal alveoloplasty, preserving as much vertical height and cortical bone as possible, is generally indicated. (Figure 13-29). After the bony recontouring and elimination of

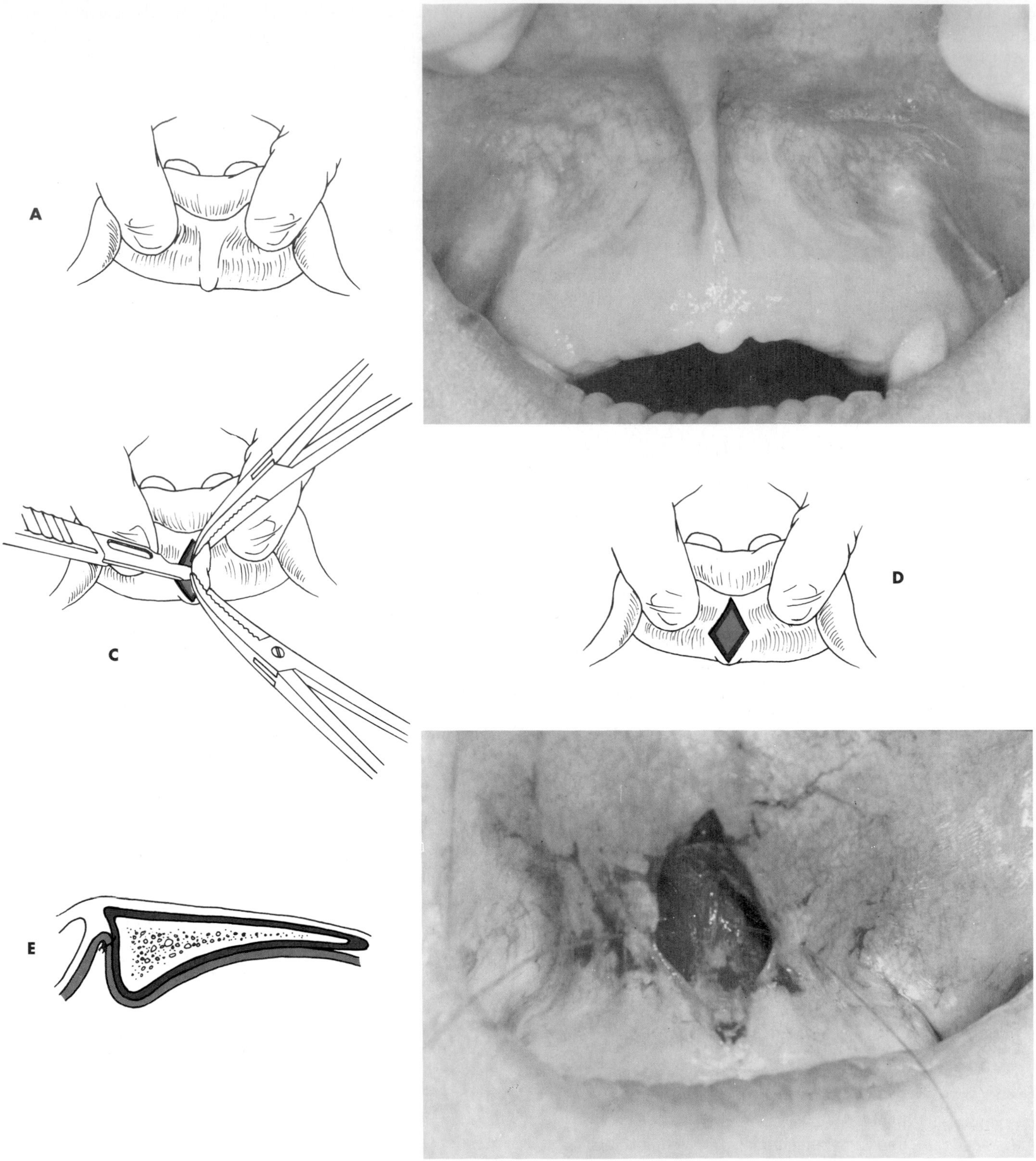

◇ Figure 13-24

Simple excision of maxillary labial frenum. **A** and **B,** Eversion and exposure of frenal attachment area. **C** and **D,** Excision along lateral margins of frenum. Tissue is removed, exposing underlying periosteum. **E** and **F,** Placement of suture through mucosal margins and periosteum, which closes mucosal margin and sutures mucosa to periosteum at depth of vestibule. *Continued*

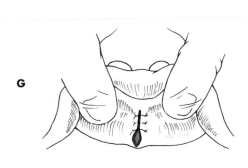

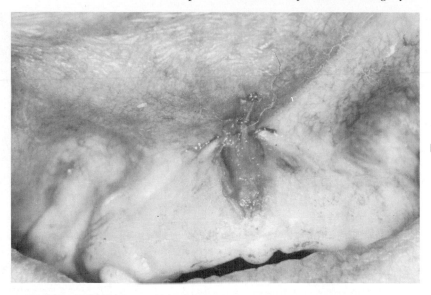

Figure 13-24, cont'd

G and **H,** Wound closure. Removal of tissue in areas adjacent to attached mucosa sometimes prevents complete primary closure at most inferior aspect of wound margin.

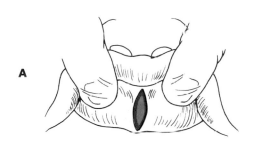

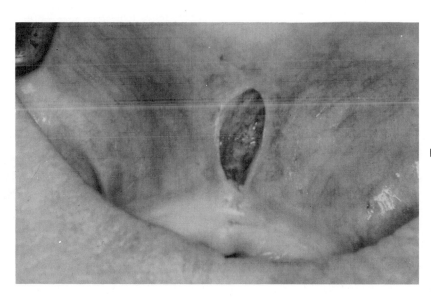

Figure 13-25

Z-plasty technique for elimination of labial frenum. **A** and **B,** Small elliptic excision of mucosa and underlying loose connective tissue.

Continued

gross irregularities is completed, the tissue is approximated with digital pressure, and the clear acrylic surgical guide constructed on the presurgical casts is inserted. Any areas of tissue blanching or gross irregularities are then reduced until the clear surgical guide is adapted to the alveolar ridge in all areas. Incisions are closed with continuous or interrupted sutures. The immediate denture with a soft liner is inserted, and the occlusal relationships are checked and adjusted as necessary. The patient is instructed to wear the denture continuously for 24 hours and to return the next day for a postoperative check. Bupivacaine or another similar long-acting local anesthetic injected at the conclusion of the surgical procedure greatly improves comfort in the first 24-hour postoperative period. At that time the denture is gently removed, and the underlying mucosa and alveolar ridge areas are inspected for any areas of excessive pressure. The denture is cleaned and reinserted, and the patient is instructed to wear the denture for 5 to 7 days and to remove it only for oral saline rinses. Sutures are generally taken out 7 days postoperatively.

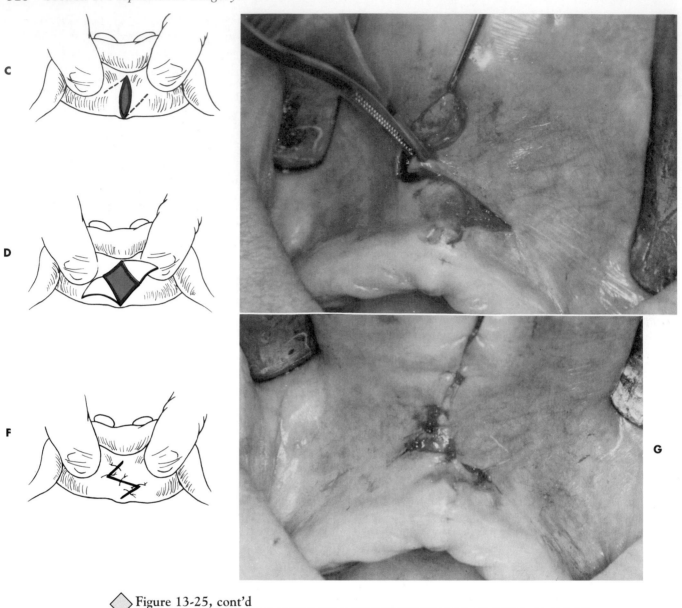

◇ Figure 13-25, cont'd

C to **E,** Flaps are undermined and rotated to desired position. **F** and **G,** Closure with interrupted sutures.

OVERDENTURE SURGERY ─◇

Alveolar bone is maintained primarily in response to stresses transferred to the bone through the teeth and periodontal ligament during mastication. By maintaining teeth wherever possible, resorption of bone under a prosthetic appliance may be minimized. An overdenture technique attempts to maintain teeth in the alveolus by transferring force directly to the bone and improving masticatory function with prosthetic restoration. The presence of teeth may also improve proprioception during function, and special retentive attachments can be incorporated into the retained teeth to improve denture retention and stability. Overdentures should be considered wherever teeth exist with adequate bone support and when good periodontal health can be maintained and the teeth can be properly restored. Because this technique also requires

endodontic and prosthetic treatment of retained teeth, financial considerations must also be taken into account.

A complete discussion of periodontal considerations is not within the scope of this chapter; however, it is extremely important to evaluate any potentially retained teeth before preparing the patient for an overdenture. Adequate clinical and radiographic evaluation of these teeth should be completed, including a clinical examination, evaluation of pocket depth around the teeth, and evaluation of the attached gingiva. Ideally, pocket depth around retained teeth should not exceed 3 mm. If excessive pocket depth is present but adequate bone support exists, every attempt should be made to retain the tooth. A gingivectomy to reduce pocket depth to the 3 mm range can be done at the time of overdenture insertion, provided that all infrabony pockets have been eliminated (Figure 13-30). Apically repositioned flaps may also be

Text continued on p. 322

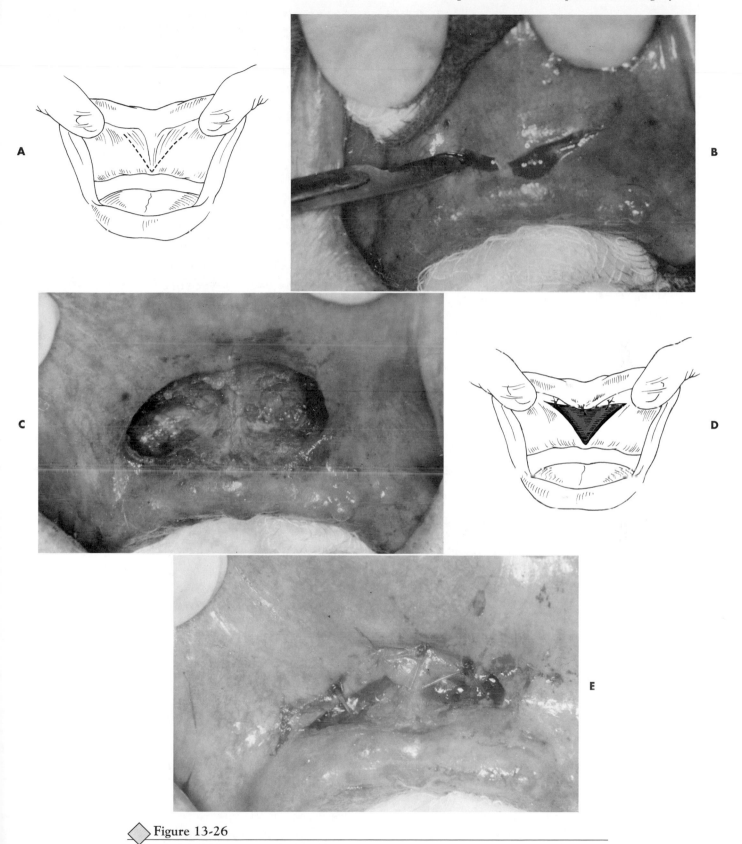

◇ Figure 13-26

Release of labial frenum with wide base. **A** and **B,** Wide V type of incision made at most inferior portion of frenal attachments in area of alveolar ridge. **C,** Supraperiosteal dissection completed, releasing mucosa and fibrous frenal attachments. **D** and **E,** Mucosal margins sutured to periosteum at depth of vestibule.

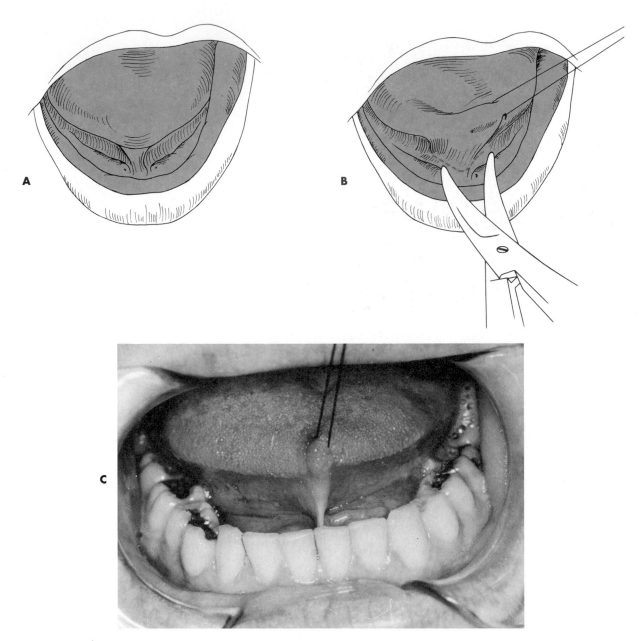

◇ Figure 13-27

Lingual frenum release. **A,** Frenal attachment connecting tip of tongue to lingual aspect of mandible. In edentulous patients, movement of tongue will dislodge denture. **B** and **C,** Retraction suture placed in tip of tongue. Horizontal incision made at superior portion of frenal attachment to inferior surface of tongue.

Continued

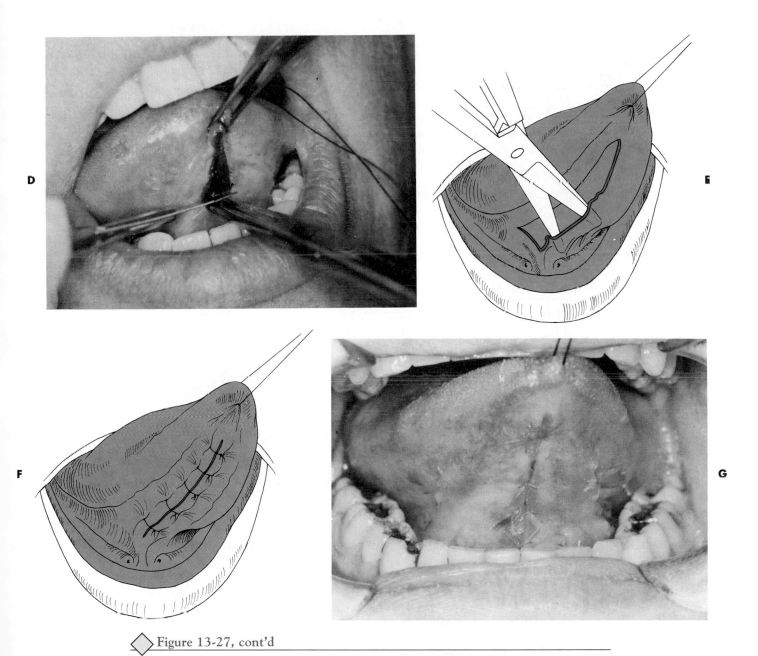

◈ Figure 13-27, cont'd

D, Improved hemostasis can be accomplished by placing hemostat across area to be incised, before severing frenal attachment. **E,** Lateral borders of wound margin are undermined. **F** and **G,** Soft tissue closure.

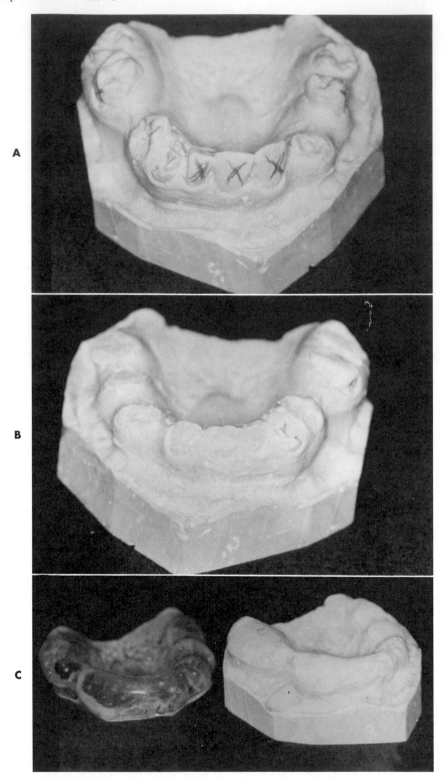

◇ **Figure 13-28**

Construction of clear acrylic surgical guide for immediate denture surgery. **A,** Presurgical cast. **B,** Cast after removal of teeth, before mock recontouring. **C,** Recontoured maxillary cast and surgical guide.

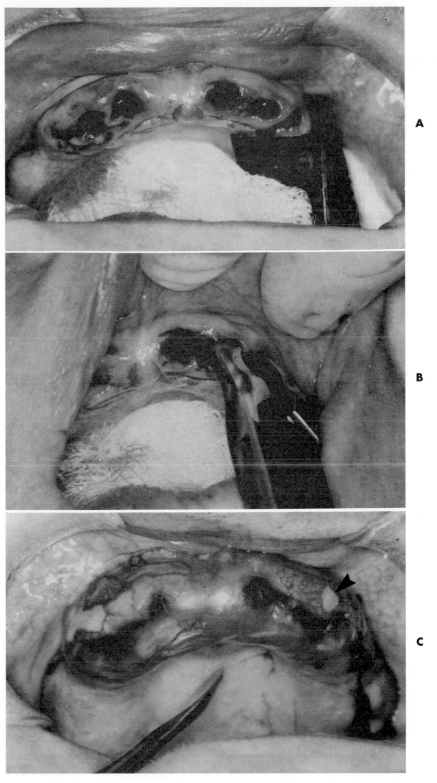

◇ Figure 13-29

A, Appearance of maxillary alveolar ridge after removal of teeth. **B,** Intraseptal removal of bone with rongeur. **C,** Clear acrylic surgical guide in place. Any areas that interfere with seating of template or cause blanching of tissue from excess bone or underlying soft tissue should be removed *(arrow).*

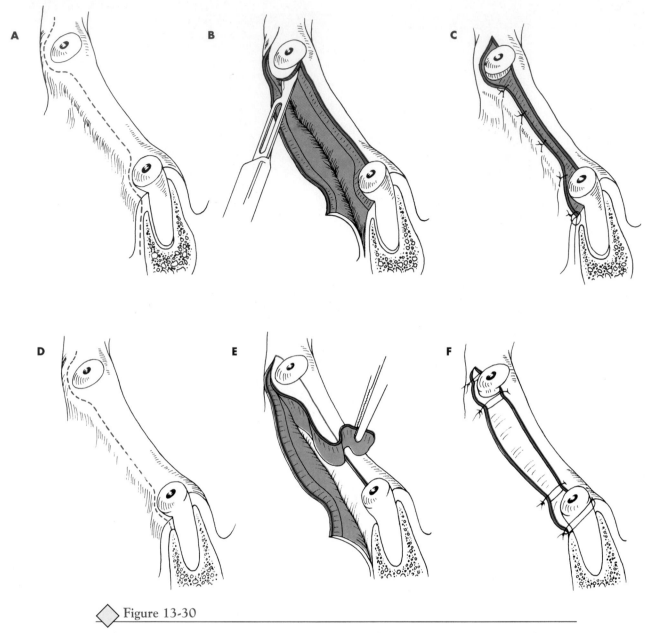

◇ Figure 13-30

A, Outline of incision for gingivectomy and split-thickness flap repositioning. **B,** Removal of gingival tissues. **C,** Repositioning of the split-thickness flap with suturing to periosteum. **D,** Incision for full-thickness flap. **E,** Removal of gingival tissue and bone recontouring. **F,** Repositioning of full-thickness flap.

considered for this purpose. A split-thickness flap is indicated when less than 3 mm of attached gingiva would be left if a gingivectomy were performed or when there is less than 3 mm of attached gingiva before surgery and when no bony recontouring is necessary at the time of surgery. A full-thickness, apically repositioned flap is indicated when very little attached gingival tissue is present and osseous defects require recontouring at the time of surgery (see Figure 13-30). If 3 to 4 mm of attached gingiva is not adjacent to retained teeth, a grafting technique, such as a split-thickness free graft

from the palate to the area deficient of attached gingiva, may be indicated.

SUMMARY

The success of preprosthetic surgical preparation depends on careful evaluation and treatment planning. In general, bony abnormalities should be managed first. Associated soft tissue correction can be delayed if possible; simultaneous bony augmentation is attempted when only bony contouring is required. Final prosthesis design and goals of long-term function, esthetic quality, and tissue maintenance must be considered during all phases of treatment.

REFERENCES

1. Bhaskar SN: *Synopsis of oral pathology,* ed 7, St Louis, 1986, Mosby.
2. Crandell CE, Trueblood SN: Roentgenographic findings in edentulous areas, *Oral Surg* 13:1343, 1960.
3. Dean OT: Surgery for the denture patient, *J Am Dent Assoc* 23:2124, 1936.
4. Guernsey LH: Reactive inflammatory papillary hyperplasia of the palate, *Oral Surg* 20:814, 1965.
5. Hartwell CM Jr: *Syllabus of complete dentures,* Philadelphia, 1968, Lea & Febiger.
6. Kalas S et al: The occurrence of torus palatinus and torus mandibularis in 2478 dental patients, *Oral Surg* 6:1134, 1953.
7. Michael CG, Barsoum WM: Comparing ridge resorption with various surgical techniques on immediate dentures, *J Prosthet Dent* 35:142, 1976.
8. Starshak TJ: Corrective soft tissue surgery. In Starshak TJ, Sanders B, editors: *Preprosthetic oral and maxillofacial surgery,* St Louis, 1980, Mosby.
9. Starshak TJ: Oral anatomy and physiology. In Starshak TJ, Sanders B, editors: *Preprosthetic oral and maxillofacial surgery,* St Louis, 1980, Mosby.
10. Weintraub JA, Burt BA: Oral health status in the United States: tooth loss and edentulism, *J Dent Educ* 49:368, 1985.

CHAPTER 14

ADVANCED PREPROSTHETIC SURGERY

MYRON R. TUCKER

After the loss of natural teeth, bony changes in the jaws begin to take place immediately. Because the alveolar bone no longer responds to stresses placed in this area by the teeth and periodontal ligament, bone begins to resorb. The specific pattern of resorption is unpredictable in a given patient because there is great variation among individuals. In many patients this resorption process tends to stabilize after a period, whereas in others a continuation of the process eventually results in total loss of alveolar bone and underlying basal bone (Figure 14-1). The results of this resorption are accelerated by wearing dentures and tend to affect the mandible more severely than the maxilla because of the decreased surface area and less favorable distribution of occlusal forces.[31]

FACTORS AFFECTING BONE RESORPTION

General systemic and local factors are responsible for the variation in the amount and pattern of alveolar bone resorption.[4] General factors include the presence of nutritional abnormalities and systemic bone disease, such as osteoporosis, endocrine dysfunction, or any other systemic condition that may affect bone metabolism. Local factors affecting alveolar ridge resorption include alveoloplasty techniques used at the time of tooth removal and localized trauma associated with loss of alveolar bone. Denture wearing also may contribute to alveolar ridge resorption because of improper ridge adaptation of the denture or inadequate distribution of occlusal forces. Variations in facial structure may contribute to resorption patterns in two ways. First, the

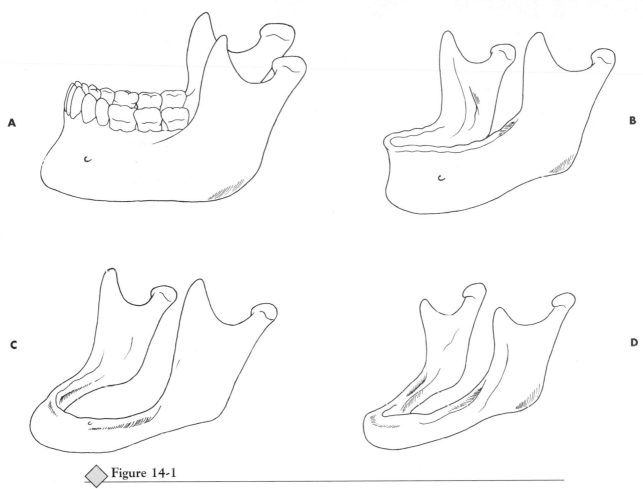

◇ **Figure 14-1**

Diagrammatic representation of progression of bone resorption in mandible after tooth extraction.

actual volume of bone present in the alveolar ridges varies with facial form.[25] Second, individuals with low mandibular plane angles and more acute gonial angles are capable of generating higher bite force, thereby placing greater pressure on the alveolar ridge areas. The long-term result of combined general and local factors is the loss of the bony alveolar ridge, increased interarch space, increased influence of surrounding soft tissue, decreased stability and retention of the prosthesis, and increased discomfort from improper prosthesis adaptation. In the most severe cases of resorption a significant increase in the risk of spontaneous mandibular fracture exists.

Goals of Advanced Preprosthetic Surgery ──◇

When severe resorption of the alveolar ridges has taken place, basic preprosthetic surgical techniques may not be adequate to modify the denture-bearing area enough to allow construction of a proper prosthesis for the patient. More complicated surgical and prosthetic procedures may be necessary to satisfy the functional, esthetic, and comfort requirements of the patient.

The principal objectives of treatment of severely atrophic alveolar ridges should include the following[7]:

1. Creation of a broad ridge form
2. Adequate fixed tissue over the denture-bearing area
3. Adequate vestibular depth for prosthesis extension
4. Proper interarch relationships
5. Added strength where mandibular fracture may occur
6. Protection of the neurovascular bundle
7. Adequate palatal vault form
8. Proper posterior tuberosity notching
9. Adequate bony support and attached soft tissue covering to facilitate implant placement when necessary

Patient Evaluation ────◇

Before considering preprosthetic surgery, a detailed history and physical examination should be completed. As stated in Chapter 13, a thorough discussion of the patient's goals and expectations for treatment should be included in this evaluation. A thorough assessment of overall general health is especially important when considering more advanced preprosthetic surgical techniques, because many of the approaches described require general anesthesia, donor-site

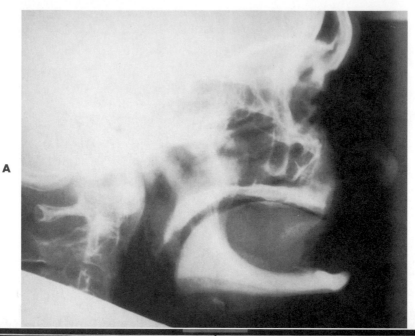

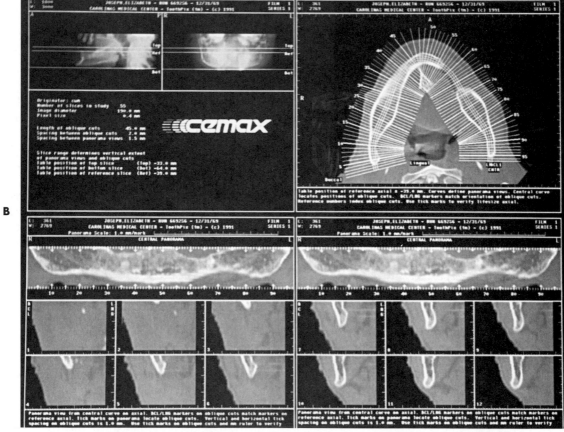

◇ Figure 14-2

A, Cephalometric radiograph. The cross-sectional anatomy of the anterior mandible can be seen easily. (Note: In this radiograph the patient is overclosed, giving the relative appearance of a class III jaw relationship.) **B,** Computerized tomography showing detailed cross-sectional anatomy of mandible.

surgery to harvest autogenous graft material, and multiple surgical procedures. Specific attention should also be given to possible systemic diseases that may be responsible for the severe degree of bone resorption. Laboratory tests, such as serum levels of calcium, phosphate, parathyroid hormone, and alkaline phosphatase, may be useful in pinpointing potential metabolic problems that may affect bone resorption.[4]

BONE EVALUATION

A clinical examination must include evaluation of the height, width, and contour of the available alveolar ridge and underlying basal bone. In the mandible it is necessary to palpate the posterior ridge area to identify concavities and to locate the mental neurovascular bundle. In the maxilla the palatal vault, ridge form, anterior nasal spine, zygomatic buttress, and posterior tuberosity notching should be assessed. Interarch relationships should be evaluated in the antero-posterior, transverse, and vertical planes of space. In partially edentulous patients the presence of hypererupted or malpositioned teeth or segments should also be noted.

Radiographs should be obtained to evaluate the bony configuration of the maxilla and mandible. A panoramic film is the most useful for a general overview of bony structures in both the maxilla and mandible.

Cephalometric radiographs may also be helpful in evaluating the cross-sectional configuration of the anterior mandibular ridge area and ridge relationships (Figure 14-2, *A*). To evaluate the ridge relationship in the vertical and antero-posterior dimensions it will be necessary to obtain the cephalometric radiograph in the appropriate vertical dimension. This may require adjusting or reconstructing dentures to this position or making properly adjusted bite rims to be used for positioning at the time the radiograph is taken.

More sophisticated radiographic studies, such as tomography or computerized tomography (CT scans), may provide further information. CT scans are particularly helpful in evaluating the cross-sectional anatomy of the maxilla, including ridge form and sinus anatomy (Figure 14-2, *B*). The cross-sectional anatomy of the mandible can be more precisely evaluated by including the location of the inferior alveolar nerve.

SOFT TISSUE EVALUATION

Results of a soft tissue evaluation are important in planning for preprosthetic surgery. A biopsy should be performed on any suspicious pathologic lesions, and they should be treated appropriately. The denture-bearing area should be evaluated to determine the amount and quality of attached mucosa in the alveolar ridge area. This may be especially important in providing fixed, keratinized tissue around areas of implant placement. The buccal and lingual vestibular areas should be examined for mucosal and muscular attachments that may affect the stability of the denture. With the patient's tongue in several positions the lingual aspect of the mandible must be examined to evaluate the area of attachment of the mylohyoid and genioglossus muscles in relation to the alveolar ridge.

TREATMENT PLANNING

When severe bony atrophy exists, treatment must be directed at correction of the bony deficiency and alteration of the associated soft tissue. When adequate bony tissue remains despite alveolar atrophy, improvement of the denture-bearing area may be accomplished either by directly treating the bony deficiency or by compensating for it with soft tissue surgery. A classification of alveolar ridges and possible treatment based on clinical and radiographic findings has been proposed (Table 14-1).[22] The most appropriate treatment plan should also consider several other factors. In an older patient in whom moderate bony resorption has taken place, soft tissue surgery alone may be sufficient for improved prosthesis function. In an extremely young patient who has undergone the same degree of atrophy, bony augmentation procedures may be indicated. The role of implants may alter the need for surgical modification of bone or soft tissue. The patient's health status must be carefully evaluated, because the surgery may require hospitalization, general anesthesia, donor-site surgery, and more than one oral surgical procedure. The patient's ability and willingness to undergo these surgical procedures, including possible long periods without dentures during healing phases, should be considered.

A definite decision on the need for bony augmentation must be made before considering soft tissue surgery. If bony or

◇ Table 14-1. Classification of alveolar ridges and treatment protocol (if considering HA augmentation)

Class	Characteristics	Treatment
I	Alveolar ridge adequate in height but inadequate in width, lateral deficiency or undercut areas	Hydroxyapatite (HA) alone
II	Alveolar ridge deficient in both height and width and has a knife-edge appearance	HA alone
III	Alveolar ridge resorbed to level of the basilar bone, producing concave form on posterior areas of the mandible and sharp, bony ridge form with bulbous, mobile soft tissue in the maxilla	HA alone or mixed with autogenous cancellous iliac bone
IV	Resorption of the basilar bone, producing pencil-thin, flat mandible or flat maxilla	HA mixed with autogenous cancellous iliac bone

Modified from Kent JN et al: Alveolar ridge augmentation using nonresorbable hydroxylapatite with or without autogenous cancellous bone, *J Oral Maxillofac Surg* 41:629, 1983.

alloplastic augmentation is indicated, maximal augmentation frequently depends on availability of adjacent soft tissue to provide tension-free coverage of the graft. Soft tissue surgery should be delayed until hard tissue grafting and appropriate healing have occurred.

Mandibular Augmentation

Augmentation grafting adds strength to an extremely deficient mandible and improves the height and contour of the available bone for implant placement on denture-bearing areas. Sources of graft material include autogenous or allogeneic bone and alloplastic materials. Historically, autogenous bone has been the most biologically acceptable material used in mandibular augmentation. Disadvantages of the use of autogenous bone include the need for donor-site surgery and extensive resorption after grafting. The use of allogeneic bone eliminates the need for a second surgical site. However, when used for large augmentations, this material often results in dehiscence of the graft and resorption similar to that of autogenous bone. During the past 15 years, hydroxyapatite (HA) alloplastic materials have become popular for use in bony augmentation of the maxilla and mandible. The material is readily available, eliminates the need for donor-site surgery, and is shown by clinical experience to provide effective long-term maintenance of height and contour. Although HA may be suitable for augmentation to support removable prostheses, the increased popularity of implants has renewed enthusiasm for use of autogenous bone grafts in areas augmented for placement of implants.

Superior Border Augmentation

Superior border augmentation with a bone graft is occasionally indicated when severe resorption of the mandible results in inadequate height and contour and potential risk of fracture or when the treatment plan calls for placement of implants in areas of insufficient bone height or width. Neurosensory disturbances from inferior alveolar nerve dehiscence at the location of the mental foramen at the superior aspect of the mandible also can be corrected with this technique (Figure 14-3).

Superior border grafting was originally described using autogenous rib grafts.[1,2] The disadvantages of this technique include the morbidity associated with removal of the ribs, the need for secondary soft tissue surgery at a later date, the necessity of the patient to forego denture wearing to allow 6 to 8 months of healing after surgery, and the possibility of significant postoperative resorption of the graft.[2] The size and shape of the rib graft also limits the possibility of implant placement in some cases. More recently, there has been a renewed interest in the use of autogenous corticocancellous blocks of ilial crest bone. In 1951, Thoma and Holland[34] proposed the use of iliac crest for superior border augmentation. However, as much as 70% resorption of iliac crest bone can occur with this technique.[10] This large amount of

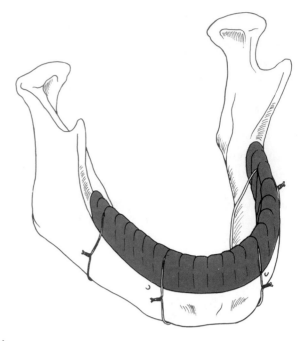

◇ **Figure 14-3**

Superior border grafting of atrophic mandible. Diagrammatic representation of rib strut scored on one side and contoured to adapt to configuration of mandible.

resorbtion may be the result of movement of the bone graft segments that were initially wired to the mandible allowing slight movement combined with the exteranl rather than internal loads placed on the graft after healing. Currently, these blocks of bone are frequently secured to the mandible with small rigid fixation screws, minimizing graft mobility. In some cases, implants can be placed at the same time the bone graft augmentation is completed.

When large segments of allogeneic bone are used for total ridge augmentation of the mandible, unpredictable resorption and graft dehiscence result. The use of small particles of freeze-dried bone to correct contour defects of the posterior mandible has been effective.[33]

Inferior Border Augmentation

Sanders and Cox[30] reported the first clinical use of an inferior border technique for augmentation of the atrophic mandible (Figure 14-4). Indications for use of this technique, in addition to atrophy of the alveolar ridge area, included the prevention and management of fractures of the atrophic mandible. However, this technique does not address abnormalities of the denture-bearing areas, such as the increased interarch distance, superior border irregularities, or exposed position of the mental nerve, which result from mandibular atrophy. These disadvantages, combined with the morbidity of rib harvesting, make this a seldom-used technique.

Pedicle or Interpositional Grafts

A pedicle graft is designed to minimize resorption after healing by maintaining a vascular supply to the augmented

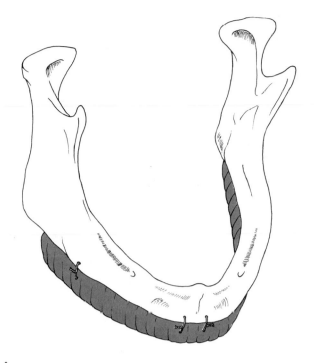

Figure 14-4

Diagrammatic representation of rib graft used for augmentation of inferior border of mandible.

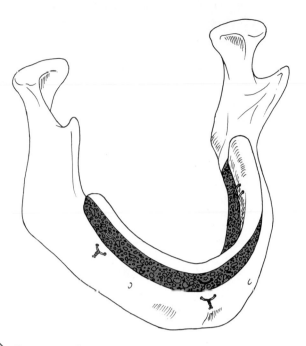

Figure 14-5

Modified visor osteotomy. Diagram of lingual portion of the mandible repositioned and stabilized in superior position.

bony area through an attached soft tissue pedicle. The visor osteotomy, first described by Harle[16] and modified by Peterson and Slade,[29] uses a pedicle of suprahyoid and genioglossus muscles to the lingual aspect of the mandible, which is repositioned on the superior portion of the anterior aspect of the mandible and effectively improves mandibular height and contour (Figure 14-5). Several modifications of this technique have been suggested, including the use of horizontal rather than vertical sagittal osteotomies and a combination of vertical osteotomies posteriorly and a horizontal osteotomy with interpositional grafting in the anterior region (Figure 14-6).[14]

Pedicle grafting techniques have several advantages, including decreased bony resorption with more stable height and contour of the mandible after surgery. Because relatively little cancellous bone is required, donor-site morbidity can also be reduced. Because of the viability of the repositioned segment and the immediate vestibuloplasty performed at the time of surgery, denture construction can usually take place within 3 to 5 months. Because this augmentation repositions the lingual aspect of the mandible, a correction of the class III ridge relationship that can result from severe bony resorption may occur.

The disadvantages of this technique include the need for hospitalization, general anesthesia, and donor-site surgery and the inability to wear dentures for 3 to 5 months after surgery. Postoperative neurosensory deficit has also been noted in many patients undergoing this type of procedure,[14] and subsequently this procedure in seldom used.

HYDROXYAPATITE AUGMENTATION OF THE MANDIBLE

The problems associated with bone grafting, including resorption, donor-site morbidity, and the need for hospitalization, have in part been responsible for the search for an alloplastic material that would function as an adequate graft material for the atrophic mandible. Hydroxyapatite (HA) is a dense biocompatible material that can be produced synthetically or obtained from biologic sources such as coral. At this time the granular, or particle, form is most commonly used for alveolar ridge augmentation. When placed in a subperiosteal environment adjacent to bone, HA bonds physically and chemically to the bone. Although some bony growth may occur adjacent to the particles at the area of the interface, the remainder of the particles not directly adjacent to the bone are primarily surrounded by fibrous tissue. Histologically, each particle appears to be surrounded in a fibrous tissue capsule, with some infiltration of vascular tissue throughout the graft material. This fibrous encapsulation of the HA particles appears to occur without the production of any significant inflammation.[22]

Indications for the use of HA for mandibular augmentation are similar to those for bone grafts. A classification of appropriate treatment based on anatomy of the existing mandible has been suggested (see Table 14-1).[23]

With the exception of the severely atrophic class IV mandible, for which donor-site surgery is necessary to obtain autogenous bone, HA augmentation of the mandible can generally be performed on an outpatient basis, using local

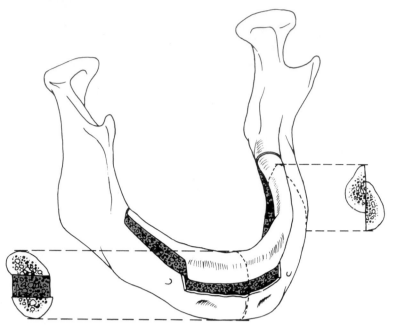

◇ Figure 14-6

Modification of visor osteotomy combining vertical osteotomies in posterior mandible with horizontal osteotomy and interpositional grafting in anterior area.

anesthetic combined with conscious sedation techniques. A subperiosteal tunnel technique is used, which exposes the entire superior aspect of the mandible in the area to be augmented but carefully avoids the neurovascular bundles. After the tunnel is created, a preloaded beveled syringe containing HA is inserted into the most posterior aspect of the tunnel, and the HA is injected until the desired height and contour of the mandible is obtained (Figure 14-7). Similarly, insertion of the HA from each lateral incision area augments the anterior area of the mandible. Some surgeons prefer splints to minimize HA displacement and to improve vestibular form during the postoperative period. The splint, constructed on a cast that has been waxed to the desired contour of the mandible after augmentation, is secured in place with circummandibular sutures for 7 to 10 days. Vestibuloplasty and skin grafting can be performed 8 to 12 weeks after augmentation. During this time the HA granules consolidate and become firmly fixed by connective tissue.

In some cases the standard subperiosteal technique may not provide the adequate soft tissue release necessary to allow for maximum augmentation. The major restricting factor in these cases is the periosteum. By combining an open submucosal dissection (transpositional flap vestibuloplasty) with a periosteal releasing incision, improved augmentation can be achieved. This technique is discussed later in this chapter (see Figure 14-17).

The advantages of HA augmentation are that donor-site surgery is eliminated and that most patients can undergo this type of procedure in an outpatient setting. Because HA is nonresorbable, no postoperative loss of the graft augmenting the mandible occurs, and vascular tissue ingrowth around the HA provides an adequate vascular bed for future soft tissue grafts if necessary. The disadvantages of HA are the difficulty sometimes encountered in containing the material within the subperiosteal tunnel and in achieving the adequate absolute height augmentation that is often desirable. Some nerve dysesthesias have also been associated with HA augmentation. Although there is evidence to suggest that some increase in mandibular strength exists as a result of HA augmentation, the material may not be as effective as a bone graft in preventing possible fracture in the severely atrophic mandible.

GUIDED BONE REGENERATION (OSTEOPROMOTION)

In guided bone regeneration a nonresorbable membrane is used to cover an area where bone graft healing or bone regeneration is desired. The concept of guided regeneration, or osteopromotion, is based on the ability to exclude undersirable cell types, such as epithelial cells or fibroblasts, from the area where bone healing is taking place.

In 1982, Nyman[26] described a technique to improve periodontal ligament regeneration using a membrane barrier to exclude undesirable cells from the area where periodontal ligament healing or regeneration was required. Dahlin et al[11] showed that bone growth around implants could be facilitated using a similar technique. By placing a membrane covering over a bone graft, faster-growing fibroblasts and epithelial cells can be walled off, allowing bone to grow in a relatively protected environment.

Many types of materials have been used as membrane coverings. Currently, expanded polytetrafluoroethylene (ePFTE) membrane is the most popular.* This membrane is

---

*WL Gore and Associates, Inc., Flagstaff, Ariz.

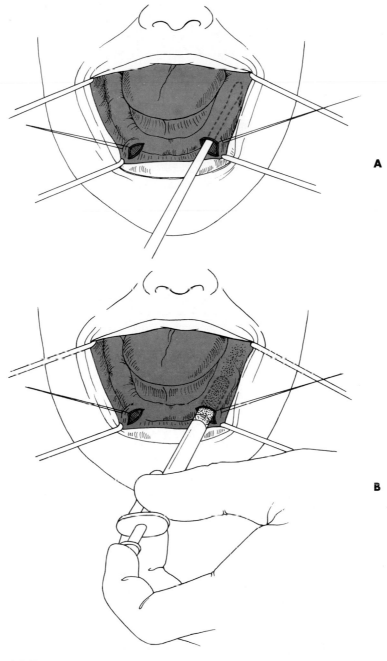

◇ Figure 14-7

Diagrammatic representation of hydroxyapatite (HA) augmentation procedure. **A,** Vertical incisions placed anterior to mental nerve area. Subperiosteal tunnels are then developed in posterior and anterior areas. Retraction sutures are used to elevate margins of incision. **B,** Injection of HA into subperiosteal tunnels.

Continued

not resorbable and must be removed after adequate bone healing occurs. Research is ongoing to develop other resorbable membranes, eliminating the need for a second surgical procedure for removal.

The membrane material can be placed over an area where bone is grafted to fill a defect or improve ridge contour (Figure 14-8, *A*). Implant placement can be facilited where inadequate bone thickness occurs by placing the implant and graft and covering the area with a membrane (Figure 14-8, *B*). The

membrane can be removed at the time of the second stage of surgery, to uncover the implant and place the transmucosal extension or healing cap. In some cases a bone graft may not be necessary if a membrane is used.[8] In this type of case the membrane material is "tented" up, using screws to maintain a space adjacent to the bone (Figure 14-8, *C*). A blood clot forms in the space, and osteoblasts eventually begin forming bone in the defect, which is protected from fibrous and epithelium ingrowth.

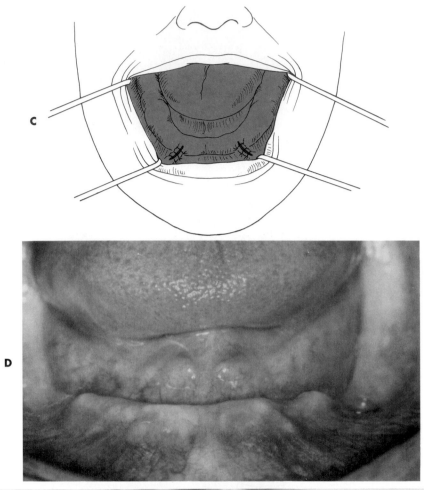

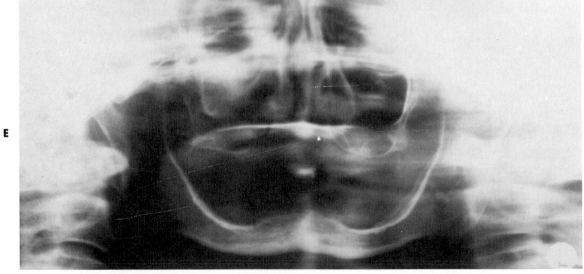

◆ Figure 14-7, cont'd

C, Soft tissue closure. **D,** Preoperative clinical photograph. **E,** Preoperative radiograph.   *Continued*

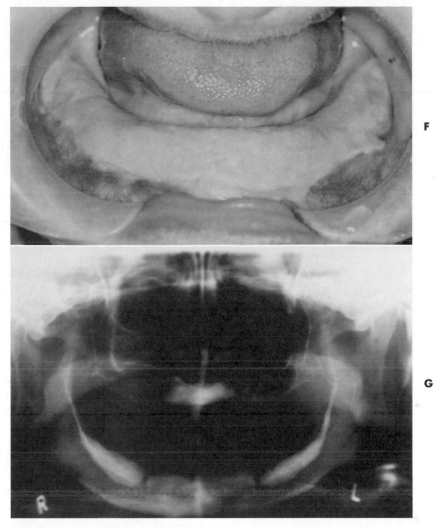

◇ Figure 14-7, cont'd

F, Postoperative clinical photograph. (Note that split-thickness skin-grafting procedure has been done after HA augmentation to improve vestibular depth.) **G,** Postoperative radiograph demonstrating improvement in height of alveolar ridge area.

The concept of guided tissue regeneraton is discussed in further detail in Chapter 15.

MAXILLARY AUGMENTATION ◇

Severe resorption of the maxillary alveolar ridge is not as common as mandibular resorption. When moderate-to-severe maxillary resorption does occur, the larger denture-bearing area of the maxilla may allow prosthetic rehabilitation without bony augmentation. In certain cases a severe increase in interarch space, loss of palatal vault, interference from the zygomatic buttress area, and absence of posterior tuberosity notching may prevent construction of proper dentures, and augmentation must be considered.

ONLAY BONE GRAFTING

Bone grafting of the edentulous atrophic maxilla with an autogenous rib was first described by Terry, Albright, and Baker.[32] Maxillary onlay bone grafting is indicated primarily when there is severe resorption of the maxillary alveolus that results in the absence of a clinical alveolar ridge and loss of adequate palatal vault form (Figure 14-9).[1] Onlay rib grafting to the maxilla requires hospitalization, general anesthesia, and the removal of two ribs in a manner similar to that described for grafting of the mandible.

The disadvantages of this technique include the need for secondary donor-site surgery, possible extensive and unpredictable postoperative resorption, the frequent need for postoperative secondary soft tissue procedures, and the delay in wearing of dentures for 6 to 8 months after graft

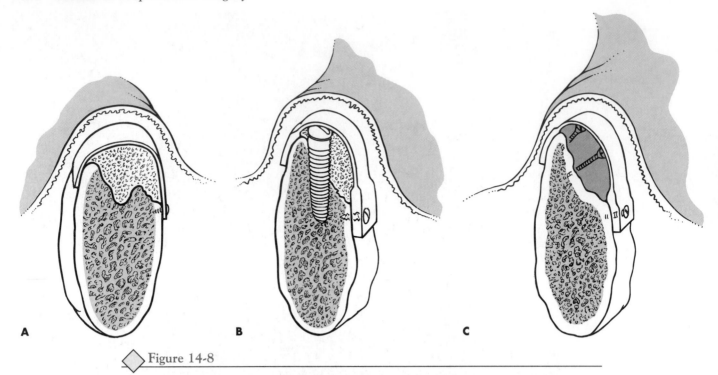

Figure 14-8

A, Alveolar ridge defect grafted with autogenous bone and covered with a membrane stabilized with a small screw. **B,** Bone graft in area of implant where alveolar ridge crest is too thin for bone coverage on facial aspect of implant. The implant and bone graft are covered with a nonresorbable membrane stabilized with a small screw. **C,** Bone defect covered with membrane supported with screws. Organized blood clot in defect is from fibrous ingrowth during osteoblastic formation of bone in defect.

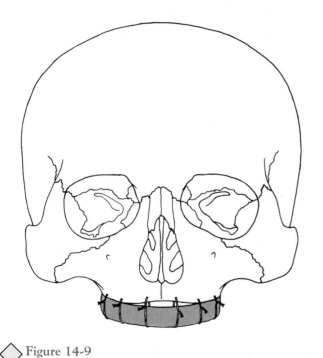

Figure 14-9

Autogenous rib graft augmentation of maxilla. Diagrammatic representation of rib graft contoured on one side and adapted to configuration of atrophic maxilla.

surgery. The size and shape of rib grafts creates difficulty with simultaneous or delayed placement of implants if desired.

Maxillary onlay grafting currently is usually accomplished using corticocancellous blocks of ilac crest bone. The blocks can be secured to the maxilla with small screws, eliminating mobility and decreasing resorption (Fig 14-10). Implants can be placed at the time of grafting in some cases but placement is often delayed to allow initial healing of the grafted bone.

INTERPOSITIONAL BONE GRAFTS

As with pedicle or interpositional bone grafts of the mandible, maxillary interpositional bone grafting maintains the blood supply to the repositioned portion of the maxilla and generally results in more predictable and less extensive resorption postoperatively. Interpositional bone grafting in the maxilla is indicated in the bone-deficient maxilla where there is adequate form to the palatal vault but insufficient ridge height, particularly in the zygomatic buttress and posterior tuberosity areas, and excessive interarch space.[6] Anteroposterior and transverse discrepancies between the maxilla and mandible can also be corrected by interpositional bone-grafting techniques (Figure 14-11).

Interpositional grafting techniques provide stable and predictable results by changing the maxillary position in the

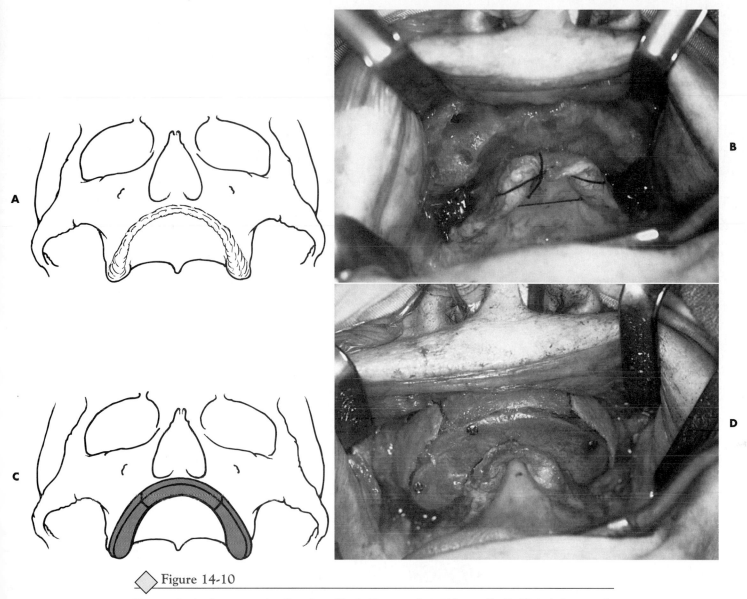

◇ Figure 14-10

Iliac crest onlay bone recontruction of maxilla. **A,** Diagram of atrophic maxilla. **B,** Clinical photograph.
C, Three segments of bone are secured in place. Small defects are filled with cancellous bone.
D, Clinical photograph.

vertical, anteroposterior, and transverse directions and may eliminate the need for secondary soft tissue procedures. Disadvantages of this type of procedure include the need to harvest bone from an iliac crest donor site and possible secondary soft tissue surgery.

MAXILLARY HYDROXYAPATITE AUGMENTATION

HA is readily available, eliminates the need for donor-site surgery, and is easily placed in an outpatient setting. HA augmentation of the maxilla is indicated when alveolar ridge resorption results in an inability to construct a denture that will provide adequate function, esthetics, and quality for the patient. HA can also be used to contour and eliminate minor ridge irregularities and undercut areas in the maxilla, as described in Chapter 13.

HA is placed into the maxilla in a technique similar to that described for mandibular augmentation. In the maxilla a single midline incision is usually sufficient for adequate access to both sides of the maxillary ridge (Figure 14-12). When access through a single incision is inadequate, bilateral vertical maxillary incisions in the canine-premolar area can be used to improve visibility and access. Subperiosteal tunnels are created over the crest of the alveolar ridge, and preloaded syringes are inserted into the most posterior aspect of these tunnels. The HA particles are injected and molded to the desired height and contour, and the incisions are closed with a horizontal mattress suture.

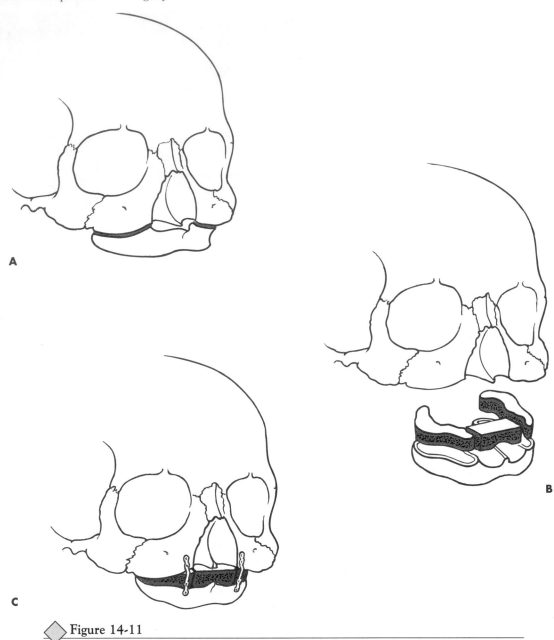

◇ Figure 14-11

Interpositional (Le Fort I) augmentation of maxilla. **A,** Diagrammatic representation of atrophic maxillary alveolar ridge. **B,** Augmentation is completed by down-fracturing maxilla and placing interpositional graft using autogenous iliac crest. The maxilla is stabilized using rigid fixation plates.

The amount of augmentation possible in the maxilla is sometimes limited by the ability to develop sufficient space for HA particles in the subperiosteal tunnels. When an extensive subperiosteal dissection allows placement of a large quantity of HA, the vestibular area may often be obliterated. A simultaneous submucosal vestibuloplasty technique combined with incision of the periosteum at the maximal extent of the vestibule may aid in attaining the desired height and contour of the maxillary alveolar ridge.

Loss of containment or displacement of HA particles can result in inadequate ridge form following HA augmentation. One recent modification of the HA augmentation technique uses a bioresorbable mesh tube to contain the HA particles.[17]

After the subperiosteal tunnels have been developed, the tube material filled with HA particles is inserted in the appropriate position along the crest of the maxillary ridge (Figure 14-13). By the time the tube material has resorbed, sufficient fibrous tissue is incorporated into the HA matrix to prevent particle displacement.

Regardless of the augmentation technique a splint is usually inserted at the time of augmentation and held in place for 7 days with suspension wires or a palatal screw. The splint can be a modification of the current denture or a prefabricated splint constructed from a cast, altered to simulate the desired postoperative height and contour. A splint technique allows upper denture wearing during most of the postoperative

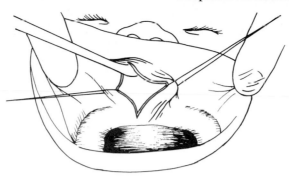

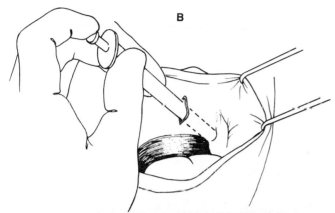

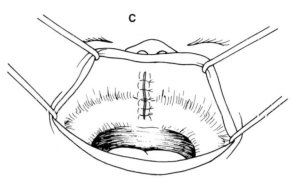

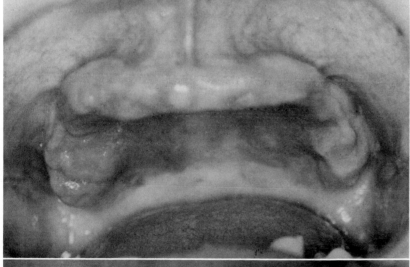

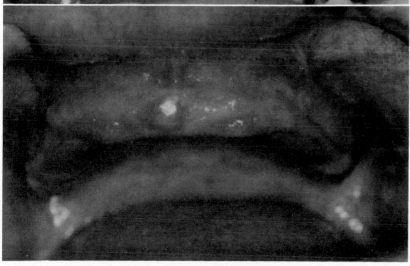

◈ Figure 14-12

HA augmentation of maxilla. **A,** Midline incision and subperiosteal tunnels used to expose areas of maxilla to be augmented. **B,** Injection of HA material into subperiosteal tunnels. **C,** Soft tissue closure. **D,** Preoperative clinical photograph showing atrophic maxillary ridge with decreased alveolar ridge height and areas of contour irregularities. **E,** One-year postoperative result demonstrating increased alveolar ridge height and improved contour.

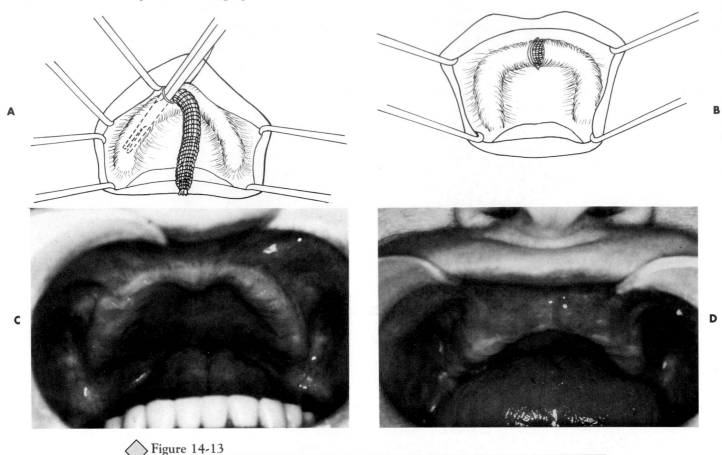

◇ Figure 14-13

Vicryl stocking technique for HA augmentation. **A,** HA particles are enclosed in bioresorbable vicryl tubing, which is inserted into subperiosteal tunnels. **B,** Diagram of HA particles and vicryl stocking after insertion and before wound closure. **C,** Preoperative photograph showing absence of maxillary alveolar ridge. **D,** Postoperative photograph.

healing period. HA augmentation can be performed in an outpatient setting with minimal postoperative morbidity, which makes it a popular technique for augmentation of the edentulous maxilla.

SINUS LIFT

Rehabilitation of the maxilla using implants is frequently problematic because of the extension of the maxillary sinus into the alveolar ridge area. In many cases the actual size and configuration of the maxilla are satisfactory in terms of height and width of the alveolar ridge area. However, extension of t he maxillary sinuses into the alveolar ridge may prevent placement of implants in the posterior maxillary area because of insufficient bony support. A sinus-lift procedure is actually a bony augmentation procedure that places graft material inside the sinus and augments the bony support in the alveolar ridge area. In this technique an opening is made in the lateral aspect of the maxillary wall, and the sinus lining is carefully elevated from the bony floor of the sinus (Figure 14-14). Alloplastic material, allogeneic bone, autogenous bone, or a combination of these materials can be used as a graft source in these areas. The current method of choice usually

incorporates some autogenous bone material in the sinus graft. The graft is allowed to heal for 4 to 6 months, after which the first stage of implant placement can begin in the usual fashion described in Chapter 15. This procedure can frequently be done as outpatient surgery and does not effect postoperative denture wearing.

TUBEROPLASTY

The tuberosity-hamular notch area prevents denture displacement and aids the peripheral seal of a maxillary denture. When the remaining alveolar ridge and palatal vault area is adequate but there is inadequate notching in the tuberosity-hamular area, a surgical procedure may improve denture retention. The tuberoplasty is designed to deepen the hamular notch by repositioning the pterygoid plate and hamulus in a posterior direction (Figure 14-15).[28]

Although a tuberoplasty can be performed on an outpatient basis, it may not be advisable to do so. During the procedure, brisk hemorrhage may be encountered when the pterygoid plates are fractured. An additional disadvantage of this procedure is the unpredictable depth of the tuberosity notch after healing.

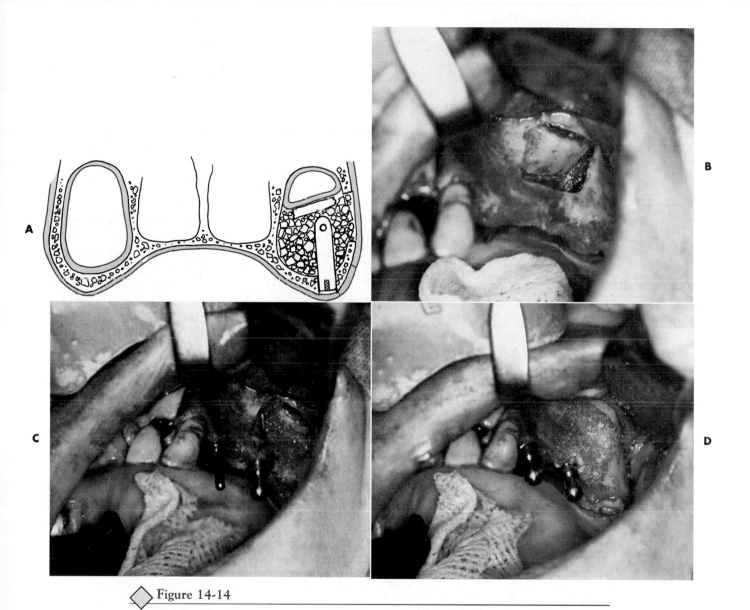

◇ Figure 14-14

Sinus-lift procedure. **A,** Cross-sectional diagram of maxilla demonstrating bone grafting to the sinus floor. Note on the left side of the diagram the sinus extending into the alveolar ridge area, which results in sufficient bone for implant placement. On the right side the lateral wall of the maxilla has been fractured inward, bone grafted in the inferior portion of the sinus, and an implant placed into the sinus floor graft. **B, C,** and **D,** Clinical photographs showing sinus opening, placement of implants, and bone graft to fill inferior portion of sinus.

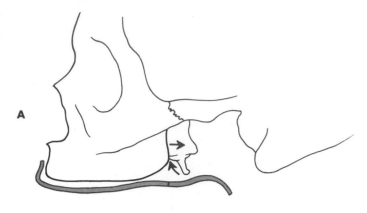

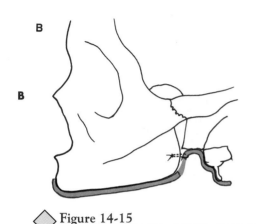

◇ **Figure 14-15**

Maxillary tuberoplasty. **A,** Representation of atrophic maxilla with inadequate tuberosity-hamular notch depth. **B,** Representation of postoperative result after fracturing of pterygoid plate and hamular notch, subsequent posterior refracturing, and soft tissue repositioning.

SOFT TISSUE SURGERY FOR RIDGE EXTENSION OF THE MANDIBLE

As alveolar ridge resorption takes place the attachment of mucosa and muscles near the denture-bearing area exerts a greater influence on the retention and stability of dentures, and the amount and quality of fixed tissue over the denture-bearing area may be decreased. Soft tissue surgery performed to improve denture stability may be carried out alone or may follow bony augmentation. In either case the primary goals of soft tissue preprosthetic surgery are to provide an enlarged area of fixed tissue in the primary denture-bearing or implant area and to improve extension in the area of the denture flanges by removing the dislodging effects of muscle attachments in the denture-bearing or vestibular areas.

TRANSPOSITIONAL FLAP VESTIBULOPLASTY (LIP SWITCH)

A lingually based flap vestibuloplasty was first described by Kazanjian.[20] In this procedure a mucosal flap pedicled from the alveolar ridge is elevated from the underlying tissue and sutured to the depth of the vestibule (Figure 14-16). The inner portion of the lip is allowed to heal by secondary epithelialization. This procedure has been modified, and the use of a technique transposing a lingually based mucosal flap and a labially based periosteal flap (transpositional flap) has become popular.[21] When adequate mandibular height exists, this procedure increases the anterior vestibular area, which improves denture retention and stability. The primary indications for the procedure include adequate anterior mandibular height (at least 15 mm), inadequate facial vestibular depth from mucosal and muscular attachments in the anterior mandible, and the presence of an adequate vestibular depth on the lingual aspect of the mandible.

The transpositional flap vestibuloplasty technique can be combined with HA augmentation procedures. After the submucosal flap is developed, the periosteum can be incised to allow a more extensive ridge augmentation without the restriction of the periosteal envelope. The mucosa is sutured to the edge of the periosteum as an enlarged tunnel for HA augmentation is created (Figure 14-17).[3]

These techniques provide adequate results in many cases and generally do not require hospitalization, donor-site surgery, or prolonged periods without a denture. Disadvantages include unpredictability of the amount of relapse of the vestibular depth, scarring in the depth of the vestibule, and problems with adaptation of the peripheral flange area of the denture to the depth of the vestibule.[18,19]

VESTIBULE AND FLOOR-OF-MOUTH EXTENSION PROCEDURES

In addition to the attachment of labial muscles and soft tissues to the denture-bearing area, the mylohyoid and genioglossus muscles in the floor of the mouth present similar problems on the lingual aspect of the mandible. Trauner[35] described detaching the mylohyoid muscles from the mylohyoid ridge area and repositioning them inferiorly, effectively deepening the floor of the mouth area and relieving the influence of the mylohyoid muscle on the denture. MacIntosh and Obwegeser[24] later described the effective use of a labial extension procedure combined with Trauner's procedure to provide maximal vestibular extension to both the buccal and lingual aspects of the mandible. The technique for extension of the labial vestibule is a modification of a labially pedicled supraperiosteal flap described by Clark.[9] Following the two vestibular extension techniques, a skin graft can be used to cover the area of denuded periosteum (Figure 14-18). The combination procedure effectively eliminates the dislodging forces of the mucosa and muscle attachments and provides a broad base of fixed keratinized tissue on the primary denture-bearing area (Figure 14-19). Split-thickness skin

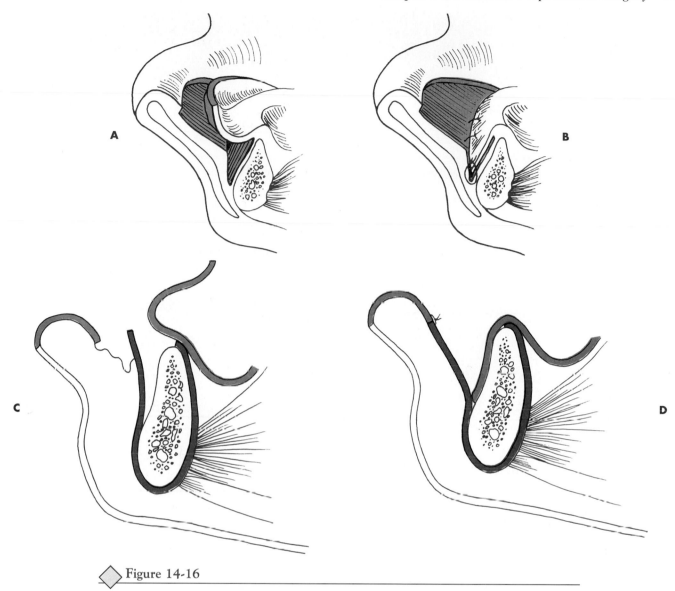

◇ **Figure 14-16**

Transpositional flap vestibuloplasty (lip switch). **A,** Incision is made in labial mucosa, and thin mucosal flap is dissected from underlying tissue. Supraperiosteal dissection is also performed on anterior aspect of the mandible. **B,** Flap of labial mucosa is sutured to depth of vestibule. Exposed labial tissue heals by secondary intention. **C,** Modification of technique by incising periosteum at crest of alveolar ridge and suturing free periosteal edge to denuded area of labial mucosa. **D,** Mucosal flap is then sutured over denuded bone to periosteal junction at depth of vestibule. *Continued*

grafting with the buccal vestibuloplasty and floor-of-mouth procedure is indicated when adequate alveolar ridge for a denture-bearing area is lost but at least 15 mm of mandibular bone height remains. The remaining bone must have adequate contour so that the form of the alveolar ridge exposed after the procedure is adequate for denture construction. If gross irregularities exist, such as large concavities in the superior aspect of the posterior mandible, they should be corrected through grafting or minor alveoloplasty procedures before the soft tissue procedure.

The technique has the advantage of early covering of the exposed periosteal bed, which improves patient comfort and allows earlier denture construction, and the long-term results of vestibular extension are predictable. The need for hospitalization and donor-site surgery combined with the moderate swelling and discomfort experienced by the patient postoperatively are the primary disadvantages. Patients rarely complain about the appearance or function of skin in the oral cavity. If the skin graft is too thick at the time of harvesting, hair follicles may not totally degenerate, and hair growth may occasionally be seen in isolated areas of the graft.

Tissue other than skin has been used effectively for grafting over the alveolar ridge. Palatal tissue offers the potential advantages of providing a firm, resilient tissue, with minimal

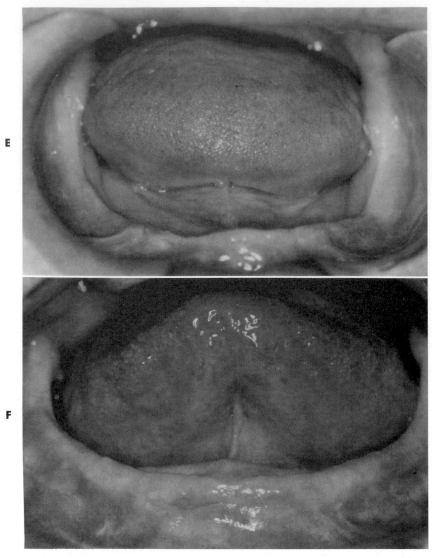

◇ **Figure 14-16, cont'd**

E, Preoperative photograph. **F,** Six-month postoperative result.

contraction of the grafted area.[15] Although palatal tissue is relatively easy to obtain at the time of surgery, the limited amount of tissue and the discomfort associated with donor-site harvesting are the primary drawbacks. In areas where only a small localized graft is required, palatal tissue is usually adequate. Figure 14-20 demonstrates palatal graft tissue used to create fixed keratinized tissue around the area of implant placement.

Full-thickness buccal mucosa harvested from the inner aspect of the cheek provides advantages similar to those of palatal tissue. However, the need for specialized mucotomes to harvest buccal mucosa and extensive buccal mucosa scarring after harvesting of a full-thickness graft are disadvantages. This mucosa does not become keratinized, is generally mobile, and often results in an inadequate denture-bearing surface.

SOFT TISSUE SURGERY FOR MAXILLARY RIDGE EXTENSION ◇

Maxillary alveolar bone resorption frequently results in mucosal and muscle attachments that interfere with denture construction, stability, and retention. Because of the large denture-bearing area of the maxilla, adequate denture construction and stability can often be achieved after extensive bone loss. However, excess soft tissue may accompany bony resorption, or soft tissue may require modification as an adjunct to previous augmentation surgery. Several techniques provide additional fixed mucosa and vestibular depth in the maxillary denture-bearing area.

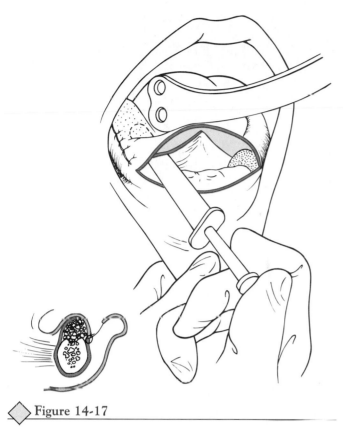

Figure 14-17

Transpositional flap vestibuloplasty and simultaneous HA augmentation. Note that the lingually based mucosa is sutured to the periosteum on the facial side of the mandible.

SUBMUCOSAL VESTIBULOPLASTY

The submucosal vestibuloplasty as described by Obwegeser[27] may be the procedure of choice for correction of soft tissue attachment on or near the crest of the alveolar ridge of the maxilla. This technique is particularly useful when maxillary alveolar ridge resorption has occurred but the residual bony maxilla is adequate for proper denture support. In this technique, underlying submucosal tissue is either excised or repositioned to allow direct apposition of the labiovestibular mucosa to the periosteum of the remaining maxilla.

To provide adequate vestibular depth without producing an abnormal appearance of the upper lip, adequate mucosal length must be available in this area. A simple test to determine whether adequate labiovestibular mucosa is present is performed by placing a dental mouth mirror under the upper lip and elevating the superior aspect of the vestibule to the desired postoperative depth (Figure 14-21). If no inversion or shortening of the lip occurs, then adequate mucosa is present to perform a proper submucosal vestibuloplasty.

The submucosal vestibuloplasty can generally be performed with local anesthetic and intravenous sedation in an outpatient setting. A midline incision is made in the anterior maxilla, and the mucosa is undermined and separated from the underlying submucosal tissue (see Figure 14-21). A

supraperiosteal tunnel is then developed by dissecting the muscular and submucosal attachments from the periosteum. The intermediate layer of tissue created by the two tunneling dissections is incised at its attachment area near the crest of the alveolar ridge. This submucosal and muscular tissue can be repositioned superiorly or excised. After closure of the midline incision a preexisting denture or prefabricated splint is modified to extend into the vestibular areas and is secured with a palatal screw or suspension wires to hold the mucosa over the ridge in close apposition to the periosteum. When healing takes place, usually within 3 weeks, the mucosa is closely adapted to the anterior and lateral walls of the maxilla at the required depth of the vestibule.

The maxillary submucosal vestibuloplasty can also be combined with HA augmentation of the alveolar ridge area. A subperiosteal tunnel can be created using a technique similar to standard maxillary HA augmentation procedures.[36] By incising the periosteum high on the lateral aspect of the mandible, the periosteal envelope can be enlarged to allow greater HA augmentation in this area (Figure 14-22).

These techniques provide a predictable increase in vestibular depth and attachment of mucosa over the denture-bearing area. A properly relined denture can often be worn immediately after the surgery or after removal of the splint, and impressions for final denture relining or construction can be completed 2 to 3 weeks after surgery.

MAXILLARY VESTIBULOPLASTY WITH TISSUE GRAFTING

When insufficient labiovestibular mucosa exists and lip shortening would result from a submucosal vestibuloplasty technique, other vestibular extension techniques must be used. In such cases a modification of Clark's vestibuloplasty technique using mucosa pedicled from the upper lip and sutured at the depth of the maxillary vestibule after a supraperiosteal dissection can be used.[28] The denuded periosteum over the alveolar ridge heals by secondary epithelialization. Moderate discomfort can occur in the postoperative period, and a longer healing time is required (6 to 8 weeks) before denture construction. Maintenance of the maxillary vestibular depth is unpredictable. The use of a labially pedicled mucosal flap combined with tissue grafting over the exposed periosteum of the maxilla provides the added benefits of more rapid healing over the area of previously exposed periosteum and more predictable long-term maintenance of vestibular depth.

CORRECTION OF ABNORMAL RIDGE RELATIONSHIPS ◇

Approximately 5% of the population has a severe skeletal discrepancy between their upper and lower jaws that results in a severe malocclusion. When the teeth are lost, an abnormal ridge relationship results that complicates construction of prosthetic appliances. When a preexisting class III ridge

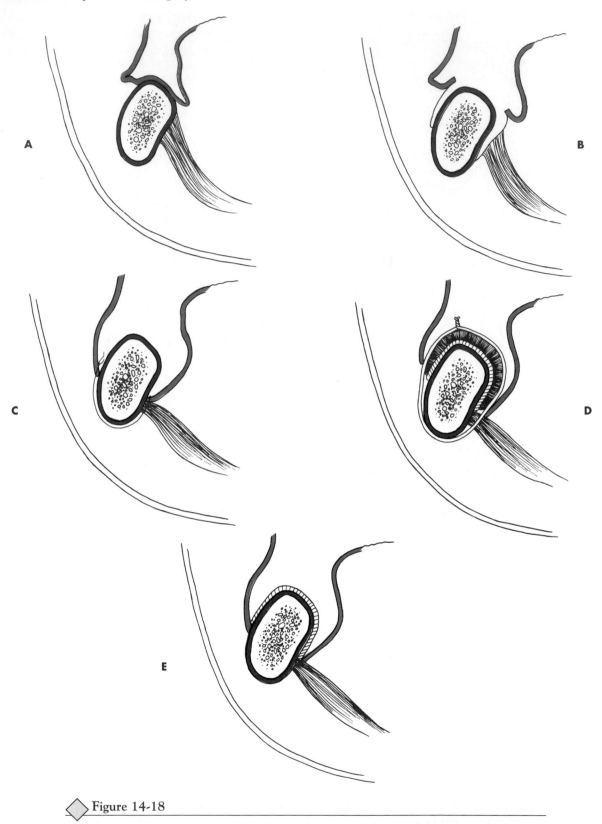

◇ **Figure 14-18**

Labial vestibuloplasty, floor-of-mouth lowering procedure, and skin grafting (Obwegeser's technique). **A,** Preoperative muscle and soft tissue attachments near crest of remaining mandible. **B,** Flaps are sutured near inferior border of mandible, with sutures passed under inferior border of mandible, tethering labial and lingual tissues near inferior border of mandible. **C,** Skin graft held in place with splint. **D,** Postoperative view of newly created vestibular depth and floor-of-mouth area.

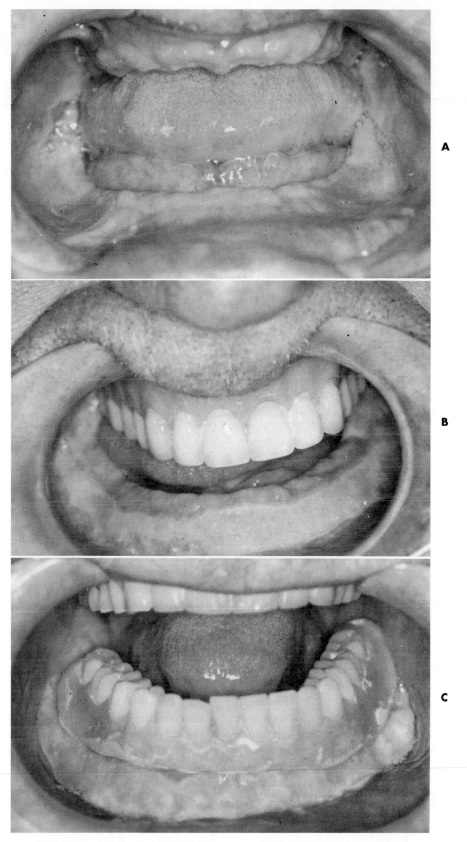

Figure 14-19

Vestibuloplasty, floor-of-mouth lowering, and skin grafting. **A,** Preoperative photograph. **B,** One-month postoperative result. **C,** Patient's old denture inserted, showing extent of previous flange area available before vestibuloplasty. Note large improvement in vestibular depth and keratinized, firmly fixed tissue over alveolar ridge denture-bearing area.

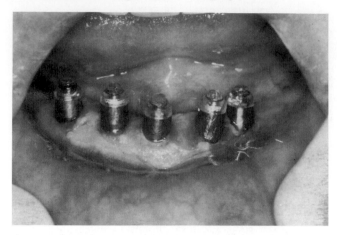

◇ **Figure 14-20**

Graft harvested from palate is used to create fixed keratinized tissue around implants.

relationship exists, loss of teeth and the pattern of bony resorption increase the severity of the class III skeletal problem. In patients with partially missing dentition the absence of opposing occlusal forces may allow the supraeruption of teeth, which may complicate subsequent prosthetic restoration.

The assessment of ridge relationships is an important, often overlooked aspect of the evaluation of patients for prosthetic treatment. In partially edentulous patients the evaluation should include an examination of the direction of the occlusal plane and a determination of interarch distances that may be affected by supraerupted teeth or segments. In totally edentulous patients the interarch space and the anteroposterior and transverse relationships of the maxilla and mandible must be evaluated with the patient's jaw at the proper occlusal vertical dimension. This determination in the diagnostic phase may require the construction of bite rims with proper lip support. Lateral cephalometric radiographs are also necessary in this evaluation, to confirm the clinical impression.

SEGMENTAL ALVEOLAR SURGERY IN THE PARTIALLY EDENTULOUS PATIENT

Supraeruption of teeth and bony segments into an opposing edentulous area may decrease interarch space and preclude the construction of an adequate fixed or removable prosthetic appliance in this area. The loss of teeth in one arch may increase the difficulty of obtaining a functional and esthetic prosthetic appliance with prosthetic teeth located properly over the underlying ridge. Several alternatives exist to restore the dentition in these patients, including extraction of teeth in the malpositioned segment or repositioning of these teeth with segmental surgery.

Preoperative considerations should include facial esthetic quality, an intraoral occlusal examination, panoramic and cephalometric radiographs, and models properly mounted on an articulator. If segmental surgery is to be considered, the models can be cut and teeth repositioned in their desired location. The dentist responsible for final prosthetic restora-

tion of the patient must make the final determination of the placement of the segments on the articulated models. Presurgical orthodontic preparation may be necessary to align teeth properly and allow proper segmental positioning. Following model surgery, a splint is fabricated to locate placement of segments precisely at the time of surgery and to provide stability during the postoperative healing period. When possible the splint should be stabilized by contacting other teeth rather than resting on soft tissue. Palatal and lingual flanges on the splint should be avoided, because pressure from the splint may interfere with blood supply important for the viability of the bone and teeth that were repositioned with segmental surgery. In some cases, construction of the splint must include contact on the alveolar ridge tissue of the opposing arch to maintain the interridge distance. The patient's deformity and the surgeon's preference and experience dictate the specific surgical procedure performed. Segmental procedures for correction of abnormalities in the maxilla and the mandible are described in Chapter 26 and in other textbooks (Figure 14-23).[5] A final fixed and removable prosthetic rehabilitation follows the surgical procedure and an adequate postoperative healing period.

CORRECTION OF SKELETAL ABNORMALITIES IN THE TOTALLY EDENTULOUS PATIENT

After the appropriate clinical and radiographic evaluation, casts should be mounted on an articulator for determination of the ideal ridge relationship. The dentist responsible for prosthetic construction should be responsible for determining the final desired position of the maxilla and mandible after surgery. In the case of the totally edentulous patient in whom the maxilla, mandible, or both are to be repositioned, the esthetic facial result must also be considered with the functional result of ridge repositioning. Casts with simulated surgical changes, cephalometric prediction tracings, and experienced clinical judgment are required to determine the desired postoperative jaw position (see Chapter 26). After an appropriate decision has been made about desired postoperative skeletal position, splints are made to allow positioning of the jaws into their proper relationship at the time of surgery (Figure 14-24). These splints must provide adequate stability over the edentulous ridge area and interdigitate with each other to maintain a proper ridge relationship (Figure 14-25). Rigid fixation techniques as discussed in Chapter 26 may be useful in stabilizing bone segments at the time of surgery and in eliminating a prolonged period of jaw immobilization. Surgical procedures for repositioning of the maxilla or mandible are described in Chapter 26.

Denture construction can begin within 3 months after surgical repositioning of the maxilla and mandible. The combination of orthognathic surgery and prosthetic rehabilitation of the patient provides satisfactory functional and esthetic results in many patients with skeletal abnormalities who would otherwise present significant problems in prosthetic reconstruction.

Text continued on p. 353

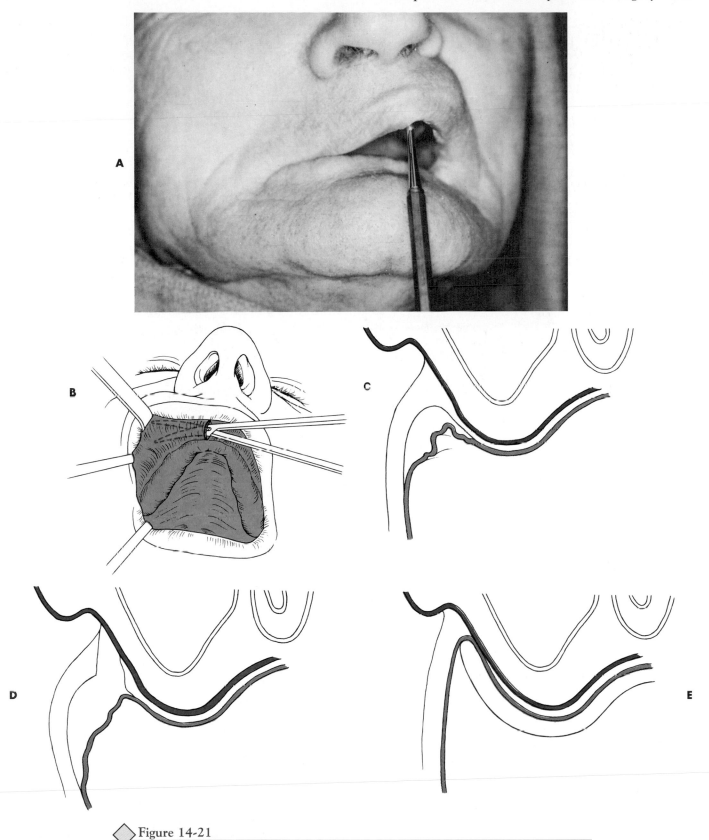

◇ Figure 14-21

Submucosal vestibuloplasty. **A,** Mouth mirror placed in maxillary vestibule under upper lip and elevated against anterior wall of maxilla to desired postoperative vestibular depth. If no abnormal lip-shortening occurs, then adequate mucosa exists to perform submucosal vestibuloplasty. **B,** Anterior vertical incision is used to create submucosal and then supraperiosteal tunnel along lateral aspects of maxilla. **C,** Cross-sectional view showing submucosal tissue layer. **D,** Excision of submucosal soft tissue layer. **E,** Splint in place holding mucosa against periosteum at depth of vestibule until healing occurs.

Continued

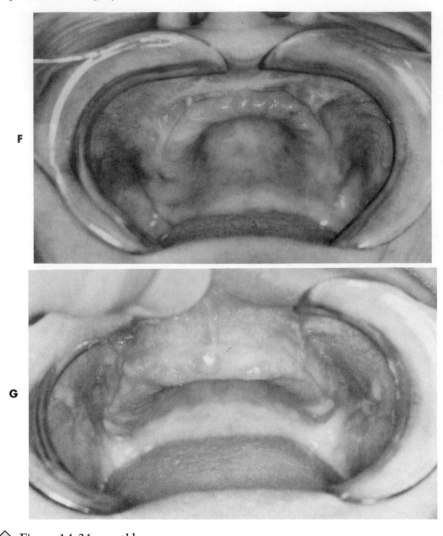

◆ Figure 14-21, cont'd

F, Preoperative photograph. **G,** Postoperative result.

◆ Figure 14-22

Diagram demonstrating cross-sectional view of maxilla with simultaneous submucosal vestibuloplasty and HA augmentation.

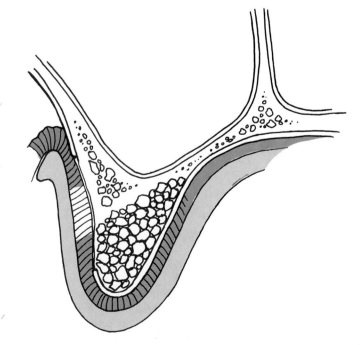

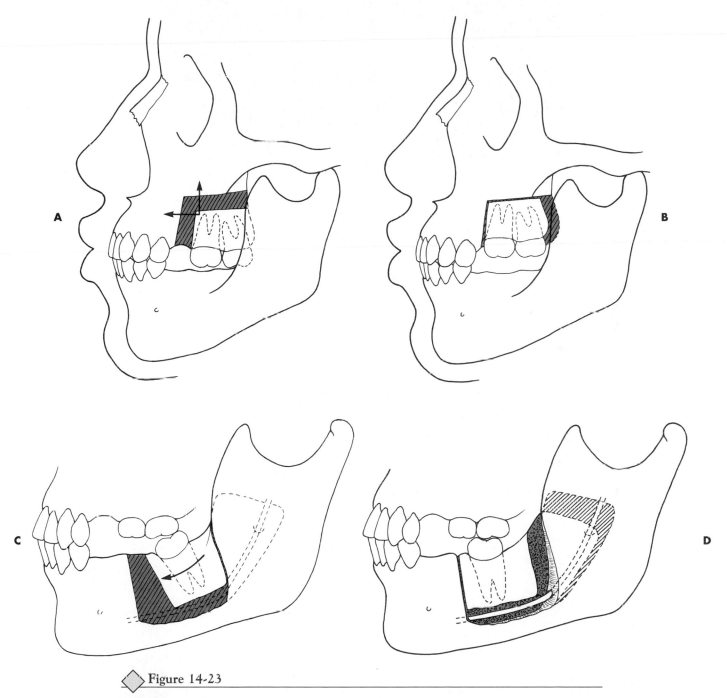

◈ Figure 14-23

Segmental osteotomies. **A** and **B,** Posterior maxillary osteotomy for superior and anterior repositioning of posterior segment of maxilla. This improves interarch space for construction of removable partial mandibular denture. **C** and **D,** Example of mandibular segmental osteotomy to reposition molar tooth to function as distal abutment for fixed prosthetic appliance or for improved support as partial denture abutment.

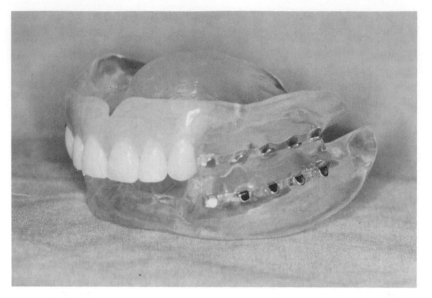

◇ Figure 14-24

Surgical splints used to properly position and to stabilize edentulous arches for orthognathic surgery.

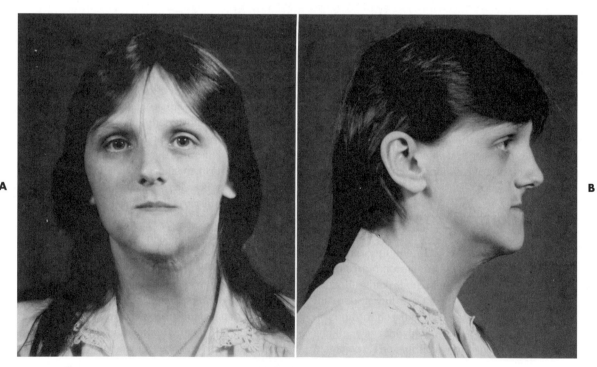

A

B

◇ Figure 14-25

A and **B,** Preoperative full-face and profile photographs.

Continued

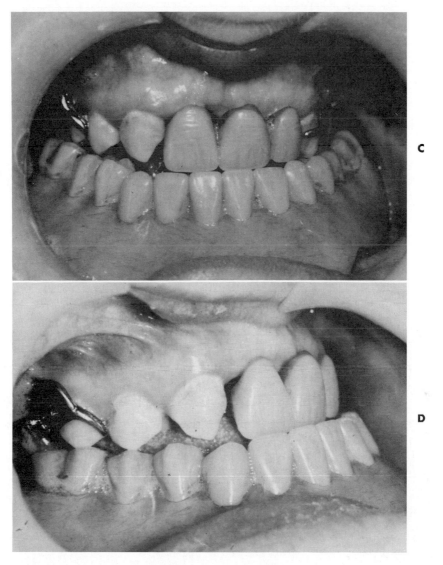

C

D

◇ Figure 14-25, cont'd

C and **D,** Preoperative photographs demonstrating poor construction of maxillary partial denture and mandibular full denture. In this case, skeletal discrepancy was too large to produce adequate occlusion with teeth placed properly over denture-bearing area. *Continued*

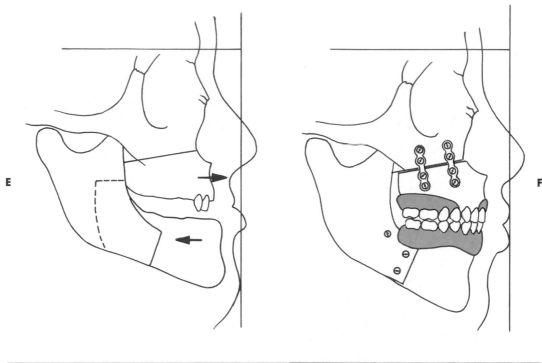

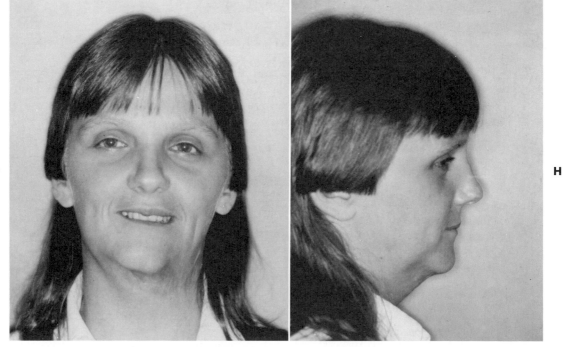

◇ Figure 14-25, cont'd

E, Diagram of preoperative condition. **F,** Diagrammatic representation of maxillary advancement and mandibular setback. **G** and **H,** Postoperative full-face and profile photographs.
Continued

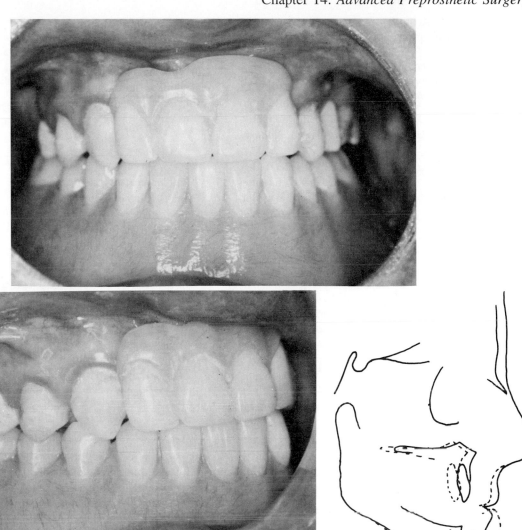

◇ **Figure 14-25, cont'd**

I and **J,** Postoperative photograph showing result after proper construction of upper partial and lower full denture. **K,** *Dashed lines,* preoperative, and *solid lines,* postoperative superimposed cephalometric tracings.

REFERENCES

1. Baker RD, Connole PW: Preprosthetic augmentation grafting: autogenous bone, *J Oral Surg* 35:541, 1977.
2. Baker RD, Terry BC, Connole PW: Long-term results of alveolar ridge augmentation, *J Oral Surg* 37:486, 1979.
3. Barsan RE, Kent JN: Hydroxyapatite reconstruction of alveolar ridge deficiency with an open mucosal flap technique, *Oral Surg* 11:113, 1985.
4. Bays RA: The pathophysiology and anatomy of edentulous bone loss. In Fonseca R, Davis W, editors: *Reconstructive preprosthetic oral and maxillofacial surgery,* Philadelphia, 1985, WB Saunders.
5. Bell WH, Proffit WR, White RP Jr: *Surgical correction of dentofacial deformities,* Philadelphia, 1980, WB Saunders.
6. Bell WH et al: Surgical correction of the atrophic alveolar ridge: a preliminary report on a new concept of treatment, *Oral Surg* 43:485, 1977.
7. Beumer J et al: Prosthodontic and surgical aspects of treatment planning for reconstructive surgery. In Fonseca R, Davis W, editors: *Reconstructive preprosthetic oral and maxillofacial surgery,* Philadelphia, 1985, WB Saunders.
8. Buser D et al: Localized ridge augmentation using guided bone regeneration. I. Surgical procedure in the maxilla, *Int J Periodont Restor Dent* 13:29, 1993.
9. Clark HB Jr: Deepening of the labial sulcus by mucosa flap advancement: report of a case, *J Oral Surg* 11:165, 1953.

10. Curtis T, Ware W: Autogenous bone graft procedures for atrophic edentulous mandibles, *J Prosthet Dent* 38:366, 1977.
11. Dahlin C et al: Generation of new bone around titanium implants using a membrane technique: an experimental study in rabbits, *Int J Oral Maxillofac Impl* 4:19, 1989.
12. Davis WH, Delo RI, Weiner JR: Transoral bone graft for atrophy of the mandible, *J Oral Surg* 28:760, 1970.
13. Fonseca RJ et al: Osseous reconstruction of edentulous bone loss. In Fonseca R, Davis W, editors: *Reconstructive preprosthetic oral and maxillofacial surgery*, Philadelphia, 1985, WB Saunders.
14. Frost DE et al: Mandibular interpositional and onlay bone grafting for treatment of mandibular bony deficiency in the edentulous patient, *J Oral Maxillofac Surg* 40:353, 1982.
15. Hall HD, O'Steen AN: Free grafts of palatal mucosa in mandibular vestibuloplasty, *J Oral Surg* 28:565, 1970.
16. Harle F: Visor osteotomy to increase the absolute height of the atrophied mandible: a preliminary report, *J Maxillofac Surg* 3:257, 1975.
17. Harle F, Kreusch TH: Augmentation of the alveolar ridge area with hydroxyapatite in a vicryl tube, Second International Congress on Preprosthetic Surgery, May 14-16, 1987, Palm Springs, Calif (abstract).
18. Hillerup S: Preprosthetic vestibular sulcus extension by the operation of Edlan and Mejchar. I. A 2-year follow-up study, *Int J Oral Surg* 8:333, 1979.
19. Hillerup S: Profile changes of bone and soft tissue following vestibular sulcus extension by the operation of Edlan and Mejchar. II. A 2-year follow-up study, *Int J Oral Surg* 8:340, 1979.
20. Kazanjian VH: Surgical operations as related to satisfactory dentures, *Dent Cosmos* 66:387, 1924.
21. Keithley JL, Gamble JW: The lip switch: a modification of Kazanjian's labial vestibuloplasty, *J Oral Surg* 36:701, 1978.
22. Kent JN, Jarcho M: Reconstruction of the alveolar ridge with hydroxyapatite. In Fonseca R, Davis W, editors: *Reconstructive preprosthetic oral and maxillofacial surgery*, Philadelphia, 1985, WB Saunders.
23. Kent JN et al: Alveolar ridge augmentation using nonresorbable hydroxyapatite with or without autogenous cancellous bone, *J Oral Maxillofac Surg* 41:629, 1983.
24. MacIntosh RB, Obwegeser HL: Preprosthetic surgery: a scheme for its effective employment, *J Oral Surg* 25:397, 1967.
25. Mercier P, Lafontant R: Residual alveolar ridge atrophy: classification and influence of facial morphology, *J Prosthet Dent* 41:90, 1979.
26. Nyman S et al: New attachment following surgical treatment of human periodontal disease, *J Clin Periodont* 9:290, 1982.
27. Obwegeser H: Die Submukose Vestibulumplastik, *Dtsch Zahnaerztl Z* 14:629, 1959.
28. Obwegeser HL: Surgical preparation of the maxilla for prosthesis, *J Oral Surg* 22:127, 1964.
29. Peterson LJ, Slade EW: Mandibular ridge augmentation by a modified visor osteotomy: preliminary report, *J Oral Surg* 35:999, 1977.
30. Sanders B, Cox R: Inferior border rib grafting for augmentation of the atrophic edentulous mandible, *J Oral Surg* 34:897, 1976.
31. Tallgren A: Continuing reduction of residual alveolar ridges in complete denture wearers: mixed longitudinal study covering twenty-five years, *J Prosthet Dent* 27:120, 1972.
32. Terry BC, Albright JE, Baker RD: Alveolar ridge augmentation in the edentulous maxilla with use of autogenous ribs, *J Oral Surg* 32:429, 1974.
33. Terry BC: Subperiosteal onlay grafts. In Stoelinga PJW, editor: *Proceedings Consensus Conference: Eighth International Conference on Oral Surgery*, Chicago, 1984, Quintessence.
34. Thoma KH, Holland DJ: Atrophy of the mandible, *Oral Surg* 4:1477, 1951.
35. Trauner R: Alveoloplasty with ridge extensions on the lingual side of the lower jaw to solve the problem of a lower dental prosthesis, *Oral Surg* 5:340, 1952.
36. Whittkamph AR: Augmentation of the maxillary alveolar ridge with hydroxyapatite in fibrin glue, *J Oral Maxillofac Surg* 46:1019, 1988.

CONTEMPORARY IMPLANT DENTISTRY

EDWIN A. MCGLUMPHY AND PETER E. LARSEN

CHAPTER OUTLINE

The dental professional must employ considerable clinical skill to help patients cope with the effects of partial or complete edentulism. Dental problems that were historically the most difficult can be solved today with the assistance of dental implants. Completely edentulous patients now enjoy the security and function of fixed restorations (Figure 15-1). Patients missing a posterior abutment, who would ordinarily require a distal extension removable partial denture, may now enjoy the benefits of a fixed restoration with dental implants (Figure 15-2). Trauma victims who are missing teeth and bone can be successfully rehabilitated with fixed restorations (Figure 15-3). Even the patient missing only a single tooth can receive a restoration more analogous to his missing natural tooth (Figure 15-4). Likewise, a patient with the available bone can receive a complete fixed implant rehabilitation (Figure 15-5). These examples illustrate advantageous and predictable alternatives to edentulism that are becoming the standard of care within the dental community.

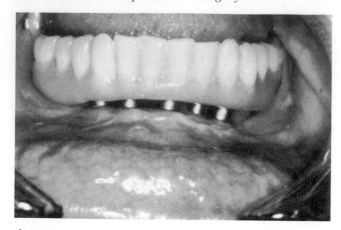

Figure 15-1

Complete-arch implant restoration supported by five implants in completely edentulous patient.

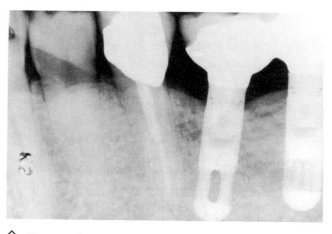

Figure 15-2

Radiograph of two-unit implant restoration used to restore dentition. Conventionally, replacement with removable partial denture would be required.

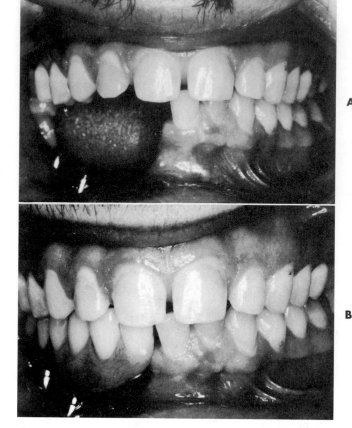

Figure 15-3

A, Twenty-six-year-old patient with large dental defect caused by shotgun wound. Three implants placed in defect. **B,** Traumatic defect restored with implant-supported hybrid restoration retained by screws.

The dental profession has not always had a positive opinion of dental implants. Implants had their beginnings around the middle of the twentieth century. Early types of dental implants came into relatively common usage during the 1960s because of patient demand, although little or no scientifically sound research had been done to characterize implant success rates.

The National Institutes of Health (NIH)-sponsored consensus development conference in 1978 sought to document the state of the art of dental implants. This conference made the first attempt to define the criteria by which the success of a dental implant could be judged (Box 15-1). However, when the consensus panel evaluated the results of research presented at the conference, it was determined that none of the available systems unequivocally met these criteria for success.[19]

In a May 1982 conference held in Toronto the North American dental profession was introduced to a body of scientific literature on Swedish research into the bone-implant interface, which is called *osseointegration*. This new concept is based on atraumatic implant placement and delayed implant loading. These factors contribute to a remarkably higher degree of implant predictably than was previously possible. The Swedish research team led by P.I. Branemark reported a 91% success in the mandible for over 15 years, which easily exceeded the criteria set by the 1978 NIH consensus conference.[2] In 1985 the American Dental Association Council on Dental Therapeutics, which had yet to approve any implant system, gave its provisional acceptance for the Branemark system. The knowledge gained from the experience of the Swedish team was also used in the development of other systems currently available on the market. Today many other systems have also been accepted by the American Dental Association.

In 1988 a second NIH consensus conference was held in Washington, D.C. This conference once again evaluated the long-term effectiveness of dental implants and this time established indications and contraindications for the various types of dental implants.[8] More stringent criteria for success were proposed and have gained general acceptance (Box 15-2). By these criteria a success rate of 85% at the end of a

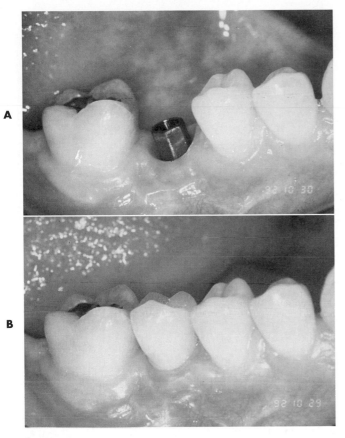

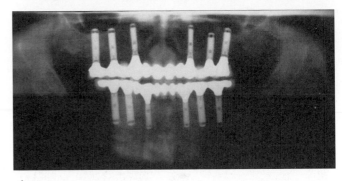

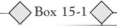

Figure 15-5

Radiograph of complete-mouth fixed implant restoration.

Figure 15-4

A, Thirty-year-old patient with missing mandibular premolar. Single dental implant has been placed in extraction site. Abutment projects through soft tissue. **B,** Single-tooth implant restored without compromising adjacent tooth structure.

◇ Box 15-1 ◇

Proposed 1978 NIH implant success criteria

1. Mobility of less than 1 mm in any direction.
2. Bone loss no greater than ⅓ of vertical height of implant.
3. Gingival inflammation amenable to treatment; absence of symptoms and infection; absence of damage to adjacent teeth; absence of paresthesia and anesthesia or violation of the mandibular canal, maxillary sinus, or floor of the nasal passage.
4. To be considered successful, the dental implant should provide functional service for 5 years and 75% of the cases.

From Adel R et al: A 15-year study of osseointegrated implants in the treatment of the edentulous jaw, *Int J Oral Surg* 10:387, 1981.

5-year observation period and 80% at the end of a 10-year period are minimal levels for success.[21]

Biologic Considerations For Osseointegration ◇

The recent success of dental implants relates directly to the discovery of methods to maximize the amount of bone-implant contact. The two basic theories regarding the bone-implant interface are fibro-osseous integration and osseointegration (Figure 15-6).[19] Fibroosseous integration is described as "tissue-to-implant contact, with healthy dense collagenous tissue between the implant and the bone."[24] Collagen fibers function similarly to the periodontal ligament in natural dentition. However, the collagen fibers around the implant are oriented differently from fibers in the periodontal ligament of natural teeth. The implant fibers are usually irregular and parallel to the implant body rather than perpendicular, as are periodontal ligament fibers. Fibro-integration is seen with implant systems that may have a good initial success rate but whose success rates drop off rapidly in

◇ Box 15-2 ◇

Proposed 1989 implant success criteria

1. The individual unattached implant is immobile when tested clinically.
2. No evidence of periimplant radiolucency is present, as assessed on an undistorted radiograph.
3. The mean vertical bone loss is less than 0.02 mm annually after the first year of service.
4. No persistent pain, discomfort, or infection is attributable to the implant.
5. The implant design does not preclude placement of a crown or prosthesis with an appearance that is satisfactory to the patient and the dentist.

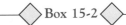

From Smith D, Zarb GA: Criteria for success for osseointegrated endosseous implants, *J Prosthet Dent* 62:567, 1989.

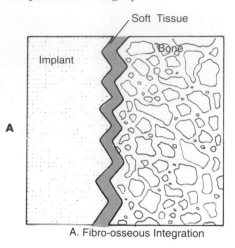
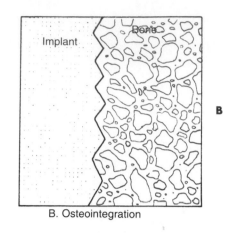

A. Fibro-osseous Integration

B. Osteointegration

◇ Figure 15-6

A, Diagrammatic representation of intervening soft tissue fibers between implant and bone, which has been termed *fibro-osseous integration*. **B,** Diagrammatic representation of direct adaptation of bone to dental implant, which has been termed *osseointegration.*

the long term. The relatively low success rates of the early root-form and blade implants were associated with the fact that the implant systems achieved fibro-osseous integration rather than osseointegration. In contrast, long-term success rates exceeding 90% have been associated with those implant systems that achieve a direct bone-to-implant interface.

Osseointegration is a histologic definition meaning "a direct connection between living bone and load-bearing endosseous implant at the light microscopic level."[2] There are four main factors necessary to achieve a successful osseointegrated bone-to-implant interface. These factors include a biocompatible material, an implant precisely adapted to the prepared bony site, atraumatic surgery to minimize tissue damage, and an immobile, undisturbed healing phase. A biocompatible material is necessary to promote healing without a foreign body rejection reaction by the host tissue. If biocompatible materials are not used, the body attempts to isolate the foreign body implant material by surrounding it with granulation and then connective tissue. It has been demonstrated that titanium and certain calcium-phosphate ceramics are both biologically inert.

The size of the gap between the implant and the bone immediately after implant placement is critical for achieving osseointegration. The gap size can be controlled primarily by the preparation of a precise surgical bed into which the implant is placed. Cylindrical preparations are the most predictably made in an accurate shape. Precision instrumentation and a technically sound surgical procedure minimize the distance between the implant and host bone.

Atraumatic surgery is required to allow minimal mechanical and thermal injury to occur. Sharp, high-quality burs that are run at low speed by high-torque drills are essential to precise atraumatic bed preparation. Copious irrigation by either internal or external methods keeps the bone temperatures to levels below 56° C, which is the level beyond which

irreversible bone damage occurs. It has been also found that bone tissue damage occurs when the bone temperature reaches 47° C for 1 to 5 minutes.[9] If the temperature rises, alkaline phosphatase within the bone is denatured, which prevents alkaline calcium synthesis. If the gap between the implant and the bone can be minimized and surgery is atraumatic, embryonic bone will rapidly be laid down between the implant and the bone and will then mature into the lamellar load-bearing bone.

It has been shown that fibrous connective tissue encapsulation will occur when an implant is loaded too soon after insertion, while a direct bone-implant interface forms when the implant is left undisturbed in the bone for a sufficient period.[5] The first month after fixture insertion is the critical period for initial healing. When loads are applied to the implants during the initial healing period, primary fixation may be destroyed. Relative motion of an implant prevents the embryonic bone from being replaced by the lamellar bone. If the direct bone-implant interface created by embryonic bone can be replaced by mature lamellar bone, osseointegration will be maintained by bone remodeling and proper loading (Figure 15-7).

Implant immobility during the healing phase is also affected by bone quality and quantity. Areas of the jaws that have a high percentage of cortical bone, such as the anterior mandible, are more likely to anchor the implant successfully. Areas of the jaws with a high percentage of cancellous bone make initial stability for the implant more difficult to achieve. It is also advantageous for initial implant stability if both the superior and inferior cortical plates can be used to stabilize the implant (Figure 15-8), which is frequently possible in the anterior mandible and the maxilla; however, the inferior alveolar canal prevents this from occurring in the posterior mandible. The minimal vertical dimension of bone for endosteal implant placement is 8 mm. It is important to leave

Osteointegration Sequence

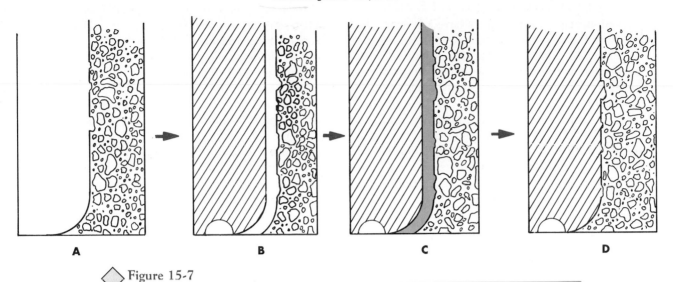

Figure 15-7

A, Implant site prepared in bone using irrigation to keep temperatures below 47° C to prevent cell death in area. **B,** Precisely machined implant placed in site. Gap between implant and bone should be less than 1 mm. **C,** If gap between implant and bone is small enough, embryonic bone will rapidly bridge gap. **D,** If implant is left undisturbed during healing phase, embryonic bone will mature to lamellar load-bearing bone.

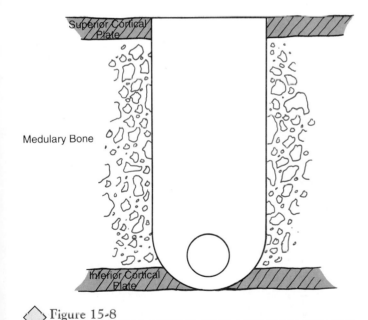

Figure 15-8

Initial implant stability can be aided if implant can engage two cortical plates of bone.

at least 2 mm of bone between the apical end of the implant and the inferior alveolar canal (Figure 15-9). Bone width is also an important consideration for successful osseointegration. Implants should have a minimum of 1 mm of bone on the buccolingual aspects of the dental implant. Therefore for a 4 mm diameter implant, 6 mm of available bone width is desirable.

Once the initial stability of the implant has been achieved, it must be maintained throughout the healing phase. Should the patient desire to continue to wear the removable prosthesis during the healing period, it is important that a soft liner be placed in the removable denture to further decrease load transfer to the implant. The bone in the mandible is generally denser than the bone in the maxilla. Therefore because the maxilla is primarily cancellous bone, osseointegration requires a longer healing period. When placing maxillary implants, it is crucial to obtain the primary stabilization for successful osseointegration.

The achievement of successful osseointegration is first assessed at the second surgery. Once the abutment is attached to the implant body, the surgeon should carefully check for any signs of clinically detectable mobility. An immobile implant at this stage indicates successful osseointegration. Detectable mobility at this stage indicates that fibrous connective tissue has encapsulated the implant. If mobility is detected, the implant should be removed at that time. The failed site is allowed to heal and another implant can be placed at a later time. Once a successful osseointegrated bone-to-implant interface has been achieved, masticatory function at least equal that of natural dentition is generally possible.

The major mechanisms for the destruction of osseointegration are similar to those of natural teeth. Disease activity in the periimplant soft tissue environment and biomechanical overload of the individual implant are the two factors most commonly associated with the potential breakdown of osseointegration.

Soft Tissue-To-Implant Interface

The successful dental implant should have an unbroken, permucosal seal between the soft tissue and the implant abutment surface. To maintain the integrity of this seal, the patient must maintain a high level of oral hygiene specific to dental implants. Clinicians, dental hygienists, and patients must understand and appreciate the necessity for a comprehensive implant maintenance program, including regularly scheduled recall visits. In the natural dentition the junctional epithelium provides a seal at the base of the gingival sulcus against the penetration of chemical and bacterial substances. It has been demonstrated that epithelial cells attach to the surface of titanium in much the same manner in which the epithelial cells attach to the surface of the natural tooth, that is, through a basal lamina and by the formation of hemidesmosomes.[13] The connection differs from that occurring with natural teeth at the connective tissue attachment level. In the natural dentition, Sharpie's fibers extend from the bundle bone of the lamina dura and insert into the cementum of the tooth root surface. Because there is no cementum or fiber insertion on the surface of an endosseous implant, the epithelial surface attachment is all important. If this seal is lost, the periodontal pocket can extend directly to the osseous structures. Therefore if the seal breaks down or is not present, the area is subject to periimplant gingival disease.

Although the abutment-to-junctional epithelium attachment is not mechanically strong, it is adequate to resist bacterial invasion, with the assistance of adequate home care. When implants are stable and they have a highly polished titanium collar transversing the tissue, gingival and periimplant health appear relatively easy to maintain. The lack of definitive gingival connective tissue attachment appears to be less of a problem in osseointegrated implants than it was in implants with fibrous connective tissue attachments. Because osseointegrated implants have a different relationship between the implant and bone, there appears to be different mechanisms working against inflammation caused by bacteria and their by-products. The pathogenicity of the bacteria seems to be particularly diminished in the completely edentulous patient restored with dental implants. Disease activity around the natural dentition in the partially edentulous patient may contribute to a slightly higher incidence of periimplant disease in these patients.

Implant survival depends on proper and timely home care and maintenance. The dentist must ensure that the patient receives thorough instruction in maintenance techniques. The goal of implant maintenance is to eradicate microbial populations. Recall visits should be scheduled at least every 3 months for the first year. The sulcular area should be débrided of calculus by using plastic or wooden scalers. Implant abutments may be polished by using a rubber cup with low abrasive polishing paste or tin oxide. Implant mobility should be evaluated and bleeding upon probing documented. Framework fit and occlusion should also be checked at recall

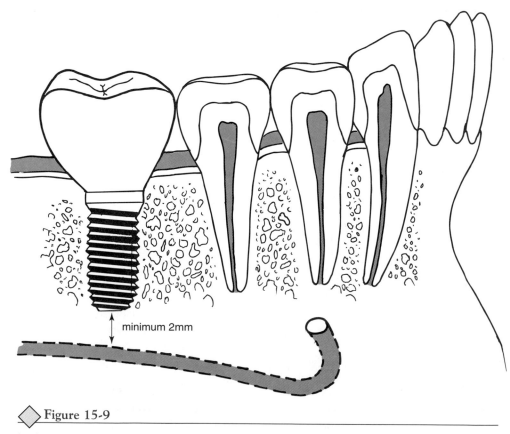

minimum 2mm

◇ **Figure 15-9**

Implants should be placed a minimum of 2 mm from inferior alveolar canal.

appointments. These biomechanical factors are as important as oral hygiene for the long-term success of the dental implant.

BIOMECHANICAL FACTORS AFFECTING LONG-TERM IMPLANT SUCCESS

Bone resorption around dental implants can be caused by premature loading or repeated overloading. Vertical or angular bone loss is usually characteristic of bone resorption caused by occlusal trauma. When pressure from traumatic occlusion is concentrated, bone resorption occurs by osteoclastic activity. In the natural dentition, bone reapposition would typically occur once the severe stress concentration is reduced or eliminated. However, in the osseointegrated implant system, after bone resorbs, it will not usually reform. Because dental implants can resist forces directed primarily in the long axis of the implant more effectively than they can resist lateral forces, lateral forces on implants should be minimized. Lateral forces in the posterior part of the mouth have higher impact and are more destructive than lateral forces in the anterior part of the mouth. When lateral forces cannot be completely eliminated from the implant prosthesis, efforts should be made to equally distribute the lateral forces over as many teeth and implants as possible.

Divergent implant placement can also increase the moment arm through which force is transferred to the bone-implant interface. Such force could potentially exceed the threshold for bone resorption. Inadequate implant distribution, which leads to excessive cantilevers, can also potentially overload individual fixtures (Figure 15-10).

Connecting a single osseointegrated implant to one natural tooth with a fixed partial denture may effectively create an excessive cantilever situation, as well. Because of the relative immobility of the osseointegrated implant compared with the functional mobility of a natural tooth, when loads are applied to the bridge, the tooth can move within the limits of its periodontal ligament. This can create stresses at the neck of the implant up to 2 times the applied load on the prosthesis

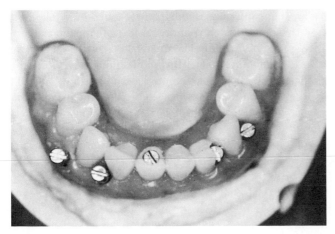

◇ **Figure 15-10**

Implants positioned outside of arch form may lead to individual fixture overload.

(Figure 15-11). Potential problems with this type of restoration are described in Box 15-3. Therefore freestanding implant restorations should be planned whenever possible.

Additionally, pathogenetic forces can be placed on implants by nonpassively fitting frameworks. If screws are tightened to close gaps between the abutment and the nonpassive framework, compressive force is placed on the interfacial bone. Excessive force of this nature can lead to implant failure (Figure 15-12).

Because osseointegrated implants feature an immobile interface between the implant and the bone, it may be necessary to incorporate some type of shock-absorbing buffer layer between the occlusal force and the implant. Occlusal collision impact force may exceed the threshold necessary to cause bone resorption. The recommended shock absorber could take the form of a specially designed element such as in the IMZ system or, as recommended in the Branemark system, acrylic resin may be used as the restoration material of choice. These recommendations are based on theoretic calculations rather than clinical data; therefore the necessity for shock-absorbing elements remains a controversial issue in implant dentistry. Many clinical problems can be avoided by joining implants to each other but not to natural teeth.

TYPES OF DENTAL IMPLANTS ────────────────◇

SUBPERIOSTEAL IMPLANTS

A subperiosteal implant is a framework specifically fabricated to fit on top of supporting areas in the mandible or maxilla under the mucoperiosteum, with permucosal extensions for support and attachment of a prosthesis (Figures 15-13 and 15-14). The technique involves an initial surgery in which flaps are reflected to expose the edentulous ridge. An impression is made of the bone at surgery, and a cast made from the impression is used to fabricate the implant framework. At the second surgery the subperiosteal implant is placed on the bony ridge, and the reflected periosteum is replaced and sutured over the framework. An implant-supported denture is fabricated to fit the intraoral projections and is retained by prosthetic clips or O-rings. Follow-up of subperiosteal implants has shown reasonable short-term success (as high as 93% over 5 years).[4] Long-term success rates often dip toward 50% as the studies approach 10 years.[1,14] Maxillary subperiosteal implants have a decidedly lower success rate than those on the mandible. Failure is usually caused by infection as a result of mobility of the implant as underlying alveolar bone resorbs. Accordingly, design changes have been made that extend the framework farther onto the lateral borders of the mandible to slow the resorption problems (Figure 15-15).

TRANSOSTEAL IMPLANTS

Transosteal implants are inserted through an extraoral incision below the chin, with a series of projections that penetrate the mandible from its inferior border and are connected by a bone

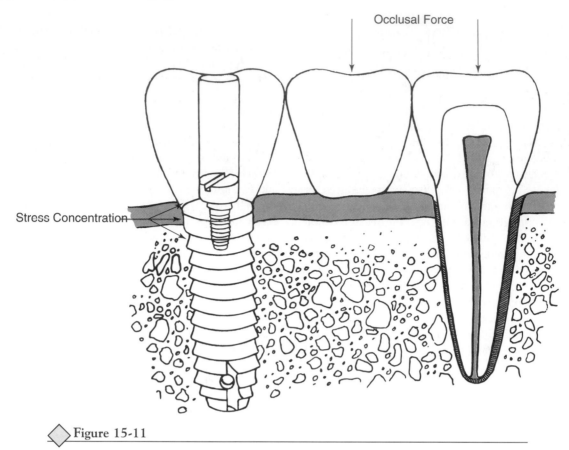

Occlusal Force

Stress Concentration

◆ Figure 15-11

When single implant is attached to natural tooth, biting forces on natural tooth and pontic cause stress to be concentrated at superior portion of implant.

─────◆ Box 15-3 ◆─────

Potential problems with tooth- and implant-supported fixed partial dentures

1. Breakdown of osseointegration
2. Cement failure on natural abutments
3. Screw or abutment loosening
4. Failure of implant prosthetic component

plate that rests on the inferior border of the mandible. Several of the projections completely transverse the mandible to enter the oral cavity and anchor the lower denture (Figures 15-13, *B* and 15-16). A series of 1437 mandibular staple bone plates has been reported in which 94% functioned well at 5 to 6 years and 87% at 10 to 15 years.[20] The transmandibular implant (TMI) has several design modifications that allow flexibility of application. Transosteal implants can only be used in the anterior mandible, and, because of the complex nature of the surgical approach, this implant modality has not enjoyed widespread popularity. The primary indication for this modality is in the very atrophic mandible in which root-form implants may further compromise the strength of the jaw.

ENDOSTEAL IMPLANTS

Endosteal implants are surgically placed within alveolar and basal bone; they are further subdivided into root-form and blade-form implants. Root-form implants are cylindrical in shape and may have an external thread. They are generally 3 to 6 mm in diameter and 8 to 20 mm in length (Figures 15-13, *C* and 15-17). Blades are wedge-shaped or rectangular in cross-section. They are generally 2.5 mm in width, 8 to 15 mm in depth, and 15 to 30 mm in length (Figures 15-13, *D* and 15-18). Endosteal implants can be used singly or in multiples. They are also categorized as *one-stage* or *two-stage*. One-stage endosteal implants are placed into the bone and project immediately through the mucosa into the oral cavity. Two-stage implants are first placed into the bone to the level of the cortical plate. The oral mucosa is then sutured over the implant and left for a prescribed healing period. The healing period depends on the quality of the bone but is usually at least 3 months and can be up to 6 to 9 months. At a second surgery the mucosa is reflected from the superior surface of the implant, and an extension collar or abutment that projects into the oral cavity is placed on the implant.

BLADE IMPLANTS.   Blade implants were the first dental implants to be used with reasonable success by many dentists. All of the original blade studies were on one-stage systems,

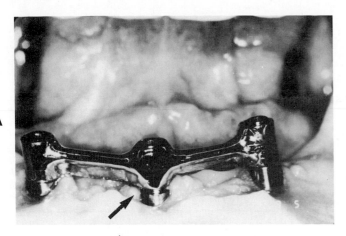
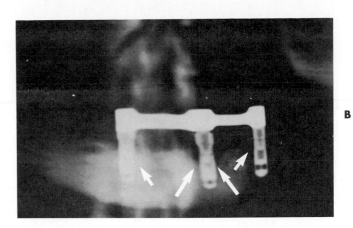

◇ Figure 15-12

A, Implant overdenture bar that does not fit passively to implant abutment (*arrow denotes gap*).
B, Stress produced by nonpassive framework can cause bone resorption at implant interface (*arrows denote bone loss*)..

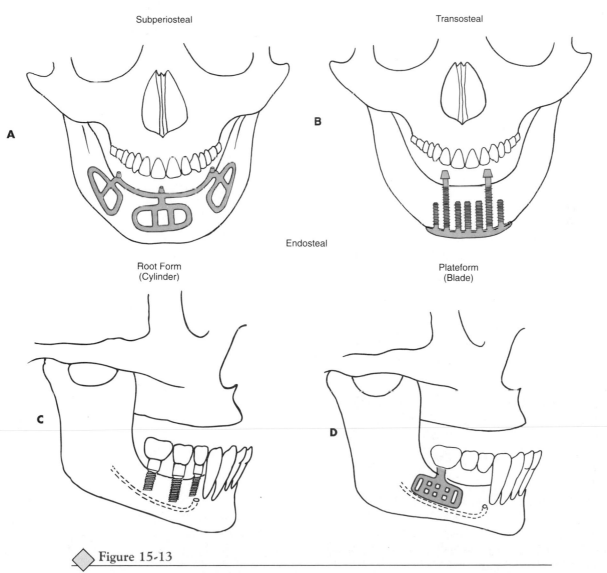

◇ Figure 15-13

Major subgroups of dental implants. **A,** Subperiosteal. **B,** Transosteal. **C,** Endosteal root-form (cylinder). **D,** Endosteal plate-form (blade).

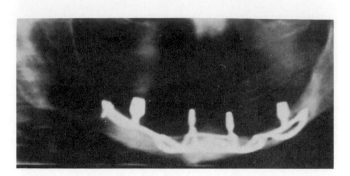

◇ **Figure 15-14**

Radiograph of one of original designs of subperiosteal implant in which force is concentrated on crest of remaining ridge.

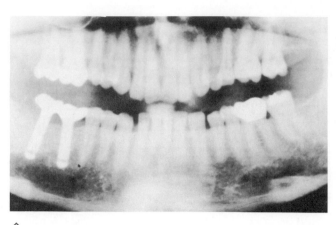

◇ **Figure 15-17**

Panoramic radiograph of root-form implants replacing teeth numbers 30 and 31.

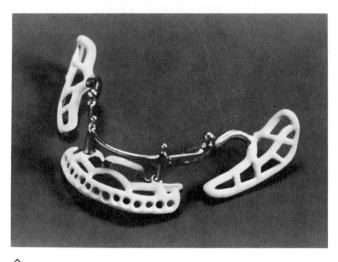

◇ **Figure 15-15**

Second-generation subperiosteal implant with framework designed to place forces more on lateral aspects of bone.

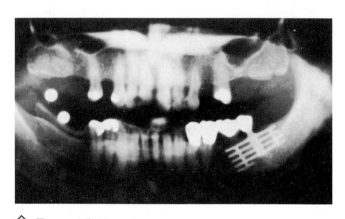

◇ **Figure 15-18**

Blade implant used to support fixed partial denture in mandibular left posterior region.

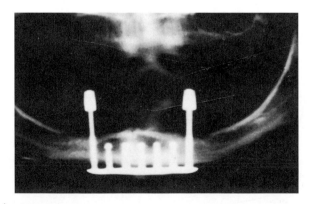

◇ **Figure 15-16**

Radiograph of transosteal implant. Two projections extend into oral cavity to anchor mandibular denture.

and success rates were well below those of current root-form systems.[6,22] It has been suggested that many of the problems of blade implants can be traced to the high temperatures at which the bone sites were prepared and to the routine immediate loading of this type of implant. Both of these practices have been linked to fibrous encapsulation, which occurs with a high percentage of blades. Accordingly, submergible titanium blades are now available. Additionally, more recent blade studies have reported success rates above 80% for 5 years.[11] The primary drawbacks to blade implants remain that it is difficult to prepare a precision slot for blade placement and that a large circumferential area of the jaw may be affected when blades fail.

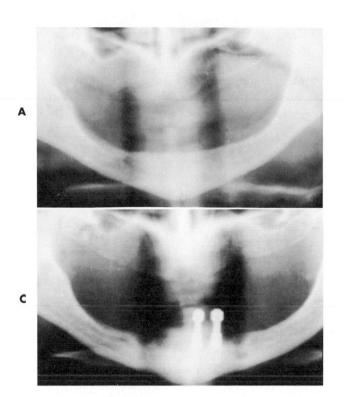
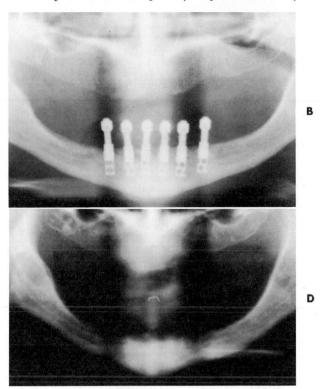

◇ Figure 15-19

A, Preoperative edentulous mandible. **B,** Six root-form implants placed in the anterior mandible. **C,** Root-form implants failed for unspecified reasons and were removed. All six implants eventually failed. **D,** Mandible after all six implants removed. Note: Vertical dimensions of mandible virtually unchanged compared with *A.*

CYLINDERS.   The history of dental implants is replete with attempts to develop a successful root-form implant. Gold, porcelain, acrylic resin, aluminum oxide, chrome cobalt, vitreous carbon, and sapphire have all been tried as root-forms, with varying degrees of success. Titanium and titanium-aluminum-vanadium alloy systems with and without hydroxyapatite (HA) coating have emerged as the systems perceived to have the best biofunctionality. Additionally, root-form implants offer the advantages of adaptability to multiple intraoral locations, uniformly precise implant site preparation, and cost of failure similar to that of tooth loss (Figure 15-19). Currently, the threaded or nonthreaded cylindrical implants of the two-stage variety enjoy the most widespread popularity.[15]

Two-stage surgical procedures with cylindrical root-form dental implants are state of the art in implant dentistry. The NIH Consensus Conference in 1988 reported that root-form implants were already 78% of the implant market.[15] The credit for this trend is given to the Branemark system, which set the precedent for the surgical techniques and restorative procedures that result in successful, predictable osseointegrated implants. It is generally believed that many of the other cylindrical implant systems will also reach this level of very high, long-term success.

CLINICAL IMPLANT COMPONENTS ————————————◇

Two-stage osseointegrated implants are generally designed to support screw-retained implant restorations. These two-stage implant systems offer many advantages over conventional dental restorations and one-stage implant systems (Box 15-4). Fabrication of screw-retained implant restorations requires the use of several component parts that heretofore had not been routinely described in conventional dental education. For the inexperienced implant clinician, the sheer number of parts within one system often creates an overwhelming obstacle to getting involved in implant dentistry. This section describes in generic terms the component parts typically necessary to restore a screw-retained, osseointegrated implant. It should be noted that the components may differ slightly in design and materials among the implant systems.

IMPLANT

The implant is the endosteal dental implant that is placed within the bone during stage I surgery. It may be either a threaded or nonthreaded cylinder. It is either titanium or titanium alloy with or without HA coating (Figure 15-20).

SEALING SCREW

A screw is placed in the implant during the healing phase following stage I surgery. This screw is usually low profile to facilitate easy suturing of the soft tissue over the implant. At stage II surgery the screw is removed and replaced with subsequent components (Figure 15-21).

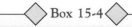

◇ Box 15-4 ◇

Advantages of two-stage osseointegrated cylinder implants

A. Surgical
   1. Documented success rate
   2. In-office procedure
   3. Adaptable to multiple intraoral locations
   4. Precise implant site preparation
   5. Reversibility in the event of implant failure

B. Prosthetic
   1. Multiple restorative options
   2. Versatility of second-stage components
      a. Angle correction
      b. Esthetics
      c. Crown contours
      d. Screw- or cement-retained restorations
   3. Retrievability in the event of prosthodontic failure

HEALING CAP

The healing cap is a dome-shaped screw that is placed after the stage II surgery and before prosthesis placement. This component may range in length from 2 mm to 10 mm and projects through the soft tissue into the oral cavity. The healing cap may screw directly into the implant or, in some systems, may screw onto the abutment immediately after stage II surgery. The cap may be made out of a resin, such as polyoxyethylene, or one of the titanium metals (Figure 15-22).

ABUTMENT

The abutment is that component of the implant system that screws directly into the implant. The abutment will eventually directly support the prosthesis. It is smooth, polished, straight-sided titanium or titanium alloy. The length may range from 1 to 10 mm (Figure 15-23).

IMPRESSION POST

The impression post facilitates the transfer of the intraoral location of the fixture or the abutment to a similar position in the laboratory cast. The impression post screws directly into the fixture or into the abutment. Once the impression post is in place an impression is made intraorally. The impression post is then removed from the mouth and joined to the laboratory analog before being transferred into the impression in the properly keyed position (Figure 15-24).

LABORATORY ANALOG

The laboratory analog is a component machined to exactly represent either the implant or the abutment in the laboratory

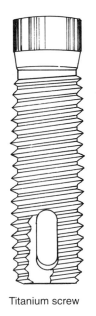
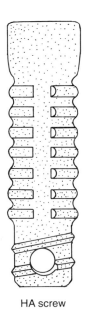
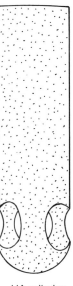
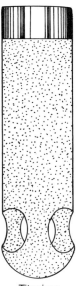

Titanium screw   HA screw   HA cylinder   Titanium plasma spray cylinder

◇ **Figure 15-20**

Four main categories of two-stage osseointegrated implants. *Left to right:* Titanium screw, hydroxyapatite (HA)-coated screw, HA-coated cylinder, titanium plasma-sprayed cylinder.

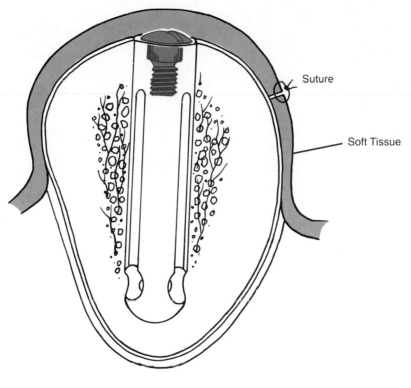

Sealing Screw

◇ **Figure 15-21**

Diagram of sealing screw in place during initial implant healing phase. Soft tissue is sutured over implant. Removable prosthesis can be worn over this area during this period.

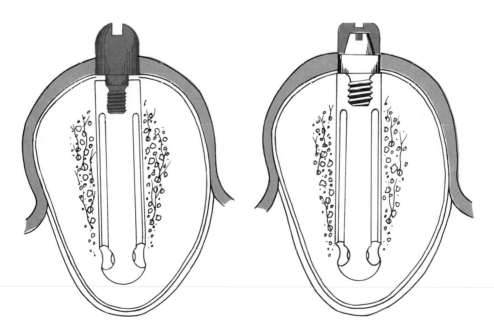

Two Types of Healing Caps

◇ **Figure 15-22**

Two types of healing caps. *Left,* Healing cap that screws directly into implant. This type may be called the *healing abutment* in some systems. *Right,* Healing cap screws into abutment. Both types allow for soft tissue healing after stage II surgery.

Abutments

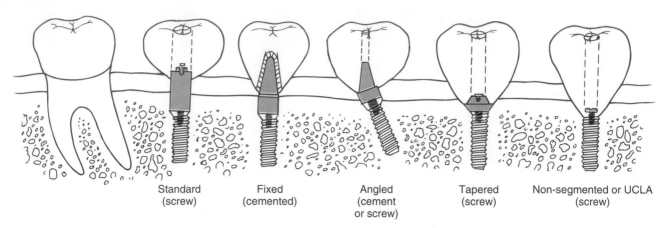

| Standard (screw) | Fixed (cemented) | Angled (cement or screw) | Tapered (screw) | Non-segmented or UCLA (screw) |

◇ **Figure 15-23**

Types of abutments (*left to right*). (1) *Standard:* Length can be selected to make margin subgingival or supergingival. (2) *Fixed:* This abutment is much like a conventional post and core. It is screwed into the implants, has a prepared finish line, and receives a cemented restoration; (3) *Angled:* Available when implant angles must be corrected for esthetic or biomechanical reasons. (4) *Tapered:* Can be used to make transition to restoration more gradual in larger teeth. (5) *Nonsegmented, or direct:* Used in areas of limited interarch distance or high esthetics demand. Restoration can be built directly on implant, so there is no intervening abutment. This direct restoration technique has been called the *UCLA abutment.*

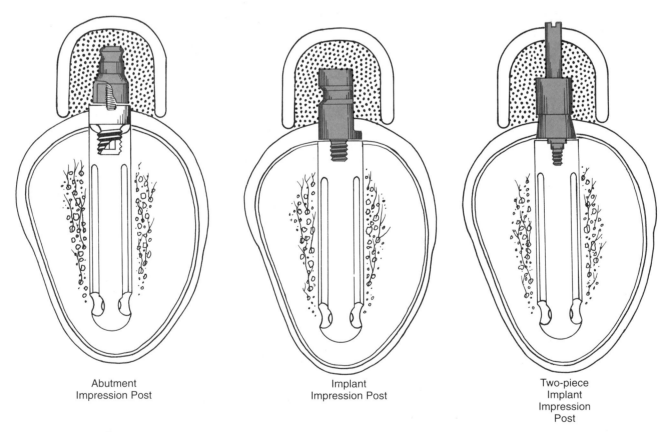

Abutment Impression Post

Implant Impression Post

Two-piece Implant Impression Post

◇ **Figure 15-24**

Types of impression posts (*left to right*). (1) *Transfer abutment post:* Used if abutment need not be changed on laboratory cast. (2) *Transfer implant post:* Used if it is desirable to change abutments on laboratory cast. This abutment should have at least one flat side to correctly orient the antirotational feature. (3) *Pickup implant impression post:* Used to orient antirotational features or to take impressions of very divergent implants.

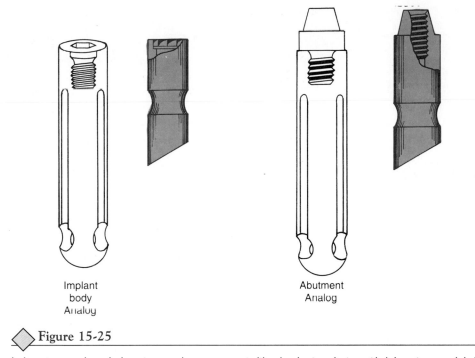

Implant
body
Analog

Abutment
Analog

◇ Figure 15-25

Laboratory analogs. Laboratory analogs represent either implant or abutment in laboratory model. *Left,*
Analog represents top of implant; *right,* analog represents top of abutment.

cast. The laboratory analog screws onto the impression post after it has been removed from the mouth and placed back into the impression before pouring (Figures 15-25 and 15-26).

Waxing Sleeve

The waxing sleeve is attached to the abutment by the prosthesis retaining screw on a laboratory model. The waxing sleeve will eventually become part of the prosthesis (Figure 15-27). It may be a plastic pattern that is "burned-out" inside the investment and replaced by a cast precious alloy, or it may be made of a precious alloy that is waxed around and "cast-to."

Prosthesis Retaining Screw

The prosthesis retaining screw penetrates the fixed restoration and secures it to the abutment. In nonsegmented restorations the screw tightens the abutment directly to the implant (Figure 15-28). The screws are tightened into place with a screwdriver. The screw can be made of titanium, titanium alloy, or gold alloy.

Implant Prosthetic Options

Completely Edentulous Patients

At least three prosthetic implant options exist for the completely edentulous patient. They include a complete implant-supported fixed rehabilitation, the all–implant-supported overdenture, and the implant- and tissue-supported overdenture.

Implant- and tissue-supported overden-ture. Completely edentulous patients have the most difficulty with the mandibular denture. Long-time denture wearers with a progressively worsening lower denture fit may derive great benefit from an implant- and tissue-supported overdenture. For this type of prosthesis, most commonly two implants are placed in the mandibular symphysis area between the mental foramina. These implants are used to retain and support the lower denture. These implants may be joined by a bar, and retention of the prosthesis is provided by a clip housed in the denture (Fig. 15-29). Implant- and tissue-supported overdentures require a very precise prosthetic technique. It is important that the retentive devices engage at the same time the posterior extensions contact the tissue and at the same time the teeth meet in occlusion. Although this option is not the answer for all patients, it provides an economic alternative for the patient who only needs additional retention and stability for a lower denture.

All–implant-supported overdenture. For those patients requiring more retention and stability for an upper and lower denture, the all–implant-supported over-denture may be the answer. For implants to support all of the load, it is recommended that a minimum of four implants be placed in the lower jaw and six implants in the upper jaw. These implants are connected by a more extensive bar design using multiple clips for retention (Figures 15-30 and 15-31). This type of prosthesis can provide the advantages of minimal tissue pressure, optimal access for hygiene, and optimal esthetics, because all metalwork is covered by the denture. In the maxilla, this prosthesis can also have the additional advantages that the palate can be removed from the denture and that all air holes can be covered, which provides the patient with a better phonetic result. The disadvantage to this prosthesis is that it is still a removable prosthesis and must be removed for cleaning and maintenance, which does not satisfy

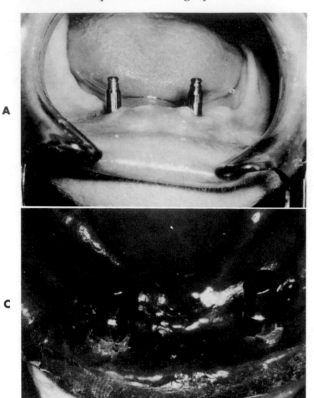

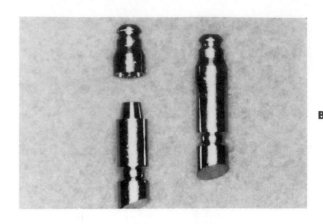

Figure 15-26

A, Impression posts screwed onto abutments intraorally. **B,** Impression post (*upper left*) unscrewed from mouth and screwed onto abutment laboratory analog (*lower left*). **C,** Laboratory analogs inverted into impression before pouring. **D,** Poured impression locating abutment analogs in cast in same position abutments were located in mouth.

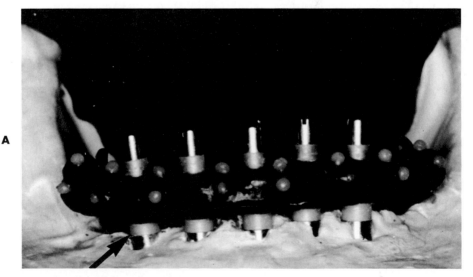

Figure 15-27

A, Five-implant framework waxed around five plastic waxing sleeves. Plastic will be "burned-out" in the investment and cast in precious alloy. Arrow denotes first plastic waxing sleeve.   *Continued*

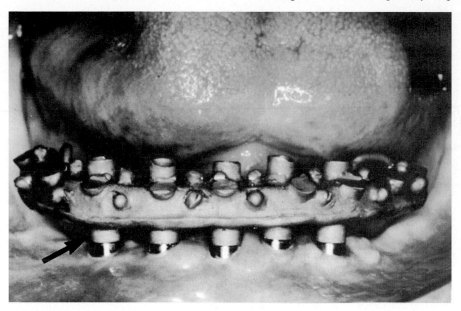

◇ Figure 15-27, cont'd

B, Five-implant framework cast in precious alloy. Note previous location of waxing sleeves.

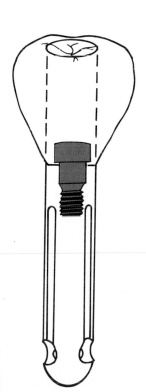
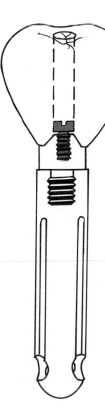

◇ Figure 15-28

Two types of prosthesis retaining screws: (*right*) crown retained on abutment, (*left*) nonsegmented crown retained to implant. The dotted lines would represent the former position of the waxing sleeve that has now become the inner wall of the screw access channel.

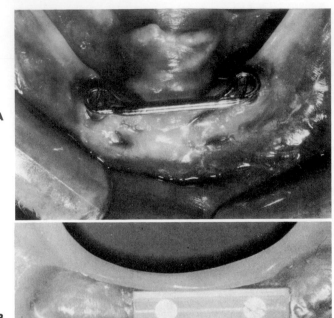

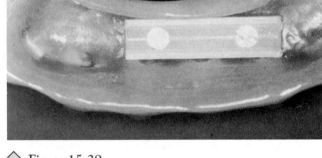

Figure 15-29

A, Two mandibular implants connected by gold bar. **B,** Plastic clip fabricated within denture and designed to snap onto single gold bar (*A*) to help support and retain denture.

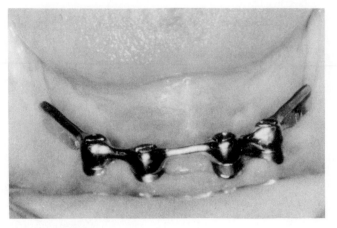

Figure 15-30

More extensive bar design with distal cantilevers joining four mandibular implants.

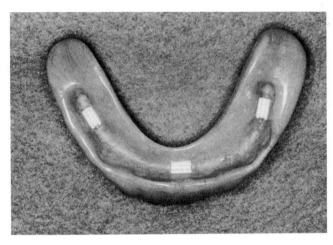

Figure 15-31

Three Hader clips in all–implant-supported overdenture.

that patient who seeks implant treatment for the psychologic benefits of having a permanently retained restoration. A further disadvantage is that clip mechanisms wear over time and must be replaced.

FIXED DETACHABLE RESTORATION. For those completely edentulous patients who require nonremovable restorations the two options are a fixed porcelain-fused-to-metal rehabilitation (Figure 15-32) or a hybrid prosthesis (Figure 15-33). The hybrid prosthesis is a cast framework with resin denture material and teeth processed to the framework. Both of these options require a minimum of 5 implants in the mandible and 6 implants in the maxilla. One major determining factor for selecting the appropriate option is the amount of bone loss. Complete-mouth fixed rehabilitation can only be made esthetically pleasing if minimal bone loss has occurred. This type of restoration is best suited for those patients who have recently lost their natural dentition. For patients who have moderate bone loss the prosthesis must replace bone and soft tissue, as well as teeth. In this case the hybrid prosthesis can best mimic soft tissue replacement. The advantages to the completely fixed restoration, either the hybrid or fixed prosthesis, is that it is completely retained by the patient at all times. Patients derive the maximal psychologic benefit by

having a restoration that is most like their natural teeth. Movement within the system is minimized, so the component parts tend to wear out less quickly. Potential disadvantages for the complete-mouth fixed rehabilitation is that implants must be very precisely placed, especially in the maxillary anterior esthetic zone, to achieve the ideal esthetic result. The relative benefit to each restorative option can be described to the edentulous patient by using Box 15-5.

PARTIALLY EDENTULOUS PATIENTS

Major advantages from implant support can be derived in the partially edentulous patient. The two main indications for implant restorations in this patient are the free-end distal extension when no terminal abutment is available and a long edentulous span. In both of these situations the conventional dental treatment plan would include a removable partial denture. In the short edentulous span, including single tooth restorations, the implant option is becoming a more popular choice. This selection is often made because natural abutments

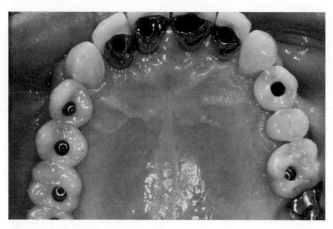

Figure 15-32

Occlusal view of porcelain-fused-to-metal implant-supported rehabilitation.

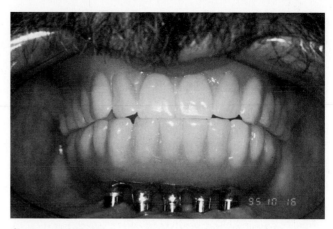

Figure 15-33

Facial view of mandibular hybrid prosthesis. This prosthesis consists of precious metal substructure with acrylic resin and denture teeth processed to it.

Box 15-5

Patient benefit scale					
0	2	4	6	8	10
No teeth	Dentures	Implant and tissue overdenture	All-implant supported overdenture	Fixed implant restoration	Natural teeth

do not have to be prepared and improved access for hygiene can be realized. If the implants are 10 mm long or less, definite consideration should be given to adding a third implant to support a three-unit fixed partial denture.

FREE-END DISTAL EXTENSION.   The implant dentist has two options in treating the patient missing terminal posterior abutments. These options include a single implant placed distal to the most posterior natural abutment and a fixed prosthesis made to connect the implant and a natural tooth abutment. Alternatively, two or more implants can be placed posterior to the most distal natural tooth, and an implant restoration can be fabricated (Figures 15-34 and 15-35).

SINGLE-TOOTH IMPLANT RESTORATIONS.   The use of single implants in restoring missing teeth is a very attractive option for the patient and the dentist. This procedure requires a careful implant placement and precise control of all prosthetic components. Single-tooth restorations supported by implants may be indicated in the following situations: (1) patients with otherwise intact dentition, (2) dentition with spaces that would be more complicated to treat with conventional fixed prosthodontics, (3) distally missing teeth when cantilevers or removable partial dentures are not indicated, and (4) patient desire for treatment that will most closely mimic the missing natural tooth. The requirements for single-tooth crown

are as follows: (1) esthetics, especially when a visible metal collar from the abutment is unacceptable; (2) antirotation to both avoid prosthetic component loosening and allow accurate transfer of angle corrections; (3) simplicity, to minimize the number of components used; (4) accessibility, so that the patient can maintain optimal oral hygiene; and (5) variability, so the clinician can easily control the height, diameter, and angulation of the implant restoration. Systems have been developed to comply with the demands of single tooth replacement. Very small teeth may be best restored with cemented crowns. Larger teeth (molars, cuspids, centrals) may be more easily restored with screw retention (Figures 15-36 and 15-37).

PREOPERATIVE MEDICAL EVALUATION OF THE IMPLANT PATIENT

As with any surgery, the implant patient must be assessed preoperatively to evaluate patient ability to tolerate the proposed procedure. The predictable risk and the expected benefit should be weighed for each patient. Surgical placement of dental implants may be associated with certain risks.

One set of concerns is the immediate surgical and anesthetic risks associated with implant placement. Because

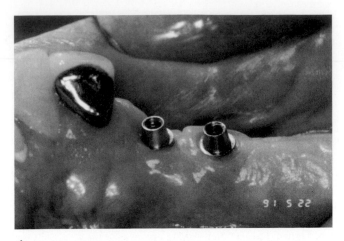

◇ **Figure 15-34**

Two implant abutments attached to implants placed distal to most posterior natural abutment.

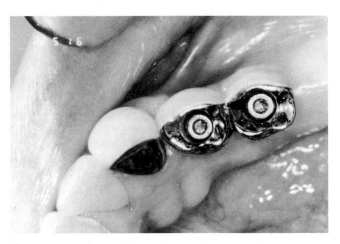

◇ **Figure 15-35**

Screw-retained prosthesis tightened to abutments with prosthesis retaining screws.

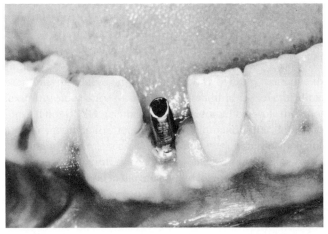

◇ **Figure 15-36**

Fixed abutment is screwed into implant and engages antirotational feature.

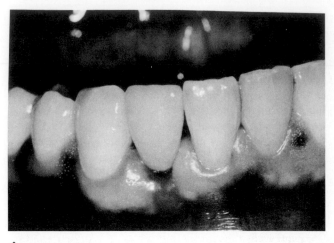

◇ **Figure 15-37**

Conventional crown is cemented over fixed implant abutment. Temporary cement can be used to maintain retrievability.

implant placement is a relatively atraumatic procedure, there is little immediate surgical risk. Absolute contraindications to implant placement on the basis of immediate surgical and anesthetic risks are limited to patients who are acutely ill, those with uncontrolled metabolic disease, and pregnant patients. These contraindications are applicable to virtually all elective surgical procedures. These conditions are also generally limited in duration, and once the illness resolves, the pregnancy is over, or the metabolic disorder controlled, the patient may become a good implant candidate. Relative contraindications may also exist. Many implant patients are elderly and have preexisting chronic systemic medical conditions, such as diabetes mellitus. The presence of a chronic medical condition is rarely a contraindication to surgical placement of implants. Each patient must be evaluated for anesthesia and surgery in light of the preexisting disease process, as discussed in Chapter 2.

Local and systemic conditions that threaten long-term retention of the implants must be evaluated. Implants may be contraindicated in patients with abnormal bone metabolism, poor oral hygiene, and previous radiation to the implant site. Studies are presently underway investigating the survival of implants placed in irradiated jaws, and protocols may be developed to allow implant placement in this group of patients.

Although osteoporosis is prevalent in the geriatric female population, there is no documented decrease in the success of implants in these patients. Other metabolic bone disorders, including osteopetrosis, fibrous dysplasia, chronic diffuse sclerosing osteomyelitis, and florid osseous dysplasia, may contraindicate implant placement.

Most patients who present for implant placement became edentulous from caries and periodontal disease resulting from poor oral hygiene. Suspicion that inadequate hygiene is likely to continue is a relative contraindication to implant placement. Patients must be motivated and educated in oral hygienic techniques as part of their preparation for implants. Some patients may not be able to improve their hygiene, such as those suffering from paralysis of the arms, debilitating arthritis, cerebral palsy, and severe mental retardation. Implants are contraindicated in these patients, unless adequate hygiene will be provided by caregivers. A summary of contraindications to implant placement is presented in Box 15-6.

Lastly, several previous authors have recommended extensive diagnostic laboratory testing as part of patient evaluation for implant placement. Blood indices and chemistry and even urinalysis have been recommended. Rather than generically recommending laboratory testing, a rational approach is preferred; that is, no laboratory tests are generally indicated unless dictated by specific underlying medical conditions for which laboratory testing will assist in safe patient management.

SURGICAL PHASE: TREATMENT PLANNING

Clinical and radiographic evaluation of the planned implant site is essential to treatment planning, to determine whether there is adequate bone and to evaluate the proximity of anatomic structures that may interfere with implant placement. The combined surgical and restorative plan and feasible nonimplant alternatives are then presented to the patient so that he or she can make an informed decision whether to proceed with treatment.

EVALUATION OF THE IMPLANT SITE

Evaluation of the planned site begins with a thorough clinical examination. Visual inspection and palpation will allow the detection of flabby excess tissue, narrow bony ridges, and sharp underlying ridges and undercuts that may limit implant placement. Clinical inspection alone may not be adequate if the thick overlying soft tissue is dense, immobile, fibrous tissue (Figure 15-38).

Radiographic evaluation is also necessary, with the best initial film being a panoramic radiograph. Because variations in magnification from 5% to 35% may occur (Figure 15-39), a small radiopaque reference object of known size placed at the area of the proposed implant placement allows correction for any magnification. A ball bearing placed in wax on a denture baseplate or within polyvinylsiloxane putty adapted to the ridge works well (Figure 15-40).

Bone width not revealed on panoramic films can be evaluated in the anterior maxilla and mandible with a lateral cephalometric film. Width of the posterior mandible and maxilla are primarily determined by clinical examination. Specialized computerized tomograms (CT scans) are useful to determine the location of the inferior alveolar canal and maxillary sinus. However, the high expense contraindicates their routine use.

◇ Box 15-6 ◇

Contraindications to implant placement (NIH Consensus Conference)

Acute illness
Terminal illness
Pregnancy
Uncontrolled metabolic disease
Tumoricidal radiation to the implant site
Unrealistic expectations
Improper motivation
Lack of operator experience
Unable to prosthodontically restore

From Dental implants. *NIH Consensus Development Conference Statement*, US Department of Health and Human Services 7(3):108, 1988.

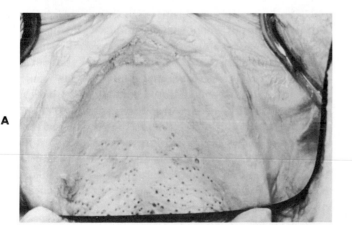 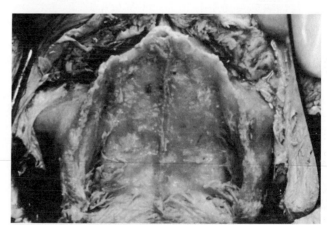

◇ Figure 15-38

A, Cadaver specimen of edentulous maxilla that appears to have adequately wide ridge. **B,** Same specimen with soft tissue removed. Note very thin and knife edge ridge that is present, which was not evident from clinical examination.

When the radiographic and clinical examination results are equivocal and further information is required, sounding of the bone with a probe can be done. Under local anesthesia a periodontal probe is used to judge the soft tissue thickness at the planned implant sites by simply pushing the probe through the tissue until it contacts bone.

BONE HEIGHT, WIDTH, AND ANATOMIC LIMITATIONS

To maximize the chance for success, there must be adequate bone width to allow 1 mm of bone on the lingual aspect and 0.5 mm on the facial aspect of the implant. There should also be adequate space between the implants. The minimal distance between implants varies slightly among implant systems, but is generally accepted as 3 mm. This minimal space is necessary to ensure bone viability between the implants and to allow adequate oral hygiene once the restorative dentistry is complete.

Specific limitations as a result of anatomic variations between different areas of the jaws must also be considered. Implant length, diameter, proximity to adjacent structures, and time required to achieve integration varies in areas within the jaws. The anterior maxilla, posterior maxilla, anterior mandible, and posterior mandible each require special consideration when placing implants. Some common guidelines for implant placement are summarized in Table 15-1.

After tooth loss, resorption of the ridge follows a pattern that results in crestal bone thinning and change in angulation of the residual ridge (Figure 15-41), which is most often a problem in the anterior mandible and maxilla. The altered

anatomy of the residual ridge may lead to intraoperative problems of achieving ideal implant angulation or lack of adequate bone along the labial aspect of the implant. Techniques for intraoperative management of these problems are discussed later, but the potential for such problems must be anticipated in the preoperative phase to allow adequate management should they arise.

The anterior maxilla must be evaluated for proximity of the nasal cavity. A minimum of 1 mm of bone should be left between the apical end of the implant and the nasal cavity. The incisive foramen may be located near the residual ridge as a

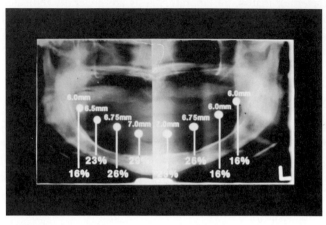

◇ **Figure 15-39**

Panoramic radiograph with standard-sized steel ball bearings placed along ridge. Magnification varies from 5% to 35%.

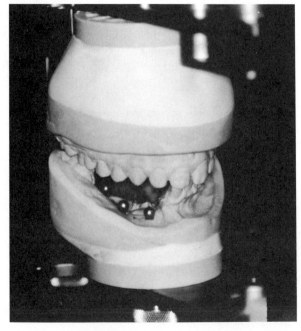

◇ **Figure 15-40**

A, Steel ball bearings of known diameter are placed on cast at points at which implants are to be placed. **B,** Polyvinylsilaoxane impression material is placed over bearings. This can be carried to mouth and used to produce a radiograph with ball bearings as a standard to calculate effect of magnification.

result of resorption of anterior maxillary bone. This is especially true in patients in whom the edentulous maxilla has been allowed to function against natural mandibular anterior dentition. Anterior maxillary implants should be located slightly off midline on either side of the incisive foramen.

Implant placement in the posterior maxilla poses two specific concerns. First, the *quality* of the bone in the maxilla, particularly the posterior maxilla, is poorer than mandibular bone. There are larger marrow spaces and thinner, less dense cortical bone that affect treatment planning, because increased time must be allowed for integration of implants. Generally, a minimum of 6 months is necessary for adequate integration of implants placed in the maxilla (Table 15-2).

The second concern is that the maxillary sinus is in close proximity to the edentulous ridge in the posterior maxilla. Frequently, as a result of resorption of bone and increased

pneumatization of the sinus, there are only a few millimeters of bone between the ridge and the sinus (Figure 15-42). In treatment planning of implants in the posterior maxilla, the surgeon should plan to leave 1 mm of bone between the floor of the sinus and the implant. This allows the implant to be anchored apically into the cortical bone of the sinus floor. Adequate bone height for implant stability can usually be found in the area between the nasal cavity and maxillary sinus (Figure 15-43). If inadequate bone exists for implant placement and support, bony augmentation through the sinus may be performed.

The posterior mandible poses some limitations on implant placement. The inferior alveolar nerve traverses the mandibular body in this region. Treatment planning of implant length

Table 15-1. Anatomic limitations to implant placement

Structure	Minimum required distance between the implant and the indicated structure
Buccal plate	0.5 mm
Lingual plate	1 mm
Maxillary sinus	1 mm
Nasal cavity	1 mm
Incisive canal	Avoid midline maxilla
Interimplant distance	3 mm between outer edge of implants
Inferior alveolar canal	2 mm from superior aspect of bony canal
Mental nerve	5 mm from anterior or bony foramen
Inferior border	1 mm
Adjacent natural tooth	0.5 mm

Table 15-2. Minimum integration times

Region of implant placement	Minimum integration time
Anterior mandible	3 months
Posterior mandible	4 months
Anterior maxilla	6 months
Posterior maxilla	6 months
Into bone graft	6-9 months

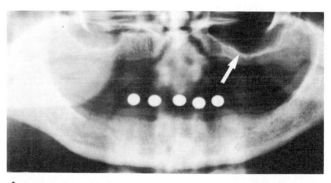

Figure 15-42

Radiograph illustrating how pneumatization of maxillary sinus and crestal bone loss together produce residual ridge that is not capable of supporting implant (*arrow*).

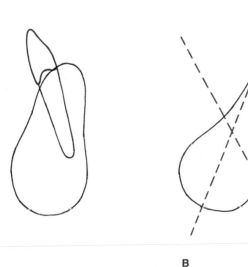

B   A

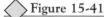

Figure 15-41

Following tooth loss, angulation of bony ridge changes as resorption occurs. Tooth had labial inclination (*line a*) at time of extraction, and remaining bone will best support implant at significantly different angulation (*line b*). Care must be taken in treatment planning to assess importance of this type of resorption on implant placement.

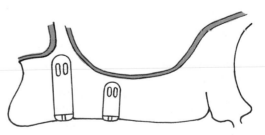

Figure 15-43

Implants should be placed so that there is a minimum of 1 mm between apical end of implant and sinus floor. Septum of bone between nasal cavity and sinus is excellent area for implant placement.

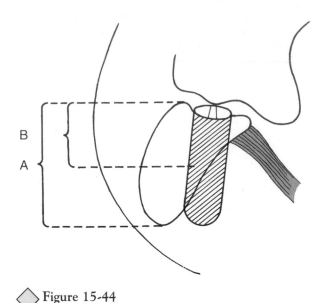

Figure 15-44

Mylohyoid muscle will maintain bone along its attachment on medial of mandibular body. There is frequently a significant depression just below this, and, if implant position and angulation do not compensate, lingual perforation may result. **A,** Apparent bone height on radiograph; **B,** actual height in desired area.

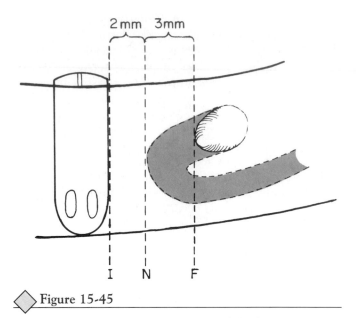

Figure 15-45

Most anterior extent of bony mental foramen (*F*) is frequently located posterior to most anterior extent of mental nerve before its exit from bone (*N*). Most posterior aspect of implant (*I*) should be placed a minimum of 2 mm from nerve. This means that implant must be placed 5 mm anterior to most anterior aspect of bony mental foramen.

must allow for a 2-mm margin from the apical end of the implant to the superior aspect of the inferior alveolar canal, which is an inviolable guideline to avoid damaging the inferior alveolar nerve and causing numbness of the lower lip. If inadequate length is present for even the shortest available implant, nerve repositioning or a conventional non–implant-borne prosthesis can be considered.

Implants placed in the posterior mandible are usually shorter, do not engage cortical bone inferiorly, and must support increased biomechanical occlusal force once loaded. As a result, slightly increased time for integration may be beneficial. Additionally, if short implants (8 to 10 mm) are used, it is advisable to "overengineer," and place more implants than usual, to withstand the occlusal load.

The width of the residual ridge must also be carefully evaluated in the posterior mandible. Attachment of the mylohyoid muscle may maintain bony width along the superior aspect of the ridge while a deep lingual depression forms immediately below (Figure 15-44). This area should be palpated at the time of evaluation and visualized at surgery.

The anterior mandible is usually the most straightforward area for treatment planning, with respect to anatomic limitations. The mandible is usually wide enough and tall enough to provide adequate bone for implant placement. The bone quality is usually excellent, which makes this the area of the jaw that requires the least time for integration to occur. When possible, the implant should be placed through the entire mandible to engage the cortex of the inferior border with the apical end of the implant. In the premolar area, care must be taken to ensure that the implant is placed anterior to the mental foramen. The inferior alveolar nerve usually courses anterior

to the mental foramen before turning posteriorly and superiorly to exit the mental foramen. Because the nerve may be as much as 3 mm anterior to the foramen, the most posterior extent of the implant should be a minimum of 5 mm anterior to the mental foramen (Figure 15-45).

INFORMED CONSENT

Once adequate information is obtained to allow formulation of a treatment plan, informed consent is obtained before surgery. This step is best accomplished using a team approach involving the surgeon and the restorative dentist. Models of various implant-supported protheses can be used to demonstrate the proposed treatment. The patient should be informed regarding the timing of surgery, the necessity of two surgical procedures, and the expected time between the initial surgery and the delivery of the finished prosthesis. The patient should also be informed concerning the necessity to leave existing dentures out and the length of time this would be necessary. The patient should be informed about potential short- and long-term risks, such as nerve injury, infection, and implant failure. Alternative treatment options, including conventional dentures or bridges, should be presented. Finally, a clear understanding of the expected cost of the proposed treatment should be reached. After this information is discussed, the patient should then sign a written informed consent document.

SURGICAL GUIDE TEMPLATE

The coordination of the surgical and prosthetic procedures through proper treatment planning is one of the most critical factors in obtaining an ideal esthetic and functional result for the implant restoration. The surgical guide template is a

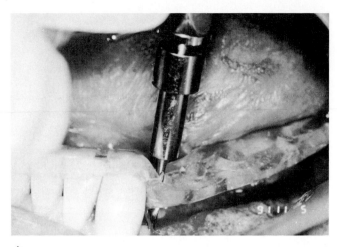

◇ Figure 15-46

Posterior surgical template used to align drill path of insertion. Individual embrasure spaces are delineated by template.

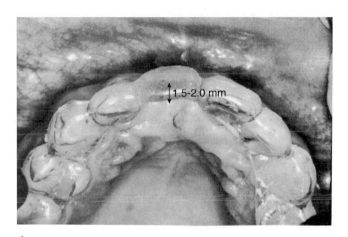

1.5-2.0 mm

◇ Figure 15-47

Anterior surgical template. Thickness should equal that of porcelain on final restoration. Distance from facial of tooth to be restored and lingual extent of template should be approximately 2 mm (*arrow*).

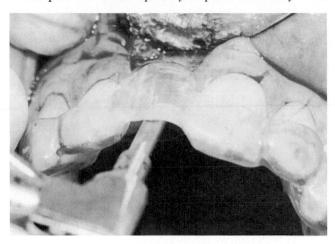

◇ Figure 15-48

With final-dimension drill, surgeon should stay as close to surgical template as possible.

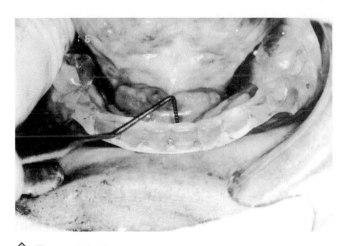

◇ Figure 15-49

Completed edentulous surgical template used to delineated arch form and facial tooth location.

critical factor for implants placed in an esthetic area, because even slight variations of angulation can have large effects on the appearance of the final restoration. The construction of the surgical guide template is nearly indispensable for those patients for whom it is necessary to optimize implant placement to ensure correct emergence profiles in the anterior esthetic zone. The objectives of using a surgical template for the partially edentulous patient are as follows: (1) delineate embrasure, (2) locate implant within tooth contour, (3) align implants with long access of completed restoration, and (4) identify level of CEJ or tooth emergence from the soft tissue (Figure 15-46). The template most useful in the anterior esthetic zone is a clear resin template, which allows a surgeon ease of access to the bone and uninterrupted visual confirmation of frontal and sagittal angulations (Figure 15-47). The surgeon stays as close as possible to the template during implant placement (Figure 15-48). The ultimate result should

allow the surgeon to place the implant optimally in bone while maintaining the angulation that will provide the least compromise of the final restoration.

In posterior edentulous areas a similar template is fabricated with directional holes drilled through the template. This type of surgical template provides the surgeon with a guide to accurately locate the implant placement and direct the long-access inclination of the implant (see Figure 15-46).

The surgical template for the completely edentulous mandible should allow the surgeon maximal flexibility to select the implant position in the resorbed bone but yet provide guidance as to the angulation requirements of the restorative dentist. A template with a labial flange that simulates the labial surface of the anticipated position of the denture teeth but that is cut out on the lingual aspect satisfies these two requirements (Figure 15-49). The surgeon places the implants within the arch form, as close to the surgical template as possible. This technique prevents the placement of the implants too far lingually or labially.

Stage I Surgery: Implant Placement

Patient Preparation

Implant surgery can be performed in an ambulatory setting with local anesthesia. Such surgery requires more time than other surgical procedures, so the use of conscious sedation is beneficial. Although implant placement is less traumatic than tooth extraction, the patient will have the expectation that it will be more so. Preoperative patient education and conscious sedation both help to lessen anxiety.

Preoperative antibiotic prophylaxis is usually recommended. An oral dose of 2 g penicillin V 1 hour preoperatively or an intravenous dose of 1 million U penicillin G immediately preoperatively are both effective. Alternative medications include 1 g cefazolin IV or 300 mg clindamycin PO. No postoperative antibiotic administration is necessary.[17]

Profound local anesthesia is required for precise implant placement. In the atrophic mandible, block anesthesia, as well as infiltration anesthesia, is sometimes required to achieve this goal. Long-acting anesthetics, such as bupivacaine, are useful when long procedures are anticipated. They also aid with early postsurgical pain control.

Adequate aseptic technique minimizes the risk for postoperative infection. The patient should rinse with 15 mL of a 0.12% chlorhexidine gluconate (Peridex) for 30 seconds immediately before the start of surgery. This significantly reduces the oral microbial count and maintains a reduced level for an hour or more.[23] A perioral facial preparation using an iodine- or chlorhexidine-based antiseptic solution may be useful. The field is then isolated with sterile towels. The surgeon and assistants should follow sound sterile techniques using masks, sterile gloves, and sterile instrumentation. A complete sterile surgical gown is not required.

Proper implant placement is a technically demanding procedure requiring precision. Therefore adequate visualization is critical. Carefully directed lighting and adequate retraction are both necessary. Self-retaining photographic cheek retractors are an effective aid in retracting the cheek and lips (Figure 15-50).

Soft Tissue Incision

Several types of incisions can be used to gain access to the residual ridge for implant placement. The incision should be designed to allow convenient retraction of the soft tissue for unimpeded implant placement. It should preserve or increase the quantity of attached tissue and preserve local soft tissue esthetics.

When the quantity of attached tissue is adequate and the underlying bone is expected to be of adequate width, a simple crestal incision is the incision of choice (Figure 15-51). Closure of the incision must be done carefully, because the implants lie directly beneath the incision.

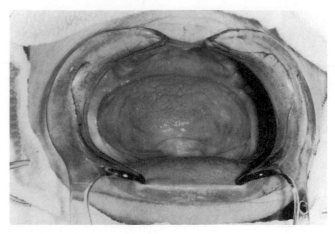

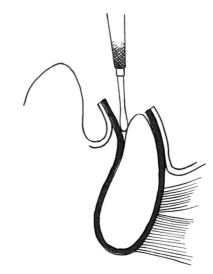

◇ **Figure 15-50**

Self-retaining photographic cheek retractors provide excellent access and soft tissue retraction.

◇ **Figure 15-51**

Crestal incision is most straightforward method of access to residual ridge for implant placement.

In the posterior mandible the incision may be placed toward the buccal aspect of the ridge to allow the flap to be retracted by the use of a tractional suture (Figure 15-52). A buccal incision has the disadvantage of placing the incision line immediately over the area where the bone may be the thinnest and where bony dehiscence may occur during surgery. An incision placed slightly palatal may be a better choice. This type of incision is particularly effective in the completely edentulous anterior maxilla (Figure 15-53).

When there has been loss of vestibular depth and of attached tissue in the edentulous mandible, periimplant soft tissue health is more likely if the tissue adjacent to the implant is nonmobile. A modification of the Kazanjian vestibuloplasty can be used to gain access to the ridge for implant placement

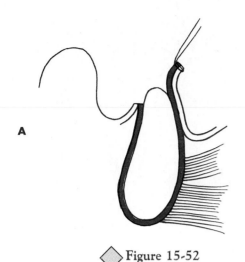

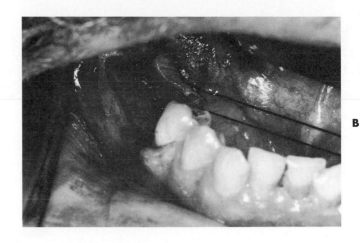

Figure 15-52

A, In posterior mandible a buccal incision avoids lingual nerve and produces excellent access for implant placement. **B,** Lingually based flap can be tied back to teeth of opposite arch to aid in retraction and access.

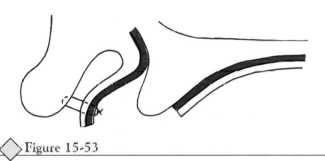

Figure 15-53

Palatal incision is very effective in anterior maxilla and when there is concern that buccal dehiscence around neck of implant may result. Flap can be sutured to lip to provide retraction.

and to increase vestibular depth and quantity of attached tissue on the residual ridge (Figure 15-54).

PREPARATION OF IMPLANT SITE

After the bone is exposed the surgical guide template is positioned, and a periodontal probe is used to make a preliminary assessment of potential implant sites (Figure 15-55). The residual ridge may have areas of unevenness or sharp ridges that are best reduced with a rongeur before implant placement.

Placement procedures for all implant systems require atraumatic preparation of the recipient site. A low-speed (1500 to 2000 rpm),[9] high-torque handpiece and copious irrigation are necessary to prevent excess thermal injury to the bone. Irrigation may be externally applied or internally directed through the drills. Recommendations of the specific implant manufacturer should be followed, because they relate to the type of irrigation and the allowable speed of the drilling equipment. Implants that are threaded require final thread preparation in the bone at very low speeds (15 rpm).

The implant recipient site is prepared by a series of gradually larger burs. All implant systems have an initial small-diameter drill that is used to mark the implant site (Figure 15-56).

The implant site is located using the surgical guide template, which may also assist in directing the angulation of the implant. With the initial drill the center of the implant recipient site is marked and the initial pilot hole is prepared. A paralleling pin is placed in the initial preparation, to check alignment and angulation (Figure 15-57).

Once the initial preparation for the implant is determined to be appropriate, it is sequentially enlarged to a dimension that precisely conforms to the dimensions of the implant. Cylindrical implant systems accomplish this with a series of progressively larger-diameter drills of the desired length. Each drill follows the path created by the previous drill.

IMPLANT PLACEMENT

After the desired depth and diameter of the recipient site is accomplished, the implant is placed. For titanium implants, an uncontaminated surface oxide layer is necessary to obtain osseointegration. Contamination by touching the implant with instruments made of a dissimilar metal or by contact with cloth, soft tissue, or even surgical gloves may affect the degree of osseointegration. HA-coated implants are also sensitive to contamination. HA is porous and will easily absorb liquids or oils and become contaminated with fibers from cloth drapes or powder from surgical gloves.

Nonthreaded implants are positioned into the recipient site and gently tapped into place with a mallet and seating instrument (Figure 15-58). Threaded implants are screwed into place, which requires an additional step to place the screw threads into the recipient-site bone (Figure 15-59). Self-tapping implants are available for use in the maxilla, where the bone is soft enough to make prethreading unnecessary.

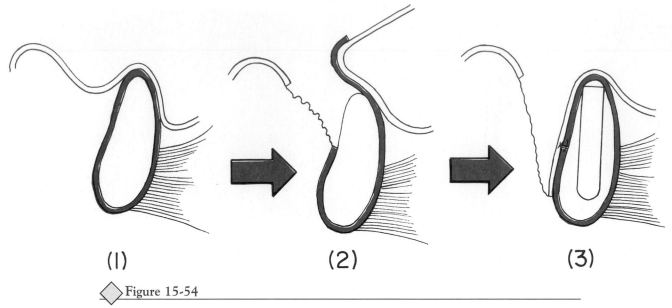

(I)   (2)   (3)

◆ **Figure 15-54**

Kazajian style of vestibuloplasty allows access for implant placement and increased vestibular depth and attached tissue, as well.

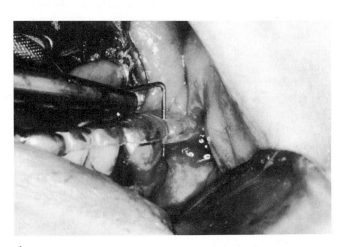

◆**Figure 15-55**

Access is gained to bone, and periodontal probe is placed through guide hole of splint and locates ideal implant position.

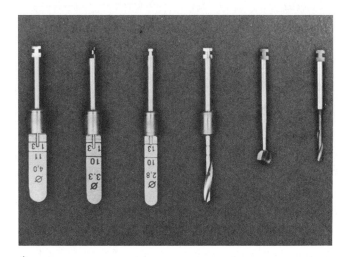

◆**Figure 15-56**

Configuration of drills differs from system to system. All cylindrical implant systems use progression of drills of increasing diameter to produce implant recipient site. Drill system shown here is part of IMZ System. *Steri-Oss, Yorba Linda, Calif.

After all implants are placed, the wound is closed. A tension-free closure is important to prevent wound dehiscence. Horizontal mattress closure with monofilament suture will produce a watertight closure.

POSTOPERATIVE CARE

A radiograph should be taken postoperatively to evaluate the position of the implant in relation to adjacent structures, such as the sinus and inferior alveolar canal, and relative to other implants.

Patients should be provided analgesics. Mild-to-moderate strength analgesics are usually sufficient. Rarely will potent oral analgesics be required. Patients should also be placed on 0.12% chlorhexidine gluconate rinses (Peridex) for 2 weeks after surgery to help keep bacterial populations at a minimum during healing. The patient is evaluated on a weekly basis until soft tissue wound healing is complete (approximately 2 to 3 weeks). If the patient wears a denture over the area of implant placement, the denture can be relined with a soft liner after 1 week and may be worn.

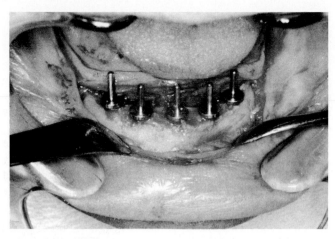

◇ Figure 15-57

Paralleling pins are placed in each hole after it is drilled and help to direct angulation of adjacent hole. This aids in producing parallelism between multiple implants.

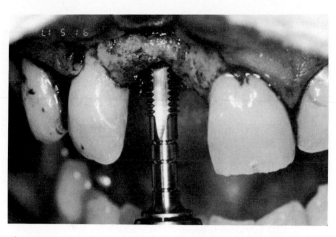

◇ Figure 15-59

Many screw type of implants require bone to be tapped to produce threads for implant to follow. This is Branemark tap being used to prepare threads for implant.

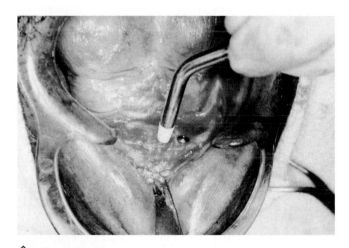

◇ Figure 15-58

Press-fit implants are driven into place with mallet and driver that is angulated to improve access and direct force along long axis of implant.

STAGE II SURGERY: IMPLANT UNCOVERING ◇

The length of time necessary to achieve integration varies from site to site and may require modification based on the individual patient. Longer times may be required if the bone quality at surgery was poor or if there was a question regarding the adequacy of bone-to-implant interface at the time of placement.

The goals of surgical uncovering are to accurately attach the abutment to the implant, preserve attached tissue, and recontour and thin tissue as necessary. This may be accomplished by one of the following three general techniques: the

tissue punch, crestal incision, or flap repositioning. Each has its own advantages and indications (Box 15-7).

The simplest method of implant uncovering is the tissue punch (Figure 15-60). This method of uncovering is easy to perform, only minimally disturbs the tissue surrounding the implant, and produces minimal patient discomfort. To use this technique, the implant must be located with certainty below the tissue. Use of the punch is contraindicated if inadequate attached tissue will remain after the punch is used. The punch also has the slight disadvantage of not allowing visualization of the bone. If a graft was placed or if there was some question regarding the relationship between the marginal bone and the implant, this technique would not allow assessment at the time of uncovering nor could nonresorbable guided tissue-regeneration membranes be removed. This technique also makes visualization of the abutment-implant body interface difficult. The operator must rely on tactile sense to determine if the abutment is completely seated on the implant body.

If the implants cannot be palpated or there is a need to visualize the marginal bone, a crestal incision over the implant is indicated. If there is sufficient attached tissue, a punch or scissors can be used to contour the edge of the flap to conform to the implant before wound closure. This technique will also heal rapidly because there is primary closure. This technique also requires adequate attached tissue.

If there is limited or inadequate attached tissue surrounding the implant, an apically repositioned flap is the uncovering method of choice. A crestal incision developed in a supraperiosteal plane is performed to develop a split-thickness flap. The flap is then sutured over the facial surface at a more apical level. Healing occurs by secondary intention. This technique requires the longest healing time and is more painful. It preserves and increases the amount of attached soft tissue. In situations in which the overlying tissue is very thick, it may be necessary to recontour tissue. Electrocautery with a

◇ Box 15-7 ◇

Indications for various uncovering techniques

Tissue punch

Requirements:

Adequate attached tissue

Implant can be palpated

Advantages:

Least traumatic

Periosteum not reflected—less bone resorption

Early impressions are possible

Disadvantages:

Sacrifice attached tissue

Unable to visualize bone

Unable to visualize implant-superstructure interface

Crestal incision

Requirements:

Adequate attached tissue

Advantages:

Does not require implants to be palpable

Easy access

Minimal trauma

Able to visualize bone

Able to visualize implant-superstructure interface

Disadvantages:

Periosteum reflected—may lead to bone loss

Apically repositioned flap

Advantages:

Improve vestibular depth, attached tissue

Disadvantages:

Longer healing time

Bone loss as a result of reflection of periosteum

Technically more difficult

---

loop attachment is quite effective. Contact of the cautery with the implant should be avoided.

After the implant is exposed the implant abutment is placed. There are two approaches to this. One approach is to place the abutment that the restorative dentist will use in the restoration. The other technique is to place a temporary healing cap that will remain until the tissue heals and will then be discarded and replaced by an abutment.

When the abutment is placed, it is important that the superstructure be completely seated on the implant body without gaps or intervening soft or hard tissue. In systems that have antirotational facets built into the implant, these must be aligned to allow complete seating of the abutment. The superstructure-implant body interface should be evaluated radiographically immediately after uncovering. If a gap is present, the superstructure must be repositioned (Figure 15-61).

COMPLICATIONS ──────◇

COMPLICATIONS OF STAGE I SURGERY

Potential complications include improper angulation or position of the implants; perforation of the inferior border, the maxillary sinus, or the inferior alveolar canal; dehiscence of the buccocortical or linguocortical plate; mandibular fracture; and soft tissue wound dehiscence.

Variation in the position or angulation of the implant results when the anatomy found at surgery requires implant placement different from that planned preoperatively. A variety of prosthodontic attachments are available to salvage implants that have nonoptional angulation.

Sinus perforation occurring during drilling for implant placement is unlikely to cause serious sequelae. Shorter implant length than planned may be necessary to prevent the implant from extending too far into the sinus. Usually, the

A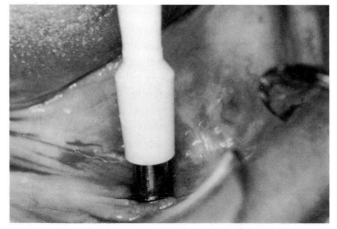

B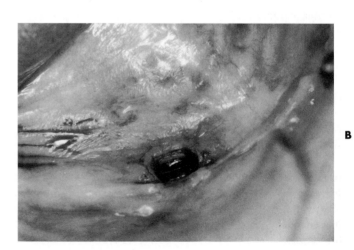

◇ Figure 15-60

A and **B,** Tissue punch removes small plug of tissue overlying implant and allows access for attachment of superstructure.

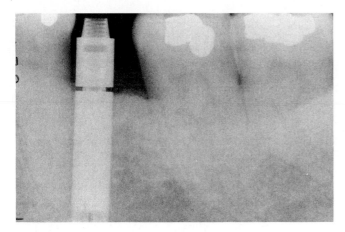

◇ Figure 15-61

Radiographs should be taken after attachment of abutments, before impressions. This radiograph shows that abutments are not properly seated on implant body, which could lead to error in fabrication of implant prosthesis if not properly seated before impression.

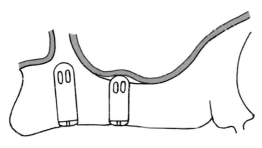

◇ Figure 15-62

If implant perforates maxillary sinus, it is unlikely that any serious sequelae will follow. Apical holes in implant body should be kept within bone and attempts made to avoid perforation of sinus membrane.

resistance provided by the cortical bone of the maxillary sinus floor is encountered before a perforation results and can serve as an indicator that maximum depth has been reached. If perforation does occur and the implant is placed only a short distance into the maxillary sinus, a problem is not likely if the retention holes in the apical end of the implant are within bone (Figure 15-62).

Similar guidelines exist for perforation of the inferior border of the mandible. The apical portion of the implant should be within the cortical bone of the inferior border.

Perforation of the inferior alveolar canal is a serious problem and requires immediate attention. If the canal is perforated at surgery, sudden increased bleeding or a sudden sharp pain may result. If this occurs, an implant shorter than planned should be used. If the implant appears to extend into the inferior alveolar canal on the postoperative radiographs (Figure 15-63), the implant should be immediately removed and a shorter implant placed. If no indication of perforation exists and no radiographic evidence of violation of the canal is noted, patients may still have postoperative neurosensory

alteration. This may be from traction on the mental nerve or from direct injury during implant placement. These patients should be followed closely. Deficits of this nature will generally resolve with time but may require surgical intervention if they persist and are bothersome to the patient.

Perforation of the buccocortical or linguocortical plates may occur when resorption has resulted in a thin ridge along the planned implant site. A simple solution is to countersink the implant until the depth of the implant recipient site is adequate for the length of the implant. This may leave excess bone height on the lingual, mesial, and distal surfaces. At the time of uncovering there may be bone growth over the implant that requires removal. If the sharp crest is generalized and several implants are to be placed, the entire crest can be reduced down to a suitable width. If a dehiscence does occur, it should be evaluated and a decision made regarding treatment. A small, 1- to 2-mm bony dehiscence on the buccal aspect of an implant will generally require no additional treatment. Larger defects, particularly if the implant is short, may compromise stability. If this results, the defect can be grafted using the principles of guided tissue regeneration (Figure 15-64).

An unusual complication of implant placement in the mandible is mandibular fracture (Figure 15-65). This is most likely when the mandible is very atrophic, when there is preexisting metabolic disease, such as osteoporosis, or when there is a history of postoperative trauma. Management may require bone grafting to increase the bone mass of the mandible.

Soft tissue wound dehiscence may occur, which allows part of the implant to become exposed. If this occurs, no attempt should be made to resuture the wound, because the only result will be increased wound dehiscence. Chlorhexidine rinses should be used until soft tissue healing has occurred. If the tissue is healthy but the implant remains exposed, a soft toothbrush dipped in chlorhexidine should be used to keep the implant clean throughout the integration period.

THE AILING OR FAILING IMPLANT

Implant failure occurs at three distinct times. A few implants will fail to integrate. This failure will be identified at the time of stage II surgery or shortly after. Failure in this period may be related to a variety of factors. Overheating of the bone during placement or failure to achieve a precise implant fit with primary stability may lead to failure of integration. Postoperative infection, excessive pressure on tissue overlying the integrating implant with movement of the implant, or wound healing problems may also jeopardize implant integration. Following loading with a prosthesis, bone loss will occur for approximately 18 months following which time a steady state will be achieved. During this 18-month period, additional implant failure may occur.[1] Failure in this period is often associated with excessive biomechanical forces on the implant or compromised periimplant soft tissue health resulting from lack of attached tissue, poor hygiene, or both. Smoking is also associated with increased failure in this period, as well as with later failures.[3] Late failure (more than

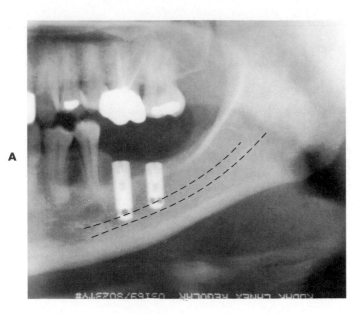
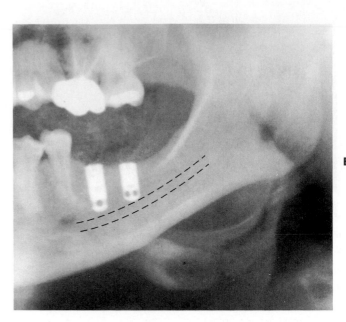

◇ **Figure 15-63**

A, Radiograph taken immediately after placement of two implants in right posterior mandible. Implants appear to violate superior border of inferior alveolar canal (*dotted line*). **B,** Implants were replaced and are above canal (*dotted line*). Patient had no permanent deficit.

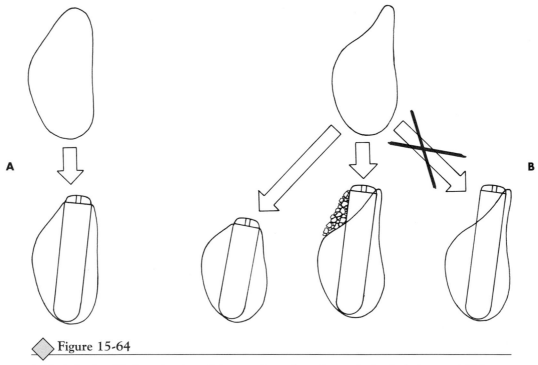

◇ **Figure 15-64**

In ideal situation (**A**), there is adequate bone on buccolingual areas for implant placement. This may not occur when there has been resorption of buccal bone (**B**). Acceptable ways to handle this include removal of sharp crest to level of adequate width for implant or placement of bone graft over buccal dehiscence that results.

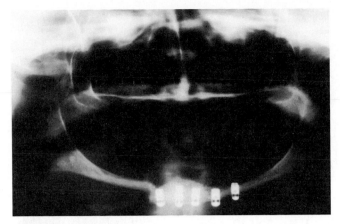

◆ **Figure 15-65**

Implants may weaken mandible and lead to fracture. This is most common in severely atrophic mandible and following trauma.

18 months following placement of the prosthesis) may also occur. This is rare, and frequently the cause is not identifiable. In general, these implants are identified as "ailing" during routine recall. Progressive bone loss in spite of rigorous hygiene measures is often seen. A combined prosthodontic and surgical intervention can often restore health to these ailing implants.

Once periimplant bone loss has been identified, efforts should initially be focused on optimizing hygiene. This may even require removal of the prosthesis to facilitate access. If bone loss is severe or progressive, surgical intervention is necessary. The implant must be exposed surgically and all soft tissue adjacent to the implant surface removed. The surface of the implant is then cleaned with hydrogen peroxide followed by citric acid. Tetracycline powder is placed along the implant surface and into the bony defect, and the defect reconstructed with a graft. Healing for a minimum of 4 months is allowed, following which the implant is uncovered and the prosthesis replaced.

ADVANCED SURGICAL TECHNIQUES ◇

GUIDED TISSUE REGENERATION

Guided tissue regeneration is a process that allows bone growth while retarding the ingrowth of fibrous connective tissue. It is well recognized that most bone defects will regenerate with new bone if the invasion of connective tissue from adjacent soft tissue can be prevented. Guided tissue regeneration uses a barrier that is placed over the bone defect and prevents fibrous tissue ingrowth while the bone underlying the barrier has time to grow and fill the defect. This technique is particularly useful in the treatment of buccal dehiscence, where labiobuccal augmentation of bone is required. Guided tissue regeneration can be performed simultaneously with implant placement or before stage I. A variety of materials may serve as barriers to fibrous tissue

ingrowth. Expanded polytetrafluoroethylene (Gore-Tex) is the most extensively tested material.[7] Resorbable materials are also now available, eliminating the necessity of removal.

POSTEXTRACTION PLACEMENT OF IMPLANTS

When implant placement is planned before extraction of the tooth, consideration should be given to the most desirable time for implant placement. The implant may be placed immediately (at the time of extraction), early (2 months following extraction), or late (more than 6 months following extraction). Each of these times has its own indications, advantages, and disadvantages.

Immediate placement allows the overall shortest healing time and combines the tooth extraction with the surgical implant placement.[12] Immediate placement can be considered if the tooth to be removed is not infected and can be removed without the loss of alveolar bone. Once the tooth is removed the implant is placed at least 4 mm apical to the apex of the tooth (Figure 15-66). The implant should be countersunk 2 mm below the height of the crestal bone to allow for resorption of the bone secondary to extraction. The gap between the implant and the residual tooth socket must be evaluated and managed according to its size. If the gap is less than 1 mm, no treatment modification is needed. If the gap is greater than 1 mm, the same type of guided tissue regeneration may be necessary.

After implant placement, every effort should be made to achieve a primary soft tissue closure. If this is not possible, a resorbable collagen pellet may be placed over the implant and held in place with a figure-eight suture. The time for integration should be extended by 1 or 2 months.

Even if the extraction site meets the requirements for immediate implant placement, it may be desirable to wait for 2 months before implant placement. During this time the overlying soft tissue will heal, and primary closure will be easier at the time of implant placement. This is generally long enough to allow remodeling of the socket and, in the case of multirooted teeth, some filling of the socket with bone. In this situation, implants are placed using the same technique described for routine implant placement. The bone in the area of surgery will be softer but generally will allow preparation of the implant recipient site with little modification. No increase in integration time is generally necessary in this situation. If teeth have been removed longer than 6 months, implant placement should proceed with no modification in technique.

MANDIBULAR ATROPHY

In the atrophic mandible (less than 8 mm of vertical height) the shortest implant may be longer than the available bone. Implants may be placed by purposefully perforating the inferior cortex. This may decrease the crown-to-root ratio or increase the risk of fracture. Recent studies have shown that following restoration of the atrophic mandible with an entirely implant-supported prosthesis, there is an increase in bone height and density, presumably as a result of the functional

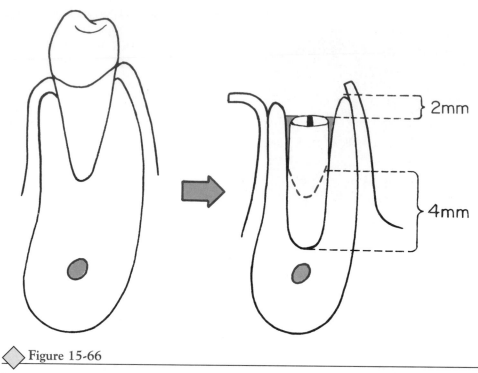

◇ Figure 15-66

Implants placed in fresh extraction sockets must have 4 mm of precise fit along apical aspect of implant. They should be countersunk 2 mm, and gap between sides of extraction socket and implant should be less than 1 mm. If gap is greater than 1 mm, grafting with demineralized allogeneic bone should be considered.

stresses that result from the prosthesis.[18] Therefore an effective approach in the atrophic mandible is to place five implants, leaving 2 to 3 mm above the height of the residual bone. An entirely implant-supported hybrid prosthesis is then fabricated. Alternatively, the transmandibular implant (TMI) has also been shown to be effective in the very atrophic mandible, with similar remodeling and formation of new bone. Either of these techniques may be considered in the atrophic mandible where there is 6 mm or more of bone height. If the bone height is less than 6 mm, augmentation of the bony height in this area with autogenous grafts may be necessary. Autogenous grafts onlayed onto the residual ridge will undergo resorption if conventional dentures are placed but are generally maintained well if an implant-borne prosthesis is placed.

TRANSANTRAL GRAFTING

Initial implant restorative approaches for the fully edentulous maxilla concentrated on implant placement in the anterior region, similar to the edentulous mandible. However, the resulting prosthesis was often unsatisfactory. If adequate space was allowed for proper hygiene, phonetics and esthetics were severely compromised. If the prosthesis was developed in such a way as to eliminate these problems, hygiene became virtually impossible. The cantilever effect of this type of prosthesis on implants placed within the compromised bone of the maxilla also resulted in increased failures. If implants are placed bilaterally in the posterior maxilla, a prosthesis with ideal esthetics, phonetics, and hygiene access can be created.

However, the bone overlying the sinus is frequently inadequate to place the implant and to allow suitable bony support. In these situations the sinus floor may be grafted to increase the quantity of bone for implant placement. Transantral grafting (sinus lift) procedures can be performed in an outpatient setting using autogenous bone or allogeneic bone. The available bone to support the implant can be significantly improved with these techniques (Figure 15-67).

NERVE REPOSITIONING

As discussed earlier the posterior mandible poses unique problems. Presence of the inferior alveolar nerve limits implant length. This, coupled with increased occlusal load, is one reason for the higher implant failure rate in this region. Overengineering with placement of more implants can improve the prognosis. When there is less than 8 mm of vertical height overlying the inferior alveolar nerve, implant success will be severely compromised. In this case, the inferior alveolar nerve may be repositioned to allow use of the entire height of the mandibular body. This procedure carries the risk of permanent anesthesia or painful dysesthesia. The advantage is that with repositioning of the nerve a longer implant can be placed, with stabilization in both the superior and inferior cortical bone.

IMPLANTS IN GROWING PATIENTS

Children may present with edentulous spaces resulting from congenital absence of teeth or loss of teeth from trauma, infection, or neoplasia. The ability to restore the lost function

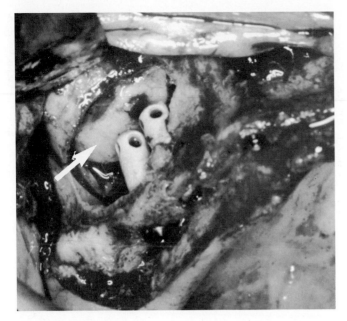

Figure 15-67

This patient had inadequate bone for implant placement without sinus perforation. Transantral graft is being performed. Bony window in lateral wall of sinus is outlined and fractured inward. Arrow points to bone that has been infractured and that will become new sinus floor.

without damage to adjacent virgin teeth that would occur from conventional restorative methods is appealing. There is evidence that implants can be successfully placed into growing patients. In the fully edentulous patient, an implant-supported prosthesis can be fabricated as soon as the patient is old enough to cooperate with hygiene requirements. This is usually defined as age 7. In patients who have lost a portion of the jaw from tumor resection or trauma, an implant-supported prosthesis can likewise be used as early as age 7. However, when the edentulous area in question is associated with unerupted natural teeth, no implants should be placed until complete eruption of the natural dentition, at approximately age 12. Implants placed before this will behave in a similar fashion to an ankylosed tooth, with progressive submersion of the implant as a result of eruption of adjacent teeth and alveolar bone growth.[16]

IMPLANTS IN IRRADIATED BONE

Cancer patients frequently suffer from surgery- and irradiation-associated soft and hard tissue defects that significantly compromise conventional prosthodontic rehabilitation. An implant-supported prosthesis could improve function and esthetics; however, concern regarding the compromised wound healing that results following tumoricidal irradiation to the jaws has contraindicated even minor surgery and implant placement in these patients. It now appears that it may be possible to place implants in this group of patients. Careful soft tissue handling and perioperative hyperbaric oxygen treatments have been used for patients receiving implants in irradiated tissue, with results comparable to that found in nonirradiated patients.[10] Little is known about the long-term

results in these patients, and there is still potential for increased failure and serious sequelae, such as osteoradionecrosis. As a result, implant placement in this group of patients should be managed by the experienced implant surgeon.

REFERENCES

1. Adel R: Long-term treatment results. In Branemark PI, Zarb G, Albrektson I, editors: *Tissue-integrated prostheses,* Chicago, 1985, Quintessence.
2. Adell R et al: A 15-year study of osseointegrated implants in the treatment of the edentulous jaw, *Int J Oral Surg* 10:387, 1981.
3. Bain CA, May PK: The association between the failure of dental implants and cigarette smoking, *Int J Oral Maxillofac Implants* 8:609, 1993.
4. Bodine RL, Yanase RF: Thirty-year report on 28 implant dentures inserted between 1952 and 1959. Presented at the International Symposium on Preprosthetic Surgery, May 16-18, 1985, Palm Springs, Calif.
5. Brunski JB et al: The influence of functional use of endosseous dental implants on the tissue implant interface. I. Histological aspects, *J Dent Res* 58:1953, 1979.
6. Cranin AN, Rabkin MF, Garfinkel L: A statistical evaluation of 952 endosteal implants in humans, *J Am Dent Assoc* 94:315, 1977.
7. Dahlin C et al: Generation of new bone around titanium implants using a membrane technique: an experimental study in rabbits, *J Oral Maxillofac Implants* 4:19, 1989.
8. Dental implants. *NIH Consensus Development Conference Statement,* US Department of Health and Human Services 7(3):108, 1988.
9. Eriksson AR, Albrektsson T: Temperature threshold levels for heat-induced bone tissue injury: a vital microscopic study in the rabbit, *J Prosthet Dent* 50:101, 1983.
10. Granstom G et al: A detailed analysis of titanium implants lost in irradiated tissue, *Int J Oral Maxillofac Implants* 9:653, 1994.
11. Kapur KK: VA cooperative dental implant study: comparisons between fixed partial dentures supported by blade-vent—1989 implants and removable partial dentures. II. Comparisons of success rates and periodontal health between two treatment modalities, *J Prosthet Dent* 6:685-702, 1989.
12. Lazzara RJ: Immediate implant placement into extraction sites: surgical and restorative advantages, *Int J Periodont Rest Dent* 9:333, 1989.
13. McKinney RV, Steflik DE, Roth DL: The biologic response to single crystal sapphire endosteal implant: SEM observations, *J Prosthet Dent* 51:372, 1984.
14. Mercier P, Cholewa J, Djokovic S: Mandibular subperiosteal implants: retrospective analysis in light of Harvard consensus, *J Can Dent Assoc* 47:46, 1981.
15. NIH Consensus Development Conference Statement on Dental Implants, June 13-15, 1988, *J Dent Educ* 12:824, 1988.
16. Perrott, DH, Shama AB, Vargerik K: Endosseous implants for pediatric patients, *Oral Maxillofac Clin N Am* 6:79, 1994.
17. Peterson LJ et al: Comparison of mandibular bone response to implant overdentures versus implant-supported hybrid, *J Dent Res* 75:333, 1996.

18. Peterson LJ et al: Long-term antibiotic prophylaxis is not necessary for placement of dental implants, *J Oral Maxillofac Surg* 54(suppl 3):76, 1996.

19. Schnitman PA, Shulman LB: Dental implants: benefits and risk, *NIH-Harvard Consensus Development Conference,* US Department of Health and Human Services 1:351, 1979.

20. Small IA: Clinical evaluation of the mandibular staple bone plate, *J Oral Maxillofac Surg* 44:60, 1986.

21. Smith D, Zarb GA: Criteria for success for osseointegrated endosseous implants, *J Prosthet Dent* 62:567, 1989.

22. Smithloff M, Fritz ME: Use of blade implants in a selected population of partially edentulous patients, *J Periodontol* 53:413, 1982.

23. Veksler AE, Kayrouz GA, Newman MG: Chlorhexidine reduces salivary bacteria during scaling and root planing, *J Dent Res* 69:240, 1990.

24. Weiss CM: Tissue integration of dental endosseous implants: description and comparative analysis of the fibro-osseous integration and osseous integration systems, *J Oral Implant* 12:169, 1986.

INFECTIONS

Odontogenic infections are usually mild and are easily treated. These infections may require only the administration of an antibiotic, may be more complex and require an incision and drainage, or may be very complicated and require that the patient be admitted to the hospital. Some infections that occur in the oral cavity are preventable if the surgeon uses appropriate antibiotic prophylaxis. This section presents the principles of infection management and infection prevention in dental patients.

Chapter 16 describes the basic management techniques, including surgery and antibiotic administration, for the treatment of odontogenic infections. It also presents the principles of antibiotic prophylaxis for prevention of both wound infection and distant metastatic infection, such as subacute bacterial endocarditis.

Chapter 17 presents an overview of complex odontogenic infections that involve fascial spaces and may require hospitalization of the patient for treatment. Osteomyelitis and other unusual infections are also discussed.

Chapter 18 presents the indications, rationale, and technical aspects of surgical endodontics. Although it is clear that periapical surgery is occasionally necessary for successful endodontic management, it is necessary for the clinician to be wise in deciding when to choose this treatment modality. Therefore the discussion of the indications and contraindications for surgical endodontic is extensive. The technical aspects of surgical endodontics are profusely illustrated.

Chapter 19 presents information about patients at risk for infection and other comprising problems that are caused by patient host-defense compromise as the result of radiotherapy or cancer chemotherapy. These patients are susceptible to a variety of problems, and the prevention and management of these problems are discussed.

Chapter 20 describes maxillary sinus problems that arise secondary to odontogenic infections and other problems. Although general practitioners rarely see these problems, they may have to diagnose them before referring the patient to the right person for definitive care.

Finally, Chapter 21 discusses salivary gland diseases, primarily the obstructive and infectious types. The major diagnostic and therapeutic modalities used in managing these problems are discussed.

CHAPTER 16

PRINCIPLES OF MANAGEMENT AND PREVENTION OF ODONTOGENIC INFECTIONS

LARRY J. PETERSON

O ne of the most difficult problems to manage in dentistry is an odontogenic infection. These infections may range from low-grade, well-localized infections that require only minimal treatment to severe, life-threatening fascial space infections. Although the overwhelming majority of odontogenic infections are easily managed by minor surgical procedures and supportive medical therapy that includes antibiotic administration, the practitioner must constantly bear in mind that these infections occasionally become severe in a very short time.

This chapter is divided into several sections. The first section discusses the typical microbiology involved in odontogenic infections. Appropriate therapy of odontogenic infections depends on a clear understanding of the causative bacteria. The second section discusses the natural history of odontogenic infections. When infections occur, they may erode through bone and into the overlying soft tissue. Knowledge of the usual pathway of infection from the teeth and surrounding tissues through the bone and into the overlying soft tissue planes is essential when planning appropriate therapy. The third section of this chapter deals with the principles of management of odontogenic infections. A series of principles are discussed, with consideration of the

microbiology and typical pathway of infection. The chapter concludes with a section on prophylaxis against infection. The prophylaxis of wound infection and of metastatic infection is discussed.

MICROBIOLOGY OF ODONTOGENIC INFECTIONS ◇

The bacteria that cause infection are most commonly part of the indigenous bacteria (that normally live on or in the host). Odontogenic infections are no exception, because the bacteria that cause odontogenic infections are those normal oral flora: those that comprise the bacteria of plaque, those found on the mucosal surfaces, and those found in the gingival sulcus. They are primarily aerobic gram-positive cocci, anaerobic gram-positive cocci, and anaerobic gram-negative rods. These bacteria cause a variety of common diseases, such as dental caries, gingivitis, and periodontitis. When these bacteria gain access to deeper underlying tissues, as through a necrotic dental pulp or through a deep periodontal pocket, they cause odontogenic infections.

Many carefully performed microbiologic studies of odontogenic infections have demonstrated the microbiologic composition of these infections. Several important factors must be noted. First, almost all odontogenic infections are caused by multiple bacteria. The polymicrobial nature of these infections makes it important that the clinician understand the variety of bacteria that are likely to cause the infection. In most odontogenic infections the laboratory can identify an average of five species of bacteria. It is not unusual for as many as eight different species to be identified in a given infection. On rare occasions a single species may be isolated.

A second important factor is the anaerobic-aerobic char-

Table 16-1. Causative organisms*

	Number of patients	Percentage
Aerobic only	28	7
Anaerobic only	133	33
Mixed	243	60

*In 404 patients; data from Aderhold L, Konthe H, Frenkel G: The bacteriology of dentogenous pyogenic infections, *Oral Surg* 52:583, 1981; Bartlett JG, O'Keefe P: The bacteriology of perimandibular space infections, *J Oral Surg* 50:130, 1980; Chow AW, Roser SM, Brady FA: Orofacial odontogenic infections, *Ann Intern Med* 88:392, 1978; Lewis MAO et al: Prevalence of penicillin resistant bacteria in acute suppurative oral infection, *J Antimicrob Chemother* 35B:785, 1995; McGowan DA: Is antibiotic prophylaxis required for dental patients with joint replacement? *Br Dent J* 158:336, 1985; Norden CW: Prevention of bone and joint infections, *Am J Med* 78:229, 1985.

Table 16-2. Microorganisms causing odontogenic infections*

Organism	Percentage
Aerobic[†]	25%
Gram-positive cocci	85
Streptococcus spp.	90
Streptococcus (group D) spp.	2
Staphylococcus spp.	6
Eikenella spp.	2
Gram-negative cocci (Neisseria spp.)	2
Gram-positive rods (*Corynebacterium* spp.)	3
Gram-negative rods (*Haemophilus* spp.)	6
Miscellaneous and undifferentiated	4
Anaerobic[‡]	75%
Gram-positive cocci	30
Streptococcus spp.	33
Peptostreptococcus spp.	65
Gram-negative cocci (*Viellonella* spp.)	4
Gram-positive rods	14
Eubacterium spp.	
Lactobacillus spp.	
Actinomyces spp.	
Clostridia spp.	
Gram-negative rods	50
Bacteroides spp.	75
Fusobacterium spp.	25
Miscellaneous	6

*In 404 patients.
[†]49 different species.
[‡]119 different species.

acteristic of the bacteria causing odontogenic infections. Because the mouth flora is a combination of aerobic and anaerobic bacteria, it is not surprising to find that most odontogenic infections have both anaerobic and aerobic bacteria. Infections caused only by aerobic bacteria probably account for 5% of all odontogenic infections. Infections caused by only anaerobic bacteria make up about 35% of the infections. Infections caused by both anaerobic and aerobic bacteria comprise about 60% of all odontogenic infections (Table 16-1).

The aerobic bacteria that cause odontogenic infections consist of many species (Table 16-2). The most common causative organisms are streptococci, which comprise about 70% of the aerobic bacterial species that cause odontogenic infections. Staphylococci are found in about 5% of the infections, and many miscellaneous bacteria contribute 1% or less. Rarely found bacteria include group D *Streptococcus* organisms, *Neisseria* spp., *Corynebacterium* spp., and *Haemophilus* spp.

The anaerobic bacteria that cause infections include an even greater variety of species (see Table 16-2). Two main groups, however, predominate. The anaerobic gram-positive cocci account for about one third of the infections. These cocci are anaerobic *Streptococcus* and *Peptostreptococcus*. The gram-positive rods *Eubacterium* and *Lactobacillus* organisms are most commonly found in this group. The gram-negative anaerobic rods are cultured in about half of the infections. The *Prevotella* and *Porphyromonas* (previously *Bacteroides*) spp. account for about 75% of these and *Fusobacterium* organisms for 25%.

Of the anaerobic bacteria, several gram-positive cocci (anaerobic *Streptococcus* and *Peptostreptococcus* spp.) *and gram-negative rods (Prevotella* and *Fusobacterium* spp.) play a more important pathogenic role. The anaerobic gram-negative cocci and the anaerobic gram-positive rods appear to have little or no role in the etiology of odontogenic infections; instead, they appear to be opportunistic organisms (Table 16-3).

The method by which mixed aerobic and anaerobic bacteria cause infections is known with some certainty.

After initial inoculation into the deeper tissues, the more invasive organisms with higher virulence (the aerobic *Streptococcus* spp.) begin the infection process, initiating a cellulitis type of infection. The anaerobic bacteria will then also grow, and as the local reduction-oxidation potential is lowered (because of the growth of the aerobic bacteria), anaerobic bacteria become more prominent. As the infection reaches a more chronic, abscess stage, the anaerobic bacteria predominate and eventually become the exclusive causative organisms. Early infections appearing initially as a cellulitis may be characterized as *aerobic streptococcal infections,* and late, chronic abscesses may be characterized as *anaerobic infections.*

Natural History of Progression of Odontogenic Infections

Odontogenic infections have two major origins: periapical, as a result of pulpal necrosis and subsequent bacterial invasion into the periapical tissue, and periodontal, as a result of a deep periodontal pocket that allows inoculation of bacteria into the underlying soft tissues. Of these two, the periapical origin is the most common in odontogenic infections.

Necrosis of the dental pulp as a result of deep caries allows a pathway for bacteria to enter the periapical tissues. Once this

Table 16-3. Bacteria responsible for odontogenic infections

Aerobic bacteria	Frequency*	Anaerobic bacteria	Frequency*
Gram-positive cocci			
Streptococcus spp.		*Streptococcus* spp.	C
α hemolytic	VC	*Peptostreptococcus* spp.	VC
β hemolytic	U		
Group D	R		
Staphylococcus spp.	R		
Gram-negative cocci			
Neisseria spp.	R	*Viellonella* spp.	U
Gram-positive bacilli			
Corynebacterium spp.	R	*Eubacterium* spp.	U
		Lactobacillus spp.	U
Gram-negative bacilli			
Haemophilus influenzae	R	*Prevotella*	VC
Eikenella corrodens	R	*Porphyromonas*	C
		Fusobacterium spp.	C

*VC, very common; C, common; U, unusual; R, rare.

tissue has become inoculated with bacteria and an active infection is established, the infection will spread equally in all directions but preferentially along the lines of least resistance. The infection will spread through the cancellous bone until it encounters a cortical plate. If this cortical plate is thin, the infection erodes through the bone and enters the soft tissues. Treatment of the necrotic pulp by standard endodontic therapy or extraction of the tooth will resolve the infection. Antibiotics alone may stop the infection, but the infection will recur when antibiotic therapy is ended.

When the infection erodes through the cortical plate of the alveolar process, it appears in predictable anatomic locations. The location of the infection from a specific tooth is determined by the following two major factors: the thickness of the bone overlying the apex of the tooth and the relationship of the site of perforation of bone to muscle attachments of the maxilla and mandible.

Figure 16-1 demonstrates how infections perforate through bone into the overlying soft tissue. In Figure 16-1, *A,* the labial bone overlying the apex of the tooth is thin compared with the bone on the palatal aspect of the tooth. Therefore as the infectious process spreads it goes into the labial soft tissues. In Figure 16-1, *B,* the tooth is severely flared, which results in thicker labial bone and a relatively thinner palatal bone. In this situation, as the infection spreads through the bone into the soft tissue, the infection is expressed as a palatal abscess.

Once the infection has eroded through the bone, the precise location of the soft tissue infection will be determined by the position of the perforation relative to the muscle attachments. In Figure 16-2, *A,* the infection has eroded through to the labial aspect of the tooth and inferior to the attachment of the buccinator muscle, which results in an infection that appears as a vestibular abscess. In Figure 16-2, *B,* the infection has eroded through the bone superior to the attachment of the buccinator muscle and will be expressed as an infection of the buccal space.

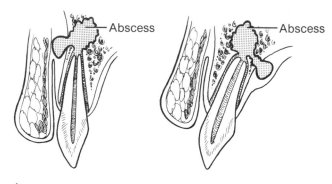

Figure 16-1

When infection erodes through bone, it will enter soft tissue through thinnest bone. *Left,* Tooth apex is near thin labial bone, so infection erodes labially; *Right,* apex is near palatal aspect, so bone will be perforated.

Infections from most maxillary teeth erode through the labiobuccocortical plate (Table 16-4). They also erode through the bone below the attachment of the muscles that attach to the maxilla, which means that most maxillary tooth abscesses appear initially as vestibular abscesses. Occasionally, a palatal abscess from a severely inclined lateral incisor or palatal root of a maxillary first molar will occur. Likewise, on occasion a long maxillary canine tooth will erode through the bone superior to the insertion of the levator anguli oris and will cause a canine space infection. More commonly, the maxillary molars will have infections that erode through the bone superior to the insertion of the buccinator muscle, which result in a buccal space infection.

In the mandible, infections of the incisors, canines, and premolars usually erode through the labiobuccocortical plate and above the associated musculature, resulting in vestibular abscesses (Table 16-4). Molar teeth infections erode through

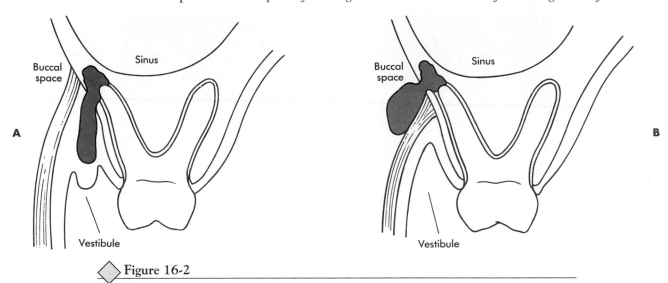

◇ **Figure 16-2**

Relationship of point of bone perforation to muscle attachment will determine fascial space involved. **A,** When tooth apex is lower than muscle attachment, vestibular abscess results. **B,** If apex is higher than muscle attachment, adjacent fascial space will be involved.

◇ **Table 16-4.** Spread of infection from the teeth

Involved teeth	Usual site of perforation of bone	Relation of perforation to muscle attachment	Determining muscle	Site of localization
Maxilla				
Central incisor	Labial	Below	Orbicularis oris	Labial vestibule
Lateral incisor	Labial	Below	Orbicularis oris	Labial vestibule
	(Palatal)*	—	—	(Palatal)
Canine	Labial	Below	Levator anguli oris	Oral vestibule
	Labial	(Above)	Levator anguli oris	(Canine space)
Premolars	Buccal	Below	Buccinator	Buccal vestibule
Molars	Buccal	Below	Buccinator	Buccal vestibule
	Buccal	Above	Buccinator	Buccal space
	(Palatal)	—	—	(Palatal)
Mandible				
Incisors	Labial	Above	Mentalis	Labial vestibule
Canine	Labial	Above	Depressor anguli oris	Labial vestibule
Premolars	Buccal	Above	Buccinator	Buccal vestibule
First molar	Buccal	Above	Buccinator	Buccal vestibule
	Buccal	Below	Buccinator	Buccal space
	Lingual	Above	Mylohyoid	Sublingual space
Second molar	Buccal	Above	Buccinator	Buccal vestibule
	Buccal	Below	Buccinator	Buccal space
	Lingual	Above	Mylohyoid	Sublingual space
	Lingual	Below	Mylohyoid	Submandibular space
Third molar	Lingual	Below	Mylohyoid	Submandibular space

Modified from Laskin DM: Anatomic considerations in diagnosis and treatment of odontogenic infections, *J Am Dent Assoc* 69:308, 1964.
*Parentheses indicate rare occurrences.

the linguocortical bone more frequently than the anterior teeth. First molar infections will drain either buccally or lingually, the second molar can perforate either buccally or lingually but usually lingually, and third molar infections almost always erode through the linguocortical plate. The mylohyoid muscle will determine whether infections that drain lingually go into the sublingual or submandibular space.

The most common odontogenic infection is a vestibular abscess (Figure 16-3). Occasionally, patients do not seek treatment for these infections, and the process will rupture spontaneously and drain, resulting in resolution of the infection. The infection will recur if the site of spontaneous drainage closes. Sometimes the abscess establishes a chronic sinus tract that drains to the oral cavity (Figure 16-4). As long

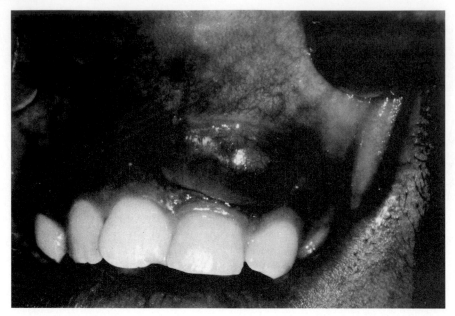

◇ **Figure 16-3**

Vestibular abscess arising from maxillary incisor. Overlying mucosa is thin because pus is near surface.

as the sinus tract continues to drain, the patient will experience no pain. Antibiotic administration will usually cause a cessation of the drainage, but when antibiotics are stopped, the drainage will recur. Definitive treatment of a chronic sinus tract requires treatment of the original problem, that is, the necrotic pulp treated by endodontic therapy or by extraction of the tooth.

PRINCIPLES OF THERAPY OF ODONTOGENIC INFECTIONS ◇

This section discusses the management of the odontogenic infection. A series of principles are discussed that are useful in treating patients who come to the dentist with infections related to the teeth and gingiva. The clinician must keep in mind the information in the preceding two sections of this chapter to understand these principles.

PRINCIPLE I: DETERMINE THE SEVERITY OF THE INFECTION

Most odontogenic infections are mild and require only minor therapy. When the patient comes for treatment the initial goal is to assess the severity of the infection. This determination is based on a complete history of the current infectious illness and a physical examination.

COMPLETE HISTORY. The history of the patient's infection follows the same general guidelines as any history. The initial purpose is to find out the patient's chief complaint. Typical chief complaints of patients with infections are "I

have a toothache," "My jaw is swollen," and "I have a gum boil in my mouth." The complaint should be recorded in the patient's own words.

The next step in taking of the history is determining how long the infection has been present. First, the dentist should inquire as to time of *onset* of the infection. How long ago did the patient first have symptoms of pain, swelling, or drainage, which indicated the beginning of the infection? The *duration* of the infection is then discussed. Have the symptoms of the infection been constant, have they waxed and waned, or has the patient steadily grown worse since the first symptoms were noted? Finally, the practitioner should determine the *rapidity* of progress of the infection. Has the infection process progressed rapidly over a few hours, or has it gradually increased in severity over several days to a week?

The next step is eliciting the patient's symptoms. Infections are actually a severe inflammatory response, and the typical signs of inflammation are clinically easily discernible. These signs and symptoms are dolor, tumor, calor, rubor, and functio laesa (loss of function.) The most common complaint is dolor (pain). The patient should be asked where the pain actually started and how the pain has spread since it was first noted. The second sign is tumor (swelling). Swelling is a physical finding that is sometimes subtle and not obvious to the practitioner, although it is to the patient. It is important that the dentist ask the patient to describe any area of swelling, where it is, and how large he or she feels it is. The third characteristic of infection is calor (warmth). The patient should be asked if the area feels hot. Rubor (erythema, or redness) of the overlying area is the next characteristic to be discussed. The patient should be asked if there has been or currently is any change in color, especially redness, over the area of the infection. Functio laesa should then be checked. When

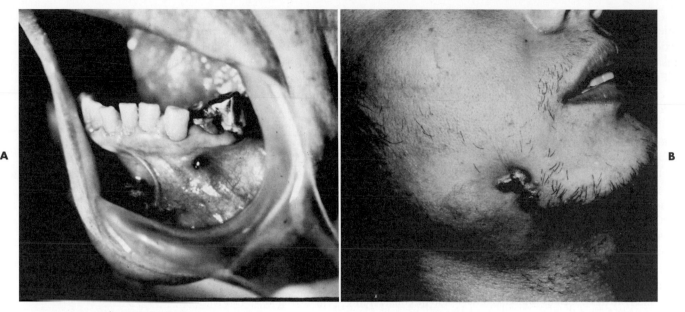

◇ Figure 16-4

Chronic drainage sinus tracts that result from low-grade infections may drain intraorally (**A**) or extraorally (**B**).

inquiring about this characteristic, the dentist asks about trismus and difficulty in swallowing, breathing, or chewing.

Finally, the dentist should ask the patient how he or she feels in general. Patients who feel fatigued, hot, sick, and generally out of sorts are said to have *malaise*. Malaise usually indicates a generalized reaction to a moderate-to-severe infection (Figure 16-5).

In the next step in taking of the history the dentist inquires about treatment. The dentist should ask about previous professional treatment and self-treatment. Many patients will "doctor" themselves with leftover antibiotics, hot soaks, and a variety of other home remedies. Occasionally, a dentist sees a patient who received treatment in an emergency room 2 or 3 days earlier and was referred to a dentist by the emergency room physician. The patient may have neglected to follow that advice until the infection became rather severe.

The patient's past medical history should be obtained in the usual manner by interview or by self-administered questionnaire.

PHYSICAL EXAMINATION.   The first step in the physical examination is to collect the patient's vital signs. This includes temperature, blood pressure, pulse rate, and respiratory rate. The need for evaluation of temperature is obvious. Patients who have systemic involvement of infection will have elevated temperatures. Patients with severe infections will have temperatures elevated to 101° to 102° F.

The patient's pulse rate will increase as the patient's temperature increases. Pulse rates of up to 100 beats per minute are not uncommon in patients with infections. If pulse rates increase above 100 beats per minute, the patient may have a severe infection and should be treated more aggressively.

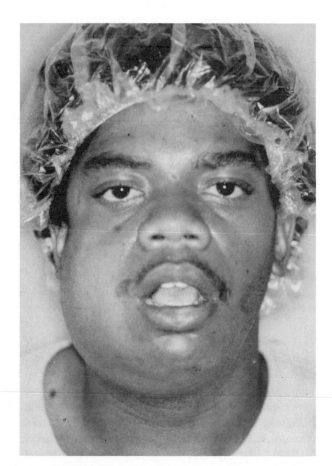

◇ Figure 16-5

Patient with severe infection and elevated temperature, pulse rate, and respiratory rate. He feels very sick and tired and has "toxic appearance."

The vital sign that varies the least with infection is the patient's blood pressure. Only if there is significant pain and anxiety will there be a mild elevation in systolic blood pressure.

Finally, the patient's respiratory rate should be closely observed. One of the major considerations in odontogenic infections is the potential for upper airway obstruction as a result of extension of the infection into fascial spaces in the area of the pharynx. As respirations are monitored, the dentist should carefully check to ensure that the upper airway is clear and that breathing is without difficulty. The normal respiratory rate is 14 to 16 breaths per minute. Patients with mild-to-moderate infections have elevated respiratory rates of up to 18 to 20 breaths per minute.

Patients who have normal vital signs with only a mild temperature elevation usually have a mild infection that can be readily treated. Patients who have abnormal vital signs with elevation of temperature, pulse rate, and respiratory rate are more likely to have serious infection and should be considered as having potential problems.

Once vital signs have been taken, attention should be turned to physical examination of the patient. The initial portion of the physical examination should be inspection of the patient's general appearance. Patients who have more than a minor, localized infection have an appearance of fatigue, feverishness, and malaise. This is a "toxic appearance" (see Figure 16-5).

The patient's head and neck should be carefully examined for signs of infection and the patient inspected for any evidence of swelling and overlying erythema. The patient should be asked to open the mouth widely, swallow, and take deep breaths so that the dentist can check for dysfunction.

Areas of swelling must be examined by palpation. The dentist should gently touch the area of swelling to check for tenderness, amount of local warmth or heat, and the character of the swelling. The character of the swelling varies from feeling very soft and almost normal through a firmer swelling (described as having a doughy feeling) to an even firmer or hard swelling (described as feeling *indurated*). An indurated swelling has the same firmness as a tightened muscle. Another characteristic swelling texture is *fluctuant*. Fluctuance is the feeling of a fluid-filled balloon. Fluctuant swelling almost always means that there is an accumulation of pus in the underlying tissues.

The dentist then performs an intraoral examination to try to find the specific cause of the infection. There may be severely carious teeth, an obvious periodontal abscess, severe periodontal disease, or combinations of caries and periodontal disease. The dentist should look and feel for areas of gingival swelling and fluctuance and for localized vestibular abscesses or draining sinus tracts.

The next step is to perform a radiographic examination. This usually consists of the indicated periapical radiographs; occasionally, however, extraoral radiographs, such as a pantogram, may be necessary because of limited mouth-opening or other extenuating circumstances.

After the physical examination, the practitioner should

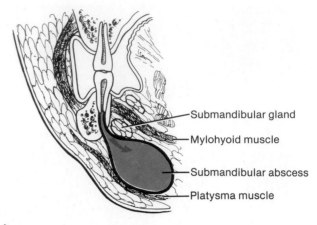

Figure 16-6

Cellulitis infection involving submandibular region. It is indurated on palpation, and patient is quite sick.

begin to have a sense of whether this particular patient has a *cellulitis* or an *abscess* (Figures 16-6 and 16-7). These two terms are typically used to describe two separate states of infection, which have distinct, unique methods of treatment. Distinctions between the cellulitis and abscess are typically in duration, pain, size, peripheral definition, texture to palpation, presence of pus, and potential danger (Table 16-5). The duration of cellulitis is usually thought to be acute and is the initial presentation of the infection. An abscess, on the other hand, is usually a chronic process. Cellulitis is usually described as more painful than an abscess, which may be the result of its acute onset and distension of tissues. The size of the cellulitic area is typically larger and more widespread than that of the abscess. The periphery of a cellulitis is usually vague and indistinct, with a diffuse border that makes it difficult to determine where the swelling begins or ends. The abscess usually has distinct and well-defined borders. Texture to palpation is one of the primary distinctions between cellulitis and an abscess. When palpated, an early cellulitis can be very soft or doughy; a severe cellulitis is almost always described as indurated or even as being "boardlike." The severity of the cellulitis increases as its firmness to palpation increases. On palpation the abscess feels fluctuant, because it is a pus-filled cavity in the tissue. Finally, a cellulitis may be innocuous in its early stages and extremely dangerous in its more advanced, indurated, rapidly spreading stages. An abscess is typically less dangerous, because it is more chronic and less aggressive. The presence of pus usually indicates that the body has walled off the infection and that the local host resistance mechanisms are bringing the infection under control. In many clinical situations the distinction between severe cellulitis and abscess may be difficult to make, especially if an abscess lies deeply within the soft tissue. In some patients an indurated cellulitis may have areas of abscess formation in it (see Chapter 17).

In summary, a cellulitis is an acute, painful infection whose swelling is larger, with diffuse borders. It can be soft-to-hard

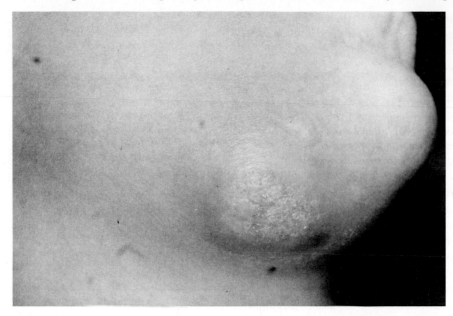

◇ Figure 16-7

Well-localized abscess has crusted surface secondary to tissue necrosis. Mass is fluctuant on palpation.

◇ Table 16-5. Differences between cellulitis and abscess

Characteristic	Cellulitis	Abscess
Duration	Acute	Chronic
Pain	Severe and generalized	Localized
Size	Large	Small
Localization	Diffuse borders	Well circumscribed
Palpation	Doughy to indurated	Fluctuant
Presence of pus	No	Yes
Degree of seriousness	Greater	Less
Bacteria	Aerobic	Anaerobic

◇ Box 16-1 ◇

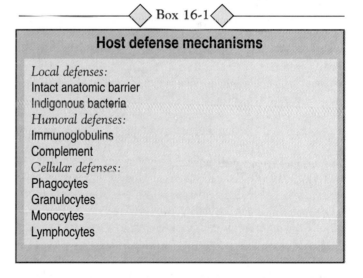

Host defense mechanisms

Local defenses:
Intact anatomic barrier
Indigenous bacteria
Humoral defenses:
Immunoglobulins
Complement
Cellular defenses:
Phagocytes
Granulocytes
Monocytes
Lymphocytes

on palpation and contains no pus. It may be a rapidly spreading process in serious infections. An abscess is a chronic infection with more localized pain, whose swelling tends to be smaller, with well-circumscribed borders. It is fluctuant on palpation, because it is a pus-filled tissue cavity. A chronic abscess is usually slow-growing and less serious than a cellulitis.

PRINCIPLE II: EVALUATE THE STATE OF THE PATIENT'S HOST DEFENSE MECHANISMS

Part of the evaluation of the patient's medical history is designed to establish the patient's ability to defend against infection. Several disease states and several types of drug usage may compromise this ability. Compromised patients are more likely to have infections, and these infections often become serious more rapidly. Therefore to manage their infections more effectively it is important to be able to discern those patients who may have a compromised host defense mechanism.

REVIEW OF HOST DEFENSE MECHANISMS. The body defends itself against bacterial invasion by the three major methods of local defenses, humoral defenses, and cellular defenses (Box 16-1).

Local defense mechanisms have two components. First, the anatomic barrier, comprised of intact skin and mucosa, prevents the invasion of bacteria into underlying tissues. Breaches in this anatomic barrier, such as by surgical incisions, deep periodontal pockets, or necrotic dental pulps, allow the entry of bacteria into underlying tissue where infections can be established. The second local defense is the population of normal indigenous bacteria. These bacteria usually live in harmony with the host and do not cause disease. However, if the normal bacteria are lost or altered, as occurs with antibiotic administration, other bacteria can populate the area previously occupied by the innocuous bacteria and cause infection. An example of this is oral thrush or candidiasis, which may follow penicillin administration. The penicillin eliminates the susceptible oral organisms, allowing the overgrowth of penicillin-resistant *Candida* organisms.

The humoral defenses are noncellular, are contained in the plasma and other body secretions, and aid in bacterial defense. The two main components are immunoglobulins and complement. The immunoglobulins are the antibodies that attach to invading bacteria and allow more active phagocytosis by leukocytes and thus more effective killing of the bacteria. The immunoglobulins are produced from plasma cells that are differentiated B lymphocytes. There are five types of immunoglobulins. IgG comprises about 75% of all the immunoglobulins. Its primary responsibility is in the defense against gram-positive bacteria. IgA makes up about 12% of the immunoglobulins. This immunoglobulin is known as the *secretory immunoglobulin,* because it is found on moist mucous membranes. Its primary activity is to prevent adhesion of bacteria to surface mucosa. IgM accounts for about 7% of the immunoglobulins and is mainly responsible for defense against gram-negative bacteria. IgE is primarily responsible for delayed hypersensitivity reactions. The function of IgD is not known at the present time.

Complement, the other humoral defense, is a complex group of serum proteins produced in the liver that must be activated to function. Activation of complement results from a multistep cascade that splits off portions of proteins that act as mediators and activators for further activated complement. First, they are important for the recognition of bacteria. Second, they increase chemotaxis, the attracting of polymorphonuclear leukocytes from the bloodstream to the area of bacterial invasion. Third, they opsonize, which helps immunoglobulins such as IgG stick to the surface of bacteria, which aids in the destruction of the bacteria. Fourth, they enhance phagocytosis as a result of the opsonization process. Finally, they increase the killing ability of the white blood cells by helping to perforate the bacterial cell wall with lysosomal enzymes.

The cellular portion of host defense mechanisms is primarily composed of phagocytes and lymphocytes. The primary phagocytes in the early phase of an infection are the polymorphonuclear leukocytes. These cells leave the bloodstream and migrate in chemotactic response to the area of the bacterial invasion. They respond rapidly, but their life span is short, and they are able to phagocytize only a small number of bacteria. This phase is followed by the egress of monocytes from the bloodstream into the tissue, where they are recognized as macrophages. Macrophages are able to phagocytize, kill, and digest multiple bacteria and live much longer than the polymorphonuclear leukocyte. Monocytes are seen more commonly in the later stages and chronic form of infection.

The second component of the cellular defenses is the population of lymphocytes. As mentioned earlier, B lymphocytes differentiate into plasma cells under the proper stimu-

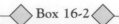

Compromised host defenses

Uncontrolled metabolic diseases:
Uremia
Alcoholism
Malnutrition
Severe diabetes
Suppressing diseases:
Leukemia
Lymphoma
Malignant tumors
Suppressing drugs:
Cancer chemotherapeutic agents
Immunosuppressives

lation and are then able to produce specific antibodies, such as IgG antibodies. T lymphocytes are primarily responsible for activities such as graft rejection and tumor surveillance. However, they do play a major role in helping B lymphocytes combat certain types of infection.

MEDICAL CONDITIONS THAT COMPROMISE HOST DEFENSES.   With the foregoing discussion in mind, it is important to delineate those medical conditions that may result in decreased host defenses. These compromises allow more bacteria to enter the tissues or to be more active, or they prevent the humoral or cellular defenses from exerting their full effect. There are several specific conditions that may compromise patients' defenses (Box 16-2).

Severe, uncontrolled metabolic diseases, such as severe diabetes, end-stage renal disease that leads to uremia, and severe alcoholism with malnutrition, result in decreased function of leukocytes, including decreased chemotaxis, phagocytosis, and bacterial killing.

The second major group of host compromisers are diseases that interfere with host defense mechanisms, such as leukemias, lymphomas, and many types of cancer. These result in decreased white cell function and decreased antibody synthesis and production.

Patients taking certain drugs are also compromised. Cancer chemotherapeutic agents decrease circulating white cell counts to extremely low levels, commonly below 1000 cells per milliliter. When this occurs, patients will be unable to defend themselves effectively against bacterial invasion. Patients on immunosuppressive therapy, usually for organ transplantation or autoimmune diseases, are compromised. The common drugs in these categories are cyclosporin, corticosteroids, and azathioprine (Imuran). These drugs decrease T- and B-lymphocyte function and immunoglobulin production. Thus patients taking these medications are more likely to have severe infections.

In summary, when evaluating a patient whose chief

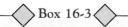

Criteria for referral to a specialist

1. Rapidly progressive infection
2. Difficulty in breathing
3. Difficulty in swallowing
4. Fascial space involvement
5. Elevated temperature (greater than 101° F)
6. Severe jaw trismus (less than 10 mm)
7. Toxic appearance
8. Compromised host defenses

complaint may be an infection, the patient's medical history should be carefully examined for the presence of diabetes, severe renal disease, alcoholism with malnutrition, leukemias and lymphomas, cancer chemotherapy, and immunosuppressive therapy of any kind. When the patient's history includes any of these, the patient with an infection must be treated much more vigorously, as the infection may spread more rapidly. Early and aggressive surgery to remove the cause and more parenteral antibiotic therapy must be considered. Additionally, when a patient with a history of one of these problems is seen for routine oral surgical procedures, it may be necessary to provide the patient with prophylactic antibiotics to prevent an infection from occurring.

PRINCIPLE III: DETERMINE WHETHER THE PATIENT SHOULD BE TREATED BY A GENERAL DENTIST OR A SPECIALIST

Most odontogenic infections seen by the dentist can be managed with the expectation of normal rapid resolution. Odontogenic infections, when treated with minor surgical procedures and commonly used antibiotics, almost always respond rapidly. However, some odontogenic infections are potentially life-threatening and require aggressive medical and surgical management. In these special situations, early recognition of the potential severity is essential, and these patients should be referred to a specialist, usually an oral-maxillofacial surgeon, for definitive management. For some patients, hospitalization will be required, whereas others will be managed as outpatients.

When a patient with an odontogenic infection comes for treatment, the dentist must have a set of criteria by which to judge the seriousness of the infection (Box 16-3). If some or all of these criteria are met, immediate referral must be considered.

Three main criteria suggest immediate referral to a specialist. The first is a history of a *rapidly progressing infection*. This means that the infection began 1 or 2 days before the interview and is growing rapidly worse, with increasing swelling, pain, and associated signs and symptoms. This type of odontogenic infection may spread to areas in which it is potentially life-threatening and therefore must be treated aggressively. The second criterion is *difficulty in*

breathing. Patients who have severe swelling of the soft tissue of the upper airway as the result of infection may have difficulty maintaining a patent airway. In these situations the patient often cannot lie down, has difficulty with speech, and is obviously distressed with the breathing difficulties. This patient should be referred directly to an emergency room, because immediate surgical attention may be necessary to maintain an intact airway. The third urgent criterion is *difficulty in swallowing*. Patients who have swelling and trismus may have difficulty swallowing their saliva. This is an ominous sign, because difficulty in swallowing frequently indicates a narrowing of the oral pharynx and potential for acute airway embarrassment. This patient should also be referred to the hospital emergency room, because surgical intervention may be required for airway maintenance.

Several other criteria should indicate referral to the specialist. Patients who have involvement of extraoral fascial spaces, such as buccal space infections or submandibular space infections, may require extraoral surgical incision and drainage, as well as hospitalization. Next, although infection almost always causes an elevated temperature, a temperature higher than 101° F indicates a greater likelihood of severe infection and the patient should be referred. Another important sign is trismus, which is the inability to open the mouth widely. In odontogenic infections, trismus results from the involvement of the muscles of mastication in the inflammatory process. A patient with mild-to-moderate trismus will be able to open his or her mouth up to 15 mm. Severe trismus—the inability to open the mouth wider than 10 mm—may be an indication of severe oral pharyngeal involvement of the infection. In this situation, referral to a specialist is necessary for evaluation of upper airway patency. Additionally, systemic involvement of an odontogenic infection is an indication for referral. Patients with systemic involvement will have a typical toxic facial appearance, glazed eyes, open mouth, and a dehydrated, sick appearance. When this is seen, the patient is usually fatigued, has a substantial amount of pain, has an elevated temperature, and is dehydrated. Finally, if the patient has readily identifiable host defenses, hospitalization is likely to be required. A specialist is usually prepared to admit the patient easily and effectively.

PRINCIPLE IV: TREAT THE INFECTION SURGICALLY

The primary principle of management of odontogenic infections is to perform surgical drainage and removal of the cause of the infection. Surgical treatment may range from something as simple as the opening of a tooth and extirpation of the necrotic tooth pulp to treatment as complex as the wide incision of soft tissue in the submandibular and neck regions for a severe infection.

The primary goal in surgical management of infection is to remove the cause of the infection, which is most commonly a necrotic pulp or deep periodontal pocket. A secondary goal is to provide drainage of accumulated pus and necrotic debris.

When a patient has a typical odontogenic infection, the most likely appearance will be a small vestibular abscess.

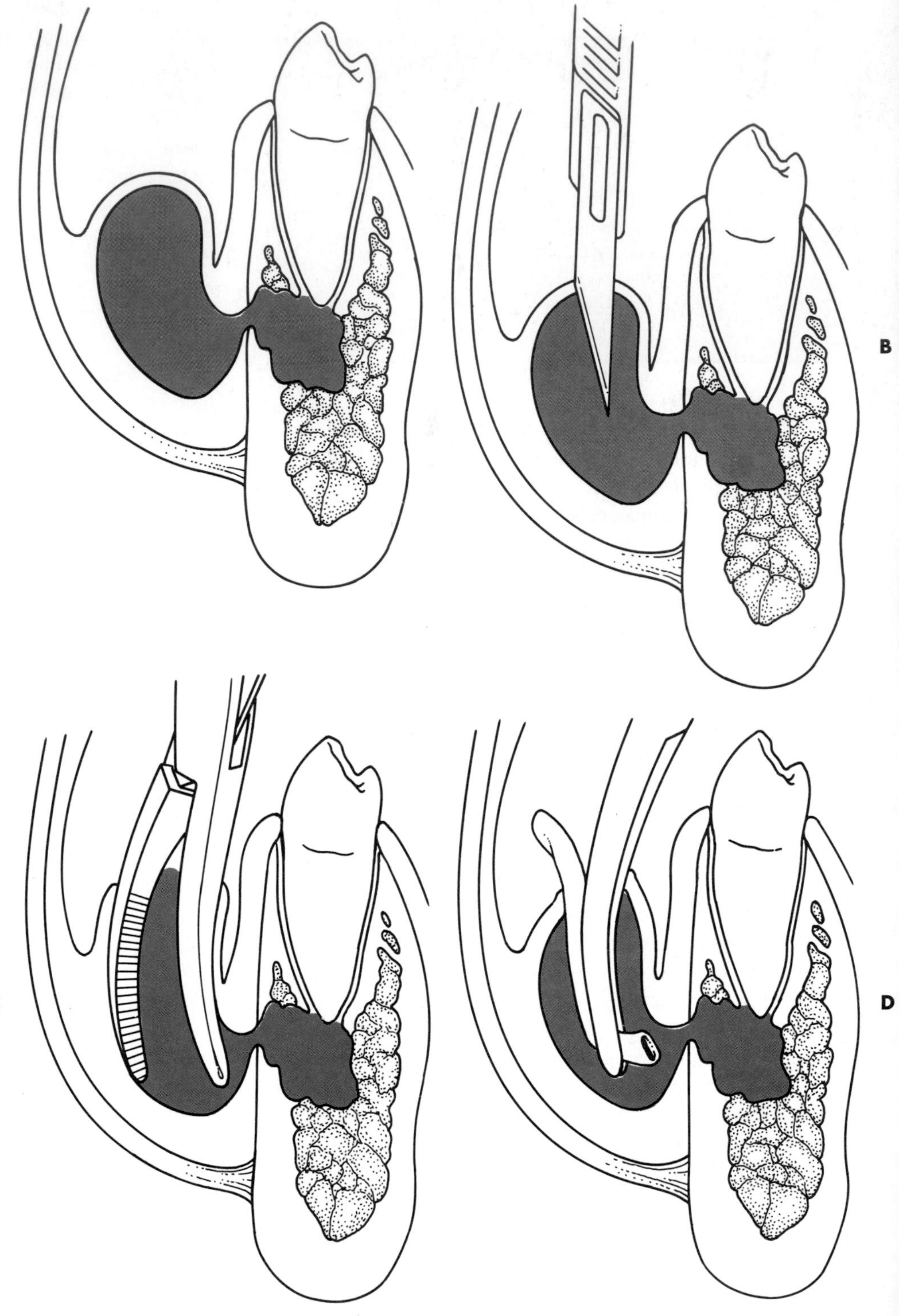

Continued

◇ Figure 16-8

A, Periapical infection of lower bicuspid extends through buccal plate and creates sizable vestibular abscess. **B,** Abscess is incised with no. 11 blade. **C,** Beaks of hemostat are inserted through incision and opened so that beaks spread to break up any loculations of pus that may exist in abscessed tissue. **D,** Small rubber drain is inserted to depths of abscess cavity with hemostat.

With this presentation the dentist has the three options for surgical management of endodontic treatment, extraction, or incision and drainage. If the tooth is not to be extracted, it should be opened and the pulp removed, which results in elimination of the cause and obtaining limited drainage. If the tooth cannot be salvaged, it should be extracted as soon as possible.

Extraction provides both removal of the cause of the infection and drainage of the accumulated pus and debris. In addition to the endodontic procedure or extraction of the tooth, an incision and drainage procedure may be required. Incision of the abscess cavity provides for drainage of the accumulated pus and bacteria from the underlying tissue. Drainage of pus provides for a reduction in tissue tension, which improves the local blood supply and increases the delivery of host defenses to the localized area. The incision and drainage procedure includes the insertion of a drain, usually made of rubber, to prevent the closure of the mucosal incision, which would

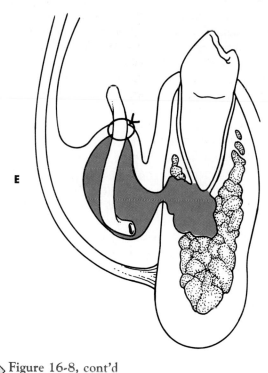

E

◇ Figure 16-8, cont'd

E, Small rubber drain is sutured into place with single black silk suture.

result in reformation of the abscess cavity. It is important to remember that the surgical goal is to achieve adequate drainage. If endodontic opening of the tooth does not provide adequate drainage of the abscess, it is essential to perform an incision and drainage.

The technique for incision and drainage of a fluctuant vestibular abscess is straightforward (Figure 16-8). The preferred site for the incision is directly over the most dependent area, to encourage drainage. (When incision and drainage procedures are performed extraorally, a more complex set of criteria must be met when selecting a site for the incision.) Once the area of incision has been selected, a method of pain control must be employed. Regional nerve block anesthesia achieved by injecting an area away from the site of the incision is preferred. Alternatively, superficial infiltration of local anesthetic solution anterior and posterior to the area to be drained can be employed.

Before the actual incision of the abscess cavity is performed, consideration must be given to obtaining a specimen of the pus for culture and sensitivity. If the decision is made to perform a culture, the procedure is carried out as the initial portion of the surgery. Once the localized area has been anesthetized, a large-gauge needle, usually 18 gauge, is used for specimen collection. A small syringe, usually 2 mL, is adequate. The surface mucosa is disinfected with a solution such as Betadine and dried with sterile gauze. The needle is then inserted into the abscess cavity, and 1 or 2 mL of pus is aspirated. The syringe is held vertically, and any air bubbles contained in the syringe are ejected from it. The tip of the needle is then capped with a rubber stopper and taken directly

to the microbiology laboratory. This method for obtaining a specimen permits both aerobic and anaerobic cultures and Gram's staining. As discussed earlier, anaerobic bacteria are almost always present in odontogenic infections, and therefore care must be taken to provide the laboratory the best opportunity to find them.

Once the culture specimen is obtained, an incision is made with a no. 11 blade just through the mucosa and submucosa into the abscess cavity (see Figure 16-8). The incision should be short, usually no more than 1 cm in length. Once the incision is completed, a closed curved hemostat is inserted through the incision into the abscess cavity. The hemostat is then opened in several directions to break up any small loculations or cavities of pus that have not been opened by the initial incision. The pus that drained out during this time should be aspirated into the suction and should not be allowed to drain into the patient's mouth.

Once all areas of the abscess cavity have been opened and all pus drained, a small rubber drain is inserted to maintain the opening. The most commonly used drain for intraoral abscesses is a ¼-in sterile Penrose drain. A frequently used substitute is a small strip of sterilized rubber dam. A piece of drain of adequate length to reach the depth of the abscess cavity is prepared and inserted into the cavity, using the hemostat. The drain is then sutured into place with a nonresorbable suture. The suture should be placed in viable tissue to prevent loss of the drain as the result of the suture tearing through nonvital tissue.

The drain should remain in place until all the drainage from the abscess cavity has stopped, usually 2 to 5 days. Removal is done by simply cutting the suture and slipping the drain from the wound.

Early-stage infections that initially appear as a cellulitis with soft, doughy, diffuse swelling do not respond to incision and drainage procedures. Surgical management of infections of this type is limited to removal of the necrotic pulp or removal of the involved tooth.

It is critical to keep in mind that the *primary* method for treating odontogenic infections is to perform surgery to remove the source of the infection and drain pus where it exists. Whenever an abscess cavity with pus is diagnosed, the surgeon must drain it. Failure to do so will result in worsening of the infection and failure of the infection to resolve, even if antibiotics are given. If there is a question as to whether pus is present, the surgeon should do a test aspiration with an 18-gauge needle. Even if the tooth can neither be opened nor extracted, incision of the abscess cavity to drain the pus should be done.

PRINCIPLE V: SUPPORT THE PATIENT MEDICALLY

Patients with odontogenic infections may have depressed host defense mechanisms as the result of the pain and swelling associated with the infection. Because of the pain from the infection, patients frequently have not had adequate fluid intake, nutritional intake, or rest. During the immediate postincision and drainage period, patients should be encouraged to drink a lot of water or juice and take high-calorie nutritional supplements. They should also be prescribed adequate analgesics for relief of pain so they can rest. Patients should be given careful postoperative instructions and should be able to manage this portion of their therapy without complications. It is the responsibility of the clinician, however, to provide careful instructions about these important issues.

PRINCIPLE VI: CHOOSE AND PRESCRIBE THE APPROPRIATE ANTIBIOTIC

Choosing the appropriate antibiotic for treating an odontogenic infection must be done carefully. When all factors are weighed, the clinician may decide that no antibiotic is necessary at all, whereas in other situations, broad-spectrum or even combination antibiotic therapy may be necessary. A variety of factors must be considered when choosing an antibiotic from the nearly 70 antibiotics currently available. Antibiotics must be viewed as a double-edged sword. Although appropriate use may result in dramatic resolution and cure of patients with infections, misuse of antibiotics provides little benefit to offset the associated risks and expense of antibiotic administration. Therefore the following guidelines are recommended for consideration when choosing a specific antibiotic.

IS ANTIBIOTIC ADMINISTRATION NECESSARY? It is a common misconception that all infections, by definition, require antibiotic administration; this is not necessarily the case. There are some situations in which antibiotics are not useful and in fact may be contraindicated. In making this determination, three factors must be considered. The first factor is the seriousness of the infection when the patient comes to the dentist. If the infection has modest swelling, has progressed rapidly, or is a diffuse cellulitis, the evidence would support the use of antibiotics in addition to surgical therapy. The second factor is whether adequate surgical treatment can be achieved. In many situations, extraction of the offending tooth may result in rapid resolution of the infection. However, in other situations, removal of the tooth may not be possible. Antibiotic therapy is important to control the infection so that the tooth can be removed. The third consideration is the state of the patient's host defenses. A young, healthy patient may be able to mobilize host defenses and need less antibiotic therapy for resolution of the infection. On the other hand, patients who have any type of decreased host resistance, such as those with severe metabolic disease or those receiving cancer chemotherapy, may require vigorous antibiotic therapy for even minor infections.

When these three factors are balanced, it becomes clear that in dentistry there are several definite indications for antibiotic usage (see Box 16-4). The first and most common indication is the presence of an acute-onset infection, with diffuse swelling and moderate-to-severe pain. This infection is usually in the cellulitis stage, and, with appropriate antibiotic therapy and treatment of the offending tooth, rapid resolution is expected. The second indication is almost any type of infection in a patient who is medically compromised. Such patients who have infections of any severity should be considered candidates for antibiotic administration. The third indication for antibiotic therapy is the presence of an infection that has progressed to involvement of extraoral fascial spaces. In these situations the infection is aggressive enough to have spread beyond the mouth, indicating that the host defenses are inadequate to contain the infection. The fourth indication is severe pericoronitis, with temperatures higher than 100° F, trismus, and some swelling of the lateral aspect of the face, which occurs most commonly around impacted mandibular third molars. Finally, the patient who has osteomyelitis requires antibiotic therapy in addition to surgical therapy to achieve resolution of the infection.

Based on the same three criteria, antibiotic therapy would not be indicated or is even contraindicated in other situations (Box 16-5). The first is a minor, chronic, well-localized abscess for which an incision and drainage and treatment of the offending tooth result in rapid resolution, assuming that the patient's host defenses are intact and that the patient has no other compromising conditions. A second, albeit similar, contraindication is a very well-localized vestibular abscess, with little or no facial swelling. In these situations the tooth can be opened and necrotic pulp removed or the tooth extracted and the abscess incised and drained, which will result in rapid resolution in most patients. Third is a localized osteitis, or dry socket. Treatment of the dry socket is primarily palliative, and it is not treated as an infection. Fourth, patients who have mild pericoronitis with minor gingival edema and

---

◇ Box 16-4 ◇

Indications for use of antibiotics

1. Rapidly progressive swelling
2. Diffuse swelling
3. Compromised host defenses
4. Involvement of fascial spaces
5. Severe pericoronitis
6. Osteomyelitis

◇ Box 16-5 ◇

Situations in which use of antibiotics is not necessary

1. Chronic well-localized abscess
2. Minor vestibular abscess
3. Dry socket
4. Mild pericoronitis

mild pain do not require antibiotics for resolution of their infection. Irrigation with hydrogen peroxide or chlorhexidine will result in resolution.

In summary, antibiotics should be used when there is clear evidence of bacterial invasion into underlying tissues that is greater than the host defenses can ward off. Patients who have an impaired ability to defend themselves against infection and patients who have infections that are not amenable to surgical treatment should be considered for antibiotic therapy. Antibiotics should not be used when there is no evidence of bacterial involvement. Antibiotics do not hasten wound healing and do not provide any benefit for nonbacterial conditions. Patients who have inflammatory pulpitis will have severe pain, but the pain results from local inflammatory reaction within the pulp, not from bacterial infection. These patients should not be given antibiotic therapy.

USE EMPIRIC THERAPY ROUTINELY. Odontogenic infections are caused by a highly predictable group of bacteria. Additionally, the antibiotic sensitivity of these organisms is well known and consistent. As a result the use of culture and sensitivity testing is not necessary for routine odontogenic infections. The bacteria that cause more than 90% of odontogenic infections are aerobic streptococci and anaerobic streptococci, peptostreptococci, prevotella, and fusobacteria. Many other species of bacteria are also involved, but they appear to be opportunistic rather than causative bacteria. Fortunately, the antibiotic susceptibility of the causative bacteria is remarkably consistent. The orally administered antibiotics that are effective against odontogenic infections include penicillin, erythromycin, clindamycin, cefadroxil, metronidazole, and the tetracyclines (Box 16-6). These antibiotics are effective against streptococci (except metronidazole) and oral anaerobes. There are several relatively important variations among the group. (See Appendix IX for detailed description of the various antibiotics.)

Because the microbiology and antibiotic sensitivity is well known, it is a reasonable therapeutic maneuver to use one of these antibiotics empirically, that is, to give the antibiotic with the assumption that an appropriate drug is being given. The drug of choice is usually penicillin. Alternative drugs for use in the penicillin-allergic patient are erythromycin and clindamycin. The cephalosporin cefadroxil is a useful drug when a broader antibacterial spectrum is necessary. The cephalosporins should be used with caution in penicillin-allergic patients, because they may also be allergic to the cephalosporins. The tetracyclines are another useful alternative, although some strains of bacteria are resistant to the tetracyclines. Metronidazole is useful only against anaerobic bacteria and should be reserved for situations in which only anaerobic bacteria are suspected.

When treating a patient with a fluctuant abscess, aspiration of a small amount of pus with a small syringe and 18-gauge needle makes it easy to perform a smear on a glass slide that can be Gram's stained for bacteria. A small amount of pus is expressed onto a glass slide and spread very thinly. This can be heat-fixed over a flame for several seconds and set aside. Should the clinician require additional information on the microbiology of a particular infection, the slide can then be taken to a microbiology laboratory for Gram's staining and interpretation.

Routine culture and sensitivity testing (C & S) is not cost-effective for the routine odontogenic infection. However, there are some cases in which the dentist should seriously consider sending a specimen for culture and sensitivity testing (Box 16-7). The first is the rapid onset of infection and its rapid spread. Delay in bacterial identification may have disastrous consequences in this situation. The second case is postoperative infection. If a patient had no signs of infection when the original surgery was done but returns 3 or 4 days later with an infection, there is an increased probability of nonindigenous bacteria causing the infection. Precise identification of the causative bacteria may be critical to facilitate resolution of the infection. The third case is an infection that is not resolving. In these situations the clinician should make every effort to obtain a specimen of pus for culture and antibiotic sensitivity testing. The fourth case is a recurrent infection. When the initial infectious problem has resolved and there has been an infection-free period of 2 days to 2 weeks, but a second infection occurs, there is a high probability that the infection is caused by bacteria that have altered antibiotic sensitivity patterns. The fifth case is the patient who has compromised host defenses. The causative bacteria are not likely to be different from the usual odontogenic infection; however, because these patients have a decreased ability to defend themselves from infection, it is advantageous to have a precise

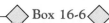

◇ **Box 16-6** ◇

Effective orally administered antibiotics useful for odontogenic infections

1. Penicillin
2. Erythromycin
3. Clindamycin
4. Cefadroxil
5. Metronidazole
6. Tetracycline

◇ **Box 16-7** ◇

Indications for culture and antibiotic sensitivity testing

1. Rapidly spreading infection
2. Postoperative infection
3. Nonresponsive infection
4. Recurrent infection
5. Compromised host defenses
6. Osteomyelitis
7. Suspected actinomycosis

diagnosis of the causative organisms for maximal effective-ness. The sixth case in which the dentist should consider sending a specimen for testing is osteomyelitis. Finally, testing should be done when chronic actinomycosis is suspected.

USE THE NARROWEST-SPECTRUM ANTIBIOTIC.
When an antibiotic is administered to a patient, all susceptible bacteria are killed. If the antibiotic is a narrow-spectrum antibiotic, it kills bacteria of a narrow range. For example, penicillin will kill streptococci and oral anaerobic bacteria but will have little effect on the staphylococci of the skin and almost no effect on gastrointestinal tract bacteria. As a result, penicillin has little or no effect on the gastrointestinal tract and does not expose a multitude of other bacteria to the opportunity to develop resistance. By contrast, drugs such as tetracycline are broad-spectrum antibiotics, killing not only the streptococci and oral anaerobes but also a variety of gram-negative rods. Thus when this antibiotic is given it has an effect on skin and gastrointestinal bacteria, which may result in problems caused by alterations of host flora and overgrowth of resistant bacteria. Also, broad-spectrum anti-biotics provide a multitude of bacteria the opportunity to develop resistance.

In summary, antibiotics that have narrow-spectrum activity against the causative organisms are just as effective as antibiotics that have broad-spectrum activity, without the problems of upsetting normal host microflora populations and increasing the chance of bacterial resistance.

USE THE ANTIBIOTIC WITH THE LOWEST INCI-DENCE OF TOXICITY AND SIDE EFFECTS.
Most antibiotics have a variety of toxicities and side effects that limit their usefulness. These range from mild to so severe that the antibiotic cannot be used in clinical practice. The antibiotics usually employed for odontogenic infections have a surprisingly low incidence of toxicity-related problems. It is important, however, for the clinician to understand the probable toxicities and side effects of the drugs they use.

Allergy is penicillin's major side effect. Approximately 2% or 3% of the total population is allergic to penicillin. Patients who have allergic reactions to penicillin, as exhibited by hives, itching, or wheezing, should not be given penicillin again. Penicillin does not have other major side effects or toxicities in the normal dosage range employed by dentists.

Erythromycin and clindamycin likewise have a low incidence of toxicity and side effects. Their side effects are mainly nausea, vomiting, abdominal cramping, and diarrhea. These side effects can be lessened by using smaller doses of the drug and by providing a small amount of food when medication is taken. Clindamycin also may cause a severe diarrheal state called *pseudomembranous colitis*. Several other drugs, such as ampicillin and the oral cephalosporins, also cause this problem; the elimination of much of the anaerobic gut flora allows the overgrowth of an antibiotic-resistant bacteria, *Clostridium difficile*. This bacteria produces metabolites that are toxic to the gut wall, which results in colitis. Patients who take clindamycin, amoxicillin, or cefadroxil should be warned of the possibility of profuse watery diarrhea and told to contact their prescribing dentist if it occurs.

The oral cephalosporins are associated with only mild toxicity problems. As with penicillin, the cephalosporins may cause allergic reactions. They should be given cautiously to patients with penicillin allergies, because these patients may be allergic to the cephalosporins also. Patients who have experienced an anaphylactic type of reaction to penicillin should *not* be given a cephalosporin because of increased chance for that life-threatening event to occur again.

The tetracyclines have minor toxicities for most patients. There are the commonly encountered gastrointestinal prob-lems of nausea, vomiting, abdominal cramping, and diarrhea, although these are not as common as with erythromycin. Some patients may develop a photosensitivity while they are taking this drug and should be warned to stay out of the sun. Finally, tetracyclines may produce tooth discoloration if given to patients who are pregnant or who are in the tooth-development stages of their lives. This discoloration is the result of chelation of the tetracycline to calcium, which results in incorporation of the tetracycline into the tooth.

Metronidazole has mild toxicities, the most prominent being the typical gastrointestinal disturbances discussed previously. The drug may also produce a disulfiram effect; that is, the patient taking metronidazole who also drinks alcohol may experience sudden violent abdominal cramping and vomiting.

Finally, antibiotics may cause effects that, strictly speaking, are not toxicity reactions but are side effects that result from interaction with other systemically administered drugs. An important example of this is the interaction of certain antibiotics with birth control pills. There is some evidence that taking antibiotics may increase the chance of failure of birth control pills to prevent pregnancy. The birth control pill is a combination of progestogen and estrogen. The estrogen in the pill causes a variety of undesirable side effects; the dosage is kept as low as possible to minimize these side effects yet provide consistent contraceptive effect. The estrogen is metabolized by the liver and excreted into the bile. It is hydrolyzed there by intestinal flora and reabsorbed into the blood stream. This enterohepatic circulation is responsible for the plasma level of estrogen. When antibiotics are given, two effects may lower the plasma concentration of the estrogen. The first is that there may be some induction of hepatic microsomal enzymes that alter the metabolism of the estrogen. The second is that the antibiotics may kill portions of the intestinal flora, thereby altering the amount of estrogen that is hydrolyzed for reabsorption. Both of these actions may lower the amount of estrogen in the plasma, rendering the patient fertile.

It is important to recognize that many other factors also may affect the plasma level of estrogen. The most important is patient compliance in routinely taking the pill. At this time there is no hard evidence that antibiotic administration will actually cause this phenomenon. The above explanation is somewhat theoretic and lacks scientific confirmation.

Antibiotics that have been implicated are rifampin, penicillin, ampicillin, amoxicillin, cephalexin, the tetracyclines, and erythromycin. Therefore it is prudent that when dentists prescribe antibiotics to patients of childbearing age who take birth control pills, they inform the patients that there may be less control of contraception during the period of antibiotic administration.

USE BACTERICIDAL ANTIBIOTIC IF POSSIBLE.

Antibiotics may either kill bacteria (bactericidal antibiotics) or interfere with reproduction (bacteriostatic antibiotics). Bactericidal antibiotics usually interfere with cell wall production of newly forming, growing bacteria. The resultant defective cell wall is not able to withstand osmotic pressure differential, and the bacteria literally explode. The antibiotic actually kills the bacteria, while host white cells, complement, and antibodies play a less important role in fighting the bacteria.

Bacteriostatic antibiotics interfere with bacterial reproduction and growth. This slowing of bacterial reproduction allows the host defenses to move into the area of infection, phagocytize the existing bacteria, and kill them. Bacteriostatic antibiotics require reasonably intact host defenses. This type of antibiotic should be avoided in patients who have compromised host defense systems.

For patients with compromised host defenses, bactericidal antibiotics should be the drug of choice. For example, the bactericidal antibiotic penicillin would be preferred over the bacteriostatic antibiotic erythromycin in a patient who is receiving cancer chemotherapy.

BE AWARE OF THE COST OF ANTIBIOTICS.

Antibiotics vary widely in their cost to patients. Newer drugs tend to be more expensive, whereas older drugs, which are made by a variety of companies, tend to be less expensive. Drugs prescribed generically also tend to be less expensive than brand name prescriptions. Generic prescriptions for newer drugs are not available. Table 16-6 includes the price of the antibiotics that are discussed in this section. For a 10-day course of therapy the range in price (in the United States) is from $3.00 for penicillin to $52.00 for cefaclor. When other factors are equal, the clinician should prescribe the less-expensive antibiotic.

SUMMARY.

Antibiotics should be used to assist the dentist in treating patients with infections. Surgical treatment of the infection remains the primary method of treatment in most patients; antibiotic therapy plays an adjunctive role. Antibiotics are especially important in patients who have infections that cannot be adequately treated by surgery alone, such as cellulitis, and in patients who have some compromise of their host defense mechanisms. When antibiotic therapy is to be used for a routine odontogenic infection, empiric antibiotic therapy is recommended, because the microbiology of odontogenic infections is well known and usually consistent from patient to patient. The antibiotic of choice for odontogenic infections is still penicillin. Penicillin is bactericidal; has a narrow spectrum that includes streptococci and the oral anaerobes, which are responsible for approximately 90% of odontogenic infections; has low toxicity; and is inexpensive. An alternative drug is erythromycin, which is a useful alternative for mild infections but cannot be used in high doses in more extensive infections. Clindamycin is also a useful alternative, but its high cost and increased toxicity make it most useful in special situations in which resistant anaerobic bacteria are suspected. The oral cephalosporins are excellent choices when the patient has a history of mild allergy to penicillin and in whom bacteria other than the normal oral flora are suspected. Tetracycline, especially doxycycline, is a good choice for mild infections but is limited in its usefulness because it is broad-spectrum and has a high incidence of resistant bacteria. Metronidazole may be a useful adjunct when only anaerobic bacteria are involved. Although slightly more than one third of all odontogenic infections are caused by only anaerobic bacteria, this cannot be predicted reliably, and therefore the use of metronidazole alone in acute infections should be somewhat limited (Table 16-6).

PRINCIPLE VII: ADMINISTER THE ANTIBIOTIC PROPERLY

Once the decision is made to prescribe an antibiotic to the patient, the drug should be administered in the proper dosage and at the proper dosage interval. The proper dosage is usually recommended by the manufacturer. It is adequate to provide plasma levels that are sufficiently high to kill the bacteria that are sensitive to the antibiotic but are not so high as to cause toxicity. The peak plasma level of the drug should usually be at least 4 or 5 times the minimal inhibitory concentration for the bacteria involved in the infection.

Likewise, the clinician must administer the antibiotic at the proper interval. This interval is usually recommended by the manufacturer and is determined by the plasma half-life of the drug. The interval is usually 4 times the plasma half-life of the drug. Strict adherence to this interval is critical with the bacteriostatic antibiotics but is much less important with bactericidal antibiotics, because bacteria exposed to bactericidal antibiotics will die from a defective cell wall, but those exposed to bacteriostatic antibiotics can resume protein synthesis once the antibiotic is gone.

When antibiotics are given, they should be given for an adequate period. The usual recommended duration of antibiotic therapy is 2 to 3 days after the infection has resolved. In clinical terms this means that the patient who has been treated with both surgery and antibiotics will usually have dramatic improvement in symptoms by the third day and by the fifth day will be reasonably asymptomatic. Antibiotics should then be administered for an additional 2 days, for a total of 7 days. Most mild odontogenic infections that are treated on an outpatient basis can usually be managed with a prescription for antibiotics sufficient for 7 days. Additional administration of antibiotics may be necessary in some infections that do not resolve as rapidly. It is important for the clinician to make it clear to the patient that the entire prescription should be taken. If for some reason the patient is advised to stop taking the antibiotic early, all remaining pills or capsules should be

◇ Table 16-6. Profile of orally useful antibiotics

	Penicillin V	Erythromycin	Clindamycin	Cephalexin	Cefadroxil	Metronidazole	Doxycycline	Amoxicillin	Nystatin
Bactericidal or bacteriostatic	Bactericidal	Bacteriostatic	Both	Bactericidal	Bactericidal	Bactericidal	Bacteristatic	Bactericidal	Bactericidal
Spectrum	Streptococci, oral anaerobes	Gram-positive cocci, oral anaerobes	Gram-positive cocci, anaerobes	Gram-positive cocci, some gram-negative rods, oral anaerobes	Gram-positive cocci, some gram-negative rods, oral anaerobes	Anaerobes	Gram-positive cocci, some gram-negative rods, oral anaerobes	Gram-positive cocci; *E. coli*, *H. influenzae*, oral anaerobes	*Candida* organisms
Dose-interval	250-500 mg qid	250-500 mg qid	150-300 mg q6h	500 mg qid	500 mg bid	250 mg qid	100 mg bid	250 mg tid	200,000 U lozenge qid
Metabolized	Kidney	Liver	Liver	Kidney	Kidney	Liver	Liver	Kidney	—
Toxicity and side effects	Allergy	Nausea, vomiting, cramping, diarrhea	Nausea, vomiting, cramping, diarrhea, antibiotic-associated colitis	Allergy, antibiotic-associated colitis	Allergy, antibiotic-associated colitis	Nausea, vomiting, cramping, diarrhea, disulfiram-like effect	Teeth discoloration, photosensitivity, nausea, vomiting, diarrhea	Allergy, antibiotic-associated colitis	—
Primary indication	Drug of choice	Useful alternative for mild infection	Useful alternative, especially for resistant anaerobes	Bactericidal drug required	Bactericidal drug required	Only anaerobic bacteria involved	Broad-spectrum in mild infections	Broader-spectrum needed	Candidosis
Cost to pharmacist for 10-day prescription*	500 qid $6	250 qid $7	150 qid $33	500 qid $18	500 bid $43	250 qid $6	100 bid $7	250 tid $5	10 qid $40

*Prices are for generic drugs when available. Price to patient will be 25% to 75% higher.

discarded. Keeping small amounts of left-over antibiotics in medicine cabinets for the anticipated sore throat next winter should be strongly discouraged. Casual self-administration of antibiotics is not useful and may be hazardous to the health of the individual and community.

PRINCIPLE VIII: EVALUATE THE PATIENT FREQUENTLY

Once the patient has been treated by surgery and antibiotic therapy has been prescribed, the patient should be followed up carefully to monitor response to treatment and complications. In most situations the patient should be asked to return to the dentist 2 days after the original therapy. Typically, the patient is much improved. If therapy is successful, there is a dramatic decrease in swelling and pain. The dentist should check the incision and drainage site to determine whether the drain should be removed at this time. Other parameters, such as temperature, trismus, swelling, and the patient's subjective feelings of improvement, should also be investigated.

If the patient has not had an adequate response to treatment, he or she should be examined carefully for clues to the reason for failure (Box 16-8). The most common cause of treatment failure is inadequate surgery. A tooth may have to be reevaluated for extraction, or a fluctuant area not obvious at the first treatment may have to be incised.

A second reason for failure is depressed host defense mechanisms. A review of the patient's medical history should be performed and more careful probing questions asked. Local defense mechanism depression by things such as dehydration and pain should also be considered and corrected if necessary.

A third reason for treatment failure is the presence of a foreign body. Although this is unlikely in an odontogenic infection, the dentist may consider taking a periapical radiograph of the area to help ensure that a foreign body is not present.

Finally, there may be problems with the antibiotic that was given to the patient. The dentist first ascertains if the patient has been compliant. The patient must have the prescription filled and take the antibiotic according to directions. Many patients fail to follow the orders of their dentists as carefully as they should. Another problem to consider is whether the antibiotic reached the infected area. Failure to reach the area may be related to inadequate surgery, inadequate blood supply to the local area, or a dose that is too low to be effective against the bacteria. Another antibiotic-related problem is an incorrect bacterial diagnosis. If a culture was not performed at the initial surgical treatment or if no surgical treatment was done at the initial therapy, the dentist should obtain a pus specimen for culture and antibiotic sensitivity testing. Finally, it is possible that the wrong antibiotic was prescribed for the infection, which may be because of an inaccurate bacterial diagnosis or because there is an unusual antibiotic resistance of typical bacteria. For example, *Prevotella* organisms are usually susceptible to penicillin, but there appears to be an increasing number of *Prevotella* spp. that resist it. Such bacteria may be causing the infection.

The clinician must also examine the patient to look

◇ Box 16-8 ◇

Reasons for treatment failure

1. Inadequate surgery
2. Depressed host defenses
3. Foreign body
4. Antibiotic problems
   a. Patient noncompliance
   b. Drug not reaching site
   c. Drug dosage too low
   d. Wrong bacterial diagnosis
   e. Wrong antibiotic

---

specifically for toxicity reactions and untoward side effects. Patients may report complaints such as nausea and abdominal cramping but may fail to associate watery diarrhea with the drug administration. Specific questioning about the expected toxicities is important to their early recognition.

The dentist should also be aware of the possibility of secondary or superinfections. The most common secondary infection encountered by dentists is oral or vaginal candidiasis. This is the result of an overgrowth of *Candida* organisms, because the normal oral flora has been altered by the antibiotic therapy. Other secondary infections may arise as normal host flora is altered, but they are not seen with any degree of frequency in the management of odontogenic infections.

Finally, the dentist should follow the patient carefully once the infection has resolved, to check for recurrent infection. This would be seen in a patient who had incomplete therapy for the infection. A variety of reasons may account for this. For example, the patient may have stopped taking the antibiotics too early. The rubber drain may have been removed too early and the drainage site sealed too early, which reestablished the infectious process. If infection does recur, surgical intervention and reinstitution of antibiotic therapy should be considered.

PRINCIPLES OF PREVENTION OF INFECTION ————————◇

The use of antibiotics to treat an established infection is a well-accepted and well-defined technique. These drugs provide major assistance for the patient in overcoming an established infection. The use of antibiotics for prevention (that is, prophylaxis) of infection is also clearly established but less widely accepted. The final section of this chapter discusses the use of antibiotics for prophylaxis of two distinct types of infection. The use of antibiotics to prevent wound infection after surgery is presented first, followed by a discussion of their use to prevent metastatic infection.

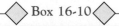

Box 16-9

Advantages of appropriate prophylactic antibiotic use

1. Reduces incidence of infection
2. Reduces health care costs
3. Reduces total antibiotic usage
4. Allows fewer resistant bacteria

Box 16-10

Disadvantages of appropriate prophylactic antibiotic use

1. Alters host flora
2. May be of no benefit
3. May encourage lax surgery
4. Cost
5. Toxicity

Box 16-11

Principles of prophylactic antibiotic use

1. Risk of infection must be significant
2. Choose correct antibiotic
3. Antibiotic level must be high
4. Time the antibiotic correctly
5. Use shortest effective antibiotic exposure

PRINCIPLES OF PROPHYLAXIS OF WOUND INFECTION

The use of antibiotics for prophylaxis of postoperative wound infections can be highly effective and desirable in certain situations. The advantages of the appropriate use of prophylactic antibiotics are clear (Box 16-9). First of all, prophylactic antibiotics reduce the incidence of patient infection and thereby reduce postoperative patient morbidity. When a patient becomes infected after surgery, wound healing and recovery are substantially delayed. Second, appropriate and effective antibiotic prophylaxis reduces the cost of health care. By decreasing the incidence of postoperative infection, the patient is saved the additional expense of returning to the dentist, buying additional antibiotics, and missing additional days of work. Third, appropriate use of prophylactic antibiotics requires a shorter-term administration than therapeutic use, thereby decreasing the total amount of antibiotics used by the population. Finally, there are fewer opportunities for resistant bacteria to arise when effective prophylactic antibiotics are used.

There are also disadvantages to the use of prophylactic antibiotics (Box 16-10). First, they may alter host flora. The body is populated with a variety of bacteria that have a symbiotic relationship with the host. When antibiotics are administered, some of these bacteria are eliminated, allowing the overgrowth of antibiotic-resistant and perhaps more pathogenic bacteria that may then cause infection. Second, the antibiotic may provide no benefit, which means that in certain situations the risk of infection is so low that the antibiotic provides no additional decrease in the incidence of infection. Third, the use of prophylactic antibiotics may encourage lax surgical technique on the part of the dentist. The attitude of

"oh well, the patient is on antibiotics" may become an excuse when principles of surgery are violated. Fourth, the cost of the antibiotic must be considered. Although for a single event for a single patient the cost may be small, the cost for many surgeries for many patients can be enormous. Finally, the toxicity of the drug to the patient must be also kept in mind. All drugs have the potential to cause injury to the patient. Although most antibiotics used by dentists have low toxicity, the possibility of toxicity is always present. The principles of prophylactic antibiotic use are summarized in Box 16-11.

PRINCIPLE I: PROCEDURE SHOULD HAVE SIGNIFICANT RISK OF INFECTION

For prophylactic antibiotics to reduce the incidence of infection, the surgical procedure must have a high enough incidence of infection to be reduced with antibiotic therapy. Clean surgery done with strict adherence to basic surgical principles usually has an incidence of infection of about 3%. Infection rates of 10% or more are usually considered unacceptable, and the use of prophylactic antibiotics must be strongly considered. For the dentist doing routine office surgery, this means that most office procedures performed on healthy patients do not require prophylactic antibiotics. The incidence of infection after tooth extraction, frenectomy, biopsy, minor alveoloplasty, and torus reduction is extremely low, and therefore antibiotics would provide no benefit.

However, there are several surgical factors that may influence the dentist to consider strongly the use of antibiotic prophylaxis (Box 16-12). The most obvious factor that may lead to infection is a bacterial inoculum of sufficient size. The usual surgical procedure performed in the mouth rarely involves sufficient bacterial inoculation to cause infection. The second factor is surgical procedures that are rather extensive and require prolonged surgery. The incidence of infection increases both with the extent of surgery and with longer surgical procedures. A third factor that may suggest the use of antibiotics is the insertion or presence of a foreign body, most commonly a dental implant. Most data seem to suggest that the use of antibiotics may decrease the incidence of infection when foreign bodies, such as dental implants, are inserted into the jaws.

The final and most important factor for most dentists in determining which patients should receive prophylactic antibiotics is whether the patient has depressed host defenses (see Box 16-12). Patients who have a compromised ability to

◇ Box 16-12 ◇

Box 16-12

Factors related to postoperative infection

1. Size of bacterial inoculum
2. Extent and time of surgery
3. Presence of foreign body
4. State of host resistance

defend themselves against infection should probably receive prophylactic antibiotics because they are likely to have a higher incidence of more severe infection. All patients receiving cancer chemotherapy or immunosuppressives should receive prophylactic antibiotics, even when minor surgical procedures are performed. Patients receiving immunosuppressives for organ transplant will be taking these drugs for the remainder of their lives and should be given preventive antibiotics accordingly. Patients receiving cancer chemotherapy will receive cytotoxic drugs for 1 year or less but should be given prophylactic antibiotics for at least 1 year after the cessation of their chemotherapy.

PRINCIPLE II: CHOOSE THE CORRECT ANTIBIOTIC

The choice of antibiotic for prophylaxis against infections after surgery of the oral cavity should be based on the following criteria. First, the antibiotic should be *effective* against the organisms most likely to cause the infection in the oral cavity. As previously discussed, these are aerobic and anaerobic streptococci and anaerobic gram-negative rods. Second, the antibiotic chosen should be a *narrow-spectrum* antibiotic. By using a narrow-spectrum antibiotic, the disadvantage of altering host flora is minimized. Third, the antibiotic should be the *least toxic* antibiotic available for the patient. Finally, the drug selected should be a *bactericidal* antibiotic. Because many of the routine uses of prophylactic antibiotics in the dental office will be for patients with compromised host defenses, it is important that the antibiotic effectively kill the bacteria.

Taking into account these four criteria, the antibiotic of choice for prophylaxis after oral surgery is penicillin. It is effective against the causative organisms, is narrow-spectrum, has a low toxicity, and is bactericidal. For patients who have had mild allergic reactions to penicillin, the drug of choice is a cephalosporin, such as cefadroxil. It is effective, nontoxic, and bactericidal, but it is a broader-spectrum antibiotic, which makes it the second-choice drug. The third choice is clindamycin. It is effective, narrow-spectrum, and bactericidal against anaerobic bacteria and quite effective against streptococci, but it has some increased toxicity. The last choice for oral administration for prophylaxis is erythromycin. It is reasonably effective against the usual organisms, is narrow-spectrum, and is mildly toxic to the gastrointestinal tract, but it is bacterio-

static. This drug is a fourth-choice drug in patients who have clear compromise of normal host defenses.

PRINCIPLE III: ANTIBIOTIC PLASMA LEVEL MUST BE HIGH

When prophylactic antibiotics are used, the antibiotic level in the plasma must be higher than when therapeutic antibiotics are used. The peak plasma levels should be high to ensure diffusion of the antibiotic into all fluid and tissue spaces where the surgery is going to be performed. The usual recommendation for prophylaxis is that the drug be given in a dosage at least *2 times* the usual therapeutic dosage. For penicillin this would mean at least 1 g; for the cephalosporins, such as cefadroxil, it would be 1 g; for clindamycin, at least 300 mg; and for erythromycin, 1 g.

PRINCIPLE IV: TIME THE ANTIBIOTIC ADMINISTRATION CORRECTLY

For the antibiotic to be maximally effective in preventing postoperative infection the antibiotic must be given *before* the surgery begins. This principle has been clearly established in many animal and human clinical trials. Antibiotic administration that occurs after surgery either is markedly decreased in its efficacy or has no effect at all on preventing infection.

If the surgery is prolonged and an additional antibiotic dose is required, intraoperative dosage intervals should be shorter, that is, one half the usual therapeutic dosage interval. Therefore penicillin should be given every 2 hours, cephalexin every 2 hours, clindamycin every 3 hours, and erythromycin every 2 hours. This ensures that the peak plasma levels will stay adequately high and avoids periods of inadequate antibiotic levels in the tissue fluids.

PRINCIPLE V: USE THE SHORTEST ANTIBIOTIC EXPOSURE THAT IS EFFECTIVE

For the antibiotic prophylaxis to be effective, the antibiotic must be given before the surgery begins, and adequate plasma levels must be maintained during the surgical procedure. Once the surgical procedure is completed, there is no additional benefit from continued antibiotic administration. Therefore the final dose of the antibiotic is usually given after the surgical operation. If the procedure is a short operation, a single preoperative dose of antibiotics is adequate. If the surgery lasts for 1 to 2 hours, the surgeon should give a second dose of antibiotics before the patient leaves the office. There is a plethora of animal and human clinical data that clearly demonstrates that the use of prophylactic antibiotics is necessary only for the time of surgery. After closure of the wounds and formation of the blood clots, migration of bacteria into the wound and underlying tissues occurs at such a low level that additional antibiotics are not necessary.

SUMMARY

The use of antibiotics for prophylaxis of postoperative wound infection can be very effective. It reduces patient pain, morbidity, cost, and total antibiotic use. Appropriate antibiotic prophylaxis does little to alter host flora and does not encourage resistant bacteria. Most dental procedures on healthy patients do not require antibiotic prophylaxis. A few select patients who are to undergo extensive or long surgical procedures or the insertion of foreign bodies, such as dental implants, should be considered for prophylaxis. Patients who have compromised host defenses because of poorly controlled metabolic diseases or certain diseases that interfere with defenses or who are taking drugs that interfere with host defenses should also be given prophylactic antibiotics. The drug of choice is a narrow-spectrum antibiotic that is effective against causative organisms, nontoxic, and bactericidal. Penicillin fits these criteria the best. When the antibiotic is given, it should be begun before the surgery begins, at a normal dosage twice that of therapeutic antibiotics. If the surgery is prolonged, interim doses of half the normal dosage interval should be used. High plasma levels should be maintained during the surgical procedure, but no additional antibiotics are necessary after surgery. A common practice is to provide a second and final dosage of antibiotic at the termination of the surgery before the patient leaves the office.

Principles of Prophylaxis of Metastatic Infection

Metastatic infection is defined as infection that occurs at a location physically separate from the portal of entry of the bacteria. The classic and most widely understood example of this phenomenon is bacterial endocarditis, which arises from bacteria that are introduced into the circulation as a result of tooth extraction. The incidence of metastatic infection can be reduced if antibiotic administration is used to eliminate the bacteria before they can establish an infection at the remote site.

For metastatic infection to occur, several conditions must be met (Box 16-13). The first and most important is that there must be a susceptible location in which an infection can be established. The deformed heart valve with its altered endothelial surface onto which a sterile vegetation has formed is an example of this.

There also must be bacterial seeding of the susceptible area. This seeding occurs as the result of a bacteremia in which bacteria from the mouth are carried to the susceptible site. There is most likely a quantitative factor involved in this seeding process, because the body has multiple episodes of small bacteremias as a result of normal daily activities. More than likely, bacteremias with large quantities of bacteria are necessary to produce metastatic infection. The duration of the bacteremia may also play a role. In some situations, such as in total joint replacement, a prolonged high-level bacteremia, or septicemia, is usually necessary to establish a metastatic infection. It is important to remember that the bacteremia following oral surgery is usually completely eliminated by the body's reticuloendothelial system within 15 minutes after completion of the surgery.

Also necessary for the establishment of metastatic infection is some impairment of the local host defenses. Once bacteria have attached to a cardiac vegetation, they are protected from white blood cell phagocytosis by a thin coating of fibrin.

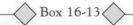

Box 16-13

Factors necessary for metastatic infection

1. Distant susceptible site
2. Hematogenous bacterial seeding
3. Impaired local defenses

Bacteria that are in close proximity to foreign bodies, such as implants, may not be easily phagocytized by white blood cells, and small numbers of bacteria may be able to establish an infection.

Prophylaxis of infectious endocarditis

Infectious endocarditis may be caused by bacteria that was introduced into the circulation as a result of oral surgery and that attached to a sterile vegetation that exists on an abnormal heart valve. This vegetation can arise because of the turbulent flow around an incompetent heart valve. The turbulent flow causes loss of the surface endocardium, which exposes the underlying collagen. Platelets aggregate on the exposed collagen and, together with precipitated fibrin, form a sterile fibrin-platelet thrombus called a *vegetation*. This vegetation presents no problems to the patient until it becomes infected with bacteria and produces bacterial endocarditis. When this occurs the patient must be treated in the hospital with high dosages of intravenous antibiotics for prolonged periods. Although initial recovery from bacterial endocarditis approaches 100%, recurrent episodes reduce the 5-year survival rate of patients with this disease to approximately 60%.

Bacterial endocarditis resulting from introduction of bacteria from an oral source is almost exclusively the result of a-hemolytic streptococci with typical antibiotic sensitivity patterns. Prophylaxis regimens against bacterial endocarditis after dental procedures are directed toward effective killing of *Streptococcus* organisms. The goals of antibiotic prophylaxis in this case are to reduce the intensity of the bacteremia, assist the reticuloendothelial system in killing the bacteria, and decrease the bacterial adherence to the damaged heart valves and vegetations.

The American Heart Association has had formal recommendations for the prevention of bacterial endocarditis after dental treatments since 1960. The latest formal recommendations appeared in June 1997.

When the dentist treats patients surgically, it is important that he specifically inquire about cardiac valvular lesions that may predispose the patient to bacterial endocarditis (Box 16-14). Antibiotic prophylaxis should be used when a dental procedure is performed that will produce bleeding of the mucosa. There are procedures that obviously cause bacteremias, such as tooth extraction and periodontal surgery, but vigorous dental prophylaxis should also be included in these considerations (Box 16-15). Some

◇ Box 16-14 ◇

Cardiac conditions associated with endocarditis

High-risk category—prophylaxis recommended
1. Prosthetic cardiac valve
2. Previous bacterial endocarditis
3. Complex cyanotic congenital heart disease
4. Surgically constructed systemic pulmonary heart

Moderate-risk category—prophylaxis recommended
1. Most other congenital malformations
2. Acquired valvar dysfunction
3. Hypertropic cardiomyopathy
4. Mitral valve prolapse *with valvar regurgitation*

Negligible-risk category—prophylaxis NOT recommended
1. Isolated secundum atrial septal defect
2. Surgical repair of atrial septal defect; patient ductus arteriosus
3. Coronary artery bypass graft
4. Mitral valve prolapse *without regurgitation*
5. Physiologic, functional, or innocent heart murmur
6. Previous rheumatic fever with valvar dysfunction

◇ Box 16-15 ◇

Dental procedures in which prophylaxis is recommended

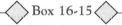

1. Dental extractions
2. Periodontal procedures
3. Dental implant placement
4. Periapical endodontic procedures
5. Initial placement of orthodontic bands but not brackets
6. Intraligamentary local anesthetic injections
7. Dental prophylaxis when bleeding is expected

◇ Box 16-16 ◇

Dental procedures in which prophylaxis is NOT recommended

1. Restorative dentistry
2. Routine local anesthetic injection
3. Intracanal endodontic therapy
4. Suture removal
5. Placement of removable appliances
6. Making impressions

icillin was not made to provide a broader antimicrobial spectrum.

For patients who are allergic to penicillin, two alternative drugs have been recommended. The first recommended drug is clindamycin, with a dosage of 600 mg orally 1 hour before the surgery. If the patient's allergy to penicillin is mild and not of an anaphylactic type, he or she can take a first-generation cephalosporin. Either cephalexin or cefadroxil is recommended. Although erythromycin is no longer recommended, the newer macrolide antibiotics azithromycin or clarithromycin are acceptable alternative drugs. Their chief disadvantage is that they are more expensive than the other regimens. If the patient is unable to take oral medication, parenteral administration can be used.

For the pediatric patient, the dosage of the drugs that are given must be reduced. The recommendations include clear guidelines for these reductions (see Box A-1).

Some patients at risk for bacterial endocarditis will be taking daily dosages of penicillin to prevent recurrence of rheumatic fever or taking an antibiotic for other reasons. In these patients the streptococci may be relatively resistant to penicillin. The recommendation is that the dentist should use clindamycin, azithromycin, or clarithromycin for endocarditis prophylaxis. The cephalosporins should be postponed because of possible cross-reference. If possible, the procedure should be postponed until 9 to 14 days after the antibiotic is completed, thus allowing normal oral flora to be reestablished.

If a particular patient requires a series of dental treatments that requires antibiotic prophylaxis, a period of 9 to 14 days between appointments is recommended. The reason for the interval is that the administration of antibiotics for several days or more continuously may allow the overgrowth of oral streptococci, which are resistant to the antibiotic being given, thus making prophylaxis more likely to fail. The 9- to 14-day antibiotic-free period allows recovery to antibiotic-sensitive organisms.

Occasionally, unexpected bleeding may occur during dental treatment in a patient who is at risk for endocarditis. In this situation, appropriate antibiotic prophylaxis should be administered as soon as possible, but definitely within 2 hours. Prophylaxis given longer than 4 hours after the bacteremia will have no prophylactic benefit.

Patients at risk for bacterial endocarditis should have a

procedures, such as supragingival tooth cleaning, placement and adjustments of orthodontic appliances, typical restorative tooth preparation procedures, and conservative nonsurgical endodontic therapy, do not require antibiotic prophylaxis (Box 16-16). These procedures do not cause bacteremias of sufficient intensity to predispose the patient to endocarditis.

Bacterial endocarditis prophylaxis is achieved for most routine conditions with the administration of 2 g of amoxicillin 1 hour before the procedure (Table 16-7). Amoxicillin is the drug of choice, because it is better absorbed from the gastrointestinal tract and provides higher and more sustained plasma levels. Amoxicillin is an effective killer of a-hemolytic (viridans) *Streptococcus,* which is the organism that most commonly causes endocarditis following dental procedures. The decision to recommend amox-

◇ **Table 16-7.** Antibiotic regimen for prophylaxis of bacterial endocarditis

Situation	Antibiotic	Regimen	
Standard prophylaxis	Amoxicillin	Adults:	2 g orally 1 hr pre-op
		Children:	50 mg/kg orally 1 hr pre-op*
Penicillin allergic	Clindamycin	Adults:	600 mg orally 1 hr pre-op
		Children:	20 mg/kg orally 1 hr pre-op*
	OR		
	Cephalexin or cefadroxil	Adults:	2 g orally 1 hr pre-op
		Children:	50 mg/kg orally 1 hr pre-op*
	OR		
	Azithromycin or clarithromycin	Adults:	500 mg orally 1 hr pre-op
		Children:	15 mg/kg orally 1 hr pre-op*
Unable to take oral medication	Ampicillin	Adults:	2 g IM or IV within 30 min before procedure
		Children:	50 mg/kg IM or IV within 30 min before procedure*
Unable to take oral medication and penicillin allergic	Clindamycin	Adults:	600 mg IV within 30 min before procedure
		Children:	20 mg/kg IV within 30 min before procedure*
	OR		
	Cefazolin	Adults:	1 g IM or IV within 30 min before procedure
		Children:	25 mg IM or IV within 30 min before procedure*

*Total children's dose should not exceed adult dose.

comprehensive prophylaxis program that includes excellent oral hygiene with excellent periodic professional care. Special care should be taken for the establishment of an effective preventive program, and all incipient dental and periodontal disease should be treated. If surgery is required, the dentist should do everything possible to keep the size of the bacteremia as small as possible. Two steps can be taken. First, the extent of the surgical procedure should be limited, which can be done by dividing the surgical procedure into two or three appointments rather than doing all of the indicated surgery at the same time. For example, if the patient requires the removal of 10 teeth, the dentist should remove three or four in each of three appointments. Second, the mouth should be rinsed preoperatively with an antibacterial agent, such as chlorhexidine. If there are fewer bacteria on and around the teeth during the surgical procedure, there will be a less intense bacteremia.

Finally, it is important for the dentist to understand that even when appropriate measures are taken to prevent bacterial endocarditis, it may still occur. Patients should be informed of this and advised to return to the dentist or to their family physician if any of the signs and symptoms of bacterial endocarditis, especially fever and malaise, occur.

Prosthetic valve endocarditis occurs when the tissue around the cardiac valve implant becomes infected. Such infections are caused by the same bacteria that cause typical native valve endocarditis. Prosthetic valve endocarditis is a much more serious illness than native valve endocarditis, because the loosening of the heart valve may result in death. The 1-year survival rate for patients who have prosthetic valve endocarditis is about 50%. The American Heart Association currently recommends that the standard 2 g of amoxicillin regimen is adequate for most patients with prosthetic heart valves.

PROPHYLAXIS IN OTHER CARDIOVASCULAR CASES

Several other cardiovascular conditions are susceptible to metastatic infection. The first is the coronary artery bypass graft (CABG). The procedure for reconstructing the coronary arteries with a vein graft does not predispose the patient to metastatic infection. Patients who have had this procedure should not be given prophylactic antibiotics if dental procedures are performed.

Patients with a transvenous pacemaker have a battery pack implanted in their chests, with a thin wire that runs through the superior vena cava into the right side of the heart. These patients usually do not require prophylactic antibiotics when dental procedures are performed. However, consultation with the patient's cardiologist is advisable to confirm that this is the best management.

Patients on renal dialysis frequently have an arteriovenous shunt appliance implanted in their forearms to provide the dialysis team ready access to the bloodstream. Metastatic infection may occur in these shunts after bacteremia. These are usually caused by staphylococci and not oral bacteria.

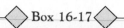

Box 16-17

Conditions placing patients at risk for prosthetic joint infection

1. Immunosuppression
2. Rheumatoid arthritis
3. Systemic lupus erythematosus
4. Insulin-dependent diabetes
5. Previous prosthetic joint infection
6. Prosthetic joint within 2 years

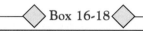

Box 16-18

Procedures that require prophylaxis

1. Dental extractions
2. Implant placement
3. Periodontal procedures
4. Periapical surgery
5. Initial placement of orthodontic bands
6. Intraligamentory local anesthetic injections

Table 16-8. Antibiotic regimen for prophylaxis of total joint replacement infection

Regimen	Drug	Dose
Standard oral prophylaxis	First generation cephalosporin	2 g 1 hr before procedure
	OR	
	Amoxicillin	2 g 1 hr before surgery
Penicillin allergic oral prophylaxis	Clindamycin	600 mg 1 hr before procedure
Parenteral prophylaxis	Cefazolin	1 g IV within 1 hr of procedure
	OR	
	Ampicillin	2 g IV within 1 hr of procedure
Penicillin allergic parenteral prophylaxis	Clindamycin	600 mg IV within 1 hr of procedure

Therefore antibiotic prophylaxis is not usually necessary. However, the dentist should contact the patient's nephrologist or renal dialysis team to discuss the best management.

Patients who have hydrocephaly may have decompression with ventriculoatrial shunts. Because these shunts may induce valvular dysfunction, antibiotic prophylaxis may be required. Consultation with the patient's neurosurgeon should be considered.

Patients who have had severe atherosclerotic vascular disease and have had alloplastic vascular grafts placed to replace portions of their arteries may be at risk for metastatic infection. After the vascular implant is in place, the interior of the graft undergoes endothelialization, a process that usually requires approximately 3 to 6 months. Until this process is complete, the alloplastic vascular implant is exposed in the lumen of the vessel. Potentially, a bacteremia of oral origin could seed the implant and cause infection. Therefore prophylactic antibiotics should be strongly considered during the first 6 months. After a 6-month interval, prophylactic antibiotics are usually not indicated. The dentist should consider consultation with the patient's vascular surgeon before performing extensive dental surgery.

PROPHYLAXIS OF TOTAL JOINT REPLACEMENT INFECTION

Patients who have undergone total replacement of a joint with a prosthetic joint may be at risk for hematogenous spread of bacteria and subsequent infection. These late prosthetic joint infections result in severe morbidity, because the implant is usually lost when infections occur. There has been great concern that the bacteremia caused by tooth extraction may result in such infections. However, the recent literature suggests that bacteremias from oral procedures do not cause prosthetic joint infections. It appears that the bacteremia following oral surgery is of a transient nature and does not expose the implant and peri-implant tissues to bacteria long enough to cause infection. Instead, it appears that the hematogenous spread of prosthetic joint infections is caused by chronic infections elsewhere in the body that result in chronic septicemias. These infections are typically urinary tract infections, pulmonary infections, and skin infections, but established odontogenic infections may also cause a septicemia of sufficient magnitude to cause a total joint infection.

In July, 1997 the American Dental Association and the American Academy of Orthopedic Surgeons issued a joint recommendation concerning the management of patients with prosthetic total joints. The recommendations of the ADA-AAOS recognize that most patients with a prosthetic joint are not at risk for joint infection following a dental surgical procedure. Rather, the guidelines identify the high-risk patients who are potentially susceptible to such infections (Box 16-17). Likewise, it identifies those procedures that are most likely to cause joint infections and therefore require prophylaxis (Box 16-18). Finally, the joint statement recommends a specific antibiotic recommendation to help prevent infection in the susceptible patient who is undergoing one of the procedures that require prophylaxis (Table 16-8).

When the dentist decides to provide antibiotic prophylaxis for a patient, the recommended antibiotics are first-generation cephalosporin and ampicillin. For patients who are allergic to penicillin, clindamycin is recommended. As with bacterial endocarditis prophylaxis, only a single preoperative dose is

---

◇ Box 16-19 ◇

Indication for parenteral regimen

1. Patient to have general anesthetic and is NPO
2. Unable to take oral medications
3. High-risk patients, such as those with history of previous BE

---

recommended, with no follow-up dosages. If patients are unable to take oral medication, a parenteral regimen is also suggested (Box 16-19).

If a patient who has a total joint replacement presents for treatment of an infection, aggressive therapy for the infection is necessary to prevent seeding of the bacteria causing odontogenic infection to the prosthetic joint. This aggressive treatment should include extraction, incision and drainage, and the use of high-dose bactericidal antibiotics, probably given intravenously. The clinician should also strongly consider performing a culture and sensitivity test, because if a prosthetic joint infection does occur, it would be useful to know which bacteria is likely the culprit and its antibiotic sensitivity.

BIBLIOGRAPHY

Aderhold L, Konthe H, Frenkel G: The bacteriology of dentogenous pyogenic infections, *Oral Surg* 52:583, 1981.

American Dental Association, Academy of Orthopedic Surgeons: Antibiotic prophylaxis dental patients with total joint replacements, *JADA* 128:1. 1997.

Antimicrobial prophylaxis for surgery, *Med Lett Drugs Ther* 27:105, 1985.

Antimicrobial prophylaxis in surgery, *Med Lett Drugs Ther* 29:91, 1987.

Bartlett JG, O'Keefe P: The bacteriology of perimandibular space infections, *J Oral Surg* 50:130, 1980.

Canner GC: The infected hip after total hip arthroplasty, *J Bone Joint Surg* 66A:1393, 1984.

Chow AW, Roser SM, Brady FA: Orofacial odontogenic infections, *Ann Intern Med* 88:392, 1978.

Conover MA, Kaban LB, Mulliken JB: Antibiotic prophylaxis for major maxillocraniofacial surgery, *J Oral Maxillofac Surg* 43:865, 1985.

Conover MA, Kaban LB, Mulliken JB: Antibiotic prophylaxis for major maxillofacial surgery: one-day vs. five-day therapy, *Otolaryngology* 95:554, 1986.

Council on Dental Therapeutics, American Heart Association: Preventing bacterial endocarditis: a statement for the dental professional, *J Am Dent Assoc* 122:87, 1991.

Dajani AS et al: Prevention of bacterial endocarditis: recommendations by the American Heart Association, *JAMA* 277:1794, 1997.

Durack DT: Current issues in prevention of infective endocarditis, *Am J Med* 78:149, 1985.

Edson RS et al: Recent experience with antimicrobial susceptibility of anaerobic bacteria: increasing resistance to penicillin, *Mayo Clin Proc* 57:737, 1982.

Field EA, Martin MV: Prophylactic antibiotics for patients with artificial joints undergoing oral and dental surgery: necessary or not? *J Oral Maxillofac Surg* 29B:341, 1991.

Heimdahl A, Nord CE: Treatment of orofacial infections of odontogenic origin, *Scand J Infect Dis* 46(suppl):101, 1985.

Jacobson JJ, Matthews LS: Bacteria isolated from late prosthetic joint infections: dental treatment and chemoprophylaxis, *Oral Surg Oral Med Oral Pathol* 63:122, 1987.

Jacobsen PL, Murray W: Prophylactic coverage of dental patients with artificial joints: a retrospective analysis of thirty-three infants in hip prosthesis, *Oral Surg* 37:407, 1979.

Jacobson JJ, Schweitzer SO, Kowalski CJ: Chemoprophylaxis of prosthetic joint patients during dental treatment: a decision-utility analysis, *Oral Surg Oral Med Oral Pathol* 72:167, 1991.

Jacobson JJ et al: Dental treatment and late prosthetic joint infections, *Oral Surg* 61:413, 1986.

Kaye D: Prophylaxis for infective endocarditis: an update, *Ann Intern Med* 104:419, 1986.

Konow LV, Nord CE, Nordenram A: Anaerobic bacteria in dentoalveolar infections, *Int J Oral Surg* 10:313, 1981.

Labriola JD, Mascaro J, Alpert B: The microbiologic flora of orofacial abscesses, *J Oral Maxillofac Surg* 41:711, 1983.

Laskin DM: Anatomic considerations in diagnosis and treatment of odontogenic infections, *J Am Dent Assoc* 69:308, 1964.

Lewis MAO, MacFarlane TW, McGowan DA: Quantitative bacteriology of acute dento-alveolar abscesses, *J Med Microbiol* 2:101, 1986.

Lewis MAO et al: A randomised trial of co-amoxiclav (*Augmentin*) versus penicillin V in the treatment of acute dentoalveolar abscess, *Br Dent J* 175:169, 1993.

Lewis MAO et al: Prevalence of penicillin-resistant bacteria in acute suppurative oral infection, *J Antimicrob Chemother* 35B:785, 1995.

Little JW: The need for antibiotic coverage for dental treatment of patients with joint replacements, *Oral Surg* 55:20, 1983.

Martin C, Karabouta I: Infection after orthognathic surgery, with and without preventative antibiotics, *Int J Oral Surg* 13:490, 1984.

McGowan DA: Is antibiotic prophylaxis required for dental patients with joint replacement? *Br Dent J* 158:336, 1985.

Nager C, Murphy AA: Antibiotics and oral contraceptive pills, *Semin Reproductive Endocrin* 7:220, 1989.

Newman MG et al: Antibacterial susceptibility of plaque bacteria, *J Dent Res* 58:1722, 1979.

Norden CW: Prevention of bone and joint infections, *Am J Med* 78:229, 1985.

Onderdonk AB: Use of an animal model system for assessing the efficacy of antibiotics in treating mixed infections, *Infect Dis Clin Prac* 3(suppl 1):S28, 1994.

Paterson SA, Curzon MEJ: The effect of amoxicillin versus penicillin V in the treatment of acutely abscessed primary teeth, *Br Dent J* 174:443, 1993.

Peterson LJ: Prophylactic antibiotics and prosthetic joints, *JAMA* 244:1782, 1980.

Peterson LJ: Antibiotic prophylaxis against wound infections in oral and maxillofacial surgery, *J Oral Maxillofac Surg* 48:617, 1990.

Peterson LJ: Microbiology of head and neck infections, *Oral Maxillofac Surg Clin North Am* 3:247, 1991.

Peterson LJ: Contemporary management of deep infections of the neck, *J Oral Maxillofac Surg* 51:226,1993.

Polk HC et al: Guidelines for prevention of surgical wound infection, *Arch Surg* 118:1213, 1983.

Quayle AA, Russell C, Hearn B: Organisms isolated from severe odontogenic soft tissue infections: their sensitivities to cefotetan and seven other antibiotics and implications for therapy and prophylaxis, *J Oral Maxillofac Surg* 25B:34, 1987.

Rubin R: Infected total hip replacement after dental procedures, *Oral Surg* 41:18, 1976.

Sabiston CB, Grigsby WR: Bacterial study of pyogenic infections of dental origin, *Oral Surg* 44:430, 1976.

Stinchfield FE: Late hematogenous infection of total joint replacement, *J Bone Joint Surg* 62A:1345, 1980.

Sullam PM: Pathogenesis of endocarditis, *Am J Med* 78:110, 1985.

Thyne GM, Ferguson JW: Antibiotic prophylaxis during dental treatment in patients with prosthetic joints, *J Bone Joint Surg* 73B:191, 1991.

COMPLEX ODONTOGENIC INFECTIONS

LARRY J. PETERSON

CHAPTER OUTLINE

Odontogenic infections are usually mild and easily treated by antibiotic administration and local surgical treatment. Abscess formation in the buccolingual vestibule is managed by simple intraoral incision and drainage procedures, occasionally including dental extraction. (The principles of management of routine odontogenic infections are discussed in Chapter 16.) Some odontogenic infections are very serious and require management by clinicians who have extensive training and experience. Even after the advent of antibiotics and improved dental health, serious odontogenic infections still sometimes result in death. These deaths occur when the infection reaches areas distant from the alveolar process. The purpose of this chapter is to present overviews of fascial space infections of the head and neck caused by odontogenic infections and several of the more frequently seen unusual infections of the oral cavity.

FASCIAL SPACE INFECTIONS

The erosion process of infections through bone into surrounding soft tissue is discussed in Chapter 16. As a general rule, infection erodes through the thinnest bone and causes infection in the adjacent tissue. Whether or not this becomes a vestibular or fascial space abscess is determined primarily by the relationship of the muscle attachment to the point at which the infection perforates. Most odontogenic infections penetrate the bone in such a way that they become vestibular abscesses. On occasion they erode into fascial spaces directly, which causes a fascial space infection (Figure 17-1). Fascial spaces are fascia-lined areas that can be eroded or distended by purulent exudate. These areas are potential spaces that do not exist in healthy people but become filled during infections. Some contain named neurovascular structures and are known as *compartments;* others, which are filled with loose areolar connective tissue, are known as *clefts.*

The spaces that are involved directly are known as the *fascial spaces of primary involvement.* The principal maxillary primary spaces are the canine, buccal, and infratemporal spaces (Box 17-1). The principle mandibular primary spaces are the submental, buccal, submandibular, and sublingual spaces. Infections can extend beyond these primary spaces into additional fascial spaces, or secondary spaces.

MAXILLARY SPACES

The canine space is a thin potential space between the levator anguli oris and the levator labii superioris muscles. The canine space becomes involved primarily as the result of infections from the maxillary canine tooth. This is the only tooth with a root sufficiently long to allow erosion to occur through the alveolar bone superior to the muscles of facial expression. The infection erodes superior to the origin of the levator anguli oris muscle and below the origin of the levator labii superioris muscle. When this space is infected there is a swelling of the anterior face that obliterates the nasolabial fold (Figure 17-2). Spontaneous drainage of infections of this space commonly occurs just inferior to the medial canthus of the eye.

The buccal space becomes involved from the maxillary teeth when infection erodes through the bone superior to the attachment of the buccinator muscle. The buccal space is bounded by the overlying skin of the face on the lateral aspect

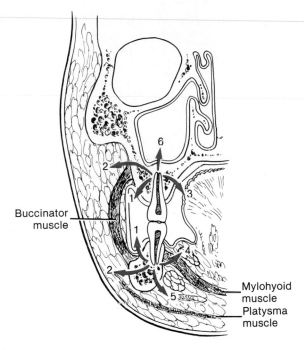

Buccinator muscle

Mylohyoid muscle

Platysma muscle

◇ Figure 17-1

As infection erodes through bone, it can express itself in a variety of places, depending on thickness of overlying bone and relationship of muscle attachments to site of perforation. This illustration notes six possible locations: (*1*), vestibular abscess; (*2*), buccal space; (*3*), palatal abscess; (*4*), sublingual space; (*5*), submandibular space; and (*6*), maxillary sinus. *(From Cummings CW et al, editors:* Otolaryngology: head and neck surgery, *vol 2, St Louis, 1986, Mosby.)*

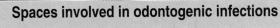
◇ Box 17-1 ◇

Spaces involved in odontogenic infections

Primary maxillary spaces
Canine
Buccal
Infratemporal
Primary mandibular spaces
Submental
Buccal
Submandibular
Sublingual
Secondary fascial spaces
Masseteric
Pterygomandibular
Superficial and deep temporal
Lateral pharyngeal
Retropharyngeal
Prevertebral

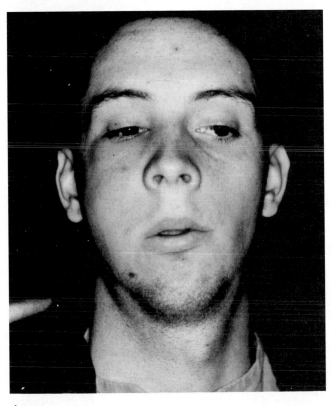

◇ Figure 17-2

Canine space infection in patient's right side resulted from infected canine tooth. Note swelling of nasolabial and infraorbital areas.

and the buccinator muscle on the medial aspect (Figure 17-3). This space may become infected from extensions of infection from either the maxillary or mandibular teeth. Most buccal space infections are caused by the maxillary teeth, most commonly the molars. Infection from the premolars may cause buccal space involvement. Involvement of the buccal space usually results in swelling below the zygomatic arch and above the inferior border of the mandible. Thus both the zygomatic arch and the inferior border of the mandible are palpable in buccal space infections.

The infratemporal space lies posterior to the maxilla. It is bounded medially by the lateral plate of the pterygoid process of the sphenoid bone and superiorly by the base of the skull. Laterally, the infratemporal space is continuous with the deep temporal space. The infratemporal space is rarely infected, but when it is, the cause is usually an infection of the maxillary third molar (Figure 17-4).

Maxillary odontogenic infections may also spread superiorly to cause secondary periorbital or orbital cellulitis or cavernous sinus thrombosis. Periorbital or orbital cellulitis rarely occurs as the result of odontogenic infection, but when either does occur, the presentation is typical: redness and swelling of the eyelids and involvement of both the vascular and neural components of the orbit. This is a serious infection

and requires aggressive medical and surgical intervention from multiple specialists.

Cavernous sinus thrombosis may also occur as the result of superior spread of odontogenic infection via a hematogenous route (Figure 17-5). Bacteria may travel from the maxilla

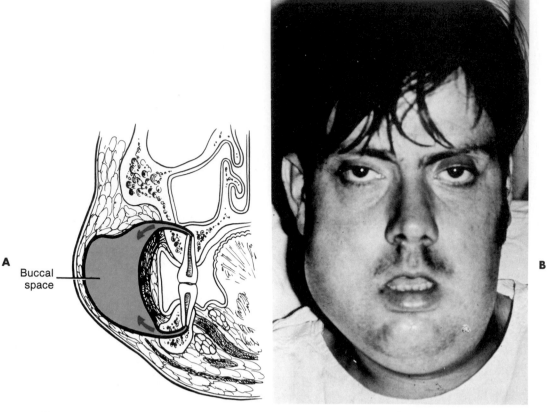

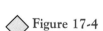 Figure 17-3

A, Buccal space lies between buccinator muscle and overlying skin and superficial fascia. This potential space may become involved via maxillary or mandibular molars. **B,** This buccal space infection was result of maxillary molar. Note typical swelling of cheek, which does not extend beyond inferior border of mandible. *(From Cummings CW et al, editors:* Otolaryngology: head and neck surgery, *vol 2, St Louis, 1986, Mosby.)*

Figure 17-4

Spaces of ramus of mandible are bounded by masseter muscle, medial pterygoid muscle, temporal fascia, and skull. Temporal space is divided into two portions, deep and superficial, by temporalis muscle. *(Redrawn from Cummings CW et al, editors:* Otolaryngology: head and neck surgery, *vol 2, St Louis, 1986, Mosby.)*

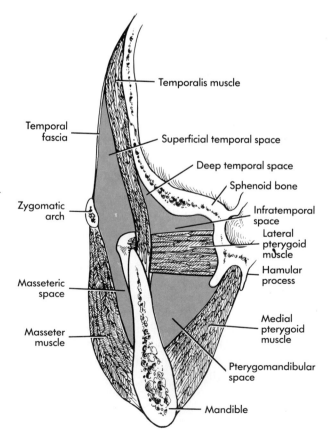

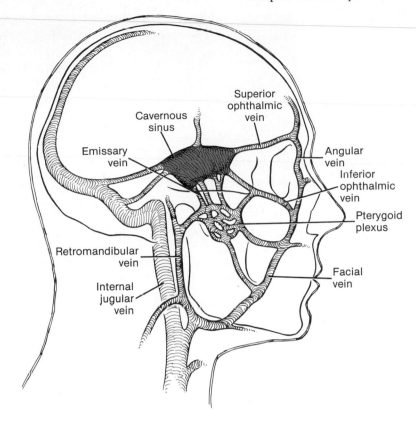

◇ Figure 17-5

Hematogenous spread of infection from jaw to cavernous sinus may occur anteriorly via inferior or superior ophthalmic vein or posteriorly via emissary veins from pterygoid plexus. *(From Cummings CW et al, editors:* Otolaryngology: head and neck surgery, *vol 2, St Louis, 1986, Mosby.)*

posteriorly via the pterygoid plexus and emissary veins or anteriorly via the angular vein and inferior or superior ophthalmic veins to the cavernous sinus. The veins of the face and orbit lack valves, which permits blood to flow in either direction. Thus bacteria can travel via the venous drainage system and contaminate the cavernous sinus, which results in thrombosis. Cavernous sinus thrombosis is an unusual occurrence that is rarely the result of an infected tooth. Like orbital cellulitis, cavernous sinus thrombosis is a serious, life-threatening infection that requires aggressive medical and surgical care. Cavernous sinus thrombosis has a high mortality even today.

MANDIBULAR SPACES

Although most infections of the mandibular teeth erode into the buccal vestibule, they may also spread into fascial spaces. There are four primary mandibular spaces.

The submental space lies between the anterior bellies of the digastric muscle and between the mylohyoid muscle and the overlying skin (Figure 17-6). This space is primarily infected by mandibular incisors, which are sufficiently long to allow the infection to erode through the labial bone apical to the attachment of the mentalis muscle. The infection is thus allowed to proceed under the inferior border of the mandible and involve the submental space. Isolated submental space infection is a rare occurrence.

The buccal space can be infected as an extension of infection from mandibular teeth, similar to the way in which it is involved from the maxillary teeth (Figure 17-3). The buccal space is most commonly infected from maxillary teeth but can also be involved from the mandibular teeth.

The sublingual and submandibular spaces have the medial border of the mandible as their lateral boundary. These two spaces are involved primarily by lingual perforation of infection from the mandibular molars, although they may be involved by premolars, as well. The factor that determines whether the infection is submandibular or sublingual is the attachment of the mylohyoid muscle on the mylohyoid ridge of the medial aspect of the mandible (Figure 17-7). If the infection erodes through the medial aspect of the mandible above this line, the infection will be in the sublingual space and is most commonly seen with premolars and the first molar. If the infection erodes through the medial aspect of the mandible inferior to the mylohyoid line, the submandibular space will be involved. The mandibular third molar is the tooth that most commonly involves the submandibular space primarily. The second molar may involve either the sublingual or submandibular space, depending on the length of the individual roots, and may involve both spaces primarily.

The sublingual space lies between the oral mucosa of the

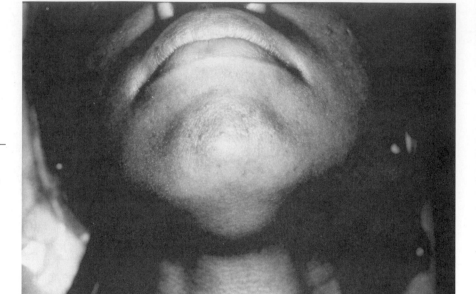

⬦ **Figure 17-6**

Submental space infection appears as discrete swelling in central area of submandibular region.

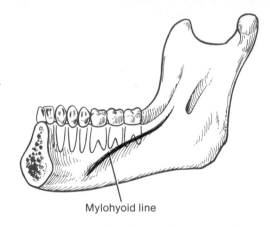

⬦ **Figure 17-7**

Mylohyoid line is area of attachment of mylohyoid muscle. Linguocortical plate perforation by infection from premolars and first molar causes sublingual space infection, whereas infection from third molar involves submandibular space. *(From Cummings CW et al, editors:* Otolaryngology: head and neck surgery, *vol 2, St Louis, 1986, Mosby.)*

Mylohyoid line

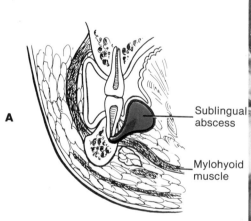

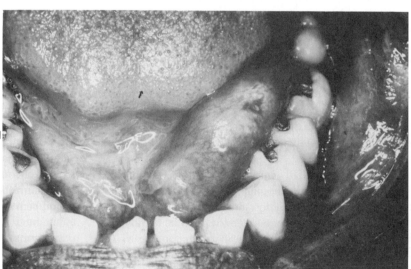

A

Sublingual abscess

Mylohyoid muscle

B

⬦ **Figure 17-8**

A, Sublingual space between oral mucosa and mylohyoid muscle. It is primarily involved by infection from mandibular premolars and first molar. **B,** This isolated sublingual space infection produced unilateral swelling of floor of mouth. *(From Cummings CW et al, editors:* Otolaryngology: head and neck surgery, *vol 2, St Louis, 1986, Mosby.)*

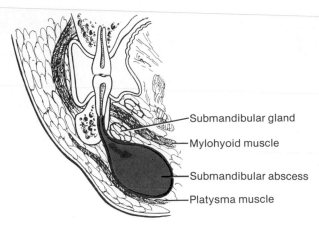

- Submandibular gland
- Mylohyoid muscle
- Submandibular abscess
- Platysma muscle

◇ **Figure 17-9**

Submandibular space lies between mylohyoid muscle and skin and superficial fascia. It is infected primarily by second and third molars. (*From Cummings CW et al, editors:* Otolaryngology: head and neck surgery, *vol 2, St Louis, 1986, Mosby.)*

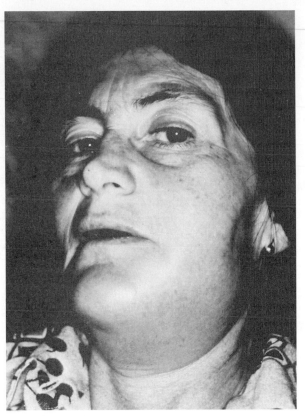

◇ **Figure 17-10**

This submandibular space infection produced large, indurated swelling of submandibular space. (*From Cummings CW et al, editors:* Otolaryngology: head and neck surgery, *vol 2, St Louis, 1986, Mosby.)*

floor of the mouth and the mylohyoid muscle (Figure 17-8, *A*). Its posterior border is open, and therefore it freely communicates with the submandibular space and the secondary spaces of the mandible to the posterior aspect. Clinically there is little or no extraoral swelling in infection of the sublingual space but much intraoral swelling of the floor of the mouth on the infected side (Figure 17-8, *B*). The infection usually becomes bilateral, and the tongue becomes elevated.

The submandibular space lies between the mylohyoid muscle and the overlying skin and superficial fascia (Figure 17-9). The posterior boundary of the submandibular space communicates with the secondary spaces of the jaw posteriorly. Infection of the submandibular space causes swelling that begins at the inferior border of the mandible and extends medially to the digastric muscle and posteriorly to the hyoid bone (Figure 17-10).

When bilateral submandibular, sublingual, and submental spaces become involved with an infection, it is known as *Ludwig's angina*. This infection is a rapidly spreading cellulitis that commonly spreads posteriorly to the secondary spaces of the mandible. There is almost always severe swelling, with elevation and displacement of the tongue, and a tense, hard induration of the submandibular region superior to the hyoid bone. The patient usually has trismus, drooling of saliva, and difficulty with swallowing and sometimes breathing. The patient often experiences severe anxiety concerning the inability to swallow and maintain an airway. This infection may progress with alarming speed and thus may produce upper airway obstruction that often leads to death. The most common cause of Ludwig's angina is an odontogenic infection, usually as the result of streptococci. This infection must be aggressively managed with vigorous incision and drainage procedures and aggressive antibiotic therapy. Special attention must be given to maintenance of the airway.

SECONDARY FASCIAL SPACES

The primary spaces discussed so far are immediately adjacent to the tooth-bearing portions of the maxilla and mandible. If proper treatment is not received for infections of the primary spaces, the infections may extend posteriorly to involve the secondary fascial spaces. When these spaces are involved, the infections frequently become more severe, cause greater complications and greater morbidity, and are more difficult to treat. Because these spaces are surrounded by a connective tissue fascia that has a poor blood supply, infections involving these spaces are difficult to treat without surgical intervention to drain the purulent exudate.

The masseteric space exists between the lateral aspect of the mandible and the medial boundary of the masseter muscle (Figure 17-4). It is involved by infection most commonly as the result of spread from the buccal space or from soft tissue infection around the mandibular third molar. When the masseteric space is involved, the area overlying the angle of the jaw and ramus becomes swollen. Because of the involvement of the masseter muscle, the patient will also have moderate-to-severe trismus caused by inflammation of the masseter muscle.

The pterygomandibular space lies medial to the mandible and lateral to the medial pterygoid muscle (Figure 17-4). This

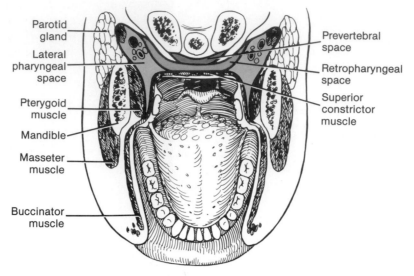

Parotid gland
Lateral pharyngeal space
Pterygoid muscle
Mandible
Masseter muscle
Buccinator muscle

Prevertebral space
Retropharyngeal space
Superior constrictor muscle

◇ Figure 17-11

Lateral pharyngeal space is located between medial pterygoid muscle on lateral aspect and superior pharyngeal constrictor on medial aspect. Retropharyngeal and prevertebral spaces lie between pharynx and vertebral column. Retropharyngeal space lies between superior constrictor muscle and alar portion of prevertebral fascia. Prevertebral spaces lie between alar layer and prevertebral fascia. *(From Cummings CW et al, editors:* Otolaryngology: head and neck surgery, *vol 2, St Louis, 1986, Mosby.)*

is the space into which local anesthetic solution is injected when an inferior alveolar nerve block is performed. Infections of this space spread primarily from the sublingual and submandibular spaces. When the pterygomandibular space alone is involved, there is little or no facial swelling, but the patient almost always has significant trismus. Therefore trismus without swelling is a valuable diagnostic clue for pterygomandibular space infection. The most common occurrence of this clinical picture is caused by needle tract infection from a mandibular block.

The temporal space is posterior and superior to the masseteric and pterygomandibular spaces (Figure 17-4). It is divided into two portions by the temporalis muscle—a superficial portion that extends to the temporal fascia and a deep portion that is continuous with the infratemporal space. The superficial and deep temporal spaces are secondarily involved rarely and usually only in severe infections. When these spaces are involved, the swelling that occurs is evident in the temporal area, superior to the zygomatic arch and posterior to the lateral orbital rim.

When taken as a group, the masseteric, pterygomandibular, and temporal spaces are known as the *masticator space,* because they are bounded by the muscles and fascia of mastication. These spaces communicate freely with one another, so when one becomes involved the others may also. The term *masticator space* does have some general clinical usefulness, but it lacks specificity and is therefore less useful than specific space designations.

CERVICAL FASCIAL SPACES

Extension of odontogenic infections beyond the primary and secondary mandibular spaces is an uncommon occurrence. However, when it does happen, spread to deep cervical spaces may have serious life-threatening sequelae. These sequelae may be the result of locally induced complications, such as upper airway obstructions, or of distant problems, such as mediastinitis.

Infection extending posteriorly from the pterygomandibular space first encounters the lateral pharyngeal space. This space extends from the base of the skull at the sphenoid bone to the hyoid bone inferiorly. It is medial to the medial pterygoid muscle and lateral to the superior pharyngeal constrictor on the medial side (Figure 17-11). It is bounded anteriorly by the pterygomandibular raphe and extends posteromedially to the prevertebral fascia. The styloid process and associated muscles and fascia divide the lateral pharyngeal space into an anterior compartment, which contains primarily muscles, and a posterior compartment, which contains the carotid sheath and several cranial nerves.

The clinical findings of lateral pharyngeal space infection include severe trismus as the result of involvement of the medial pterygoid muscle; lateral swelling of the neck, especially inferior to the angle of the mandible; and swelling of the lateral pharyngeal wall, toward the midline. Patients who have lateral pharyngeal space infections have difficulty swallowing and usually have a high temperature and become quite sick.

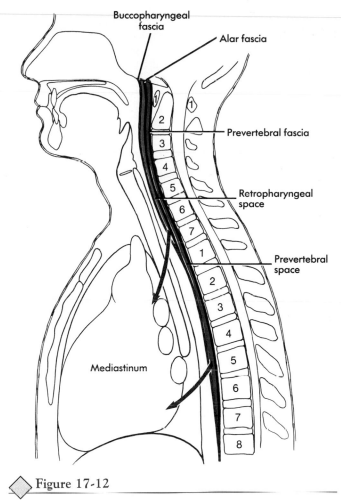

Figure 17-12

If retropharyngeal space is involved, posterosuperior mediastinum may also become infected secondarily. If prevertebral space is infected, inferior boundary is diaphragm, so entire mediastinum is at risk. *(From Cummings CW et al, editors: Otolaryngology: head and neck surgery, vol 2, St Louis, 1986, Mosby.)*

Patients who have infection of the lateral pharyngeal space have several serious potential problems. When the lateral pharyngeal space is involved, the odontogenic infection is severe and may be progressing at a rapid rate. Another possible problem is the direct effect of the infection on the contents of the space, especially those of the posterior compartment. These problems include thrombosis of the internal jugular vein, erosion of the carotid artery or its branches, and interference with cranial nerves IX through XII. A third serious complication arises if the infection progresses from the lateral pharyngeal space to the retropharyngeal space.

The retropharyngeal space lies behind the soft tissue of the posterior aspect of the pharynx. It is bounded anteriorly by the superior pharyngeal constrictor muscle and its investing fascia and posteriorly by the alar layer of prevertebral fascia (Figure 17-11). The retropharyngeal space begins at the base of the skull and extends inferiorly to the level of vertebra C7 or T1, where the alar fascia fuses anteriorly with the buccopharyngeal fascia (Figure 17-12). The retropharyngeal space has

few contents, and therefore infection in this space does not carry some of the grave problems that involvement of the lateral pharyngeal space does. However, when the retropharyngeal space becomes involved, the major concern is that the infection can extend inferiorly to the posterosuperior mediastinum relatively rapidly. Should infection spread by this route, the result may be extension of the infection into the mediastinum, which is a serious complication.

When a patient has extension of infection into the cervical region, the retropharyngeal space must be evaluated with lateral radiographs of the neck to determine if the space is enlarged and thereby compromising the airway (Figure 17-13).

A final danger of retropharyngeal space infection is progressive involvement of the prevertebral space. The prevertebral space is separated from the retropharyngeal space by the alar layer of prevertebral fascia. If this fascia is perforated, the prevertebral space can become involved. The prevertebral space extends from the pharyngeal tubercle on the base of the skull to the diaphragm. Infection of this space can extend rapidly inferior to the level of the diaphragm (Figure 17-12) and can involve the thorax and mediastinum along the way.

When the retropharyngeal and/or prevertebral fascial spaces are involved as a result of odontogenic infection, the patient is almost always seriously ill. The following are the three greatest potential complications: (1) the serious possibility of upper airway obstruction as a result of anterior displacement of the posterior pharyngeal wall into the oral pharynx; (2) rupture of the retropharyngeal space abscess, with aspiration of pus into the lungs and subsequent asphyxiation; and (3) spread of the infection from the retropharyngeal spaces into the mediastinum, which results in severe infection in the thorax.

MANAGEMENT OF FASCIAL SPACE INFECTIONS

Management of infections, mild or severe, always has the following same general goals: (1) medical support of the patient, with special attention to correcting host defense compromises where they exist; (2) administration of proper antibiotics in appropriate dosages; (3) surgical removal of the source of infection as early as possible; (4) surgical drainage of the infection, with placement of proper drains; and (5) constant reevaluation of the resolution of the infection. The principles of surgical and medical management of fascial space infections are the same as those for less serious infections. However, fascial space infections require more extensive and aggressive treatment.

Medical management of the patient with a serious infection must include a thorough assessment and support of host defense mechanisms, including analgesics, fluid requirements, and nutrition. High-dosage bactericidal antibiotics are usually necessary and are almost always administered intravenously. Additionally, the patient's airway must be continually monitored, and a surgical airway established if warranted.

Surgical management of fascial space infections almost

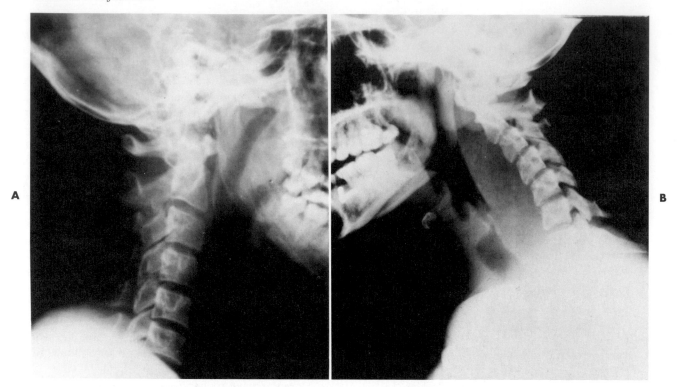

Figure 17-13

A, Retropharyngeal soft tissue shadow is narrow (3 to 4 mm) and located at C2 and at C6. Retrotracheal soft tissue is usually 14 to 15 mm. **B,** When retropharyngeal space is involved, soft tissue becomes substantially thicker, and width of oropharyngeal air shadow decreases. *(From Cummings CW et al, editors:* Otolaryngology: head and neck surgery, *vol 2, St Louis, 1986, Mosby.)*

always requires a generous incision and aggressive exploration of the involved fascial spaces with a hemostat. One or more drains are usually required to provide adequate drainage and decompression of the infected area. Because incision and drainage must be extensive, they are usually done in an operating room, with the patient under general anesthesia. The locations of various incision and drainage sites are depicted in Figure 17-14. Ample clinical experience and experimental evidence indicate that, although no pus formation can be documented by palpation or even by needle aspiration, even the serious cellulitis will resolve more rapidly if incised. The surgeon must not wait until there is unequivocal evidence of pus formation. In the preantibiotic era, surgical treatment was the only method of therapy for infections, and early and aggressive surgical therapy was frequently curative for these severe infections. It is important to remember that aggressive surgical exploration is still the primary method of therapy for serious odontogenic infections of the head and neck.

OSTEOMYELITIS

The term *osteomyelitis* literally means "inflammation of the bone marrow." Clinically, osteomyelitis usually implies an infection of the bone. It usually begins in the medullary cavity, involving the cancellous bone, and then extends and spreads to the cortical bone and eventually to the periosteum. Invasion of bacteria into the cancellous bone, which causes inflammation and edema in the marrow spaces, results in compression of the blood vessels in the bone and subsequent severe compromise of the blood supply. The failure of microcirculation in the cancellous bone is a critical factor in the establishment of osteomyelitis, because the involved area becomes ischemic and bone becomes necrotic. Bacteria can then proliferate, because normal blood-borne defenses do not reach the tissue, and the osteomyelitis spreads until it is stopped by medical and surgical therapy.

Although the maxilla can also become involved in osteomyelitis, it does so rarely compared with the mandible. The primary reason for this is that the blood supply to the maxilla is much richer and is derived from several arteries, which form a complex network of feeder vessels. Because the mandible tends to draw its primary blood supply from the inferior alveolar artery, and because the dense overlying cortical bone of the mandible prevents penetration of periosteal blood vessels, the mandibular cancellous bone is more likely to become ischemic and therefore infected.

Osteomyelitis of the jaws is relatively uncommon in contemporary, developed countries, primarily because of the use of antibiotics in the management of odontogenic infections. However, it is occasionally seen and requires vigorous

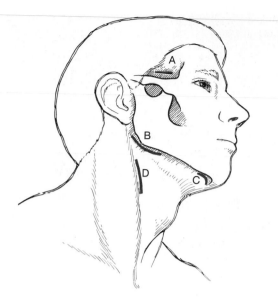

Figure 17-14

Typical incision and drainage sites for various fascial space infections. **A,** Superficial and deep temporal space; **B,** submandibular masseteric and pterygomandibular spaces; **C,** submental space; **D,** lateral pharyngeal and retropharyngeal spaces. *(From Cummings CW et al, editors:* Otolaryngology: head and neck surgery, *vol 2, St Louis, 1986, Mosby.)*

management to prevent its spread and the potentially disabling and disfiguring sequelae of loss of major portions of the mandible.

Osteomyelitis of the jaws is classified into two major types. Acute suppurative osteomyelitis is a process that occurs shortly after the predisposing event and will either resolve or progress to the more chronic stage, depending on treatment. The second type of osteomyelitis is chronic suppurative osteomyelitis. This form persists for longer periods, because the diagnosis is usually not made until the process has been present for several weeks or because the infection has been resistant to previous treatment.

Considering the opportunities that bacteria have to enter into the cancellous bone, osteomyelitis of the mandible rarely occurs if the body's host defenses are reasonably intact. The major predisposing factors for osteomyelitis of the jaws are preceding odontogenic infections and fractures of the mandible. Even these two events rarely cause infections of the bone unless the host defenses are suppressed by problems such as the alcoholism malnutritional syndrome, diabetes, intravenous drug abuse, and myeloproliferative diseases, such as the leukemias, sickle cell disease, and chemotherapy-treated cancer.

Recent carefully performed investigations on the microbiology of osteomyelitis of the mandible have adequately demonstrated that the primary bacteria of concern are similar to those causing odontogenic infections, that is, streptococci, anaerobic cocci such as *Peptostreptococcus* spp., and gram-negative rods such as those of the genera *Fusobacterium* and *Prevotella.* Traditional investigation of the microbiology of osteomyelitis of the jaws has used culture specimens from surface drainage of pus (contaminated with *Staphylococcus* organisms) and not anaerobic culture techniques (and thereby have not grown anaerobes). Thus osteomyelitis of the mandible differs substantially from osteomyelitis of other bones in which staphylococci are the predominant bacteria.

The clinical findings in patients who have acute suppurative osteomyelitis of the mandible are typically deep, severe pain and tenderness, swelling, and, on occasion, fever and malaise. There is almost always a clearly identifiable cause, such as a preceding odontogenic infection or jaw fracture.

The signs and symptoms are different in chronic suppurative osteomyelitis. Teeth in the area of the infection tend to become loose and sensitive to palpation and percussion. Pus is usually seen exuding from mucosal or cutaneous sinus tracts. The patient usually has pain and tenderness to palpation. High fever is not common in the chronic disease.

Acute suppurative osteomyelitis shows little or no radiographic change, because 10 to 12 days are required for lost bone to be detectable radiographically. Chronic osteomyelitis usually demonstrates bony destruction in the area of infection (Figure 17-15). The appearance is one of increased radiolucency, which may be uniform in its pattern or patchy, with a "moth-eaten" appearance. There may also be areas of radiopacity within the radiolucency. These radiopaque areas represent islands of bone that have not been resorbed and are known as *sequestra.* In long-standing chronic osteomyelitis there may actually be an area of increased radiodensity surrounding the area of radiolucency. This is the result of an osteitis type of reaction in which bone production increases as a result of the inflammatory reaction.

Treatment of osteomyelitis is both medical and surgical. Because patients with osteomyelitis almost always have depressed host defense mechanisms, the clinician must take these compromises into account during the treatment and seek medical consultation when necessary.

Acute osteomyelitis of the jaws is primarily managed by the administration of appropriate antibiotics. The precipitating event and/or condition must also be carefully managed. If the event is a fracture of the mandible, careful attention must be given to its treatment. The antibiotic of choice is penicillin, because it is effective against streptococci and the anaerobes that are usually involved in osteomyelitis. If the patient has a serious acute osteomyelitis, hospitalization may be required for administration of intravenous antibiotics. If the patient is allergic to penicillin, the drug of second choice is clindamycin. Clindamycin is preferred because it is an excellent drug for both streptococci and the usual causative anaerobes. Surgical treatment of acute suppurative osteomyelitis is usually limited. It consists primarily of removing obviously nonvital teeth in the area of the infection, wires or bone plates that may have been used to stabilize a fracture in the area, or any obviously loose pieces of bone. For acute osteomyelitis that results from jaw fracture, the surgeon must stabilize the mobile segments of the mandible with tight intermaxillary fixation or some other technique.

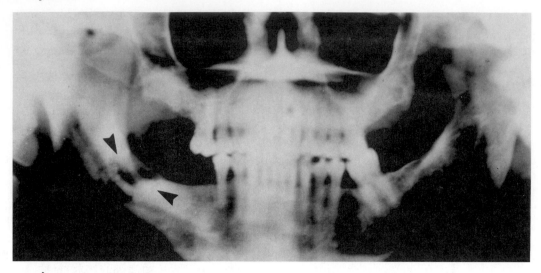

⬦ Figure 17-15

This chronic osteomyelitis resulted from surgical extraction of a tooth.

Chronic osteomyelitis requires not only aggressive antibiotic therapy but also aggressive surgical therapy. Because of the severe compromise in the blood supply to the area of osteomyelitis, the patient is usually admitted to the hospital and given high-dose intravenous antibiotics to control the initial symptoms. Penicillin is the drug of choice and clindamycin the drug of second choice. An effort should be made to obtain culture material at the time of surgery so that the selection of an antibiotic can be based on the specific microbiology of the infection.

Surgical management of chronic osteomyelitis must be aggressive, because there are large areas of ischemia and necrotic bone. Tissues with compromised vascularity must be removed and tissue with an adequate blood supply preserved to allow delivery of antibiotics and host defenses to the local area. Generous extraoral incisions are usually required, and all nonvital bone is removed. Obvious sequestra are lifted from the area of the infection (sequestrectomy), and all nonvital bone is removed with a rongeur or a drill with a large round bur (decortication and saucerization). Bone is removed until vital bleeding areas of bone are reached in all directions. The wound is irrigated thoroughly, and care is taken to ensure that all loose pieces of nonvital bone have been removed. Primary closure is usually performed at this time. Irrigation and suction drains may be placed during this surgery. The patient remains in the hospital for 6 to 18 days, during which time intravenous antibiotics are continued. If therapy is successful, there will be primary wound healing without any discharge or further wound-healing problems (Figure 17-16).

Therapy of both acute and chronic osteomyelitis, most authorities agree, should ensure that antibiotics are continued for a much longer time than is usual for odontogenic infections. For mild acute osteomyelitis that has responded well, antibiotics should be continued for at least 4 weeks. For severe chronic osteomyelitis that has been difficult to control, antibiotic administration may continue for up to 6 months.

Osteomyelitis of the mandible is a severe infection that may result in loss of a large portion of the mandible. Therefore this infection should be managed by a clinician who has the training and experience to handle the problem expeditiously. In addition, it is likely that medical consultation will be required, to help correct any underlying compromise of host defenses.

ACTINOMYCOSIS

Actinomycosis is a relatively uncommon infection of the soft tissues of the jaws. It is usually caused by *Actinomyces israelii* but may also be caused by *A. naeslundii* or *A. viscosus*. *Actinomyces* is an endogenous bacterium of the oral cavity that was once thought to be an anaerobic fungus. However, it has now been clearly established that actinomycetes are anaerobic bacteria.

Actinomycosis is a relatively uncommon disease, because the bacteria have a low degree of virulence. For the infection to become established, the bacteria must be inoculated into an area of injury or locally increased susceptibility, such as areas of recent tooth extraction, severely carious teeth, or minor oral trauma. The infection is primarily one of soft tissue and progresses by direct extension into adjacent tissues. Unlike other infections, actinomycosis does not follow usual anatomic planes but rather burrows through them and becomes a lobular "pseudotumor." If the infection erodes through a cutaneous surface, which is common with orofacial actinomycosis, multiple sinus tracts typically develop. Once drainage is established, the patient has minimal pain, although the sinus tracts will continue to drain spontaneously until the infection is brought under control (Figure 17-17).

Thus actinomycosis may be seen either as a tumorlike mass associated with the jaw or, as it is usually seen in the well-established phase, with chronic purulent drainage from the sinus tracts. The exudate classically contains sulfur

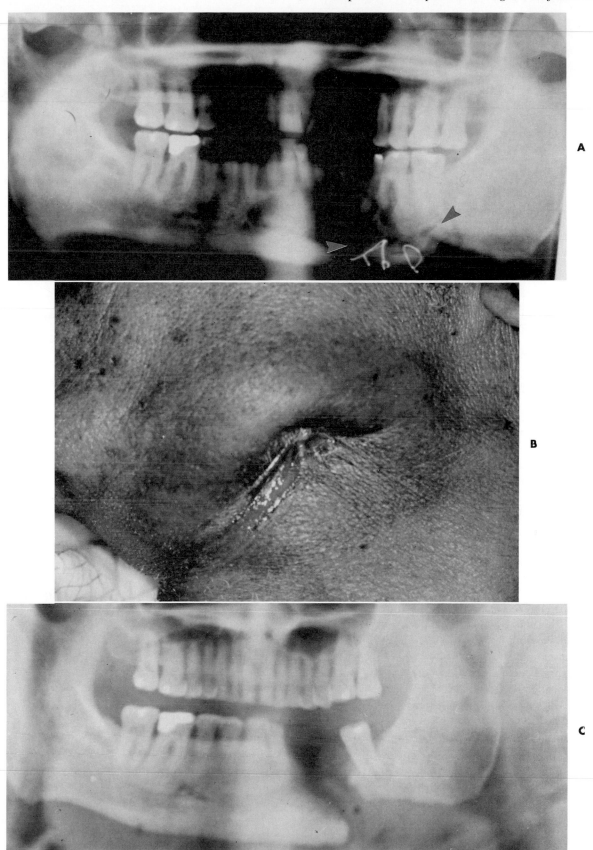

◇ Figure 17-16

A, Following complex fracture of mandible, this osteomyelitis developed. Patient was poorly nourished alcoholic. **B,** Cutaneous draining sinus tract. **C,** After multiple surgical treatments and prolonged antibiotic treatment, there is substantial loss of mandible.

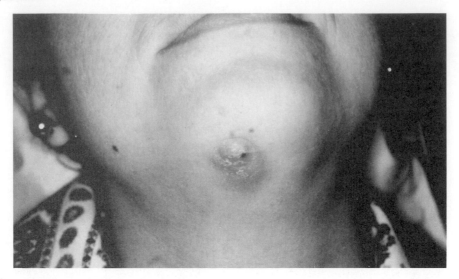

◇ **Figure 17-17**

This actinomycosis had multiple recurrences. There is small amount of swelling with multiple small sinus tracts.

granules. These are collections of microcolonies of the organisms that are approximately 1 to 2 mm in size. On Gram's stain, careful examination will reveal clusters of gram-positive branching rods. The presence of sulfur granules in the exudate leads to the presumptive diagnosis of actinomycosis. However, a definitive diagnosis depends on laboratory identification. *Actinomyces* is an anaerobic bacterium and therefore must be incubated in an anaerobic environment, usually on brain-heart agar or blood agar, for 4 to 6 days.

In up to 50% of all actinomycotic infections the organism is not grown. However, the clinical presentation of the patient with actinomycosis is characteristic. The patient has an atypical infection of the jaws that responds well to antibiotic therapy initially; however, after the antibiotic is stopped, the infection recurs. The patient with this disease frequently has had multiple episodes of recurrent infection in the same area. This clinical presentation is so characteristic that the presumptive diagnosis of actinomycosis can be made by the patient's history.

Therapy of actinomycosis includes surgical incision and drainage and excision of all sinus tracts. This portion of the treatment is important, to ensure that adequate amounts of antibiotic are actually delivered to the infected area.

The antibiotic of choice for actinomycosis is penicillin in the nonallergic patient. The dose varies with the seriousness of the disease. If the patient has had a serious infection or the bone of the jaws is involved, high doses of penicillin should be given parenterally while the patient is hospitalized. Intravenous administration of 10 million U of penicillin daily in divided doses is continued until the disease is clinically cured. This ranges from 3 to 14 days. The patient is then discharged from the hospital, and a course of oral penicillin is begun. The usual recommended dose is 500 mg 4 times a day for at least 3 months. The reason for the prolonged administration of the antibiotic is to prevent the recurrence of the infection.

The drug of second choice is tetracycline, with doxycycline or minocycline being the preferred drugs. These two tetracyclines are preferred because they can be administered once per day during the long-term antibiotic administration.

In summary, actinomycosis is an indolent infection that tends to erode through tissues rather than follow typical fascial planes and spaces. It is difficult to eradicate using short-term antibiotic regimens. Therefore incision and drainage of any accumulation of pus and excision of chronic sinus tracts must be accomplished. Finally, high-dose antibiotic administration is recommended for initial control of the infection, with long-term antibiotic therapy to prevent recurrence of actinomycosis.

CANDIDOSIS

The organism *Candida albicans* is a naturally occurring fungus in the oral cavity. It rarely causes disease unless the patient's health becomes compromised. The two most common causes of compromise are administration of antibiotics, especially penicillin, for prolonged periods and chemotherapy for leukemias and other forms of cancer. In these situations *Candida* organisms overgrow the oral cavity and cause a superficial infection, which usually appears intraorally as distinct white patches that can be easily rubbed off with gauze to expose an underlying red, raw surface (Figure 17-18). *Candida* spp. can be easily cultured and diagnosed by their typical appearance on Gram's stain.

Angular cheilitis can be aggravated by the presence of

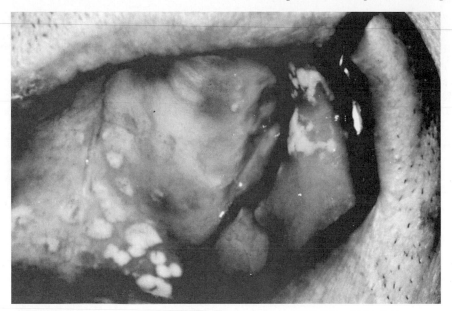

◇ **Figure 17-18**

Candidiasis of oral cavity appears as white patches on oral mucosa.

Candida organisms. Most patients who have this problem are edentulous and overclosed and have a resultant chronic wetness at the corner of the mouth and subsequent yeast growth.

Therapy for oral candidosis can usually be delivered by topical antifungal agents. The two most commonly used drugs for this purpose are nystatin and clotrimazole. Both of these drugs are prepared as lozenges and are delivered by sucking on the lozenge until it is totally dissolved. Nystatin is the preferred drug, because essentially none of the drug is absorbed and the chances for adverse reactions are essentially zero. Clotrimazole has a quite small risk of toxicity and therefore is usually viewed as being a drug of second choice. The usual dosage of either preparation is one lozenge 4 or 5 times per day for 2 weeks. Patients usually experience rapid resolution of the signs and symptoms of candidosis but must be informed that there will be a recurrence of the infection unless they continue the therapy for the entire 14 days. If the patient has a denture, the denture should be soaked in chlorhexidine overnight for the entire treatment.

Oral candidosis can also be treated by systemically administered drugs, such as fluconazole. This antifungal drug is quite effective, especially in oropharyngeal candidosis, which is not responsive to topical therapy.

It is important to remember that candidosis usually occurs only in medically compromised patients. Patients without histories of recent antibiotic therapy, cancer chemotherapy, or other types of immunocompromise should be suspected of having an underlying, undiagnosed immunocompromising disease. Predominant among these is acquired immunodeficiency syndrome (AIDS).

BIBLIOGRAPHY

Barratt GE, Koopmann CF, Coulthand SW: Retropharyngeal abscess: a ten-year experience, *Laryngoscope* 94:455, 1984.

Beck HJ et al: Life-threatening soft tissue infections of the neck, *Laryngoscope* 94:354, 1984.

Bennhoff DF: Actinomycosis: diagnosis and therapeutic considerations and a review of 32 cases, *Laryngoscope* 94:1198, 1984.

Dzyak WR, Zide MF: Diagnosis and treatment of lateral pharyngeal space infections, *J Oral Maxillofac Surg* 42:243, 1984.

Fielding AF et al: Cavernous sinus thrombosis: report of a case, *J Am Dent Assoc* 106:342, 1983.

Finkelstein M, Vincent S: Management of mucosal and related dermatologic disorders. In Peterson LJ, editor: *Principles of oral and maxillofacial surgery,* Philadelphia, 1992, JB Lippincott.

Giordano AM et al: Chronic osteomyelitis following mandibular fracture and its treatment, *Arch Otolaryngol* 108:30, 1982.

Hall BB, Fitzgerald RH, Rosenblatt JE: Anaerobic osteomyelitis, *J Bone Joint Surg* 64A:30, 1983.

Haug RH, Picard U, Indresano AT: Diagnosis and treatment of the retropharyngeal abscess in adults, *J Oral Maxillofac Surg* 28B:34, 1990.

Karlin RJ, Robinson WA: Septic cavernous sinus thrombosis, *Ann Emerg Med* 13:449, 1984.

Marciani RD: Clinical considerations in head and neck infections. In Peterson LJ, editor: *Principles of oral and maxillofacial surgery,* Philadelphia, 1992, JB Lippincott.

Meanier F, Aoun M, Gerard M: Therapy for oropharyngeal candidiasis in the immunocompromised host: a randomized double blind study of fluconazole vs. ketoconazole, *Rev Infect Dis* 12:5364, 1990.

Patterson HC, Kelly JH, Strome M: Ludwig's angina: an update, *Laryngoscope* 92:370, 1982.

Peterson LJ: Principles of antibiotic therapy. In Topazian RG, Goldberg MH, editors: *Management of oral and maxillofacial infections,* ed 2, Philadelphia, 1987, WB Saunders.

Peterson LJ: Odontogenic infections of the head and neck. In

Cummings CW et al, editors: *Otolaryngology: head and neck surgery,* ed 2, St Louis, 1992, Mosby.

Range A, Ruud A: Osteomyelitis of the jaws, *Int J Oral Surg* 7:523, 1978.

Schechtman LV et al: Clotrimazole treatment of oral candidiasis in patients with neoplastic disease, *Am J Med* 76:91, 1984.

Virolainen E et al: Deep neck infections, *Int J Oral Surg* 8:407, 1979.

PRINCIPLES OF ENDODONTIC SURGERY

RICHARD E. WALTON

CHAPTER OUTLINE ⬦

E ndodontic surgery is the management or prevention of periradicular pathosis by a surgical approach. In general, this includes abscess drainage, periapical surgery, corrective surgery, intentional replantation, and root removal (Box 18-1).

Surgery has traditionally been an important part of endodontic treatment. However, until recently, there was little research on indications and contraindications, techniques, success and failure (long-term prognosis), wound healing, and materials and devices to augment procedures. Because of this lack of information, many surgeries were performed for the wrong reasons, such as the routine correcting of failed root canal treatment, removing of large lesions believed to be cysts, or the performing of single-visit root canal treatment. Indeed, there are clear *indications* for a surgical approach, but there are few *situations* in which surgery is required. Other modalities, such as root canal treatment or retreatment, may be preferred. However, when surgery is required, it must adhere to basic endodontic principles, that is, the assessing and obtaining of adequate débridement and/or obturation of the canal(s).[9]

Root canal treatment is generally a successful procedure when there is accurate diagnosis and careful technique. A common misconception is that if conventional root canal treatment fails, surgery is indicated for correction. Usually this is not true; most failures are better managed by retreatment.[2,23] At other times, surgery is necessary to correct a failure or, for other reasons, may be the only alternative to extraction.

The purpose of this chapter is to present the indications and contraindications for endodontic surgery, the diagnosis and treatment planning, and the basics of endodontic surgical techniques. Most of the procedures presented should be performed by experienced generalists or specialists. However, the general dentist must be skilled in diagnosis and treatment planning, as well as able to recognize which procedures are indicated in particular situations. In addition, the generalist should assist in the follow-up care and long-term assessment of treatment outcomes.

The procedures discussed in this chapter are drainage of an abscess, apical surgery, and corrective surgery.

DRAINAGE OF AN ABSCESS ⬦

Drainage releases purulent or hemorrhagic transudates and exudates from a focus of liquefaction necrosis (abscess). Draining the abscess relieves pain and increases circulation, as well as removes a potent irritant. The abscess may be confined to bone or may have eroded through bone and periosteum to invade soft tissue. Managing these intraoral or extraoral swellings by incision for drainage is reviewed in Chapters 16 and 17.

An abscess in bone may be drained by two methods. One is by opening into the offending tooth to obtain drainage through the canal. The abscess often does not communicate with the apex. A method to manage this is *trephination*. This is done by creating a pathway with a rotary instrument through gingiva and cortical bone directly into the abscess (Figure 18-1).

PERIAPICAL SURGERY

Periapical surgery includes resection of a portion of the root that contains undébrided/unobturated canal space and/or to reverse filling and sealing of the canal when conventional root canal treatment is not feasible. It is often performed in conjunction with apical curettage for reasons explained later in this chapter.

Box 18-1

Categories of endodontic surgery

Abscess drainage
Periapical surgery
Hemisection/root amputation
Intentional replantation
Corrective surgery

INDICATIONS

The success of apical surgery varies considerably, depending on the reason for and nature of the procedure.[7] With failed root canal treatment, often retreatment is not possible or a better result cannot be achieved by a coronal approach.[16] If an etiology for failure cannot be identified, surgical exploration may be necessary (Figure 18-2). On occasion, an unusual entity in the periapical region requires surgical removal and biopsy for identification. Those indications for periapical surgery are discussed below. (See Box 18-2.)

ANATOMIC PROBLEMS.   Calcifications or other blockages, severe root curvatures, or constricted canals (calcific metamorphosis) may compromise root canal treatment, that is, prevent instrumentation and/or obturation (Figure 18-3). Because a canal is always present (even if very small), failure to débride and obturate may lead to failure. Although the outcome may be questionable, it is preferable to attempt conventional root canal treatment or retreatment before apical surgery. If this is not possible, removing or resecting the uninstrumented and unfilled portion of the root and placing a root-end filling may be necessary (Figure 18-4). An anatomic perforation of the root apex through the bone may necessitate removal of that portion of the extruded apex following treatment. This is corrected by beveling the root apex to within the confines of the overlying bone.

Occasionally, adequate débridement and obturation is not possible because of extensive apical root resorption. In these cases it may be necessary to resect the root to include the resorbed area, then place a root-end filling.

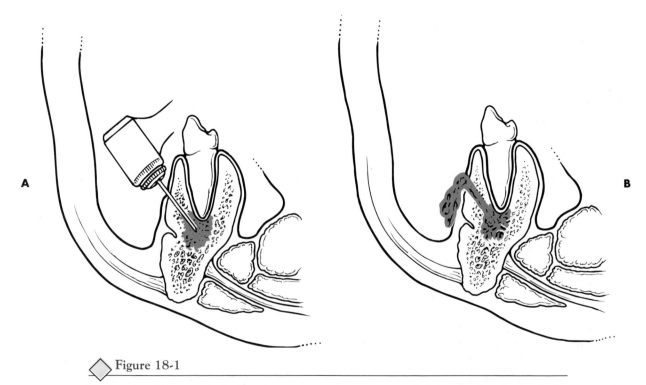

Figure 18-1

Trephination. **A,** Penetration is through mucosa and bone and into apical abscess. An effective device is Stabident Perforator. **B,** Purulence is released, and pressure and pain are relieved.

RESTORATIVE CONSIDERATIONS. Root canal treatment may be risky because of problems that may occur from attempting access through a restoration, such as through a crown on a mandibular incisor. An opening could compromise retention of the restoration or perforate the root. Rather than attempt the root canal treatment, root resection and root-end filling to seal in irritants is preferred.

A common requirement for surgery is failed treatment on a tooth that has been restored with a post and core (Figure 18-5). Many posts are difficult to remove or may cause root fracture during removal.

◇ Box 18-2 ◇

Indications for periapical surgery

Anatomic problems preventing complete débridement/ obturation

Restorative considerations that compromise treatment

Horizontal root fracture with apical necrosis

Irretrievable material preventing canal treatment or retreatment

Procedural errors during treatment

Large periapical lesions that do not resolve with root canal treatment

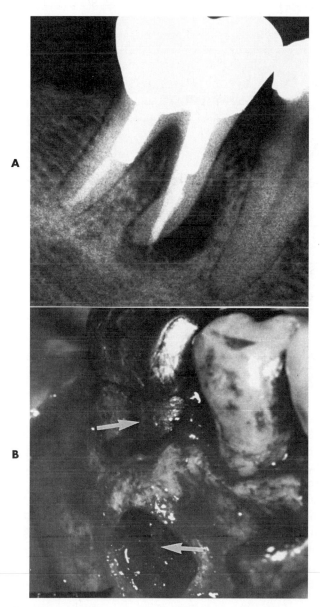

◇ Figure 18-2

Surgical exploration. **A,** Periradicular lesion on mesial root may be caused by post perforation in furcation, incomplete débridement/ apical perforation, or vertical root fracture. **B,** Visualization after flap reflection shows vertical root fracture (*arrow*); root must be removed or tooth extracted.

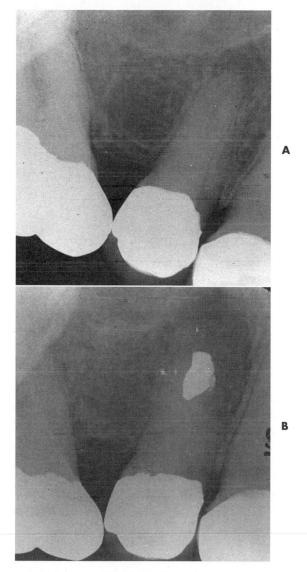

◇ Figure 18-3

A, Very small canal (calcific metamorphosis) with pulp necrosis and apical pathosis. Canal could not be located with occlusal access. **B,** Apical resection and root-end retrograde amalgam to seal in irritants.

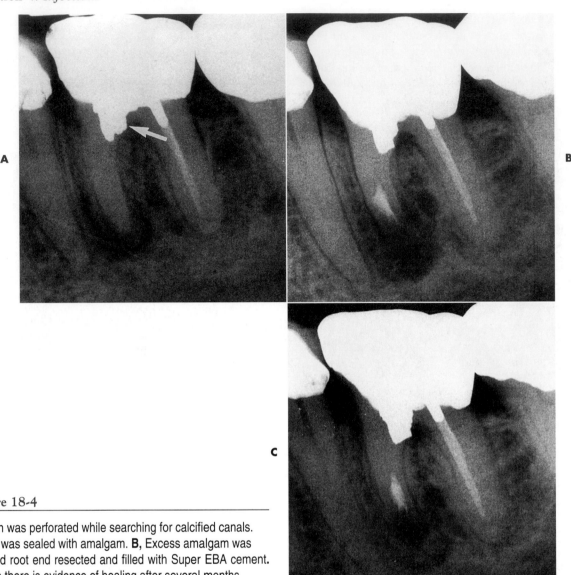

A, Furcation was perforated while searching for calcified canals. Perforation was sealed with amalgam. **B,** Excess amalgam was trimmed and root end resected and filled with Super EBA cement. **C,** Although there is evidence of healing after several months, long-term prognosis is still questionable.

HORIZONTAL ROOT FRACTURE. Occasionally, following a traumatic root fracture the apical segment undergoes pulp necrosis. Because this cannot be predictably treated from a coronal approach, the apical segment is removed surgically following root canal treatment of the coronal portion (Figure 18-6).

IRRETRIEVABLE MATERIAL IN CANAL. Canals are occasionally blocked by objects such as separated instruments (Figure 18-7), restorative materials, segments of posts, or other foreign objects. If there is evidence of apical pathosis, those materials must be removed surgically, usually with a portion of the root (Figure 18-8).

PROCEDURAL ERROR. Broken instruments, ledging, perforations, and gross overfills (Figure 18-9) may result in failure. Although overfilling is not in itself an indication for removal of the material, surgical correction is frequently necessary in these situations.

LARGE, UNRESOLVED LESIONS FOLLOWING ROOT CANAL TREATMENT. Occasionally, very large periradicular lesions do not heal or may even enlarge following adequate débridement/obturation. These are generally best resolved with decompression[18] and not curettage, which may damage adjacent structures (Figure 18-10). Often, decompression alone is sufficient to manage these lesions; surgical correction (removal) is unnecessary.[18]

CONTRAINDICATIONS (OR CAUTIONS)
There are reasons why periapical surgery is not the preferred choice or should be avoided if other options are available (Box 18-3).

UNIDENTIFIED CAUSE OF TREATMENT FAILURE. Relying on surgery to try to correct all root canal treatment failures could be labeled indiscriminate. An important consideration is to identify the cause of failure, then design an appropriate corrective treatment plan. Usually, retreatment is

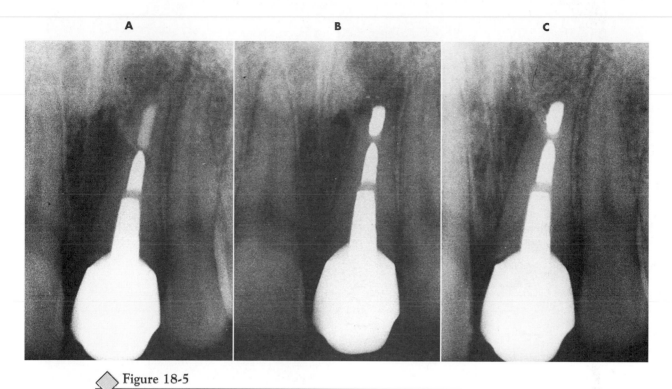

◇ Figure 18-5

A, Irretrievable fractured post and apical pathosis. **B,** Root-end resection and filling with amalgam to seal in irritants, likely from coronal leakage. **C,** Regeneration of bone is evident after several months; prognosis is good.

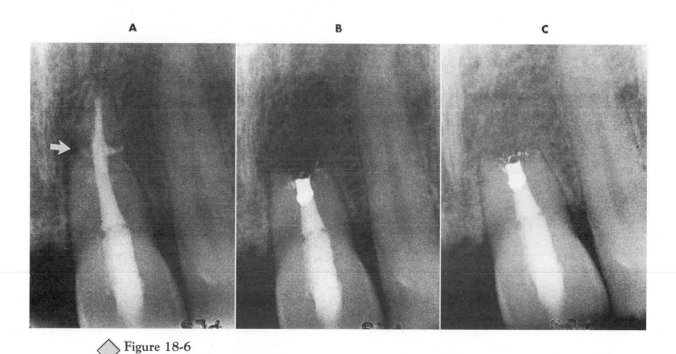

◇ Figure 18-6

A, Horizontal root fracture, with failed attempt to treat both segments. **B,** Apical segment is removed surgically and retrograde amalgam placed. **C,** Healing is complete after 1 year.

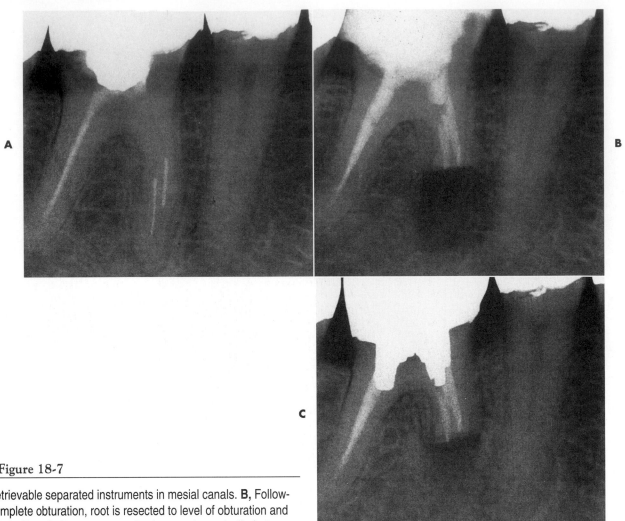

◆ **Figure 18-7**

A, Irretrievable separated instruments in mesial canals. **B,** Following complete obturation, root is resected to level of obturation and to include files. **C,** Bone regeneration is occurring apically, but additional monitoring is necessary.

indicated and will give the best chance of success.[11] Surgery to correct a treatment failure for which the cause cannot be identified is often unsuccessful. Surgical management of all periapical pathoses and/or large periapical lesions is often not necessary because they will resolve following appropriate root canal treatment. This includes lesions that may be cystic; these also usually heal following root canal treatment.

WHEN CONVENTIONAL ROOT CANAL TREATMENT IS POSSIBLE.

In most situations, orthograde conventional root canal treatment is preferred (Figure 18-11). Also, there is no increased incidence of posttreatment complications or compromised long-term healing if treatment is done in a single appointment.[19] Surgery is not indicated just because débridement and obturation are in the same visit.

SIMULTANEOUS ROOT CANAL TREATMENT AND APICAL SURGERY.

Few situations occur in which simultaneous root canal therapy and apical surgery is indicated. Usually, there are no advantages to an approach that includes both of these as a single procedure. It is preferable and likely will result in better success to perform only the conventional treatment without the adjunctive apical surgery.

ANATOMIC CONSIDERATIONS.

Most oral structures do not interfere with a surgical approach but must be considered. An example is the maxillary sinus, which may become exposed. Creating a sinus opening is neither unusual nor dangerous. However, caution is necessary to not introduce foreign objects into the opening and to remind the patient not to exert pressure by forcibly blowing the nose until the surgical wound has healed (in 1 to 2 weeks). Bony structures generally do not contraindicate surgery, with the exception of the external oblique ridge over the mandibular second and third molars. In most cases this structure prevents adequate access to the root apices; periapical surgery of these teeth is not feasible. Other approaches, such as intentional replantation (Figure 18-12), may be indicated. The zygomatic

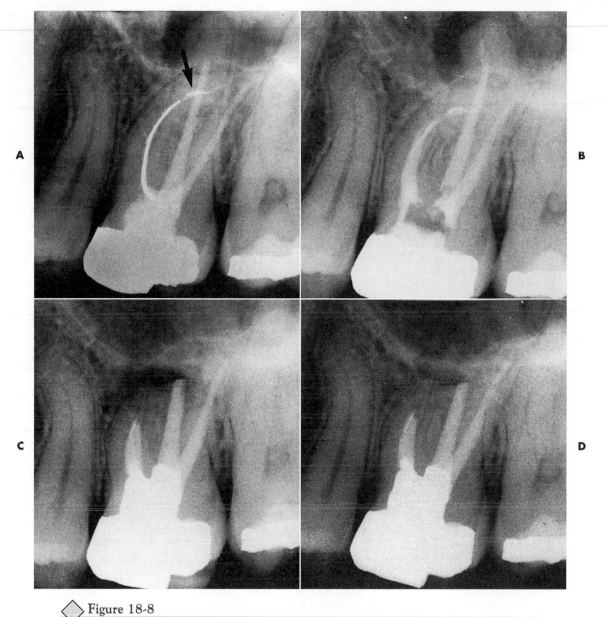

◈ Figure 18-8

A, Irretrievable material in mesial and lingual canals and apical pathosis. **B,** Canals are retreated, but there is failure to heal. **C,** Treatment is root-end resection to level of gutta percha in the mesial and lingual aspects. **D,** After 2 years, healing is complete.

buttress may inhibit access to maxillary molar apices. A prominent chin creates a shallow vestibule with limited access to mandibular anteriors.

Poor crown/root ratio. Teeth with very short roots have compromised bony support and are poor candidates for surgery; root resection in such cases may compromise stability. However, shorter roots may support a relatively long crown if the surrounding cervical periodontium is healthy (see Figure 18-6).

MEDICAL (SYSTEMIC) COMPLICATIONS. The general health and condition of the patient are always essential considerations. There are no specific contraindications for

endodontic surgery that would not be similar to other types of oral surgical procedures.

SURGICAL PROCEDURE

The following sequence, with modifications as appropriate, is typical: (1) flap design, (2) incision and reflection, (3) access to the apex, (4) curettage, (5) root and resection, (6) root-end preparation and filling, (7) radiographic verification, (8) flap replacement and suturing, (9) postoperative instructions, and (10) suture removal and evaluation. This sequence is shown in Figure 18-13.

FLAP DESIGN. A properly designed and carefully reflected flap will result in good access and uncomplicated

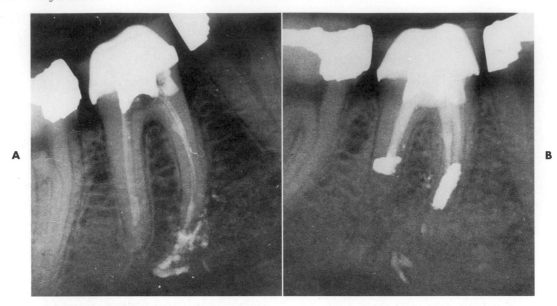

◇ Figure 18-9

A, Overfill of injected obturating material has resulted in pain and paresthesia as a result of damage to inferior alveolar nerve. **B,** Corrected by retreatment, then apicectomy, curettage, and a root-end amalgam fill.

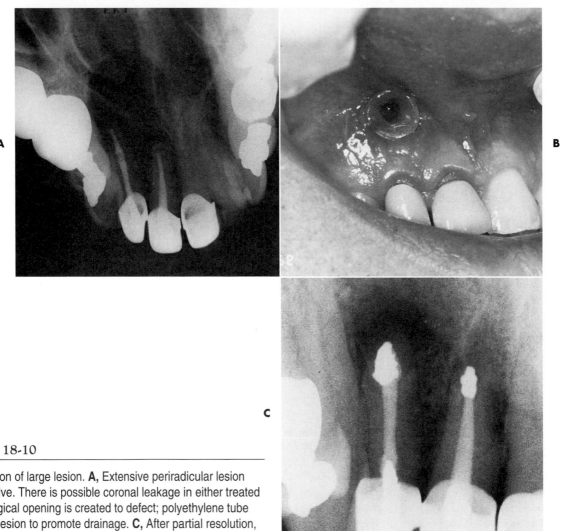

◇ Figure 18-10

Decompression of large lesion. **A,** Extensive periradicular lesion failed to resolve. There is possible coronal leakage in either treated tooth. **B,** Surgical opening is created to defect; polyethylene tube extends into lesion to promote drainage. **C,** After partial resolution, apicoectomy and restoration are performed.

◇ Box 18-3 ◇

Contraindications for periapical surgery

Unidentified cause of root canal treatment failure
When conventional root canal treatment is possible
Combined coronal treatment/apical surgery
When retreatment of a treatment failure is possible
Anatomic structures (adjacent nerves and vessels, etc.) are in
　jeopardy
Structures interfere with access and visibility
Compromise of crown/root ratio
Systemic complications (bleeding disorders, etc.)

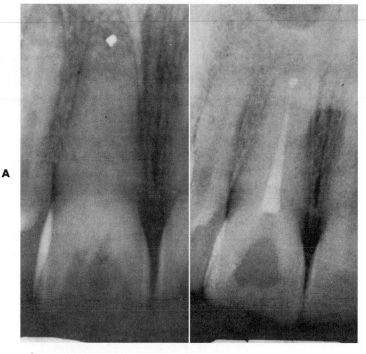

A　　　　　　　　　　　　　　　　　　　　　　　B

◇ Figure 18-11

This case is poorly done and for wrong reasons. **A,** Inadequate root-end resection and root-end filling does not seal apex. **B,** Root-canal treatment is readily accomplished, with better chance of success.

healing.[12] The basic principles of flap design should be followed; these are detailed in Chapter 8. Although there are several possibilities, the three most common incisions are submarginal curved (semilunar), submarginal, and full mucoperiosteal (sulcular). The submarginal and full mucoperiosteal incision will have either a three-corner (triangular) or four-corner (rectangular) design.

Semilunar incision.   This is a slightly curved half-moon horizontal incision in the alveolar mucosa (Figure 18-14). Although the location allows easy reflection, there is restricted access to the apex. There are other disadvantages to this incision, including excessive hemorrhage, delayed healing, and scarring; this design is contraindicated for endodontic surgery.

Submarginal incision.   The horizontal component is in attached gingiva with one or two accompanying vertical incisions (Figure 18-15). Generally, the incision is scalloped in the horizontal line, with obtuse angles at the corners. It is used most successfully in the maxillary anterior region or, occasionally, with maxillary premolars with crowns. Because of the design, prerequisites are at least 4 mm of attached gingiva and good periodontal health.

The major advantage is esthetics. Leaving the gingiva intact around the margins of crowns is less likely to result in bone resorption with tissue recession and crown margin exposure. Compared with the semilunar incision, the submarginal provides less risk of incising over a bony defect with better access and visibility. Disadvantages include hemorrhage along the cut margins into the surgical site and occasional healing by scarring, compared with the full mucoperiosteal sulcular incision.

Full mucoperiosteal incision.   This is an incision into the gingival sulcus, extending to the gingival crest (Figure 18-16). This procedure includes elevation of interdental papilla, free gingival margin, attached gingiva, and alveolar mucosa. One or two vertical relaxing incisions may be used, creating a three- or four-corner design. When feasible the full mucoperiosteal design is preferred over the other two techniques. The advantages include maximum access and

visibility, not incising over the lesion or bony defect, less tendency for hemorrhage, complete visibility of the root, allowance of root planing and bone contouring, and reduced likelihood of healing with scar formation. The disadvantages are somewhat more difficult to replace and to suture; also there frequently is gingival recession, exposing crown margins and/or cervical root surfaces.

ANESTHESIA.   For most surgical procedures, anesthetic approaches are conventional. In most regions a block is administered, followed by local infiltration to enhance hemostasis. Frequently, the patient is sensitive to curettage of the inflammatory tissue, particularly toward the lingual aspect. Some of the sensitivity may be decreased by a preemptive periodontal ligament or intraosseous injection, using a device specifically designed for this purpose.

A long-acting anesthetic agent is recommended, such as bupivacaine or etidocaine. Bupivacaine 0.5 % with epinephrine 1:200,000 has been shown to give long-lasting anesthesia, followed by a lingering analgesia.[4]

INCISION AND REFLECTION.   A firm incision should be made through periosteum to bone. It is important to incise and reflect a full-thickness flap to minimize hemorrhage and to prevent tearing of the tissue. Elevation is with a sharp periosteal elevator beginning in the vertical incisions, then raising the horizontal component. To reflect the periosteum the

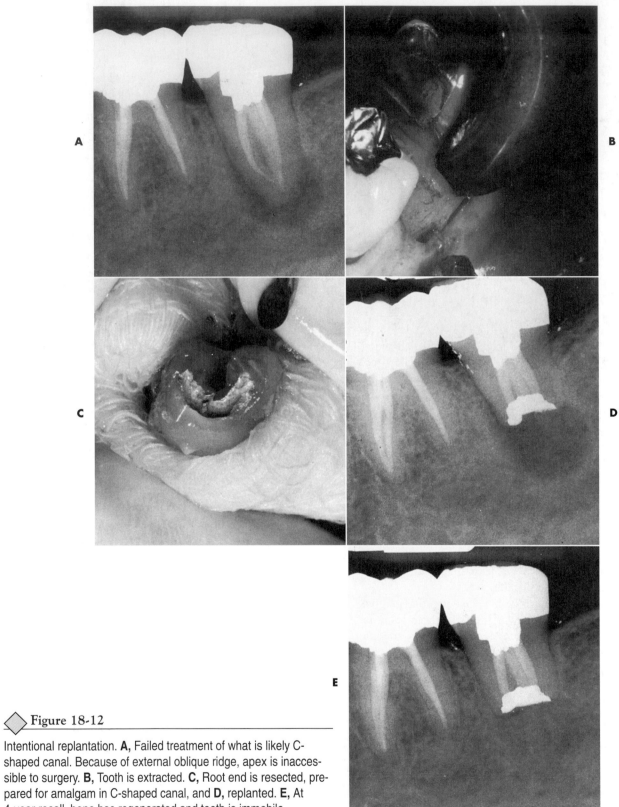

◇ **Figure 18-12**

Intentional replantation. **A,** Failed treatment of what is likely C-shaped canal. Because of external oblique ridge, apex is inaccessible to surgery. **B,** Tooth is extracted. **C,** Root end is resected, prepared for amalgam in C-shaped canal, and **D,** replanted. **E,** At 4-year recall, bone has regenerated and tooth is immobile.

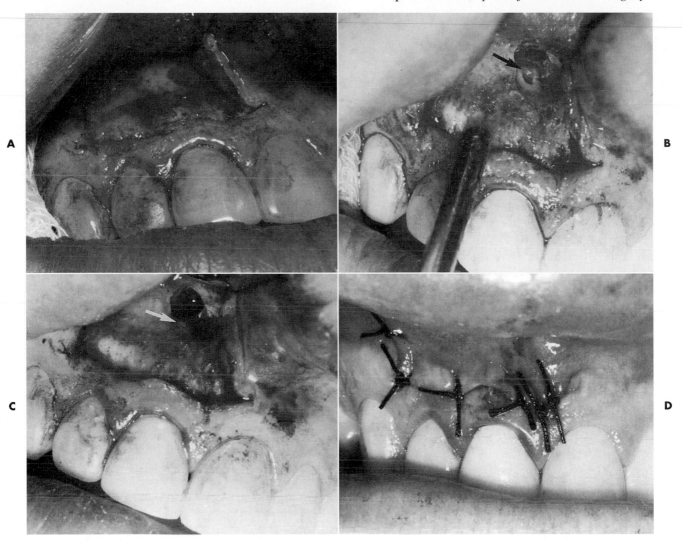

Periapical surgical procedure. **A,** Submarginal incision, three-corner (triangular), reflected flap. **B,** Root end is resected and prepared *(arrow)* for fill. **C,** Amalgam (*arrow*) has been condensed. **D,** Flap is replaced, compressed, and sutured (interrupted).

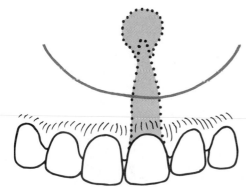

Semilunar flap incision, primarily horizontal and in alveolar mucosa. Because of limitations of access and poorer healing, this design is contraindicated.

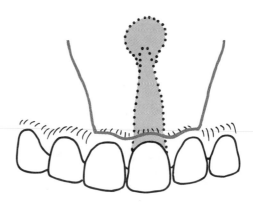

Submarginal incision is a scalloped horizontal line in attached gingiva, with one or two vertical components. This incison is usually confined to maxillary anterior region.

elevator must firmly contact bone as the tissue is raised (Figure 18-17). Reflection is to a level adequate for access to the surgical site while allowing a retractor to have contact with bone.

PERIAPICAL EXPOSURE.   Frequently, the cortical bone overlying the apex has been resorbed, exposing a soft tissue lesion. If the opening is small, it should be enlarged using a large surgical round bur, until approximately half the root and the lesion are visible (Figure 18-18). With a limited bony opening, radiographs are used in conjunction with root and bone topography to locate the apex. A measurement may be made with a periodontal probe on the radiograph, then transferring to the surgical site to determine the apex location.

To avoid air emphysema, the use of handpieces that direct pressurized air, water, and abrasive particles (or combinations)

should not be used.[3] Vented high-speed handpieces or electrical surgical handpieces are preferred during osseous entry and/or root-end resection. Sealed-end air-pressurized handpieces also direct air away from the surgical site. Irrespective of the handpiece used, there should be copious irrigation with sterile saline solution.[5] Enough overlying bone should be removed to expose the area around the apex and at least half the length of the root. Good access and visibility are important.

CURETTAGE.   Most of the granulomatous inflamed tissue surrounding the apex should be removed (Figure 18-19) to gain access and visibility of the apex, obtain a biopsy for histologic examination, and minimize hemorrhage.

If possible, the tissue should be enucleated in one piece with a suitably sized sharp curette, although total lesion removal usually does not occur. A cleaner bony cavity will have the least hemorrhage and the best visibility. Tissue removal should not jeopardize the blood supply to an adjacent tooth. Also, some areas of the lesion may be inaccessible to the curettes, such as on the lingual aspect of the root. Portions of inflamed tissue or epithelium may be left, without compromising healing; total removal is not necessary.[15] If hemorrhage from soft or hard tissue is excessive to the extent that visibility is compromised, homeostatic agents or other control techniques are useful.[14]

ROOT-END RESECTION.   Root-end resection is often, but not always, indicated. It is useful in the following two situations: (1) to gain access to the canal for examination and placement of a root-end restoration and (2) to remove an undébrided/unobturated portion of a root. This may be necessary in cases with dilacerated roots, ledged or blocked canals, or apical canal space that is inaccessible because of restorations and in accessing of lingual structures.

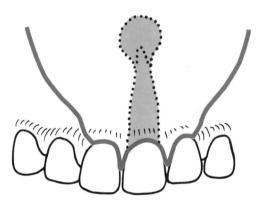

◇ Figure 18-16

Full mucoperiosteal (sulcular) incision. Horizontal incision is into sulcus, accompanied by one (three-corner) or two (four-corner) vertical components.

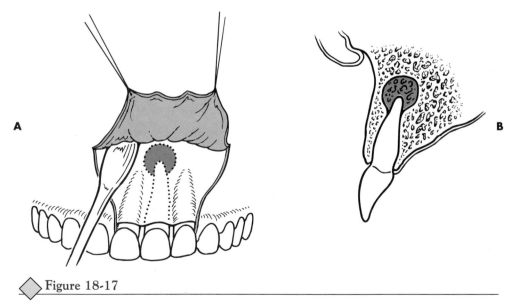

◇ Figure 18-17

Full-thickness flap is raised with sharp elevator in firm contact with bone. Enough tissue is raised to allow access and visibility to apical area. **A,** Frontal view. **B,** Cross-section.

Before sectioning, a trough is created around the apex with a tapered fissure bur to expose and isolate the root end. The resecting is with the same tapered fissure bur. Depending on the location and whether a root-end preparation is to be placed, a bevel of varying degrees is made in a faciolingual direction (Figure 18-20). The amount of root removed depends on the reason for performing the resection. Sufficient root apex must be removed to provide a larger surface and to expose additional canals. In general, approximately one half to one third of the root is resected—more if necessary for apical access, less if too much removal would further compromise stability of an already short root.

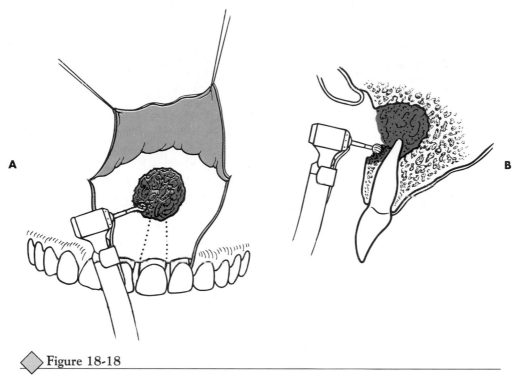

◆ **Figure 18-18**

Apical exposure. Large round bur is used to "paint" bony window. Enough is removed to give good visibility, and access to lesion and apex. **A,** Frontal view. **B,** Cross-section.

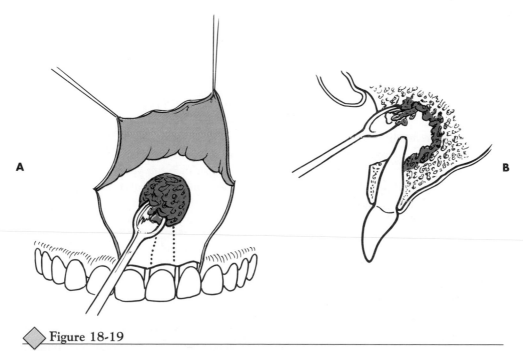

◆ **Figure 18-19**

Curettage. Much of lesion that is accessible is removed with large curettes. Usually, remnants of tissue remain, which is not a problem. **A,** Frontal view. **B,** Cross-section.

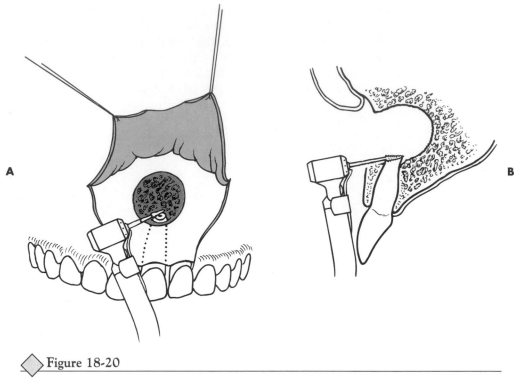

◈ Figure 18-20

Root-end resection. Approximately one third of apex is removed with tapered bur. Amount removed and degree of bevel varies according to situation. **A,** Frontal view. **B,** Cross-section.

ROOT-END PREPARATION AND RESTORATION. This is indicated if there likely is an inadequate apical seal. A class 1 type of preparation should extend 3 to 4 mm into the root to include the canal. The shape of the preparation should mimic the shape of the cut surface of the root. The outline should include other canals and aberrations, such as an isthmus. Root-end preparation may be done by slow-speed, specially designed micro-handpieces (Figure 18-21) or by ultrasonic tips (Figure 18-22). Ultrasonic instruments offer some advantages of control and ease of use, as well as permitting less apical root removal in certain situations (Figure 18-23).[26]

The root-end filling material is placed into a dry cavity preparation (Figure 18-24). These materials should be tissue tolerant, nonresorbable, easily inserted, minimally affected by moisture, and visible radiographically.

Amalgam (preferably zinc-free) and Super EBA (ethoxybenzoic acid) cement are commonly used materials.[25] Gutta percha, composite resin, glass ionomer cement, IRM, Cavit, and mineral trioxide aggregate (MTA) cement have also been recommended; these materials have less clinical documentation of success.[10] However, MTA has shown favorable biologic and physical properties and ease of handling; it may become a widely used material in the future.[24] As yet, no root-end filling material demonstrates superiority in both biologic acceptability and long-term stability.

FLAP REPLACEMENT AND SUTURING. The flap is returned to its original position and held with moderate digital pressure and moistened gauze. This expresses hemorrhage from under the flap and gives initial adaptation and more accurate suturing. Silk sutures are generally used, although other materials are suitable, including 4-0 absorbable suture. Interrupted sutures are common, although both horizontal and vertical mattress and sling sutures are applicable in certain situations. Following suturing, the flap should again be compressed digitally with moistened gauze to express more hemorrhage. This encourages less postoperative swelling and more rapid healing.

POSTOPERATIVE INSTRUCTIONS. Both oral and written information should be supplied in simple, straightforward descriptions. The wording should minimize anxiety arising from normal postoperative sequelae by describing the ways in which the patient can promote healing and comfort. Instructions inform the patient of what to expect (swelling, discomfort, possible discoloration, and some oozing of blood) and the ways in which these sequelae can be prevented and/or managed. The surgical site should not be disturbed, and pressure should be maintained (cold packs over the surgical area until bedtime might help). Oral hygiene procedures are indicated everywhere except the surgical site; careful brushing and flossing may begin after 24 hours. Proper nutrition and fluids are important but should not traumatize the area.

Analgesics are recommended, although pain is frequently minimal; strong analgesics are not required. There is no preferred category of pain medications; selection depends on the clinician and the patient. Analgesics for moderate pain will

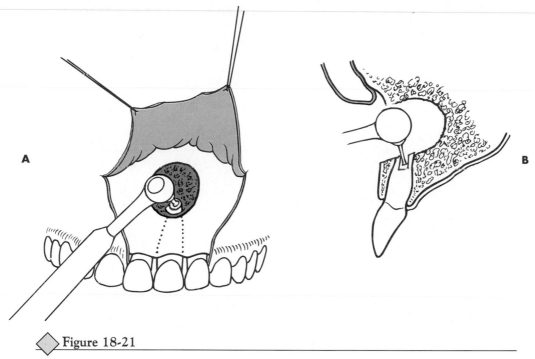

◇ Figure 18-21

Root-end preparation. Micro-handpiece with small round or inverted cone bur should prepare several millimeters into root. **A,** Frontal view. **B,** Cross-section.

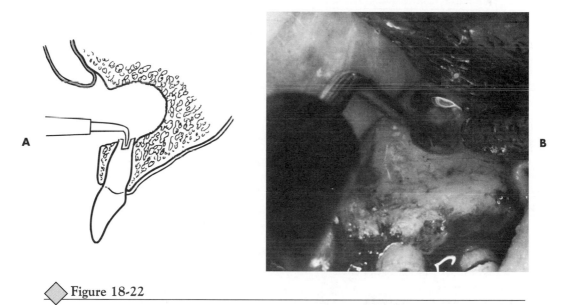

◇ Figure 18-22

A, Ultrasonic tips are good alternative for root-end preparation. **B,** These permit preparation with better control and less root removal.

usually suffice and are most effective if administered before the surgery or at least before the anesthetic wears off. Antibiotics are not indicated even with a localized abscess, and there is no demonstrated benefit to the prescribing of steroids.[6]

The patient is instructed to call if he or she experiences excessive swelling or pain. Postoperative complications are a response to injury from the procedure; infection following this type of surgical procedure is rare. However, the patient should be evaluated in person if he or she is having difficulties. Occasionally, sutures have torn loose, a foreign body (such as a cotton pellet) is under the flap, or there is simply an overreaction of the soft tissues. Again, antibiotics would not be indicated; palliative or corrective treatment will usually suffice.

SUTURE REMOVAL AND EVALUATION. Sutures ordinarily are removed in 3 to 6 days, with shorter periods being preferred to enhance healing. By 3 days, swelling and discomfort should be decreasing. Also, there should be evidence of primary wound closure; tissues that were reflected should be in apposition. Occasionally, a loose or torn suture may result in nonadapted tissue. In these cases, the margins are readapted and resutured.

CORRECTIVE SURGERY

Corrective surgery is managing defects that have occurred by a biologic response (resorption) or iatrogenic (procedural) error. These may be anywhere on the root, from cervical margin to apex. Many are accessible; others are difficult to

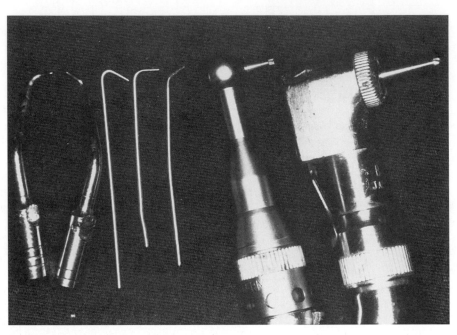

◇ **Figure 18-23**

Ultrasonic preparation tips are available in several designs and shapes for different applications. On right are micro-handpiece and conventional handpiece.

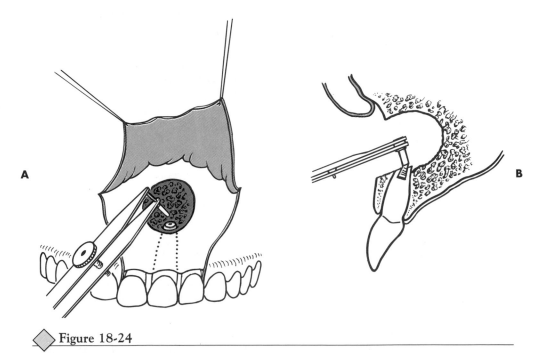

◇ **Figure 18-24**

Special small amalgam carriers are used to place material, which is then packed with small condensers. Other, cement type of materials are carried and compacted with paddles and burnishers. **A,** Frontal view. **B,** Cross-section.

reach or are in virtually inaccessible areas. Usually, an injury or defect has occurred on the root. In response to the injury, there may be an inflammatory lesion or one may develop in the future. A corrective procedure is necessary. Generally, the procedure involves exposing, preparing, then sealing the defect. Usually included are removal of irritants and rebuilding the root surface (Box 18-4).

INDICATIONS

PROCEDURAL ERRORS.   Procedural errors are created by the operator, typically during access, canal instrumentation or post-space preparation (Figure 18-25). The result is perforation, which presents a difficult surgical challenge, more so than repairing damage to a root-end. Perforations often require restorative management and completion of the root canal treatment, usually in conjunction with the surgical phase. The location of the perforation influences success; some are virtually inaccessible. If the defect is on the interproximal, in the furcation, or close to adjacent teeth or to the lingual, repair may not be possible or is compromised. Defects that are too far posterior (particularly on the distal or lingual aspects) may be very difficult to reach. The nature and location of the perforation should be determined with angled radiographs before the decision is made whether to repair surgically, remove the involved root, or extract.[8]

RESORPTIVE PERFORATIONS.   Resorptive perforations may be internal or external in origin (Figure 18-26). Generally, a communication is established between pulp and periodontium. A more serious defect is one that extends to include cervical exposure to the oral cavity. There are several etiologies for these resorptions, but most include inflammation from an irritant. These irritants include sequelae to trauma, internal bleaching procedures, orthodontic tooth movement, restorative procedures, or other factors causing pulp or periradicular inflammation. There are occasional resorptions that are idiopathic, with no demonstrable etiology.

As with procedural errors, the considerations as to treatability and surgical approach are similar.

CONTRAINDICATIONS

ANATOMIC CONSIDERATIONS.   Consideration must be given to structural impediments to a surgical approach.

There are few, and most can be managed or avoided. Included are various nerve and vessel bundles and bony structures, such as the external oblique ridge.

LOCATION OF PERFORATION.   As mentioned above, the defect must be accessible surgically. This means the clinician must be able to locate and, ideally, to readily visualize the surgical area.

ACCESSIBILITY.   A handpiece or an ultrasonic instrument generally is necessary to prepare the defect. Therefore the defect must be reachable, without impedance by structures or lack of visibility.

CONSIDERATIONS

Repair presents a unique set of problems. The defect may wrap from facial to proximal to lingual, creating not only difficulties in visualization but also problems with access and hemostasis. A general guideline is that the defect is larger and more complex than it appears on a radiograph.

Generally, the defect must be enlarged to provide a sound cavosurface margin and to avoid knife-edge margins. Occasionally, the repair is internal (from inside the canal), with material being extruded through the defect. The excess is removed and contoured with burs or sharp instruments. The objective is to seal and stabilize the defect with a restorative material.

External repair is often with amalgam or, if the field is dry, glass ionomer or dentin bonding agent with composite resin. Other materials have been suggested, such as mineral trioxide aggregate or Super EBA; these have not had the test of time but are promising materials.[13] If a post or other material is perforating the root, it must be reduced with burs to within root structure and a cavity prepared. Then the defect is restored with one of the materials mentioned above.

Repairs in the cervical third or furcation have the poorest prognosis. Communication often is eventually established with the junctional epithelium, which will result in periodontal breakdown and pocket formation. This would mean that a periodontal procedure (such as crown lengthening) would be required in conjunction with the defect repair.

SURGICAL PROCEDURE

The basic approaches with periapical surgery are followed with corrective surgery. Flap designs are similar but are more limited. A sulcular incision is usually required, with at least one vertical incision to form a three-cornered flap. A full-thickness flap is reflected and bone removed to expose the defect (Figure 18-27). Bone removal should be adequate to allow maximal visualization and access. If possible, a rim of cervical bone should be retained to support the flap and possibly to enhance reattachment; this frequently is not possible with cervical defects.

The preparation of a facial or lingual defect is similar to that of a class I cavity preparation (Figure 18-28). An interproximal defect resembles a class II preparation, with an opening from the facial (or lingual) aspect and including the interproximal wall but leaving a lingual wall (if possible).

◇ Box 18-4 ◇

Corrective surgery

Indications
Procedural errors (perforations, etc.)
Resorptive defects
Contraindications
Anatomic impediments
Inaccessible defect
Repair would create periodontal defect

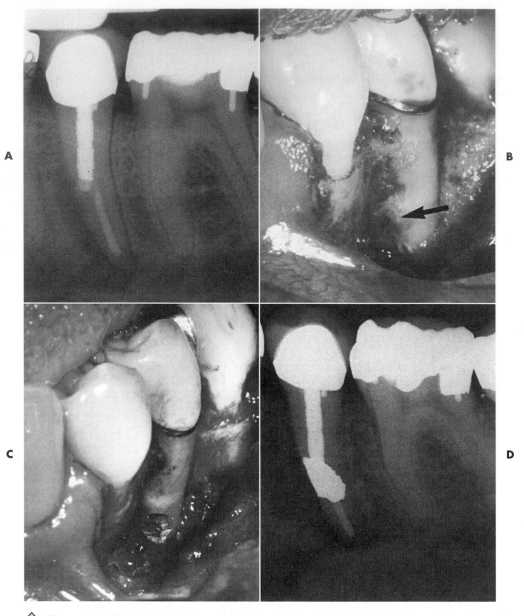

Figure 18-25

Post perforation repair. **A,** Lesion developing lateral to off-centered post suggests perforation that (**B**) is identified (*arrow*) on flap reflection. **C,** Post is reduced to within root and cavity filled with amalgam (**D**).

The facial or lingual cavity is then filled by direct placement of the material. A class II (interproximal, or furcation) cavity requires a matrix. For example, an amalgam matrix band is held in position with fingers or a wedge, then material is packed into the cavity preparation. This matrix is less critical if amalgam is not used. The material is carved flush with the cavity margins. Flap replacement, suturing, and digital pressure are as described earlier. Suture removal should be within 3 to 6 days. Postoperative instructions are similar to those following periapical surgery.

HEALING

Healing after endodontic surgery is rapid because most tissues being manipulated are healthy, with a good blood supply, and tissue replacement enables healing by primary intention.[22] Both soft tissues (periosteum, gingiva, alveolar mucosa, and periodontal ligament) and hard tissues (dentin, cementum, and bone) are involved. Time and mode of healing varies with each, but involve similar processes. The specifics of short-term healing of soft and hard tissues are discussed in Chapter 4.

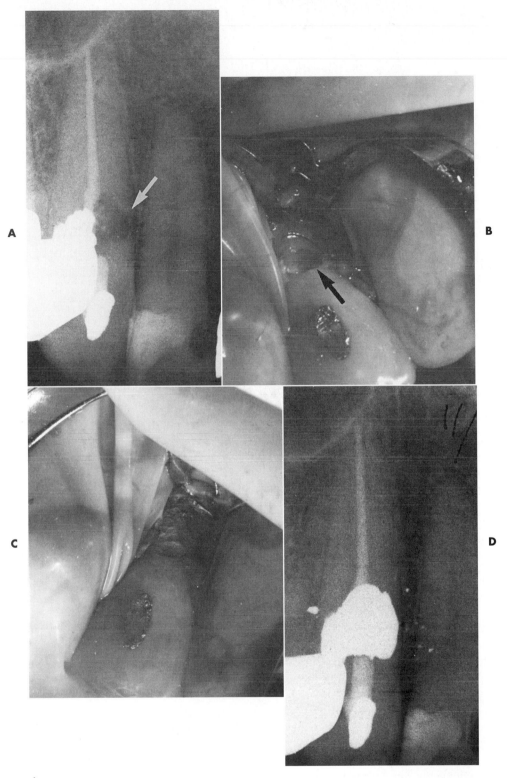

◇ Figure 18-26

External resorption repair. **A,** Mesially angled radiograph shows defect (*arrow*) to be lingual. **B,** After flap reflection, crestal bone reduction, and rubber dam isolation, defect is prepared (*arrow*). Margins must be in sound tooth structure. **C,** Cavity is filled with amalgam and flap apically positioned. **D,** Long-term radiographic and clinical evaluation is necessary; at times, resorption recurs.

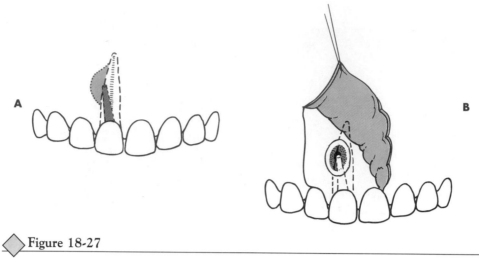

◈ Figure 18-27

A, Misdirected post is perforating distal. **B,** Full mucopercosteal (sulcular incision) three-corner flap is raised and bone removed to expose defect.

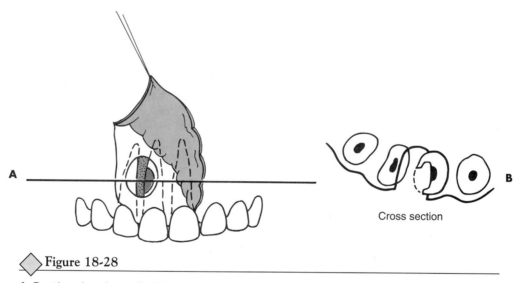

Cross section

◈ Figure 18-28

A, Post is reduced to well within root and cavity is prepared. **B,** In this cross-section through defect, there is a lingual wall to the preparation.

Recall evaluations to assess long-term healing are important. Some failures following surgery are evidenced only by radiographic findings. A 1-year follow-up is generally a good indicator. If, after 1 year, there is no radiographic evidence of decrease in lesion size or there is an increase, these generally indicate a failure and persistent inflammation.[21] A decrease in lesion size, (indicating hard tissue formation) may lead to complete healing and requires evaluation at 6 to 12 months. Of course, persistent symptoms, such as pain and/or swelling, presence of sinus tract, deep probing defects, or other adverse findings would also indicate failure. Healing by scar tissue following surgery occurs primarily in the maxillary incisors (Figure 18-29). This is an unusual occurrence and has a unique radiographic appearance. Healing by scar tissue is considered to be a successful outcome.[17]

Frequently, structures that appear normal do not regenerate over the apex. At times, connective tissue or bony arrange-ments over the apex leave a slightly "widened" periodontal ligament space. This should have relatively distinct, corticated margins and not be diffuse (which indicates inflammation and a failure).[16]

ADJUNCTS

Newer devices and materials have enhanced and in some cases improved surgical procedures. These include the surgical microscope and techniques of guided tissue regeneration.

SURGICAL MICROSCOPE

Relatively recently, the microscope has been adapted and used for surgery, as well as for other diagnostic and treatment procedures in endodontics (Figure 18-30). Advantages of the microscope include magnification and in-line illumination. These enhance the view of the surgical field and help identify

A   **B**   **C**

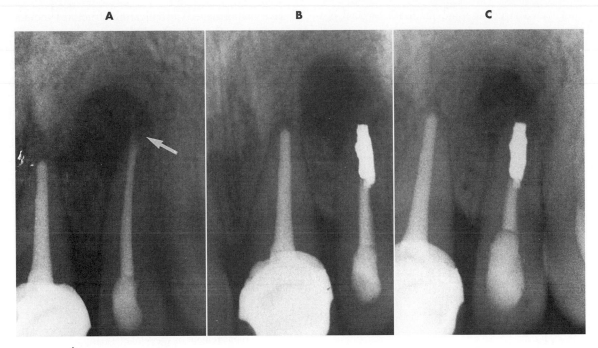

◇ **Figure 18-29**

Healing by scar tissue. **A,** Failed treatment because of transportation and perforation, leaving area of canal (*arrow*) undébrided and unobturated. **B,** Root-end resection, curettage, and root-end filling. **C,** After 2 years, there is an area of radiolucency. Sharp border, separation from apex, and distinct radiolucency show this to be a scar.

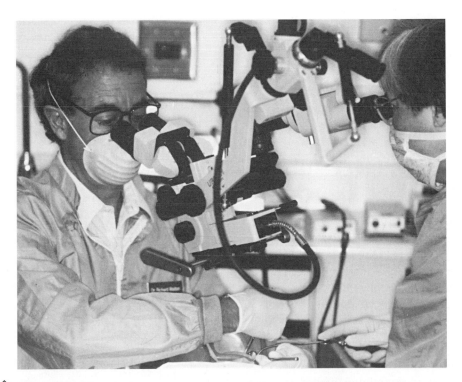

◇ **Figure 18-30**

Surgical microscope has been adapted for endodontic procedures, including surgery. Magnification and in-line illumination enhance visualization for diagnosis and treatment. Add-on binoculars for dental assistant are useful adjunct.

previously undetected structures and facilitate surgical procedures. Although there are advocates for and excitement about the use of these microscopes, as yet there have not been demonstrated substantial clinical benefits through long-term controlled studies. However, it is likely that as more information becomes available these microscopes will expand and improve on surgical techniques and outcomes.

GUIDED TISSUE REGENERATION

Originally intended for periodontal surgery, guided tissue regeneration also has been applied to endodontic surgery. The membranes used in this procedure are applied where defects have extended to cervical margins or as a covering of large defects surrounded by bone.[20] These membranes, particularly those that are resorbable, may prove useful in selected situations. However, as yet there is incomplete evidence as to their effectiveness in endodontic surgery.

WHEN TO CONSIDER REFERRAL

Although many of the procedures presented in this chapter appear relatively straightforward, endodontic surgery is often complex and difficult to perform. Clinicians should carefully consider the problems before undertaking such surgeries.

TRAINING AND EXPERIENCE

Most generalists do not have the advanced training, including didactic and clinical experience, necessary to perform surgical procedures. These procedures are a unique discipline and require special skills in diagnosis, treatment planning, and management. Also important are skill in long-term evaluation and resolving of failures or other complications. With increased emphasis on standards of care and litigation problems coupled with the availability of experienced specialists, general dentists should consider their own expertise, as well as case difficulty. These procedures are often the last hope of tooth retention. Lack of training may result in inadequate or inappropriate surgery and loss of a particular tooth and possible damage to other structures.

DETERMINE THE ETIOLOGY OF ROOT CANAL TREATMENT FAILURE

Critical to success, particularly with surgery being considered, are identification of the cause of failure and design of the treatment plan. Frequently, surgery is not the best choice but when necessary must be done appropriately. A specialist is better able to identify these etiologies and approach their resolution. If an etiology for failure cannot be identified, these cases should be considered for referral.

SURGICAL DIFFICULTIES

In many situations, surgical accessibility is limited and even hazardous. For example, the neurovascular bundle near mandibular posterior teeth and maxillary palatal root apices presents the potential for creating paraesthesia and/or excessive hemorrhage. Complicating structures include overlying bone throughout the mandible and in the palate, the frena and other muscle attachments, fenestrations of cortical bone, and sinus cavities. These structures necessitate care and require proper instruments and surgical skill. In summary, most of these procedures discussed in this chapter require greater training and experience than are provided in an undergraduate dental education program. If the clinician has not had additional postgraduate training and experience, referral should be considered for most of these procedures.

REFERENCES

1. Andreassen J, Rud J: Correlation between histology and radiography in the assessment of healing after endodontic surgery in 70 cases, *Int J Oral Surg* 1:161, 1972.
2. Allen RK, Newton CW, Brown CE: A statistical analysis of surgical and nonsurgical endodontic retreatment cases, *J Endodon* 15:261, 1989.
3. Battrum DE, Gutmann JL: Implications, prevention, and management of subcutaneous emphysema during endodontic treatment, *Endodon Dent Traumatol* 11:109, 1995.
4. Davis W, Oakley J, Smith E: Comparison of the effectiveness of etidocaine and lidocaine as local anesthetic agents during oral surgery, *Anesth Prog* 31:159, 1984.
5. Fister J, Gross BD: A histologic evaluation of bone response to bur cutting with and without water coolant, *Oral Surg Oral Med Oral Pathol* 49:105, 1980.
6. Fouad A, Rivera E, Walton R: Penicillin as a supplement in resolving the localized acute apical abscess, *Oral Surg Oral Med Oral Path Oral Radiol Endodon* 81:590, 1996.
7. Friedman S, Stabholz A: Endodontic retreatment-case selection and technique. I, Criteria for case selection, *J Endodon* 12:28, 1986.
8. Fuss Z, Trope M: Root perforations: classification and treatment choices based on prognostic factors, *Endodon Dent Traumatol* 12:255, 1996.
9. Grung B, Molven O, Halse A: Periapical surgery in a Norwegian county hospital: follow-up findings of 477 teeth, *J Endodon* 16:411, 1990.
10. Harrison JW, Johnson SA: Excisional wound healing following the use of IRM as root-end filling materials, *J Endodon* 23:19, 1997.
11. Kaufman AY, Keila S: Conservative treatment of root perforations using apex locator and thermatic compactor: case study of a new method, *J Endodon* 15:267, 1989.
12. Kramper BJ et al: A comparative study of the wound healing of three types of flap design used in periapical surgery, *J Endodon* 10:17, 1984.
13. Lee S, Monsef M, Torabinejad M: Sealing ability of a mineral trioxide aggregate for repair of lateral root perforations, *J Endodon* 19:541, 1993.
14. Lemon R, Steele P, Jeansonne B: Ferric sulfate hemostasis: effect on osseous wound healing, *J Endodon* 19:170, 1993.
15. Lin LM, Gaengler P, Langeland K: Periradicular curettage, *Int Endodon J* 29:220, 1996.
16. Molven O, Halse A, Grung B: Surgical management of endodontic failures: indications and treatment results, *Int Dent J* 46:33, 1991.
17. Molven O, Halse A, Grung B: Incomplete healing (scar

tissue) after periapical surgery: radiographic findings 8 to 12 years after treatment, *J Endodon* 22:264, 1996.

18. Neaverth EJ, Burg HA: Decompression of large periapical cystic lesions, *J Endodon* 8:175, 1982.

19. Pekruhn RB: The incidence of failure following single-visit endodontic therapy, *J Endodon* 12:68, 1986.

20. Rankow H, Krasner P: Endodontic applications of guided tissue regeneration in endodontic surgery, *J Endodon* 22:34, 1996.

21. Rud J, Andreassen J, Moller J: A multivariate analysis of the influence of various factors upon healing after endodontic surgery, *Int J Oral Surg* 1:258, 1972.

22. Selvig, K, Torabinejad M: Wound healing after mucoperiosteal surgery in the cat, *J Endodon* 22:507, 1996.

23. Taintor JF, Ingle JI, Fahid A: Retreatment versus further treatment, *Clin Prev Dent* 5:8, 1983.

24. Torabinejad M et al: Investigation of mineral trioxide aggregate for root-end filling in dogs, *J Endodon* 21:603, 1995.

25. Trope M et al: Healing of apical periodontitis in dogs after apicoectomy and retrofilling with various filling materials, *Oral Surg Oral Med Oral Pathol Oral Radiol Endodon* 81:221, 1996.

26. Wuchenich G, Meadows D, Torabinejad M: A comparison between two root end preparation techniques in human cadavers, *J Endodon* 20:279, 1994.

BIBLIOGRAPHY

El Deeb, ME, Tabibi A, Jensen MR Jr: An evaluation of the use of amalgam, cavit and calcium hydroxide in the repair of furcation perforations, *J Endodon* 8:459, 1982.

El-Swiah JM, Walker RT: Reasons for apicectomies: a retrospective study, *Endodon Dent Traumatol* 12:185, 1996.

Gutmann JL, Harrison JW: Posterior endodontic surgery: anatomical consideration and clinical techniques, *Int Endodon J* 18:8, 1985.

Gutmann JL, Harrison JW: *Surgical endodontics*, Boston, 1994, Blackwell Scientific.

Gutmann JL et al: *Problem solving in endodontics: prevention, identification, and management*, ed 3, St Louis, 1997, Mosby.

Harrison JW, Jurosky KA: Wound healing in the periodontium following endodontic surgery. I, The incisional wound, *J Endodon* 17:425, 1991.

Harrison JW, Jurosky KA: Wound healing in the periodontium following endodontic surgery. II, The dissectional wound, *J Endodon* 17:544, 1991.

Harrison JW, Jurosky KA: Wound healing in the tissues of the periodontium following endodontic surgery. III, The osseous excisional wound, *J Endodon* 18:76, 1992.

Lubow RM, Wayman BE, Cooley RL: Endodontic flap design: analysis and recommendation for current usage, *Oral Surg Oral Med Oral Pathol* 58:207, 1984.

McDonald N, Hovland E: Surgical endodontics. In Walton R, Torabinejad M, editors: *Principles and practice of endodontics*, Philadelphia, 1996, WB Saunders.

Skoner JR et al: Blood mercury levels with amalgam retroseals: a longitudinal study, *J Endodon* 22:140, 1996.

Stromberg T, Hasselgren G, Bergstedt H: Endodontic treatment of traumatic root perforations in man: a clinical and roentgenological follow-up study, *Swen Tandlak* 65:457, 1972.

Witherspoon D, Gutmann J: Haemostasis in periradicular surgery, *Int Endod* J 29:135, 1996.

Management of the Patient Undergoing Radiotherapy or Chemotherapy

Edward Ellis III

Dental Management of Patients Undergoing Radiotherapy to the Head and Neck ──────◇

Radiotherapy (radiation therapy, x-ray treatment) is a common therapeutic modality for malignancies of the head and neck. Approximately 30,000 cases of head and neck cancer occur each year. Many of these are managed by therapeutic irradiation. Its use is *ideally* predicated on the ability of the radiation to destroy neoplastic cells while sparing normal cells. In practice, however, this is never actually achieved, and there is always some undesirable effect on normal tissues. Any neoplasm can be destroyed by radiation if the dose delivered to the neoplastic cells is sufficient. The limiting factor is the amount of radiation that the surrounding tissues can tolerate.

Radiotherapy destroys neoplastic (and normal) cells by interfering with nuclear material necessary for reproduction, cell maintenance, or both. The faster the cellular turnover, the more susceptible the tissue is to the damaging effects of radiation. Thus neoplastic cells, which are usually reproducing at higher rates than normal tissue, are selectively destroyed (relatively). In practice, normal tissues with rapid turnover rates are also affected to some degree. Therefore hematopoietic cells, epithelial cells, and endothelial cells are affected soon after treatments with radiotherapy begin.

Early in the course of radiotherapy the oral mucosa shows the effects of treatment. The changes in and around the oral cavity as the result of destruction of the fine vasculature are most notable to dentistry. Salivary glands and bone are relatively radioresistant, but because of the intense vascular compromise resulting from radiotherapy, these tissues bear a considerable hardship in the long run.

RADIATION EFFECTS ON ORAL MUCOSA

The initial effect of radiotherapy on the oral mucosa, which is seen in the first 1 or 2 weeks, is an erythema that may progress to a severe mucositis with or without ulceration. Pain and dysphagia may be severe and make adequate nutritional intake difficult. These mucosal reactions begin to subside after completion of the course of radiotherapy. The taste buds, also comprised of epithelial cells, show similar reactions. Clinically, loss of taste is a prominent complaint early in treatment and gradually returns, depending on the quantity and quality of saliva that remains after treatment.

The long-term effects of radiotherapy to the oral mucosa are characterized by a predisposition to breakdown and delayed healing, even after minor insult. The epithelium is thin and less keratinized, and the submucosa is less vascular, which gives a pale appearance to the tissue. Radiotherapy induces submucosal fibrosis, which makes the mucosal lining of the oral cavity less pliable and less resilient. Minor trauma may create ulcerations that take weeks or months to heal. These ulcerations are often difficult to differentiate from recurrent malignant disease.

RADIATION EFFECTS ON SALIVARY GLANDS

Salivary gland epithelium has a very slow turnover rate; therefore the salivary glands might be expected to be radioresistant. However, because of the destruction of the fine vasculature by the radiation, the salivary glands show considerable damage, with resultant atrophy, fibrosis, and degeneration. This manifests clinically as xerostomia (the decreased production of saliva) and gives the patient a "dry mouth." The severity of xerostomia depends on which salivary glands were within the field of radiation. A dry mouth may be the patient's most significant complaint.

The effects of xerostomia on the oral cavity are devastating. Because saliva is the principal protector of the oral tissues, absence results in serious complications. Rampant "radiation caries" can swiftly destroy the remaining dentition and predispose the patient to severe infections of the jaws. Teeth thus affected exhibit decay around the entire circumference of the cervical portion (Figure 19-1). Periodontitis is also accelerated in the absence of saliva. Dysgeusia, dysphonia, and dysphagia are also caused by xerostomia.

TREATMENT OF XEROSTOMIA

After radiotherapy, patients often complain of chronic dry mouth. At present, there is no general agreement on how to prevent these changes. Unfortunately, in many cases, xerostomia never improves substantially, and exogenous replacement of saliva is necessary. For the most simple form of replacement, water can be sipped throughout the day. There are also several saliva substitutes on the market that can be obtained without a prescription at the pharmacy. These substitutes contain several of the ions in saliva and other ingredients (for example, glycerine) to mimic the lubricating action of saliva. Unfortunately, artificial salivas on the market do not possess the protective proteins that are present in the salivary secretions. The patients are therefore still prone to the problems induced by xerostomia. For comfort, however, many patients seem to be just as satisfied with plain water as artificial salivas and keep small quantities available at all times to sip.

Efforts to stimulate the patient's residual saliva have met with some success. Recently, the Food and Drug Administration approved the use of oral pilocarpine HCl to relieve symptoms of xerostomia for head and neck cancer patients. Pilocarpine HCl is a parasympathomimetic agent that functions primarily as a muscarinic agonist, causing stimulation of exocrine glands. This can increase the production of saliva, even in patients whose salivary glands have been exposed to radiation. An oral dosage of 5 mg 3 times each day has been shown to improve many symptoms of radiation-induced xerostomia without significant drug related side effects.[17] This may prove to be a beneficial treatment for some patients with postradiation xerostomia.

RADIATION EFFECTS ON BONE

One of the most severe and complicating sequelae of radiotherapy for patients with head and neck cancer is osteoradionecrosis (Figure 19-2). Basically, osteoradionecrosis is devitalization of the bone by cancericidal doses of radiation. The bone within the radiation beam becomes virtually nonvital from an endarteritis that results in elimination of the fine vasculature within the bone. The turnover rate of any remaining viable bone is slowed to the point of being ineffective in self-repair. The continual process of remodeling normally found in bone does not occur, and sharp areas on the alveolar ridge will not smooth themselves, even with considerable time. The bone of the mandible is denser and has a poorer blood supply than that of the maxilla. Thus the mandible is the jaw most commonly affected with nonhealing ulcerations and osteoradionecrosis.

OTHER EFFECTS OF RADIATION

Patients undergoing radiotherapy may have an alteration in the normal oral flora, with overgrowth of anaerobic species and fungi. Most researchers feel that oral flora colonizing the mucous membranes play an important role in the severity of mucositis and subsequent healing process.[26,27] *Candida albicans* commonly thrives in the oral cavities of patients who have been irradiated. It is not known whether the alteration in the flora is caused by the radiation itself or the resultant xerostomia. Patients frequently require the application of topical antifungal agents, such as nystatin, to help control the amount of *Candida* organisms present. Another oral rinse frequently prescribed is 0.1% chlorhexidine (Peridex). This agent has been shown to have potent in vitro antibacterial and antifungal effects. When used throughout the course of radiation treatment, it has been shown in at least one study to greatly reduce the prevalence and symptoms associated with radiation-induced mucositis.[21] It's use in other studies has been equivocal.[11,26]

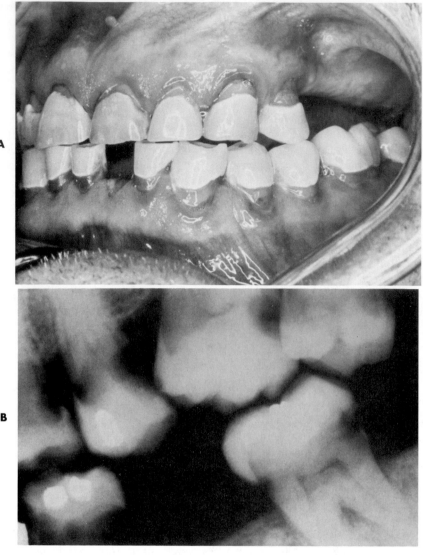

◇ Figure 19-1

A, Typical clinical appearance of radiation caries. **B,** Typical radiographic appearance of radiation caries. Note the erosion around the cervical portion of the teeth.

EVALUATION OF THE DENTITION BEFORE RADIOTHERAPY

The most feared side effect of radiotherapy is osteoradionecrosis. Most patients who develop this complication have residual teeth throughout the course of radiotherapy. Thus the clinician may wonder what to do with the teeth before irradiation. Should teeth be extracted? This question has no categorical answer; however, several factors must be considered.[3,4,6] For a more thorough discussion of the following topics, the reader is referred to the excellent articles by Beumer, Curtis, and Harrison.[4,5]

CONDITION OF THE RESIDUAL DENTITION. *All* teeth with a questionable or poor prognosis should be extracted before radiotherapy. The more advanced the periodontal condition, the more likely the patient is to develop caries and continued periodontitis. Although this may not be in keeping with usual dental principles, *if in doubt, extract.* Extraction in these cases may spare the patient months or years of suffering from osteoradionecrosis.

PATIENT'S DENTAL AWARENESS. The present state of the dentition and periodontium is a good clue to the past care they have received. In patients with excellent oral hygiene and oral health, the clinician should retain as many of the teeth as possible. Conversely, in patients who have neglected oral health for years, the chances are that they will continue to do so, especially in the face of severe xerostomia and oral pain, which will make oral hygiene even more difficult. Preradiotherapy patient preparation is similar to preorthodontic patient preparation. If an individual cannot or will not care for his or her mouth before the application of the braces,

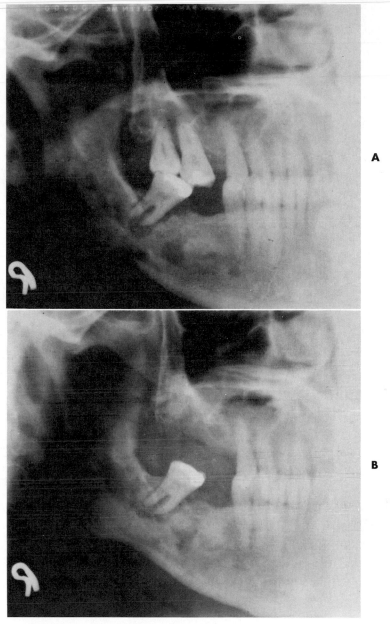

◇ Figure 19-2

Progressive course of osteoradionecrosis. **A,** Radiograph showing radiolucencies in right mandible and around apex of molar tooth. **B,** Six months later, during which time antibiotics and local irrigations were used, radiolucent process is spreading into ramus. Molar was removed at this time. *Continued*

it will be impossible for him or her to do so when faced with future obstacles.

IMMEDIACY OF RADIOTHERAPY.   If the radiotherapist feels that therapy must be instituted urgently, there may not be time to perform the necessary extractions and allow for initial healing of the extraction sites. In this instance the dentist may elect to maintain the dentition but must work closely with the patient throughout the course of radiotherapy and thereafter in an attempt to maintain oral health as optimally as possible.

RADIATION LOCATION.   The more salivary glands and bone involved in the field of radiation, the more severe will be the resultant xerostomia and vascular compromise of the jaws. Thus the dentist should discuss with the radiotherapist the locations of the radiation beams and estimate the severity of the probable xerostomia and bone changes. Xerostomia by itself may not result in severe problems if the dentition can be maintained, because the bone is still healthy. It is the combination of xerostomia and irradiated bone that usually causes the problem. In individuals who will have radiation to

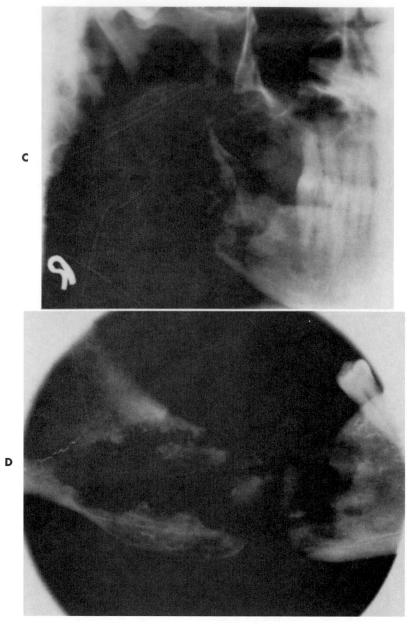

◇ Figure 19-2, cont'd

C, Five months after tooth removal, extraction site did not heal and destructive process spread, resulting in pathologic fracture of mandible. **D,** Radiograph following removal of devitalized bone, showing extent of process. *(Courtesy Dr. Richard Scott, University of Michigan, Ann Arbor.)*

the major salivary glands *and* a portion of the mandible, preirradiation extractions should be considered. Frequently, the radiotherapist agrees to delay the institution of irradiation for 1 to 2 weeks if the dentist feels that time is necessary to allow the extraction sites to begin to heal.

RADIATION DOSE.   The higher the radiation dose, the more severe is normal tissue damage. The radiotherapist should discuss with the dentist the amount of radiation planned for the individual. Frequently, the dosage is not maximal, and tissue damage may be minimized. This tends to

make the dentist more conservative in preirradiation extraction considerations. Squamous cell carcinomas of the oral cavity make up approximately 90% of malignant tumors for which radiation therapy is employed. Unfortunately, this cancer requires a very large dose of radiation (greater than 6000 rads [60 Gy]) to effect a result. Other malignancies, such as lymphoma, require much less radiation for a response, and the oral cavity will therefore be less affected. When the total dose falls below 5000 rads (50 Gy), long-term side effects, such as xerostomia and osteoradionecrosis, are dramatically decreased.

PREPARATION OF THE DENTITION FOR RADIOTHERAPY AND MAINTENANCE AFTER IRRADIATION

Every tooth to be maintained must be carefully inspected for pathologic conditions and restored to the best state of health obtainable. A thorough prophylaxis and topical fluoride application should be performed before radiotherapy. Oral hygiene measures and instructions should be demonstrated and reinforced. Any sharp cusps should be rounded to prevent mechanical irritation. Impressions for dental casts should be obtained for fabrication of custom fluoride trays to be used during treatment. Because tobacco use and alcohol consumption irritate the mucosa, the patient should be encouraged to stop these before commencement of radiation therapy.

During radiation treatment the patient should rinse the mouth at least 10 times a day with saline rinses. The patient should be placed on chlorhexidine mouthrinses twice a day to help minimize the bacterial and fungal levels within the mouth. The patient should be seen by the dentist each week during the radiotherapy for observation and oral hygiene evaluations. If an overgrowth of *Candida albicans* occurs, nystatin or clotrimazole topical applications will bring this under control relatively rapidly. The ability of the patient to open the mouth should be carefully monitored throughout the course of radiation treatment. Radiation causes a progressive fibrosis within the muscles of mastication that makes it difficult for the patient to adequately open the mouth. Patients should be instructed in physiotherapy exercises to maintain the preradiation-treatment interincisal dimension. All patients must be weighed weekly to determine whether they are maintaining an adequate nutritional status. The combination of mucositis and xerostomia makes oral intake an extremely uncomfortable endeavor. However, malnutrition causes further difficulties by delaying healing of the oral tissues and giving the patient an overall feeling of generalized illness. In severe cases it may be necessary to feed the patient via nasogastric tube to maintain a reasonable nutritional status.

Following radiation treatment the patient should be seen by the dentist every 3 to 4 months. A prophylaxis is performed during these postirradiation visits, and topical fluoride applications are made. The patient should be fitted with custom trays to deliver topical fluoride applications. The patient should be instructed in the use of the trays and in *daily* self-administration of topical fluoride applications. The use of a 1% fluoride rinse for 5 minutes each day has been found to decrease the incidence of radiation caries.[9] Over-the-counter fluoride rinses currently available can be used without a customized delivery splint with good success and seem to have better patient acceptance.

METHOD OF PERFORMING PREIRRADIATION EXTRACTIONS

If the decision has been made to extract some or all teeth before radiotherapy, the question becomes, "How should the teeth be extracted?" In general, the principles of atraumatic exodontia apply. However, the concepts of bone preservation are disregarded, and an attempt is made to remove a good portion of the alveolar process along with the teeth and achieve a primary soft tissue closure. With the onset of radiotherapy the normal remodeling process is inhibited, and, if there are any sharp areas of bone, ulceration occurs with bone exposure. Thus the teeth are usually removed in a surgical manner, with flap reflection and generous bone removal. Atraumatic handling of the mucoperiosteal flaps is necessary to ensure a rapid soft tissue healing. Burs or files should be used to smooth the bony edges under copious irrigation, because the remodeling capability of the tissues is greatly decreased after radiotherapy. Prophylactic antibiotics are indicated under these circumstances. *Remember: the dentist is in a race against time. If the wound fails to heal, the radiotherapy will be delayed, or if the radiation is delivered anyway, the wound will take months or even years to heal.*

INTERVAL BETWEEN PREIRRADIATION EXTRACTIONS AND THE BEGINNING OF RADIOTHERAPY

There is no categoric answer to the question of how much time should be allowed after extractions before beginning radiotherapy. Obviously, the sooner radiotherapy is begun, the more beneficial it may be. Thus when the soft tissues have healed sufficiently, radiotherapy may begin. Traditionally, 7 to 14 days between tooth extraction and radiotherapy have been suggested.[2,3,28] Most authors base their recommendations on the clinical impression that reepithelialization has occurred in this period. However, radiotherapy should be delayed for 3 weeks after extraction if possible. This helps to ensure that sufficient soft tissue healing has occurred. The radiotherapy should be delayed further, if possible, if a local wound dehiscence has occurred. In this instance, daily local wound care with irrigations and postoperative antibiotics are mandatory until the soft tissues have healed.

IMPACTED THIRD MOLAR REMOVAL BEFORE RADIOTHERAPY

If the patient has a partially erupted mandibular third molar, removal may be prudent to prevent pericoronal infection. In general, however, allowing a tooth that is totally impacted within the bone of the mandible to remain in place is more expeditious than removing it and waiting for it to heal.

METHOD OF DEALING WITH CARIOUS TEETH AFTER RADIOTHERAPY

Teeth that develop postradiotherapy caries must be immediately cared for in an attempt to prevent further spread of infection. Composites and amalgam are the materials of choice to repair the defects caused by decay. Full crowns are probably not warranted, because recurrent decay is more difficult to detect under such restorations. Oral hygiene measures, including fluoride application, must be reinforced in any patient who develops postirradiation caries.

If a tooth has necrotic pulp, endodontic intervention with systemic antibiotics can be carefully performed and the tooth ground out of occlusion and maintained. Frequently, root canal treatment is difficult because of a progressive sclerosis of the pulp chamber that occurs in irradiated teeth. In such instances the tooth can simply be amputated above the gingiva and left in place.

TOOTH EXTRACTION AFTER RADIOTHERAPY

Can teeth be extracted after radiotherapy and, if so, how? These are probably the most difficult questions to answer. Each dentist has a view on this subject, and the literature is contradictory. Postirradiation extractions are also the most undesirable extractions the dentist will ever perform, because the outcome is always uncertain.

The answer to the question of whether extractions *can* be done after radiotherapy is certainly *yes*. The more important question is "how"? If the tooth is to be extracted, the dentist can either perform a simple extraction without primary soft tissue closure or a surgical extraction with alveoloplasty and primary closure. Either of these techniques yields similar results, with a certain concomitant incidence of osteoradionecrosis. The use of systemic antibiotics is recommended.

Another technique that has been shown to be effective and that is gaining in popularity is the use of hyperbaric oxygen *before* and *after* tooth extraction. Hyperbaric oxygen therapy is the administration of oxygen under pressure to the patient. It has been shown to increase the local tissue oxygenation and vascular ingrowth into the hypoxic tissues.[18,19] In a prospective clinical trial comparing this regimen with the use of prophylactic antibiotics before dental extraction without hyperbaric oxygenation, Marx, Johnson, and Kline[20] found a significant decrease in the incidence of osteoradionecrosis (5.4% compared with 30%).

Because considerable controversy exists over how to manage an extraction surgically in a patient who has undergone irradiation, because few hyperbaric oxygenation chambers are available for use, and because the incidence of severe complications is relatively high, it is recommended that the patient who has received irradiation and requires extrac tions be managed by an oral and maxillofacial surgeon.

DENTURE WEAR IN POSTIRRADIATION EDENTULOUS PATIENTS WHO HAVE RECEIVED RADIOTHERAPY

Patients who were edentulous before radiotherapy manage very nicely with well-constructed dentures. However, patients rendered edentulous just before or after radiotherapy exhibit more problems with mucosal ulcerations and subsequent osteoradionecrosis. The normal remodeling process of the alveolar bone cannot smooth even the most minor irregularities left by extraction. With denture wear, these minor irregularities cause ulceration of the mucosa.

Soft denture liners might seem an ideal solution for patients who have received irradiation. However, the silicone soft liners proved to be not particularly useful for several reasons.

At present, patients are probably best served with ordinary dentures.

Denture fabrication for patients who were previously edentulous should be deferred until *at least* 6 months after the completion of radiotherapy.[6] For patients who underwent extractions just before or after radiotherapy, it is prudent to wait at least 1 year or more. Patients who can tolerate being without dentures (especially the lower) are probably best advised never to wear lower dentures, because the risk of mucosal breakdown is high.

When dentures are constructed, the dentist must be certain that the denture base and occlusal table are designed so that forces are distributed evenly throughout the alveolar ridge and that lateral forces on the denture are eliminated.

USE OF DENTAL IMPLANTS IN IRRADIATED PATIENTS

The dental rehabilitation of the edentulous patient who has received radiation therapy is one of the greatest challenges facing the reconstructive dentist. Many patients who have had ablative surgery for malignancy do not have the normal anatomy that makes denture wear possible. There may be no vestibules to accommodate a denture flange. Often, portions of the tongue have been removed. There may be hard and soft tissue defects and deficits. When reconstructed, the bone may have poor form for support of a tissue-borne prosthesis. Frequently, such patients have thick, nonpliable soft tissue flaps that have been grafted from distant areas and are not adherent to the underlying bone. All of these combine to make conventional denture fabrication extremely challenging. In such instances, the use of *implant*-borne prostheses are preferred from a functional standpoint.

For years, however, a history of irradiation has been a relative contraindication to the placement of dental implants.[16] The effects of radiation on bone and soft tissue present a formidable challenge to the use of implanted metallic devices. Not surprising, success rates for implants placed into radiated tissues are reported to be lower than implants placed into nonirradiated tissues.[13,31] However, the benefits that can accrue from providing this group of patients a functional and esthetic dental reconstruction are great. Such patients have been through a great deal of hardship. They have lost portions of their anatomy, are frequently deformed, and feel the uncomfortable effects of the radiation therapy, such as xerostomia, dysphagia, and dysgeusia. They relish the thought of being able to chew solid food with a functional dentition. Implant-borne prostheses can help achieve this goal in these difficult situations. However, the unpredictable reaction of soft and hard tissue in an irradiated patient and the surgical trauma of treatment have all combined to promote caution in such cases.

Many variables must be evaluated when considering placement of dental implants into irradiated bone, including the radiation type, dosage, sites, elapsed time since the treatment, protection provided to the bone during treatment, and the patient's own physiologic responses (which themselves are affected by age, sex, genetics, smoking, and other systemic considerations). Other critical factors are whether the implants will be placed into irradiated host mandibular bone, irradiated bone grafts, or bone that has been transplanted after the radiation therapy. In the latter instance, if the mandible was reconstructed using a microvascular graft, in which the blood supply to the bone is brought in from a distant source and has not been altered by the previous radiation therapy, no adverse tissue reaction should be expected after placement of dental implants.

When dental implants are to be placed into irradiated host or grafted bone, the dentist must proceed with caution. Consultation with the radiotherapist is recommended to determine the amount of radiation that has occurred to the area of the jaws where the proposed implants will be placed. It has been demonstrated that the success of implant retention is directly and positively correlated with the amount of radiation to which the bone was exposed.[31] If the amount of radiation is less than approximately 4500 rads (45 Gy), implants may be placed with care. When the amount of radiation exceeds this amount, preoperative and postoperative hyperbaric oxygen treatments should be considered. Hyperbaric oxygen treatments have been shown to be beneficial in such patients.[12]

The time required for osseointegration will be prolonged in irradiated patients because of the lower metabolic activity in the bone, so the implants should not be loaded for at least 6 months after placement. The dentist must pay particular attention to oral hygiene in such patients, because their tissues will not be as able to resist bacterial invasion as tissues in patients who have not been irradiated. The prosthetic design should therefore be made as cleansible as possible, with frequent use of over-dentures. These patients will require more careful follow-up and hygiene measures.

In spite of the fear that implants placed into irradiated bone will lead to osteoradionecrosis, it is uncommonly reported in the literature.[1,29] However, there has been an insufficient duration of experience to predict the long-term outcome of implant prosthetics in the patient who has undergone radiation.

MANAGEMENT OF PATIENTS WHO DEVELOP OSTEORADIONECROSIS

Most mucosal breakdown and subsequent osteoradionecrosis occur in the mandible. They occur most often in mandibles that have received radiation in excess of 6500 rads (65 Gy) and do not usually occur in mandibles that have received radiation doses below 4800 rads (48 Gy).[7,23,24] Severe pain may follow. The patient should discontinue wearing any prosthesis and try to maintain a good state of oral health. Irrigations should be instituted to remove necrotic debris (Figure 19-3). Only occasionally are systemic antibiotics necessary, because osteoradionecrosis is not an infection of the bone but rather a nonhealing hypoxic wound.[19] Because of the decreased vascularity of the tissues, systemic antibiotics do not gain ready access to the area to perform the function for which they are intended. However, in acute secondary infections, antibiotics may be useful to help prevent spread of the infection. Any loose sequestra are removed, but no attempt is made

initially to close the soft tissues over the exposed bone. Most wounds smaller than 1 cm eventually heal, although it may take weeks to months.

For nonhealing wounds or extensive areas of osteoradionecrosis, surgical intervention may be indicated. In this instance, resection of the exposed bone and a margin of unexposed bone followed by primary soft tissue closure can be attempted (Figure 19-4). This is successful in many cases. Greatly improved results have recently been obtained by the use of hyperbaric oxygen therapy in conjunction with surgical intervention.[18] Reconstructive efforts with bone grafts used for continuity defects can also be undertaken successfully in many patients who have undergone irradiation. Free microvascular grafting techniques are becoming more popular for restoring continuity defects in patients who have received radiotherapy. These bone grafts have their own blood supply from a reconnection of blood vessels and are therefore less dependent on the local tissues for incorporation and healing.

DENTAL MANAGEMENT OF PATIENTS ON SYSTEMIC CHEMOTHERAPY FOR MALIGNANT DISEASE

Destruction of malignant cells by tumoricidal chemotherapeutic drugs has proved an effective treatment for a variety of malignancies. Like radiotherapy, the antitumor effect of cancer chemotherapeutic agents is based on their ability to destroy or retard the division of rapidly proliferating cells, such as tumor cells, nonspecifically. Unfortunately, normal host cells that have a high mitotic index are also adversely affected. Normal cells most affected are the epithelium of the gastrointestinal tract (including oral cavity) and the cells of the bone marrow.

EFFECTS ON ORAL MUCOSA

Many chemotherapeutic agents reduce the normal turnover rate of oral epithelium, which results in atrophic thinning of the oral mucosa manifested clinically as painful, erythematous, and ulcerative mucosal surfaces in the mouth. The effects are most noted on the unattached mucosa and rarely seen on gingival surfaces. These changes are seen within 1 week of the onset of the administration of the antitumor agents. The effects are usually self-limiting, and spontaneous healing occurs in 2 to 3 weeks after cessation of the agent.

EFFECTS ON HEMATOPOIETIC SYSTEM

Myelosuppression, as manifested by leukopenia, neutropenia, thrombocytopenia, and anemia, is a common sequela of several forms of cancer chemotherapy. Within 2 weeks of the beginning of chemotherapy administration, the white blood cell count falls to an extremely low level. The effect of myelosuppression in the oral cavity is marginal gingivitis. Mild infections may develop, and bleeding from the gingiva

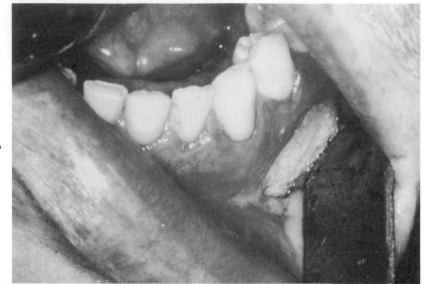

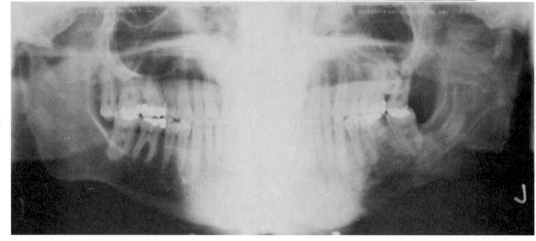

Figure 19-3

A, Typical appearance of an area of mucosal breakdown and exposure of underlying bone. This bone is devitalized and painful and has not responded to local wound care. **B,** Radiograph showing diffuse radiolucency of left mandibular body region. *(Courtesy Dr. Richard Scott, University of Michigan, Ann Arbor.)*

is common. If the neutropenia is severe and prolonged, severe infections may develop. The microorganisms involved in these infections may be overgrowths of the usual oral flora, especially fungi; however, other microorganisms may be causative. Thrombocytopenia can be marked, and spontaneous bleeding may occur. This is especially common in the oral cavity after oral hygiene measures. Recovery from myelosuppression is usually complete 3 weeks after cessation of chemotherapy.

It is important to find out the type of neoplasm for which the patient is being treated. The type of neoplasm dictates the type of chemotherapeutic agents to be used. Many hematologic neoplasms (leukemia, for example) are treated with chemotherapeutic agents that result in profound alterations in the function and number of bone marrow elements. Comparatively, chemotherapeutic manage-

ment of some nonmarrow solid tumors may not be associated with as severe a marrow aplasia as is found in patients with hematologic neoplasms.

EFFECTS ON ORAL MICROBIOLOGY

Chemotherapeutic agents, because of their immunosuppressive side effect, cause profound changes in the oral flora. For example, overgrowth of indigenous microbes, superinfection with gram-negative bacilli, and opportunistic infections are all common sequelae and lead to patient discomfort and morbidity. Systemic infections are responsible for about 70% of the deaths in patients receiving myelosuppressive cancer chemotherapy.[14,22] *Oral* microorganisms have been shown to be a common source of bacteremia in these patients.[14] Thus most patients who are on chemotherapy are treated concomitantly with systemic antimicrobial agents.

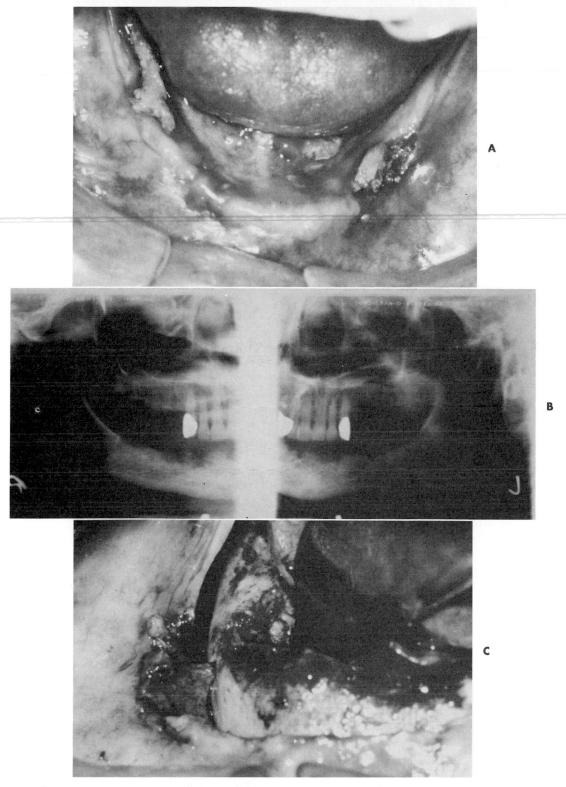

Figure 19-4

A, Large areas of osteoradionecrosis in edentulous mandible that did not respond to conservative therapy. This patient was debilitated from pain. **B,** Radiographic appearance. Twenty hyperbaric oxygen sessions were performed, without healing of oral wounds. **C,** Surgical exposure of mandible at time of alveolectomy. Note mental neurovascular bundle as it exits mandible and ragged appearance of alveolar crest.

Continued

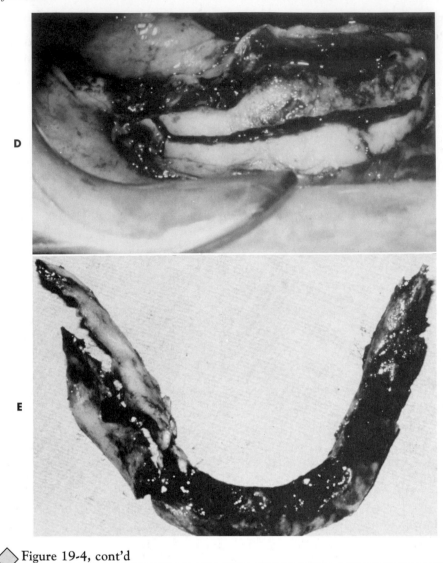

◇ **Figure 19-4, cont'd**

D, Osteotomy cuts made to remove alveolar crest. **E,** Specimen following removal. Wound was closed primarily, and 20 more hyperbaric oxygen sessions were instituted. *Continued*

However, in spite of these regimens, patients frequently develop overgrowth of some organisms, most commonly the *Candida* spp.[10,15,25]

GENERAL DENTAL MANAGEMENT

In general, the principles of dental management for the patient who has had or will have radiotherapy apply equally well to the patient who has had or will have chemotherapy.[8,32] However, because of the intermittent nature of the chemotherapy delivered in many instances, the minimal effects on the vasculature, and the almost normal state of the individual between chemotherapeutic administrations, dental management can be much easier. The effects of the chemotherapy are almost always only temporary, and, with the passage of time, systemic health improves to optimal levels, which allows almost routine dental management.

Primary concerns for the dentist should be the severity and duration of bone marrow suppression. The dentist must be aware of the dates of chemotherapy and the hematologic status of the patient before beginning dental care. If the patient is being treated for a hematologic neoplasm (for example, leukemia), *both* the disease *and* the chemotherapy lead to decreases in the functional blood elements. Therefore these patients may be at great risk for infection and hemorrhage at any time in the course of their disease. Consultation with the patient's physician in these instances is mandatory. In most cases of nonhematopoietic neoplasm the patient is at risk for infection and hemorrhage only during the course of the chemotherapy, after which recovery of the blood elements occurs.

The decision of when to extract teeth before treatment is based on the condition of the residual dentition, the patient's past dental hygiene practices, the immediacy of the need for chemotherapy, and the overall prognosis of the malignant disease. Prechemotherapy dental measures that should routinely be performed are a thorough prophylaxis, fluoride

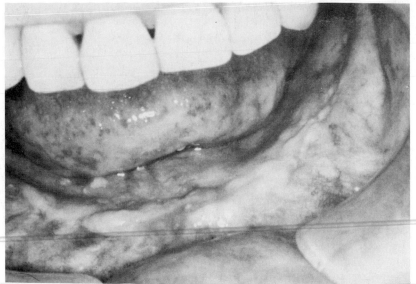

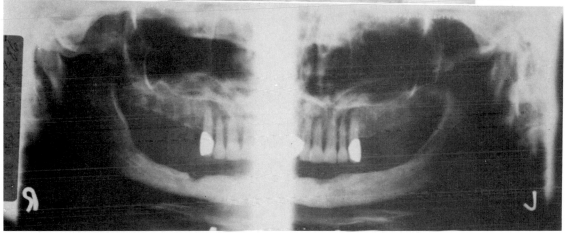

◇ Figure 19-4, cont'd

F, Clinical appearance of mandible 6 months after alveolectomy. **G,** Radiographic appearance of mandible at same time. *(Courtesy Dr. Richard Scott, University of Michigan, Ann Arbor.)*

treatment, and any necessary scaling. Unrestorable teeth should be removed before chemotherapy begins.

Patients who have begun chemotherapy must maintain scrupulous oral hygiene. This is difficult in the face of mucositis and ulceration, which frequently occur. No dental procedures should be performed on any patient receiving chemotherapy whose white blood cell and platelet status is unknown. In general, patients who have a white blood cell count greater than or equal to 2000 mm³, with at least 20% polymorphonuclear leukocytes, and a platelet count greater than or equal to 50,000 mm³, can be treated in routine fashion. Prophylactic antibiotics should be administered if the patient has had chemotherapy within 3 weeks of dental treatment. If the white blood cell count and platelet levels fall below those specified, minimal oral care should be practiced, because infection, severe bleeding, or both can occur. The patient may even need to avoid flossing and to use an extremely soft toothbrush during these periods. Any removable dental appliance should be left out at these times to prevent ulceration of the fragile mucosa.

TREATMENT OF ORAL CANDIDOSIS

Initial treatment of candidosis is with topical application of an antifungal medication.[10] The advantage of using topical medication is that systemic side effects are minimized. Similarly, in patients with persistent infection, advantage can be gained by continuing topical agents in addition to systemic medications. The use of this combination may allow a reduced dose and duration of systemic administration of the antifungal medication and also may reduce the potential side effects.

Topical agents are available as oral rinses, oral tablets, and creams. In general, oral rinses provide a short contact time for the drug and are therefore of less efficacy. The tablets are one of the most accepted forms of topically treating candidiasis, because they can be dissolved slowly in the mouth and provide increased exposure time of the drug with the oral flora. The cream forms of topical antifungals are helpful for candida of the oral commissures or for application to the oral surfaces of prosthetic devices to prolong medication exposure.

The most commonly administered topical medication for oropharyngeal *Candida* infections is nystatin. It is available in several forms and should be applied 4 times daily. Therapy should continue 2 weeks following cessation of clinical signs and symptoms. An alternate drug is clotrimazole. Troches of these medications are available and can be dissolved in the mouth 4 or 5 times a day. For more stubborn cases, ketoconazole or fluconazole (systemic antifungal medications) can be prescribed. However, the dentist must be careful with systemic administration of antifungal medications because of their toxic side effects. These vary widely with the type of medication and can be serious.

Another widely prescribed medication for oral candidosis is chlorhexidine mouthrinse. Chlorhexidine (Peridex) has been shown to have potent antibacterial and antifungal properties in vitro. Its in vivo effects are less well documented, especially for use against *Candida* spp. in immunosuppressed individuals.[26,30] However, it is used in most of such patients on the basis that it probably does no harm and may prove beneficial in many instances.

REFERENCES

1. Albrektsson T: A multicenter report on osseointegrated oral implants, *J Prosthet Dent* 60:75-94, 1988.
2. Bedwinek JM et al: Osteonecrosis in patients treated with definitive radiotherapy for squamous cell carcinomas of the oral cavity and naso and oropharynx, *Radiology* 119:665, 1976.
3. Beumer J, Brady F: Dental management of the irradiated patient, *Int J Oral Surg* 7:208, 1978.
4. Beumer J, Curtis T, Harrison RE: Radiation therapy of the oral cavity. I. Sequelae and management, *Head Neck Surg* 1:301, 1979.
5. Beumer J, Curtis T, Harrison RE: Radiation therapy of the oral cavity. II. Sequelae and management, *Head Neck Surg* 1:392, 1979.
6. Beumer J, Curtis TA, Morrish RB: Radiation complications in edentulous patients, *J Prosthet Dent* 36:193, 1976.
7. Beumer J et al: Postradiation dental extractions: a review of the literature and a report of 72 episodes, *Head Neck Surg* 6:581-586, 1983.
8. DePaola LG et al: Dental care for patients receiving chemotherapy, *J Am Dent Assoc* 112:198, 1986.
9. Driezen S et al: Prevention of xerostomia-related dental caries in irradiated cancer patients, *J Dent Res* 56:99, 1977.
10. Epstein JB: Antifungal therapy in oropharyngeal mycotic infections, *Oral Surg* 69:32-41, 1990.
11. Ferretti GA, Raybould TP, Brown AT et al: Chlorhexidine prophylaxis for chemotherapy- and radiation-induced stomatitis: a randomized double-blind trial, *Oral Surg Oral Med Oral Path* 70:331-338, 1990.
12. Granström G, Jacobsson M, Tjellström A: Titanium implants in the irradiated tissue. Benefits from hyperbaric oxygen, *Int J Oral Maxillofac Implants* 7:15-25, 1992.
13. Granström G, Tjellström A, Branemark P-I et al: Bone-anchored reconstruction of the irradiated head and neck cancer patient, *Otolaryngol Head Neck Surg* 108:334-343, 1993.
14. Greenberg MS et al: The oral flora as a source of septicemia in patients with acute leukemia, *Oral Surg* 53:32-39, 1982.
15. Heimdahl A, Nord CE: Oral yeast infections in immunocompromised and seriously diseased patients, *Acta Odontol Scand* 48:77-84, 1990.
16. Hobo S, Ichida E, Garcia LT: *Osseointegration and occlusal rehabilitation.* Tokyo, 1989, Quintessence.
17. Khan Z, Jacobsen CS: Oral pilocarpine HCl for post-irradiation xerostomia in head and neck cancer patients. *Proceedings of the First International Congress on Maxillofacial Prosthetics,* New York, 1995, Memorial Sloan-Kettering Cancer Center.
18. Marx RE: A new concept in the treatment of osteoradionecrosis, *J Oral Maxillofac Surg* 41:351, 1983.
19. Marx RE: Osteoradionecrosis: a new concept in its pathophysiology, *J Oral Maxillofac Surg* 41:283, 1983.
20. Marx RE, Johnson RP, Kline SN: Prevention of osteoradionecrosis: a randomized prospective clinical trial of hyperbaric oxygen versus penicillin, *J Am Dent Assoc* 111:49, 1985.
21. Matheis MJ, Rybicki LA, Waskowski J et al: Evaluation of oral mucositis in patients receiving radiation therapy for head and neck cancer: a pilot study of 0.12% chlorhexidine gluconate oral rinse. *Proceedings of the First International Congress on Maxillofacial Prosthetics,* New York, 1995, Memorial Sloan-Kettering Cancer Center.
22. McElroy TH: Infection in the patient receiving chemotherapy: oral considerations, *J Am Dent Assoc* 109:454-460, 1984.
23. Murray CG, Herson J, Daly TE et al: Radiation necrosis of the mandible: a 10-year study. I. Factors influencing the onset of necrosis, *Int J Radiat Oncol Biol Phys* 6:543-548, 1980.
24. Murray CG, Herson J, Daly TE et al: Radiation necrosis of the mandible: a 10-year study. II. Dental factors: onset, duration, and management of necrosis, *Int J Radiat Oncol Biol Phys* 6:549-553, 1980.
25. Odds FC, Kibbler CC, Walker E et al: Carriage of *Candida* species and *C. albicans* biotypes in patients undergoing chemotherapy or bone marrow transplantation for haematological disease, *J Clin Pathol* 42:1259-1266, 1989.
26. Spijkervet FKL: *Irradiation mucositis,* Copenhagen, 1991, Munksgaard.
27. Spijkervet FK, van Saene HK, van Saene JJ et al: Effect of selective elimination of the oral flora on mucositis in irradiated head and neck cancer patients, *J Surg Oncol* 46:167-173, 1991.
28. Starcke EN, Shannon IL: How critical is the interval between extractions and irradiation in patients with head and neck malignancy? *Oral Surg* 43:333, 1977.
29. Taylor TD, Worthington P: Osseointegrated implant rehabilitation of the previously irradiated mandible: results of a limited trial at 3 to 7 years, *J Prosthet Dent* 69:60-69, 1993.
30. Thurmond JM, Brown AT, Sims RE et al: Oral *Candida albicans* in bone marrow transplant patients given chlorhexidine rinses: occurrence and susceptibilities to the agent, *Oral Surg* 72:291-295, 1991.
31. Visch LL, Levendag PC, Denissen HW: Five-year results of 227 HA-coated implants in irradiated tissues. *Proceedings of the First International Congress on Maxillofacial Prosthetics,* New York, 1995, Memorial Sloan-Kettering Cancer Center.
32. Wright WE et al: An oral disease prevention program for patients receiving radiation and chemotherapy, *J Am Dent Assoc* 110:43, 1985.

ODONTOGENIC DISEASES OF THE MAXILLARY SINUS

STERLING R. SCHOW

CHAPTER OUTLINE

EMBRYOLOGY AND ANATOMY

The maxillary sinuses are air-containing spaces that occupy the maxillary bone bilaterally. They are the first of the paranasal sinuses (maxillary, ethmoid, frontal, and sphenoid) to develop embryonically and begin as a mucosal invagination that grows laterally from the middle meatus of the nasal cavity at approximately the seventieth day of gestation. At birth the sinus cavity is still somewhat less than a centimeter in any dimension.

After birth the maxillary sinus expands by pneumatization into the developing alveolar process and extends anteriorly and inferiorly from the base of the skull, closely matching the growth rate of the maxilla and the development of the dentition. As the dentition develops, portions of the alveolar process of the maxilla, vacated by the eruption of teeth, become pneumatized. By the time a child reaches age 12 or 13, the sinus will have expanded to the point at which its floor will be on the same horizontal level as the floor of the nasal cavity. Expansion of the sinus normally ceases after the

eruption of the permanent teeth but will, on occasion, pneumatize further, after the removal of one or more posterior maxillary teeth, to occupy the residual alveolar process. The sinus may then extend virtually to the crest of the edentulous ridge. In adults the apices of the teeth may extend into the sinus cavity and may be identified readily in the dry skull lying in the sinus floor.

The sinuses are lined by respiratory epithelium—a mucus-secreting, pseudostratified, ciliated, columnar epithelium—and periosteum. The cilia and mucus are necessary for the drainage of the sinus, because the sinus opening, or ostium, is not in a dependent position but lies two thirds of the distance up from the inferior part of the medial wall and drains into the nasal cavity. The maxillary sinus opens into the posterior, or inferior, end of the semilunar hiatus, which lies in the middle meatus of the nasal cavity, between the inferior and middle nasal conchae. The ostium remains at the level of the original lateral extension from the nasal cavity from which the sinus began formation in the embryo and the location of which is close to the roof of the sinus (Figure 20-1). Beating of the cilia moves the mucus produced by the lining epithelium and any foreign material contained within the sinus toward the ostium, from which it drains into the nasal cavity.

The maxillary sinus is the largest of the paranasal sinuses. It may be described as a four-sided pyramid, with the base lying vertically on the medial surface and forming the lateral nasal wall. The apex extends laterally into the zygomatic process of the maxilla. The upper wall, or roof, of the sinus is also the floor of the orbit. The posterior wall extends the length of the maxilla and dips into the maxillary tuberosity. Anteriorly and laterally the sinus extends to the region of the first bicuspid or cuspid teeth. The floor of the sinus forms the base of the alveolar process. The adult maxillary sinus averages 34 mm in anteroposterior direction, 33 mm in height, and 23 mm in width. Its volume is approximately 15 cc (Figure 20-2).

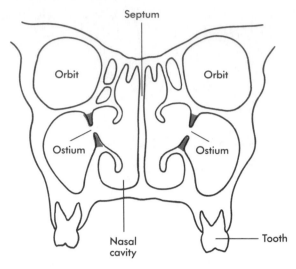

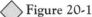

Figure 20-1

Frontal diagram of midface at ostium or opening of maxillary sinuses into middle meatus of nasal cavity. Ostium is in upper third of sinus cavity.

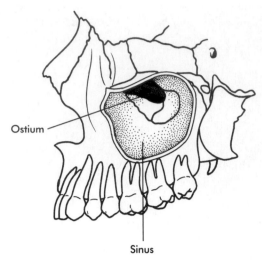

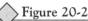

Figure 20-2

Lateral diagram of right maxillary sinus with zygoma removed. Medial sinus wall (lateral nasal wall) is seen in depth of sinus, as is ostium. Maxillary sinus is pyramidal, with its apex directed into base of zygoma.

CLINICAL EXAMINATION OF THE MAXILLARY SINUS

Clinical examination of the patient with suspected maxillary sinus disease should include tapping of the lateral walls of the sinus externally over the prominence of the cheekbones and palpation intraorally on the lateral surface of the maxilla between the canine fossa and the zygomatic buttress. The affected sinus may be markedly tender to gentle tapping or palpation. Further examination may include transillumination of the maxillary sinuses. In unilateral disease, one sinus may be compared with the sinus on the opposite side. The involved sinus shows decreased transmission of light secondary to the accumulation of fluid, debris, and pus and the thickening of the sinus mucosa. Transillumination of the maxillary sinus is done by placing a bright flashlight or fiberoptic light against the mucosa on the palatal or facial surfaces of the sinus and observing the transmission of light through the sinus in a darkened room. These simple tests help to distinguish sinus disease, which may cause pain in the upper teeth, from abscess or other pain of dental origin associated with the molar and bicuspid teeth.

RADIOGRAPHIC EXAMINATION OF THE MAXILLARY SINUS

Radiographic examination of the maxillary sinus may be accomplished with a wide variety of exposures readily available in the dental office or radiology clinic. These exposures include periapical, occlusal, and panoramic views, which will, in most instances, provide adequate information to either confirm or rule out pathologic conditions of the sinus. If additional radiographic information is required, Waters' radiographs (Figure 20-3) are usually diagnostic. Rarely, linear tomography (Figure 20-4) and computed axial tomography (Figure 20-5) of the structures in question may be necessary.

Interpretation of radiographs of the maxillary sinus is not difficult. The findings in the normal antrum are those to be expected of a rather large, air-filled cavity surrounded by bone and dental structures. The body of the sinus should appear radiolucent and should be outlined in all peripheral areas by a well-demarcated layer of cortical bone. It is helpful to compare one side to the other when examining the radiographs. There should be no evidence of thickened mucosa on the bony walls (usually indicative of chronic sinus disease) (Figure 20-3), air-fluid levels (caused by accumulation of mucus, pus, or blood) (Figure 20-6), or foreign bodies lying free. Frequently, the apices of the roots of the posterior maxillary teeth and impacted third molars may be seen to project into the sinus floor (Figure 20-7). In edentulous areas the sinus may be pneumatized into the alveolar process and extend almost to the alveolar crest. Complete opacification of the maxillary sinus may be caused by the mucosal hypertrophy and fluid accumulation of sinusitis, by filling with blood secondary to trauma, or by neoplasia (Figure 20-8). Disruption of the cortical outline may be a result of trauma, tumor formation, or surgical procedures that violate the sinus walls.

Radiographic changes are to be expected with acute maxillary sinusitis and are secondary to filling of a normal, air-containing cavity with thickened mucosal sinus lining and accumulated mucus and/or pus. Mucosal thickening secondary to odontogenic infections may obstruct the ostium of the sinus and allow accumulation of mucus, which will become

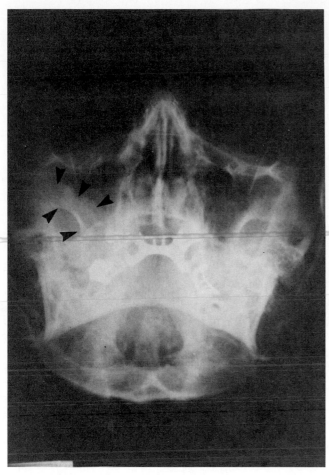

◇ Figure 20-3

Waters' radiograph showing mucosal thickening on right maxillary sinus floor and lateral wall. Patient had oroantral fistula secondary to removal of first molar tooth and symptoms of chronic maxillary sinusitis.

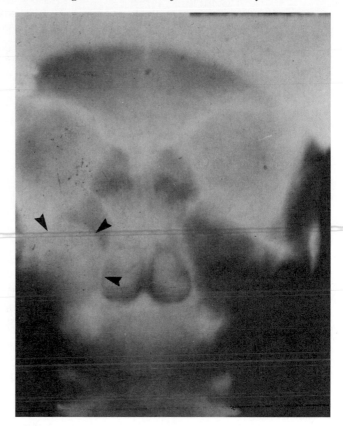

◇ Figure 20-4

Tomogram of midface taken in frontal plane. Large, cystlike radiolucent lesion is seen to occupy bulk of right maxillary sinus.

infected and produce pus. The characteristic radiographic changes may include an air-fluid level in the sinus (Figure 20-6), thickened mucosa on any or all of the sinus walls (Figure 20-3), or complete opacification of the sinus cavity (Figure 20-8).

The radiographic changes indicative of chronic maxillary sinusitis include mucosal thickening, sinus opacification, and nasal or antral polyps. Air-fluid levels in the sinuses are more characteristic of acute sinus disease but may be seen in chronic sinusitis in periods of acute exacerbation (Figure 20-9).

Dental pathologic conditions such as cysts or granulomas may produce radiolucent lesions that extend into the sinus cavity. They may be distinguished from normal sinus anatomy by their association with the tooth apex, the clinical correlation with the dental examination, and the presence of a cortical osseous margin on the radiograph, which generally separates the area in question from the sinus itself (Figure 20-10).

Periapical, occlusal, and, occasionally, panoramic radiographs are of value in locating and retrieving foreign bodies within the sinus—particularly teeth, root tips, or osseous

fragments—that have been displaced by trauma or during tooth removal (Figure 20-11). These radiographs should also be used for the careful planning of surgical removal of teeth adjacent to the sinus.

ODONTOGENIC INFECTIONS OF THE MAXILLARY SINUS ◇

The mucosa of the sinus is susceptible to infectious, allergic, and neoplastic diseases. Inflammatory diseases of the sinus, such as infection or allergic reactions, cause hyperplasia and hypertrophy of the mucosa and produce the signs and symptoms of sinusitis, as well as the radiographic changes seen with these conditions. If the ostium of the sinus becomes obstructed, the mucus produced by the secretory cells lining the walls is collected over long periods. Bacterial overgrowth may then produce an infection.

When inflammation develops in any of the paranasal sinuses, whether caused by infection or allergy, the condition is described as *sinusitis.* Inflammation of most or all of the paranasal sinuses simultaneously is known as *pansinusitis* and is usually caused by infection. Similar conditions of individual sinuses are known, for example, as *maxillary sinusitis* or *frontal sinusitis.* Maxillary sinusitis is commonly odontogenic in nature because of the anatomic juxtaposition of the teeth

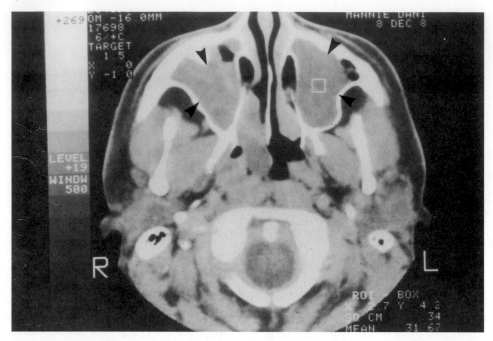

◇ **Figure 20-5**

Computed axial tomogram of head in coronal plane. Both maxillary sinuses are almost totally opacified by mucosal lesions, as is right nasopharynx. Such lesions are typical of allergic disease or chronic sinusitis.

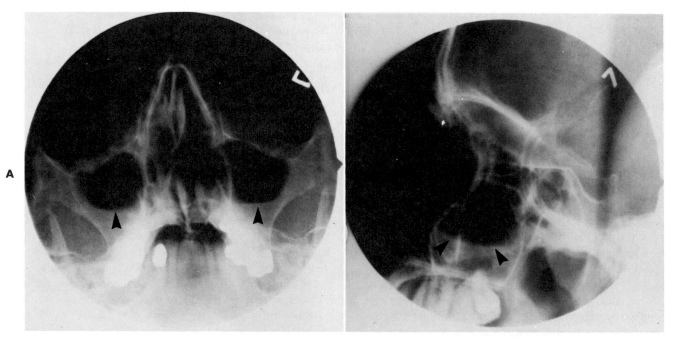

◇ **Figure 20-6**

A, Waters' radiograph demonstrating bilateral maxillary sinus air-fluid levels. **B,** Lateral radiograph demonstrating air-fluid levels in maxillary sinus.

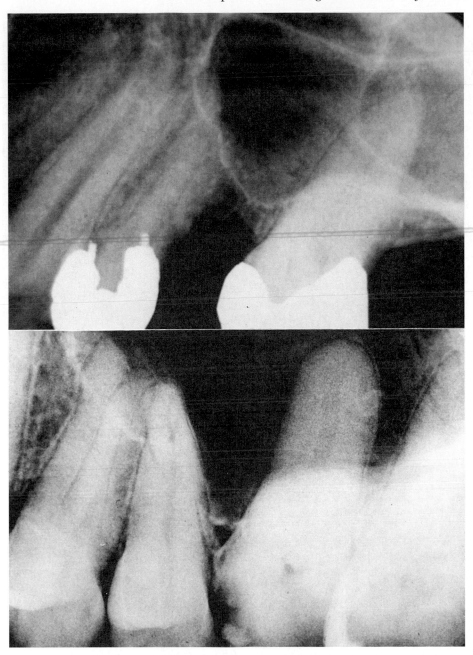

◇ Figure 20-7

Maxillary molar roots appear to be "in" sinus, because sinus has pneumatized around roots.

and the maxillary sinus. This condition may readily spread to involve the other paranasal sinuses if it is left untreated or inadequately treated or is fulminant or chronic in nature. Like infections, maxillary sinusitis may be acute or chronic.

Odontogenic infections that may involve the maxillary sinus include acute and chronic periapical disease and periodontal disease. Infection and sinusitis may also result from trauma to the dentition or from surgery in the posterior maxilla, including removal of teeth, alveolectomy, tuberosity reduction, or other procedures that cause communications between the oral cavity and the maxillary sinus.

Acute maxillary sinusitis may occur at any age. Its onset is usually described by the patient as a rapidly developing sense of pressure, pain, or fullness in the vicinity of the affected sinus. The discomfort rapidly increases in intensity and may be accompanied by facial swelling and erythema, malaise, fever, and drainage of foul-smelling mucopurulent material into the nasal cavity and nasopharynx.

Chronic maxillary sinusitis is a less common result of odontogenic infection. It is usually a result of bacterial or fungal infections that are low-grade and recurrent in nature, obstructive nasal disease, or allergy. It is characterized by

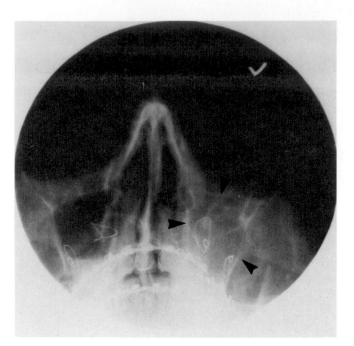

◇ **Figure 20-8**

Waters' radiograph showing opacification of left maxillary sinus by hypertrophied tissue and purulent material. Patient was previously treated with Le Fort I osteotomy.

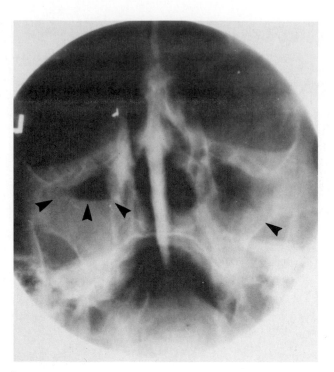

◇ **Figure 20-9**

Waters' radiograph showing air-fluid level in left maxillary sinus and mucosal thickening in right maxillary sinus.

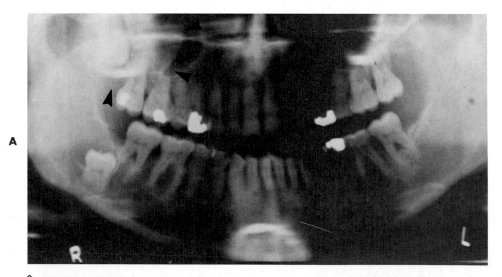

◇ **Figure 20-10**

A, Panoramic radiograph showing large odontogenic keratocyst associated with impacted right maxillary third molar tooth. Cyst has impinged on right maxillary sinus as it expanded. Sinus cavity is almost totally obstructed by lesion. Another odontogenic keratocyst is seen associated with impacted right mandibular third molar. *Continued*

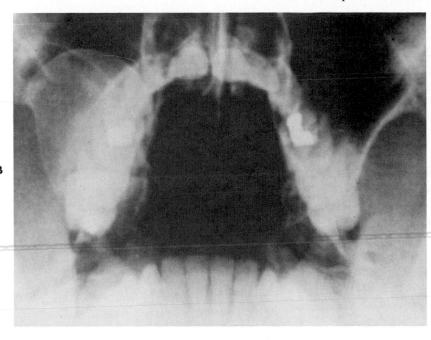

B

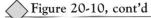

B, Waters' radiograph of the odontogenic keratocyst seen in **A.** Lesion is also seen to have expanded lateral wall of right maxillary sinus.

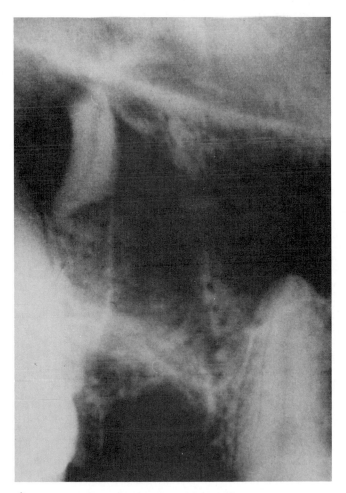

Figure 20-11

Periapical radiograph showing apical one third of palatal root of maxillary first molar, which was displaced into maxillary sinus during removal of tooth.

episodes of sinus disease that respond initially to treatment, only to return, or that remain symptomatic in spite of treatment.

Infections of the maxillary sinuses may be caused by aerobic, anaerobic, or mixed bacteria. The normal healthy maxillary sinus has a small population of bacteria that is composed mainly of aerobic streptococci and anaerobic gram-negative rods of the genera *Porphyromonas, Prevotella,* and *Fusobacterium.* In maxillary sinusitis of nonodontogenic origin, the causative bacteria are primarily aerobic, with a few anaerobes. The important aerobes are *Streptococcus pneumoniae, Haemophilus influenzae,* and *Staphylococcus aureus. Porphyromonas, Prevotella, Peptococcus,* and *Fusobacterium* spp. are the common anaerobes.

Maxillary sinus infections of odontogenic origin are more likely to be caused by anaerobic bacteria as is the usual odontogenic infection. Rarely does *H. influenzae* or *S. aureus* cause odontogenic sinusitis. The predominant organisms are aerobic streptococci and anaerobic *Peptococcus, Peptostreptococcus, Porphyromonas, Prevotella,* and *Eubacterium* spp.

This information is important to the selection of an antibiotic. The otolaryngologist usually chooses a drug that is effective against *H. influenzae* and *S. aureus,* which is not usually necessary for odontogenic sinusitis. Drugs such as penicillin, erythromycin, and clindamycin are effective for sinusitis of odontogenic origin.

However, because of the wide variety of microorganisms that can be participants in infections of the maxillary sinus, it is important to obtain purulent material for culture and sensitivity testing whenever possible. Sensitivity testing may suggest a change to another antibiotic if resistant organisms are cultured from the sinus and if the infection is failing to respond to appropriate initial treatment. As many as 25% of the organisms cultured from acute sinus infections are

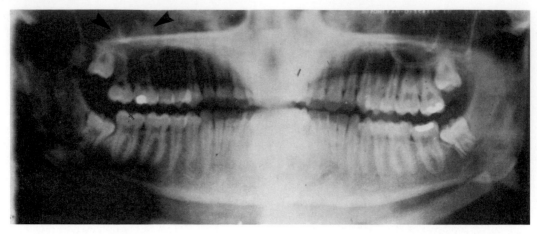

◇ **Figure 20-12**

Panoramic radiograph showing mucus-retention phenomenon in right maxillary sinus.

b-lactamase producers, and many may be anaerobic, especially if the infection is odontogenic in origin.

TREATMENT OF MAXILLARY SINUSITIS

Early treatment of maxillary sinusitis consists of humidification of inspired air to loosen and aid in the removal of dried secretions from the nasal passage and the sinus ostium. Also required are antibiotics, systemic decongestants, and topically applied decongestants to decrease mucosal edema and inflammation and to promote drainage of the sinus through its natural opening. On occasion, surgical drainage of the sinus is indicated. The cause of the sinusitis should be diagnosed, treated, and eliminated.

Treatment is directed at relief of pain, and narcotic analgesics are usually required. A nasal spray containing vasoconstrictors, such as 2% ephedrine or 0.25% phenylephrine, is prescribed, as are orally administered antihistamines, such as pseudoephedrine (Sudafed). Antibiotics, selected empirically as described above, are prescribed for a period of 10 to 14 days. Purulent material is submitted for culture and sensitivity testing using both aerobic and anaerobic techniques.

If the patient fails to respond to this initial treatment regimen within 72 hours, it is necessary to reassess the treatment and the antibiotic. If the cause of the problem has not been identified and eliminated, this should be accomplished. The results of the culture and sensitivity tests should be evaluated, and changes should be made if indicated. If the organism(s) causing the infection is a β-lactamase producer, another antibiotic, such as the combination agent trimethoprim-sulfamethoxazole (Bactrim, Septa), may be effective. Cefaclor or a combination of amoxicillin and potassium clavulanate (Augmentin) have also been shown to be effective.

Acute maxillary sinusitis is a painful, potentially serious condition that requires immediate attention and aggressive medical and surgical care. Patients suspected of having maxillary sinusitis should be referred to an oral and maxillofacial surgeon or another specialist, such as an otolaryngologist. Radiographs, the results of clinical procedures, the results of culture and sensitivity tests of purulent drainage, and any other pertinent diagnostic information should be sent to the surgeon by the referring clinician.

Diagnosis and treatment of chronic maxillary sinusitis is difficult and may include allergy testing, nasal or septal surgery, surgical débridement of the sinuses with a Caldwell-Luc procedure, or sinus trephination and irrigation.

Untreated maxillary sinusitis may progress to a variety of serious complications if inadequately treated. These potential problems include orbital cellulitis, cavernous sinus thrombosis, meningitis, osteomyelitis, intracranial abscess, and death.

MUCUS-RETENTION PHENOMENON

The mucus-retention phenomenon (mucocele, mucosal cyst) of the maxillary sinus (Figure 20-12) is a chronic, expansile secretory cyst that is lined with respiratory epithelium. The cause of this lesion is not certain, but it probably represents a collection of mucus within the sinus membrane caused by cystic dilation of a mucous gland. Mucoceles are not unusual within the maxillary sinus and may be seen in pantographic radiographs in 1% to 3% of the adult population. Radiographically, the mucosal cyst is a homogenous, curved radiopaque area that is oval or dome-shaped. The base of its attachment may be broad or narrow. The cyst has a smooth, uniform outline. Most mucosal cysts arise from the floor of the sinus. They vary in size from a few millimeters to occupying the majority of the sinus cavity.

Mucosal cysts are rarely symptomatic in the maxillary sinus and generally require no treatment beyond observation. Radiographs taken several months after diagnosis commonly show resolution of the lesion. If, however, there are symptoms of sinus disease that cannot be attributed to other factors, these patients should be referred to a specialist for further treatment.

Mucosal cysts should be differentiated from other conditions that produce a similar radiographic picture. These conditions include cysts of odontogenic origin, antral polyps, and benign or malignant neoplasms. On rare occasions, secondary infection may produce a pyocele—a symptomatic lesion that may invade associated structures with symptoms of acute maxillary sinusitis. These patients should also be referred to an oral-maxillofacial surgeon for medical and surgical management.

OROANTRAL COMMUNICATIONS

An opening may be made into the maxillary sinus when teeth are removed and, occasionally, as a result of trauma. This sinus perforation happens particularly when a maxillary molar with widely divergent roots that is adjacent to edentulous spaces requires extraction. In this instance the sinus is likely to have become pneumatized into the edentulous alveolar process surrounding the tooth, which weakens the entire alveolus and brings the tooth apices into a closer relationship with the sinus cavity. Other causes of perforation into the sinus include destruction of a portion of the sinus floor by periapical lesions, perforation of the floor and sinus membrane with injudicious use of instruments, forcing a root or tooth into the sinus during attempted removal, and removal of large cystic lesions that encroach on the sinus cavity.

The treatment of oroantral communications is accomplished either immediately, when the opening is created, or later, as in the instance of a long-standing fistula or failure of an attempted primary closure.

IMMEDIATE TREATMENT

The best treatment of a potential sinus exposure is avoiding the problem through careful observation and treatment planning. Evaluation of high-quality radiographs before surgery begins usually reveals the presence or absence of an excessively pneumatized sinus or widely divergent or dilacerated roots, which have the potential of having a communication with the sinus or causing fractures in the bony floor of the antrum during removal (Figure 20-7). If this observation is made, surgery may be altered to section the tooth and remove it one root at a time (see Chapter 8).

When exposure and perforation of the antrum result, the least invasive therapy is indicated initially. If the opening to the sinus is small and the sinus is disease-free, efforts should be made to establish a blood clot in the extraction site and preserve it in place. Additional soft tissue flap elevation is not

required. Sutures are placed to reposition the soft tissues, and a gauze pack is placed over the surgical site for 1 to 2 hours. The patient is instructed to use nasal precautions for 10 to 14 days. These include opening the mouth while sneezing, not sucking on a straw or cigarettes, and avoiding nose-blowing and any other situation that may produce pressure changes between the nasal passages and oral cavity. The patient is placed on an antibiotic, usually penicillin; an antihistamine; and a systemic decongestant for 7 to 10 days to prevent infection, to shrink mucous membranes, and to lessen nasal and sinus secretions. The patient is seen postoperatively at 48- to 72-hour intervals and is instructed to return if an oroantral communication becomes evident by leakage of air into the mouth or fluid into the nose or if symptoms of maxillary sinusitis appear.

The majority of patients treated in this manner heal uneventfully if there was no evidence of preexisting sinus disease. If larger perforations occur, the patient should be referred to an oral and maxillofacial surgeon for immediate treatment.

TREATMENT OF LONG-STANDING COMMUNICATIONS

Successful treatment and closure of the oroantral communication requires extensive surgery. Aggressive antibiotic treatment is also necessary. If the fistula has developed next to the root of an adjacent tooth, closure is further complicated and, to be successful, removal of the tooth may be necessary.

Surgeons use various techniques to close oroantral fistulas or communications. Some techniques involve mobilization and rotation of large mucosal flaps to cover the osseous defect with soft tissues, the margins of which are sutured over and therefore supported by intact bone. The mucosal flaps must be designed to have a good blood supply and to alter the surrounding anatomy to the smallest extent possible. If sinus disease exists, it may be necessary to remove diseased tissues from the sinus using a Caldwell-Luc procedure through the lateral maxillary wall above the apices of the remaining teeth. The Caldwell-Luc procedure includes the creation of an opening into the nose at the level of the sinus floor beneath the inferior turbinate to allow drainage of secretions of the sinus mucosa into the nasal cavity. This portion of the procedure is a nasal antrostomy.

Other methods of closing oroantral fistulae include buccal flap advancement (Figure 20-13), palatal flap advancement (Figure 20-14), and advancement of both palatal and facial flaps over a metallic foil plate. This plate is adapted to the contour of the alveolar process in the fistulous tract area and interposed between the alveolar bone and overlying mucosal flaps (Figure 20-15). The metal foil technique provides a physical barrier over the osseous defect and also a more stable platform to support the mucosal flaps.

Regardless of the technique used, it must be remembered that the osseous defect surrounding the fistula is always much larger than the clinically apparent soft tissue deformity. Surgical planning of closure technique must be adjusted accordingly.

Text continued on p. 485

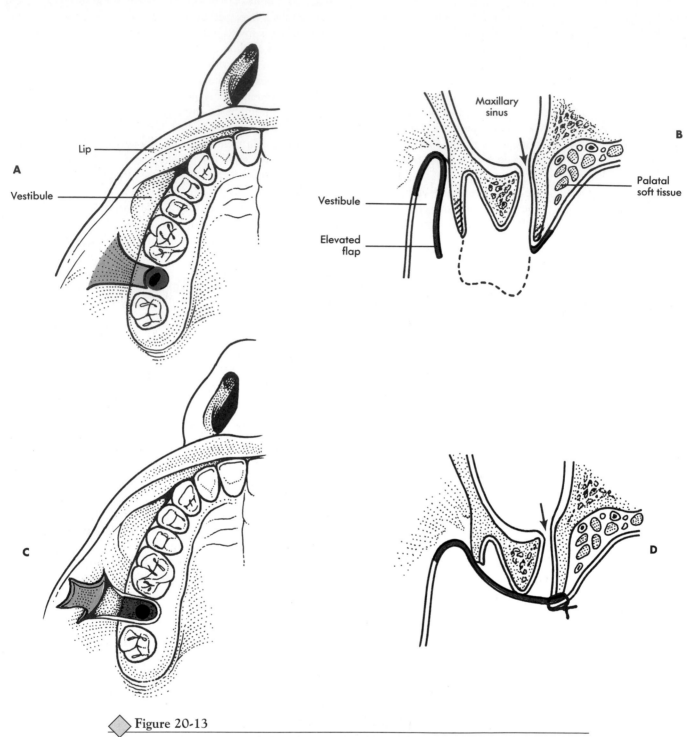

◈ Figure 20-13

A, Diagrammatic illustration of oroantral fistula in second molar region of right maxillary alveolar process. Incision for closure of fistula with buccal flap advancement procedure is outlined. Note that fistulous tract itself will be excised. Also note that margins of flap are wide enough to rest on bone when advanced to cover osseous defect. **B,** Elevated buccal flap. Flap is released to depth of labial vestibule. If necessary, periosteum may be incised on deep surface of flap to allow advancement of soft tissue to cover osseous defect without placing flap under tension. **C,** Advanced and sutured buccal flap. Flap must be positioned with minimal tension and its margins supported by underlying bone to ensure adequate closure of fistulous defect. **D,** Cross-section of buccal flap closure of oroantral fistula. Buccal flap has been elevated and underlying periosteum incised to improve mobility of flap. *Continued*

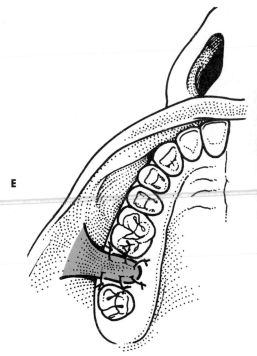

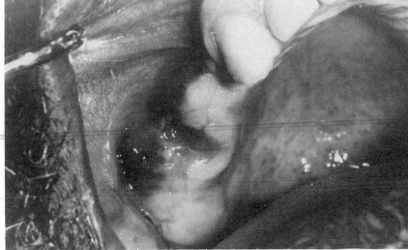

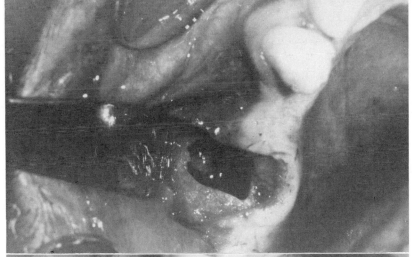

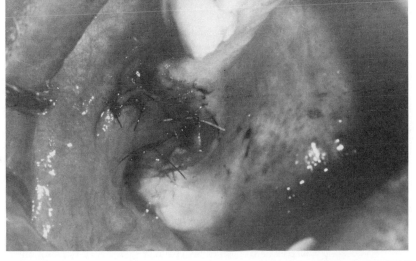

◇ Figure 20-13, cont'd

E, Buccal flap has been advanced over alveolar process and sutured to palatal mucosa to close fistulous tract. Note reduction of alveolar bone accomplished on facial surface of alveolus, which allows more passive approximation of flap in its new position. Disadvantage of buccal flap closure is loss of labiovestibular depth illustrated in diagram. **F,** Clinical photograph of small oroantral defect created during removal of right maxillary second bicuspid tooth. **G,** Buccal flap has been elevated, which reveals residual underlying alveolar process and oroantral osseous defect. **H,** Buccal flap has been advanced to cover osseous defect in alveolar process and sutured to palatal mucosa. Margins of flap are supported by intact alveolar bone. Note loss of vestibular depth, which is result of mobilization and advancement of buccal flap.

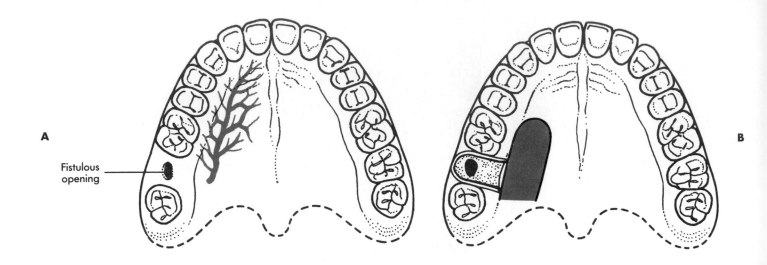

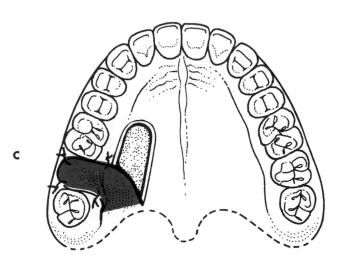

⬦ Figure 20-14

Palatal flap closure of oroantral communications. **A,** Diagrammatic illustration of oroantral fistulous tract in right maxillary alveolar process in region of second molar, which is to be closed with rotation of palatal flap. Anterior palatine artery must be included in flap to provide adequate blood supply to transpositioned soft tissues. **B,** Soft tissues surrounding oroantral opening are excised, exposing underlying alveolar bone around osseous defect. Palatal flap is outlined, incised, and elevated from anterior to posterior. Flap should be full thickness of mucoperiosteum, should have broad posterior base, and should include anterior palatine artery. Its width should be sufficient to cover entire defect around oroantral opening, and its length must be adequate to allow rotation of flap and repositioning over defect without placing undue tension on flap. **C,** Palatal flap has been rotated to cover osseous defect in alveolar process and sutured in place. Exposed bone on palate, which remains after rotation of flap, will heal by secondary intention with minimal discomfort to patient and little or no alteration in normal soft tissue anatomy.

Continued

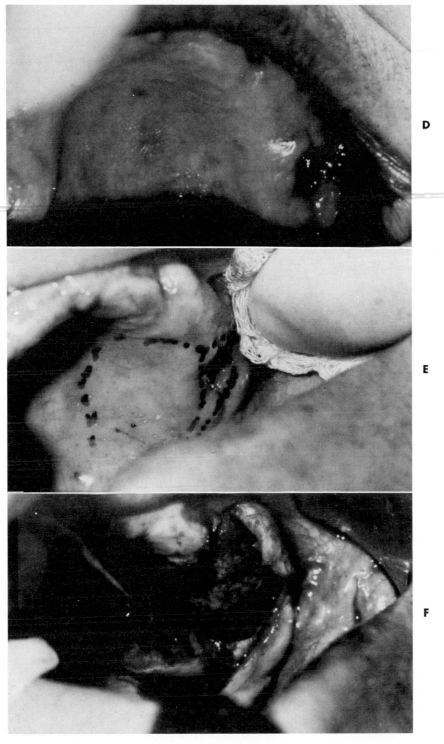

◇ Figure 20-14, cont'd

D, Large oroantral communication in left maxilla that developed following removal of second molar tooth. **E,** Palatal flap outlined. Flap is posteriorly based and receives its blood supply from anterior palatine neurovascular bundle. Width of flap is much larger than clinical oroantral communication. **F,** Palatal flap is elevated and readied for transposition laterally to cover osseous oroantral defect. Buccal mucosa has also been elevated to facilitate suturing of flap. Note large size of osseous defect.

Continued

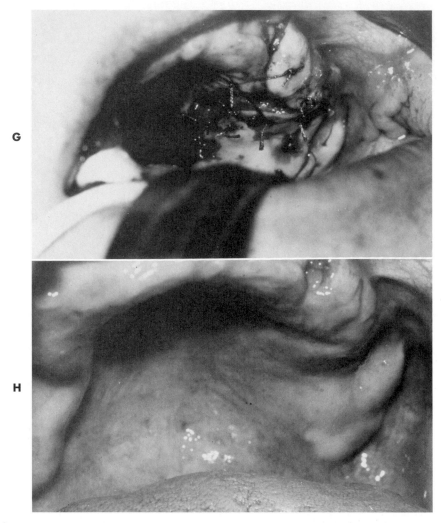

◇ **Figure 20-14, cont'd**

G, Palatal flap has been rotated laterally and sutured in place. Osseous defect is well covered. Small area of exposed bone near palatal midline will heal by secondary intention. **H,** Well-closed oroantral communication 4 weeks after rotation of palatal flap. Vestibular depth is maintained with this procedure. Metallic foil closure of oroantral communications.

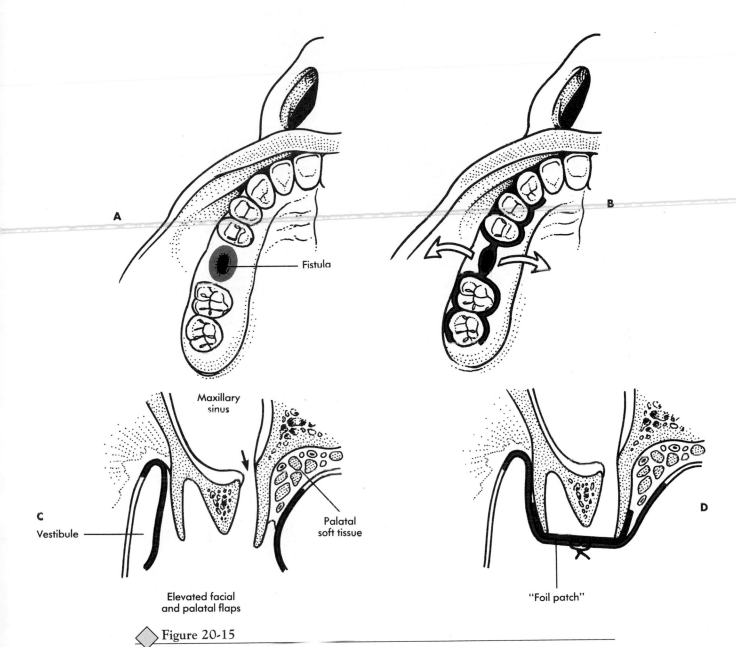

A

Fistula

B

Maxillary
sinus

C

Vestibule

Palatal
soft tissue

D

Elevated facial
and palatal flaps

"Foil patch"

◇ **Figure 20-15**

Metallic foil closure of oroantral communications. **A,** Diagrammatic illustration of oroantral fistula in right maxillary alveolar process in region of missing first molar tooth, which is to be closed with subperiosteal placement of metallic foil "patch." **B,** Both facial and palatal mucoperiosteal flaps are developed. When elevated, these provide ample exposure of underlying alveolar process and fistulous tract. Fistulous tract is excised. Osseous margins must be exposed 360 degrees around bony defect to allow placement of metallic foil patch beneath mucoperiosteal flaps. Flap is supported on all sides by underlying bone. **C,** Metallic foil patch has been adapted to cover osseous defect and positioned between alveolar process and overlying buccal and palatal mucoperiosteal flaps. Foil should be supported on all its margins by sound underlying bone. Mucoperiosteal flaps have been repositioned and sutured over foil. **D,** Cross-sectional diagram of metallic foil closure technique. Both buccal and palatal mucoperiosteal flaps are elevated to expose osseous defect and large area of underlying alveolar bone around oroantral communication.

Continued

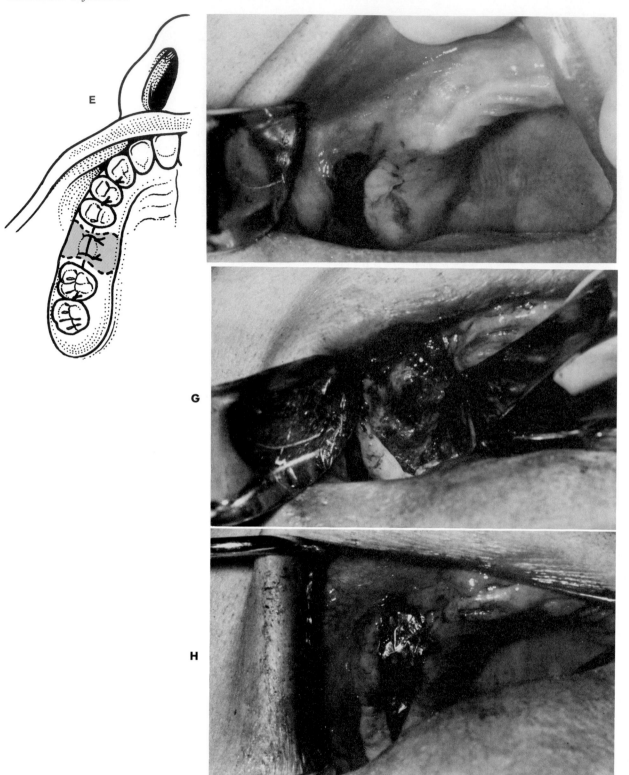

⬦ Figure 20-15, cont'd

E, Metallic foil "patch" has been positioned between alveolar process and deep surface of buccal and palatal mucoperiosteal flaps. Foil is entirely supported on its margins by underlying bone. Mucoperiosteal flaps are repositioned and approximated over foil. **F,** Oroantral fistula of several weeks' duration in right posterior maxilla that developed secondary to removal of retained first molar tooth root. **G,** Elevation of large buccal and palatal mucoperiosteal flaps has been completed. Note large size of exposed alveolar osseous defect. **H,** Titanium foil patch has been adapted over defect in alveolar process. Foil is inserted beneath facial and palatal mucosa and covers minimum of 5 mm of alveolar bone on all sides of osseous defect.

Continued

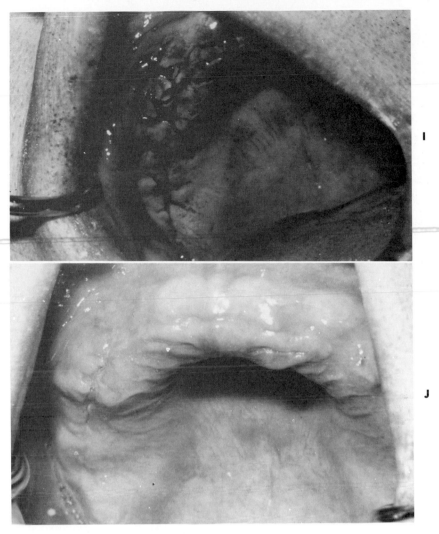

◇ **Figure 20-15, cont'd**

I, Palatal and buccal mucosal flaps are sutured in place over metallic foil patch. Flaps are minimally advanced, and no real attempt is made to close mucosa primarily over foil. **J,** Four weeks after closure of right maxillary oroantral defect with the foil patch procedure. Area is well healed. Normal vestibular depth and palatal anatomy are maintained.

BIBLIOGRAPHY

Bergeron RT, Osborn AG, Som PM, editors: *Head and neck imaging,* St Louis, 1984, Mosby.

Ritter FN: *The paranasal sinuses: anatomy and surgical technique,* St Louis, 1978, Mosby.

Scott JH, Dixon AD: *Anatomy for students of dentistry,* Baltimore, 1972, Williams & Wilkins.

Sicher H, editor: *Orban's oral histology and embryology,* St Louis, 1961, Mosby.

Sicher H, DuBrul EL: *Oral anatomy,* St Louis, 1970, Mosby.

Topazian RG, Goldberg MH: *Management of infections of the oral and maxillofacial regions,* ed 2, Philadelphia, 1987, WB Saunders.

CHAPTER 21

DIAGNOSIS AND MANAGEMENT OF SALIVARY GLAND DISORDERS

STERLING R. SCHOW
MICHAEL MILORO

CHAPTER OUTLINE

The clinician is frequently confronted with the necessity of assessing and managing salivary gland disorders. A thorough knowledge of the embryology, anatomy, and pathophysiology is necessary to treat patients appropriately. This chapter examines the etiology, diagnostic methodology, radiographic evaluation, and management of a variety of salivary gland disorders, including sialolithiasis and obstructive phenomena (mucocele and ranula), acute and chronic salivary gland infections, traumatic salivary gland disorders, Sjögren's syndrome, necrotizing sialometaplasia, and benign and malignant salivary gland tumors.

EMBRYOLOGY, ANATOMY, AND PHYSIOLOGY

The salivary glands can be divided into two groups, the minor and major glands. All salivary glands develop from the embryonic oral cavity as buds of epithelium that extend into the underlying mesenchymal tissues. The epithelial ingrowths branch to form a primitive ductal system that eventually becomes canalized to provide for drainage of salivary secretions. The minor salivary glands begin to develop around the fortieth day in utero, whereas the larger major glands begin to develop slightly earlier, at about the thirty-fifth day in utero. At around the seventh or eighth month in utero, secretory cells called *acini* begin to develop around the ductal system. The acinar cells of the salivary glands are classified as either *serous cells,* which produce a thin, watery serous secretion, or *mucous cells,* which produce a more thick, viscous mucous secretion. The minor salivary glands are well developed and functional in the newborn infant. The acini of the minor salivary glands primarily produce mucous secretions, although some are made up of serous cells, as well. The major salivary glands are paired structures and are the parotid, submandibular, and sublingual glands. The parotid glands contain primarily serous acini with few mucous cells. Conversely, the sublingual glands are for the most part composed of mucous cells. The submandibular glands are mixed glands, made up of approximately equal numbers of serous and mucous acini. Between 800 and 1000 minor salivary glands are found throughout the portions of the oral cavity that are covered by mucous membranes, with a few exceptions, such as the anterior third of the hard palate, the attached gingiva, and the dorsal surface of the anterior third

Table 21-1. Salivary gland embryology and anatomy

	Minor salivary glands	Major salivary glands
In utero development	Day 40	Day 35
Number	800-1000	6
Types	Labial	Parotid
	Buccal	Submandibular
	Palatine	Sublingual
	Tonsillar	
	• Weber's glands	
	Retromolar	
	• Carmalt's glands	
	Lingual	
	• Inferior apical (Glands of Blandin Nuhn)	
	• Taste buds (von Ebner's glands)	
	• Posterior lubricating glands	

of the tongue. The minor salivary glands are referred to as the *labial, buccal, palatine, tonsillar (Weber's glands), retromolar (Carmalt's glands),* and *lingual glands,* which are divided into three groups: inferior apical (glands of Blandin Nuhn), taste buds (von Ebner's glands), and the posterior lubricating glands (Table 21-1).

The parotid glands, the largest salivary glands, lie superficial to the posterior aspect of the masseter muscle and the ascending ramus of the mandible. Peripheral portions of the parotid gland extend to the mastoid process, along the anterior aspect of the sternocleidomastoid muscle, and around the posterior border of the mandible into the pterygomandibular space (Figure 21-1). The major branches of the seventh cranial (facial) nerve roughly divide the parotid gland into a superficial lobe and a deep lobe while coursing anteriorly from their exit at the stylomastoid foramen to innervate the muscles of facial expression. Small ducts from various regions of the gland coalesce at the anterosuperior aspect of the parotid to form Stenson's duct, which is the major duct of the parotid gland. Stenson's duct is about 1 to 3 mm in diameter and 6 cm

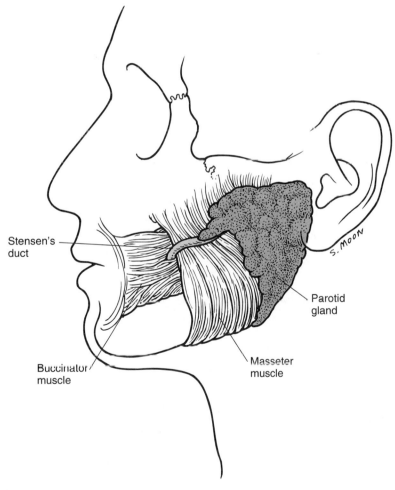

Stensen's duct

Buccinator muscle

Parotid gland

Masseter muscle

S. MOON

◆ Figure 21-1

Diagram of parotid gland anatomy. Note that the course of Stensen's duct runs superficial to the masseter muscle, and then curves sharply anteriorly to pierce the buccinator muscle fibers and enter the oral cavity.

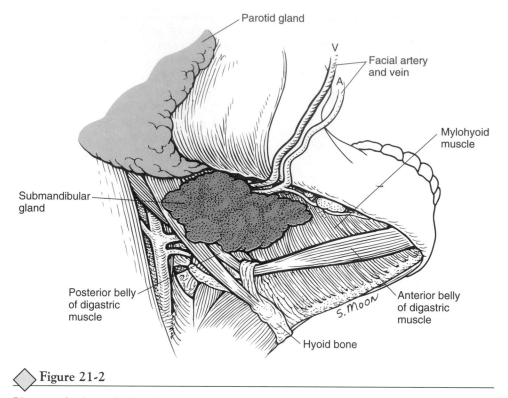

Parotid gland

Facial artery
and vein

Mylohyoid
muscle

Submandibular
gland

Posterior belly
of digastric
muscle

Anterior belly
of digastric
muscle

Hyoid bone

◇ **Figure 21-2**

Diagram of submandibular gland anatomy. Note that the submandibular triangle is formed by the
anterior and posterior bellies of the digastric muscles and the inferior border of the mandible.

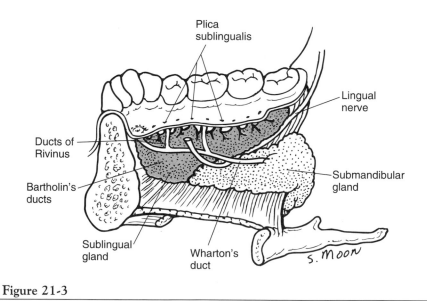

Plica
sublingualis

Lingual
nerve

Ducts of
Rivinus

Submandibular
gland

Bartholin's
ducts

Sublingual
gland

Wharton's
duct

◇ **Figure 21-3**

Diagram of sublingual gland anatomy. Note the interrelationships between the ductal systems of the
submandibular and sublingual glands and the relationship of the lingual nerve to Wharton's duct.

in length. Occasionally, a normal anatomic variation occurs in which there is an accessory parotid duct that may aid Stensen's duct in drainage of salivary secretions. Additionally, an accessory portion of the parotid gland may be present somewhere along the course of Stensen's duct. The duct runs anteriorly from the gland and is superficial to the masseter muscle. At the location of the anterior edge of the masseter muscle, Stenson's duct turns sharply medial and passes through the fibers of the buccinator muscle. The duct opens into the oral cavity through the buccal mucosa, usually adjacent to the maxillary first or second molar tooth. The parotid gland receives innervation from the ninth cranial (glossopharyngeal) nerve via the auriculotemporal nerve from the otic ganglion.

◇ Table 21-2. Composition of normal adult saliva

	Parotid gland	Submandibular gland
Sodium (Na$^+$)	23 mEq/L	21 mEq/L
Potassium (K$^+$)	20 mEq/L	17 mEq/L
Chloride (Cl$^-$)	23 mEq/L	20 mEq/L
Bicarbonate (HCO$_3^-$)	20 mEq/L	18 mEq/L
Calcium (Ca^{2+})	2.0 mEq/L	3.6 mEq/L
Phosphate (PO$_4^{2-}$)	6.0 mEq/L	4.5 mEq/L
Magnesium (Mg^{2+})	0.2 mEq/L	0.3 mEq/L
Urea	15 mg/dl	7.0 mg/dl
Ammonia	0.3 mg/dl	0.2 mg/dl
Uric acid	3 mg/dl	2 mg/dl
Glucose	<1 mg/dl	<1 mg/dl
Cholesterol	<1 mg/dl	<1 mg/dl
Fatty acids	1 mg/dl	<1 mg/dl
Amino acids	1.5 mg/dl	<1 mg/dl
Proteins	250 mg/dl	150 mg/dl

◇ Box 21-1 ◇

Daily saliva production by salivary gland

Submandibular gland	70%
Parotid gland	25%
Sublingual gland	3%-4%
Minor glands	Trace

The submandibular glands are located in the submandibular triangle of the neck, which is formed by the anterior and posterior bellies of the digastric muscles and the inferior border of the mandible (Figure 21-2). The posterosuperior portion of the gland curves upward around the posterior border of the mylohyoid muscle and gives rise to the major duct of the submandibular gland known as *Wharton's duct*. This duct passes forward along the superior surface of the mylohyoid muscle in the sublingual space, adjacent to the lingual nerve. The anatomic relationship is such that the lingual nerve loops under Wharton's duct, from lateral to medial, in the posterior floor of the mouth. Wharton's duct is about 5 cm in length, and the diameter of its lumen is 2 to 4 mm. Wharton's duct opens into the floor of the mouth via a punctum located close to the incisors at the most anterior aspect of the junction of the lingual frenum and the floor of the mouth. The punctum is a constricted portion of the duct, and it functions to limit retrograde flow of bacteria-laden oral fluids. This particularly limits those bacteria that tend to colonize around the ductal orifices.

The sublingual glands lie on the superior surface of the mylohyoid muscle, in the sublingual space, and are separated from the oral cavity by a thin layer of oral mucosa (Figure 21-3). The acinar ducts of the sublingual glands are called *Bartholin's ducts* and in most instances coalesce to form 8 to 20 ducts of Rivinus. These ducts of Rivinus are short and small in diameter, and either open individually directly into the anterior floor of the mouth on a crest of mucosa known as the *plica sublingualis* or open indirectly through connections to the submandibular duct, and then into the oral cavity via Wharton's duct. The sublingual and submandibular glands are innervated by the facial nerve through the submandibular ganglion via the chorda tympani nerve.

The functions of saliva are to provide lubrication for speech and mastication, to produce enzymes for digestion, and to produce compounds with antibacterial properties (Table 21-2). The salivary glands produce approximately 1000 to 1500 mL of saliva per day, with the highest flow rates occurring during meals. The relative contributions of each salivary gland to total daily production varies, with the submandibular gland providing 70%, the parotid gland 25%, the sublingual gland 3% to 4%, and the minor salivary glands contributing only trace amounts of saliva (Box 21-1). The electrolyte composition of saliva also varies between salivary glands, with parotid gland concentrations generally higher than the submandibular gland, except for submandibular calcium concentration, which is approximately twice the concentration of parotid calcium (Table 21-2). The relative viscosities of saliva vary according to gland and correspond to the percentage of mucous and serous cells; therefore the highest viscosity is in the sublingual gland, followed by the submandibular gland, and, lastly, the parotid gland, which is composed mainly of serous cells. Interestingly, the daily production of saliva begins to decrease gradually after the age of 20.

DIAGNOSTIC MODALITIES ◇
HISTORY AND CLINICAL EXAMINATION

The most important component of diagnosis in salivary gland disorders, as with most other disease processes, is the patient history and the clinical examination. In most cases the patient will guide the doctor to the diagnosis merely by relating the events that have occurred in association with the presenting complaint. The astute clinician must perform a thorough evaluation, and, in many instances, the diagnosis can be determined without the necessity of further diagnostic evaluation. At the very least, the clinician may be able to categorize the problem as reactive, obstructive, inflammatory, infectious, metabolic, neoplastic, developmental, or traumatic in origin and guide further diagnostic testing. Occasionally, the clinician may find it necessary to use any of several diagnostic modalities.

SALIVARY GLAND RADIOLOGY

PLAIN FILM RADIOGRAPHS. The primary purpose of plain films in the assessment of salivary gland disease is to identify salivary stones (calculi), although only 80% to 85% of all stones are radiopaque and therefore visible radiographically. The incidence of radiopaque stones varies depending on the specific gland involved (Box 21-2). A mandibular occlusal film is most useful for detecting sublingual and submandibular gland calculi in the anterior floor of the mouth (Figure 21-4, *A*). A "puffed cheek view," in which the patient forcibly blows the cheek laterally to distend the soft tissues overlying the lateral ramus, can demonstrate parotid stones. Panoramic radiographs can reveal stones in the parotid gland, as well as posteriorly located submandibular stones (Figure 21-5). Periapical radiographs can show calculi in each salivary gland or duct, including minor salivary glands, depending on film placement. In most instances, the radiographic image corresponds in size and shape to the actual stone (Figure 21-4, *B*).

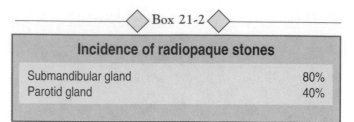

◇ Box 21-2 ◇

Incidence of radiopaque stones

Submandibular gland	80%
Parotid gland	40%

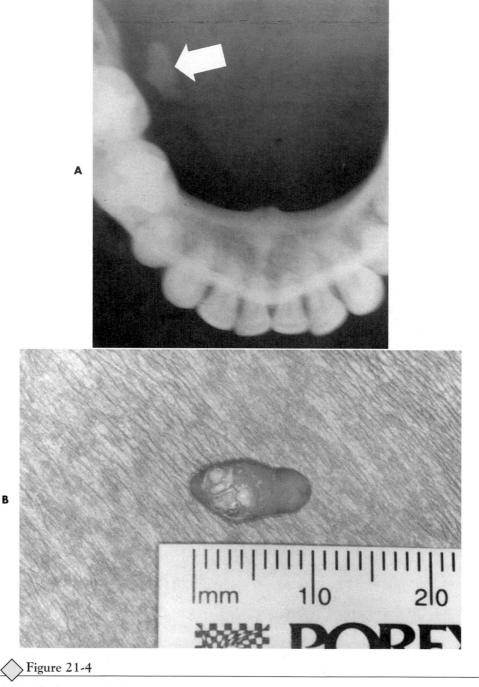

◇ **Figure 21-4**

A, Mandibular occlusal radiograph showing a radiopaque sialolith (*arrow*). **B,** Submandibular sialolith following intraoral removal.

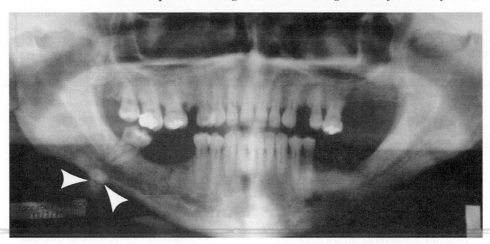

◇ Figure 21-5

Panoramic radiograph demonstrating a right submandibular sialolith (*arrowheads*).

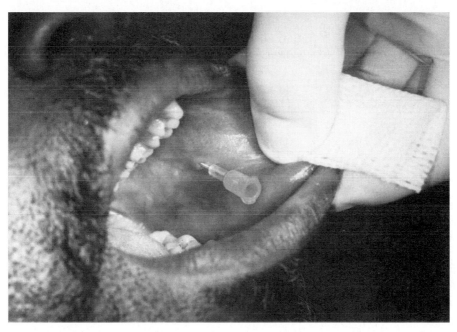

◇ Figure 21-6

Cannulation of Stensen's duct with a plastic catheter.

SIALOGRAPHY. The gold standard in diagnostic salivary gland radiology may be the sialogram. Sialography is indicated as an aid in the detection of radiopaque stones and the 15% to 20% of stones that are radiolucent and in the assessment of the extent of destruction of the salivary duct and/or gland as a result of obstructive, inflammatory, traumatic, and neoplastic diseases. In addition to its diagnostic role, sialography may be used as a therapeutic maneuver, because the ductal system is dilated during the study, and small mucous plugs or necrotic debris may be cleared during injection of contrast.

Sialography is a technique in which the salivary duct is cannulated with a plastic or metal catheter (Figure 21-6), a radiographic contrast medium is injected into the ductal system and the substance of the gland, and a series of radiographs are obtained during this process. Approximately 0.5 to 1 mL of contrast material can be injected into the duct and gland before the patient begins to experience pain. The two types of contrast media available for sialographic studies are water-soluble and oil-based. Both types of contrast material contain relatively high concentrations of iodine (25% to 40% iodine). Most clinicians prefer to use water-soluble media, which are more miscible with salivary secretions, more easily injected into the finer portions of the ductal system, and more readily eliminated from the gland after the study is completed, either by drainage through the duct or systemic

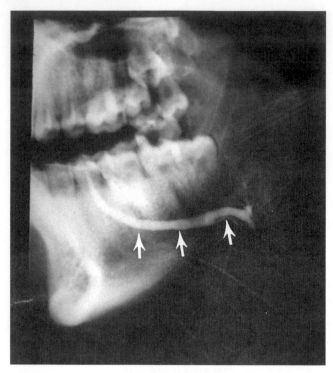

Figure 21-7

Ductal phase of a submandibular sialogram, showing contrast contained only within the main salivary ducts (*arrows*).

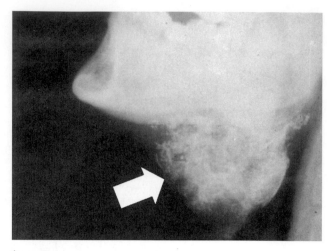

Figure 21-8

Acinar phase of a submandibular sialogram, showing normal arborization of the entire ductal system of the gland (*arrow*).

absorption from the gland and excretion through the kidneys. The oil-based media are more viscous and require a higher injection pressure to visualize the finer ductules than do the water-soluble media. As a result, they usually produce more discomfort to the patient during injection. Oil-based media are poorly eliminated from the ductal system and may cause iatrogenic ductal obstruction. Residual oil-based contrast medium is not absorbed by the gland and may produce severe foreign body reactions and glandular necrosis. Additionally, if there is ductal disruption secondary to chronic inflammatory changes, the extravasation of oil-based media may cause significantly more soft tissue damage than water-soluble material.

A complete sialogram consists of three distinct phases, depending on the time at which the radiograph is obtained following injection of the contrast material. These phases are the ductal phase (Figure 21-7), which occurs almost immediately after injection of contrast material and allows visualization of the major ducts; the acinar phase (Figure 21-8), which begins after the ductal system has become fully opacified with contrast and the gland parenchyma becomes filled subsequently; and the evacuation phase, which assesses normal secretory clearance function of the gland to determine if there is any evidence of retention of contrast in the gland and/or ductal system following the sialogram. The retention of contrast in the gland and/or ductal system beyond 5 minutes is considered abnormal. A normal sialogram shows a large primary duct branching gradually and smoothly into secondary and terminal ductules. Evenly distributed contrast will result in opacification of the acinoparenchyma that will outline the gland and its lobules. When a stone obstructs a salivary duct, continued secretion by the gland produces distension of the ductal system proximal to the obstruction and finally leads to pressure atrophy of the parenchyma of the gland (Figure 21-9).

Sialodochitis is a dilation of the salivary duct secondary to epithelial atrophy as a result of repeated inflammatory or infectious processes, with irregular narrowing caused by reparative fibrosis ("sausage-link" pattern) (Figure 21-10). Sialadenitis represents inflammation mainly involving the acinoparenchyma of the gland. There is saccular dilation of the acini of the gland secondary to acinar atrophy and infection, which results in "pruning" of the normal arborization of the small ductal system of the gland. Centrally located lesions or tumors that occupy a part of the gland or impinge on its surface displace the normal ductal anatomy. On sialography, ducts adjacent to the lesion are curvilinearly draped and stretched around the mass, producing a characteristic "ball-in-hand" appearance (Figure 21-11).

Sialograms are specialized radiologic studies performed by oral and maxillofacial surgeons and some interventional radiologists trained in the technique. This examination should not be attempted by those inexperienced in its performance or its proper interpretation. The three contraindications to performing a sialogram are acute salivary gland infections, because a disrupted ductal epithelium may allow extravasation of contrast into the soft tissues and cause severe pain and possibly a foreign body reaction; patients with a history of iodine sensitivity, especially a severe allergic reaction following a previous radiologic examination using contrast; and before a thyroid gland study, because retained iodine in the salivary gland or ducts may interfere with the thyroid scan.

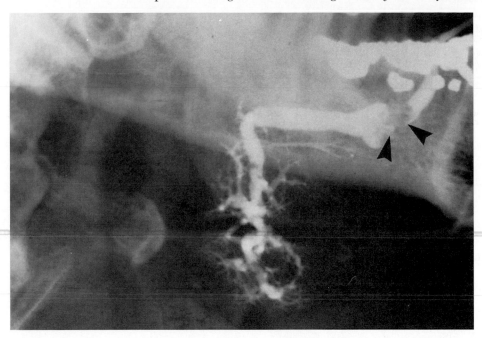

Figure 21-9

Sialogram of right submandibular gland. Obstruction of duct by a radiolucent sialolith (*arrows*) has caused dilation of the duct and loss of normal parenchyma of the gland.

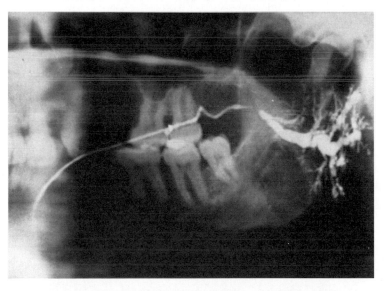

Figure 21-10

Sialogram of right parotid gland, showing the characteristic "sausage link" appearance of the duct, which indicates ductal damage from obstructive disease, with irregular narrowing of duct caused by reparative fibrosis.

COMPUTED TOMOGRAPHY, MAGNETIC RESO-NANCE IMAGING, AND ULTRASOUND. The use of computed tomography (CT) scan technology has been generally reserved for the assessment of mass lesions of the salivary glands. Although CT scanning results in radiation exposure to patients, it is less invasive than sialography and does not require the use of contrast material. Additionally, CT scanning can demonstrate salivary gland calculi, especially

submandibular stones that are located posteriorly in the duct, at the hilum of the gland, or in the substance of the gland itself (Figure 21-12).

Magnetic resonance imaging (MRI) is superior to CT scanning in delineating the soft tissue detail of salivary gland lesions, specifically tumors, with no radiation exposure to the patient or the necessity of contrast enhancement.

Ultrasonography is a relatively simple, noninvasive imag-

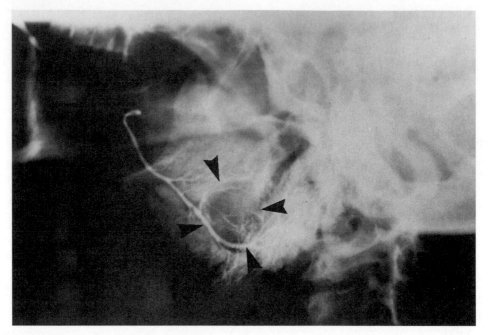

◇ Figure 21-11

Sialogram of right parotid gland illustrating "ball-in-hand" phenomenon (*arrows*). The filling defect in this sialogram locates a tumor of the gland with displacement of normal surrounding ductal anatomy.

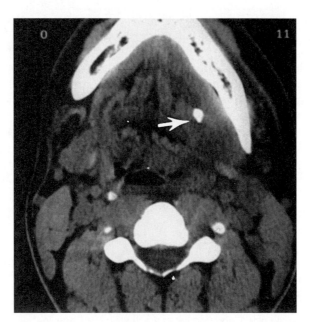

◇ Figure 21-12

CT scan of the mandible and floor of mouth, showing a posterior submandibular sialolith (*arrow*).

ing modality, with poor detail resolution. The primary role of ultrasonography is in the assessment of superficial structures to determine whether a mass lesion that is being evaluated is solid or cystic (fluid-filled) in nature.

SALIVARY SCINTIGRAPHY (RADIOACTIVE ISOTOPE SCANNING). The use of nuclear imaging in the form of

radioactive isotope scanning, or salivary scintigraphy, allows a thorough evaluation of the salivary gland parenchyma, with respect to the presence of mass lesions and the function of the gland itself. This study uses a radioactive isotope (usually, technetium-99m) injected intravenously, which is distributed throughout the body and taken up by a variety of tissues, including the salivary glands. The major limitation of this study, aside from patient radiation exposure, is the poor resolution of the images obtained. Salivary gland scintigraphy may demonstrate increased uptake of radioactive isotope in an acutely inflamed gland or decreased uptake in a chronically inflamed gland, as well as the presence of a mass lesion, either benign or malignant.

SIALOCHEMISTRY

An examination of the electrolyte composition of the saliva (Table 21-2) of each gland may indicate a variety of salivary gland disorders. Principally, the concentrations of sodium and potassium, which normally change with salivary flow rate, are measured. Certain changes in the relative concentrations of these electrolytes are seen in specific salivary gland diseases. For example, an elevated sodium concentration with a decreased potassium concentration may indicate an inflammatory sialadenitis.

FINE-NEEDLE ASPIRATION BIOPSY

The use of fine-needle aspiration biopsy in the diagnosis of salivary gland tumors has been well documented. This procedure has a high accuracy rate for distinguishing between benign and malignant lesions in superficial locations. Fine needle aspiration biopsy is performed using a syringe with a 20-gauge or smaller needle. Following local anesthesia the needle is advanced into the mass lesion, the plunger is activated to create a vacuum in the syringe, and the needle is moved back and forth throughout the mass, with pressure maintained on the plunger. The pressure is then released, the needle is withdrawn, and the cellular material and fluid is expelled onto a slide and fixed for histologic examination. This allows an immediate determination of benign vs. malignant disease, as well as the possibility of providing a tissue diagnosis, especially if the oral surgeon and oral pathologist are experienced in performing and interpreting this examination and its results.

SALIVARY GLAND BIOPSY

A salivary gland biopsy, either incisional or excisional, can be used to diagnose a tumor of one of the major salivary glands, but it is usually performed as an aid in the diagnosis of Sjögren's syndrome. The lower lip labial salivary gland biopsy has been shown to demonstrate certain characteristic histopathologic changes that are seen in the major glands in Sjögren's syndrome. The procedure is performed using local anesthesia, and approximately 10 minor salivary glands are removed for histologic examination (Figure 21-13).

OBSTRUCTIVE SALIVARY GLAND DISEASE ——————◇

SIALOLITHIASIS

The formation of stones, or calculi, may occur throughout the body, including the gallbladder, urinary tract, and salivary glands. The occurrence of salivary gland stones is twice as common in males, with a peak incidence between ages 30 and 50. Multiple stone formation occurs in approximately 25% of patients. The pathogenesis of salivary calculi progresses through a series of stages beginning with an abnormality in calcium metabolism and salt precipitation, with formation of a nidus that subsequently becomes layered with organic and inorganic material to form a calcified mass.

The incidence of stone formation varies depending on the specific gland involved (Box 21-3). The submandibular gland is involved in 85% of cases, which is more common than all other glands combined. A variety of factors contribute to the higher incidence of submandibular calculi. Salivary gland secretions contain water, electrolytes, urea, ammonia, glucose, fats, proteins, and other substances, and, in general, parotid secretions are more concentrated than those of the other salivary glands. The main exception is the concentration of calcium, which is about twice as abundant in submandibular saliva as in parotid saliva (Table 21-2). Also, the alkaline pH of submandibular saliva may further support stone formation. In addition to salivary composition, several anatomic factors of the submandibular gland and duct are important. Wharton's duct is the longest salivary duct and therefore saliva has a greater distance to travel before being emptied into the oral cavity. In addition, the duct of the submandibular gland has two sharp curves in its course. The first occurs at the posterior border of the mylohyoid muscle, and the second is near the ductal opening in the anterior floor of the mouth. Finally, the punctum of the submandibular duct is smaller than the opening of Stenson's duct. These features contribute to a slowed salivary flow and provide potential areas of stasis of salivary flow, or obstruction, that is not found in the parotid or sublingual ductal systems. Precipitated material, mucous, and cellular debris are more easily trapped in the tortuous and lengthy submandibular duct, especially when its small orifice is its most elevated location and its flow therefore occurs against the force of gravity. The precipitated material forms the nidus of mucous plugs and either radiopaque or radiolucent sialoliths that may eventually enlarge to the point of obstructing the flow of saliva from the gland to the oral cavity.

The clinical manifestations of the presence of submandibular stones become apparent when acute ductal obstruction occurs at mealtime, when saliva production is at its maximum and salivary flow is stimulated against a fixed obstruction. The resultant swelling is sudden and is usually very painful (Figure 21-14). Gradual reduction of the swelling follows, but swelling reoccurs repeatedly when salivary flow is stimulated. This process may continue until complete obstruction and/or infection occurs. Obstruction, with or without infection, causes atrophy of the secretory cells of the involved gland. Infection of the gland manifests itself by swelling in the floor of the mouth, erythema, and an associated lymphadenopathy. Palpation of the gland and simultaneous examination of the duct and its opening may reveal the total absence of salivary flow or the presence of purulent material.

The management of submandibular gland calculi depends on the duration of symptoms, the number of repeated episodes, the size of the stone, and, perhaps most importantly, the

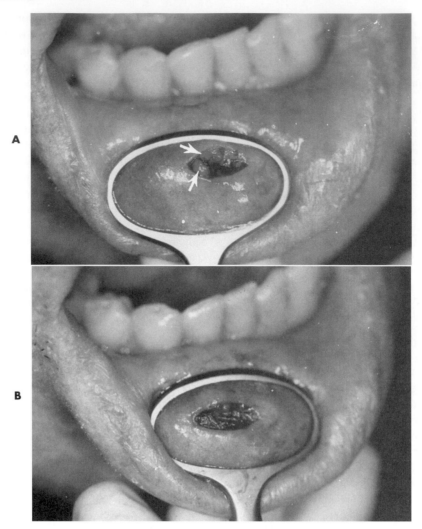

Figure 21-13

A, Labial salivary gland biopsy. The lower lip is everted and controlled with a chalazion clamp. An incision through mucosa permits visualization of the minor salivary glands (*arrows*). **B,** The minor salivary glands are removed and submitted for histopathologic assessment.

location of the stone. Submandibular stones are classified as either *anterior* or *posterior* stones, in relation to a transverse line between the mandibular first molars. Stones that occur anterior to this line are generally well visualized on a mandibular occlusal radiograph and may be amenable to intraoral removal. Small anteriorly located stones may be retrieved through the ductal opening following dilatation of the orifice. Occasionally, it becomes necessary to remove submandibular stones via an incision made in the floor of the mouth to expose the duct and the stone. A longitudinal incision is then made in the duct, the stone is retrieved, and the ductal lining is sutured to the mucosa of the floor of the mouth. Saliva will then flow out the revised duct. This procedure, known as a *sialodochoplasty* (revision of the salivary duct), eliminates many of the factors that contributed to formation of the stone. The entire length of the duct is decreased, the opening created is now larger, and there is less contribution of gravity to salivary stasis. Regardless of the procedure performed,

patients are encouraged to maintain ample salivary flow by using salivary stimulants, such as citrus fruits, flavored candies, or glycerin swabs. Posterior stones occur in up to 50% of cases and may be located at the hilum of the gland or within the substance of the gland itself. A routine occlusal film will likely not demonstrate the stone, and a panoramic radiograph (Figure 21-5) or a CT scan (Figure 21-12) may be necessary to localize the stone. In cases of posterior stones that cannot be palpated intraorally and in many instances of repeated stone formation, the submandibular gland, as well as the stone, should be removed by an extraoral approach (Figure 21-15).

Salivary gland calculi occur much less commonly in the parotid gland. In general, parotid gland infection usually leads to stone formation; the opposite, however, is the case for the submandibular gland. The parotid gland is examined by inspection and palpation of the gland extraorally over the ascending mandibular ramus. Stenson's duct and its orifice can be examined intraorally. Palpation of the gland and simulta-

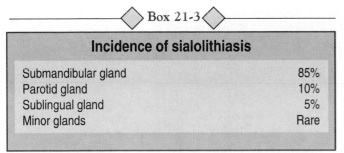

Box 21-3

Incidence of sialolithiasis

Submandibular gland	85%
Parotid gland	10%
Sublingual gland	5%
Minor glands	Rare

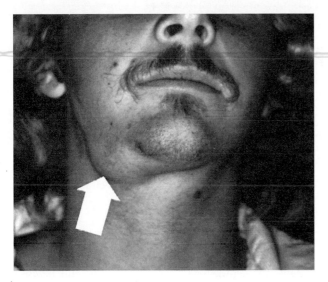

Figure 21-14

Clinical photograph of a patient with a right submandibular swelling (*arrow*) secondary to obstruction from a submandibular sialolith.

neous observation of the duct allow observation of salivary flow or the production of other material, such as purulence, from the punctum of the duct. Parotid sialoliths found in the distal third of Stenson's duct that can be palpated intraorally may be removed following dilatation of the duct orifice, or, if slightly more proximal, may require surgical exposure to gain access to the stone. On rare occasion the presence of a parotid stone at the hilum of the gland or in the gland itself may necessitate an extraoral approach to remove the stone and the superficial lobe of the parotid gland.

The sublingual gland is examined by observation and bimanual palpation of the anterior third of the floor of the mouth. The minor salivary glands are examined by observation and palpation of the mucosal surfaces of the lips, buccal mucosa, palate, and floor of the mouth. Obstruction of the sublingual gland is unusual, but if it occurs, it is usually secondary to obstruction of Wharton's duct on the same side of the oral cavity. Although stone formation is rare in the sublingual and minor salivary glands the treatment is simple excision of the stone and associated gland.

MUCOUS-RETENTION/ EXTRAVASATION PHENOMENA
MUCOCELE

Salivary ducts, especially those of the minor salivary glands, are occasionally traumatized, commonly by lip biting, and severed beneath the surface mucosa. Subsequent saliva production may then extravasate beneath the surface mucosa

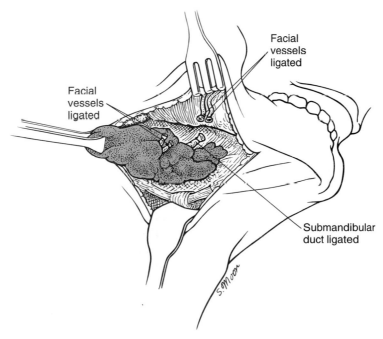

Figure 21-15

Extraoral technique for removal of the submandibular gland.

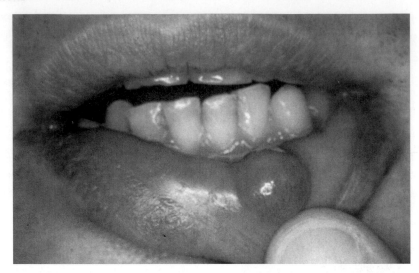

◇ **Figure 21-16**

Mucocele of left lower lip. Accumulation of minor salivary gland secretions in soft tissues from ruptured minor salivary duct.

into the soft tissues. Over time, secretions accumulate within the tissues and produce a pseudocyst (without a true epithelial lining) that contains thick, viscous saliva. These lesions are most common in the mucosa of the lower lip and are known as *mucoceles* (Figure 21-16). The second most common site of mucocele formation is the buccal mucosa. Mucocele formation results in an elevated, thinned, stretched overlying mucosa that appears as a vesicle filled with a clear or blue-gray mucous. The patient frequently relates a history of the lesion filling with fluid, rupture of the fluid collection, and refilling of these lesions. Many instances of mucocele formation regress spontaneously without surgery. For persistent or recurrent lesions the preferred treatment consists of excision of the mucocele and the associated minor salivary glands that contributed to its formation (Figure 21-17).

RANULA

The most common lesion of the sublingual gland is the ranula, which may be considered a mucocele of the sublingual salivary gland. The two types of ranulas are the simple ranula and the plunging ranula. Ranulas result from either mucous retention in the sublingual gland ductal system or mucous extravasation as a result of ductal disruption. The simple ranula is confined to the area occupied by the sublingual gland in the sublingual space, superior to the mylohyoid muscle (Figure 21-18, *A*). The progression to a plunging ranula occurs when the lesion extends beyond the level of the mylohyoid muscle into the submandibular space. Ranulas may reach a larger size than mucoceles, because their overlying mucosa is thicker and because trauma that would cause their rupture is less likely in the floor of the mouth. As a result a plunging ranula has the potential to extend into the neck and compromise the air-

way, resulting in a medical emergency. The usual treatment of the ranula is marsupialization, in which a portion of the oral mucosa of the floor of the mouth is excised, along with the superior wall of the ranula (Figure 21-18, *B*). Subsequently, the ranula wall is sutured to the oral mucosa of the floor of the mouth and allowed to heal by secondary intention (Figure 21-18, *C*). The preferred treatment for recurrent or persistent ranulas is excision of the ranula and sublingual gland via an intraoral approach (Figure 21-19); several recent studies have indicated that this might be appropriate for initial therapy.

SALIVARY GLAND INFECTIONS ◇

Infections of the major salivary glands can be acute or chronic and are commonly, but not always, related to obstructive disease, especially in the submandibular gland (obstruction leads to infection). The etiology of acute suppurative sialadenitis of the parotid gland usually involves a change in fluid balance that is likely to occur in patients who are elderly, debilitated, malnourished, dehydrated, or plagued with chronic illness. In these cases, gland infections are usually bilateral. There is a slight male predilection, and the mean age of occurrence of infections is 60 years. Salivary gland infections may be caused by a variety of organisms, including aerobic and anaerobic bacteria, viruses, fungal organisms, and mycobacteria. In most cases, mixed bacterial flora is responsible for sialadenitis. The single most common organism implicated in salivary gland infection is *Staphylococcus aureus*. This is because this organism normally colonizes around ductal orifices, and, during instances of decreased or

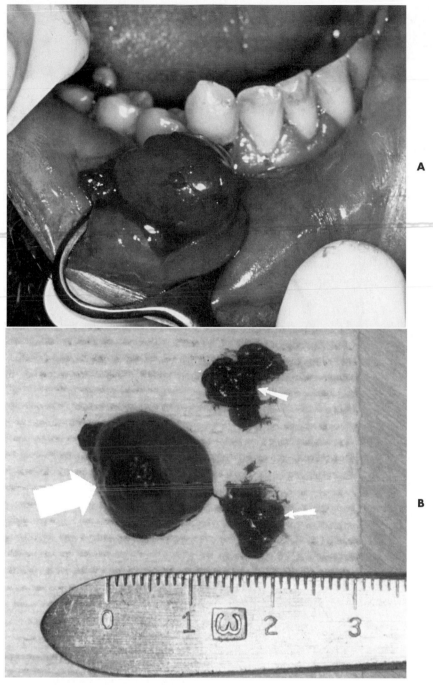

◇ Figure 21-17

A, Excision of mucocele of right lower lip. **B,** Gross specimen of intact mucocele (*large arrow*) and associated minor salivary gland tissue (*small arrows*).

slowed salivary flow (that is, obstruction or dehydration), retrograde influx of *S. aureus* into the ductal system and gland occurs and results in infection.

The clinical characteristics of acute bacterial salivary gland infections include rapid onset of swelling in the preauricular (parotid gland) or submandibular regions, with associated erythema and pain (Figure 21-20). Palpation of the involved gland will reveal no flow or elicit a thick, purulent discharge from the orifice of the duct (Figure 21-21). Treatment of bacterial salivary gland infections includes symptomatic and supportive care, including intravenous fluid hydration, antibiotics, and analgesics. Initial empiric antibiotics should be aimed at the most likely causative organism, *S. aureus*, and should include a cephalosporin (first-generation) or an

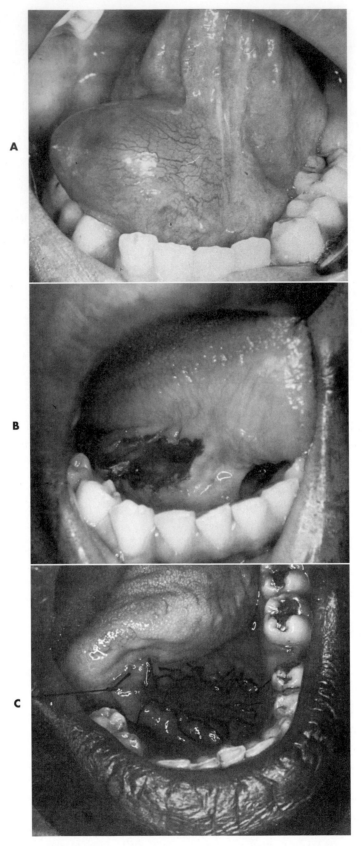

Figure 21-18

A, Ranula in the right floor of mouth caused by accumulation of sublingual gland secretions in soft tissues secondary to rupture of salivary duct. **B,** Marsupialization of ranula, with excision of oral mucosa and superior wall of ranula. **C,** Completion of marsupialization of left floor of mouth ranula with placement of circumferential sutures.

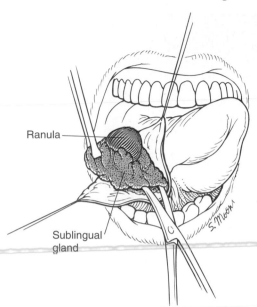

Figure 21-19

Intraoral sublingual gland and ranula removal.

antistaphylococcal semisynthetic penicillin (oxacillin or dicloxacillin). Culture and sensitivity studies of purulent material should be obtained to aid in selecting the most appropriate antibiotic for each patient. Antibiotics should be administered intravenously in high doses for the majority of these patients, who ordinarily require hospitalization. On most occasions, surgery consisting of incision and drainage becomes necessary in the management of salivary gland infections. Untreated infections may progress rapidly and can cause respiratory obstruction, septicemia, and, eventually, death. In some instances of recurrent salivary gland infection the repeated insults result in irreversible functional impairment of gland function, and excision of the gland may be indicated.

Viral parotitis, or mumps, is an acute, nonsuppurative communicable disease. Before routine vaccination (measles, mumps, rubella vaccine) against the disease began, viral parotitis occurred in epidemics during the winter and spring. It is important to differentiate viral from bacterial salivary gland infection, because viral infections are not the result of obstructive disease and require different treatment, not including antibiotics. Mumps is characterized by a painful, nonerythematous swelling of one or both parotid glands that begins 2 to 3 weeks after exposure to the virus (incubation period). This disease occurs most commonly in children between ages 6 and 8. The signs and symptoms of mumps include preauricular pain and swelling, fever, chills, and headache. Viral parotitis usually resolves in 5 to 12 days following its onset. Viral parotitis is treated by providing supportive and symptomatic care for fever, headache, and malaise with antipyretics, analgesics, and adequate hydration. Complications of the disease include meningitis, pancreatitis, nephritis, orchitis, testicular atrophy, and sterility in approximately 20% of young males affected.

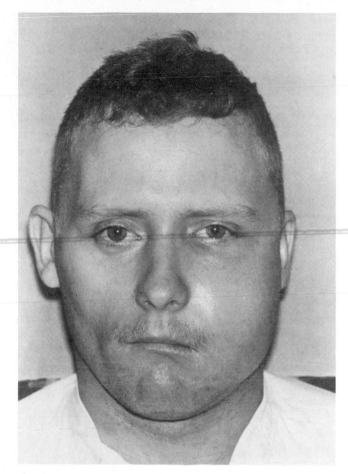

Figure 21-20

Patient with left parotid gland infection. These infections are extremely painful and may indicate other serious illness. Treatment requires hospitalization, intravenous antibiotics, and possibly surgical drainage.

NECROTIZING SIALOMETAPLASIA

Necrotizing sialometaplasia is a reactive, nonneoplastic inflammatory process that usually affects the minor salivary glands of the palate. However, it may involve minor salivary glands in any location. Necrotizing sialometaplasia is of unclear etiology but is thought to be secondary to vascular infarction of the salivary gland lobules. Potential causes of diminished blood flow to the affected area include trauma, local anesthetic injection, smoking, diabetes mellitus, vascular disease, and pressure from a denture prosthesis. The usual age range of affected patients is between 23 and 66 years. Lesions usually appear as large (1 to 4 cm), painless or painful, deeply ulcerated areas lateral to the palatal midline and near the junction of the hard and soft palate (Figure 21-22). Although lesions are usually unilateral, bilateral involvement may occur. Some patients may report a prodromal flulike illness before the onset of the ulceration.

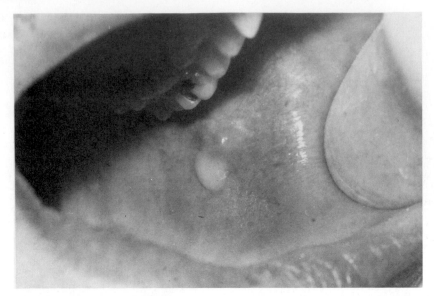

◇ **Figure 21-21**

Purulent discharge from left parotid duct in patient with infection involving parotid gland (*arrow*).

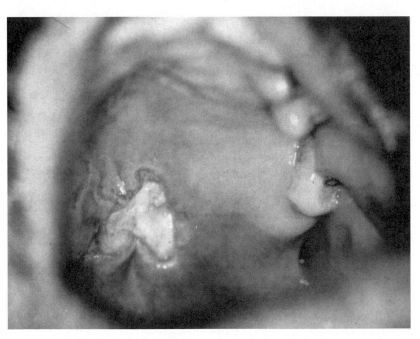

◇ **Figure 21-22**

Necrotizing sialometaplasia of posterior palate with ulceration.

This condition is of considerable concern because, both clinically and histologically (Figure 21-23), it resembles a malignant carcinoma (squamous cell or mucoepidermoid carcinoma). The appropriate diagnosis and management of this disease relies on evaluation by an oral surgeon and pathologist who are familiar with this entity, because the result of a misdiagnosis may be extensive, unwarranted surgical resection. Helpful histologic criteria for distin-

guishing necrotizing sialometaplasia from a malignant process include the maintenance of the overall salivary lobular morphology, the generally nondysplastic appearance of the squamous islands or nests, and evidence of residual ductal lumina within the epithelial nests. The ulcerations of necrotizing sialometaplasia usually heal spontaneously within 6 to 10 weeks following their onset and require no surgical management.

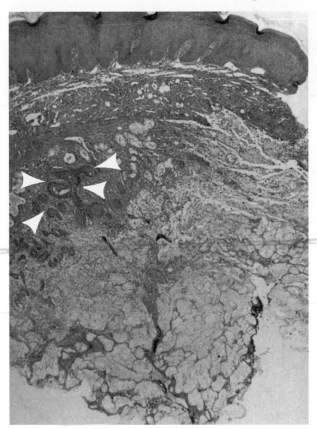

◇ **Figure 21-23**

Histopathology of necrotizing sialometaplasia, showing pseudo-epitheliomatous hyperplasia (*arrowheads*) that appears similar to infiltration of a squamous cell carcinoma.

SJÖGREN'S SYNDROME ———◇

Sjögren's syndrome (SS) is a multisystem disease process with a variable presentation. The two types of Sjögren's syndrome are primary SS, or sicca syndrome, characterized by xerostomia (dry mouth) and keratoconjunctivitis sicca (dry eyes), and secondary SS, which is composed of primary SS and an associated connective tissue disorder, most commonly rheumatoid arthritis. Although the etiology of SS is unknown, there appears to be a strong autoimmune influence. There is a female predilection of 9:1, with over 80% of affected individuals being females with a mean age of 50 years. Generally, the first symptoms to appear are arthritic complaints, followed by ocular symptoms, and, late in the disease process, salivary gland symptoms. The involvement of the salivary and lacrimal glands results from a lymphocytic replacement of the normal glandular elements. The xerostomia results from a decreased function of both the major and minor salivary glands, with the parotid gland being the most sensitive. The diagnosis of SS is suggested by the patient's complaints, as well as by a variety of abnormal immunologic laboratory tests. The oral component of SS may be diagnosed using salivary flow rate studies and sialography, but the use of

a labial minor salivary gland biopsy (Figure 21-13) currently is considered to be highly accurate in aiding the diagnosis. The histopathologic changes seen in the minor glands are similar to those in the major glands (parotid). Keratoconjunctivitis sicca is suggested by the patient's complaints and a Schirmer's test for lacrimal flow (Figure 21-24). The treatment for SS includes symptomatic care with artificial tears for the dry eyes and salivary substitutes for the dry mouth. Additionally, the medication pilocarpine (Salagen) may be useful to stimulate salivary flow from the remaining functional salivary gland tissue.

TRAUMATIC SALIVARY GLAND INJURIES ———◇

Traumatic injuries, particularly lacerations, involving the salivary glands and their ducts may accompany a variety of facial injuries, including fractures. Injuries that occur in close proximity to one of the major salivary glands or ducts require careful evaluation. Facial lacerations may involve not only the gland and its ductal system, but also branches of the facial nerve and branches of major facial vessels. These structures require meticulous attention for appropriate diagnosis and prompt repair. Repair may include ductal anastomoses, in which the proximal and distal portions of the duct are identified, a plastic or metal catheter is placed as a stent, and the duct is sutured over the stent (Figure 21-25). The catheter usually remains in place for 10 to 14 days for epithelialization of the duct to occur. Additionally, nerve anastomoses may be required and performed by placing epineurial sutures, using magnification, to reapproximate the nerve stumps. The lacerations are closed in a usual layered fashion, following débridement of the soft tissue wounds to cleanse the site of entrapped particles, such as glass or dirt. Potential sequelae of trauma involving the major salivary glands include infection, facial paralysis, cutaneous salivary gland fistula, sialocele formation, and duct obstruction as a result of scar formation, with eventual glandular atrophy and decreased function. The involved gland may eventually require surgical removal.

NEOPLASTIC SALIVARY GLAND DISORDERS ———◇

Although a comprehensive discussion of salivary gland neoplasms is beyond the scope of this chapter and many other sources are available for this information, a brief review of several important aspects of the more common lesions is warranted. Salivary gland tumors occur much more commonly in the major glands (80% to 85%), as opposed to the minor glands (15% to 20%) (Table 21-3). Additionally, between 75% and 80% of major gland tumors are benign, whereas 50% to 55% of minor gland tumors are benign. The overwhelming majority of salivary tumors occur in the parotid gland, and the majority of those are benign (mostly pleomorphic adenomas).

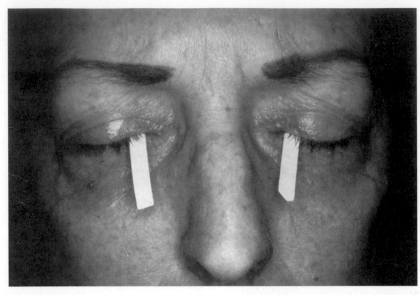

◇ **Figure 21-24**

Schirmer's test for dry eyes in a patient with Sjögren's disease. Filter paper is placed in the ocular fornix and observed for "wetting" to a certain distance within a specific time limit.

◇ **Table 21-3.** Salivary gland tumor distribution

Major glands	**80%-85%**
Parotid gland	85%-90%
Submandibular gland	5%-10%
Sublingual gland	Rare
Minor glands	**15%-20%**
Palate	55%
Lips	15%
Remainder	Rare

BENIGN SALIVARY GLAND TUMORS

The pleomorphic adenoma, or benign mixed tumor, is the most common salivary gland tumor. The mean age of occurrence is 45 years, with a male-to-female ratio of 3:2. In the major glands, the parotid gland is involved in over 80% of cases; in the minor glands, the most common intraoral site is the palate (Figure 21-26). Pleomorphic adenomas are usually slow-growing, painless masses. The histopathology shows two cell types: the ductal epithelial cell and the myoepithelial cell, which may differentiate along a variety of cell lines (*pleomorphic* means many forms). There is a connective tissue capsule, which may be incomplete. The treatment involves complete surgical excision with a margin of normal uninvolved tissue. Parotid lesions are treated with removal of the involved lobe along with the tumor. There is a small risk of recurrence, as well as a small (5%) risk of malignant transformation to a carcinoma-ex-pleomorphic adenoma.

Warthin's tumor, or papillary cystadenoma lymphomatosum, almost exclusively affects the parotid gland, specifically the tail of the parotid gland (Figure 21-27). The peak incidence is in the sixth decade of life, with a male-to-female ratio of 7:1. This lesion presents as a slow-growing, soft, painless mass. Warthin's tumor is believed to be caused by entrapped salivary epithelial rests within developing lymph nodes. The histopathology shows two components: an epithelial component in a papillary pattern and a lymphoid component with germinal centers. The treatment of this lesion is simple surgical excision, and recurrence is rare.

The monomorphic adenoma is an uncommon solitary lesion composed of one cell type, affecting predominantly the upper lip minor glands (canalicular adenoma) (Figure 21-28) and the parotid gland (basal cell adenoma). The mean age of occurrence is 61 years, and the lesion usually presents as an asymptomatic, freely movable mass. The histopathology reveals an encapsulated lesion composed of one type (monomorphic) of salivary ductal epithelial cell. The treatment is simple surgical excision.

MALIGNANT SALIVARY GLAND TUMORS

The mucoepidermoid carcinoma is the most common malignant salivary gland tumor. It comprises 10% of major gland tumors (mostly parotid) (Figure 21-29) and 20% of minor gland tumors (mostly palate) (Figure 21-30). This lesion may occur at any age, but there is a mean age of 45 years. The male-to-female ratio is 3:2. The clinical presentation is a submucosal mass that may be painful or ulcerated. The mass may appear to have a bluish tinge because of the mucous content contained within the lesion. An intraosseous form of mucoepidermoid carcinoma may present as a multilocular radiolucency of the posterior mandible. The histopathology shows three cell types: mucous cells, epidermoid cells, and intermediate (clear) cells. The proportion of each cell type helps to grade the mucoepidermoid carcinoma as high-, intermediate-, or low-grade lesions. The higher the grade, the

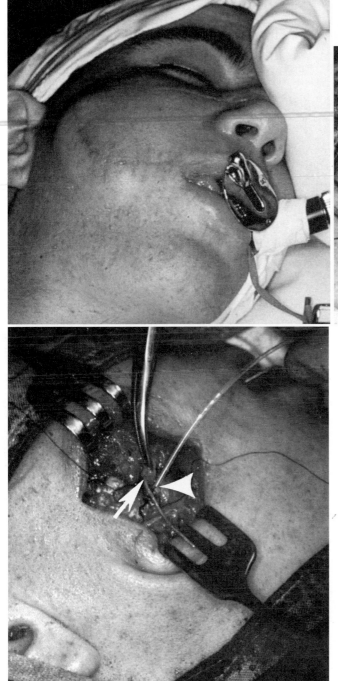

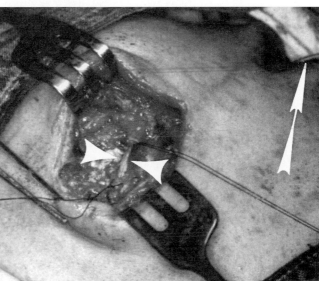

◇ **Figure 21-25**

A, Patient who had cheek laceration repaired with failure to appreciate a Stensen's duct laceration, who subsequently developed a sialocele (localized collection of saliva). **B,** Operative repair of Stensen's duct laceration with a metal probe in the distal duct (*arrow*), and a plastic catheter (*arrowheads*) placed into the proximal portion of the duct. **C,** Repair of Stensen's duct laceration via suturing over a plastic stent (*arrowheads*) placed via intraoral cannulation of Stensen's duct (*arrow*).

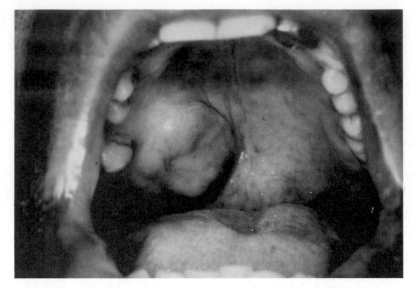

Figure 21-26

Pleomorphic adenoma of the right palate.

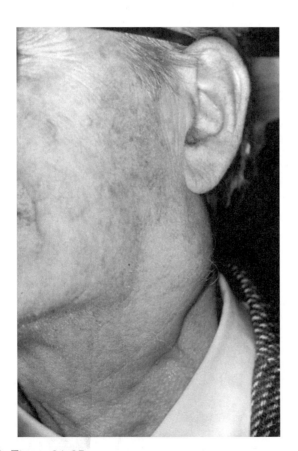

Figure 21-27

Warthin's tumor of the tail of the left parotid gland.

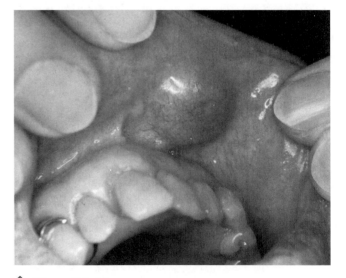

Figure 21-28

Monomorphic (canalicular) adenoma of the left upper lip.

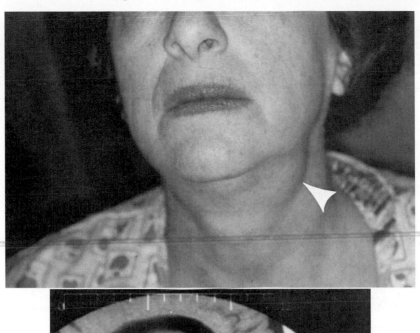

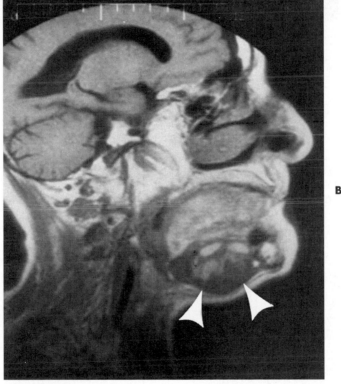

Figure 21-29

A, Mucoepidermoid carcinoma of the left submandibular gland (*arrowhead*). **B,** MRI showing the mucoepidermoid carcinoma of the left submandibular gland (*arrowheads*).

more predominance of epidermoid cells and pleomorphism, lack of mucous cells and cystic areas, and overall more aggressive behavior. The treatment of low-grade lesions is wide surgical excision with a margin of uninvolved normal tissue; high-grade lesions require more aggressive surgical removal with margins, and, possibly, local radiation therapy. The low-grade lesions have a 95% 5-year survival rate, whereas the high-grade lesions have less than a 40% 5-year survival rate.

The polymorphous low-grade adenocarcinoma is the second most common intraoral salivary gland malignancy. This lesion was first described in 1983, and, before its identification, many cases were probably misdiagnosed as adenoid cystic carcinoma. The most common site is the junction of the hard and soft palates (Figure 21-31). The male-to-female ratio is 3:1, with a mean age of 56 years. These tumors present as slow-growing, asymptomatic masses that may be ulcerated. The histopathology shows many cell

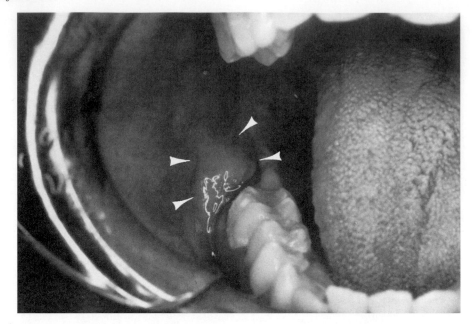

◇ **Figure 21-30**

Mucoepidermoid carcinoma of the right retromolar pad minor salivary glands (*arrowheads*).

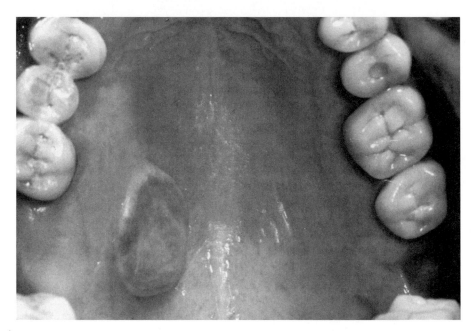

◇ **Figure 21-31**

Polymorphous low-grade adenocarcinoma of the right palate.

shapes and patterns (polymorphous). There is an infiltrative proliferation of ductal epithelial cells in an "Indian file" pattern. This lesion shows a predilection for invasion of surrounding nerves. The treatment of this tumor is wide surgical excision, and there is a relatively high recurrence rate of 14%.

The adenoid cystic carcinoma is the third most common intraoral salivary gland malignancy, with a mean age of 53 years and a male-to-female ratio of 3:2. Approximately 50%

of these tumors occur in the parotid gland, whereas the other 50% occur in the minor glands of the palate (Figure 21-32). These present as slow-growing, nonulcerated masses, with an associated chronic dull pain. Occasionally, parotid lesions may result in facial paralysis as a result of facial nerve involvement. The histopathology demonstrates an infiltrative proliferation of basaloid cells arranged in a cribriform ("Swiss cheese") pattern. As seen in the polymorphous low-grade adenocarcinoma, there may be perineural invasion. The

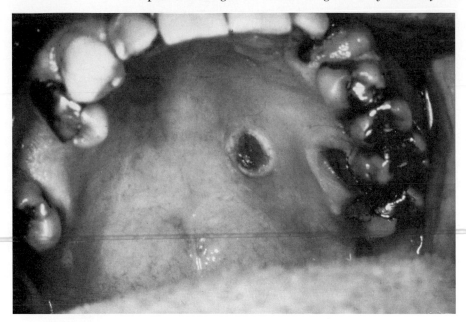

◇ Figure 21-32

Adenoid cystic carcinoma of the left palate.

treatment is wide surgical excision, followed in some cases by radiation therapy. The prognosis is poor despite aggressive therapy.

BIBLIOGRAPHY

Abaza NA, Miloro M: The role of fine-needle aspiration in oral and maxillofacial diagnosis. In Gold L, editor: Diagnosis and management of oral pathologic lesions, *Oral Maxillofac Surg Clin North Am* 6(3):401-420, 1994.

Abaza N et al: The role of labial salivary gland biopsy in the diagnosis of Sjögren's syndrome: report of three cases, *J Oral Maxillofac Surg* 51(5):574-580, 1993.

Baurmash HD: Marsupialization for treatment of oral ranula: a second look at the procedure, *J Oral Maxillofac Surg* 50:1274, 1992.

Berry RL: Sialadenitis and sialolithiasis: diagnosis and management, *Oral Maxillofac Surg Clin North Am* 7:479, 1995.

Carlson ER: Salivary gland tumors: classification, histogenesis, and general considerations, *Oral Maxillofac Surg Clin North Am* 7:519, 1995.

Curtin HD: Assessment of salivary gland pathology, *Otolaryngol Clin North Am* 21:547, 1988.

Delbalso A: Salivary imaging, *Oral Maxillofac Surg Clin North Am* 7:387, 1995.

Goldberg MH, Bevilacqua RG: Infections of the salivary glands, *Oral Maxillofac Surg Clin North Am* 7:423, 1995.

Lustmann J, Regev E, Melamed Y: Sialolithiasis: a survey on 245 patients and a review of the literature, *Int J Oral Maxillofac Surg* 19:135-138, 1990.

Mandel ID: Sialochemistry in diseases and clinical situations affecting salivary glands, *Crit Rev Clin Lab Sci* 12:321, 1980.

Regezzi JA, Sciubba JJ: Salivary gland diseases. In Regezzi JA, Sciubba JJ, editors: *Oral pathology: clinical-pathologic correlations,* Philadelphia, 1989, WB Saunders.

Topazian RG, Goldberg MH: *Management of infections of the oral and maxillofacial regions,* ed 2, Philadelphia, 1987, WB Saunders.

Van der Akker HP: Diagnostic imaging in salivary gland disease, *Oral Surg Oral Med Oral Pathol* 66:625, 1988.

VanSickels JE, Alexander JM: Parotid duct injuries, *Oral Surg* 52:364, 1981.

Yoshimura Y et al: A comparison of three methods used for treatment of ranula, *J Oral Maxillofac Surg* 53:280-282, 1995.

Youngs RP, Walsh-Waring GP: Trauma to the parotid region, *Laryngol Otol* 101:475, 1987.

MANAGEMENT OF ORAL PATHOLOGIC LESIONS

The dentist in general practice has a more thorough and continuous exposure to his or her patients' oral cavities and perioral areas than any other health care provider. Therefore the dentist is responsible for maintaining the overall health and well-being of these structures. Whether directly involved in the surgical management of pathologic entities or indirectly involved through referral to another health care provider, the dentist is the individual who provides the needed continuity of care to help ensure adequate patient follow-up and dental reconstructive efforts.

The unique role of general dentists as oral health experts requires them to be constantly on the lookout for pathologic lesions during the everyday care of patients. General dentists must be aware of the natural history of the more common maxillofacial disease processes and must be astute diagnosticians. As with any disease process in dentistry and medicine, prevention is the best form of therapy, and early diagnosis and treatment is the best way of managing pathologic entities.

The following two chapters describe the role that the general dentist should assume in the management of a patient's pathologic conditions. The most important aspect of this care begins with a thorough patient examination and an accurate diagnosis of disease. Chapter 22 covers these topics in detail and in a fashion meaningful to the general dentist. Chapter 23 describes the surgical management of pathologic diseases of the oral cavity and contiguous structures. Details of surgical technique are provided in depth for lesions that the general dentist may encounter. The surgical management of major pathologic conditions and tumors of the oral and maxillofacial region is also presented, but the emphasis is on the general dentist's role in overall patient management.

CHAPTER 22

PRINCIPLES OF DIFFERENTIAL DIAGNOSIS AND BIOPSY

EDWARD ELLIS III

EXAMINATION AND DIAGNOSTIC METHODS

Lesions of the oral cavity and perioral areas *must* be identified and characterized so that specific therapy can lead to elimination of the lesion. When a lesion is discovered, several important, orderly steps should be undertaken to identify and characterize it (Figure 22-1). These steps include the health history, history of the specific lesion, clinical examination, radiographic examination, laboratory investigation, and, if indicated, surgical procedures to obtain a specimen for pathologic examination.

When the patient or dentist discovers a lesion, the dentist must be careful how this information is discussed with the patient. The words *lesion, tumor, growth,* and *biopsy* carry terrifying connotations to many patients. The empathetic dentist can spare patients from anxiety and frustration by carefully wording the discussion of the lesion. It behooves the dentist to remember and make the patient aware that the vast majority of lesions discovered in the oral and maxillofacial area are benign.

HEALTH HISTORY

The overall medical status of the patient is of paramount importance when investigating a lesion. There are two basic reasons why an accurate health history and, if needed, a thorough clinical evaluation or consultation with medical

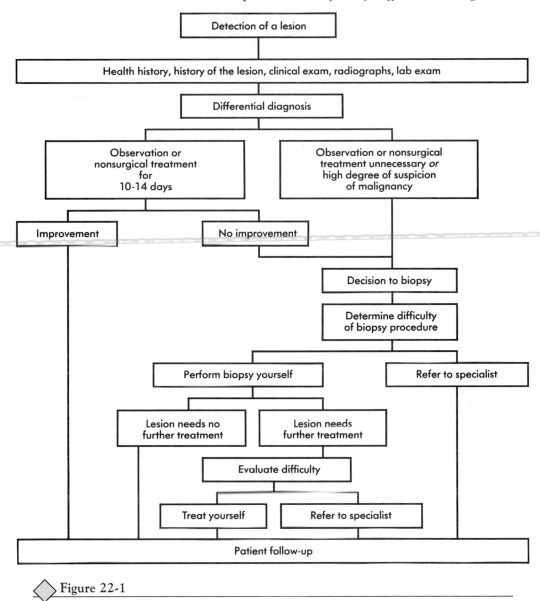

Detection of a lesion

Health history, history of the lesion, clinical exam, radiographs, lab exam

Differential diagnosis

Observation or nonsurgical treatment for 10-14 days

Observation or nonsurgical treatment unnecessary *or* high degree of suspicion of malignancy

Improvement

No improvement

Decision to biopsy

Determine difficulty of biopsy procedure

Perform biopsy yourself

Refer to specialist

Lesion needs no further treatment

Lesion needs further treatment

Evaluate difficulty

Treat yourself

Refer to specialist

Patient follow-up

◇ Figure 22-1

Decision tree for treatment of oral lesions.

specialists are mandatory. The first reason is that a preexisting medical problem may affect or be affected by the dentist's treatment of the patient. As outlined in Chapters 1 and 2, patients with certain medical conditions, such as congenital heart defects, coagulopathies, and hypertension, may require special precautions when any surgical treatment is required. Furthermore, surgical intervention may upset the delicate balance between health and disease in a poorly controlled diabetic or immunocompromised person.

The second reason for a thorough knowledge of the patient's overall health status is that the lesion under investigation may be an oral manifestation of a systemic disease. For instance, a patient with agranulocytosis or Crohn's disease may present with oral lesions. An ulceration in a chronic smoker should alert the dentist to the possibility of carcinoma. Literally hundreds of systemic disease pro-

cesses can present orally, so the dentist should be aware of them and cognizant of any of their oral presentations.

HISTORY OF THE LESION

It is generally accepted that 85% to 90% of systemic diseases can be discovered by a thorough and properly gathered health history. The same can be true of many lesions of the oral cavity when the diagnostician knows the natural history of the more common disease processes. The patient should be questioned for the following:

1. *How long has the lesion been present?* The duration of the lesion may provide valuable clues to its nature. For instance, a lesion that has been present for several years may be congenital. Establishing the duration of a lesion provides much more information when taken in concert with the change in its size.

2. *Has the lesion changed in size? If so, at what rate and to what magnitude?* The change in the size of a lesion is one of the most important pieces of information the dentist can obtain. A rapidly growing lesion is more likely to be aggressive, whereas a slow-growing lesion may indicate a more benign process. Similarly, by combining this information with that on the duration of the lesion, a more accurate assessment of the true nature of the lesion can be ascertained. For instance, a lesion that has been present for several months and has not changed in size might indicate a benign process. On the other hand, a fast-growing lesion that has existed for only a short time might indicate a more serious process.

3. *Has the lesion changed in character (that is, did a lump become an ulcer; did an ulcer begin as a vesicle)?* A change in the physical character of a lesion may assist in the diagnostic process. For example, if a lesion presents to the dentist as an ulcer, but the patient says that it began as a vesicle, a more thorough search for other signs or symptoms of a vesiculobullous or viral disease may be indicated.

4. *What symptoms are associated with the lesion (for example, pain, abnormal sensations, anesthesia, a feeling of swelling, bad taste or smell, dysphagia, swelling or tenderness of adjacent lymph nodes)? If painful, what is the character of the pain? What exacerbates and what diminishes the pain?* Pain is most often associated with lesions that contain an inflammatory component. Cancer, although feared as a painful lesion, often is not. Numbness in the distribution of one of the sensory nerves usually indicates an inflammatory or malignant process, unless other physical causes can be ascertained. Dysphagia indicates that the muscles of deglutition or the contents of the floor of the mouth or parapharyngeal areas are involved. Swelling may be one of the more common symptoms associated with oral lesions, which indicates nothing more than an expansile process that can result from a variety of causes. It is important to note that the patient may feel a sensation of swelling or fullness before the clinician can actually identify swelling by clinical examination. In general, tender lymph nodes indicate an inflammatory or infectious cause of the lesion. Thus clues to the nature of the lesion should be sought and the patient carefully questioned about associated symptoms.

5. *Are there any associated constitutional symptoms (for example, fever, nausea, anorexia)?* With this question, the dentist is looking for a possible systemic manifestation of a systemic disease. For example, systemic viral illnesses (such as measles and mononucleosis) can cause oral manifestations along with the systemic illness.

6. *Is there any historic reason for the lesion (for example, trauma to the area, a recent toothache)?* One of the first things the dentist should do when a lesion is discovered is seek an explanation based on the patient's history. Frequently, lesions in and around the oral cavity are caused by habits, hard or hot foods, application of medicines not intended for topical use, and recent trauma. Additionally, the dentition should always be examined very carefully when a lesion is found in the general area, because many such lesions have some relationship to the teeth.

CLINICAL EXAMINATION

When a lesion is discovered, it must be carefully examined for clues to its nature. Furthermore, a thorough examination of the areas around the lesion, including the regional lymph nodes, is mandatory. Once the examination is complete, a detailed description of the findings is placed in the patient's chart. It is very helpful to draw the lesion in the chart or on a schematic of the oral cavity and perioral areas (Figure 22-2). A description and illustration allow the dentist to follow the course of the lesion over time and to determine whether it is resolving or changing in nature.

An examination classically includes inspection, palpation, percussion, and auscultation. In the oral-maxillofacial region, inspection and palpation are the most commonly used diagnostic modalities, with percussion usually being reserved for examination of the dentition. Although auscultation is infrequently used, it is an important diagnostic tool when examining suspected vascular lesions. Inspection is *always* performed before palpation, which allows the dentist to describe the lesion before it is handled, because some lesions are extremely friable and/or fragile. Manipulation of such a lesion may precipitate hemorrhage or may rupture a fluid-filled lesion, which then makes accurate inspection more difficult. The following are some of the more important points to be evaluated.

1. *The anatomic location of the mass.* Lesions may arise from any tissue within the oral cavity, including epithelium, subcutaneous and submucosal connective tissue, muscle, tendon, nerve, bone, blood vessels, and salivary glands. The dentist should ascertain as much as possible which tissues are contributing to the lesion. The exact anatomic location of the lesion should aid in this determination. For example, if a mass is present on the dorsum of the tongue, the dentist must consider an epithelial, connective tissue, or muscle origin for the mass. Similarly, a swelling on the inner aspect of the lower lip should prompt the dentist to include a salivary gland etiology in the differential diagnosis. Whenever a lesion is discovered, the dentist should always try to elucidate the cause of the lesion based on its anatomic location. The etiologic role of trauma in oral lesions should always be entertained and a search for a source of trauma undertaken. Ill-fitting prosthetic devices, chronic cheek-biting and other habits, sharp teeth, and so on are common causes of oral lesions. Periapical and periodontal dental pathologic conditions also cause a high percentage of oral lesions.

2. *The overall physical character of the lesion.* The lesion should be described in proper medical terminology, because lay terminology is sometimes misleading. For example, a "swelling" may be interpreted in many ways. Box 22-1 lists the more common physical descriptions that are useful in describing oral pathologic entities. A

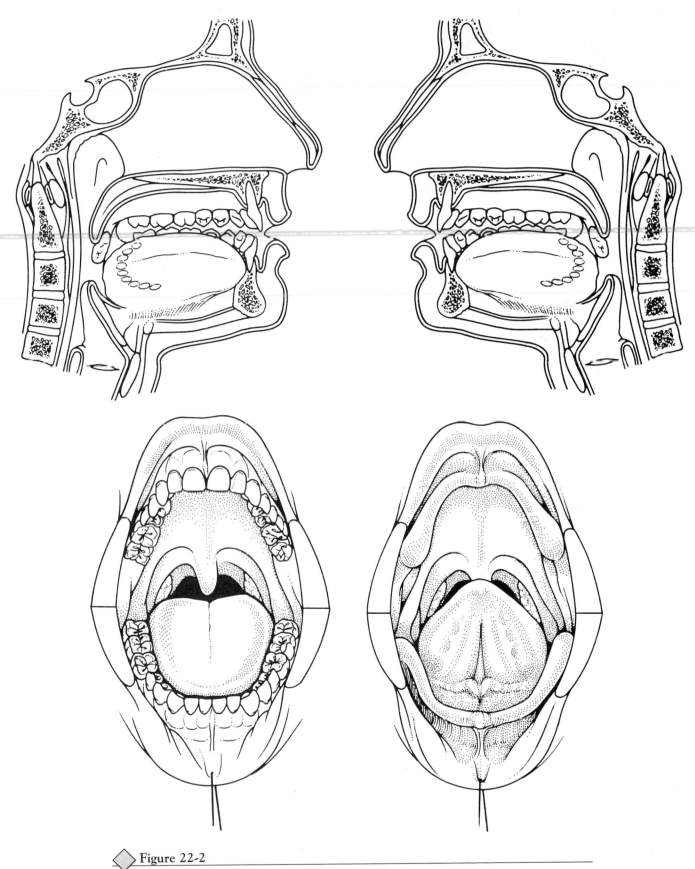

◇ Figure 22-2

Illustrations of oral cavity and perioral areas, which are useful for indicating size and location of oral lesions.

Continued

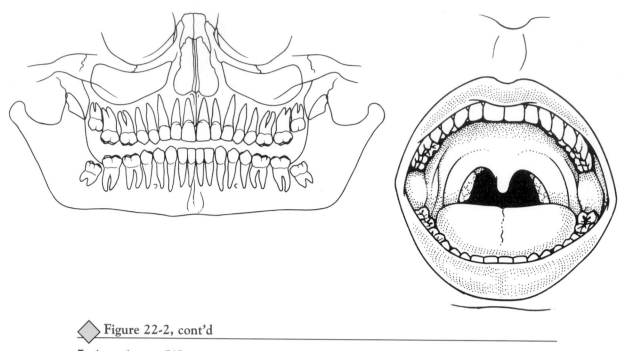

◆ Figure 22-2, cont'd

For legend see p. 515.

───── ◆ Box 22-1 ◆ ─────

Physical types of lesions

Bulla (pl. bullae): Loculated fluid in or under the epithelium of skin or mucosa; a large blister

Crusts: Dried or clotted serum protein on the surface of skin or mucosa

Erosion: Superficial ulcer (excoriation)

Macule: Circumscribed area of color change without elevation

Nodule: Large palpable mass, elevated above the epithelial surface

Papule: Small palpable mass, elevated above the epithelial surface

Plaque: Flat elevated lesion; the confluence of papules

Pustule: Cloudy or white vesicle, the color of which results from the presence of polymorphonuclear leukocytes (pus)

Scale: Macroscopic accumulation of keratin

Ulcer: Loss of epithelium

Vesicle: Small loculation of fluid in or under the epithelium; a small blister

lesion's physical characteristics should always be categorized as (at least) one of the several types of lesions listed.

3. *The size and shape of the lesion.* Accurate recordings of these two basic physical characteristics should be made for future reference.

4. *Single versus multiple lesions.* The presence and location of multiple lesions is an important diagnostic sign. When multiple areas of ulceration are found within the mouth, the dentist can begin to rank the differential diagnostic possibilities. It is unusual to find multiple areas of carcinoma in the mouth, whereas a vesiculobullous disease commonly presents with such a pattern. Similarly, an ulcerated lesion on the lip and tip of the tongue (the so-called kissing ulcers) may indicate an infectious process whereby one lesion infects the tissue with which it comes into contact.

5. *The surface of the lesion.* The surface may be smooth, lobulated, or irregular. If ulceration is present, the characteristics of the ulcer base should be recorded. Ulcer beds can be smooth; full of granulation tissue; covered with a slough, membrane, or scab; or fungating, such as is seen with some malignancies.

6. *The color of the lesion.* The color or colors are an important consideration. A bluish swelling that blanches on pressure may indicate a vascular lesion, whereas a bluish lesion that does not blanch may indicate a mucus-containing lesion. A pigmented lesion of the oral mucosa may carry more importance than a lesion of normal color. An erythematous lesion may be more ominous than a white lesion. Some lesions may have more than one color, and this should be noted in detail. Frequently, inflammation is superimposed on areas of the lesion because of mechanical trauma or ulceration, which gives a varied picture from one time to the next.

7. *The sharpness of the boundaries of the lesion.* If a mass is present, is it fixed to surrounding deeper tissues or is it freely movable? The determination of the boundaries will aid in establishing whether the mass is fixed to bone, arising from the bone and extending into soft tissues, or of an infiltrating nature. The same applies to an ulceration; however, a description of the boundaries should include

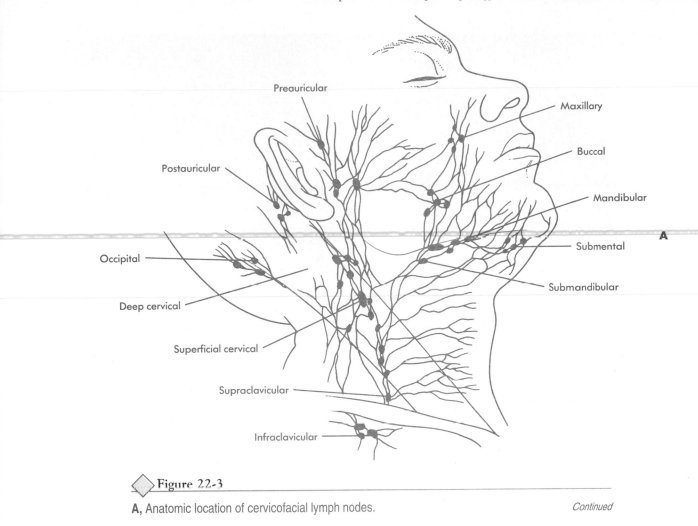

◇ **Figure 22-3**

A, Anatomic location of cervicofacial lymph nodes.   *Continued*

a physical description of the margins. The margin of an ulcer may be flat, rolled, raised, or everted.

8. *The consistency of the lesion to palpation.* The consistency of lesions is described as *soft,* as in the case of a lipoma; *firm,* which is the consistency of a fibroma; or *hard,* as in the case of an osteoma or tori. *Indurated* simply means firm or hard.

9. *Presence of fluctuation.* Fluctuation is the term given to a wavelike motion felt on palpating a mass or cavity with nonrigid walls, which contains fluid. This is a valuable physical sign, because it usually indicates fluid within the mass. It can be elicited by palpating with two or more fingers in a rhythmic fashion, such that as one finger exerts pressure, the other finger feels the impulse transmitted through the fluid-filled cavity.

10. *Presence of pulsation.* Palpation of a mass may reveal a pulsatile quality, which indicates a large vascular component. This is especially important in bony lesions. A *thrill* is the name given to the palpable vibration accompanying a vascular murmur or pulsation. If a thrill is palpable, auscultation with a stethoscope may reveal a *bruit,* or audible murmur. Lesions with palpable thrills or

audible bruits should be referred to a specialist for treatment, because life-threatening hemorrhage can arise when biopsy is attempted.

11. *Lymph node examination.* No evaluation of an oral lesion is complete without a thorough regional lymph node examination. Before *any* biopsy procedure, it is particularly important to perform a thorough examination of the regional lymph nodes. Sometimes lymphadenitis develops in regional nodes following a biopsy procedure. The enlargement of these nodes as a result of inflammation may pose a problem in differentiating infection or inflammation from metastatic spread of tumor. Figure 22-3 illustrates the important and more common lymph nodes in the maxillofacial region.

In recording findings, the following five characteristics should routinely be included: location; size, preferably giving the diameter in centimeters; tenderness (painful versus nonpainful); degree of fixation, that is, movable, matted, or fixed; and texture, that is, soft, hard, or firm. Normal lymph nodes are not palpable. However, nodes enlarge with inflammation and may be palpable as a result. Cervical nodes up to 1 cm in

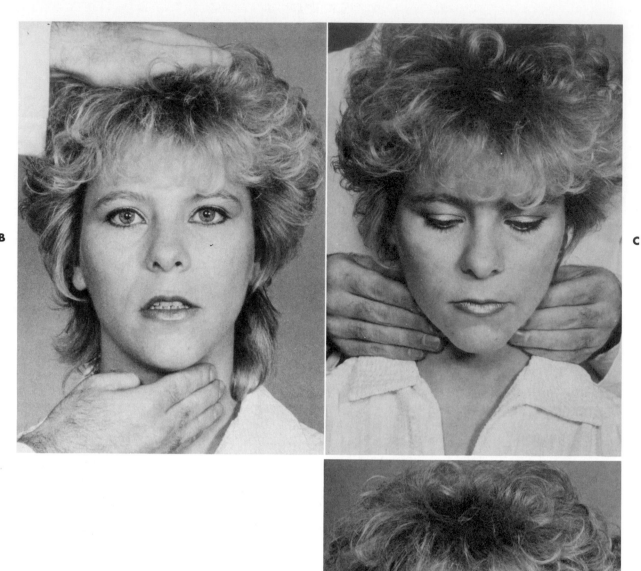

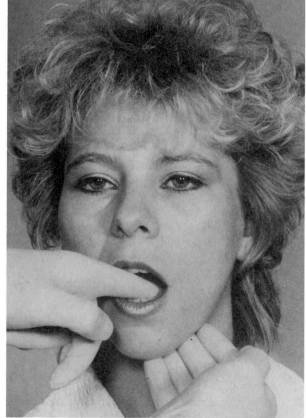

◇ Figure 22-3, cont'd

B, Anterior approach to cervical lymph node examination. Fingers are gently moved in circular motion along full length of sternocleidomastoid muscle. **C,** Posterior approach to cervical lymph node examination. It is generally helpful for patient to move head from side to side and to tilt head forward to make lymph nodes more palpable. **D,** Bimanual palpation of floor of mouth and submandibular lymph nodes.

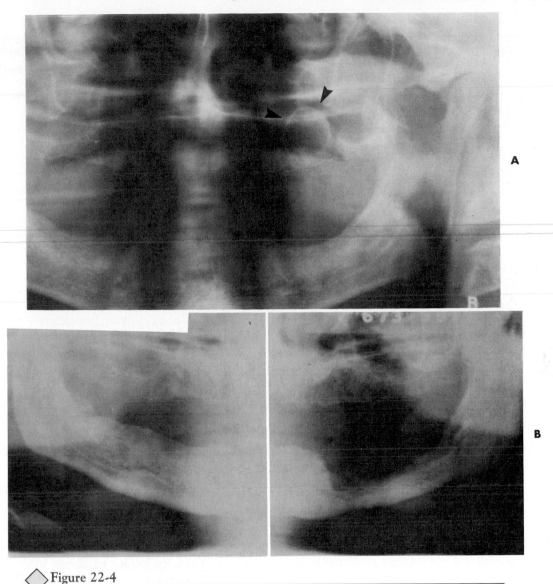

◇ **Figure 22-4**

A, Radiographic appearance of cyst (*arrows*). Note peripheral condensing osteitis around radiolucent center. **B,** Radiographic appearance of bone destruction by malignancy (*right*). Squamous cell carcinoma has eroded into mandible. Note ragged appearance.

diameter are almost always felt in the cervical region of children up to age 12 and are not an abnormal finding. The standard examination of the lymph nodes requires only simple inspection and palpation. It is always useful to compare sides by using the middle three fingers for palpation. This examination is methodical and proceeds downward as follows: (1) occipital and postauricular; (2) submandibular and submental; (3) anterior cervical triangle (upper end of deep cervical chain); (4) downward along sternocleidomastoid muscle (superficial cervical nodes); (5) posterior triangle (lower end of deep cervical chain); and (6) supraclavicular. Movements during palpation should be slow and gentle; the fingers move across each area examined in vertical and horizontal directions followed by rotary motion.

RADIOGRAPHIC EXAMINATION

Radiographs are useful as diagnostic adjuncts to the clinical examination and history of lesions within or adjacent to bone. When lesions within the soft tissues are proximal to bone, radiographs may elucidate whether the lesion is causing an osseous reaction or eroding into the bone. A variety of radiographic projections may be used, depending on the anatomic location of the lesion. Most pathologic conditions of the mandible or maxilla can be satisfactorily demonstrated by routine radiography, but, occasionally, special imaging techniques are required to elucidate some particular facet of the case under investigation.

The radiographic appearance frequently gives clues to the true nature of a lesion. For example, a cyst usually appears as a radiolucency with sharp radiographic borders (Figure 22-4,

◇ Box 22-2 ◇

Indications for biopsy

1. Any lesion that persists for more than 2 weeks with no apparent etiologic basis
2. Any inflammatory lesion that does not respond to local treatment after 10 to 14 days (that is, after removing local irritant)
3. Persistent hyperkeratotic changes in surface tissues
4. Any persistent tumescence, either visible or palpable beneath relatively normal tissue
5. Inflammatory changes of unknown cause that persist for long periods
6. Lesions that interfere with local function (e.g., fibroma)
7. Bone lesions not specifically identified by clinical and radiographic findings
8. Any lesion that has the characteristics of malignancy (see Box 22-3)

◇ Box 22-3 ◇

Characteristics of lesions that raise the suspicion of malignancy

1. *Erythroplasia:* Lesion is totally red or has a speckled red and white appearance.
2. *Ulceration:* Lesion is ulcerated or presents as an ulcer.
3. *Duration:* Lesion has persisted more than 2 weeks.
4. *Growth rate:* Lesion exhibits rapid growth.
5. *Bleeding:* Lesion bleeds on gentle manipulation.
6. *Induration:* Lesion and surrounding tissue is firm to the touch.
7. *Fixation:* Lesion feels attached to adjacent structures.

A). Conversely, a ragged radiolucency may indicate a more aggressive lesion, such as a malignancy (Figure 22-4, *B*). Any time an intraosseous lesion is suspected by radiographic evaluation, the dentist must always determine whether the lesion is in fact a normal anatomic structure. This is especially true in radiographs of the maxilla, in which the complex anatomy of the nasal and paranasal cavities can produce extremely misleading radiographic images.

In special instances, radiopaque dyes or instruments can be useful in conjunction with routine or special radiographs. Sialography, the injection of a radiopaque dye into the duct of a salivary gland to outline the ductal structures, can be used to provide an indirect image of the glandular architecture and any pathologic processes within it. Injection of a cyst with a radiopaque dye allows a much more accurate radiographic image of the true extent of the cyst. Radiopaque probes (needles) can be used to localize a foreign object or pathologic entity.

LABORATORY INVESTIGATION

Several oral lesions may be manifestations of systemic diseases. For instance, multiple lytic lesions and loss of lamina dura bone suggest the possibility of hyperparathyroidism. Serum levels of calcium, phosphorus, and alkaline phosphatase should identify this metabolic abnormality. A patient with multiple radiolucencies of the jaws or other bones may also have multiple myeloma. Serum protein analysis can be useful for identifying this disease process.

In most instances, laboratory investigations are unnecessary in evaluation of oral lesions, because they generally are low yield and nondiagnostic for most oral lesions, and because biopsy yields more accurate results. They play an important role, however, once a biopsy yields a tissue diagnosis of a tumor, such as central giant cell granuloma. This histologic

picture may be the result of a solitary nonsystemic lesion or of hyperparathyroidism. In this instance the dentist should determine serum calcium, phosphorus, and alkaline phosphatase levels to rule out the possibility that the lesion is an oral manifestation of a systemic disease.

SURGICAL SPECIMEN FOR PATHOLOGIC EXAMINATION

Once the preceding steps have been accomplished, the dentist should compile a differential diagnosis. In most instances the data obtained from the history and the clinical and radiographic examinations provide enough information for a tentative diagnosis. Lesions that appear traumatic in origin may be initially treated nonsurgically by elimination of any continued source of irritation (for example, relieve or reline dentures or smooth a sharp tooth or appliance). Observation for 10 to 14 days will verify the presumptive diagnosis in these cases; that is, the lesion should heal if trauma is a cause.

When these steps have not provided an accurate diagnosis of a lesion that is thought to be nontraumatic in origin, observation of the lesion for 7 to 10 days may be prudent, unless the clinician strongly suspects significant disease. The patient should be *closely* examined initially, with accurate recording of the exact size and characteristics of the lesion. Comparison at the later date indicates whether improvement has occurred. If no improvement in the lesion is obvious, obtaining tissue for histopathologic analysis is the next and most definitive step. Lesions on which biopsies should be performed are listed in Box 22-2. The typical characteristics of lesions that should raise the clinician's suspicion of malignancy are listed in Box 22-3.

PRINCIPLES OF BIOPSY ◇

Biopsy is the removal of tissue from a living individual for diagnostic examination. It is the least equivocal (most diagnostic) of all the diagnostic procedures performed in the laboratory and should be carried out whenever a definitive diagnosis cannot be obtained using less invasive diagnostic modalities. The four major types of biopsy in and around the oral cavity are cytology, aspiration biopsy, incisional biopsy, and excisional biopsy.

ORAL CYTOLOGY

Cytologic examination for tumor cells was first described as a diagnostic procedure for detection of uterine cervical malignancy. Although application to the oral cavity has been advocated, it should be used as an adjunct to, not a substitute for, biopsy. Studies have shown oral cytology to be unreliable (having an unacceptable number of false negatives), especially when the specimen is examined by pathologists who lack expertise in oral cytology. Cytology allows examination of individual cells but cannot provide the histologic architecture so important to an accurate diagnosis.

INDICATIONS.   When large areas of mucosal change must be monitored for dysplastic change, such as postradiation changes, herpes, and pemphigus, cytology may be helpful.

TECHNIQUE.   The lesion is scraped repeatedly and firmly with a moistened tongue depressor or cement spatula. The cells obtained are smeared evenly on a glass slide, and the slide is immediately immersed in a fixing solution or sprayed with a fixative (hair spray works well). The cells are stained, and the cellular characteristics examined under the microscope.

ASPIRATION BIOPSY

Aspiration biopsy is the use of a needle and syringe to penetrate a lesion for aspiration of its contents. Although no tissue (that is, a collection of cells with an architecture) is obtained with aspiration, it is included here because it is a biopsy in the broadest sense of the word and because it is used frequently for lesions in and around the oral cavity. Inability to aspirate fluid or air indicates that the mass is probably solid. Aspiration biopsy can yield extremely valuable information about the nature of a lesion while causing little patient discomfort. A radiolucent lesion in the jaw that yields straw-colored fluid on aspiration is most likely a cystic lesion. If pus is aspirated, an inflammatory or infectious process should be considered (abscess). Air on aspiration may indicate that a traumatic bone cavity has been entered. Blood on aspiration could represent several lesions, the most important of which is a vascular malformation in the jaw. However, other vascular lesions may produce blood on aspiration. Aneurysmal bone cysts, central giant cell granulomas, and other lesions can produce a bloody aspirate. A fluctuant mass in the soft tissues should also be aspirated to determine its contents before definitive treatment. *Any* radiolucency in the bone of the jaws should be aspirated before surgical intervention to rule out a vascular lesion that could result in life-threatening hemorrhage if incised. Material obtained by aspiration biopsy can be submitted for pathologic examination, chemical analysis, or microbiologic culturing.

INDICATIONS.   Aspiration biopsy should be carried out on all lesions thought to contain fluid (with the possible exception of a mucocele) or any intraosseous lesion before surgical exploration.

TECHNIQUE.   An 18-gauge needle is connected to a 5- or 10-mL syringe. The area is anesthetized and the 18-gauge needle inserted into the depth of the mass during aspiration. The tip of the needle may have to be repeatedly repositioned in an effort to locate a fluid center. For intraosseous lesions, if expansion and thinning of the cortical plates has occurred, the needle may be firmly applied directly through mucoperiosteum to the bone and twisted until it perforates the cortical plate. If this fails, a small mucoperiosteal flap may be elevated and a bur used to penetrate the cortical plate. The needle is then advanced through the cortical hole.

INCISIONAL BIOPSY

An incisional biopsy is a biopsy that samples only a particular or representative part of the lesion. If the lesion is large or has different characteristics at different locations, more than one area of the lesion may require sampling.

INDICATIONS.   If the area under investigation appears difficult to excise because of its extensive size (larger than 1 cm in diameter) or hazardous location or whenever there is a great suspicion of malignancy, incisional biopsy is indicated.

PRINCIPLES.   A biopsy in wedge fashion should be performed on representative areas of the lesion. The biopsy site should be selected in an area that shows complete tissue changes (the lesion extends into normal tissue at the base and/or margin of the lesion). Necrotic tissue should be avoided, because it is useless in diagnosis. The material should be taken from the edge of the lesion to include some normal tissue. However, care must be taken to include an adequate amount of abnormal tissue. It is much better to take a deep, narrow biopsy rather than a broad, shallow one, because superficial changes may be quite different from those deeper in the tissue.

EXCISIONAL BIOPSY

An excisional biopsy implies removal of the entire lesion at the time the surgical diagnostic procedure is performed. A perimeter of normal tissue surrounding the lesion is also excised to ensure total removal. Not only is the entire lesion made available for pathologic examination, but complete excision may constitute definitive treatment.

INDICATIONS.   Excisional biopsy should be employed with smaller lesions (less than 1 cm in diameter) that on clinical examination appear to be benign. Any lesion that can be removed completely without mutilating the patient is best treated by excisional biopsy. Pigmented and small vascular lesions should also be removed in their entirety.

PRINCIPLES.   The entire lesion, along with 2 to 3 mm of normal appearing surrounding tissue, is excised.

Table 22-1. Armamentarium for biopsy

Instruments for soft tissue biopsy	Additional instruments for hard tissue biopsy or biopsy of soft tissue within bone	Instruments for aspiration biopsy
Local anesthetic equipment	Periosteal elevator	5 or 10 mL syringe
Scalpel (no. 15 blade)	Rongeur	18-gauge needle
Scissors with pointed tips	Bur and rotary handpiece	
Fine tissue forceps	Sterile saline irrigation	
Small hemostat	Curettes	
Gauze sponges (suction if necessary)		
Needle holder, needle, and suture		
Biopsy bottle containing 10% formalin		
Biopsy data sheet		

SOFT TISSUE BIOPSY TECHNIQUE AND SURGICAL PRINCIPLES

Oral soft tissue biopsy is a technique that every dentist should be competent to perform. Performed properly, it is a simple and painless procedure that can be done quickly in the dental office with common, simple instrumentation (Table 22-1). The entire oral mucosa is amenable to biopsy, and the technique only differs according to local anatomy and the size and type of lesion.

The surgical principles presented in Chapter 3 apply to biopsy technique, as well as to any other surgical procedure within the oral cavity. These principles are briefly outlined below.

ANESTHESIA

Block local anesthetic techniques are employed when possible. The anesthetic solution should not be injected within the tissues to be removed, because it can cause artifactual distortion of the specimen. When blocks are not possible, infiltration of local anesthetic may be used, but the solution should be injected at least 1 cm away from the lesion (field block).

TISSUE STABILIZATION

Soft tissue biopsies in the oral cavity are frequently performed on movable structures, such as the lips, soft palate, and tongue. Accurate surgical incisions are easiest to perform on tissues that are properly stabilized. Several methods are available in the dental office to achieve tissue stabilization. The lips can be immobilized by an assistant's fingers pinching the lip on both sides of the biopsy area (Figure 22-5, *A*). This method also aids

in hemostasis by compressing the labial arteries. Instruments are available to perform this same function (see Figure 22-5, *B*). Heavy retraction sutures or towel clips can be used to aid immobilization of the tongue or soft palate (Figure 22-5, *C*). When used, the sutures should be placed deeply into the substance of the tissue, away from the proposed biopsy site. In this way they will be useful for secure stabilization, without pulling through the tissue.

HEMOSTASIS

The use of a suction device for aspiration of surgical hemorrhage during biopsy should be avoided. This is especially true of the high-volume evacuators available in most dental offices. Small surgical specimens can be easily aspirated into these devices and lost. Gauze wrapped over the tip of a low-volume suction device or simple gauze compresses are adequate in most cases, unless severe hemorrhage is encountered.

INCISION

A sharp scalpel should be used to incise tissues for biopsy. The use of electrosurgical equipment is much less desirable. This equipment causes destruction of tissue adjacent to the incision line and may distort the histologic architecture of the specimen. Two incisions forming an ellipse at the surface and converging to form a V at the base of the lesion provide a good specimen and leave a wound that is easy to close (Figure 22-6). Modification of the size of the ellipse and the convergence of the V portion of the incisions depend on the suspected depth of the lesion. Palpation gives clues to the size of the lesion beneath the mucosa. In excisional biopsies the initial incisions should be gauged to exceed the total depth of the lesion slightly. In incisional biopsies the depth into the lesion that provides sufficient material for histopathologic evaluation is adequate. Thin, deep specimens are preferable to broad, shallow specimens (Figure 22-7). An attempt should be made to keep incisions parallel to the normal course of nerves, arteries, and veins. This will preclude, as much as possible, their injury. A periphery of normal-appearing tissue should be included in excisional biopsy specimens. If the lesion appears benign, 2 to 3 mm of peripheral tissue is adequate. If the lesion appears malignant, pigmented, vascular, or with diffuse borders, 5 mm of peripheral tissue should be submitted with the specimen. More than one incisional biopsy may be necessary if the lesion's characteristics vary from one area to another (Figure 22-8).

HANDLING OF TISSUE

Any tissue specimen removed must be in a condition that readily lends to histopathologic examination. Crushed specimens may be nondiagnostic and only delay definitive diagnosis and therapy because of the necessity of performing a repeat biopsy. Extreme care must be exercised when removing the surgical specimens. Liberal use of tissue forceps on the specimen will severely damage the cellular architecture, especially in small biopsies. Once a tissue forceps is applied to the specimen, repeated releasing and replacing of

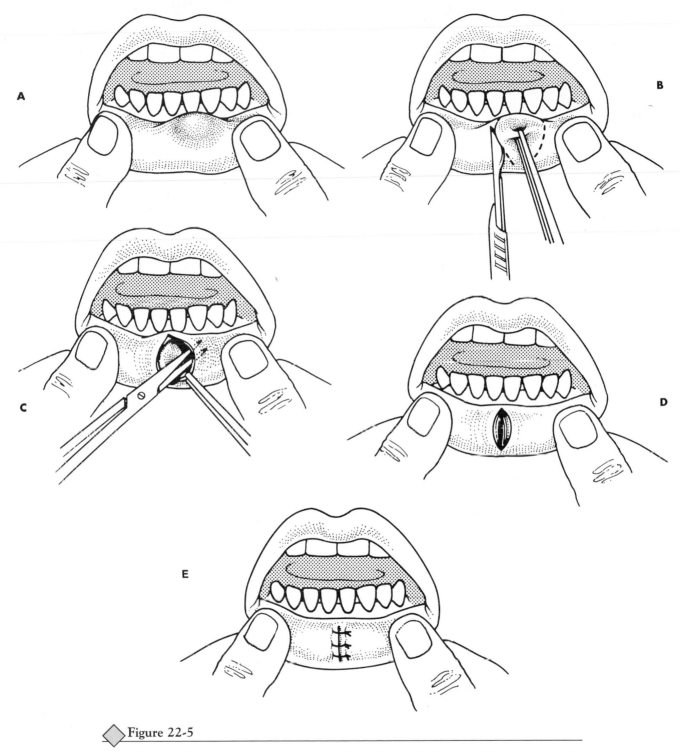

◇ **Figure 22-5**

A, Stabilization of tissue before biopsy, using assistant's fingers. **B,** Excisional biopsy of mucocele. Elliptic incision is made around lesion, followed by submucosal excision of associated minor salivary glands (**C**). Mucosa is undermined and closed (**D** and **E**). *Continued*

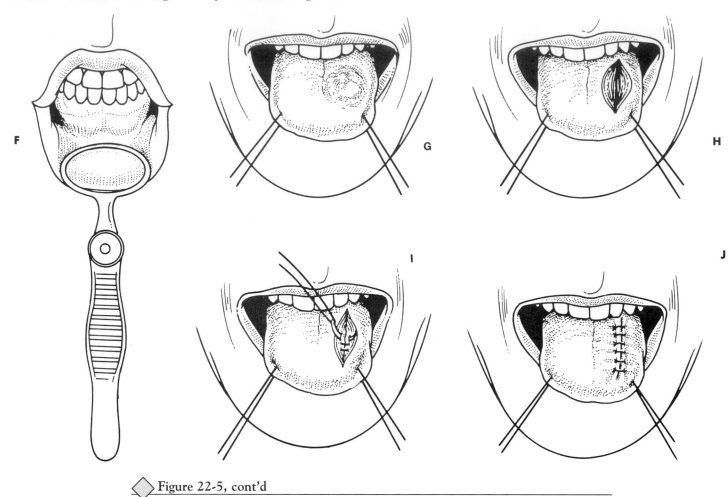

◇ **Figure 22-5, cont'd**

F, Stabilization of tissue with mechanical device. **G,** Stabilization of tissue with traction sutures. Two silk sutures are used to stabilize tongue before excisional biopsy. They are placed through substance of tongue (both mucosa and muscle) to prevent pulling through tissue. Elliptic incision is made around lesion, and lesion is removed (**H**). Resorbable sutures are placed to approximate muscle (**I**) before closing of mucosa (**J**).

the instrument should be avoided. The use of a traction suture through the specimen is an excellent method for avoiding specimen trauma (Figure 22-9).

IDENTIFICATION OF SURGICAL MARGINS

When the dentist suspects anything but a benign process, the margins of the biopsy specimen should be marked with a silk suture to orient the specimen for the pathologist. If the lesion is diagnosed as requiring additional treatment, the pathologist can determine which margins, if any, had residual tumor. Future surgical intervention can then be confined to the margins with residual tumor. The orientation of the lesion and the method by which the specimen was marked should be illustrated on the pathology data sheet.

SPECIMEN CARE

After removal the tissue should be immediately placed in 10% formalin solution (4% formaldehyde) that is at least 20 times the volume of the surgical specimen. The tissue *must* be totally

immersed in the solution, and care should be taken to be sure that the tissue has not become lodged on the wall of the container above the level of the formalin. Wound closure can then proceed.

SURGICAL CLOSURE

Once the specimen is removed, primary closure of the elliptic wound is usually possible. The mucosa is undermined first by placing the closed tips of pointed scissors well into the submucosal area and spreading the tissues by opening the scissor tips (Figure 22-10). The submucosa is loose tissue that allows the mucosa to be easily undermined. The extent to which the margins should be undermined depends on the anatomic location and size of the wound. In the lip, cheek, floor of mouth, and soft palate, undermining of the wound margins by at least the width of the ellipse *in each direction* is easily performed and allows approximation of the tissues with little tension on the suture line. The incision is then closed with just enough sutures to obtain primary closure. Elliptic

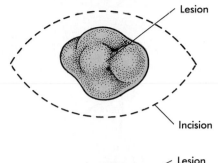

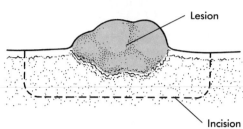

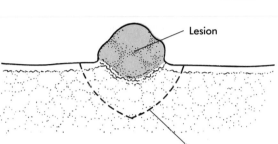

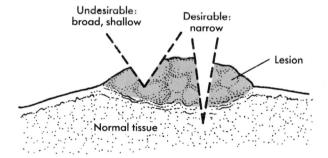

◇ Figure 22-6

Illustration of excisional biopsy of soft tissue lesion. **A,** Surface view. Elliptic incision is made around lesion, at least 3 mm away from lesion. **B,** Side view. Incision is made deep enough to remove lesion completely. **C,** End view. Incisions are made convergent to depth of wound. If excision is made in this manner, closure will be facilitated.

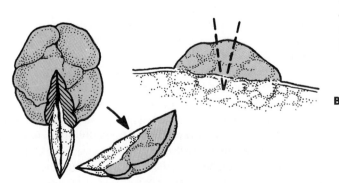

◇ Figure 22-7

A, Illustration showing desirability of obtaining deep specimen rather than broad and shallow specimen when incisional biopsy is performed. If malignant cells are present only at base of lesion, broad and shallow biopsy might not obtain these diagnostic cells. **B,** Illustration showing desirability of obtaining incisional biopsy at margin of soft tissue lesion. Junction of lesion with normal tissue frequently provides pathologist with more diagnostic information than if biopsy were taken only from center of lesion.

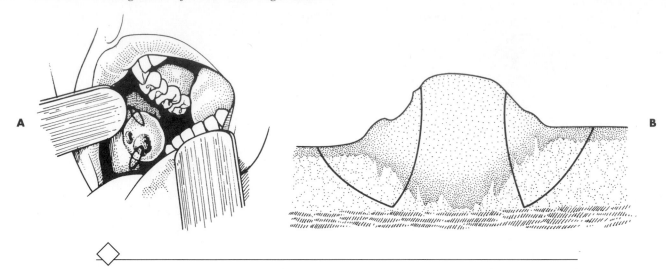

Illustration demonstrating desirability of obtaining more than one incisional biopsy if characteristics of lesion differ from one area to another. Frequently, one area of lesion appears histologically different from another (**A**). When obtaining biopsy on buccal or labial mucosa, incision is usually carried to depth of musculature (**B**).

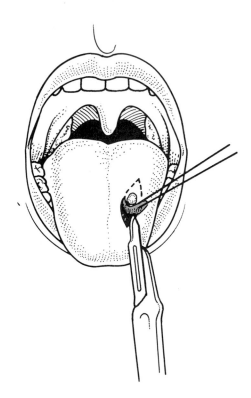

◆ Figure 22-9

Illustration showing use of traction suture placed through specimen. While lesion is incised, traction suture is used to lift specimen from wound bed. Suture can then be tied and left attached to lesion to identify margin of specimen.

incisions on attached mucosal surfaces, such as gingiva and palate, are not closed but rather allowed to heal by secondary intention. Periodontal dressings can be applied to large wounds of the gingiva or palate for patient comfort and to promote healing. Frequently, palatal biopsies of any size are

best managed postoperatively with the use of an acrylic splint, which can be secured to adjacent teeth once it has been lined with a dressing. Biopsy wounds on the dorsum or lateral border of the tongue require sutures to be placed *deeply* and *at frequent intervals* into the substance of the tongue to retain closure (Figure 22-5, *C*). The constant movement of the tongue makes suture retention difficult.

BIOPSY DATA SHEET

All specimens must be carefully labeled and identified with demographic data of both the patient and the dentist's office on a biopsy data sheet (Figure 22-11). The pathology laboratory will supply the dentist with specimen bottles and the biopsy data sheet. All pertinent history and a clinical description of the lesion must be conveyed to the pathologist on this form. Because radiographs of the lesion are useful to the pathologist when dealing with hard tissue lesions, the dentist should submit a copy of them along with the specimen. Inadequate information can waste time and lead to inaccurate diagnoses. The pathologist should receive as much assistance as possible from the dentist to arrive at a diagnosis based on complete data. A complicated biopsy with margin identification or the obtaining of multiple biopsies should be noted carefully. The lesion margins and the location from which the specimen was obtained are identified on the illustration (Figure 22-12). Each specimen should be sent in its own properly labeled bottle.

Once the biopsy has been performed, the dentist should make a follow-up appointment with the patient for 10 days to 2 weeks after surgery. Most pathology laboratories will have the report of a soft tissue biopsy back in this time. The surgical site can be examined at the follow-up appointment, and the report can be discussed with the patient.

It should be emphasized that the final diagnosis should correspond to the clinical course before *and* after biopsy. If the lesion that was reported as benign is suspect and behaves

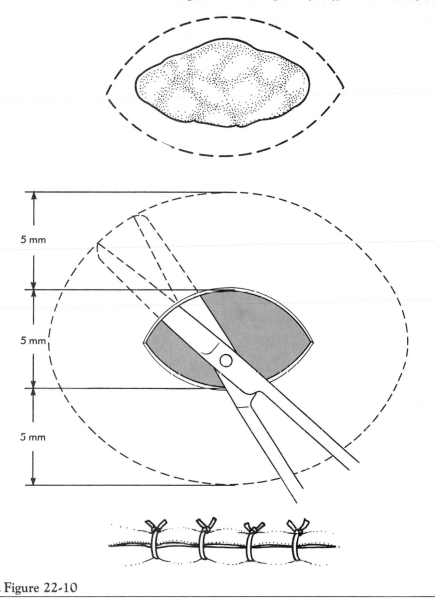

◇ **Figure 22-10**

Illustration showing principles used in closing an elliptic biopsy wound. Mucosa should be undermined bluntly with scissors to width of original ellipse *in each direction.* This allows approximation of wound margins without tension.

clinically as if it were malignant, the dentist should search for further information. A negative pathology report for cancer should not lull the dentist into a false sense of security when the clinical characteristics of the lesion still indicate malignant potential. *If the pathology report does not corroborate the clinical impression of the lesion, the biopsy procedure should be repeated.* The area biopsied may have been nondiagnostic or nonrepresentative of the entire lesion, or the pathologist may have been unfamiliar with the appearance of oral lesions. Always keep in mind that a pathologist's report can be in error. Several types of benign oral pathologic conditions may be read as malignant by general pathologists unfamiliar with oral tissues, which is why many head and neck surgeons repeat the biopsy procedure of oral lesions before performing ablative surgery. The second specimen is sent to a pathologist who has expertise in oral pathology. It is important that

the dentist completely understand the terminology in the pathology report. If unsure or unfamiliar with any terminology, the dentist should contact the pathologist to discuss the findings.

A reported diagnosis of cancer should be handled definitively but very carefully. It is the dentist's responsibility to refer the patient to another clinician or a treatment center for definitive therapy. This referral is an important step, and the dentist must make the patient aware of the significance of the condition. Procrastination on the part of either the dentist or the patient only delays definitive treatment and worsens the prognosis. On the other hand, patients can become irrationally distraught with the bad news and thrown into a state of depression. Thus each dentist must carefully handle these instances in his or her own way and never forget to keep the patient's best interests in mind.

YOUR LOCAL BIOPSY SERVICE
999 City Ave.
Date: _____   Anytown, USA 90909

Patient Name: John Doe
        Address: 1234 Anystreet, Anytown, USA 90909

Submitted by Doctor: Toothache
        Address: 6789 Anyroad, Anytown, USA 90909
Date of Birth: 7-17-53   Occupation: plumber
Sex: male   Race: white

History: 29 yr. old white plumber with 2 month history of asymptomatic
        white plaque on left lateral border of tongue. He noticed it at
        that time and came in for an examination. It was observed for 2
        weeks without a change in its appearance. An incisional biopsy
        was taken and was reported as mild epithelial dysplasia. The
        patient does not know how long it was there prior to his
        noticing it. The last time he saw a dentist was several years
        ago. He denies a history of smoking, drinking, oral habits and
        has had no recent changes in his activities. He cannot recall
        any traumatic episode or oral pain. The patient's past medical
        history is unremarkable. He claims there are no other lesions
        elsewhere on his body.

Clinical Appearance of Lesion: A 3x5cm white, ragged plaque on the left
        lateral border of the tongue which extends onto the dorsum in
        one area, and slightly down onto the floor of the mouth in
        another (see illustration). The lesion is not ulcerated in any
        area and feels "leathery and tough". The incisional biopsy site
        has healed well and cannot be identified at present. There are
        no local factors apparent which may have contributed to the
        lesion. There are no other lesions within the oral cavity or on
        the skin. There is no lymphadenopathy present.

Nature of Treatment: Excisional biopsy

Comments: The anterior margin is marked with one suture, the superior
        margin with two sutures, and the posterior margin with three
        sutures. One centimeter clinical margins were obtained at
        surgery.

◇ Figure 22-11

A, Biopsy data sheet. Such sheets vary from one laboratory to the next; the one listed here represents several. Information provided on this data sheet describes lesion shown in Figure 22-12.

Continued

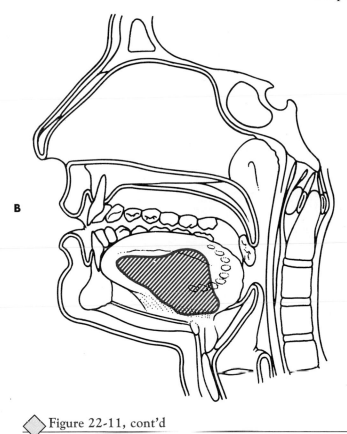

B

⬦ Figure 22-11, cont'd

B, Drawing of lesion, which is to be sent with data sheet.

Intraosseous, or Hard Tissue, Biopsy Technique and Surgical Principles ⬦

A lesion either on or within the osseous tissues of the jaws requires investigation. Frequently, problems related to the dentition are the primary cause, and osseous lesions resolve with proper dental treatment. However, any lesion that seems unrelated to the dentition or does not respond to the customary treatment of the dentition should have tissue removed for definitive diagnosis.

The most common intraosseous lesions the dentist will encounter are periapical granulomas and cysts of the jaws. Because these have a characteristic radiographic appearance and are usually asymptomatic, a presumptive diagnosis is frequently possible. However, treatment may involve surgical removal of the cyst in the form of an excisional biopsy. When a lesion is large, perforating into soft tissues, or suspected of malignancy, incisional biopsy is indicated.

Before performing hard tissue biopsy, the dentist should carefully palpate the area of the jaws where the suspect lesion is located. Comparison with the opposite side is helpful. Bone that feels smooth and firm to palpation usually indicates that the lesion has not expanded or eroded the cortical plate. A

spongy feel to the jaw when compressed indicates erosion or thinning of the cortical plates. This knowledge may change the approach to treatment, as is discussed later.

Hard tissue biopsies are no different in their surgical and pathologic principles from soft tissue biopsies; however, their location mandates some special considerations.

Aspiration Biopsy of Radiolucent Lesions

Any radiolucent lesion that requires biopsy should undergo aspiration biopsy before surgical exploration. This provides the dentist with valuable diagnostic information regarding the nature of the lesion. The results of aspiration biopsy may make the dentist decide to refer the patient to another clinician. For example, brisk, pulsating blood may indicate a vascular lesion, which should not undergo surgical exploration by the general dentist. The return of straw-colored fluid would corroborate the presumptive diagnosis of a cyst, and surgical removal can then be undertaken without hesitation. The aspiration of air may indicate that the needle tip is within the maxillary sinus or a traumatic bone cavity. The technique for aspiration biopsy was outlined previously.

Mucoperiosteal Flaps

Because of their location within or proximal to the jaws, most lesions of hard tissue must be approached through a mucoperiosteal flap. Several varieties of mucoperiosteal flaps are available; the choice depends chiefly on the size and location of the lesion. The principles of flap design outlined in Chapter 8 are the same for surgery for an impacted tooth or an osseous biopsy. The size of the lesion dictates how much access is necessary when excisional biopsy is indicated. Access may necessitate extension of the mucoperiosteal flap. The location of the lesion dictates where the flap incisions are to be made. It is important to avoid major neurovascular structures when possible and to keep incisions over sound bone for closure. Optimally, the flap design should provide 4 to 5 mm of sound bone around the anticipated surgical margins. A central lesion that may have eroded the cortical plate of the jaw is always approached with flap elevation in an area away from the lesion and over sound bone. This technique allows establishment of the proper tissue plane for dissection. As the lesion is approached, fusion of the periosteum to the expanding lesion can more readily be ascertained. All mucoperiosteal flaps for biopsies in or on the jaws should be full thickness and incised through mucosa, submucosa, and periosteum. The dissection to expose the bone is always performed subperiosteally.

Osseous Window

Lesions within the jaws (central lesions) require the use of a cortical window. If expansion of a central lesion has eroded the cortical plate to the point that there is an osseous void once the flap has been elevated, this window (if necessary) can be enlarged with rongeurs or burs. If the cortical plate is intact, a rotating bur should be employed to remove an osseous

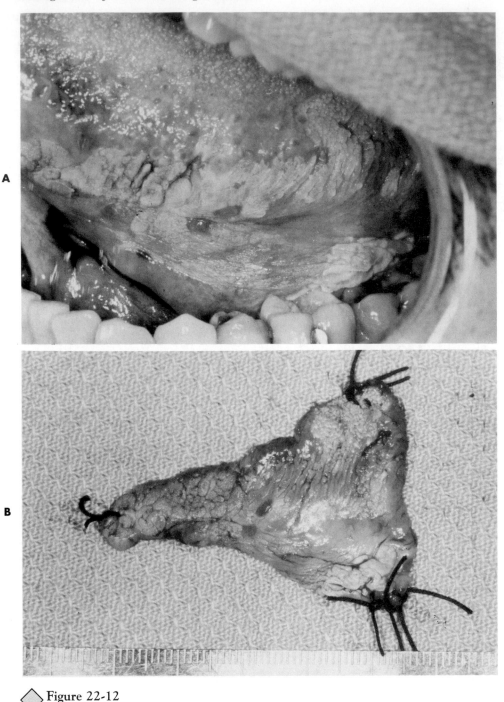

◇ Figure 22-12

A, Lesion described in Figure 22-11. **B,** Specimen after removal. Note marking of margins with sutures to orient pathologist.

window (Figure 22-13). The size of the window depends on the size of the lesion and the proximity of the window to normal anatomic structures such as roots and neurovascular bundles. A trephine bur (Figure 22-14) can also be used to create the initial access opening. Once the window has been created it can be enlarged with a rongeur. The osseous window specimens should always be submitted for histopathologic examination along with the primary specimen.

REMOVAL OF SPECIMEN

The technique for removal of the biopsy specimen depends on the nature of the biopsy (excisional versus incisional) and the consistency of the tissue encountered. Most small lesions that have a connective tissue capsule (such as cysts) can be removed in their entirety. A dental curette is used to peel the connective tissue wall of the specimen from surrounding bone. The concave surface of the instrument should always be kept

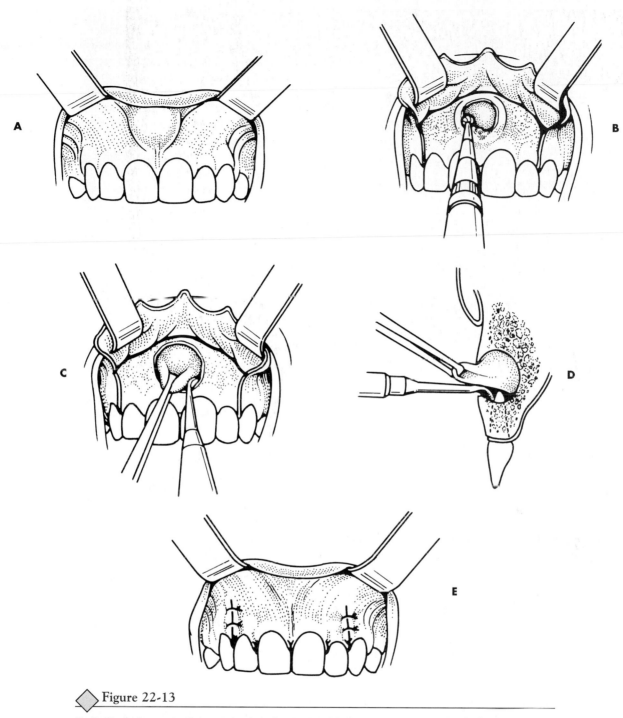

◇ Figure 22-13

Illustrations demonstrating enucleation of cyst. **A,** Mild swelling in area of periapical cyst. **B,** Muco-periosteal flap is elevated from around necks of teeth, and bur is used to remove thinned cortical bone overlying cyst. Care is taken to prevent rupturing cystic contents during this and following steps. **C** and **D,** Spoon type of curette is used to strip cyst from bone. Note concave side of curette is kept in contact with bone. Convex surface is working end of instrument. **E,** Closure.

in contact with the osseous surfaces of the bone cavity (Figure 22-13). The convex surface of the instrument is the portion that actually separates the specimen from surrounding bone. This technique is used until the specimen is free and removed. The bony cavity is inspected after irrigation with sterile saline. Any residual fragments of soft tissue within the cavity should

be removed with curettes. Once the cavity is devoid of residual pathologic tissue, it is irrigated and the flap is replaced and sutured in its proper location. If the dentist is performing an excisional biopsy and encounters a soft tissue specimen that appears solid and poorly separable from surrounding bone, the same procedure as just outlined is performed but followed

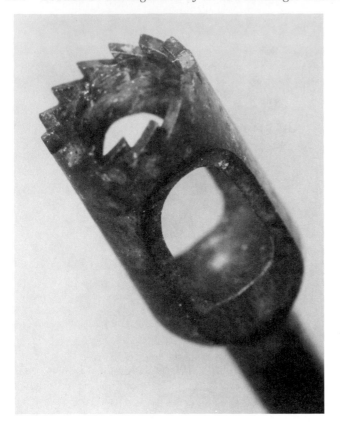

◇ Figure 22-14

Trephine bur, which can be used to create opening into osseous tissue.

by curettage of the bony cavity. Curettage is performed in a similar manner on tooth root surfaces, where the dentist tries to remove a millimeter of adjacent osseous tissue in all directions after the bulk of the lesion is removed. When performing incisional biopsies a section of the tissue is removed and the remaining lesion left undisturbed.

SPECIMEN CARE

The specimen should be handled exactly as outlined for soft tissue biopsies. The pathologist should be made aware that both hard and soft tissues have been submitted. Radiographs should always be included with the specimen.

It may take 2 weeks or longer before the pathology report is available because of the delay required for decalcification of tissue. For any benign process excised with the biopsy procedure, the dentist must follow the patient with serial radiographs to monitor osseous healing. In a lesion that had only an incisional biopsy performed or in a lesion that requires further intervention, the dentist must see that definitive treatment of the lesion (if necessary) is undertaken.

REFERRALS FOR BIOPSY ——◇

As with any dental procedure, clinicians vary in their surgical interests and skills. Some dentists are adept and comfortable in performing almost any biopsy on their patients, whereas others refer all lesions. This variation has as much to do with personal preferences as it does with level of skills. However, the dentist may use certain criteria to determine which biopsies to perform personally and which to refer. These can be summarized into the following categories.

HEALTH OF PATIENT

Dentists frequently encounter patients who have systemic conditions or disease processes that make any surgical treatment either difficult to perform or a hazard to the patient's health. Several systemic conditions discussed in Chapters 1 and 2 complicate routine surgical procedures. If the dentist feels uncomfortable about or is unprepared for managing patients who require special medical precautions, referral should not be delayed.

SURGICAL DIFFICULTY

Biopsies vary in surgical difficulty. If any of the basic surgical principles outlined in Chapter 3 (such as access, lighting, anesthesia, tissue stabilization) are problematic to achieve in a given patient, the biopsy procedure is more complicated. Similarly, as the size of the lesion increases, as its position encroaches on normal anatomic structures, and as its potential for surgical complications (such as bleeding) increases, so does the difficulty of biopsy. Each dentist must decide whether the indicated biopsy is within the general scope of his or her surgical skills. If not, it should be referred.

POTENTIAL FOR MALIGNANCY

The dentist who suspects malignancy has two choices. First, a biopsy can be performed *after* a thorough clinical examination, including examination of regional lymph nodes. Secondly, the patient can be referred *before* biopsy to a clinician who can treat the patient definitively in the event that the lesion is malignant. This latter choice may provide better service if the clinician who treats the patient definitively can see the patient immediately. It is much easier for this clinician to evaluate the lesion thoroughly before surgical manipulation. Biopsy can distort the lesion locally and produce palpable, inflamed lymph nodes. Allowing the clinician to evaluate the patient before biopsy may improve the initial data base and allow a more accurate diagnosis and formulation of treatment. However, if a dentist works in an area where the patient must travel a long distance to see a clinician who can provide definitive treatment or if the clinician cannot be seen for several days, biopsy should not be delayed.

CHAPTER 23

SURGICAL MANAGEMENT OF ORAL PATHOLOGIC LESIONS

Edward Ellis III

The specific surgical techniques for treatment of oral pathologic lesions can be as varied as those for surgical management of any other entity. Each clinician surgically treats his or her patients with techniques based on previous training, biases, experience, personal skill,

intuition, and ingenuity. The purpose of this chapter is not to describe the specifics of surgical techniques for management of individual oral pathologic lesions but to present basic principles that can be applied to a variety of techniques to satisfactorily treat patients. Discussion of this topic is made easier by the fact that many different lesions can be treated in much the same manner, as is outlined later.

BASIC SURGICAL GOALS ◇
ERADICATION OF PATHOLOGIC CONDITION

The therapeutic goal of any extirpative surgical procedure is to remove the entire lesion and leave no cells that could proliferate and cause a recurrence of the lesion. The methods used to achieve this goal vary tremendously and depend on the nature of the pathologic condition of the lesion. Excision of an oral carcinoma necessitates an aggressive approach that must sacrifice adjacent structures in an attempt to remove the lesion thoroughly. Using this approach on a simple cyst would be a tragedy. It is therefore imperative to identify the lesion histologically with a biopsy before undertaking any major surgical extirpative procedure. Only then can the appropriate surgical procedure be chosen to eradicate the lesion with as little destruction of adjacent normal tissue as is feasible.

FUNCTIONAL REHABILITATION OF PATIENT

As just noted the primary goal of surgery to remove a pathologic condition is total removal of the lesion. Although eradication of disease may be the most important goal of treatment, by itself it is frequently inadequate in the comprehensive treatment of patients. The second goal of any treatment used for eradication of disease is an allowance for the functional rehabilitation of the patient. After the primary objective of eradicating a lesion has been achieved, the most important consideration is dealing with the residual defects resulting from the extirpative surgery. These defects can range from a mild obliteration of the labial sulcus secondary to the elimination of an area of denture epulis to a defect in the alveolus following removal of a benign odontogenic tumor or to a hemimandibulectomy defect resulting from carcinoma resection. The best results are obtained when future reconstructive procedures are considered before excision of lesions. Methods of grafting, fixation principles, soft tissue deficits, dental rehabilitation, and patient preparation must be thoroughly evaluated and adequately handled preoperatively.

SURGICAL MANAGEMENT OF CYSTS AND CYSTLIKE LESIONS OF THE JAWS ◇

Surgical management of oral pathologic lesions can best be discussed by broadly classifying pathologic lesions into the following major categories: cysts and cystlike lesions of the jaws, benign tumors of the jaws, malignant tumors, and benign lesions of oral soft tissues.

A cyst is defined generally as an epithelium-lined sac filled with fluid or soft material. The prevalence of cysts in the jaws can be related to the abundant epithelium that proliferates in bone during the process of tooth formation and along lines where the surfaces of embryologic jaw processes fuse. Cysts of the jaws may be divided into two types, those arising from odontogenic epithelium (odontogenic cysts) and those from oral epithelium that is trapped between fusing processes during embryogenesis (fissural cysts). The stimulus that causes resting epithelial cells to proliferate into the surrounding connective tissue has not been determined. Inflammation seems to play a major role in those cysts arising in granulomas from infected dental pulps.

Residual fragments of cystic membrane tend to produce recurrent cysts, which necessitates complete excision of the epithelial lining of the cyst at the time of operation. Some cysts (such as keratocysts) behave more aggressively in both destructive characteristics and recurrence rates. Cysts have been known to destroy large portions of the jaws and to push teeth into remote areas of the jaws (mandibular condyle or angle and coronoid process) (Figure 23-1). Enlargement of cysts is caused by a gradual expansion, and most are discovered on routine dental radiographs. Cysts are usually asymptomatic unless they are secondarily infected. The overlying mucosa is normal in color and consistency; there are no sensory deficits from encroachment on nerves. If the cyst has not expanded or thinned the cortical plate, normal contour and firmness are noted. Palpation with firm pressure may indent the surface of an expanded jaw with characteristic rebound resiliency. If the cyst has eroded through the cortical plate, fluctuance may be noted on palpation.

The radiographic appearance of cysts is characteristic and exhibits a distinct, dense periphery of reactive bone (condensing osteitis) with a radiolucent center (Figure 23-2). Most

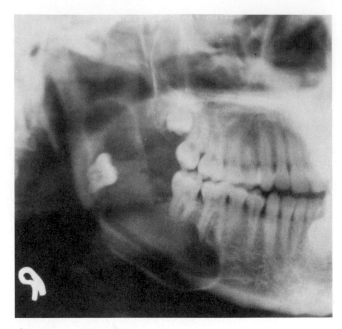

◇ **Figure 23-1**

Mandibular third molar displaced by cyst.

cysts are unilocular in nature; however, multilocularity is often seen in some keratocysts and cystic ameloblastomas (Figure 23-3). Cysts do not usually cause resorption of the roots of teeth; therefore when resorption is seen the clinician should suspect a neoplasm. The epithelial lining of cysts on rare occasions undergoes ameloblastic or malignant changes. Therefore all excised cystic tissue must be submitted for pathologic examination.

Although cysts are broadly classified as odontogenic and fissural, this classification is not relevant to the discussion of surgical techniques to remove cysts. The surgical treatment of cysts is discussed without regard to type of cyst, except for types that warrant special consideration. The principles of surgical management of cysts are also important for managing the more benign odontogenic tumors and other oral lesions.

Cysts of the jaws are treated in one of the following four basic methods: enucleation, marsupialization, a staged combination of the two procedures, and enucleation with curettage.

ENUCLEATION

Enucleation is the process by which the total removal of a cystic lesion is achieved. By definition, it means a *shelling-out of the entire cystic lesion without rupture*. A cyst lends itself to the technique of enucleation because of the layer of fibrous connective tissue between the epithelial component (which lines the interior aspect of the cyst) and the bony wall of the cystic cavity. This layer allows a cleavage plane for stripping the cyst from the bony cavity and makes enucleation similar to stripping periosteum from bone.

Enucleation of cysts should be performed with care, in an attempt to remove the cyst in one piece without fragmentation,

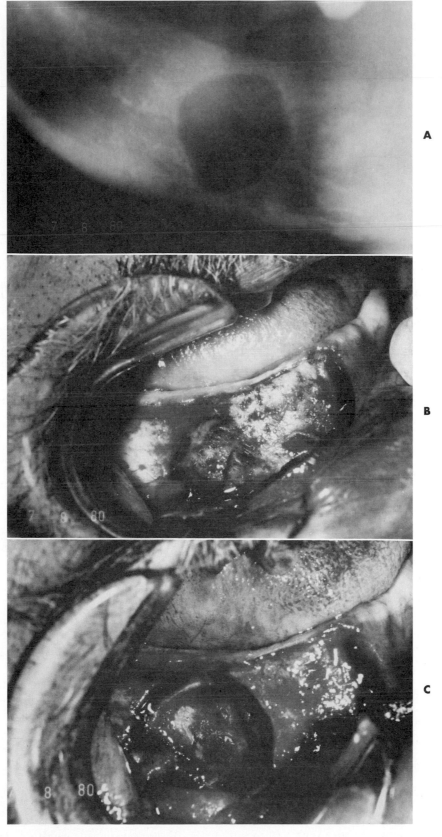

◇ Figure 23-2

A, Typical radiographic appearance of cyst. Note radiolucent center surrounded by zone of reactive bone. **B,** Expansion of buccal bone caused by underlying cyst. Note proximity to mental neurovascular bundle (on distal and inferior aspect of cystic expansion). **C,** Cystic cavity after removal of cyst. Mental nerve left intact. Note amount of osseous tissue destroyed by cyst. *Continued*

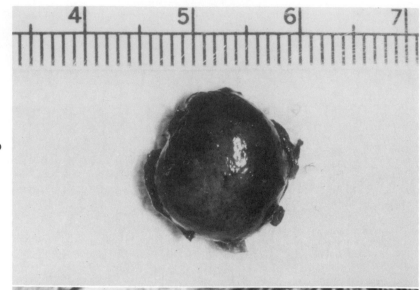

D

◇ Figure 23-2, cont'd

D, Cyst with buccal bone still attached. **E,** Mucosal closure.

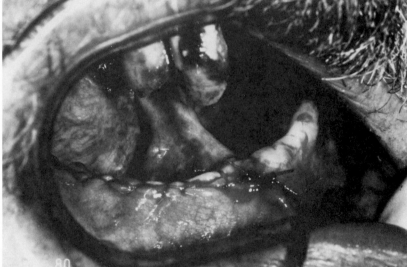

E

◇ Figure 23-3

Multilocular appearance of cyst. This lesion was diagnosed histologically as odontogenic keratocyst.

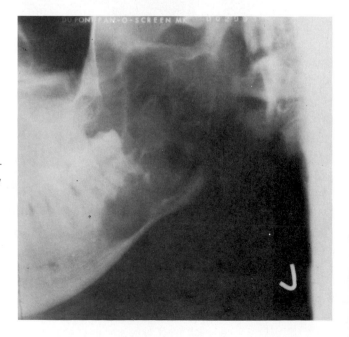

which reduces the chances of recurrence by increasing the likelihood of total removal. In practice, however, maintenance of the cystic architecture is not always possible, and rupture of the cystic contents may occur during manipulation.

INDICATIONS.   Enucleation is the treatment of choice for removal of cysts of the jaws and should be employed with any cyst of the jaw that can be safely removed without unduly sacrificing adjacent structures.

ADVANTAGES.   The main advantage to enucleation is that pathologic examination of the entire cyst can be undertaken. Another advantage is that the initial excisional biopsy (enucleation) has also appropriately treated the lesion. The patient does not have to care for a marsupial cavity with constant irrigations. Once the mucoperiosteal access flap has healed, the patient is no longer bothered by the cystic cavity.

DISADVANTAGES.   If any of the conditions outlined under the section on indications for marsupialization exist (see p. 540), enucleation may be disadvantageous. For example, normal tissue may be jeopardized, fracture of the jaw could occur, devitalization of teeth could result, or associated impacted teeth that the clinician may wish to save could be removed. Thus each cyst must be addressed individually, and the clinician must weigh the pros and cons of enucleation vs. marsupialization (with or without enucleation; see discussion of marsupialization and enucleation).

TECHNIQUE.   The technique for enucleation of cysts was described in Chapter 22; however, the clinician must address special considerations. The use of antibiotics is unnecessary unless the cyst is large or the patient's health condition warrants it (see Chapters 1 and 2).

The periapical (radicular) cyst is the most common of all cystic lesions of the jaws and results from inflammation or necrosis of the dental pulp. Because it is impossible to determine whether a periapical radiolucency is a cyst or a granuloma, removal at the time of the tooth extraction is recommended. If, on the other hand, the tooth is restorable, endodontic treatment followed by periodic radiographic follow-up will allow assessment of the amount of bone fill. If none occurs or the lesion expands in size, the lesion probably represents a cyst and should be removed by periapical surgery. When extracting teeth with periapical radiolucencies, enucleation via the tooth socket can be readily accomplished using curettes when the cyst is small (Figure 23-4). Caution is used in teeth whose apices are close to important anatomic structures, such as the inferior alveolar neurovascular bundle or the maxillary sinus, because the bone apical to the lesion may be very thin or nonexistent. With large cysts, a mucoperiosteal flap may be reflected and access to the cyst obtained through the labial plate of bone, which leaves the alveolar crest intact to ensure adequate bone height after healing.

Once access to a cyst has been achieved through the use of an osseous window, the dentist should begin to enucleate the cyst. A thin-bladed curette is a very suitable instrument for cleaving the connective tissue layer of the cystic wall from the bony cavity. The largest curette that can be accommodated by the size of the cyst and of the access should be employed. The concave surface should always be kept facing the bony cavity—the edge of the convex surface performs the stripping of the cyst. Care must be exercised to avoid tearing the cyst

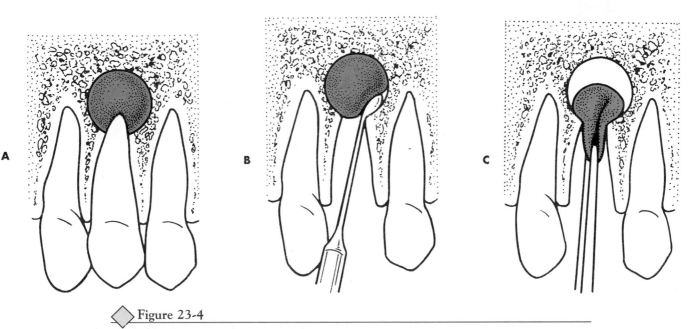

◇ Figure 23-4

Apical cystectomy performed at time of tooth removal. **A** to **C,** Removal with curette via tooth socket. This must be performed with care because of proximity of apices of teeth to other structures, such as maxillary sinus and inferior alveolar canal.

Continued

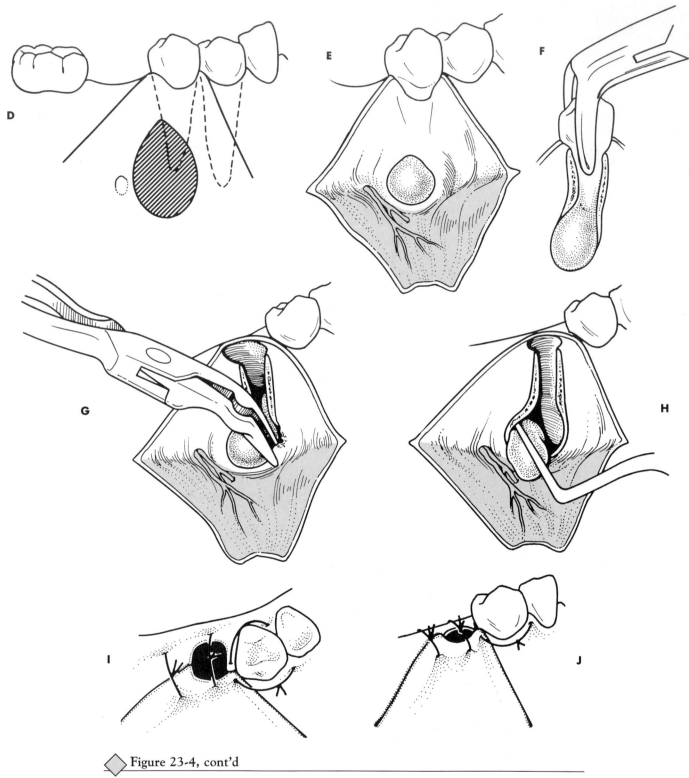

◇ Figure 23-4, cont'd

D to **J,** Removal of apical cyst by flap reflection and creation of osseous window at time of tooth removal.

and allowing the cystic contents to escape, because margins of the cyst are easier to define if the cystic wall is intact. Furthermore, the cyst separates more readily from the bony cavity when the intracystic pressure is maintained.

In large cysts or cysts proximal to neurovascular structures, nerves and vessels are usually found pushed to one side of the

cavity by the slowly expanding cyst and should be avoided or handled as atraumatically and as little as possible. Once the cyst has been removed, the bony cavity should be inspected for remnants of tissue. Irrigating and drying the cavity with

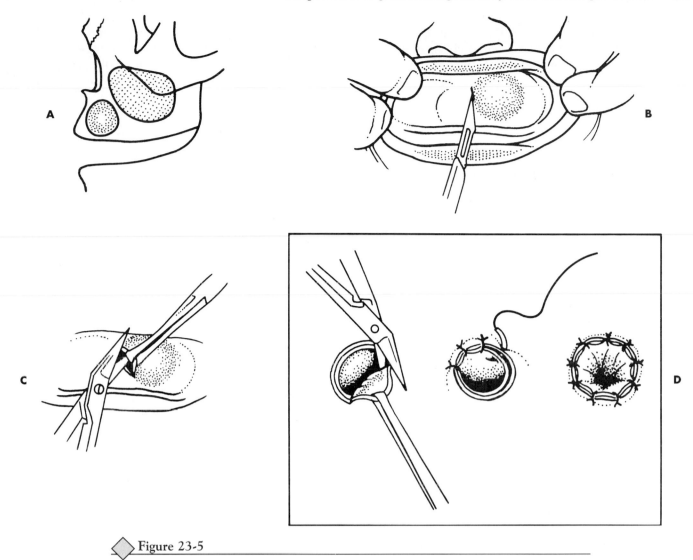

Figure 23-5

Illustration of marsupialization technique. **A,** Cyst within maxilla. **B,** Incision through oral mucosa and cystic wall into center of cyst. **C,** Scissors used to complete excision of window of mucosa and cystic wall. **D,** Oral mucosa and mucosa of cystic wall sutured together around periphery of opening.

gauze will aid in visualizing the entire bony cavity. Residual tissue is removed with curettes. The bony edges of the defect should be smoothed with a file before closure.

Cysts that surround tooth roots or are in inaccessible areas of the jaws require aggressive curettage, which is necessary to remove fragments of cystic lining that could not be removed with the bulk of the cystic wall. Should obvious devitalization of teeth occur during a cystectomy, endodontic treatment of the teeth may be necessary in the near future, which may help to prevent odontogenic infection of the cystic cavity from the necrotic dental pulp.

After enucleation, a watertight primary closure should be made with appropriately positioned sutures. The bony cavity fills with a blood clot, which then organizes over time. Radiographic evidence of bone fill will take 6 to 12 months. Jaws that have been expanded by cysts slowly remodel to a more normal contour.

If the primary closure should break down and the wound dehisce, the bony cavity should then be packed open to heal by secondary intention. The wound should be irrigated with sterile saline, and an appropriate length of strip gauze lightly impregnated with an antibiotic ointment should be gently packed into the cavity. This procedure is repeated every 2 to 3 days, gradually reducing the amount of packing until no more is necessary. Granulation tissue is seen on the bony walls in 3 to 4 days and slowly obliterates the cavity and obviates the need for packing. The oral epithelium then closes over the top of the opening, and osseous healing will progress.

MARSUPIALIZATION

Marsupialization, decompression, and the Partsch operation all refer to creating a surgical window in the wall of the cyst, evacuating the contents of the cyst, and maintaining continuity between the cyst and the oral cavity, maxillary sinus, or nasal cavity (Figure 23-5). The only portion of the cyst that is removed is the piece removed to produce the window. The remaining cystic lining is left in situ. This process decreases intracystic pressure and promotes shrinkage of the cyst and bone fill. Marsupialization can be used either as the sole therapy for a cyst or as a preliminary step in management, with enucleation deferred until later.

INDICATIONS. The following factors should be considered before deciding whether a cyst should be removed by marsupialization:

1. *Amount of tissue injury.* Proximity of a cyst to vital structures can mean unnecessary sacrifice of tissue if enucleation is employed. For example, if enucleation of a cyst would create oronasal or oroantral fistulae or cause injury to major neurovascular structures (such as the inferior alveolar nerve) or devitalization of healthy teeth, marsupialization should be considered.
2. *Surgical access.* If access to all portions of the cyst is difficult, portions of the cystic wall may be left behind, which could result in recurrence. Marsupialization should therefore be considered.
3. *Assistance in eruption of teeth.* If an unerupted tooth that is needed in the dental arch is involved with the cyst (that is, a dentigerous cyst), marsupialization may allow its continued eruption into the oral cavity (Figure 23-6).
4. *Extent of surgery.* In an unhealthy or debilitated patient, marsupialization is a reasonable alternative to enucleation, because it is simple and may be less stressful for the patient.
5. *Size of cyst.* In very large cysts, there is a risk of jaw fracture during enucleation. It may be better to marsupialize the cyst and defer enucleation until after considerable bone fill has occurred.

ADVANTAGES. The main advantage of marsupialization is that it is a simple procedure to perform. It may also spare vital structures from damage should immediate enucleation be attempted.

DISADVANTAGES. The major disadvantage of marsupialization is that pathologic tissue is left in situ, without thorough histologic examination. Although the tissue taken in the window can be submitted for pathologic examination, there is a possibility of a more aggressive lesion in the residual tissue. Another disadvantage is that the patient is inconvenienced in several respects. The cystic cavity must be kept clean to prevent infection, because the cavity frequently traps food debris. In most instances this means that the patient must irrigate the cavity several times every day with a syringe. This may continue for several months, depending on the size of the cystic cavity and the rate of bone fill.

TECHNIQUE. Prophylactic systemic antibiotics are not usually indicated in marsupialization, although they should be used if the patient's health condition warrants it (see Chapters 1 and 2). Following anesthetization of the area, the cyst is aspirated as discussed in Chapter 22. If the aspirate confirms the presumptive diagnosis of a cyst, the marsupialization procedure may proceed (Figure 23-7). The initial incision is usually circular or elliptic and creates a large (1 cm or larger) window into the cystic cavity. If the bone has been expanded and thinned by the cyst, the initial incision may extend through the bone into the cystic cavity. If this is the case, the tissue contents of the window are submitted for pathologic examination. If the overlying bone is thick, an osseous window is removed carefully with burs and rongeurs. The cyst is then incised to remove a window of the lining, which is submitted for pathologic examination. The contents of the cyst are evacuated, and, if possible, visual examination of the residual lining of the cyst is undertaken. Irrigation of the cyst removes any residual fragments of debris. *Areas of ulceration or thickening of the cystic wall should alert the clinician to the possibility of dysplastic or neoplastic changes in the wall of the cyst.* In this instance, enucleation of the entire cyst or incisional biopsy of the suspicious area(s) should be undertaken. If there is ample thickness to the cystic lining and if access permits, the perimeter of the cystic wall around the window can be sutured to the oral mucosa. Otherwise, the cavity should be packed with strip gauze impregnated with tincture of benzoin or an antibiotic ointment. This packing must be left in place for 10 to 14 days to prevent the oral mucosa from healing over the cystic window. By 2 weeks the lining of the cyst should be healed to the oral mucosa around the periphery of the window. Careful instructions to the patient regarding cleansing of the cavity are necessary.

When marsupializing cysts of the maxilla, the clinician has two choices of where the cyst will become exteriorized. The cyst may be surgically opened into the oral cavity, as just described, or into the maxillary sinus or nasal cavity. For cysts that have destroyed a large portion of the maxilla and encroached on the antrum or nasal cavity, the cyst may be approached from the facial aspect of the alveolus, as just described. Once a window into the cyst has been made, a second unroofing can be widely performed into the adjacent maxillary antrum or nasal cavity. (If access permits, the entire cyst can be enucleated at this point, which allows the cystic cavity to become lined with respiratory epithelium that migrates from the adjoining maxillary sinus or nasal cavity.) The oral opening is then closed and permitted to heal. The cystic lining is thereby continuous with the lining of the antrum or nasal cavity.

Marsupialization is rarely used as the sole form of treatment for cysts. In most instances, marsupialization is followed by enucleation. In the case of a dentigerous cyst, however, there may not be any residual cyst to remove once the tooth has erupted into the dental arch. Also, if further surgery is contraindicated because of concomitant medical problems, marsupialization may be performed without future enucleation. The cavity may or may not obliterate totally with time. If it is kept clean, the cavity should not become a problem.

MARSUPIALIZATION FOLLOWED BY ENUCLEATION

Marsupialization is frequently followed by enucleation at a later date. Initial healing is rapid after marsupialization, but the size of the cavity may not decrease appreciably past a

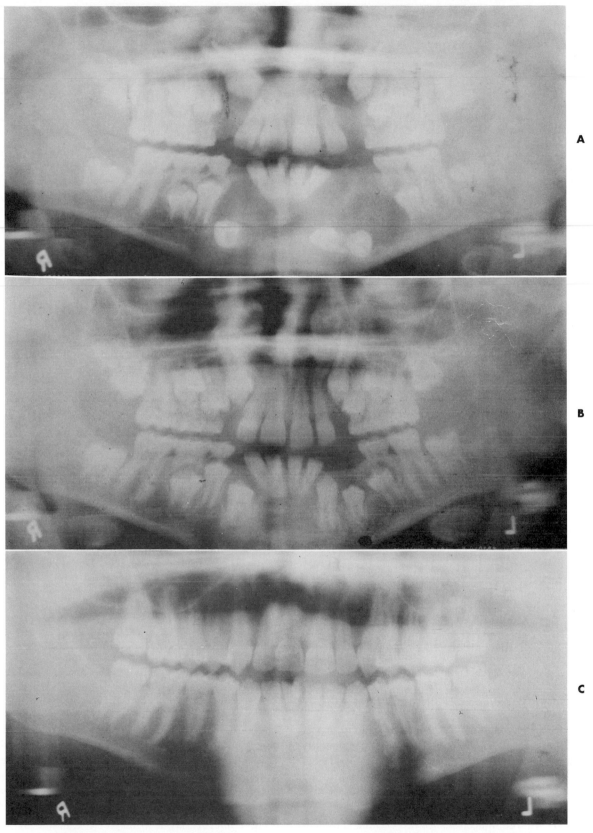

◇ **Figure 23-6**

Marsupialization of multiple dentigerous cysts. **A,** Radiographic appearance before marsupialization. Marsupialization was carried out along crest of alveolar process on both sides. **B,** One year later. Note uprighting and eruption of teeth. **C,** Three years later. No orthodontic assistance was required. *(From Ellis E, Fonseca RJ: Therapy of cysts and odontogenic tumors. In Thawley SE et al, editors: Comprehensive management of head and neck tumors, Philadelphia, 1987, WB Saunders; courtesy Dr. Timothy Pickens, Ypsilanti, Mich.)*

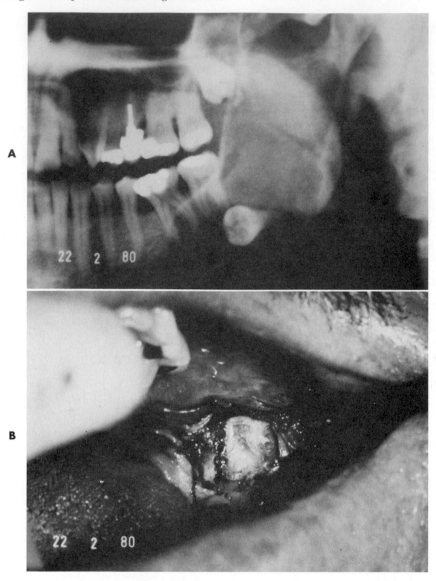

⬦ **Figure 23-7**
_____

This case combined marsupialization with subsequent enucleation. **A,** Radiographic appearance of lesion and displaced tooth on initial examination. **B,** Mucosa reflected from anterior border of ascending ramus. Osseous window created by use of round bur; bone was gently removed, exposing underlying fibrous cystic wall (white membrane). Circular piece of this cystic wall was removed, exposing cystic lumen. Cystic mucosa was then sutured to oral mucosa around periphery of osseous window. Osseous window and cystic specimen were submitted for pathologic examination.

Continued

certain point. The objectives of the marsupialization procedure have been accomplished at this time, and a secondary enucleation may be undertaken without injury to adjacent structures. The combined approach reduces morbidity and accelerates complete healing of the defect.

INDICATIONS. The indications for this combined modality of surgical therapy are the same as those listed for the technique of marsupialization. These indications are predicated on a thorough evaluation of the amount of tissue injury enucleation would cause, the degree of access for enucleation, whether or not impacted teeth associated with the cyst would

benefit from eruptional guidance with marsupialization, the medical condition of the patient, and the size of the lesion. However, if the cyst does not totally obliterate following marsupialization, enucleation should be considered. Another indication for enucleation of a previously marsupialized cyst is a cystic cavity that the patient is finding difficult to cleanse. The clinician may also desire to examine the entire lesion histologically.

ADVANTAGES. The advantages of combined marsupialization and enucleation are the same as those listed for marsupialization *and* enucleation. In the marsupialization

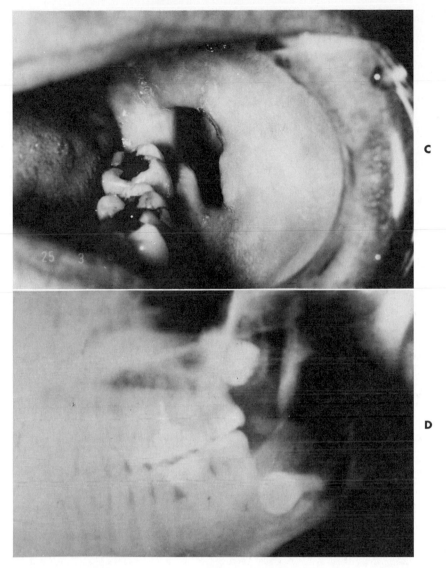

◇ **Figure 23-7, cont'd**

C, Appearance at 13 months of opening created into cyst. The patient had irrigated lumen twice a day. **D,** Radiographic appearance at 13 months. Note extent of bone regeneration (compare with Figure 23-7, **A**). There is now ample osseous tissue surrounding inferior alveolar neurovascular bundle to prevent damage during enucleation. *Continued*

phase, the advantage is that this is a simple procedure that spares adjacent vital structures. In the enucleation phase, the entire lesion becomes available for histologic examination. Another advantage is the development of a thickened cystic lining, which makes the secondary enucleation an easier procedure.

DISADVANTAGES. The disadvantages of this modality of surgical intervention are the same as those for marsupialization. The total cyst is not removed initially for pathologic examination. However, subsequent enucleation may then detect any occult pathologic condition.

TECHNIQUE. The cyst is first marsupialized, and osseous healing is then allowed to progress. Once the cyst has

decreased to a size that makes it amenable to complete surgical removal, enucleation is performed as the definitive treatment. The appropriate time for enucleation is when bone is covering adjacent vital structures, which prevents their injury during enucleation, and when adequate bone fill has provided enough strength to the jaw to prevent fracture during enucleation. (See Figure 23-7.)

The initial incisions for enucleation of the cyst differ, however, from those when the cyst is not first marsupialized. The cyst has a common epithelial lining with the oral cavity following marsupialization. The window initially made into the cyst contains the epithelial bridge between the cystic cavity and the oral cavity. This epithelium *must* be removed completely with the cystic lining; an elliptic incision completely encircling the window must be made down to sound

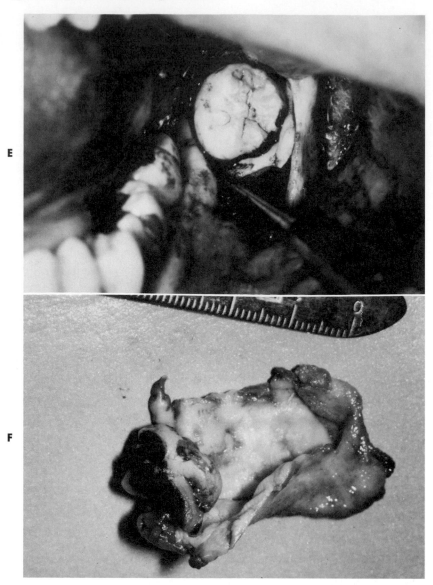

◇ Figure 23-7, cont'd

E, Cystectomy easily performed 13 months after initial marsupialization. Tooth being removed with cystic wall. Note thickness of cystic wall. **F,** Specimen after removal.

bone. The clinician then has the opportunity to begin stripping the cyst from the window into the cystic cavity. The plane of dissection is easily established with this approach, and the cyst can be enucleated without difficulty.

Once the cyst has been enucleated, the oral soft tissues must be closed over the defect if possible, which may require the development and mobilization of soft tissue flaps that can be advanced and sutured in a watertight manner over the osseous window. If complete closure of the wound cannot be achieved, packing the cavity with strip gauze impregnated with an antibiotic ointment is acceptable. This packing must be changed repeatedly with cleansing of the cavity until granulation tissue has obliterated the opening and epithelium has closed over the wound.

ENUCLEATION WITH CURETTAGE

Enucleation with curettage means that after enucleation a curette or bur is used to remove 1 to 2 mm of bone around the entire periphery of the cystic cavity. This is done to remove any remaining epithelial cells that may be present in the periphery of the cystic wall or bony cavity. These cells could proliferate into a recurrence of the cyst.

INDICATIONS.   There are two instances in which the clinician should perform curettage with enucleation. If the clinician is removing an odontogenic keratocyst, the more aggressive approach of enucleation with curettage should be used, because odontogenic keratocysts exhibit aggressive clinical behavior and a markedly high rate of recurrence.[2]

Reported recurrence rates have been between 20% and 60%.[5] Reasons for locally aggressive behavior are based on the increased mitotic activities and cellularity of the odontogenic keratocyst's epithelium.[4,6,7] Daughter, or satellite, cysts, found in the periphery of the main cystic lesion, may be incompletely removed, which contributes to the increased rate of recurrence. The cystic lining is usually very thin and readily fragmented and makes thorough enucleation difficult. Therefore when an odontogenic keratocyst is clinically suspected the minimal treatment should be careful enucleation with aggressive curettage of the bony cavity. Should the lesion recur, treatment must be predicated on the following factors: if the area is accessible, another attempt at enucleation could be undertaken; if inaccessible, bony resection with 1 cm margins should be considered. Whatever the treatment the patient must be followed closely for recurrence, because odontogenic keratocysts have recurred years after treatment.

The second instance in which enucleation with curettage is indicated is with any cyst that recurs after what was deemed a thorough removal. The reasons for curettage in this case are the same as those outlined previously.

ADVANTAGES.　If enucleation leaves epithelial remnants, curettage may remove them, thereby decreasing the likelihood of recurrence.

DISADVANTAGES.　Curettage is more destructive of adjacent bone and other tissues. The dental pulps may be stripped of their neurovascular supply when curettage is performed close to the root tips. Adjacent neurovascular bundles can be similarly damaged. Curettage must always be performed with great care to avoid these hazards.

TECHNIQUE.　After the cyst has been enucleated and removed, the bony cavity is inspected for proximity to adjacent structures. A sharp curette or a bone bur with sterile irrigation can be used to remove a 1- to 2-mm layer of bone around the complete periphery of the cystic cavity. This should be done with extreme care when working proximal to important anatomic structures. The cavity is then cleansed and closed.

PRINCIPLES OF SURGICAL MANAGEMENT OF JAW TUMORS ◇

A discussion of the surgical management of jaw tumors is made easier by the fact that many tumors behave similarly and therefore can be treated in a similar manner. The three main modalities of surgical excision of jaw tumors are enucleation (with or without curettage), marginal (segmental) or partial resection, and composite resection (Box 23-1). Many benign tumors behave nonaggressively and are therefore treated conservatively with enucleation and/or curettage (Table 23-1).

Another group of benign oral tumors behaves more

◇ Box 23-1 ◇

Types of surgical operations used for the removal of jaw tumors

A. Enucleation and/or curettage: Local removal of tumor by instrumentation in direct contact with the lesion. Used for very benign types of lesions.

B. Resection: Removal of a tumor by incising through uninvolved tissues around the tumor, thus delivering the tumor without direct contact during instrumentation (also known as *en bloc resection*).

1. **Marginal (segmental) resection:** Resection of a tumor without disruption of the continuity of the bone.
2. **Partial resection:** Resection of a tumor by removing a full-thickness portion of the jaw. (In the mandible, this can vary from a small continuity defect to a hemimandibulectomy. Jaw continuity is disrupted.)
3. **Total resection:** Resection of a tumor by removal of the involved bone (for example, maxillectomy and mandibulectomy).
4. **Composite resection:** Resection of a tumor with bone, adjacent soft tissues, and contiguous lymph node channels. (This is an ablative procedure used most commonly for malignant tumors.)

---

aggressively and requires margins of uninvolved tissue to lessen the chance of recurrence. Marginal (segmental) or partial resection is used for removal of these lesions (Figure 23-8). The last group of tumors includes the malignant varieties. These tumors require more radical intervention, with wider margins of uninvolved tissue. Surgery may include the removal of adjacent soft tissues and dissection of lymph nodes. Radiotherapy and/or chemotherapy, either alone or in addition to surgery, may be used.

Besides cysts, the most common jaw lesions the dentist encounters either are inflammatory in nature or benign neoplasms. Most of them lend themselves to removal by simple excisional biopsy techniques. However, more aggressive lesions are occasionally encountered, and several factors must be used to determine the most appropriate type of therapy. The most important of these factors is the aggressiveness of the lesion. Other factors that must be evaluated before surgery are the anatomic location of the lesion, its confinement to bone, the duration of the lesion, and the possible methods for reconstruction following surgery.

AGGRESSIVENESS OF LESION

Surgical therapy of oral lesions ranges from enucleation and/or curettage to composite resection. Histologic diagnosis positively identifies and therefore directs the treatment of the lesion. Because of the wide range in behavior of oral lesions, the prognosis is related more to the histologic diagnosis,

Table 23-1. Types of jaw tumors and primary treatment modalities

Enucleation and/or curettage	Marginal or partial resection	Composite resection*
Odontogenic tumors		
Odontoma	Ameloblastoma	Malignant ameloblastoma
Ameloblastomic fibroma	Calcifying epithelial odontogenic tumor	Ameloblastic fibrosarcoma
Ameloblastic fibroodontoma	Myxoma	Ameloblastic odontosarcoma
Adenomatoid odontogenic tumor	Ameloblastic odontoma	Primary intraosseous carcinoma
Calcifying odontogenic cyst	Squamous odontogenic tumor	
Cementoblastoma		
Central cementifying fibroma		
Fibroosseous lesions		
Central ossifying fibroma	Benign chondroblastoma	Fibrosarcoma
Fibrous dysplasia (if necessary)		Osteosarcoma
Cherubism (if necessary)		Chondrosarcoma
Central giant-cell granuloma		Ewing's sarcoma
Aneurysmal bone cyst		
Osteoma		
Osteoid osteoma		
Osteoblastoma		
Other lesions		
Hemangioma	Hemangioma	Lymphomas
Eosinophilic granuloma		Intraosseous salivary gland malignancies
Neurilemmoma		Neurofibrosarcoma
Neurofibroma		Carcinoma that has invaded jaw
Pigmented neurectodermal tumor		

NOTE: These are generalities. Treatment is individualized for each patient and each lesion.

*These lesions are malignancies and may be treated variably. For lesions totally within the jaw, partial resection may be performed without adjacent soft tissue and lymph node dissections. Radiotherapy and chemotherapy may also play a role in the overall therapy.

which indicates the biologic behavior of the lesion, than to any other single factor.

ANATOMIC LOCATION OF LESION

The location of a lesion within the mouth or perioral areas may severely complicate surgical excision and therefore jeopardize the prognosis. A nonaggressive, benign lesion in an inaccessible area, such as the pterygomaxillary fissure, presents an obvious surgical problem. Conversely, a more aggressive lesion in an easily accessible and resectable area, such as the anterior mandible, often offers a better prognosis.

MAXILLA VERSUS MANDIBLE. Another important consideration with some oral lesions, such as the more aggressive odontogenic tumors and carcinomas, is whether they are within the mandible or the maxilla. The adjacent maxillary sinuses and nasopharynx allow tumors of the maxilla to grow asymptomatically to large sizes, with symptoms occurring late. Thus maxillary tumors produce a poorer prognosis than those within the mandible.

PROXIMITY TO ADJACENT VITAL STRUCTURES. The proximity of benign lesions to adjacent neurovascular structures and teeth is an important consideration, because preservation of these structures should be attempted. Frequently, the apices of adjacent tooth roots are completely uncovered during a surgical procedure. The dental pulps are stripped of their blood supply. These teeth should be considered for endodontic treatment to prevent an odontogenic infection, which would complicate healing and

jeopardize the success of bone grafts placed in an adjacent area.

SIZE OF TUMOR. The amount of involvement within a particular site, such as the body of the mandible, has a bearing on the type of surgical procedure necessary to obtain a cure with the more aggressive lesions. When possible, the inferior border of the mandible is left intact to maintain continuity. This can be accomplished by marginal resection of the involved area. When the tumor extends through the entire thickness of the involved jaw, a partial resection becomes mandatory.

INTRAOSSEOUS VERSUS EXTRAOSSEOUS LOCATION. An aggressive oral lesion confined to the interior of the jaw, without perforation of the cortical plates, offers a better prognosis than one that has invaded surrounding soft tissues. Invasion of soft tissues indicates a more aggressive tumor, which, because of its presence in soft tissues, makes complete removal more difficult and sacrifices more normal tissues. In the latter case the soft tissue in the area of the perforation should be locally excised. A supraperiosteal excision of the involved jaw should be undertaken if the cortical plate has been thinned to the point of being eggshell in nature without obvious perforation.

DURATION OF LESION

Several oral tumors exhibit slow growth and may become static in size. The odontomas, for example, may be discovered in the second decade of life, and their size may remain

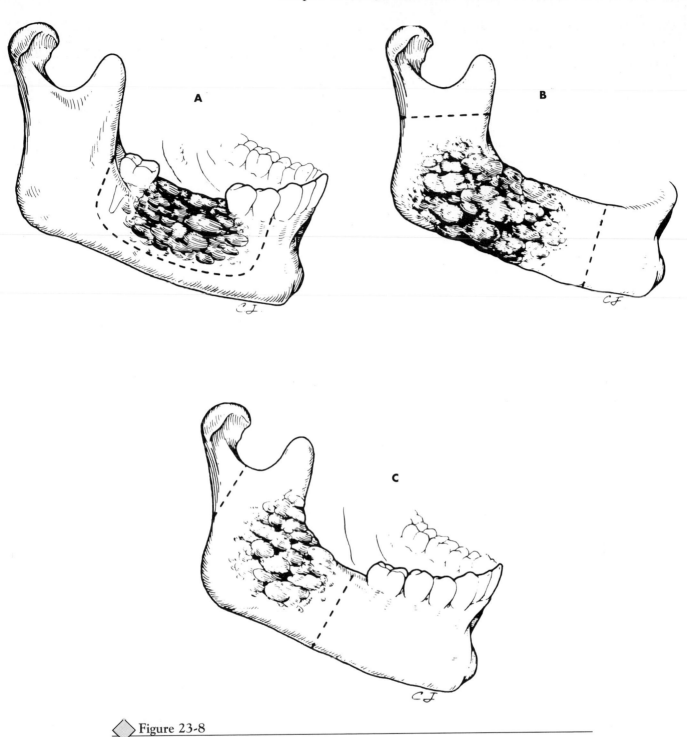

◇ **Figure 23-8**

Common types of mandibular resection. **A,** Marginal or segmental resection, which does not disrupt mandibular continuity. **B** and **C,** Partial mandibular resections, which disrupt mandibular continuity. Note attempts to leave mandibular condyle to facilitate reconstruction.

unchanged for many years. The slower-growing lesions seem to follow a more benign course, and treatment should be individually tailored to each case.

RECONSTRUCTIVE EFFORTS

As previously noted, the goal of any surgical procedure to remove a pathologic lesion should not only be the eradication of disease but also the facilitation of the patient's functional well-being. Thus reconstructive procedures should be planned and anticipated *before* initial surgery is performed. Frequently, the goals of reconstruction dictate a surgical technique that is just as effective as another technique in the removal of the disease but more optimal for facilitating future reconstructive efforts.

Jaw Tumors Treated with Enucleation and/or Curettage

Most jaw tumors with a low rate of recurrence can be treated with enucleation and/or curettage; for example, most of the odontogenic tumors, including odontomas, ameloblastic fibromas, ameloblastic fibro-odontomas, keratinizing and calcifying odontogenic cysts, adenomatoid odontogenic tumors, cementoblastomas, and central cementifying (ossifying) fibromas. Table 23-1 lists other lesions that are treated in this manner.

TECHNIQUE. The technique for enucleation and/or curettage of jaw tumors is not unlike that described for cysts. However, additional procedures, such as sectioning large calcified masses with burs in odontomas and cementomas, may be required. In these instances the principles discussed in Chapter 9 for the removal of impacted teeth are used.

Jaw Tumors Treated with Marginal or Partial Resection

When the lesion is known to be aggressive, either by histopathologic determination or by its clinical behavior, or is of such a consistency that total removal by enucleation and/or curettage would be difficult, removal may be facilitated by resecting the lesion with adequate bony margins. Odontogenic lesions treated in this manner are the ameloblastoma, the odontogenic (fibro-) myxoma, the calcifying epithelial odontogenic tumor (Pindborg), the squamous odontogenic tumor, and the ameloblastic odontoma. Table 23-1 lists other lesions treated in this manner.

TECHNIQUE. As a general principle, the resected specimen should include the lesion and 1-cm bony margins around the radiographic boundaries of the lesion. If this can be achieved with the inferior border of the mandible left intact, marginal resection is the preferred method. Reconstruction will then be limited to replacing the lost osseous structure, including the alveolus (Figure 23-9). If the lesion is close to the inferior border, the full thickness of the mandible must be included in the specimen, which disrupts mandibular continuity (Figure 23-10). Reconstruction in this instance is much more difficult, because the remaining mandibular fragments must be secured in their proper relationship to one another for proper function and symmetry to be restored.

The surgical technique for marginal (segmental) resection is relatively straightforward. A full-thickness mucoperiosteal flap is developed and stripped from the bone to be removed. Air-driven surgical saws or burs are then used to section the bone in the planned locations, and the segment is removed. Whenever marginal or partial resection is used, the clinician must determine whether the tumor has perforated the cortical plates and invaded adjacent soft tissues, in which case it is necessary to sacrifice a layer of soft tissue to eradicate the tumor, and a supraperiosteal dissection of the involved bone is performed. Immediate reconstruction is more difficult, because there may not be enough remaining soft tissues to close over bone grafts.

If there is any question as to the adequacy of the soft tissue surgical margins around a lesion when surgery is being performed in a hospital setting, specimens along the margins can be removed and sent immediately to the pathologist for histopathologic examination. This process is performed in approximately 20 minutes by freezing the tissue in liquid carbon dioxide or nitrogen and then sectioning and staining the tissue for immediate examination. The accuracy of "frozen-section" examination is good when used for detecting adequacy of surgical margins. However, it is less accurate when trying to diagnose a lesion histopathologically for the first time.

Malignant Tumors of the Oral Cavity ———◇

Malignancies of the oral cavity may arise from a variety of tissues, such as salivary gland, muscle, and blood vessels, or may even present as metastases from distant sites. Most common, however, are epidermoid carcinomas of the oral mucosa, which are the form of cancer that the dentist is in a position to discover first by doing thorough oral examinations. The seriousness of an oral malignancy can vary from the necessity for a simple excisional biopsy to composite jaw resection with neck dissection (removal of the lymph nodes and other visceral structures adjacent to lymph node channels in neck) to effect a cure. Because of the variation in clinical presentation, *clinical staging* is usually undertaken before a treatment plan is formulated.

Clinical staging refers to assessing the extent of the disease before undertaking treatment and has as its purposes (1) selection of the best treatment and (2) meaningful comparison of the end results reported from different sources. Clinical staging of the lesion is performed for several varieties of oral malignancies, including epidermoid carcinomas and oral lymphomas. Staging is performed differently for each type of malignancy and may involve extensive diagnostic tests, such as radiographs, blood tests, and even surgical exploration of other body areas to evaluate the extent of possible tumor metastasis. Once the tumor is staged, treatment is formulated. Several types of malignancies have well-defined treatment protocols that have been designed by surgeons and oncologists in an effort to study the effectiveness of treatment regimens more carefully.

Treatment Modalities for Malignancies

Malignancies of the oral cavity are treated with surgery, radiation, chemotherapy, or a combination of these modalities. The treatment for any given case depends on several factors, including the histopathologic diagnosis, the location of the tumor, the presence and degree of metastasis, the radiosensitivity or chemosensitivity of the tumor, the age and general physical condition of the patient, the experience of the

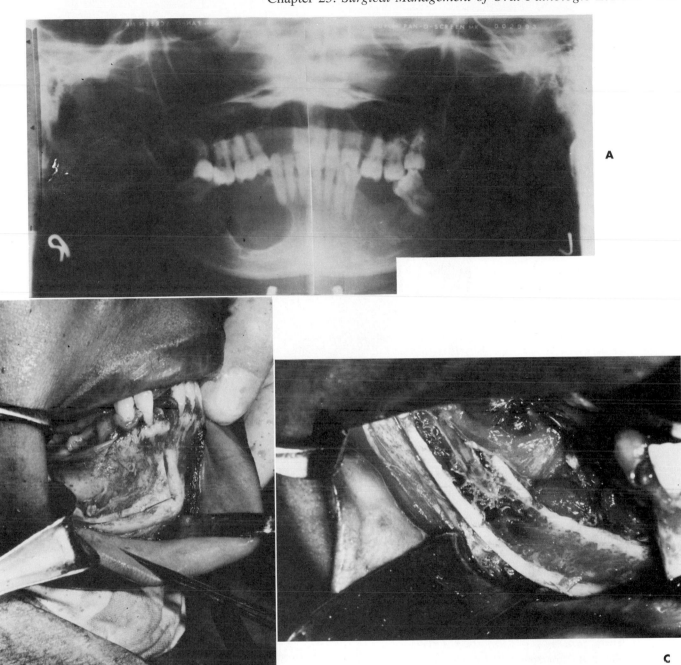

Figure 23-9

Marginal or segmental resection of ameloblastoma. **A,** Radiographic appearance of lesion. Note its relationship to inferior border of mandible. **B,** Intraoral exposure of mandible and osseous cuts made around lesion leave inferior border intact. **C,** Intraoral defect after removal of lesion. *(From Ellis E, Fonseca RJ: Therapy of cysts and odontogenic tumors. In Thawley SE et al, editors:* Comprehensive management of head and neck tumors, *Philadelphia, 1987, WB Saunders.)*   *Continued*

treating clinicians, and the wishes of the patient. In general, if a lesion can be completely excised without mutilating the patient, this is the preferred modality. If spread to regional lymph nodes is suspected, radiation may be employed before or after surgery to help eliminate small foci of malignant cells in the adjacent areas. If widespread systemic metastasis is detected or if a tumor, such as a lymphoma, is especially chemosensitive, chemotherapy is used with or without surgery and radiation.

Currently, malignancies are often treated in an institution

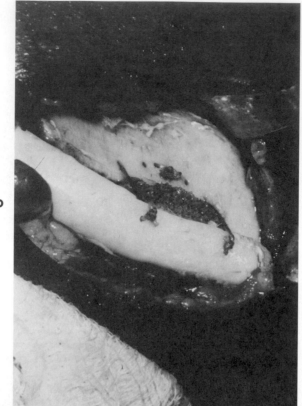

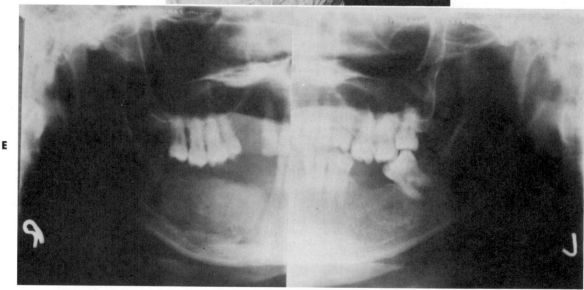

◇ **Figure 23-9, cont'd**

D, Extraoral exposure and placement of bone graft to reconstruct mandibular alveolus. **E,** Radiographic appearance immediately after graft placement.

where several specialists evaluate each case and discuss treatment regimens. These "tumor boards" include at least a surgeon, a chemotherapist, and a radiotherapist. Most head and neck tumor boards also include a general dentist, a maxillofacial prosthodontist, a nutritionist, a speech pathologist, and a sociologist and/or psychiatrist.

RADIOTHERAPY. Radiotherapy for treatment of malignant neoplasms is based on the fact that tumor cells in stages of active growth are more susceptible to ionizing radiation than adult tissue. The faster the cells are multiplying or the more undifferentiated the tumor cells, the more likely that radiation is to be effective. Radiation prevents the cells from multiplying by interfering with their nuclear material. Normal host cells are also affected by radiation and must be protected as much as possible during treatment.

Radiation can be delivered to the patient in several forms, including implantation of radioactive material into the tumor.

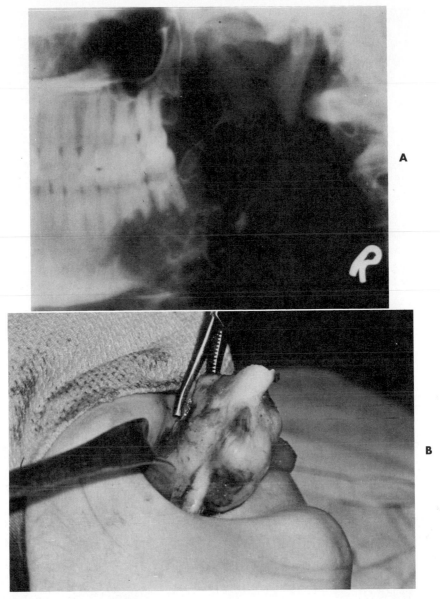

Continued

Figure 23-10

Partial mandibular resection of myxoma. **A,** Radiographic appearance on initial presentation. **B,** Photograph of intraoral resection of tumor (surgical resection similar to that shown in Figure 23-8, **B**). *(From Ellis E, Fonseca RJ: Therapy of cysts and odontogenic tumors. In Thawley SE et al, editors: Comprehensive management of head and neck tumors, Philadelphia, 1987, WB Saunders.)*

Most commonly, however, radiation is delivered externally by the use of large x-ray generators. The amount of radiation that a person may normally tolerate is not exceeded, and adjacent uninvolved areas are spared by the use of protective shielding. The patient's host tissues in the immediate area of the tumor are spared the total effect of the radiation by two mechanisms of delivery, fractionation and multiple ports. *Fractionation* of the delivery of radiation means that instead of giving the maximal amount of radiation a person can withstand at one time, smaller increments of radiation (fractions) are given over several weeks, which allows the healthier normal tissues time to recover between doses. The tumor cells, however, are less able to recover between doses. The second method employs *multiple ports* for radiation exposure. Instead of delivering the entire dosage through one beam (port), multiple beams are used. All beams are focused on the tumor but from different angles. Thus the tumor is exposed to the entire dosage of radiation. However, because different beams are used, the normal tissues in the path of the x-ray beams are spared maximal exposure and instead receive only a fraction of the tumor dose.

CHEMOTHERAPY. Chemicals that act by interfering with rapidly growing tumor cells are used for treating many types

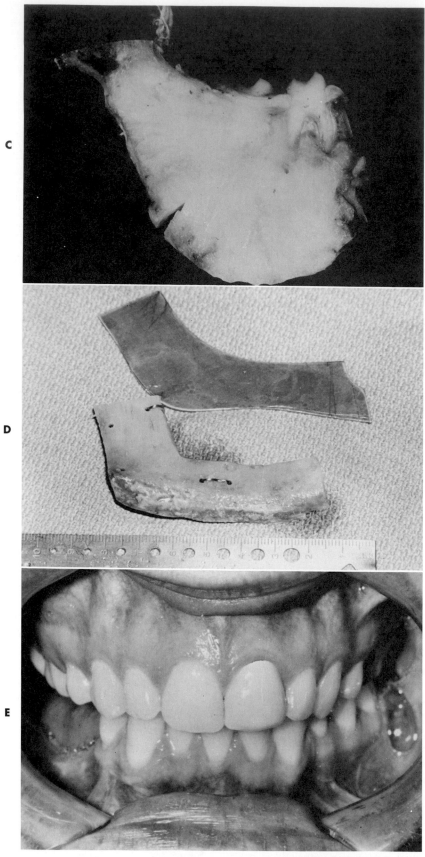

◇ Figure 23-10, cont'd

C, Lesion after sectioning. **D,** Template same size as removed specimen used to harvest similarly sized and shaped bone graft. **E,** Intraoral appearance of patient 1 year postoperatively. *Continued*

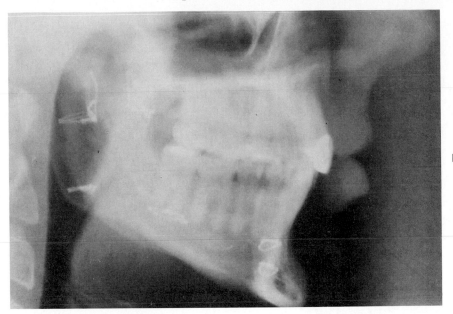

F

◇ Figure 23-10, cont'd

F, Radiographic appearance 1 year postoperatively.

of malignancies. As with radiation, the chemicals are not totally selective but affect normal cells to some extent. Most of these agents are given intravenously; recently, however, injections into the arteries feeding the tumor have been used. Because the agents are delivered systemically, they adversely affect many body systems; most notable is the hematopoietic system, which is considerably affected because of its rapid rate of cellular turnover. Thus patients who are undergoing chemotherapy are in a delicate balance between effectiveness in killing the tumor cells and anemia, neutropenia, and thrombocytopenia (see Chapter 19). Infections and bleeding are therefore common complications in these patients.

To reduce the toxicity of a single agent given in large quantities, multiple-agent therapy is frequently administered. Many patients are given three to five agents at the same time. Each may work at a different point in the life cycle of the tumor cell, thus increasing effectiveness with less toxicity to the host.

SURGERY.   The surgical procedures for excision of oral malignancies vary with the type and extent of the lesion. Small epidermoid carcinomas that are in accessible locations (for example, the lower lip) and are not associated with palpable lymph nodes can be excised (Figure 23-11). A larger lesion associated with palpable lymph nodes or a similar lesion in the area of the tonsillar pillar may require extensive surgery to adequately remove it and its local metastases.

Malignancies of the oral cavity that have either suspected or proven lymph node involvement are candidates for composite resection in which the lesion, surrounding tissues, and lymph nodes of the neck are totally removed. This procedure may produce large defects of the jaws and extensive loss of soft tissues, which make functional and esthetic rehabilitation a long, involved process.

SURGICAL MANAGEMENT OF BENIGN LESIONS IN ORAL SOFT TISSUES ◇

Superficial soft tissue lesions of the oral mucosa are usually benign and in most instances lend themselves to simple surgical removal using biopsy techniques (see Chapter 22). They include fibromas, pyogenic granulomas, papillomas, peripheral giant cell granulomas, verruca vulgaris, mucoceles (mucous extravasation phenomena), and epulis fissuratum. All of these lesions are overgrowths of the normally present histologic elements in the oral mucosa and submucosa. The principles of removal are the same as those outlined previously and include the use of elliptic, wedge type of incisions during removal. In the case of lesions that appear associated with the dentition (i.e., pyogenic granuloma), the associated tooth or teeth should be thoroughly curetted and polished to remove any plaque, calculus, or foreign material that may have played a role in the lesion's development and that may cause a recurrence if not removed.

RECONSTRUCTION OF JAWS AFTER REMOVAL OF ORAL TUMORS ◇

Osseous defects may occur following removal of oral tumors. These defects may range from loss of alveolar bone to loss of major portions of the jaw and may cause the patient concern on a functional or cosmetic basis. The treatment of oral

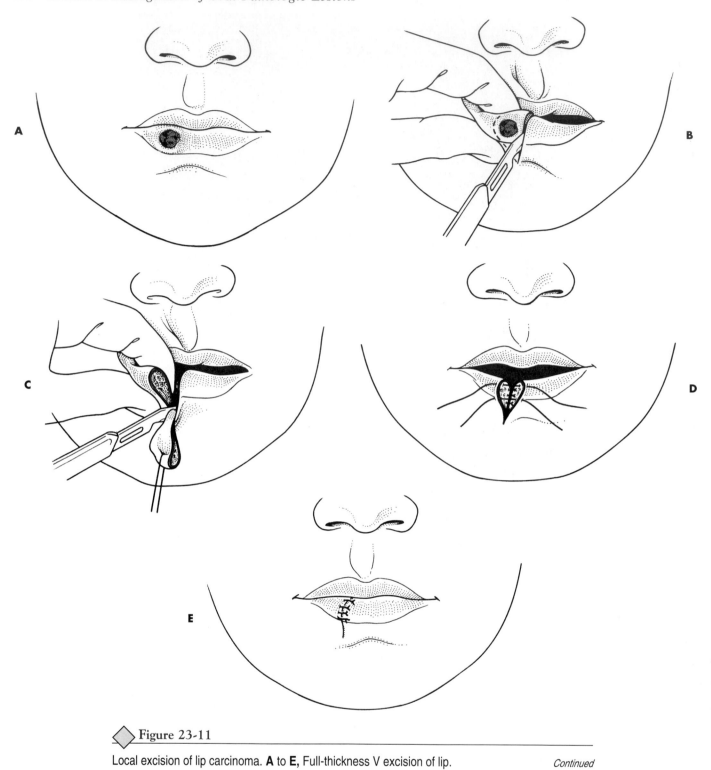

Local excision of lip carcinoma. **A** to **E,** Full-thickness V excision of lip. *Continued*

pathologic entities should always include immediate or future plans for reconstruction that have been made *before* the surgical procedure to remove the lesion, to afford the patient optimal reconstructive results.

The general dentist plays a crucial role in the functional and cosmetic rehabilitation of the patient by providing dental replacements for teeth that have been surgically removed. However, before dental rehabilitation is pursued, the under-

lying skeleton of the jaws should be reconstructed, if necessary. Frequently, surgical removal of a lesion involves removal of a portion of the alveolus, which presents the dentist with an obvious problem: any bridge across the site or any complete or partial denture will have no osseous base on which to rest. In these cases the patient would be well served to undergo ridge augmentation before dental restorative treatment. This augmentation can be in the form of bone

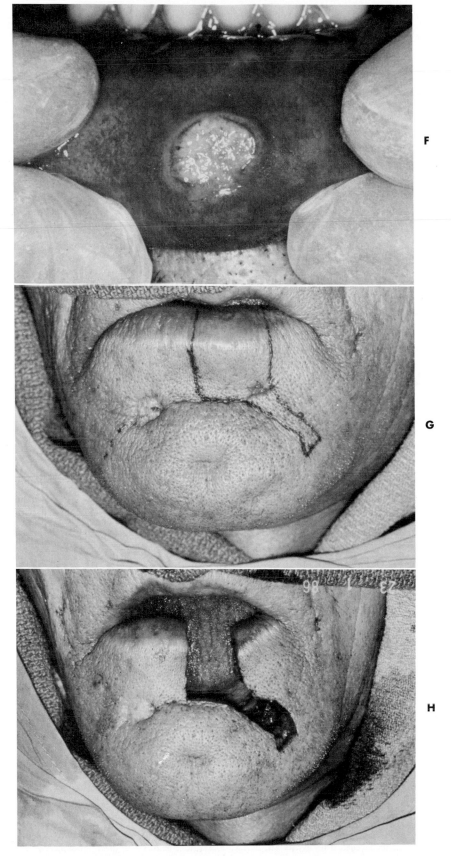

◇ Figure 23-11, cont'd

F, Carcinoma of lower lip. **G,** Surgical incisions outlined. **H,** Lip after excision of specimen.

Continued

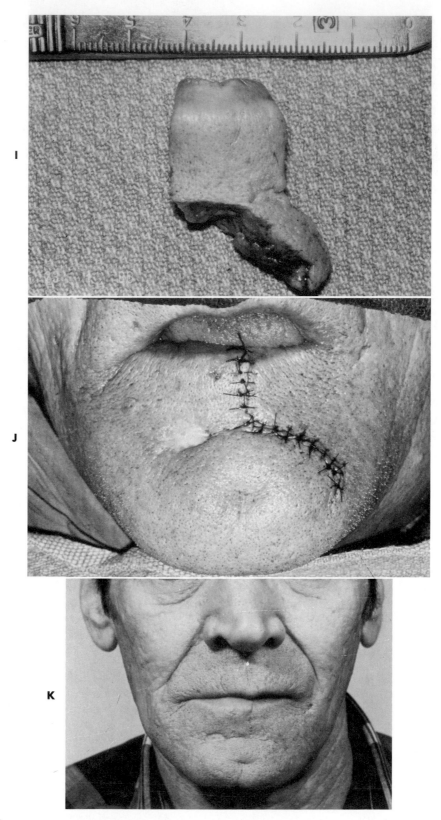

◇ Figure 23-11, cont'd

I, Specimen. **J,** Closure. **K,** Appearance after healing.

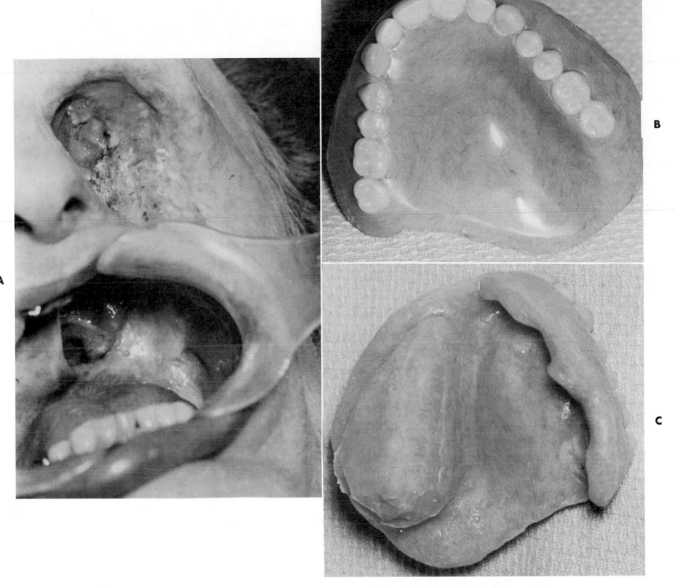

⬦Figure 23-12

Maxillofacial prosthetic reconstruction of patient who had left eye and palate removed because of tumor. **A,** Photograph showing defect in palate and loss of eye. **B** and **C,** Denture with obturator.

Continued

grafts, synthetic bone grafts, or a combination of these materials. Optimal dental restorations can then be completed.

When the patient has lost a portion of the maxilla, the maxillary sinuses or nasal cavity may be continuous with the oral cavity, which presents great difficulties for the patient in speaking and eating. Defects of the maxilla can be managed in one of two ways. The first is with surgery. Defects that are not excessive may be closed with available soft tissues of the buccal mucosa and palate. Bone grafts may also be used to provide the patient with a functional alveolar process. Very large defects or defects in patients who are poor surgical risks may require prosthetic obliteration in which a partial or complete denture extends into the maxillary sinus or nasal

cavities and effectively partitions the mouth from these structures (Figure 23-12).

The reconstruction of a defect caused by resection of the mandible or a portion thereof can be performed immediately (at the time of the surgical removal of the lesion) or may be delayed until a later date. In general, benign processes of the jaws are reconstructed immediately, whereas malignancies are reconstructed later. There are several reasons for delaying reconstruction after the surgical removal of a malignancy. Radiation is frequently used adjunctively with surgery and may jeopardize the survival of bone grafts. Another reason for delay is that soft tissue deficits may result after removal of the malignancy, and additional soft tissues may be required before

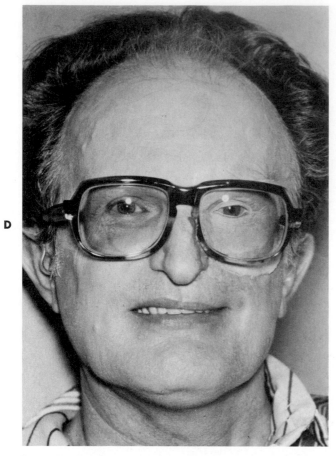

D

◇ Figure 23-12, cont'd

D, Patient with prosthetic eye and denture in place.

osseous reconstruction can be performed. A very important reason, however, is that recurrence of the malignancy may require further extirpative surgery that will negate the reconstructive efforts.

Several surgeons also delay reconstruction of defects caused by removal of benign tumors. They suggest that the presence of a simultaneous intraoral-extraoral defect, which frequently is necessary to remove the tumor, contraindicates an immediate reconstruction of the mandible. Instead, a space-maintaining device is placed at the time of resection, and a secondary reconstruction is performed weeks to months later.[1,3] When delayed reconstruction is decided upon, consideration should be given to maintaining the residual mandibular fragments in their normal anatomic relationship with intermaxillary fixation, external pin fixation, splints, internal fixation, or a combination of these modalities. This technique prevents cicatricial and muscular deformation and

displacement of the segments and simplifies secondary reconstructive efforts.

Clinical results have shown that immediate reconstruction is a viable option and has the advantages of requiring a single surgical procedure and having an early return to function with a minimal compromise to facial esthetics.[1] A possible disadvantage is loss of the graft from infection. The risk of infection may be higher when a graft is placed transorally or in an extraoral wound that was orally contaminated during the extirpative surgery. Because the recurrence rate is substantial in some tumors, prudent planning and meticulous surgery are mandatory before reconstruction is attempted. These measures minimize the risk of failure as a result of recurrence. Three choices for immediate reconstruction are possible. One is to perform the entire surgical procedure intraorally by first removing the tumor and then grafting the defect. Another method is to perform the tumor removal by a combined intraoral-extraoral route. A watertight oral closure is obtained, which is followed immediately by grafting the defect through the extraoral incision. The third method is useful when the tumor has not destroyed the alveolar crestal bone and when no extension of the tumor into oral soft tissues has occurred. In this case the involved teeth are extracted. A waiting period of 6 to 8 weeks is allowed for healing of the gingival tissues. The tumor is then removed and the defect grafted through an extraoral incision, with care taken to avoid perforation of the oral soft tissues. This procedure is the only type of *immediate* reconstruction with which oral contamination can be avoided.

REFERENCES

1. Adekeye EO: Reconstruction of mandibular defect by autogenous bone grafts: a review of 37 cases, *J Oral Surg* 36:125, 1978.
2. Eversole LR, Sabes WR, Rovin S: Aggressive growth and neoplastic potential of odontogenic cysts with special reference to central epidermoid and mucoepidermoid carcinomas, *Cancer* 35:270, 1975.
3. Kluft O, Van Dop F: Mandibular ameloblastoma (resection with primary reconstruction): a case report with concise review of the literature, *Arch Chir Neerl* 28:289, 1976.
4. Main DMG: Epithelial jaw cysts: a clinicopathological reappraisal, *Br J Oral Surg* 8:114, 1970.
5. Shafer WG, Hine MK, Levy BM: *A textbook of oral pathology,* ed 4, Philadelphia, 1983, WB Saunders.
6. Toller PA: Autoradiography of explants from odontogenic cysts, *Br Dent J* 131:57, 1971.
7. Wysocki GP, Sapp JP: Scanning and transmission electron microscopy of odontogenic keratocysts, *Oral Surg* 40:494, 1975.

ORAL AND MAXILLOFACIAL TRAUMA

One of the most rewarding and demanding aspects of dental and surgical practice is the management of the patient who has suffered facial trauma. The abruptness of the injury can cause intense emotional distress, even when only minor injuries are present. The perception of the injury by the patient or family and their reaction to the trauma may seem out of proportion to the degree of injury. The patient and the family may be highly anxious and fearful, and they depend heavily on the clinician to make an accurate diagnosis, communicate that diagnosis to them, offer hope for a successful outcome, and perform the treatment necessary to repair the injury. Therefore the clinician must effectively deal with both the patient's physical injuries and the patient's emotional state. Few conditions in clinical practice demand such compassion, competence, and attention to detail.

Whenever a maxillofacial injury is sustained the patient goes abruptly from a normal state to a state of tissue disruption. Patients usually expect that treatment of the injury will make them appear as they did before the trauma. Unfortunately, this is rarely achieved. The clinician cannot repair or heal the injuries; the most the clinician can do is provide the individual with the most favorable physical circumstances for optimal healing. The clinician accomplishes this by cleaning, debriding, and replacing tissues into their former positions. The resultant appearance of the patient therefore depends on the site, type, and degree of injury; the ability of the clinician to perform the tissue repositioning; and the ability of the patient's tissues to heal the wounds. The dentist's approach with the patient should be hopeful yet realistic.

The next two chapters discuss the diagnosis and management of injuries to the maxillofacial region. In Chapter 24 the injuries that dentists see with some frequency are discussed in detail. These include injuries to the teeth, the alveolar process, and the surrounding soft tissues. In Chapter 25 an overview of the management of more severe maxillofacial injuries is presented.

SOFT TISSUE AND DENTOALVEOLAR INJURIES

EDWARD ELLIS III

Dentoalveolar and perioral soft tissue injuries frequently occur and are caused by many types of trauma. The most common causes are falls, motor vehicle accidents, sports injuries, altercations, child abuse, and playground accidents. Many injuries are caused by falling, which starts when a child begins to walk and peaks just before school age.[3] The dentist is likely to be called by a frantic parent whose child has just fallen and is bleeding from the mouth. It is important for dentists to be familiar with dentoalveolar injuries so that they can effectively manage them when they occur.

Dentoalveolar injuries may be caused by a force directly on a tooth or an indirect force, most commonly transmitted through overlying soft tissues, such as the lip. Injuries of the surrounding soft tissues almost always accompany injuries to the dentoalveolus. For example, gingival tissues may be torn; the lower lip may have been caught between the teeth during the injury, creating a full-thickness laceration; or the floor of the mouth may be lacerated. Knowledge of management techniques for injuries to both the dentoalveolus and the soft tissues is necessary to allow the dentist to treat these

injuries effectively. The first part of this chapter discusses injuries to the teeth and alveolar process; the second portion discusses injuries to the perioral soft tissues, irrespective of whether they were caused by concomitant dentoalveolar injury.

MANAGEMENT OF DENTOALVEOLAR INJURIES ◇

Injuries to the teeth and alveolar process are common and should be considered emergency conditions, because a successful outcome depends on prompt attention to the injury. Because proper treatment can be given only after an accurate diagnosis, the diagnostic process should commence immediately.

HISTORY

The first step in any diagnostic process should be to secure an accurate history. A comprehensive history of the injury should be obtained from the patient, incorporating information on who, when, where, and how. The dentist must ask the following questions to the patient, parent, or a reliable respondent:

1. *Who is the patient?* Included here should be the patient's name, age, address, phone number, and other pertinent demographic data. It is imperative that this data be obtained quickly and time not be wasted.
2. *When did the injury occur?* This is one of the most important questions to ask, because studies have shown that the sooner an avulsed tooth can be repositioned, the better the prognosis.[4] Similarly, the results of treating displaced teeth, crown fractures (with and without exposed dental pulps), and alveolar fractures may be influenced by a delay in treatment.[1,3]

3. *Where did the injury occur?* This question may be important, because the possibility and degree of bacterial or chemical contamination should be ascertained. For example, if a child falls on the playground and gets dirt in the wound, a tetanus prophylaxis history should be carefully established. On the other hand, if an injury occurs from a clean object held in the mouth, gross bacterial contamination from external sources is not expected.

4. *How did the injury occur?* The nature of the trauma provides valuable insight into what the resultant tissue injury is likely to be. For example, an unrestrained car passenger who is thrown forward into the dashboard with sufficient force to damage several teeth may also have sustained occult injuries to the neck. The manner in which the injury occurred is valuable information and should make the clinician investigate the possibility of further injuries. Additional information that can be gained from this question may relate to the cause of the injury. If a patient cannot remember what happened, a preexisting medical condition, such as a seizure disorder, may have caused the accident producing the injury. Injuries caused by possible negligence by others are open for litigation. These considerations should caution the clinician to document the findings carefully and word any discussions with the patient thoughtfully. One other thought that must be kept in the clinician's mind when examining children whose injuries do not seem to be a likely result of the injury described by the parent is child abuse. Unfortunately, child abuse has become more prevalent in recent years, and a high degree of suspicion may be the only manner by which it can be discovered by health care providers.

5. *What treatment has been provided since the injury (if any)?* This question elicits important information regarding the original condition of the injured area. Was a partially avulsed tooth replanted by the patient or parent? How was the avulsed tooth stored before presentation to the dentist?

6. *Did anyone note teeth or pieces of teeth at the site of the accident?* Before an accurate diagnosis and treatment plan are made, it is imperative that each tooth the patient had before the accident be accounted for. If, during the clinical examination a tooth or crown is found missing and no history suggests that it was lost at the scene, radiographic examinations of the perioral soft tissues, the chest, and the abdominal region is necessary to rule out the presence of the missing piece within the tissues or other body cavities (Figure 24-1).

7. *What is the general health of the patient?* It is essential that a succinct medical history be taken; it should not be ignored in the dentist's haste to replant an avulsed tooth. It can, however, be performed concomitantly with treatment or immediately thereafter. A history that touches on drug allergy, heart murmur, bleeding disorder, other systemic disease, and current medications should be taken before treatment, because their existence affects the treatment the dentist will provide.

8. *Did the patient have nausea, vomiting, unconsciousness, amnesia, headache, visual disturbances, or confusion after*

the accident? An affirmative answer to any of these questions may indicate intracranial injury and direct the dentist to obtain medical consultation immediately after completing treatment. If the patient is still having any of the symptoms or if the patient does not feel or look well, immediate referral should be made. The patient's life should not be jeopardized to save an avulsed tooth.

9. *Is there a disturbance in the bite?* An affirmative answer to this question may indicate tooth displacement or dentoalveolar or jaw fracture.

CLINICAL EXAMINATION

The clinical examination is perhaps the most important part of the diagnostic process. A thorough examination of a patient who has had injury to the dentoalveolar structures should not focus only on that structure. Concomitant injuries may also be present; the history may direct the dentist to examine other areas for signs of injury. Vital signs such as pulse rate, blood pressure, and respiration should be measured. Such tests can usually be obtained during the taking of the history. The mental state of the patient is also assessed throughout the taking of the history and while performing the clinical examination by observation of the manner in which the patient reacts to the examination and responds to the questioning. During the clinical examination, the following areas should routinely be examined:

1. *Extraoral soft tissue wounds.* Lacerations, abrasions, and contusions of the skin are all common with dentoalveolar injuries and should be noted. If a laceration is present, the depth of it should also be determined. Does the laceration extend through the entire thickness of the lip or cheek? Are there any vital structures, such as the parotid duct or facial nerve, crossing the line of the laceration? Major lacerations such as these are best treated by an oral and maxillofacial surgeon.

2. *Intraoral soft tissue wounds.* Injuries to the oral soft tissues are very commonly associated with dentoalveolar injuries. Before a thorough examination, it may be necessary to remove blood clots, irrigate with sterile saline, and cleanse the oral cavity. Areas of bleeding usually respond to pressure applied under gauze sponges. Soft tissue injuries should be noted, and an examination should ascertain whether there are any foreign bodies, such as tooth crowns or teeth, within the substance of the lips, floor of mouth, cheeks, or other areas. The dentist should also note areas of extensive loss of soft tissues; blood supply to a segment of tissue may thereby be lost.

3. *Fractures of the jaws or alveolar process.* Fractures of the jaws are most readily found on palpation. However, because pain may be severe following the injury, examination can be difficult. Bleeding into the floor of the mouth or into the labial vestibule may indicate a fracture of the jaw. Segments of alveolar process that have been fractured are readily detected by visual examination and palpation.

4. *Examination of the tooth crowns for the presence of fractures or pulp exposure.* For adequate examination the teeth should be cleansed of blood. Any fractures should be

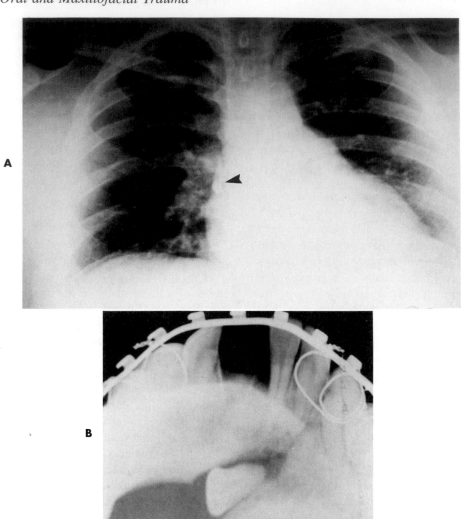

◇ Figure 24-1

Teeth displaced into abnormal locations. **A,** Chest radiograph showing maxillary canine tooth in right main-stem bronchus after traumatic displacement. **B,** Incisor tooth in line of fracture following reduction.

noted. It is important to note the depth of the fracture. Does it extend into dentin or into the pulp?

5. *Displacement of teeth.* Teeth can be displaced in any direction. Most commonly they are displaced in a buccolingual direction, but they may also be extruded or intruded. In the most severe type of displacement the teeth are avulsed—that is, totally displaced out of their alveolar process. Observation of the dental occlusion may provide assistance in determining minimal degrees of tooth displacement.

6. *Mobility of teeth.* All teeth should be checked for mobility in both the horizontal and vertical directions. A tooth that does not appear to be displaced but that has considerable mobility may have sustained a root fracture. If adjacent teeth move with the tooth being tested, a dentoalveolar fracture (in which a segment of alveolar bone and teeth are separated from the remainder of the jaw) should be suspected.

7. *Percussion of teeth.* When a tooth does not appear to be displaced, yet there is pain in the region, percussion determines whether the periodontal ligament has undergone some injury.

8. *Pulp testing of teeth.* Although rarely used in acute injuries, vitality tests (which induce a reaction from the teeth) may direct the type of treatment the teeth will receive once the injury is over. False-negative results may occur, so the teeth should be retested several weeks later and before endodontic therapy is performed.

RADIOGRAPHIC EXAMINATION

A host of radiographic techniques are available to evaluate dentoalveolar trauma. Most can be readily performed in the dental office with available equipment. Most commonly a combination of occlusal and periapical radiographs are used. The radiographic examination should provide the following information[5]:

1. Presence of root fracture
2. Degree of extrusion or intrusion
3. Presence of preexisting periapical disease
4. Extent of root development
5. Size of the pulp chamber and root canal
6. Presence of jaw fractures
7. Tooth fragments and foreign bodies lodged in soft tissues

A single radiograph may not be sufficient to demonstrate a root fracture.[3] For a radiograph to demonstrate a fractured root, the central beam of the x-ray must be parallel to the line of fracture; otherwise the fracture may not be clearly seen (Figure 24-2). Multiple views with differing vertical and horizontal angulations of the central ray may be necessary.

Displaced teeth may show a widening of the periodontal ligament space or displacement of the lamina dura. Extruded teeth may demonstrate a conical periapical radiolucency (Figure 24-3). Intruded teeth may show minimal radiographic findings because of the continued close adaption of the laminal dura and the root surface. Frequently, however, intruded teeth show an absence of the periodontal ligament space.

Radiographic evaluation for foreign bodies within the soft tissues of the lips or cheeks are taken with the radiographic film placed inside the soft tissues to be examined, labial to the alveolus (Figure 24-4, *A*). A reduced radiographic exposure time is used (approximately one third of normal). Foreign bodies in the floor of the mouth are viewed with cross-sectioned occlusal radiographs, also with reduced radiographic exposure time (Figure 24-4, *B*).

CLASSIFICATION OF TRAUMATIC INJURIES TO THE TEETH AND SUPPORTING STRUCTURES

Many systems are used for the description of dentoalveolar injuries, all of which have advantages and disadvantages. A relatively simple yet useful classification was presented by Sanders, Brady, and Johnson.[5] Their method is based entirely on a description of the injury sustained during the traumatic episode, describing the tooth structures involved, the type of displacement, and the direction of crown or root fracture. The following is a modification of their list of things to look for when classifying dentoalveolar injuries.

A. Crown craze or crack (Figure 24-5)
   1. Crack or incomplete fracture of the enamel without a loss of tooth structure
   2. Horizontal or vertical
B. Crown fracture (Figure 24-6)
   1. Confined to enamel
   2. Enamel and dentin involved
   3. Enamel, dentin, and exposed pulp involved

   4. Horizontal or vertical
   5. Oblique (involving the mesioincisal or distoincisal angle)
C. Crown-root fracture (Figure 24-7)
   1. No pulp involvement
   2. Pulp involvement
D. Horizontal root fracture (Figure 24-8)
   1. Involving apical third
   2. Involving middle third
   3. Involving cervical third
   4. Horizontal or vertical
E. Sensitivity (concussion)
   1. Injury to the tooth-supporting structure, resulting in sensitivity to touch or percussion, but without mobility or displacement of the tooth
F. Mobility (subluxation or looseness)
   1. Injury to the tooth-supporting structure, resulting in tooth mobility but without tooth displacement
G. Tooth displacement (Figure 24-9)
   1. Intrusion (displacement of tooth into its socket—usually associated with compression fracture of socket)
   2. Extrusion (partial displacement of tooth out of its socket—possibly no concomitant fracture of alveolar bone)
   3. Labial displacement (alveolar wall fractures probable)
   4. Lingual displacement (alveolar wall fractures probable)
   5. Lateral displacement (displacement of tooth in mesial or distal direction, usually into a missing tooth space—alveolar wall fractures probable)
H. Avulsion
   1. Complete displacement of tooth from its socket (may be associated with alveolar wall fractures)
I. Alveolar process fracture

TREATMENT OF DENTOALVEOLAR INJURIES

Following a thorough history and clinical and radiologic examinations the dentist should be able to determine whether the treatment plan for the patient's type of injury is within his or her range of expertise. There may be several circumstances that render an otherwise minor injury untreatable by the dentist alone. A problem the dentist frequently encounters is the uncooperative patient, most commonly a child. The combination of the traumatic episode and the child's fear of the dentist may render a simple surgical procedure impossible without general anesthesia. Another difficulty is the patient with multiple medical problems. When dentists do not feel they can effectively manage a patient because of surgical difficulty, anesthesia requirement, concomitant medical problems, or other reasons, an oral and maxillofacial surgeon should immediately be consulted for assistance with treatment.

The goal in the treatment of dentoalveolar injuries is reestablishing normal form and function of the masticatory apparatus. When the pulp is directly involved, treatment

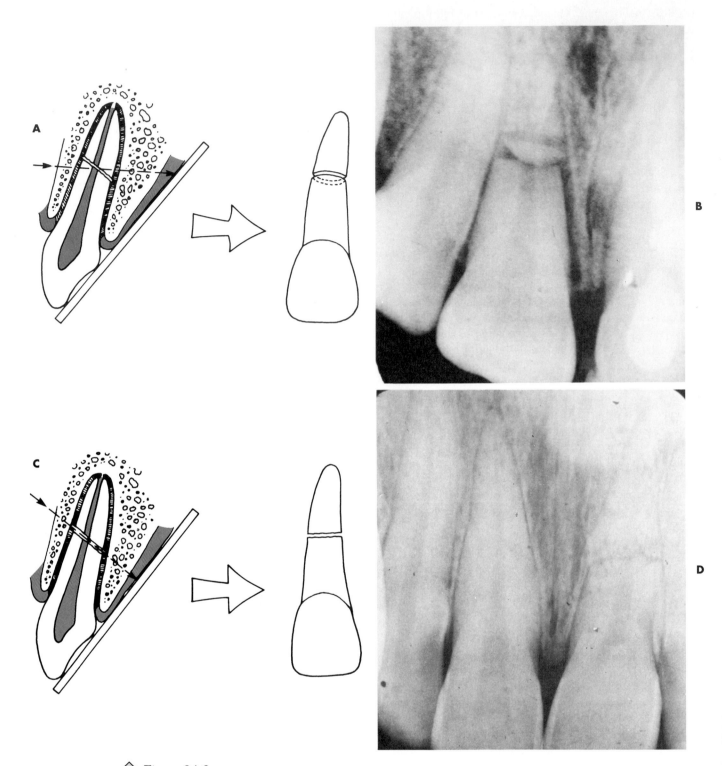

◈ Figure 24-2

Illustrations showing manner in which changing vertical angulation of central x-ray beam can affect detection of horizontal root fracture. When central ray is not parallel to fracture (**A**), either a double fracture or no fracture at all may be observed on radiograph. **B,** Shows single fracture but looks like double fracture on radiograph. When central ray is parallel to fracture (**C**), fracture appears on radiograph (**D**).

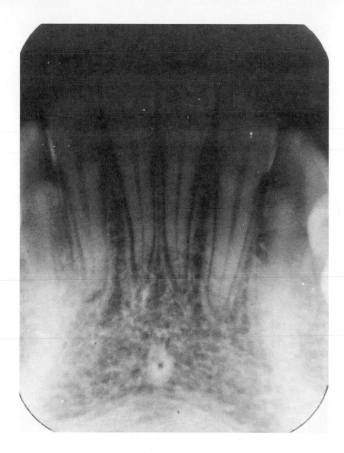

 Figure 24-3

Radiograph showing widened periodontal ligament spaces around several teeth that are displaced coronally.

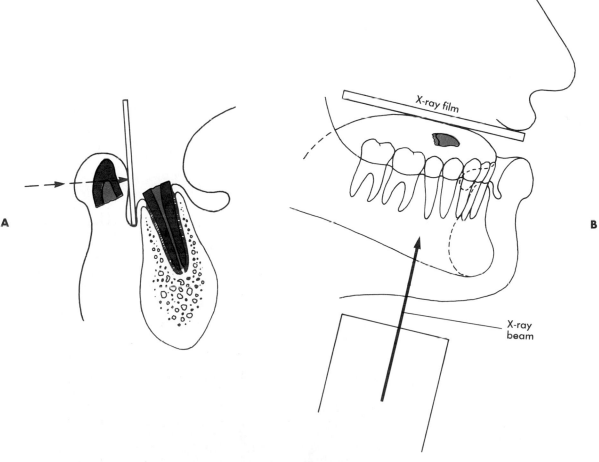

Figure 24-4

Illustrations showing radiographic technique to detect foreign bodies within lip (**A**) and tongue (**B**). The clinician should use one half to one third of normal exposure for soft tissue radiography.

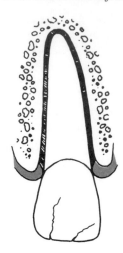

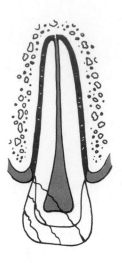

◇ **Figure 24-5**

Illustration showing crown cracks, or crazes. These usually extend only into enamel.

◇ **Figure 24-6**

Illustration of coronal fractures involving enamel, dentin, and pulp.

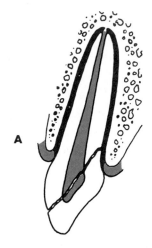

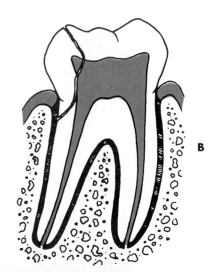

A

B

◇ **Figure 24-7**

Crown-root fractures. **A** and **B,** Illustrations of crown-root fractures in incisor and molar, respectively. Note that fractures extend below alveolar crest of bone. **C,** Clinical photograph of crown-root fracture in molar.

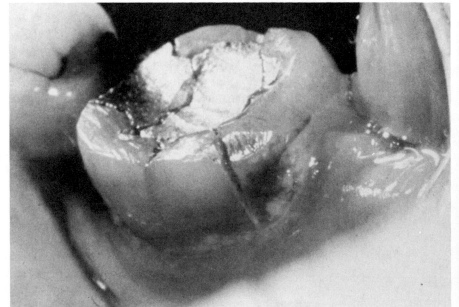

C

differs from that of tooth injuries in which the pulp is not involved. Because of the training in operative dentistry and endodontics, a dentist has the knowledge, the instrumentation, and the medications routinely available to manage cases of tooth fracture. The treatment regimen for these injuries is therefore outlined only briefly. More severe injuries, such as tooth dislocations or avulsions and dentoalveolar fractures, are fields in which the dentist may have had little training; these are presented in greater detail.

Primary teeth that have been injured are generally treated in a manner similar to that for permanent teeth.

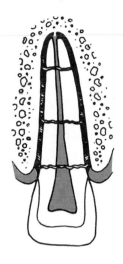

◇ Figure 24-8

Illustration of horizontal root fractures at apical, middle, and coronal levels of root (*top, middle,* and *bottom,* respectively).

However, in many instances, the lack of cooperation by the child results in treatment compromises and, frequently, extraction of the damaged tooth. If this occurs, the dentist should consider space-maintenance measures in the near future where indicated.

CROWN CRAZE OR CRACK. No treatment is usually indicated. However, because any force to the tooth can result in injury to the pulp and periodontal tissues, periodic follow-up examinations are valuable. (See Figure 24-5.)

CROWN FRACTURE. The treatment of crown fractures is determined by the depth of tooth tissue involvement. For fractures that are only through the enamel or those with minimal amounts of dentin involvement, no acute treatment other than smoothing off the sharp edges is warranted. If reshaping the teeth would leave a noticeable deformity, replacement of the missing enamel by acid-etched composite resin techniques is indicated. The sooner they are treated, the better is the prognosis, because inflammatory hyperemia of the pulp will be decreased. Periodic follow-up examinations are necessary to monitor pulp and periodontal health. (See Figure 24-6.)

If there is a considerable amount of dentin exposed, the pulp must be protected. Measures to seal the dentinal tubules and promote secondary dentin deposition by the pulp can be undertaken. Calcium hydroxide has been the traditional material applied to the exposed dentin before the fractured part is covered with a suitable restoration, most commonly a composite with or without acid etching. A celluloid crown can also be used as a temporary measure. More recently, glass ionomer cements have been used to line the exposed dentin.[6]

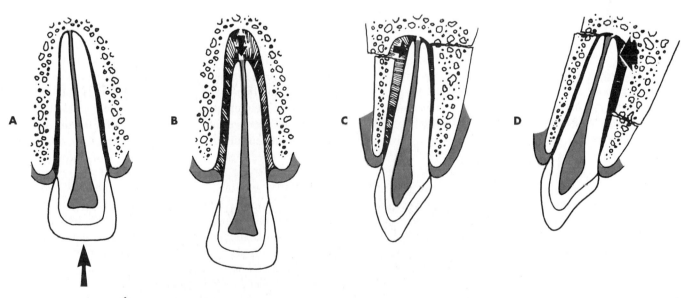

◇ Figure 24-9

Illustrations of tooth displacement. **A,** Intruded tooth. Note absence of periodontal ligament space along apex. **B,** Tooth displaced from its socket in coronal direction (extruded). **C** and **D,** Displacement of incisor tooth crown buccally and lingually, respectively. Note associated alveolar wall fractures, which are frequently present.

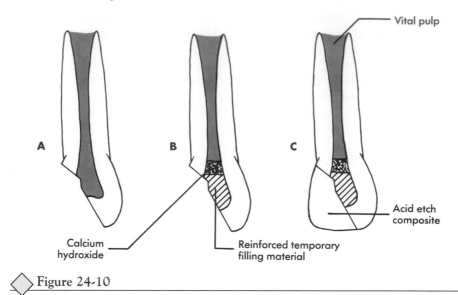

Vital pulp

A

B

C

Calcium hydroxide

Reinforced temporary filling material

Acid etch composite

◇ Figure 24-10

Illustration showing pulpotomy technique. **A,** Apically immature tooth with coronal fracture involving pulp. **B,** Coronal pulp removed aseptically, followed by application of calcium hydroxide solution over exposed pulp. Reinforced filling material can then be used to fill remainder of coronal pulp chamber, and temporary or permanent (composite) filling is placed (**C**).

This cement chemically binds to dentin, facilitating placement and restoration. The remainder of the missing tooth structure can then be repaired by composite. The status of pulp vitality at periodic follow-up visits dictates what the final treatment plan will be. If pulp and periodontal health are satisfactory, no more intervention is necessary other than for esthetic reasons.

If the pulp is exposed, the aim of treatment is to preserve it in a vital, healthy state. This can usually be accomplished by pulp capping if (1) the exposure is very small, (2) the patient is seen soon after injury, (3) there are no root fractures, (4) the tooth has not been displaced, and, (5) there are no large or deep fillings that might indicate chronic inflammation within the pulp. The most common injury for which pulp capping is instituted is in a tooth in which a single pulp horn was exposed with a crown fracture. The more apically immature the tooth, the more favorable is the response the dentist can expect from pulp-capping. As with any operative procedure on the dental pulp, isolation with a rubber dam is recommended. After application of calcium hydroxide, a water-tight restoration is placed.

A pulpotomy involves aseptic removal of damaged and inflamed pulp tissue to the level of clinically healthy pulp, followed by calcium hydroxide application. It is usually implemented in larger exposures in which the apex is not closed. In these instances a pulpotomy should be only a temporary measure to maintain the vitality of the radicular pulp until the apex is closed. Endodontic therapy should then be instituted. The technique is illustrated in Figure 24-10.

Periodic follow-up examinations are mandatory after any pulpal procedure. The final restorative decision will be based on the pulpal health of the tooth. Because the prognosis is guarded, endodontic treatment may be necessary if the pulp degenerates.

CROWN-ROOT FRACTURE. The treatment of crown-root fractures depends on the location of the fracture and local anatomic variance. If the coronal fragment is still in place, it must be removed to assess the depth to which the fracture has gone. If the fracture does not descend too far apically and the tooth is therefore restorable and if the pulp has not been exposed, the tooth is treated as already discussed for crown fracture. Depending on the apical extent of the fracture, it may be necessary to perform periodontal procedures to make the apical margin of the fracture accessible for restorative procedures. Alternatively, orthodontic extrusion of the root can make it accessible for restorative procedures. If the pulp is involved and the tooth is restorable, endodontic treatment is implemented. If, on the other hand, the tooth is not restorable, removal is indicated. If there is a concomitant alveolar fracture, the extraction may be delayed for several weeks to permit the fracture to heal and thus prevent undue loss of alveolar bone at the time of extraction. (See Figure 24-7.)

HORIZONTAL ROOT FRACTURE. When a horizontal or oblique fracture of the root occurs, the main factor in determining the prognosis and therefore in directing treatment is the position of the fracture in relation to the gingival crevice. If the fracture is above or close to the gingival crevice, either the tooth should be removed or the coronal fragment should be removed and endodontic treatment performed on the root. The root can then be restored with a post and core restoration. Fractures in the middle-to-apical one third of the root have a good prognosis for survival of the pulp and healing of the root fragments to one another. These fractures should be treated with repositioning (if any mobility is detectable), followed by firm immobilization for 2 to 3 months (techniques are described later). During this time, bridging of the fracture with calcified tissue usually occurs, and the tooth remains vital. (See Figures 24-2 and 24-8).

SENSITIVITY (CONCUSSION). No acute treatment is recommended other than symptomatic relief, such as relieving the tooth from occlusal contact. Follow-up examinations should be instituted to monitor periodontal and pulpal health.

MOBILITY. If the tooth is only mildly mobile, relieving the occlusal contact is effective treatment. Most mobile teeth stabilize ("tighten up") with time. If the tooth is extremely mobile, splinting it to adjacent teeth is recommended (described later). Periodic observation is then necessary.

INTRUSION. Traumatic intrusion of teeth indicates that the alveolar socket has sustained a compression fracture to permit the new tooth position. On percussion the tooth emits a metallic sound similar to an ankylosed tooth—distinguishing it from a partially erupted or unerupted tooth. The intrusion may be so severe that the tooth actually appears to be missing on clinical examination. Traumatic tooth intrusion is less frequent than lateral displacements; when seen, it usually involves maxillary teeth. This type of nonavulsive tooth displacement has the worst prognosis. (See Figure 24-9, *A*.)

The treatment of intruded teeth is controversial. Some clinicians favor surgically repositioning and splinting them; however, this treatment has resulted in serious periodontal and pulpal consequences. Others feel that, if left alone, intruded teeth will reerupt. Others use orthodontic forces to assist reeruption of the tooth (Figure 24-11). Andreasen[3] suggests that the chances of ankylosis are decreased when the tooth is left in place for 4 to 6 days and then orthodontically extruded. Once the tooth is in position within the dental arch, it is splinted for 2 to 3 months. Recent evidence suggests that *immediate* application of orthodontic force is necessary to prevent ankylosis in the intruded position.[8] The decision to perform endodontic treatment is based on the follow-up findings of each individual case. However, if the intrusion occurred in an apically mature tooth, pulpal degeneration is likely and endodontic treatment should be performed as described later.

If a deciduous tooth has been intruded to the point that it is touching the follicle of a succedaneous tooth, the deciduous tooth should be removed as atraumatically as possible. If the deciduous tooth is not in direct proximity to the succedaneous tooth, a period of observation should be followed, because reeruption is common. If the dentist is in doubt about the position of a deciduous tooth, removal is a sound prophylactic approach that helps to ensure the health of the succedaneous tooth.

EXTRUSION. Extruded teeth can usually be manually seated back into their sockets if the injury was very recent. After replacement of the tooth within the socket, splinting for 1 to 3 weeks is usually necessary, as is endodontic treatment (discussed later) (Figure 24-12). (See Figure 24-9, *B*).

LATERAL DISPLACEMENT. If a tooth is minimally displaced, the accompanying alveolar wall fractures may not be grossly displaced. In this case, manual repositioning of the tooth followed by splinting for several weeks is indicated. When substantial tooth displacement has occurred, displaced alveolar bone fractures have also been sustained (Figure 24-9, *C* and *D*). Gingival lacerations frequently accompany this type of injury. The tooth and the alveolar bone must be manually repositioned, the tooth splinted, and soft tissues sutured (Figure 24-13). Postsurgical follow-up examinations will determine the state of the pulp and periodontal damage.

AVULSION. Total avulsion from its socket is the most grave situation for a tooth, because the health of both the pulp and the periodontal tissues is in severe jeopardy. The factors most important for determining how successful treatment measures will be are the length of time the tooth has been out of the socket, the state of the tooth and periodontal tissues, and the manner in which the tooth was preserved before replantation. The sooner the tooth can be replanted, the better the prognosis.[4] Therefore when the dentist receives a call from a patient, parent, teacher, or other responsible person regarding a totally avulsed tooth, the dentist should direct the caller to rinse the tooth immediately with the patient's saliva, tap water, or saline solution and replant the tooth. The patient should hold the tooth by the crown, while trying to not touch the root, and then hold the tooth in place and go immediately to the dentist. If the patient cannot replace the tooth, it should be held in the buccal vestibule if the patient is responsible enough to keep from swallowing or aspirating the tooth or in the buccal vestibule of their parent or companion while they are on their way to the dentist's office. Saliva is an excellent transport medium and as effective as saline, as opposed to tap water, which destroys the health of the periodontal ligament. It does not matter if the tooth is stored in another's saliva. Milk is also an excellent storage medium because it is usually readily available, it has a pH and osmolarity compatible to vital cells, and it is relatively free of bacteria.[7] A commercially available tooth preservation system that contains Hanks Balanced Salt Solution can be kept available at schools and sporting events, in ambulances, and so on.[*]

When the patient gets to the dentist's office, the dentist must decide whether the tooth is salvageable. If it has already been replanted and seems to be in good position, it should be radiographed and then splinted for 7 to 10 days. If the tooth is carried into the office, it should be immediately rinsed in saline and replanted by the dentist. It is not necessary to remove all of the blood clot from within the socket; however, careful suctioning and gentle irrigation with sterile saline will remove the bulk of the clot. The root surface and tooth socket should never be scraped, "sterilized," or manipulated before replantation, because this destroys viable periodontal tissue.

Stabilization of an avulsed tooth can be achieved using a variety of materials, such as wires (Figure 24-14), arch bars

---

*Save-A-Tooth, Biologic Rescue Products, Conshohocken, Pa.

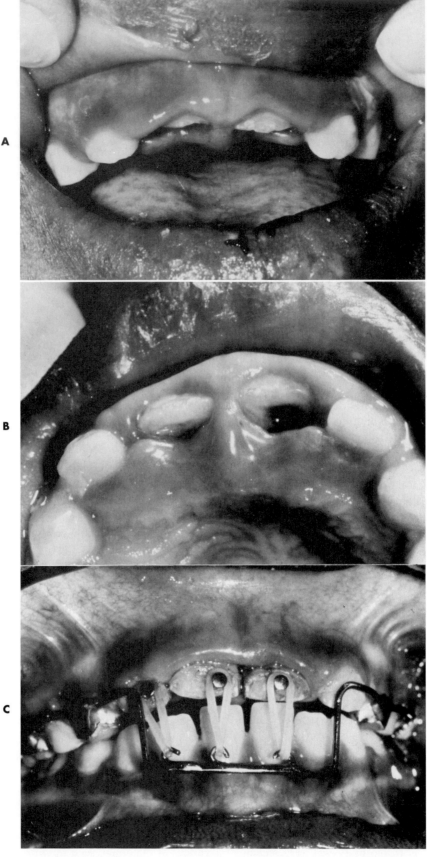

◈ **Figure 24-11**

Treatment of intruded maxillary incisors with immature apices. **A,** Buccal and **B,** palatal views of intruded maxillary incisor teeth. **C,** Orthodontic traction instituted to extrude teeth a few weeks after traumatic episode.

Continued

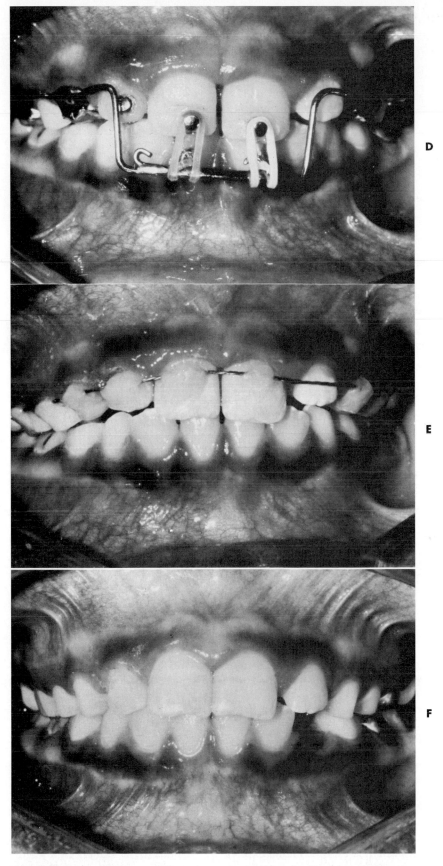

◇ Figure 24-11, cont'd

D, Appearance after 6 weeks of traction. **E,** Stabilization of teeth following orthodontic-guided reeruption with acid-etch technique for 11 weeks. **F,** Appearance after 1 year. This patient had calcium hydroxide pulpectomies and apexification during period of orthodontic extrusion; she subsequently had root canals. *(From Spalding PM et al:* The changing role of endodontics and orthodontics in the management of traumatically intruded permanent incisors. *Pediatr Dent 7:104, 1985.)*

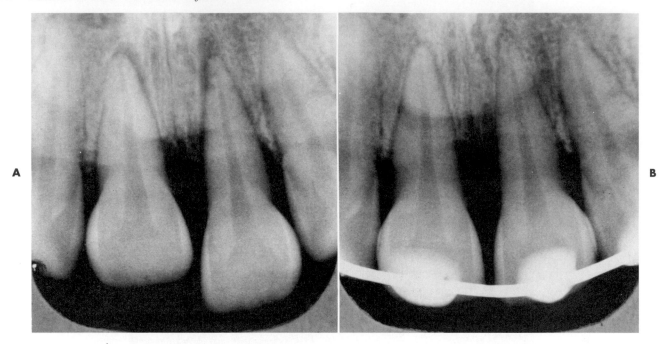

◇ **Figure 24-12**

Radiographs of extruded tooth before (**A**) and after (**B**) repositioning and stabilization with acid-etch composite technique.

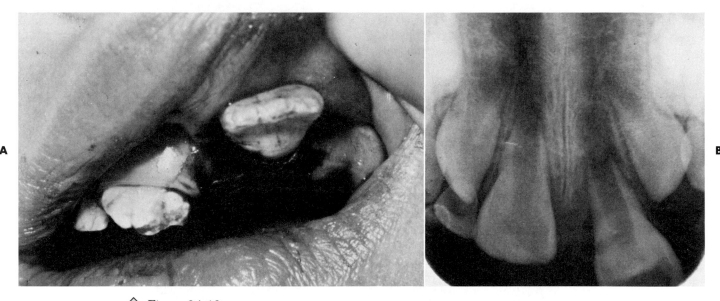

◇ **Figure 24-13**

Treatment of laterally displaced central incisor in apically immature tooth. **A,** Appearance on presentation. **B,** Radiograph showing position. *Continued*

(Figure 24-15), and splints. However, there are several factors to be considered. The stabilizing device should be as hygienic as possible and should be positioned away from the gingiva and tooth roots if possible. During the healing response, inflammation must be kept to a minimum, or inflammatory root resorption will be favored, which is one of the drawbacks to interdental wiring and cold-cured acrylic splints. It is very difficult for patients to cleanse teeth that are covered with

wires or splints. Furthermore, wire can slip apically around the cervical aspect and damage the cementum. The stabilization applied to the tooth need not be absolutely rigid, for this may predispose to ankylosis. Physiologic movements of the tooth are thought by some to promote fibrous (desired) instead of osseous (tending toward ankylosis) attachment of the root to the alveolar bone. The stabilization device should also be easy to apply and remove with readily available instruments.

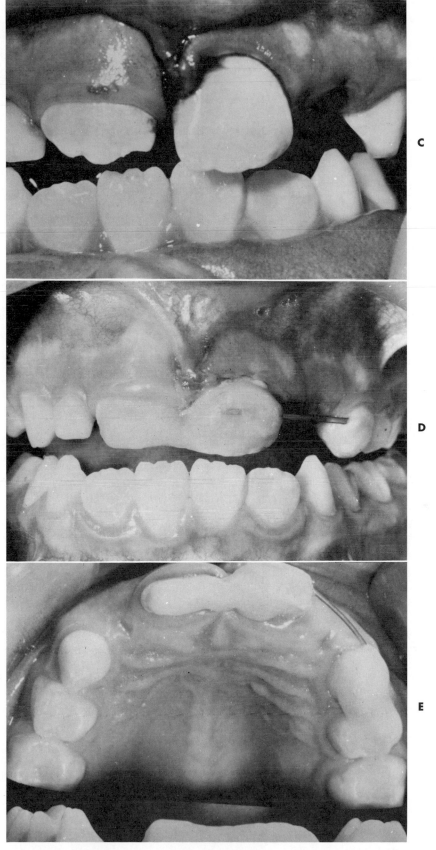

◇ Figure 24-13, cont'd

C, Position of tooth after digital reduction. **D** and **E,** Appearance of tooth after acid-etch composite stabilization to adjacent teeth.   *Continued*

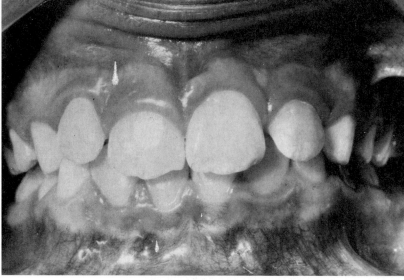

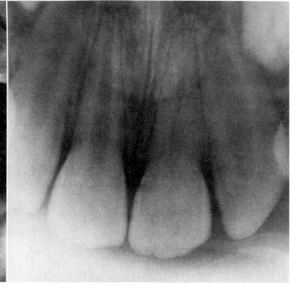

◇ **Figure 24-13, cont'd**

F, Radiograph of tooth after removal of stabilizing appliance. **G,** Appearance of tooth 1 year after trauma. **H,** Radiograph of tooth 1 year after trauma. No root canal treatment was performed because of immature nature of apex at time of displacement. *(Courtesy Dr. Peter Spalding, University of Nebraska, Lincoln.)*

◇ **Figure 24-14**

Illustration showing use of Essig wiring technique to stabilize unstable tooth. Long loop is placed around several teeth (above cingula), and several interdental wires are placed so that they pass around buccal and lingual Essig wires. Interdental wires are tightened slightly until tooth is stabilized.

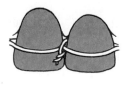

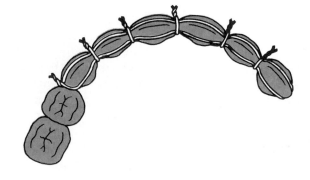

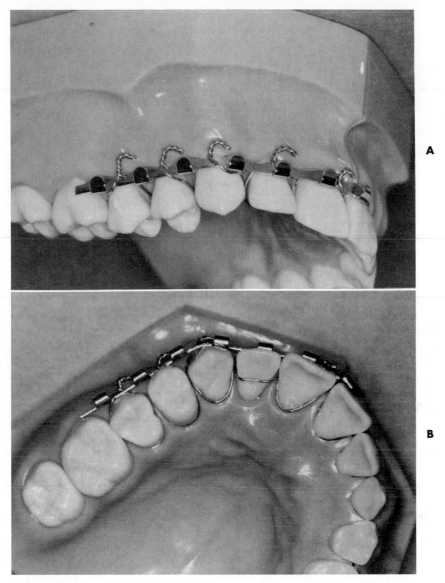

A

B

◇ Figure 24-15

Lateral (**A**) and palatal (**B**) views of arch-bar stabilization of maxillary right lateral incisor tooth. Note that wire is apical to height of contour on all teeth *except* reduced lateral incisor. Wire is coronal to cingulum on this tooth, so that intrusive force is imparted to tooth when circumdental wire is tightened.

A technique that serves admirably for the stabilization of avulsed teeth is the use of an acid-etched composite system (Figures 24-11 to 24-13, 24-16, and 24-17). A wire of moderate stiffness yet that still has some flexibility, such as braided orthodontic wire, is adapted to the facial surfaces of one or two teeth on each side of the avulsed tooth. The fewer teeth required to stabilize the avulsed tooth, the more physiologic movement that can be imparted to the replanted tooth during function. If braided orthodontic wire is unavailable, any wire—even a paper clip—will suffice. The facial surfaces of both the avulsed and the adjacent teeth are acid-etched, and the wire is cemented to them with composite. This technique makes cleansing the teeth easy, because the wire is away from the gingiva. The wire can be readily removed, and most dentists have the necessary supplies and instrumentation available for its use.

The duration of stabilization (Table 24-1) should be as short a time as necessary for the tooth to become reattached, usually 7 to 10 days. Studies have shown that the more rigid and the longer the stabilization, the more root resorption that can be expected.[2,3] On removal of the stabilization device, the tooth will still be quite mobile. It is therefore important that the stabilization device be removed with great care and the patient be instructed to avoid this region during mastication. If, however, the apical foramen is wide open, there is a chance that pulp will survive and revascularize. To promote this possibility, the tooth is usually stabilized for 3 to 4 weeks instead of the shorter time for apically mature teeth.

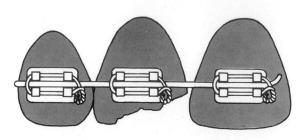

Illustration of bonded orthodontic brackets and orthodontic wire to stabilize traumatized tooth. Wire should be of light gauge. Braided wire serves purpose well and allows some physiologic motion of stabilized tooth.

Patients who have no recollection of a tetanus booster within the past 5 to 10 years should be referred to their physician for one. The use of antibiotics (penicillin) for 7 to 10 days is appropriate.

The patient should be told that several outcomes are possible after replantation. The best result to be expected is a relatively normal, functional tooth that will in most instances require endodontic therapy (described later). However, varying amounts of root resorption and ankylosis may occur. The development of these signs will determine the prognosis of the tooth. Acute dental infection is rare; it can lead to loss of the replanted tooth. These patients must be followed carefully at regular and frequent intervals for some time after replantation. Andreasen[1] lists the following factors to be considered before replanting avulsed teeth:

1. The avulsed tooth should have no advanced periodontal disease.

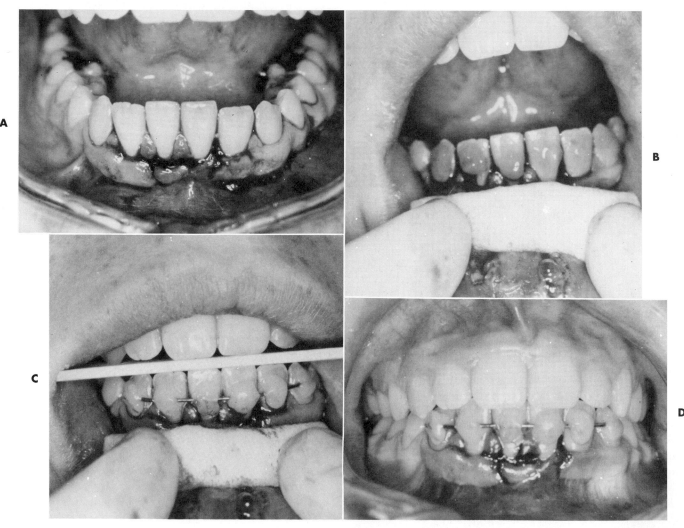

◇ **Figure 24-17**

Technique of acid-etch composite stabilization of displaced teeth. **A,** Lower incisor teeth displaced lingually. **B,** After digital repositioning, acid is applied to facial surfaces of displaced incisors and one or two teeth on each side following isolation and drying. **C,** Composite material and wire applied. **D,** Occlusion checked during *and* after stabilization.

2. The alveolar socket should be reasonably intact to provide a seat for the avulsed tooth.

3. There should be no orthodontic contraindications, such as significant crowding of teeth.

4. The extraalveolar period should be considered; periods exceeding 2 hours are usually associated with poor results. If the tooth is replanted within the first 30 minutes, excellent results can be expected.

5. The stage of root development should be evaluated. Survival of the pulp is possible in teeth with incomplete

root formation if replantation is accomplished within 2 hours after injury.

If the tooth to be replanted is not favorable for replantation, as determined by these factors, the patient should be made aware that the prognosis will be worse.

ALVEOLAR FRACTURES. Small fractures through the alveolar process, as mentioned previously, frequently accompany injuries to the teeth. However, injuries to the alveolar process often occur independently and can be challenging to manage. In most instances the segment of bone contains at least one tooth but more frequently several. There may be concomitant injuries, such as crown fractures, root fractures, and soft tissue injuries.

The treatment of this type of injury, as for any fracture, is first to place the segment into its proper position and then to stabilize it until osseous healing occurs. This procedure may be very simply performed with digital pressure applied after an appropriate anesthetic is administered (Figure 24-18). Frequently, however, splintering of the dento-osseous segment

◇ **Table 24-1.** Stabilization periods for dentoalveolar injuries

Dentoalveolar injury	Duration of immobilization
Mobile tooth	3-4 weeks
Tooth displacement	3-4 weeks
Root fracture	2-4 months
Replanted tooth (mature)	7-10 days
Replanted tooth (immature)	3-4 weeks

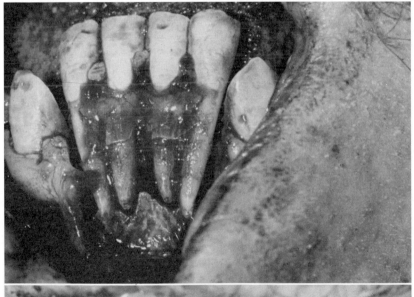

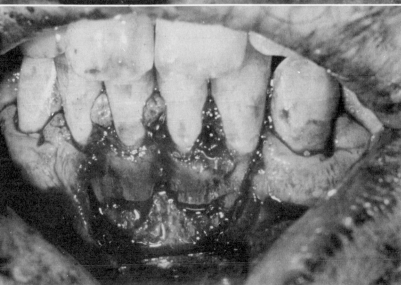

A

B

◇ Figure 24-18

Treatment of dentoalveolar fracture. **A,** Clinical appearance of fracture involving four mandibular incisors. Note that teeth are apically mature and have minimal bone around lateral and apical areas. **B,** Clinical appearance after digital reduction of fracture. Note that occlusal relationship is verified before stabilization of these teeth. *(Courtesy Dr. Stephen Feinberg, University of Michigan, Ann Arbor.)* *Continued*

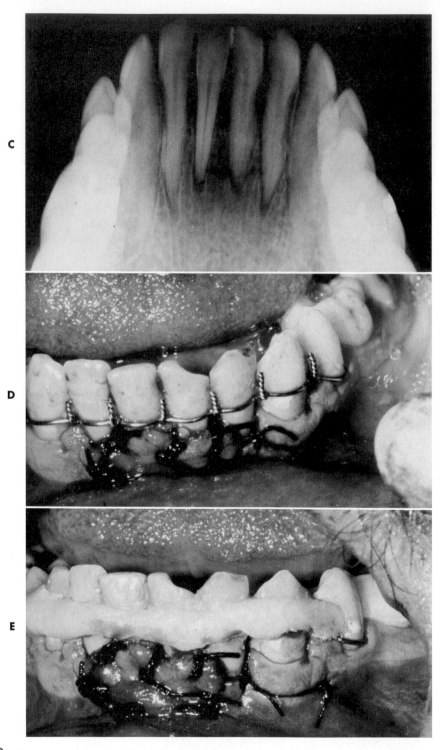

◇ **Figure 24-18, cont'd**

C, Radiographic appearance of teeth after digital reduction. **D,** Appearance after application of Essig wire and suturing of mucosa. **E,** Cold-curing acrylic added for rigidity. Because of maturity of apices, root canal treatment should be performed on these teeth in 1 to 2 weeks after trauma.

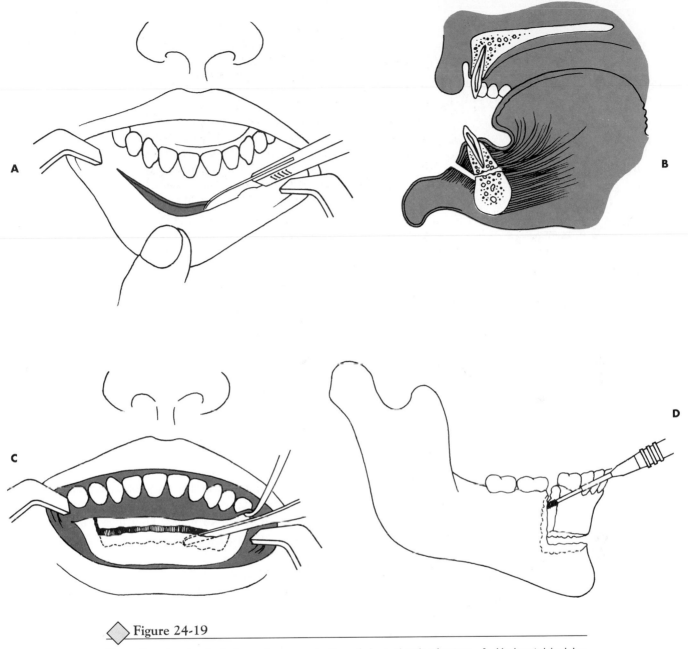

⬥ Figure 24-19

Illustration showing technique of open reduction of dentoalveolar fracture. **A,** Horizontal incision through mucosa, submucosa, mentalis muscle, and periosteum, exposing bone (**B**). **C** and **D,** Periosteal elevator used to pry alveolar segment into position or to disimpact it. Lingual plate of bone is usually fractured at different level than buccal plate, and irregularities to bone surfaces are the rule. These small spicules may prevent simple reduction of alveolar segment, and smoothing may be necessary. Clinician must take care to avoid roots of teeth when performing open reduction.

Continued

margins makes repositioning extremely difficult. In this instance it may be necessary to incise the soft tissues, develop a flap to gain access to the osseous tissues, and use instruments to reposition the segment with gentle force (Figure 24-19). The flap used for access must not jeopardize the blood supply to the dento-osseous segment. In general, the soft tissues must be left attached to the lingual portion of the alveolar process,

with exposure on the facial aspect. Exposure is most commonly made through a horizontal incision in the depth of the vestibule, with care taken not to transect the mental neurovascular elements (when in the mandible). Before incising the facial tissues, however, the clinician must verify that the lingual soft tissues are not lacerated or pulled from their bony attachments; otherwise, the blood supply will be compromised.

Once the flap is developed, examination of the dento-

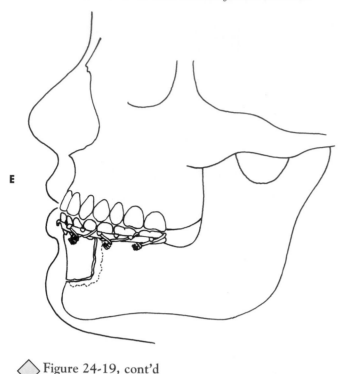

◇ **Figure 24-19, cont'd**

E, Once properly reduced, segment should be stabilized with whatever means are available, including arch-bar, orthodontic appliances, acid-etch wiring, or dental splint. Occlusion must be checked to verify that proper reduction has been achieved.

osseous segment and surrounding bone is carefully performed. The clinician should note whether the apices of the roots have been exposed, severing the vascular supply to the pulp. Occasionally, root fractures will have occurred, with the root tips remaining within the stable portion of the jaw. These should be retrieved before positioning the alveolar segment. Endodontic treatment should be performed in 1 to 2 weeks to help prevent inflammatory root resorption and infection if the apical blood supply to the teeth has obviously been interrupted.

The lateral aspects of the dento-osseous segment should also be explored to ensure that the roots of the teeth adjacent to the fracture have not been vertically fractured. The degree of bone denudation from their roots should also be ascertained to assess the potential for future periodontal problems if osseous reattachment is not complete. Even teeth that are mobile can usually be retained with a good chance of survival.

The segment should then be manipulated with digital pressure to determine where areas of resistance exist. If an irregular area of bone is sprung and inhibits repositioning, it may be removed with rongeurs or burs. Frequently, the alveolar segment can be pried into position with a thin instrument, such as a periosteal elevator, used with the adjacent basal bone as a fulcrum (Figure 24-19, *C* and *D*). Once the alveolar segment appears to be in its proper place, a careful examination of the occlusal relationship must be performed to ensure proper alignment of the dentition. Slight misalignment along the base of the alveolar segment is acceptable, as long as the occlusal relationship is accurate.

The dento-osseous segment must then be stabilized for approximately 4 weeks to allow osseous healing. There are several acceptable methods of stabilizing the segment. The simplest is to ligate an arch bar to the teeth both mesial and distal to the segment and within the fractured alveolar segment. The teeth immediately adjacent to the fracture are frequently not wired to the arch bar, so these teeth are more amenable to oral hygienic measures. Not wiring them also helps to prevent their loosening from the forces placed by the wire. The use of an acid-etched arch wire, as just described, is also acceptable. A cold-cured acrylic splint can be made either in situ or on casts obtained by taking an impression immediately after repositioning the alveolar segment. The splint can be wired to adjacent teeth and to teeth within the fractured segment.

Patients with difficult dentoalveolar injuries may require treatment by an oral and maxillofacial surgeon. This is especially true for fractures associated with other more serious injuries.

TREATMENT OF THE PULP. The dental pulp may be damaged during any of the tooth injuries just described, as a result of direct exposure, the inflammatory response of near exposure, concussive effects, or disruption of the pulp's nutrient artery. In any injury to the tooth the possibility for pulpal degeneration is real, and early detection is imperative. If a pulp degenerates, an inflammatory response occurs that leads to tooth resorption and ankylosis (Figure 24-20). Therefore for all injuries described the status of the pulp must be ascertained. Because it is difficult to establish the health status of the pulp immediately after injury, the dentist must assume that if the apex of a mature tooth has moved more than 1 mm in any direction, pulpal degeneration will occur.

Root canal treatment should not be performed at the time of tooth repositioning or replantation, because the extra time necessary to perform this treatment is not warranted and exposes the tooth to more chance of external damage. However, in all teeth with closed apical foramina, endodontic treatment should be instituted after approximately 2 weeks. This treatment helps minimize inflammatory root resorption by eliminating devital tissue from the pulp. A standard biomechanical preparation of the root canal system is then performed. However, instead of filling the root canal with gutta-percha, the clinician treats the canal in a manner similar to an apexification technique; that is, a 1:1 mixture of calcium hydroxide and barium sulfate is placed within the canal for 6 to 12 months. The barium sulfate allows radiographic evaluation of the amount of calcium hydroxide present, because it slowly dissipates within the root canal following placement. Periodic radiographic evaluations should be performed, and the calcium hydroxide should be replaced every 3 months if noted to be absent from the root canal system. A conventional root canal can be performed when successive radiographs indicate no further root resorption. This regimen should be used instead of placing a permanent

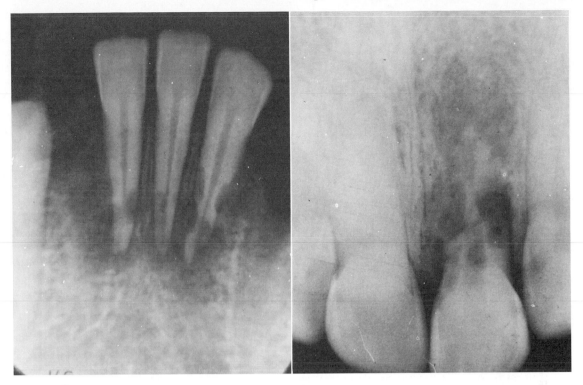

◇ **Figure 24-20**

Two cases of inflammatory root resorption that occurred several months after dentoalveolar trauma without root canal treatment.

endodontic filling soon after biomechanical preparation because it appears to minimize inflammatory root resorption.

In teeth with apical foramina that are wide open, endodontic treatment may be delayed for several weeks while careful follow-up examinations, including pulp vitality tests, determine its necessity. There is a good chance that revascularization of the root canal system will occur when the apices are open. If root canal therapy appears necessary, apexification procedures with use of calcium hydroxide, can be used before filling of the root canal system with a permanent filling material. The technique of apexification is illustrated in Figure 24-21.

SOFT TISSUE INJURIES ——◇

The types of soft tissue injuries the dentist may see in practice vary considerably. However, it is fair to assume that given the current availability of other health care providers, the dentist will probably not be involved in the management of severe soft tissue injuries around the face. Those seen with some frequency are the ones associated with concomitant dentoalveolar trauma or those that the dentist may inadvertently cause in practice.

In the following descriptions of the wounds the dentist may see in practice and their management, it must be remembered that patients may present with combinations of these injuries, and management may therefore be more complicated.

ABRASION

An abrasion is a wound caused by friction between an object and the surface of the soft tissue. This wound is usually superficial, denudes the epithelium, and occasionally involves deeper layers. Because abrasions involve the terminal endings of many nerve fibers, they are quite painful. Bleeding is usually minor, because it is capillary in nature and responds well to application of gentle pressure.

The type of abrasions most commonly seen by lay people are the scrapes that children sustain on their elbows and knees from rough play. If the abrasion is not particularly deep, reepithelialization occurs without scarring. When the abrasion extends down into the deeper layers of the dermis, healing of the deeper tissues occurs with the formation of scar tissue, and some permanent deformity can be expected.

The dentist may see abrasions on the tip of the nose, lips, cheeks, and chin in patients who have sustained dentoalveolar trauma (Figure 24-22). The abraded areas should be thoroughly cleansed to remove foreign material. Surgical hand soap is useful for this purpose, followed by copious saline irrigation. All particles of foreign matter must be removed. If these particles are allowed to remain within the tissue, a permanent "tattoo" that is difficult to treat will result. In deep abrasions that are contaminated with dirt or other material, it may be necessary to anesthetize the area and use a surgical scrub brush (or toothbrush) to remove the debris completely.

Once the wound is free of debris, topical application of an

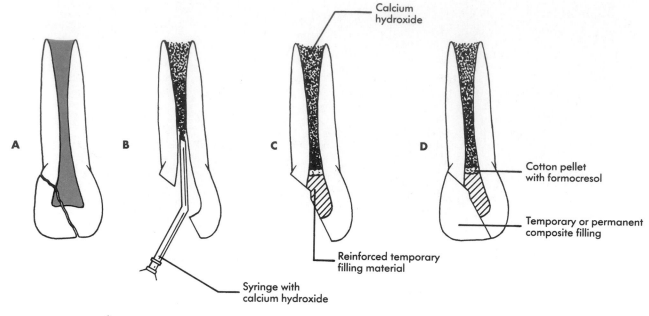

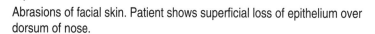

◇ Figure 24-21

Illustration showing apexification procedure. **A,** Coronal fracture involving pulp of apically immature tooth. **B,** Removal of entire pulp followed by filling with calcium hydroxide solution. This can be either injected from syringe or spun in with spiral on rotating instrument. **C,** Cotton pledget (with or without formocresol) is then placed, followed by filling of coronal pulp chamber with reinforced filling material. **D,** Temporary or permanent composite filling is then placed. Calcium hydroxide solution may require replacing every 3 months until apex is closed.

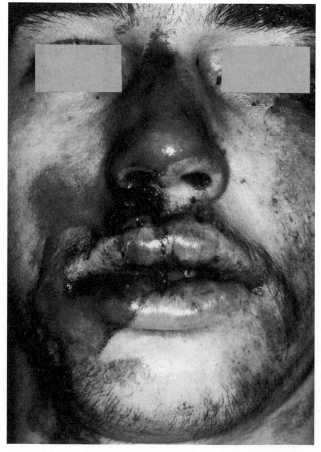

◇ Figure 24-22

Abrasions of facial skin. Patient shows superficial loss of epithelium over dorsum of nose.

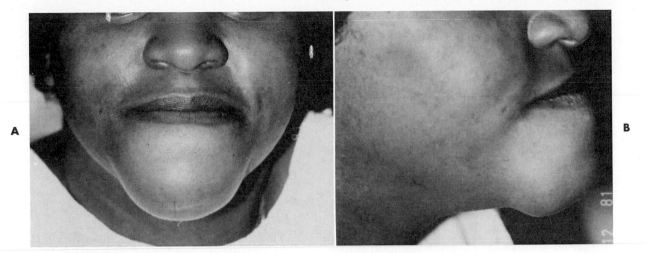

Figure 24-23

Frontal (**A**) and lateral (**B**) views of patient who sustained contusion of chin in motor vehicle accident. Note gross swelling that has resulted from disruption of subdermal tissue.

antibiotic ointment is adequate treatment. A loose bandage can be applied if the abrasion is deep but is unnecessary in superficial abrasions. Systemic antibiotics are not usually indicated. Over the next week, reepithelialization will occur under the eschar, which is a crust of dried blood and serum that develops following an injury to soft tissue (a scab). The eschar will then drop off.

If a deep abrasion on the skin surface is discovered after wound cleansing, referral to an oral and maxillofacial surgeon is indicated, because skin grafting may be necessary to prevent excessive amounts of scar formation.

The dentist may create abrasions iatrogenically, as occurs when the shank of a rotating bur touches the oral mucosa or when a gauze pack or other fabric (such as absorbent triangular pads) abrades the mucosa during removal from the mouth. Fortunately, the oral epithelium regenerates rapidly, and no treatment other than routine oral hygiene is indicated.

CONTUSION

A contusion is more commonly called a *bruise* and indicates that some amount of tissue disruption has occurred within the tissues, which resulted in subcutaneous or submucosal hemorrhage without a break in the soft tissue surface (Figure 24-23). Contusions are usually caused by trauma inflicted with a blunt object but are also frequently found with concomitant dentoalveolar injuries or facial bone fractures. In this instance the trauma to the deeper tissues (floor of mouth, labial vestibule, and so on) has occurred from the disrupting effect of the fractured bones. The importance of contusions from a diagnostic point of view is that when they are seen a search for osseous fractures should be made.

A contusion generally requires no surgical treatment. Once the hydrostatic pressure within the soft tissues equals the pressure within the blood vessels (usually capillaries), bleeding ceases. If a contusion is seen early, the application of ice or pressure dressings may help constrict blood vessels and therefore decrease the amount of hematoma that forms. If a

contusion does not stop expanding, it is likely that there is a hemorrhaging artery within the wound. The hematoma may require surgical exploration and ligation of the vessel.

Because there has been no disruption of the soft tissue surfaces, the hemorrhage formed within a contusion will in time be resorbed by the body, and the normal contour will be reestablished. In the next several days, however, the patient can expect areas of ecchymosis (purplish discoloration caused by extravasation of blood into the skin or mucosa; a "black-and-blue mark"), which will turn a variety of colors (blue-green-yellow) before fading. These areas may extend down below the clavicles and cause alarm, but they are innocuous.

When there has been no break in the surface of the soft tissue, infection is unlikely and systemic antibiotics are not indicated. If, however, the contusion is secondary to dentoalveolar trauma, there is a good chance of communication existing between the oral cavity and the submucosal hematoma. In this case, systemic antibiotics are warranted, because coagulated blood represents an ideal culture medium.

LACERATION

A laceration is a tear in the epithelial and subepithelial tissues. It is perhaps the most frequent type of soft tissue injury and is caused most commonly by a sharp object, such as a knife or a piece of glass. If the object is not sharp, the lacerations created may be jagged because the tissue is literally torn by the force of the blow (Figure 24-24). As with abrasions the depth of a laceration can vary. Some lacerations involve the external surface only, but others extend deeply into the tissue, disrupting nerves, blood vessels, muscle, and other major anatomic cavities and structures.

The dentist frequently encounters lacerations of the lips, floor of mouth, tongue, labial mucosa, and gingiva caused by trauma. Lip lacerations are commonly seen with dentoalveolar trauma, but in many instances of trauma the teeth are uninjured, because the force of the blow has been absorbed by the soft tissues.

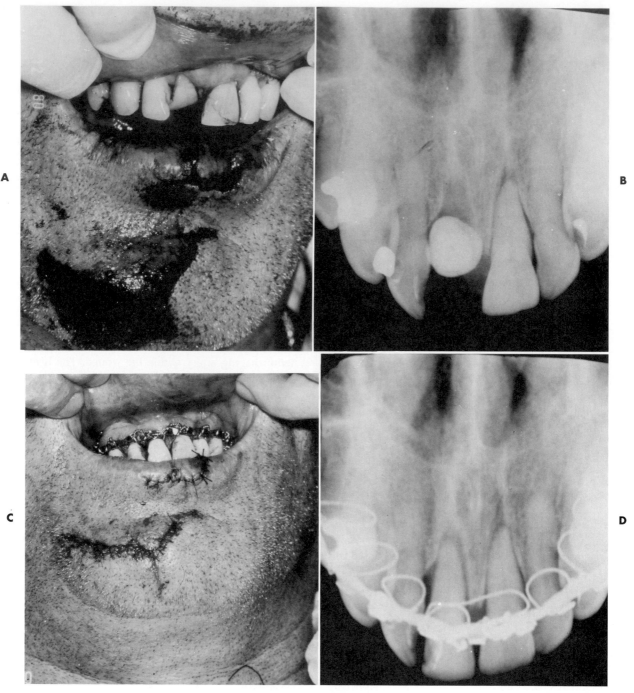

A, Clinical appearance of patient who sustained lingual displacement of tooth no. 8 and lacerations of lip in fall from ladder. **B,** Radiographic appearance of tooth. **C,** Clinical appearance of patient after repositioning of tooth, stabilization with arch bar, and closure of lip lacerations. **D,** Radiographic appearance of repositioned tooth. Because this tooth is apically mature, root canal was performed 2 weeks after trauma.

Soft tissue wounds associated with dentoalveolar trauma are always treated *after* management of the hard tissue injury. If the soft tissue is sutured first, time is wasted because the sutures are likely to be stressed too much and pulled out of the tissue during the intraoral manipulation necessary to replant an avulsed tooth or treat a dentoalveolar fracture. Further-

more, once sutures have been pulled out of the tissues, the tissues will be more difficult to close on the second attempt.

There are four major steps in the surgical management of lacerations: cleansing, débridement, hemostasis, and closure. These steps apply to lacerations anywhere in the body, including the oral cavity and perioral areas.

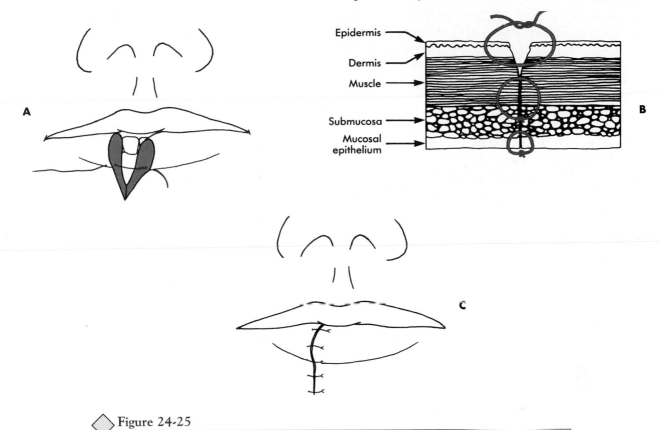

Epidermis
Dermis
Muscle
Submucosa
Mucosal
epithelium

◇ Figure 24-25

Illustration showing closure of lip laceration or incision. **A,** First suture is placed at mucocutaneous junction. It is extremely important to realign this, or cosmetic deformity will be noticeable. Lip is then closed in three layers: oral mucosa, muscle, and dermal surface (**B** and **C**). Choice of suture for oral and dermal surfaces varies with surgeon; however, muscle layer should be closed with either chromic or plain catgut suture (resorbable).

CLEANSING OF THE WOUND.   Mechanical cleansing of the wound is necessary to prevent debris from remaining. It can be performed with surgical soap and may necessitate the use of a brush. An anesthetic is usually necessary. Copious saline irrigation is then used to remove all water-soluble material.

DÉBRIDEMENT OF THE WOUND.   Débridement refers to the removal of contused and devitalized tissue from a wound. In the maxillofacial region, which enjoys a rich blood supply, the amount of débridement should be kept to a minimum. Only tissue that is obviously not vital is excised. For most of the lacerations a dentist encounters, no débridement is necessary except for minor salivary gland tissue (discussed later).

HEMOSTASIS IN THE WOUND.   Before closure, hemostasis must be achieved. Continued bleeding might jeopardize the repair by creating a hematoma within the tissues that can break the tissues open once they are sutured closed. If any bleeding vessels are identified, they should be either clamped and tied with ligatures or cauterized with an electrocoagulation unit. The largest vessel the dentist will probably encounter is the labial artery, which runs horizontally across the lip just beneath the labial mucosa. Because of its position the labial artery is frequently involved in vertical lip lacerations. This artery is approximately 1 mm in diameter and usually can be clamped and tied or clamped and electrocoagulated.

CLOSURE OF THE WOUND.   Once the wound has been cleansed and débrided and hemostasis has been achieved, the laceration is ready to be closed with sutures. However, not every laceration in the oral cavity must be closed with sutures. For example, a small laceration in the palatal mucosa caused by falling on an object extending from the mouth need not be closed. Similarly, a small laceration on the inner aspect of the lip or tongue caused by entrapment between the teeth during a fall usually does not require closure. These small wounds heal well by secondary intention and are best left to do so.

If closure of a laceration is deemed appropriate, the goal during closure is proper positioning of all tissue layers. The manner in which closure proceeds depends totally on the location and depth of the laceration.

When lacerations of the gingiva and alveolar mucosa (or floor of mouth) are noted, they are simply closed in one layer. If a patient has a laceration of the tongue or lip that involves muscle, resorbable sutures should be placed to close the muscle layer(s), followed by suturing of the mucosa. Minor salivary gland tissue protruding into a wound can be judiciously trimmed to allow for a more favorable closure.

In lacerations extending through the entire thickness of the lip, a triple-layered closure is necessary (Figure 24-25). If the laceration involves the vermilion border, the first suture placed should be at the mucocutaneous junction. It is imperative to align this junction of skin and mucosa perfectly, or it can result in a noticeable deformity that can be seen from a distance. Once this suture is placed, the wound is closed in layers *from the inside out.* The oral mucosa is first closed with either silk or resorbable suture. The orbicularis oris muscle is then sutured with interrupted resorbable sutures. Finally, the dermal surface of the lip is sutured with 5-0 or 6-0 nylon sutures. The wound will look as good at the completion of suturing as it ever will. If the alignment of tissues appears poor, consideration should be given to removing the sutures and replacing them in a more favorable manner. The dermal surface should then be covered with an antibiotic ointment.

Once a laceration is closed, the clinician must consider what supportive therapy can be instituted to bring about uneventful healing. Systemic antibiotics (such as penicillin) should be considered whenever a laceration extends through the full substance of the lip. In superficial lacerations, antibiotics are not indicated. The patient's tetanus status should be ascertained; if in doubt, patients should be referred to their physicians. Patients should also be instructed in postsurgical diet and wound care.

In general, facial skin sutures should be removed 4 to 6 days postoperatively. Adhesive strips can be placed at the time of suture removal to give external support to the healing wound.

REFERENCES

1. Andreasen JO, Hjorting-Hansen E: Replantation of teeth. I. Radiographic and clinical study of 110 human teeth replanted after accidental loss, *Acta Odontol Scand* 24:263, 1966.
2. Andreasen JO: Etiology and pathogenesis of traumatic dental injuries, *Scand J Dent Res* 78:339, 1970.
3. Andreasen JO: The effect of splinting upon periodontal healing after replantation of permanent incisors in monkeys, *Acta Odontol Scand* 33:313, 1975.
4. Andreasen JO: *Traumatic injuries of the teeth,* ed 2, Copenhagen, 1981, Munksgaard.
5. Sanders B, Brady FA, Johnson R: Injuries. In Sanders B, editor: *Pediatric oral and maxillofacial surgery,* St Louis, 1979, Mosby.
6. Rauschenberger CR, Hovland EJ: Clinical management of crown fractures, *Dent Clin North Am* 39:25-51, 1995.
7. Trope M: Clinical management of the avulsed tooth, *Dent Clin North Am* 39:93, 1995.
8. Turley PK, Joiner MW, Hellstrom S: The effect of orthodontic extrusion on traumatically intruded teeth, *Am J Orthod* 85:47, 1984.

MANAGEMENT OF FACIAL FRACTURES

MYRON R. TUCKER

CHAPTER OUTLINE ⟶ ◇

Trauma to the facial region frequently results in injuries to soft tissue, teeth, and major skeletal components of the face, including the mandible, maxilla, zygoma, naso-orbital ethmoid complex, and supraorbital structures. In addition, these injuries frequently occur in combination with injuries to other areas of the body.[7] Participation in the management and rehabilitation of the patient with facial trauma involves a thorough understanding of the types of, principles of evaluation for, and surgical treatment of facial injuries. This chapter outlines the fundamental principles for management of the patient with facial trauma.

EVALUATION OF PATIENTS WITH FACIAL TRAUMA ⟶ ◇

IMMEDIATE ASSESSMENT

Before completing a detailed history and physical evaluation of the facial area, injuries that demand immediate attention must be addressed. The first step in evaluating a trauma patient is to assess the patient's cardiopulmonary stability by ensuring that the patient has a patent airway and is adequately ventilated. Vital signs, including respiratory and pulse rates and blood pressure, should be recorded. During this initial assessment, other potentially life-threatening problems, such as excessive bleeding, should also be addressed. Immediate measures such as pressure dressings, packing, and clamping of briskly bleeding vessels should be accomplished as quickly as possible. An assessment of the patient's neurologic status and an evaluation of the cervical spine should be completed next. Injuries severe enough to cause fractures of the facial skeleton are often transmitted to the cervical spine. The neck should be temporarily immobilized until neck injuries have been ruled out. Careful palpation of the neck to assess possible areas of tenderness and cervical spine radiographs should be completed as soon as possible.

Treatment of head and neck injuries generally should be deferred until a thorough assessment and examination of the patient has been completed. However, some initial treatment is often necessary to stabilize the patient. Management of the patient's airway is of vital importance. Frequently, fractures of the facial bones severely compromise the patient's ability to maintain the airway, particularly when the patient is unconscious. Severe mandible fractures, especially bilateral fractures, cause gross posterior displacement of the mandible and tongue, which results in obstruction of the upper airway (Figure 25-1). Simply repositioning and stabilizing the mandible into a more anterior position may eliminate this problem. Placement of a nasopharyngeal or an oropharyngeal airway may also be sufficient to maintain a patent airway temporarily. In some cases, endotracheal intubation may be necessary. Any prosthetic devices, avulsed teeth, pieces of completely avulsed bone, or other debris may also contribute to airway occlusion and must be removed immediately. Any areas of bleeding should be quickly examined and managed with packing, pressure dressings, or clamping. All excess saliva and blood must be suctioned from the pharynx.

Injuries to the facial region may involve not only bones of the face but also soft tissue, such as the tongue or upper neck areas, or they may be associated with injuries such as a fractured larynx. In some cases an emergency tracheostomy may be necessary to provide an adequate airway.

HISTORY AND PHYSICAL EXAMINATION

After the patient has been initially stabilized, as complete a history as possible should be obtained. This history should be obtained from the patient; however, because of loss of consciousness or impaired neurologic status, information must often be obtained from witnesses or accompanying family members. Important questions to consider are: (1) How did the accident occur? (2) When did the accident occur? (3) What are the specifics of the injury, including the type of object contacted, the direction from which contact was made, and similar logistic considerations? (4) Was there a loss of consciousness? (5) What symptoms are now being experienced by the patient, including pain, altered sensation, visual changes, and malocclusion? A complete review of systems, including information about allergies, medications, and previous tetanus immunization, should be obtained.

Physical evaluation of the facial structures should be completed only after an overall physical assessment that addresses cardiopulmonary and neurologic functions and other areas of potential trauma, including the chest, abdomen, and pelvic areas. Because patients with multiple severe injuries frequently require evaluation and treatment by several

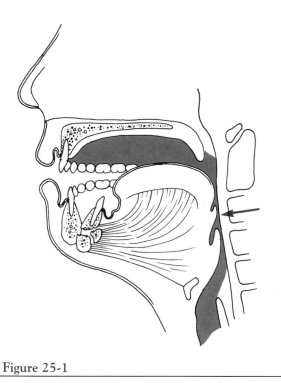

◇ Figure 25-1

Posterior displacement of tongue and occlusion of upper airway resulting from bilateral mandible fractures.

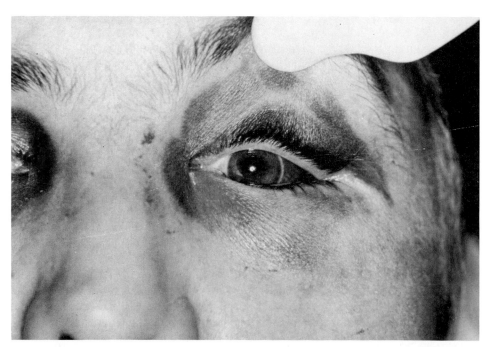

◇ Figure 25-2

Periorbital ecchymosis and subconjunctival hemorrhage associated with zygomatic complex fracture.

specialists, *trauma teams* have become standard in the emergency rooms of major hospitals. These teams usually include general surgeons and specialists in cardiothoracic surgery, vascular surgery, orthopedic surgery, neurosurgery, and anesthesiology; these specialists are on call to provide immediate attention to emergency room patients. Other trauma team specialists include oral and maxillofacial surgeons, ophthalmologists, urologists, otolaryngologists, and plastic surgeons. The combined efforts of these specialists are frequently required to assess the patient's injuries properly.

Evaluation of the facial area should be performed in an organized and sequential fashion. The face and cranium should be carefully inspected for evidence of trauma, including lacerations, abrasions, contusions, areas of edema or hematoma formation, and possible contour defects. Areas of ecchymosis should be carefully evaluated. Periorbital ecchymosis, especially with subconjunctival hemorrhage, is often indicative of orbital rim or zygomatic complex fractures (Figure 25-2). Bruises behind the ear, or Battle's sign, suggest a skull fracture. Ecchymosis in the floor of the mouth may indicate an anterior mandibular fracture.

A neurologic examination of the face should include careful evaluation of all cranial nerves. Vision, extraocular movements, and pupillary reaction to light should be carefully evaluated. Visual or pupillary changes may suggest intracranial (cranial nerve II, III, IV, or VI) or orbital trauma. Abnormalities of ocular movements may also indicate either central neurologic problems or mechanical obstruction of the movements of the eye muscles, resulting from fractures around the orbital area (Figure 25-3). Motor function of the facial muscles (cranial nerve VII) and muscles of mastication (cranial nerve V) and sensation over the facial area (cranial nerve V) should be evaluated. Any lacerations should be carefully cleaned and evaluated for possible transection of major nerves or ducts, such as the facial nerve or Stensen's duct.

The mandible should be carefully evaluated by extraorally palpating all areas of the inferior and lateral borders and the temporomandibular joint, paying particular attention to areas of point tenderness. The occlusion should be examined, and step deformities along the occlusal plane and lacerations of gingival areas should be assessed (Figure 25-4). Bimanual palpation of the suspected fracture area should be performed by placing firm pressure over the mandible posterior and anterior to the fracture area in an attempt to manipulate and elicit mobility in this area. The occlusion should be reexamined after this maneuver. Mobility of the teeth in the area of a possible fracture should also be noted.

The evaluation of the midface begins with an assessment of the mobility of the maxilla either as an isolated structure or in combination with the zygoma or nasal bones. To assess maxillary mobility, the patient's head should be stabilized by using pressure over the forehead with one hand. With the thumb and forefinger of the other hand, the maxilla is grasped; firm pressure should be used to elicit maxillary mobility (Figure 25-5). The upper facial and midfacial regions should be palpated for step deformities in the forehead, orbital rim, or nasal or zygoma areas. Firm digital pressure over these areas is used to evaluate the bony contours carefully and may be difficult when these areas are grossly edematous. An evaluation of the nose and paranasal structures includes measurement of the intercanthal distance between the innermost portions of the left and right medial canthus. Frequently, naso-orbital ethmoid injuries cause spreading of the nasal

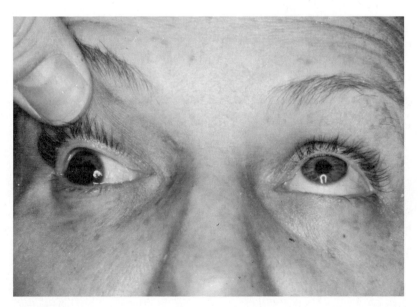

◇ Figure 25-3

Example of entrapment of inferior rectus muscle resulting from impingement in area of orbital floor fracture. In this case, patient is unable to rotate eye superiorly.

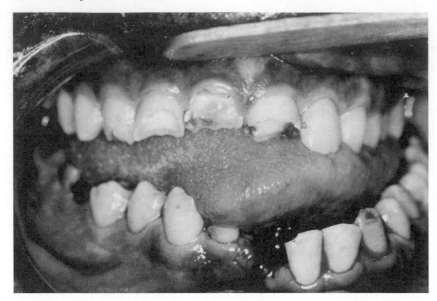

◇ **Figure 25-4**

Irregularity of plane of occlusion and small laceration in gingival area indicating likelihood of mandibular fracture in this area.

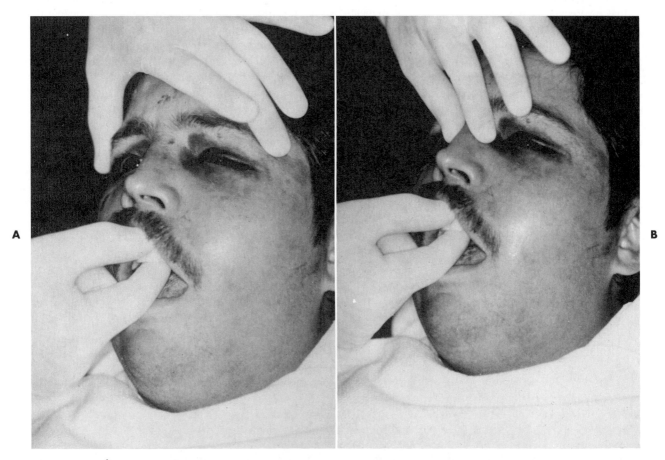

A

B

◇ **Figure 25-5**

Examination of maxilla for mobility. **A,** Firm pressure on forehead is used to stabilize patient's head. Pressure is placed on maxilla in attempt to elicit mobility. **B,** Stabilizing hand can also evaluate mobility in area of nasal bones.

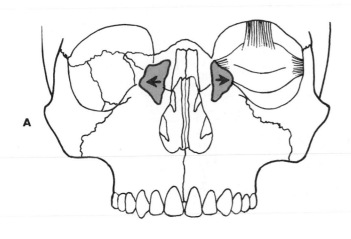

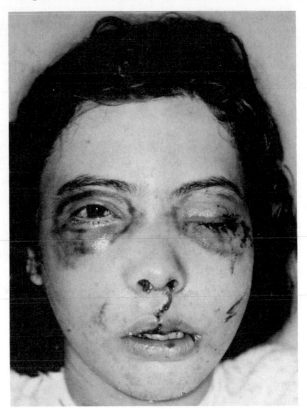

◇ Figure 25-6

A, Injury to naso-orbital ethmoid complex, resulting in detachment of medial canthal ligaments and widening of intercanthal distance (traumatic telecanthas). **B,** Clinical photograph.

bones and detachment of the medial canthal ligaments, resulting in traumatic telecanthus (widening of the medial intercanthal distance) (Figure 25-6). The nose should also be evaluated for symmetry. The bony anatomy of the nose should be evaluated by palpation. A nasal speculum is used to visualize internal aspects of the nose to locate excessive bleeding or hematoma formation, particularly in the area of the nasal septum.

Intraoral inspection should include an evaluation of areas of mucosal laceration or ecchymosis in the buccal vestibule or along the palate and an examination of the occlusion and areas of loose or missing teeth. These areas should be assessed before, during, and after manual manipulation of the mandible and midface.

RADIOGRAPHIC EVALUATION

Following a careful clinical assessment of the facial area, radiographs should be taken to provide additional information about facial injuries.[8] In cases of severe facial trauma, cervical spine injuries should be ruled out with a complete C-spine series before any manipulation of the neck. The facial radiographic examination should depend to some degree on the clinical examination and the suspected injury. Haphazard or excessive radiographic examination is generally not warranted. In the patient with facial trauma the

purpose of radiographs should be to confirm the suspected clinical diagnosis, obtain information that may not be clear from the clinical examination, and more accurately determine the extent of the injury. Radiographic examination should also document fractures from different angles or perspectives.

Radiographic evaluation of the mandible generally requires two or more of the following radiographic views: posteroanterior view, lateral oblique view, Towne view, and panoramic view (Figure 25-7). Occasionally, even these radiographs do not provide adequate information; therefore, supplemental radiographs, including occlusal or periapical views, may be helpful.[1] Computed tomography (CT) scans may provide information not obtainable from plain radiographs. Because many patients with facial trauma often receive a CT scan to rule out neurologic injury, this scan can also be used to supplement the radiographic evaluation.

Evaluation of midface fractures is generally supplemented with radiographic views, including Waters' view, lateral skull view, posteroanterior skull view, and submental vertex view (Figure 25-8). However, because of the difficulty of interpreting plain radiographs of the midface, more sophisticated techniques are generally used. This often includes CT scans done in several planes of space or three-dimensional reconstruction (Figure 25-9).

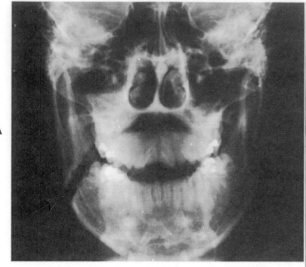

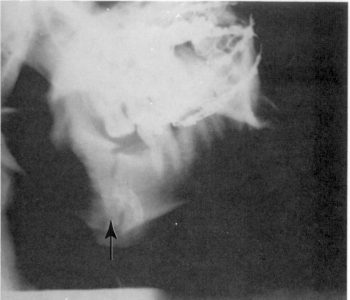

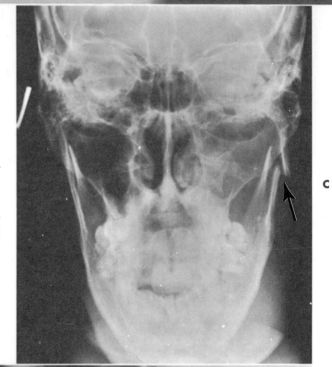

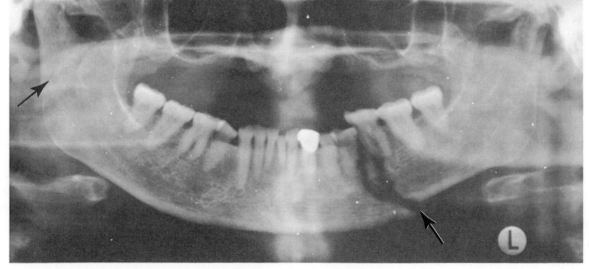

◇ Figure 25-7

A, Posterior-anterior view demonstrating fracture in body area of mandible. **B,** Lateral oblique view showing fracture in angle area. **C,** Towne view showing displacement of condylar fracture. **D,** Panoramic view showing displaced fracture of left mandibular body and right subcondylar fracture.

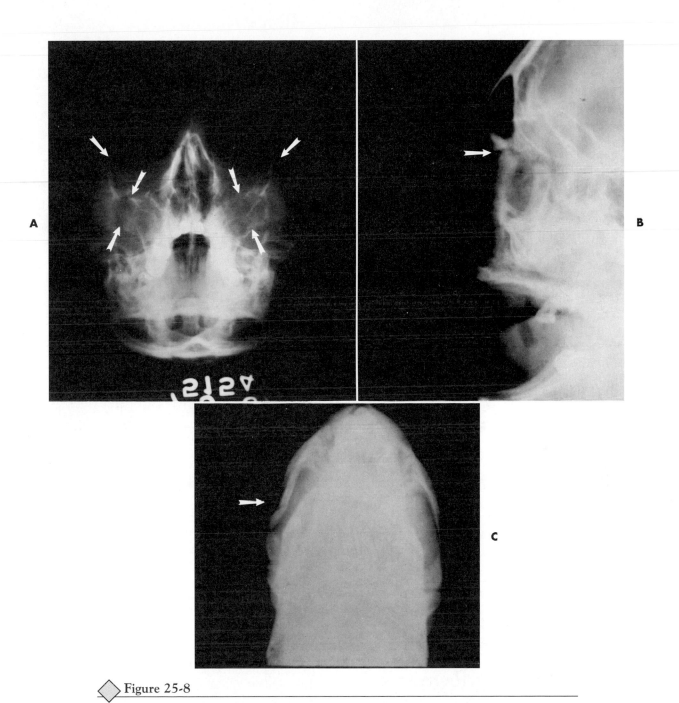

◇ Figure 25-8

A, Waters' view showing fractures of orbital rim areas. **B,** Lateral skull view illustrating a Le Fort III fracture, or craniofacial separation. Arrows denote fracture line separating midface from cranium. **C,** Submental vertex demonstrating zygomatic arch fracture.

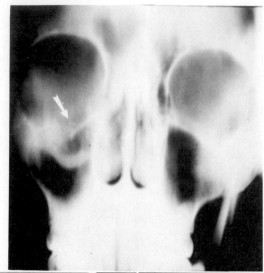

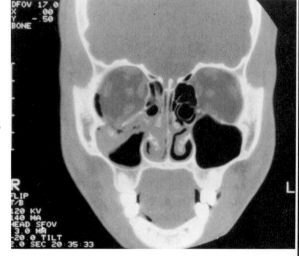

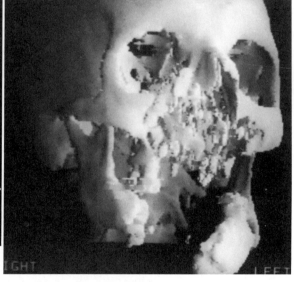

◇ Figure 25-9

A, Tomographic view demonstrating disruption of orbital floor. **B,** CT scan showing disruption of medial and inferior floor of orbit. **C,** 3-D reconstruction of shotgun wound resulting in avulsion of mandible and midface structures. *(Courtesy Dr. Mark W. Ochs.)*

ETIOLOGY AND CLASSIFICATION OF FACIAL FRACTURES ◇

CAUSES OF FACIAL FRACTURES

The major causes of facial fractures include motor vehicle accidents and altercations. Other causes of injuries include falls, sports-related incidents, and work-related accidents.[1,6] Facial fractures resulting from motor vehicle accidents are far more frequent in people who were not wearing restraints at the time of the accident.

MANDIBULAR FRACTURES

Depending on the type of injury and the direction and force of the trauma, fractures of the mandible commonly occur in several locations. One classification of fractures describes mandibular fractures by anatomic location. Fractures are designated as occurring in the condylar, angle, body, symphyseal, alveolar, ramus, and coronoid process areas. Figure 25-10 illustrates the location and frequency of different types of mandibular fractures.[13]

Another system of classification of mandibular fractures categorizes the type of fracture as *greenstick, simple, comminuted,* and *compound* fractures (Figure 25-11). These categories describe the condition of the bone fragments at the

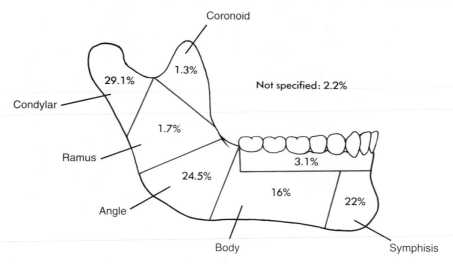

Coronoid

1.3%

29.1%

Not specified: 2.2%

Condylar

1.7%

Ramus

3.1%

24.5%

16%

22%

Angle

Body

Symphisis

◇ Figure 25-10

Anatomic distribution of mandibular fractures. *(From Olson RA et al:* Fractures of the mandible: a review of 580 cases, *J Oral Maxillofac Surg 40:23, 1982.)*

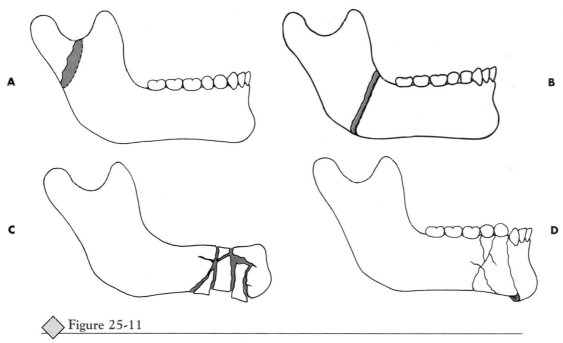

A

B

C

D

◇ Figure 25-11

Types of mandible fractures classified according to extent of injury in area of fracture site. **A,** Greenstick. **B,** Simple. **C,** Comminuted. **D,** Compound.

fracture site and possible communication with the external environment. Greenstick fractures are those involving incomplete fractures with flexible bone. Greenstick fractures generally exhibit minimal mobility when palpated. A simple fracture is a complete transection of the bone with minimal fragmentation at the fracture site. In a comminuted fracture the fractured bone is left in multiple segments. Gunshot wounds and other high-impact injuries to the jaws frequently result in comminuted fractures. A compound fracture results in communication of the margin of the fractured bone with the external environment. In maxillofacial fractures, communication with the oral or external environment may result from mucosal tears, perforation through the gingival sulcus and periodontal ligament, communication with sinus linings, and lacerations in the overlying skin.

Fractures of the mandible are referred to as *favorable* or *unfavorable,* depending on the angulation of the fracture and the force of the muscle pull proximal and distal to the fracture. In a favorable fracture, the fracture line and the muscle pull resist displacement of the fracture (Figure 25-12). In an unfavorable fracture, the muscle pull results in displacement of the fractured segments.

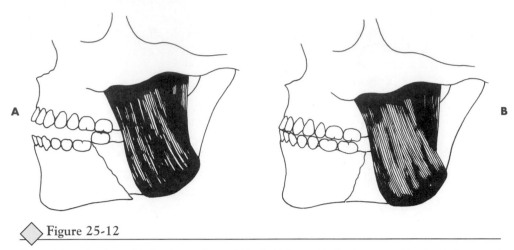

◇ Figure 25-12

Favorable and unfavorable fractures of mandible. **A,** Unfavorable fractures resulting in displacement at fracture site caused by pull of masseter muscle. **B,** Favorable fracture in which direction of fracture and angulation of muscle pull resists displacement.

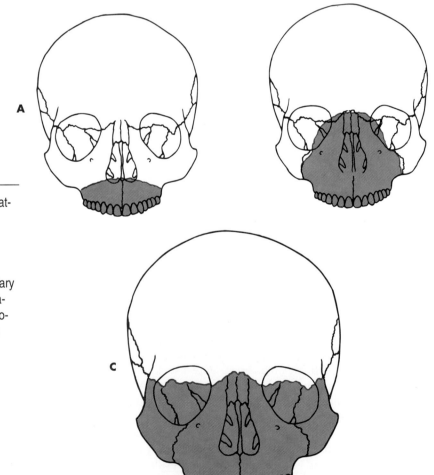

◇ Figure 25-13

Le Fort midfacial fractures. **A,** Le Fort I fracture separating inferior portion of maxilla in horizontal fashion, extending from piriform aperture of nose to pterygoid maxillary suture area. **B,** Le Fort II fracture involving separation of maxilla and nasal complex from cranial base, zygomatic orbital rim area, and pterygoid maxillary suture area. **C,** Le Fort III fracture (craniofacial separation) is complete separation of midface at level of naso-orbital ethmoid complex and zygomaticofrontal suture area. Fracture also extends through orbits bilaterally.

MIDFACE FRACTURES

Midfacial fractures include fractures affecting the maxilla, the zygoma, and the naso-orbital ethmoid complex. Midfacial fractures can be classified as *Le Fort I, II,* or *III fractures, zygomaticomaxillary complex fractures, zygomatic arch fractures,* or *naso-orbital ethmoid fractures.* These injuries may be isolated or occur in combination.

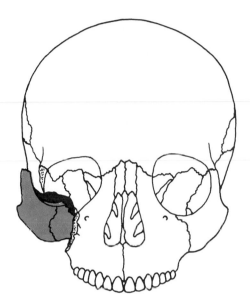

◇ **Figure 25-14**

Zygomatic complex fracture. *(Modified from Kruger E, Schilli W:* Oral and maxillofacial traumatology, *vol 1, Chicago, 1982, Quintessence.)*

The Le Fort I fracture frequently results from the application of horizontal force to the maxilla, which separates the maxilla from the pterygoid plates and nasal and zygomatic structures (Figure 25-13, *A*). This type of trauma may separate the maxilla in one piece from other structures, split the palate, or fragment the maxilla. Forces that are applied in a more superior direction frequently result in LeFort II fractures, which is the separation of the maxilla and the attached nasal complex from the orbital and zygomatic structure (Figure 25-13, *B*). A Le Fort III fracture results when horizontal forces are applied at a level superior enough to separate the naso-orbital ethmoid complex, the zygomas, and the maxilla from the cranial base, which results in a so-called craniofacial separation (Figure 25-13, *C*).

The most common type of midfacial fracture is the zygomatic complex fracture (Figure 25-14). This type of fracture results when an object, such as a fist or a baseball, impacts over the lateral aspect of the cheek. Similar trauma can also result in isolated fractures of the nasal bones, the orbital rim, or the orbital floor areas. The zygomatic arch may also be affected, either alone or in combination with other injuries (Figure 25-15).

TREATMENT OF FACIAL FRACTURES ◇

Whenever facial structures are injured, the goals of the treatment must be maximal rehabilitation of the patient. For facial fractures, goals of treatment include rapid bone healing, a return of normal ocular, masticatory, and nasal function,

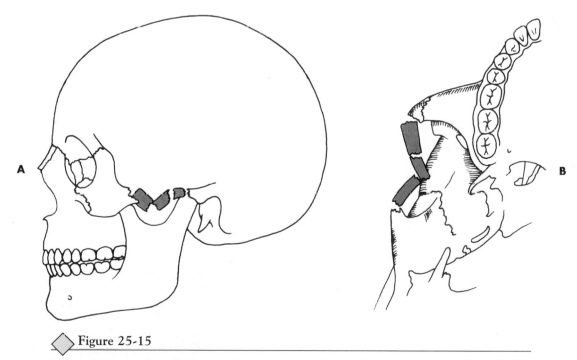

◇ **Figure 25-15**

A, Isolated zygomatic arch fracture. **B,** Lateral view. *(Modified from Kruger E, Schilli W:* Oral and maxillofacial traumatology, *vol 1, Chicago, 1982, Quintessence.)*

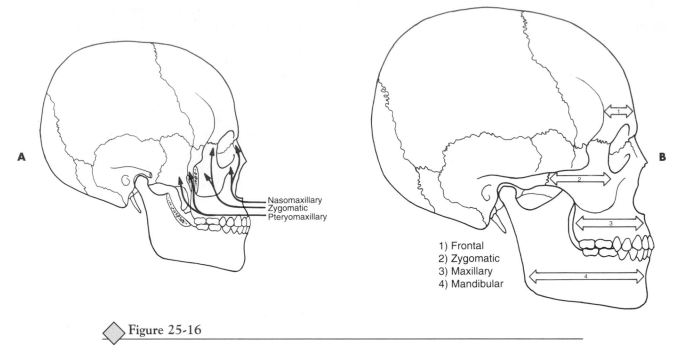

◆ Figure 25-16

A, Facial buttresses responsible for vertical support: nasomaxillary, zygomatic, and pterygomaxillary.
B, Anterior-posterior buttresses: frontal, zygomatic, maxillary, and mandibular.

restoration of speech, and an acceptable facial and dental esthetic result. During the treatment and healing phases it is also important to minimize the adverse effect on the patient's nutritional status and achieve treatment goals with the least amount of discomfort and inconvenience possible.

To achieve these goals, the following basic surgical principles should serve as a guide for treatment of facial fractures: reduction of the fracture (restoration of the bony segments to their proper anatomic location), fixation and stabilization of the bony segments, and immobilization of segments at the fracture site. In addition, the preoperative occlusion must be restored, and infection in the area of the fracture must be eradicated or prevented.

The timing of treatment of facial fractures depends on many factors. In general, it is always better to treat an injury as soon as possible. Evidence shows that the longer open or compound wounds are left untreated, the greater is the incidence of infection. In addition, a delay of several days or weeks makes an ideal anatomic reduction of the fracture difficult if not impossible. Additionally, edema worsens progressively over 2 to 3 days after an injury and frequently makes treatment of a fracture more difficult. There are, however, several reasons why treatment of facial fractures is frequently delayed. In many cases, patients have other injuries that demand more immediate treatment. An injury such as severe neurologic trauma that precludes presurgical stabilization of the patient and increases anesthetic and surgical risks should obviously be managed before facial fractures. In some cases a delay of 1 or 2 days results in the presence of tissue edema that makes a further wait of 3 to 4 days necessary for elimination of the edema and easier fracture treatment. In all cases, facial fractures should be treated as soon as the patient's

condition permits. No matter what the circumstances, a thorough evaluation of the patient, an assessment of the injury, and a treatment plan should be developed before surgical therapy is begun.

Although treatments of maxillary and mandibular fractures frequently have many aspects in common, these types of fractures are addressed separately in this chapter. Traditionally, the plan for treatment of most facial fractures was to begin with reduction of mandibular fractures and work superiorly through the midface. The rationale was that the mandible could be most easily stabilized, and the occlusion and remainder of the facial skeleton could be set to the reduced mandible. However, with the advent of and improvement in rigid fixation techniques, facial fracture treatment generally begins in the area where fractures can be most easily stabilized and progresses to the most unstable fracture areas.

In approaching facial fractures the surgeon attempts to rebuild the face based on the concept that certain bony structures within the face provide the primary support in the vertical and anteroposterior directions. Vertically, there are three buttresses existing bilaterally that form the primary vertical supports of the face. These include the nasomaxillary, zygomatic, and pterygomaxillary buttresses (Figure 25-16).[9] The structures that support the facial projection in an anterior-posterior direction include the frontal bar, zygomatic arch and zygoma complex, maxillary alveolus and palate, and the basal segment of the mandible.[10] Regardless of the type of facial fracture or the surgical approach used, the initial procedure should be to place the teeth in the proper occlusion, followed by the appropriate reduction of bony fractures. Bony repair should also precede soft tissue repair.

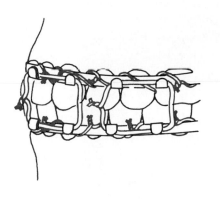

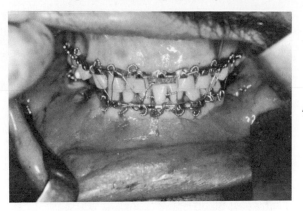

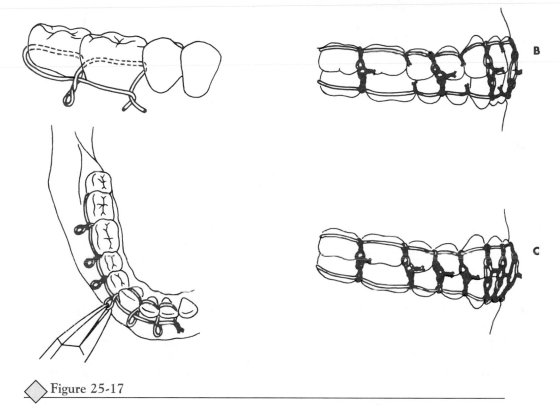

◇ Figure 25-17

Maxillomandibular fixation wiring techniques. **A,** Arch bar intermaxillary fixation. **B,** Ivy loop wiring technique. **C,** Continuous loop wiring technique. *(Modified from Kruger E, Schilli W: Oral and maxillofacial traumatology, vol 1, Chicago, 1982, Quintessence.)*

MANDIBULAR FRACTURES

The first and most important aspect of surgical correction is to reduce the fracture properly or place the individual segments of the fracture into the proper relationship with each other. In the proper reduction of fractures of tooth-bearing bones, it is most important to place the teeth into the preinjury occlusal relationship. Merely aligning and interdigitating the bony fragments at the fracture site without first establishing a proper occlusal relationship rarely results in satisfactory postoperative functional occlusion.

Establishing a proper occlusal relationship by wiring the teeth together is termed *intermaxillary fixation (IMF)* or *maxillomandibular fixation.* Several techniques have been advocated for IMF (Figure 25-17). The most common technique includes the use of a prefabricated arch bar that is adapted and wired to teeth in each arch; the maxillary arch bar is wired to the mandibular arch bar, thereby placing the teeth in their proper relationship. Other wiring techniques, such as Ivy loops or continuous loop wiring, have also been used for the same purpose.[2] When fractures have not been treated for several days or are grossly displaced, it may be difficult to place the fractured segments immediately into their proper position and into adequate IMF. Heavy elastic traction can be used to pull the bony segments into their proper positions

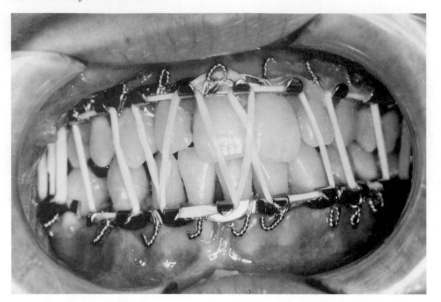

◇ **Figure 25-18**

Arch bars and heavy interarch elastics used to pull teeth and bony segments into proper occlusal relationship.

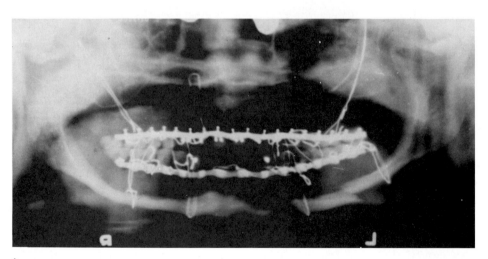

◇ **Figure 25-19**

Radiograph showing mandibular dentures secured with circumandibular wiring, maxillary denture secured in place, and intermaxillary wires used as closed reduction and stabilization technique for edentulous mandible fracture.

gradually over several hours or a few days (Figure 25-18). Treatment of fractures using only IMF is called *closed reduction,* because it does not involve direct opening, exposure, and manipulation of the fractured area.

In the case of a fracture of an edentulous patient, the mandibular dentures can be wired to the mandible with circummandibular wiring, and the maxillary denture can be secured to the maxilla using either wiring techniques or bone screws to hold the denture in place. The maxillary and mandibular dentures can then be wired together, which produces a type of IMF (Figure 25-19). A splinting technique that can be used for dentulous patients involves the use of a lingual or occlusal splint (Figure 25-20). This technique is particularly useful in treatment of mandibular fractures in children in whom placement of arch bars is difficult because of the configuration of the deciduous teeth and because patient understanding and cooperation is difficult to obtain.

After completing a closed reduction of the mandible and placing the dental component or alveolar process into the proper relationship with the maxilla, the necessity for an open reduction (direct exposure and reduction of the fracture through a surgical incision) must be determined. If adequate bony reduction has occurred, IMF may provide adequate stabilization during the initial bony healing phase of approxi-

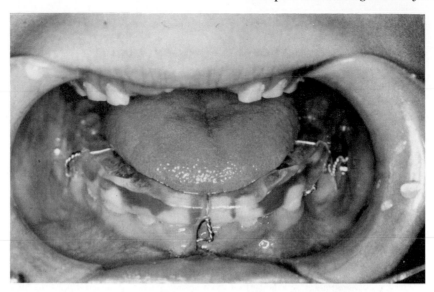

◇ Figure 25-20

Occlusal splint wired in place with circummandibular wires reducing and stabilizing fractured mandible.

mately 6 weeks. Indications for open reduction include continued displacement of the bony segments or an unfavorable fracture, such as in an angle fracture (Figure 25-12), in which the pull of the masseter and medial pterygoid muscles can cause distraction of the proximal segment of the mandible. Even when an unfavorable fracture appears to be adequately reduced with closed reduction, the muscular forces placed on the bone segment can result in subsequent segment displacement such that there is little or no contact of the bone in the fracture area, resulting in malunion or nonunion. With the advent of rigid fixation techniques, patients can be allowed to heal without undergoing IMF or at least a decreased time of IMF. This alone may be an important factor in the decision to perform an open reduction.

In some cases it is not feasible to expect an anatomic reduction of the fracture area. This is especially true of the condylar fracture. In this fracture, minimal or moderate displacement of the condylar segment generally results in adequate postoperative function and occlusion but only if a proper occlusal relationship was established during the period of healing of the fracture site. In these cases, IMF is used for a maximum of 2 to 3 weeks in adults and 10 to 14 days in children, followed by a period of aggressive functional rehabilitation.

When open reduction is performed, direct surgical access to the area of the fracture must be obtained. This access can be accomplished through several surgical approaches, depending on the area of the mandible fractured. Both intraoral and extraoral approaches are possible. Generally, the symphysis and anterior mandible areas can be easily approached through an intraoral incision (Figure 25-21), whereas posterior angle or ramus and condylar fractures are more easily visualized and treated through an extraoral approach (Figure 25-22). In some cases, posterior body and angle fractures can be treated

through a combination approach using an intraoral incision combined with insertion of a small trocar through the skin to facilitate fracture reduction and fixation (Figure 25-23). In either case a surgical approach should avoid vital structures such as nerves, ducts, and blood vessels and should result in as little scarring as possible.

The traditional method of bone stabilization after open reductions has been the placement of direct intraosseous wiring combined with a period of IMF ranging from 3 to 8 weeks. This method of stabilization can be accomplished through a variety of wiring techniques (wire osteosynthesis) and is often sufficient to maintain the bony segments in the proper position during the time of healing (Figure 25-24). If wire osteosynthesis is used for fixation and stabilization of the fracture site, continued immobilization with intermaxillary fixation is required until adequate healing has occurred in the area of the fracture.

More recently, techniques for rigid internal fixation have gained popularity for treatment of fractures.[2,3,5,12] These methods use bone plates, bone screws, or both to fix the fracture more rigidly and stabilize the bony segments during healing (Figure 25-25). Even with rigid fixation, a proper occlusal relationship must be established before reduction stabilization and fixation of the bony segments. Advantages of rigid fixation techniques for treatment of mandibular fractures include decreased discomfort and inconvenience to the patient because IMF is eliminated or reduced, improved postoperative nutrition, improved postoperative hygiene, greater safety for seizure patients, and, frequently, better postoperative management of patients with multiple injuries.

Other types of rigid stabilization have also been used, including external skeletal fixation appliances. An example of this type of appliance is a Joe Hall Morris appliance, which is constructed by placing four large bone screws that penetrate

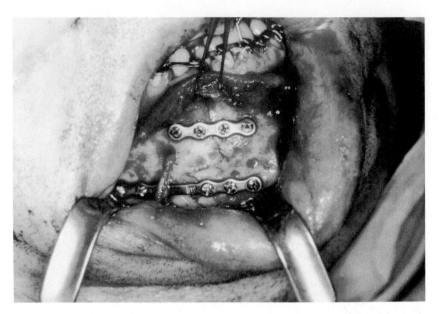

◇ Figure 25-21

Intraoral exposure of fracture in mandibular parasymphysis area. Note preservation of mental nerve.

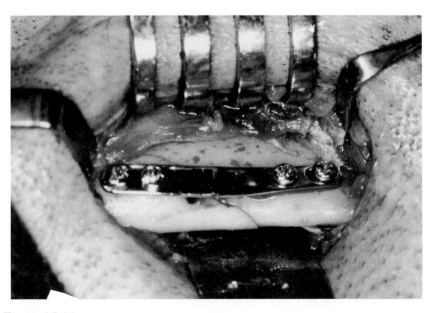

◇ Figure 25-22

Extraoral exposure of angle fracture.

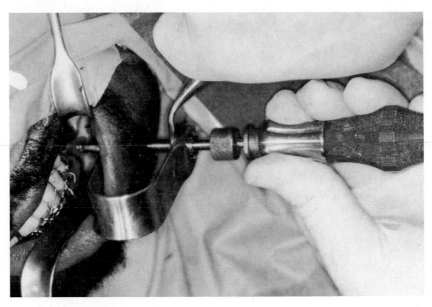

◇ Figure 25-23

Use of intraoral incision combined with percutaneous trocar placement for access to mandibular angle region.

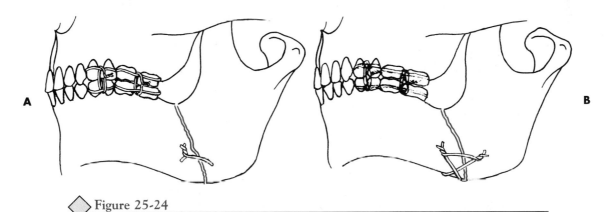

◇ Figure 25-24

A and **B,** Diagrammatic presentation of surgical wiring of fracture sites for reduction and stabilization of mandible fractures (with wire osteosynthesis of fracture sites, patients must be maintained in IMF during the healing period).

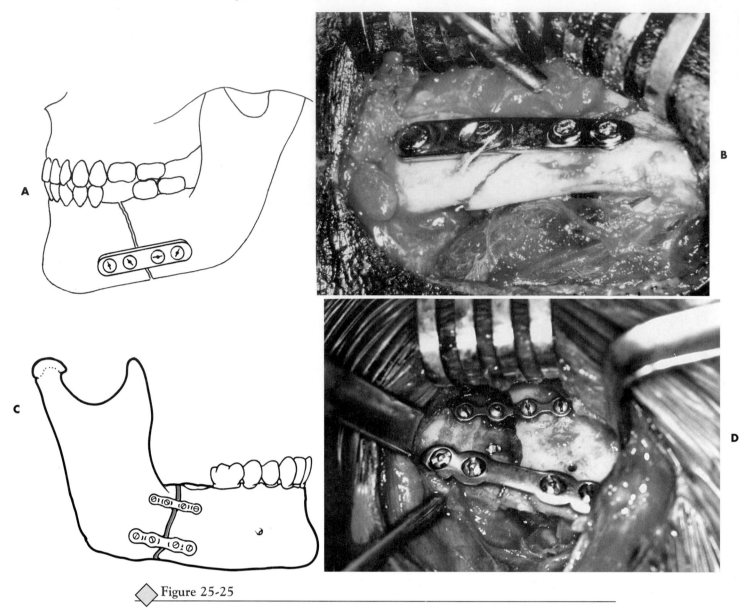

◇ Figure 25-25

A, Bone plate used for stabilization of mandible fractures. **B,** Clinical photograph of bone plate used for internal fixation of mandible fracture. **C,** Two bone plates used to stabilize fracture. **D,** Clinical photograph.   *Continued*

the skin, two on each side of the fracture site. A cold-cure acrylic bar is constructed to hold the screws in proper relationship with the fracture in the reduced position[11] (Figure 25-26). The obvious disadvantage is the appearance and inconvenience of this type of appliance. The advantages of this type of appliance are that it allows the patient to function during the time of fracture healing and that it can stabilize comminuted fractures that are best treated without opening the area, removing periosteum, and thereby denuding multiple bony segments. This type of appliance is also useful for treatment of a fracture that is infected and often best managed without placing any type of foreign material, such as a wire or a bone plate, directly in the area of the infected fracture.

MIDFACE FRACTURES

Treatment of fractures of the midface can be divided into those fractures that affect the occlusal relationship, such as Le Fort I, II, or III fractures, and those fractures that do not necessarily affect the occlusion, such as fractures of an isolated zygoma, zygomatic arch, or naso-orbital ethmoid complex.

In zygoma fractures, isolated zygomatic arch fractures, and naso-orbital ethmoid fractures, treatment is primarily aimed at the restoration of normal ocular, nasal, and masticatory function and adequate facial esthetics. In an isolated zygoma fracture (the most common midfacial injury), an open reduction is generally performed through some combination of intraoral, eyebrow, and infraorbital approaches. An instru-

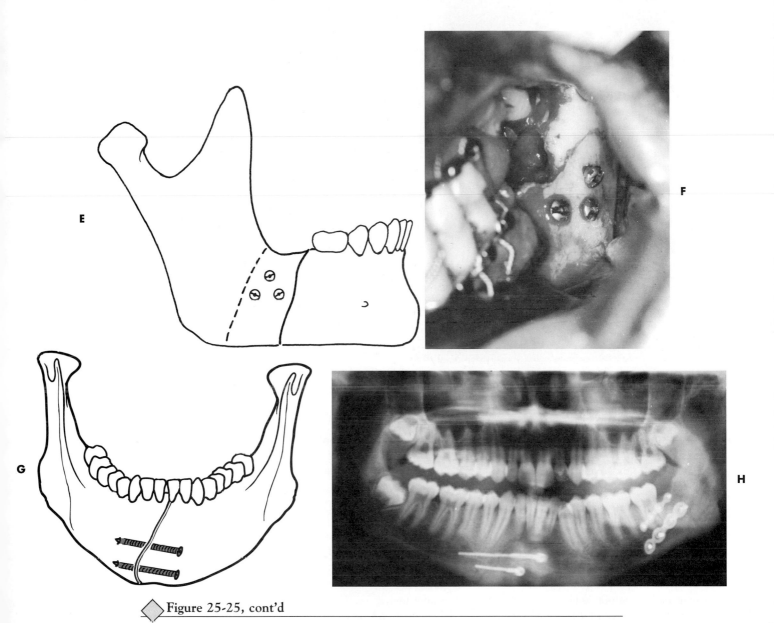

◇ Figure 25-25, cont'd

E, Diagram of oblique fracture of mandible stabilized with three lag screws. **F,** Clinical photograph of screw fixation of mandible fracture. **G,** Two screws placed tangentially across symphysis, stabilizing anterior mandible by engaging facial cortex on both sides of fracture and applying compression across fracture site with lag screws. **H,** Radiograph.

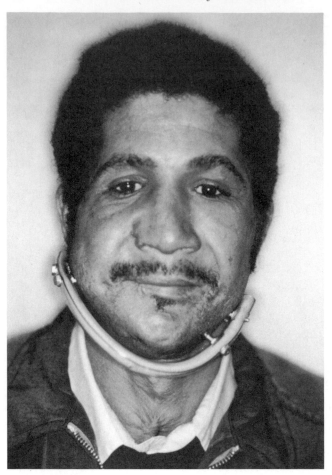

Figure 25-26

External skeletal fixation (Joe Hall Morris appliance).

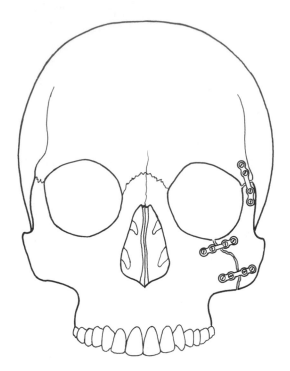

Figure 25-27

Diagram of plate stabilization of zygomatic complex fracture. Plates stabilize fractures at the zygomatic buttress, infraorbital rim, and zygomaticofrontal suture area.

ment is used to elevate and place the zygoma into the proper position. If adequate stabilization is not possible by simple manual reduction, bone plating of the zygomaticomaxillary buttress, zygomaticofrontal area, and the orbital rim area may be necessary (Figure 25-27).

In a zygomatic arch fracture, either an extraoral or an intraoral approach can be used to elevate the zygomatic arch and return it to its proper configuration. In addition to restoring adequate facial contour, this eliminates the impingement on the coronoid process of the mandible and the subsequent reduction in mandibular opening.

The goal of treatment for naso-orbital ethmoid fractures is to reproduce normal nasolacrimal and ocular function while repositioning the nasal bones and medial canthal ligaments into an appropriate position to ensure normal postoperative esthetics. In these situations, open reduction of the naso-orbital ethmoid area is usually necessary. Wide exposure to the supraorbital rim and nasal, medial canthal, and infraorbital rim areas can be achieved through a variety of surgical approaches. The most popular approach currently in use is the bicoronal flap, which allows exposure of the entire upper facial and nasoethmoidal complex through a single incision

that can be easily hidden in the hairline (see Figure 25-30).[14] Small bone plates appear to be most effective in stabilizing and maintaining bony segments in these types of injuries.

In midface fractures involving a component of the occlusion, as in mandibular fractures, it is extremely important *to reestablish a proper occlusal relationship* by placing the maxilla into the proper occlusion with the mandible. This step is accomplished by methods identical to the various types of intermaxillary fixation for mandibular fractures. However, as with mandibular fractures, reestablishing the occlusal relationship may not provide adequate reduction of the fractures in all areas. In addition to the need for anatomic reduction, additional stabilization of the fracture sites is often required.

When adequate bony reduction occurs following intermaxillary fixation but the fracture remains unstable, direct wiring, suspension wiring techniques, or bone plates may be used to stabilize the fracture. An example of such a case is a Le Fort I, II, or III midfacial fracture with an intact mandible. By placing the patient in IMF, movement of the mandible tends to dislodge the midfacial bones during any mandibular movement. Direct wiring techniques attempt to use wire osteosynthesis to directly stabilize the individual fractures (Figure 25-28).

Suspension wiring is sometimes used in addition to direct wiring. The purpose of suspension wiring is to provide stabilization of bones below the fracture site by suspending them to a more stable bone superiorly.[4] Suspension wiring

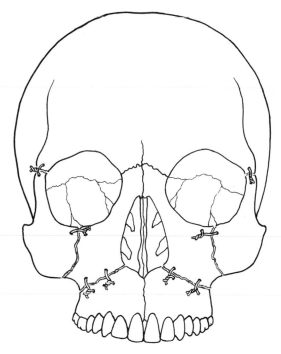

Figure 25-28

Diagram of wire placement used to stabilize various types of midfacial fractures.

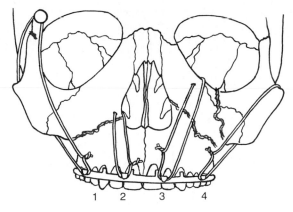

Figure 25-29

Diagram of suspension wiring techniques. *1,* Frontal bone suspension; *2,* piriform rim wiring; *3,* infraorbital rim wiring; *4,* circumzygomatic suspension.

techniques include those with wires attached to the piriform rim area, infraorbital rims, zygomatic arch, or frontal bone area (Figure 25-29). The fixation wires can be connected directly to the maxillary arch wire, interocclusal splint, or mandible. These suspension wires prevent movement of the maxilla caused by the inferior pull of the mandible during attempted opening. The use of direct and suspension wire fixation does have significant limitations in many cases. The limited rigidity of wires may make it difficult to reconstruct and maintain the appropriate anatomic contours, particulary in concave and convex areas, such as orbital rims and the prominence of the zygoma. Wires may not provide adequate resistance to muscular forces during the entire healing period, eventually resulting in some fracture displacement.

The recent development and improvement in miniaturized bone plate systems has greatly enhanced the treatment of midfacial fractures. Each of the advantages listed for rigid fixation of mandibular fractures applies to midface fractures. In addition to these advantages, small bone plates have greatly improved the ability to obtain proper bony contours at the time of surgery. When limited to the use of direct wiring or suspension wiring techniques, reestablishing curve configurations of bony anatomy is nearly impossible, particularly in the areas of severely comminuted small bone fragments. Severely comminuted unstable midface fractures can now routinely be treated by wide exposure of all fractured segments combined with the use of bony plates to reestablish the facial pillars, develop adequate contours, and stabilize as many facial bone fragments as possible (Figure 25-30). Use of

bone plates and screws has also facilitated the use of immediate bone grafting to replace comminuted or missing bone segments at the time of surgery and to improve stabilization of comminuted segments.

LACERATIONS

The general guidelines for management of facial lacerations are outlined in Chapter 24. Frequently, fractures of the facial bones are associated with severe facial lacerations. The principles of laceration repair remain the same regardless of how small or large the injury.

Cleansing of the laceration and examination of the area for disruption of any vital structures is extremely important. Possible injuries include lacerations of Stensen's duct, the facial nerve, or major vessels. In these cases, attempts must be made to reanastomose the duct, identify and perform a primary repair of the severed nerve, or manage all associated bleeding (Figure 25-31).

The lacerations should be closed from the inside out, that is, from the oral mucosa to the muscle to the subcutaneous tissue and skin. All closures should be completed in layers to orient tissues properly and to eliminate any dead space within the wound to prevent hematoma formation. Easily identifiable landmarks, such as the vermilion border of the lip, ala of the nose, or areas of the laceration that can be easily identified and properly repositioned, should be sutured first (Figure 25-32), followed by closure of areas where wound margins are not so clearly reapproximated. All wounds should be cleansed periodically with hydrogen peroxide. Some surgeons advocate including the use of antiobiotic ointment in wound care. However, use of dry occlusive dressings, such as steristrip coverings can be equally effective. Sutures from facial wounds are generally removed in 4 to 7 days, depending on the location of the wound and the amount of tension necessary to provide adequate wound closure.

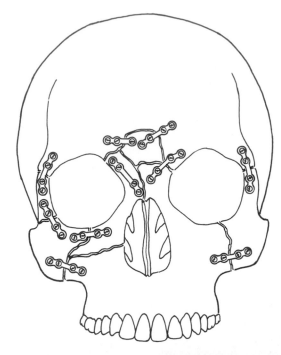

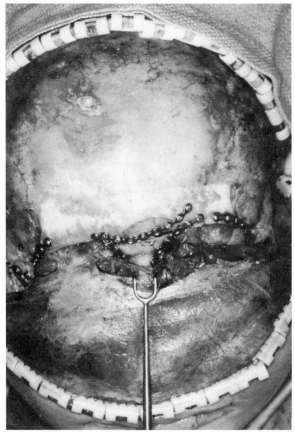

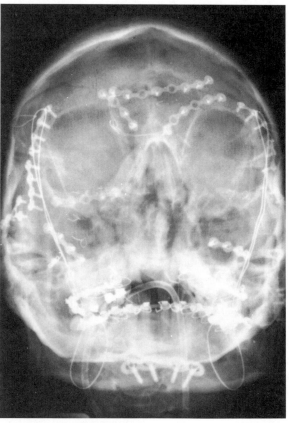

◆ **Figure 25-30**

Plate stabilization of severe midface fracture. **A,** Diagrammatic representation. **B,** View of supraorbital area after stabilization of fragments with small bone plates. **C,** Postoperative radiograph. *(Courtesy Dr. Mark W. Ochs.)*

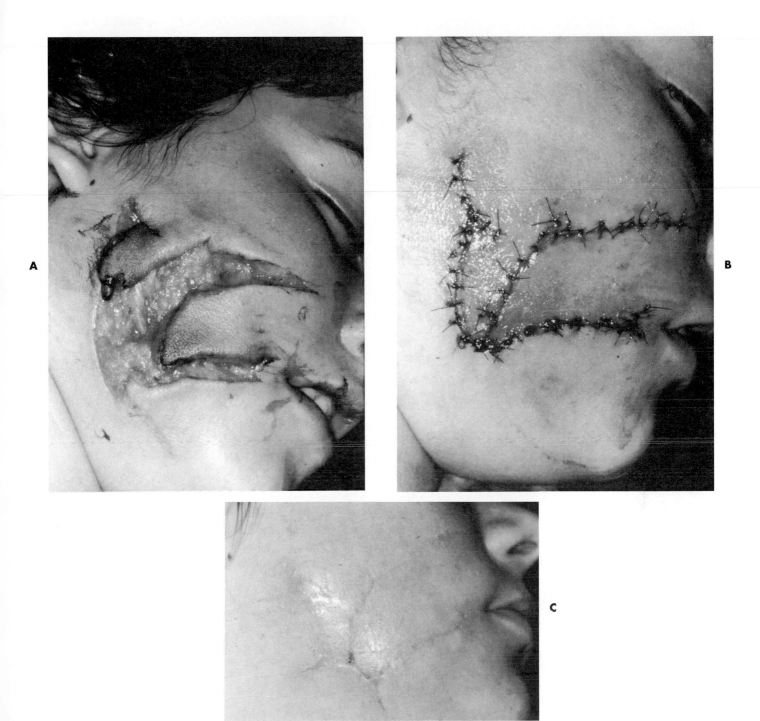

◇ Figure 25-31

A, Large laceration over the area of the facial nerve and parotid duct. Exploration may be necessary to locate and repair these structures. **B,** Immediate postoperative view. **C,** Two weeks postoperatively. Note small area of wound breakdown resulting from necrosis of severely damaged flap margin.

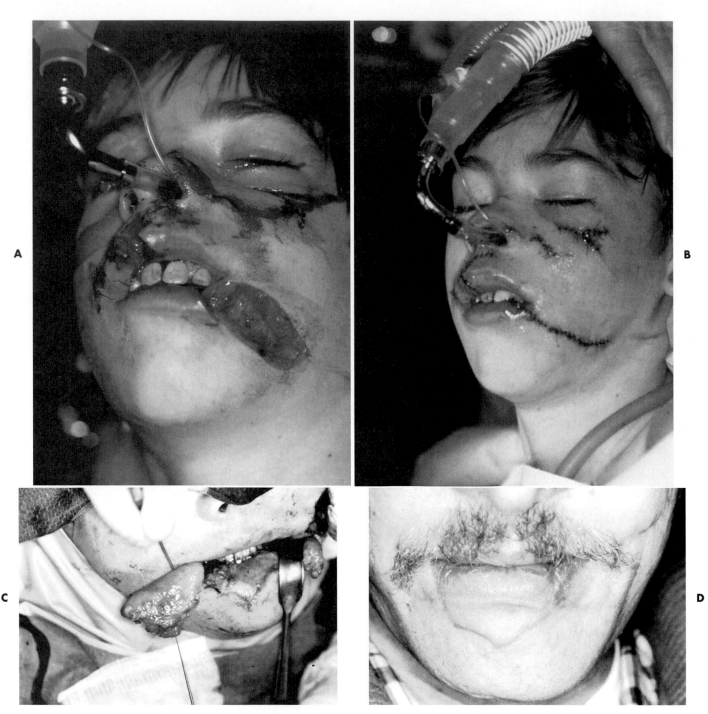

◇ Figure 25-32

A, Multiple facial lacerations through the upper lip, left commisure, and left infraorbital/paranasal area. **B,** Closure of lacerations with careful attention given to alignment of lip margins. **C,** Large laceration nearly resulting in avulsion of lower lip. Preservation of the labial artery allows large flap of lip tissue to remain viable despite small pedicle base. **D,** Appearance of lower lip 6 weeks after injury and initial repair.

REFERENCES

1. Afzelius L, Rosen C: Facial fractures: a review of 368 cases, *Int J Oral Surg* 9:25, 1980.
2. Batters BTJ: The plating of mandibular fractures, *Br J Oral Surg* 4:194, 1967.
3. Becker R: Stable compression plate fixation of mandibular fractures, *Br J Oral Surg* 12:13, 1974.
4. Bowerman JE: Fractures of the middle third of the facial skeleton. In Rowe NL, Williams JI, editors: *Maxillofacial injuries,* vol 1, New York, 1984, Churchill Livingstone.
5. Champy M et al: Mandibular osteosynthesis by miniaturized screw plates by a buccal approach, *J Maxillofac Surg* 6:14, 1978.
6. Ellis E, El-Attar A, Moos K: An analysis of 2067 cases of zygomatical orbital fractures, *J Oral Maxillofac Surg* 43:417, 1985.
7. Ellis E, Moos K, El-Attar A: Ten years of mandibular fractures: an analysis of 2137 cases, *Oral Surg* 59:120, 1985.
8. Gerlock AJ, Sinn DP, McBride KL: *Clinical and radiographic interpretation of facial fractures,* Boston, 1981, Little, Brown.
9. Manson PM, Hoopes JE, Su CT: Structural pillars of the facial skeleton: an approach to the management of Le Fort fractures, *Plast Reconstr Surg* 60:54, 1980.
10. Markowitz BL, Manson PM: Panfacial fracture: organization of treatment, *Clin Plast Surg* 16:105, 1989.
11. Morris JH: Biphase connector external skeletal pin for reduction and fixation of mandibular fractures, *Oral Surg* 2:1382, 1949.
12. Ochs MW, Tucker MR: Current concepts in management of facial trauma, *J Oral Maxillofac Surg* 51:42, 1993.
13. Olsen RA et al: Fractures of the mandible: a review of 580 cases, *J Oral Maxillofac Surg* 40:23, 1982.
14. Van Sickels JE, White RP Jr: Rigid fixation for maxillofacial surgery. In Tucker MR et al, editors: *Rigid fixation for maxillofacial surgery,* Philadelphia, 1991, JB Lippincott.

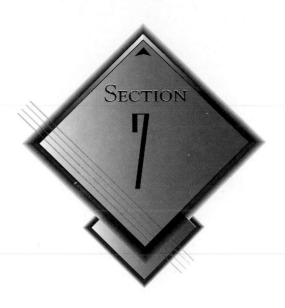

DENTOFACIAL DEFORMITIES

Patients with congenital or acquired abnormalities of facial bones and soft tissue generally require the assistance of many medical and dental specialists to achieve maximal rehabilitation. Patients with malocclusions and facial abnormalities resulting from an abnormal growth of facial bones usually require the services of general dentists, prosthodontists, periodontists, orthodontists, and oral and maxillofacial surgeons. The care of patients with cleft lips and palates involves all of the dental specialists, as well as pediatricians, plastic surgeons, otolaryngologists, speech and hearing therapists, and psychologists. Chapters 26 and 27 outline the treatments available for these patients, the sequence of treatment, and the need for participation of dental generalists and specialists.

Facial trauma and pathology often result in the loss of large portions of the jaws and associated structures. Reconstruction of missing portions of the jaws and associated facial bones and soft tissues usually necessitates comprehensive and often multiple surgical treatments to rehabilitate the patient adequately. Chapter 28 discusses the principles of maxillofacial reconstruction.

CORRECTION OF DENTOFACIAL DEFORMITIES

MYRON R. TUCKER

E pidemiologic surveys demonstrate that a large percentage of the United States' population has a significant
malocclusion. Many of these cases are severe enough to
affect facial proportions, and approximately 5% may be
classified as handicapping.[3] Approximately 10% of the
population has a class II malocclusion, 1% of which require
surgical advancement of the mandible to correct the skeletal
deficiency. A similar percentage of the population requires
surgical correction of anteroposterior maxillary excess to treat
their class II malocclusions most satisfactorily. Class III
malocclusions occur in 2.5% of the population, with 40% of
these cases being severe enough to require surgical correction
to obtain the best occlusal and esthetic result. In most class III
malocclusions the deformities can be attributed to abnormal
skeletal position of the mandible; however, 30% to 40% may
be at least partially caused by maxillary deficiency.

Historically, treatment of dentofacial deformities has been
aimed at correction of dental abnormalities, with little
attention to the accompanying deformity of the facial skeleton.
In the last 30 years, surgical techniques have been developed
to allow positioning of the entire midface complex, mandible,
or dentoalveolar segments to any desired position. The
combining of surgical and orthodontic procedures for
dentofacial deformities has become an integral part of the
correction of malocclusions and facial abnormalities.

CAUSES OF DENTOFACIAL DEFORMITY

Malocclusion and associated abnormalities of the skeletal
components of the face can be classified as either *acquired* or
developmental. Acquired deformities result from trauma or
other external influences that alter facial morphology. Developmental deformities result from abnormal growth of facial
structures. Although it is not within the scope of this book to
present a detailed discussion of facial growth, an understanding of basic principles as they relate to the development of
dentofacial deformities is essential. Enlow's *Handbook of
Facial Growth*[7] should be reviewed for a more complete
discussion of the principles of facial growth.

GENERAL PRINCIPLES OF FACIAL GROWTH

The development of proper facial form and function is a complex process affected by many factors. The primary sites of growth in the face and cranium are the free margins of the bony surfaces, sutures, synchondroses, and mandibular condyle. In the area of the craniofacial complex, there are areas that appear to have their own intrinsic growth potential, including the spheno-occipital and sphenoethmoidal synchondroses and the nasal septum. In addition, the majority of growth of the bones of the face occurs in response to adjacent soft tissue and the functional demands placed on the underlying bone. This theory, called the *functional matrix theory,* explains the dimensions of these growth patterns.[13]

The general direction of the growth of the face is downward and forward. Both the maxilla and the mandible appear to grow by differential apposition and resorption of bone, producing changes in these two directions. Enlow[8] describes this phenomenon as *area relocation,* with the maxillary-mandibular complex enlarging in the downward and forward direction as an "expanding V" (Figure 26-1). The direction and amount of growth characterize an individual's growth pattern. Alterations in the pattern of growth or in the rate at which this growth occurs may result in

abnormal skeletal morphology of the face and an accompanying malocclusion.

GENETIC AND ENVIRONMENTAL INFLUENCE

Genetic influence certainly plays a role in dentofacial deformities. Patterns of inheritance, such as a familial tendency toward a prognathic or deficient mandible, are often seen in a patient with a dentofacial deformity. However, the multifactorial nature of facial development precludes the prediction of an inherited pattern of a particular facial abnormality.

Environmental influences also play a role in the development of dentofacial deformities. As early as the prenatal stage, intrauterine molding of the developing fetal head may result in a severe mandibular deficiency. Abnormal function following birth also may result in altered facial growth. Respiratory difficulty, mouth breathing, and abnormal tongue and lip postures can adversely influence facial growth. Back braces with cervical support place pressure on the chin that can produce severe occlusal changes and alterations in the form of facial bones. This is primarily the result of forced changes in the direction of growth during a time in which growth is continuing.

Trauma to the bones of the face can obviously result in

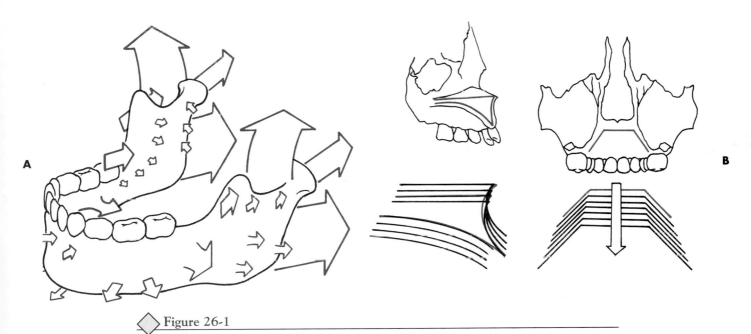

◇ Figure 26-1

A, Mandibular growth resulting from apposition and resorption of bone. Primary areas of bony apposition include superior surface of alveolar process and posterior and superior surfaces of mandibular ramus. **B,** Forward and downward growth of nasal complex and maxilla in "expanding V." Resorption of bone at superior surface of palate occurs simultaneously with apposition at inferior surfaces of palate and alveolar processes. Also, growth in posterior area of maxilla results in downward and forward expansion of maxilla. *(From Enlow DH:* Handbook of facial growth, *Philadelphia, 1975, WB Saunders.)*

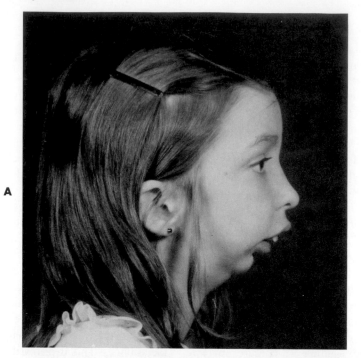

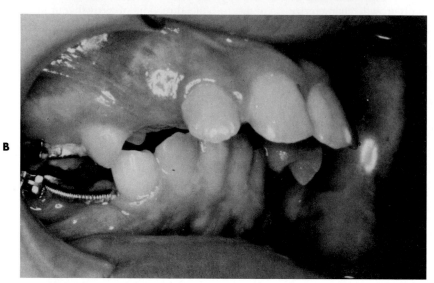

◇ Figure 26-2

Ankylosis resulting from trauma to TMJ. Damage to condylar growth center or limitation in function and resulting soft tissue influence on developing bone are responsible for resulting mandibular deficiency. **A,** Abnormal appearance of facial skeleton with severe mandibular deficiency. **B,** Severe class II malocclusion resulting from skeletal abnormality.

severe abnormalities of both the facial skeleton and the occlusion. In addition to the abnormality that occurs as an immediate result of trauma, further effects on the development of facial bones may occur, which is most evident when ankylosis of the mandibular condyle occurs as a result of trauma. In the case of temporomandibular joint (TMJ) ankylosis in a growing child, alteration of growth may result from destruction of the area of growth in the TMJ cartilage, as well as from limitation in function, which decreases the influence of soft tissues on developing bone (Figure 26-2).

EVALUATION OF PATIENTS WITH DENTOFACIAL DEFORMITY ◇

In the past, patients with dentofacial deformities were often treated by individual practitioners. Some patients have been treated with orthodontics alone, with a resultant acceptable occlusion but a compromise in facial esthetics. Other patients have had surgery without orthodontics in an attempt to correct

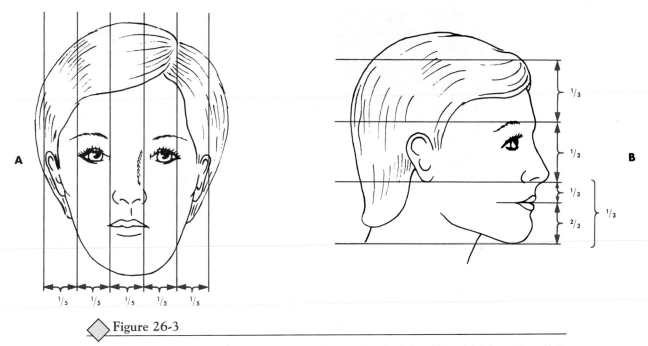

◇ Figure 26-3

Normal facial proportions. **A,** Representation of proportional relationships of full-face view. Note relationships of medial intercanthal distance, alar base width, and lip proportions to remainder of facial structures. **B,** Normal profile proportions demonstrating relationships of upper, middle, and lower thirds of face and proportional relationships of lip and chin morphology within lower third of face.

a skeletal deformity, which resulted in improved facial esthetics but a less-than-ideal occlusion. In addition to orthodontic and surgical needs, these patients often have many other problems requiring periodontic, endodontic, complex restorative, and prosthetic considerations.

Many areas of dental practice, in addition to orthodontics and surgery, must be integrated to address the complex problems of patients with dental deformities. This integrated approach, used throughout the evaluation, presurgical, and postsurgical phases of patient care, provides the best possible results for these patients.[19]

The most important phase in patient care centers on evaluation of the existing problems and definition of treatment goals. At the initial appointment a thorough interview should be conducted with the patient to discuss the patient's perception of the problems and the goals of any possible treatment. The patient's current health status and any medical or psychologic problems that may affect treatment are also discussed at this time.

The involved orthodontist and oral and maxillofacial surgeon should conduct a thorough examination of facial structure, with consideration of full-face and profile esthetics.

Evaluation of facial esthetics in the full-face view should assess the presence of asymmetries and evaluate overall facial balance. The evaluation should include assessment of the position of the forehead, eyes, infraorbital rims, and malar eminences; configuration of the nose, including the width of the alar base; paranasal areas; lip morphology; relationship of the lips to incisors; and overall

proportional relationships of the face in the vertical and transverse dimensions. Figure 26-3 demonstrates normal facial proportions. The profile evaluation allows an assessment of the anteroposterior and vertical relationships of all components of the face. The soft tissue configuration of the throat should also be evaluated. Photographic documentation of the pretreatment condition of the patient should be a standard part of the evaluation. Video/digital computerized images have recently been introduced as an additional aid in evaluating facial morphology.

A complete dental examination should include assessment of dental arch form, symmetry, tooth alignment, and occlusal abnormalities in the transverse, anteroposterior, and vertical dimensions. The muscles of mastication and TMJ function should also be evaluated. A screening periodontal examination, including probing, should assess the patient's hygiene and current periodontal health status. Impressions and a bite registration for dental cast construction and evaluation should also be obtained at this time.

Lateral cephalometric and panoramic radiographs, as well as posteroanterior facial films and TMJ films when indicated, are an important part of the initial assessment. The cephalometric radiograph can be evaluated by several techniques to aid in the determination of the nature of the skeletal abnormality[4,17] (Figure 26-4) (Table 26-1). It is important to note, however, that cephalometric radiographs are only a part of the evaluation process. Cephalometric evaluation should be combined with clinical assessment of the patient's facial structure and occlusion when the nature of the deformity is

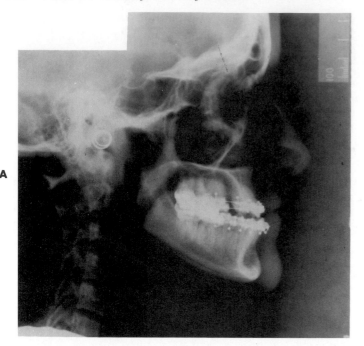

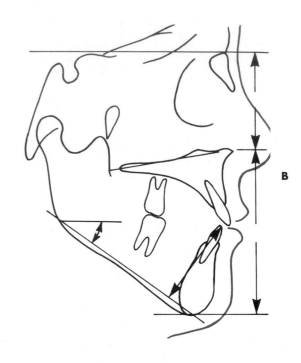

Figure 26-4

A, Lateral cephalometric radiograph. **B,** Tracing of lateral cephalometric head film, with landmarks identified for evaluating facial skeletal and dental abnormalities, using system of cephalometrics for orthognathic surgery (see Table 26-1). *(B from Burstone CJ et al: Cephalometrics for orthognathic surgery,* J Oral Surg *36:269, 1978.)*

Table 26-1. Orthognathic cephalometric analysis

	Standard (male)	Standard (female)
Horizontal (skeletal)		
N-A-Pg (angle)	3.9 degrees	2.6 degrees
N-A (∥ HP)	0.0 degrees	−2.0 degrees
N-B (∥ HP)	−5.3 degrees	−6.9 degrees
N-Pg (∥ HP)	−4.3 degrees	−6.5 degrees
Vertical (skeletal, dental)		
N-ANS (HP)	54.7 mm	50.0 mm
ANS-Gn (HP)	68.6 mm	61.3 mm
PNS-N (HP)	53.9 mm	50.6 mm
MP-HP (angle)	23.0 degrees	24.2 degrees
1-NF (NF)	30.5 mm	27.5 mm
1-MP (MP)	45.0 mm	40.8 m
6-NF (NF)	26.2 mm	23.0 mm
6-MP (MP)	35.8 mm	32.1 mm
Maxilla, mandible		
PNS-ANS (∥ HP)	57.7 mm	52.6 mm
Ar-Go (linear)	52.0 mm	46.8 mm
Go-Pg (linear)	83.7 mm	74.3 mm
Ar-Go-Gn (angle)	119.1 degrees	122.0 degrees
Dental		
OP upper-Hp (angle)	6.2 degrees	7.1 degrees
OP lower-HP (angle)	—	—
A-B (∥ OP)	−1.1 mm	−0.4 mm
1-NF (angle)	111.0 degrees	112.5 degrees
1-MP (angle)	95.9 degrees	95.9 degrees

Modified from Burstone CJ et al: Cephalometrics for orthognathic surgery, *J Oral Surg* 36:269, 1978.

determined and possible treatment is planned. Computerized video/digital technology is currently available that helps to integrate the cephalometric data with digital images of the face to improve evaluation of the relationship of the underlying facial skeleton and overlying soft tissue. After careful clinical assessment and evaluation of the diagnostic records, a problem list and treatment plan should be developed. These combine opinions from all practitioners participating in the patient's care, including the orthodontist, oral and maxillofacial surgeon, periodontist, and restorative dentist.

PRESURGICAL TREATMENT PHASE

PERIODONTAL CONSIDERATIONS

As the first step in treatment, gingival inflammation must be controlled and the patient's cooperation ensured. In patients who are unwilling or unable to clean their teeth properly before the placement of orthodontic appliances, oral hygiene procedures will be even less effective when complicated by orthodontic band placement. Periodontal therapy includes oral hygiene instruction, scaling, and root planing; in certain instances, flap surgery to gain access for root planing may be necessary to provide proper tissue health. Whenever possible it is desirable to delay comprehensive treatment until adequate patient compliance and control of inflammation are achieved.

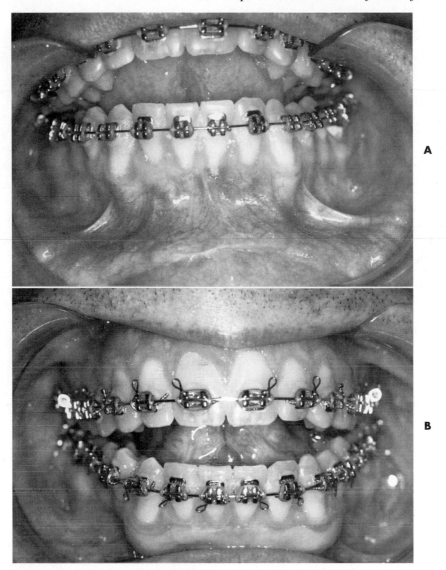

◇ Figure 26-5

A, Presurgical appearance of gingival tissue labial to lower anterior teeth. Note inadequate area of attachment and keratinization. **B,** After free gingival grafting, there is significant improvement in attachment and keratinization of labial gingival tissue.

As a result of the periodontal examination findings and proposed orthodontic-surgical plan, mucogingival surgery is often accomplished during this initial phase of therapy to provide a zone of attached keratinized tissue that is more resistant to potential orthodontic and surgical trauma. Soft tissue grafting is indicated in areas that have no keratinized gingiva or where there is only a thin band of keratinized tissue with little or no attachment when an increase in the amount of tissue trauma is likely (Figure 26-5). Such trauma to these areas includes labial orthodontic movement of teeth or a surgical procedure such as an inferior border osteotomy or segmental osteotomies in interdental areas.

RESTORATIVE CONSIDERATIONS

During the presurgical restorative phase, the patient is evaluated for carious lesions and faulty restorations. Teeth should be evaluated endodontically and periodontally for restorability, and any nonrestorable teeth should be extracted before surgical intervention. All carious lesions must be restored early in the presurgical treatment phase. Existing restorations must function for 18 to 24 months during the orthodontic and surgical treatment phases, requiring that more durable restorative materials (amalgam and composite resin) are employed, even though they may be replaced during the definitive postsurgical treatment phase. It is wise to delay final restorative treatment until the proper skeletal relationships are achieved and the finishing orthodontics completed.

In the edentulous or partially edentulous patient, particular attention is paid to residual ridge shape and contour in denture-bearing areas. The distance between the maxillary tuberosity, posterior mandible, and ramus areas must be evaluated to ensure that adequate space is present for partial

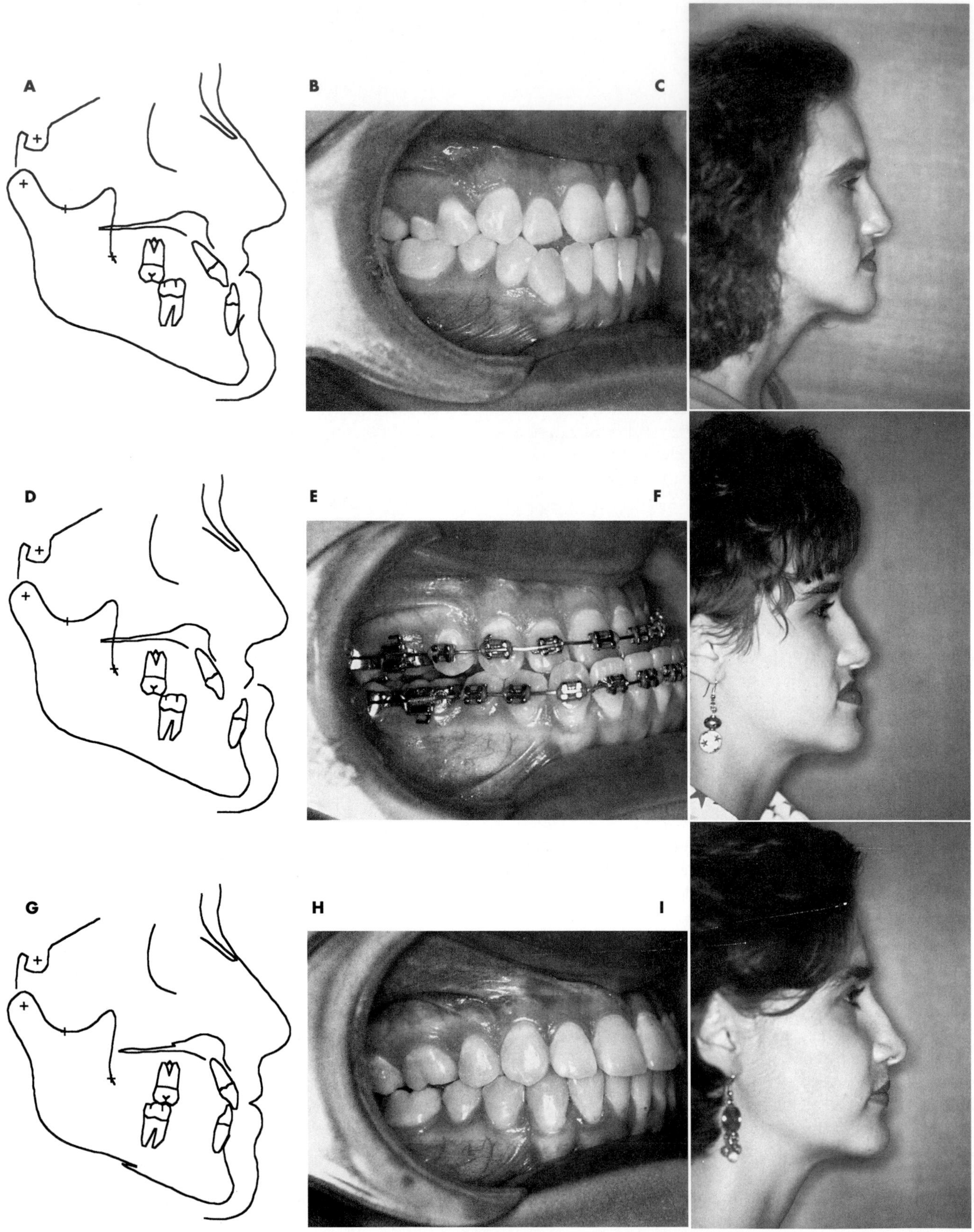

Figure 26-6

For legend see page 621.

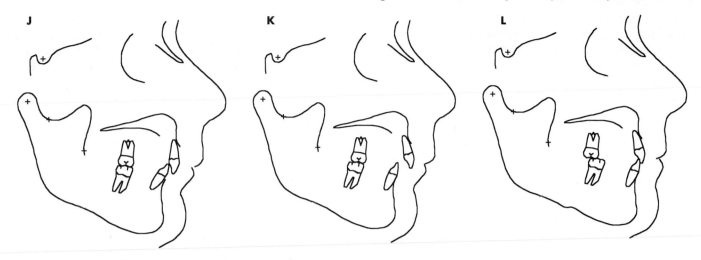

J   K   L

◇ Figure 26-6, cont'd

A, Class III skeletal malocclusion with maxillary deficiency and mandibular excess. **B,** Dental compensation includes retroclined lower incisors and proclined upper incisors. **C,** Facial profile. **D,** After initial orthodontic treatment before surgery. **E,** Dental compensation is removed with proclination of lower incisors and retroclination of upper incisors. This obviously increases the severity of malocclusion and facial discrepancy. **F** and **G,** Surgical correction with posterior positioning of mandible and advancement of maxilla. **H,** Ideal occlusion. **I,** Facial profile. **J,** Class II occlusion with compensation demonstrating proclination of lower incisors and upright upper incisors. **K,** After orthodontic decompensation. **L,** After surgical correction with mandibular advancement.

or complete dentures. Teeth that serve as removable partial denture abutments should be evaluated for potential retentive undercuts. If undercuts can be enhanced by minor orthodontic movement, this information is conveyed to the orthodontist.

PRESURGICAL ORTHODONTIC CONSIDERATIONS

It is obvious that not all malocclusions require correction with surgery. When the skeletal discrepancy is minimal and orthodontic compensation does not adversely affect dental or facial esthetics or posttreatment stability, orthodontic treatment alone may be the treatment of choice. However, in some cases an adequate occlusal relationship cannot be achieved because of the skeletal discrepancy. There are also some cases that may be treated with orthodontic compensation for a skeletal abnormality, resulting in an adequate occlusion but poor facial or dental esthetics or a poor long-term prognosis for posttreatment retention. These cases should be considered for surgery combined with orthodontic treatment.

TREATMENT TIMING. Treatment of the stable adult deformity can be started without delay, but questions often arise about how to best manage the growing child who is identified as having a developing dentofacial deformity. If the facial pattern is favorable and adequate growth potential remains, growth modification with functional appliances may be the preferred approach to dentofacial problems. Surgery usually is reserved for patients who do not respond to growth modification. As a general guideline, orthognathic surgery should be delayed until growth is complete in patients who

have problems of excess growth, although surgery can be considered earlier for patients with growth deficiencies.

ORTHODONTIC TREATMENT OBJECTIVES. Undesirable angulation of the anterior teeth occurs as a compensatory response to a developing dentofacial deformity. Patients with maxillary deficiency and/or mandibular excess often have flared upper incisors and retroclined lower incisors (Figure 26-6, *A, B,* and *C*). Dental compensations for the skeletal deformity are corrected before surgery by orthodontically repositioning teeth properly over the underlying skeletal component, without considerations for the bite relationship to the opposing arch. This presurgical orthodontic movement accentuates the patient's deformity but is necessary if normal occlusal relationships are to be achieved when the skeletal components are properly positioned at surgery (Figure 26-6, *D, E,* and *F*). The surgical treatment then results in a more ideal position of the skeletal and dental components (Figure 26-6, *G, H,* and *I*). The opposite dental compensation may occur in maxillary protrusion and/or mandibular deficiency (Figure 26-6, *J, K,* and *L*). Again, the decompensation is aimed at improving angulation of teeth over underlying bone and is followed by skeletal correction.

The essential steps in orthodontic preparation are to align the arches individually, achieve compatibility of the arches or arch segments, and establish the proper anteroposterior and vertical position of the incisors. The amount of presurgical orthodontics can vary, ranging from only appliance placement in a few patients to approximately 12 months of appliance therapy in those with severe crowding and incisor malposition.

As the patient is approaching the end of orthodontic preparation for surgery, it is helpful to take impressions and examine the hand-articulated models for occlusal compatibility. Minor interferences that exist can be corrected easily with arch wire adjustment and significantly enhance the postsurgical occlusal result. After any final orthodontic adjustments have been made, large stabilizing arch wires are inserted into the brackets, which provide the strength necessary to withstand the forces resulting from intermaxillary fixation and surgical manipulation.

FINAL TREATMENT PLANNING

After the completion of the presurgical periodontics, restorative dentistry, and orthodontics, the patient returns to the oral and maxillofacial surgeon for final presurgical planning. The evaluation completed at the initial patient examination is repeated. The patient's facial structure and the malocclusion are reexamined. Presurgical photographs, radiographs, and presurgical models are taken, a centric relation bite registration and face-bow recording for model mounting are completed, and computer images are obtained when available.

Mock surgery on a duplicated set of presurgical dental casts determines the exact surgical movements necessary to accomplish the desired postoperative occlusion (Figure 26-7). Prediction tracings of the anticipated surgical movements provide a visual treatment objective of the desired skeletal movements and resulting postoperative soft tissue changes from the lateral perspective (Figure 26-8).

One of the most recent adjuncts to treatment planning for patients with dentofacial deformity is computerized imaging. This technology allows computerized digital images of the patient's face to be superimposed over bony landmarks obtained from the cephalometric radiograph. Cephalometric

treatment planning can be completed with computer assistance. The computer can then produce a digital image that represents the facial esthetic result produced by the associated facial skeletal change (Figure 26-9). The advantage of using this type of technology is the ability to more accurately predict the facial changes that may result from a particular surgical correction. The facial images are also more easily evaluated by patients, allowing them to assess the predicted results and provide input into the surgical treatment plan. The disadvantage of the technology is related to the computer's inability to accurately predict every type of surgical change for every patient. Different muscle tone and skin thickness and variable soft tissue response to bone change, for example, make it impossible for the computer to precisely predict each individual variation. However, with continued development, this technology will most likely become more common in the treatment planning and presurgical education for patients with dentofacial deformity.

After completion of the model surgery, prediction tracings, and computer imaging evaluation, the orthodontist and/or general dentist are often consulted to ensure that the predicted occlusal result is acceptable to all practitioners involved in the patient's treatment. Any orthodontic or restorative changes necessary to improve postsurgical position should be planned at this time.

SURGICAL TREATMENT PHASE ◇

Dentofacial abnormalities can frequently be treated by isolated procedures in the mandible or maxilla/midface area. Because abnormalities can obviously occur in both the max-

Text continued on p. 626

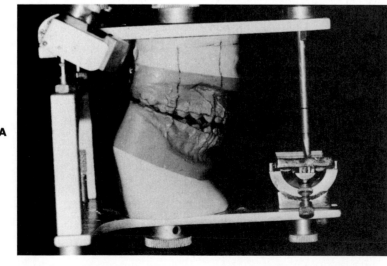

◇ Figure 26-7

Model surgery used to determine direction and distance of surgical movement necessary to achieve desired postoperative occlusion and facial esthetics. **A,** Casts mounted on semiadjustable articulator.

Continued

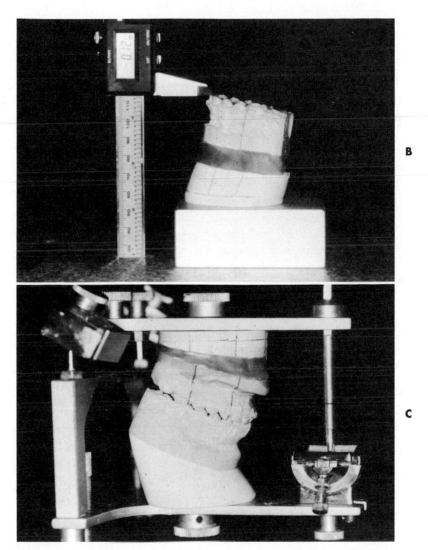

⬦ Figure 26-7, cont'd

B, Repositioning of maxillary casts using precision measuring instrument. Distances of mock surgical movements are coordinated between desired facial esthetics and movements necessary to create ideal postoperative occlusion. **C,** Maxillary casts remounted on semiadjustable articulator after precision movements have been completed and verified. Intraocclusal wafer is constructed on this final occlusal setup to be used at time of surgery to align osteotomies and dental segments into desired postsurgical position.

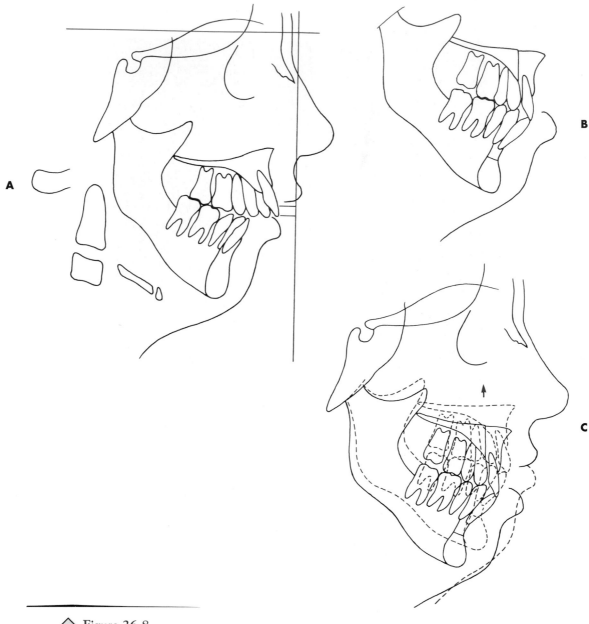

◇ Figure 26-8

Cephalometric prediction tracing to determine desired postoperative facial esthetics. **A,** Presurgical cephalometric radiograph tracing with appropriate landmarks. **B,** Overlay templates of maxilla and mandible. These are to be moved to desired postsurgical position. **C,** Tracing of predicted postoperative position of bone and overlying soft tissue (postoperative prediction [*dotted line*] demonstrating superior maxillary repositioning and mandibular advancement).

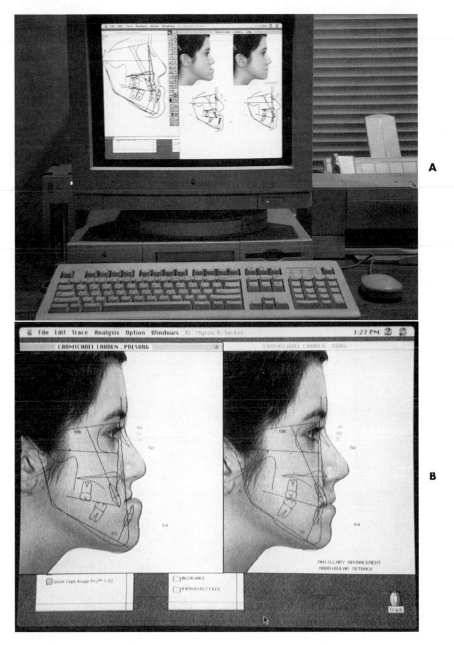

◈ Figure 26-9

Computerized imaging for dentofacial surgical treatment planning. Video image is obtained, converted to digital information, and placed in computer's memory. Landmarks from cephalometric tracing are superimposed over video image of face. Portions of cephalometric radiograph can be moved in manner similar to that used for prediction tracing (Figure 26-8). Computer then manipulates image to depict soft tissue changes. **A,** Digital images displayed on computer monitor showing predicted facial changes.*
B, Close-up view showing presurgical and predicted final images that would result from antici-pated surgical procedure (in this case, maxillary advancement and mandibular setback).

*Quick Ceph Image System.

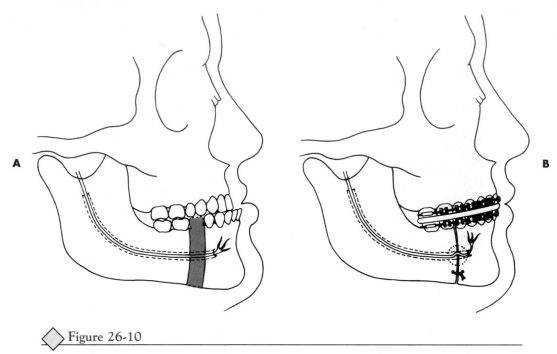

◈ Figure 26-10

Body ostectomy with resection of portion of body of mandible followed by posterior repositioning of anterior segment. **A,** Preoperative view. **B,** Postoperative view.

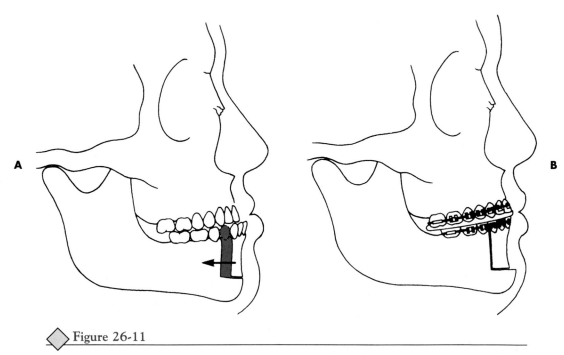

◈ Figure 26-11

Anterior mandibular subapical osteotomy. **A,** Removal of premolar teeth and bone in area of extraction sites. **B,** After separation, anterior dentoalveolar segment is repositioned posteriorly, extraction sites are closed, and anterior reverse overjet relationship is corrected.

illa and the mandible, surgical correction frequently requires a combination of surgical procedures. The following sections describe a variety of surgical procedures completed either as isolated osteotomies or as combination procedures.

MANDIBULAR EXCESS

Excess growth of the mandible frequently results in an abnormal occlusion with class III molar and cuspid relationships and a reverse overjet in the incisor area. An obvious facial deformity may also be evident. Facial features associ-

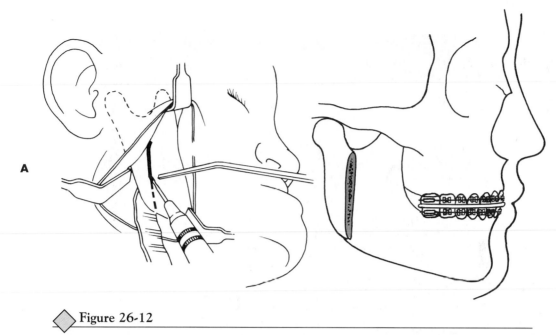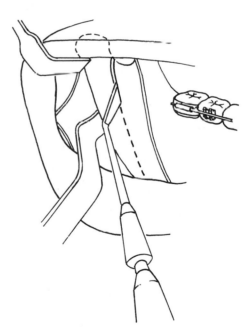

◇ **Figure 26-12**

Extraoral approach for vertical ramus osteotomy. **A,** Submandibular approach to lateral aspect of ramus showing vertical osteotomy from sigmoid notch area to angle of mandible. **B,** Overlapping of segments after posterior repositioning of anterior portion of mandible. Proximal segment containing condyle is overlapped on lateral aspect of anterior portion of ramus.

ated with mandibular excess include a prominence of the lower third of the face, particularly in the area of the lower lip and chin in the anteroposterior and vertical dimensions. In severe cases the large reverse overjet may preclude the patient's ability to obtain adequate lip closure without abnormal strain of the orbicularis oris muscles.

Mandibular excess was one of the first dentofacial deformities recognized as being best treated by a combination of orthodontics and surgery. Although surgical techniques for correction of mandibular excess were reported as early as the late 1800s, widespread use of currently acceptable techniques began in the middle of this century. Early techniques for treatment of mandibular prognathism dealt with the deformity by removing sections of bone in the body of the mandible, which allowed the anterior segment to be moved posteriorly (Figure 26-10). When the reverse overjet relationship is isolated to the anterior dentoalveolar area of the mandible, a subapical osteotomy technique can be used for correction of mandibular dental prognathism.[1] In this technique, bone is removed in the area of an extraction site of a bicuspid or molar tooth, and the anterior dentoalveolar segment of the mandible is moved to a more posterior position (Figure 26-11).

In the early 1950s, Caldwell and Letterman[5] popularized an osteotomy performed in the ramus of the mandible for the correction of mandibular excess. In this technique the lateral aspect of the ramus is exposed through a submandibular incision, the ramus is sectioned in a vertical fashion, and the entire body and anterior ramus section of the mandible are moved posteriorly, which places the teeth in proper occlusion (Figure 26-12). The proximal segment of the ramus (the portion attached to the condyle) overlaps the anterior segment,

◇ **Figure 25-13**

Intraoral technique for vertical ramus osteotomy through use of angulated oscillating saw.

and the jaw is stabilized during the healing phase with wiring of the bone segments combined with jaw immobilization using intermaxillary fixation. A similar technique is currently performed with an intraoral incision and an angulated oscillating saw (Figure 26-13).[10] The design of the osteotomy

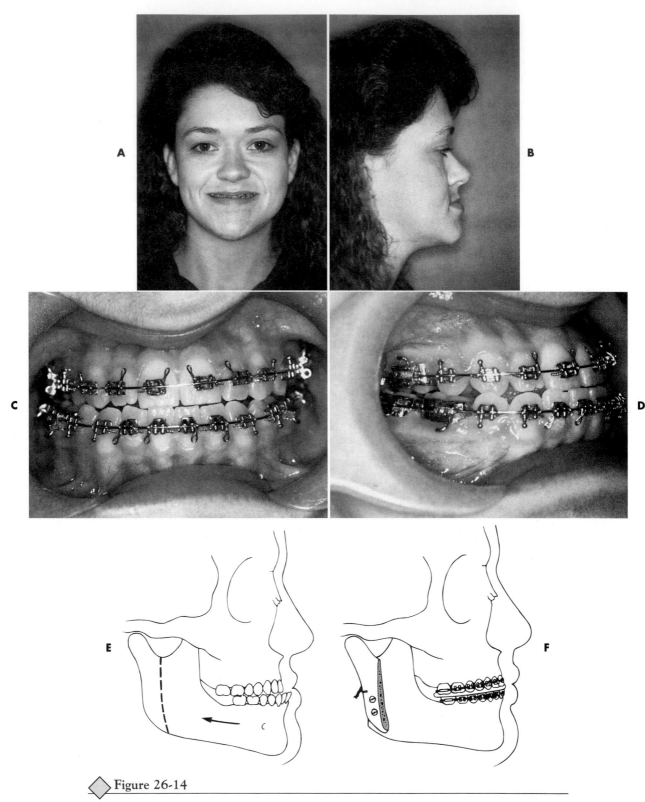

◈ Figure 26-14

Case report of mandibular excess. **A** and **B,** Preoperative facial esthetics demonstrating typical
features of class III malocclusion resulting from mandibular excess. **C** and **D,** Presurgical occlusal
photos. **E** and **F,** Diagram of intraoral vertical ramus osteotomy with posterior positioning of mandible.

Continued

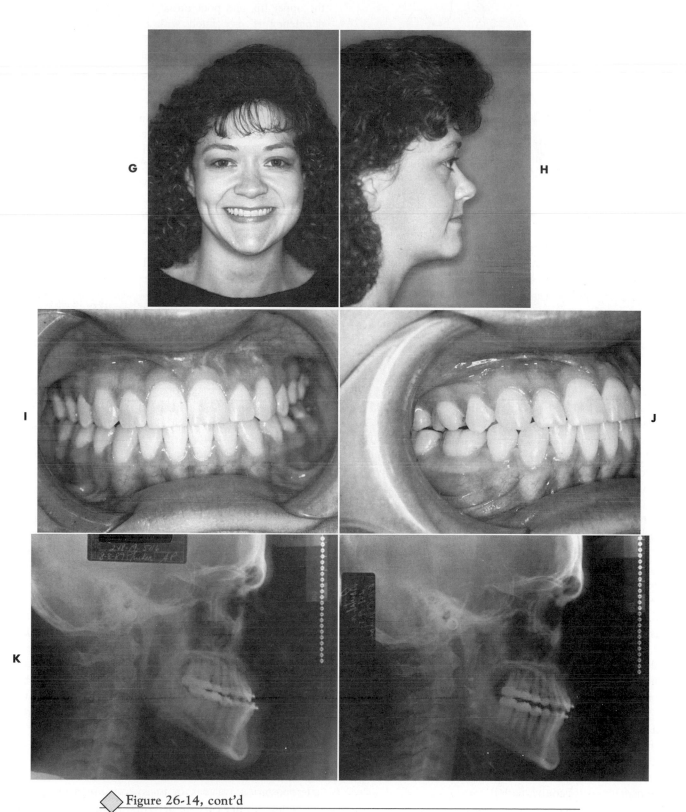

◇ Figure 26-14, cont'd

G and **H,** Postoperative facial appearance. **I** and **J,** Postoperative occlusion. **K** and **L,** Preoperative and postoperative radiographs.

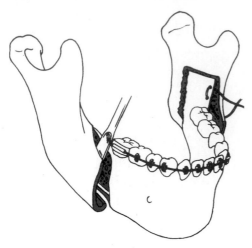

Sagittal split osteotomy. Ramus of mandible is divided by creation of horizontal osteotomy on medial aspect and vertical osteotomy on lateral aspect of mandible. These are connected by anterior ramus osteotomy. Lateral cortex of mandible is then separated from medial aspect, and mandible can be advanced or set back for correction of mandibular deficiency or prognathism, respectively.

is identical to that performed through an extraoral incision. The bone segments can be stabilized using IMF, with or without direct wiring of the segments or using rigid fixation with bone plates or screws, eliminating the need for IMF. The advantages of the intraoral technique include elimination of the need for skin incision and decreased risk of damage to the mandibular branch of the facial nerve. Figure 26-14 demonstrates the clinical results of a patient treated with an intraoral vertical ramus osteotomy to correct mandibular excess.

Another popular technique for correction of mandibular prognathism is the bilateral sagittal split osteotomy (BSSO) first described by Trauner and Obwegeser[18] and later modified by Dalpont,[6] Hunsick,[11] and Epker.[9] The BSSO is accomplished through a transoral incision similar to that for the intraoral vertical ramus osteotomy. The osteotomy splits the ramus and posterior body of the mandible in a sagittal fashion, which allows either setback or advancement of the mandible (Figure 26-15). The telescoping effect in the area of the osteotomy produces large areas of bony overlap that have the flexibility necessary to move the mandible in several directions. The BSSO technique has become one of the most popular methods for treatment of both mandibular deficiency and mandibular excess. Disadvantages include potential trauma of the inferior alveolar nerve with subsequent decreased sensation in the area of the lower lip and chin during the immediate postoperative period.

MANDIBULAR DEFICIENCY

The most obvious clinical feature of mandibular deficiency is the retruded position of the chin as viewed from the profile aspect. Other facial features often associated with mandibular deficiency may include an excess labiomental fold with a procumbent appearance of the lower lip, abnormal posture of the upper lip, and poor throat form. Intraorally, mandibular deficiency is associated with class II molar and cuspid relationships and an increased overjet in the incisor area.

Surgical correction of mandibular deficiency was described as early as 1909. However, early results with surgical advancement of the mandible before the 1950s were extremely disappointing. In 1957, Robinson[14] described surgical correction of mandibular deficiency using a vertical osteotomy and iliac crest bone grafts in the area of the osteotomy defect (Figure 26-16, *A*). Several modifications of this technique were made over subsequent years, including the development of the C osteotomy combined with sagittal splitting of the inferior border portion of the mandible (Figure 26-16, *B*). These techniques, which require an extraoral incision, provide increased bony overlap, improve healing, and give better postoperative stability for mandibular advancement. However, the extraoral incisions had the disadvantages of scar formation and potential damage to branches of the facial nerve.

Currently, the BSSO, described earlier in this chapter, is the most popular technique for mandibular advancement (Figure 26-17). This procedure is easily accomplished through an intraoral incision (see Figure 26-30, *C*). The significant bony overlap produced with the BSSO allows for adequate bone healing and improved postoperative stability. The osteotomy is frequently stabilized with rigid fixation plates or screws, eliminating the need for IMF.

If the anteroposterior position of the chin is adequate but a class II malocclusion exists, a total subapical osteotomy may be the technique of choice for mandibular advancement (Figure 26-18). By combining the osteotomy with interpositioned bone grafts, this technique can be used to increase lower facial height.

When a proper occlusal relationship exists or when anterior positioning of the mandible would not be sufficient to produce adequate projection of the chin, an inferior border osteotomy (genioplasty) with advancement may also be performed. This technique is usually performed through an intraoral incision. The inferior portion of mandible is osteotomized, moved forward, and stabilized (Figure 26-19, *A, C,* and *D*). In addition to anterior or posterior repositioning of the chin, vertical reduction or augmentation and correction of asymmetries can also be accomplished with inferior border osteotomies. Alloplastic materials can occasionally be used to augment chin projection; the material is onlaid in areas of bone deficiencies (Figure 26-19, *B*).

MAXILLARY EXCESS

Excessive growth of the maxilla may occur in the anteroposterior, vertical, or transverse dimensions. Surgical correction of dentofacial deformities with total maxillary surgery (Le Fort I) has only become popular since the early 1970s. Before that time, maxillary surgery was performed on a limited basis, and most techniques repositioned only portions of the maxilla with segmental surgery. During the early years of maxillary surgery, many techniques were

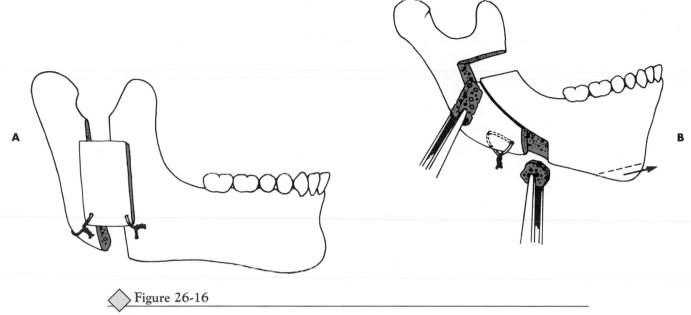

◇ Figure 26-16

Mandibular advancement techniques. **A,** Mandibular advancement using vertical osteotomy and iliac crest bone grafts in osteotomy defect. **B,** Modified C osteotomy with sagittal splitting of inferior border of mandible combined with iliac crest bone grafts.

performed in two stages. Facial or buccal cuts were performed during one operative procedure, followed by sectioning of palatal bone 3 to 4 weeks after the initial surgery. This staging was done under the assumption that it was necessary to maintain adequate vascular supply to the osteotomized segment. As experience and understanding of these techniques increased, several procedures for anterior and posterior segmental surgery evolved that used single-stage techniques.[12,15,22] In the early 1950s and 1960s, one of the more popular techniques for correction of maxillary excess was the anterior maxillary osteotomy. Several techniques have been described for repositioning of the anterior maxilla.[21,22] Anteroposterior excess of the maxilla in the anterior region can be easily and effectively treated by extracting bicuspid or molar teeth and posteriorly repositioning the anterior portion of the maxilla (Figure 26-20).

In the early 1970s, research by Bell[2] demonstrated that total maxillary surgery could be performed without jeopardizing the vascular supply to the maxilla. This work showed that the normal blood flow in the bony segments from larger feeding vessels could be reversed under certain surgical conditions. If a soft tissue pedicle is maintained in the palate and gingival area of the maxilla, the transosseous and soft tissue collateral circulation and anastomosing vascular plexi of the gingiva, palate, and sinus can provide adequate vascular supply, which allows mobilization of the total maxilla. Total maxillary osteotomies are currently the most common procedures performed for correction of anteroposterior, transverse, and vertical abnormalities of the maxilla.

Vertical maxillary excess may result in associated facial characteristics, including elongation of the lower third of the face; a narrow nose, particularly in the area of the alar base;

excessive incisive and gingival exposure; and lip incompetence (Figure 26-21). These patients may exhibit class I, class II, or class III dental malocclusions. A transverse maxillary deficiency with a posterior cross-bite relationship, constricted palate, and narrow arch form is often seen with this deformity.

Vertical maxillary excess is frequently associated with an anterior open-bite relationship (apertognathia). This results from excessive downward growth of the maxilla causing downward rotation of the mandible as a result of premature contact of posterior teeth. To correct this problem the maxilla is repositioned superiorly, particularly in the posterior area. This allows the mandible to rotate upward and forward, establishing contact in all areas of the dentition. In some cases the occlusal plane of the maxilla is level following orthodontic preparation, and the open bite can be corrected by repositioning the maxilla in one piece (Figure 26-22, *A* through *D*). In other cases, there is a step in the occlusal plane that must be leveled to achieve the desired occlusion. This requires repositioning of the maxilla in segments (Figure 26-22, *E* through *H*).

Anteroposterior maxillary excess results in a convex facial profile usually associated with incisor protrusion and a class II occlusal relationship. Total maxillary surgery can be completed to correct this problem. In some cases the entire maxilla can be moved in one piece in a posterior direction. In addition to procedures in which the maxilla is moved in one piece, the bone can be sectioned into dentoalveolar segments to allow repositioning in the anteroposterior, as well as the superior and inferior, directions or to allow expanding in the transverse direction. Figure 26-23 demonstrates a three-piece maxillary osteotomy performed to correct anteroposterior maxillary excess combined with slight vertical deficiency.

Text continued on p. 645

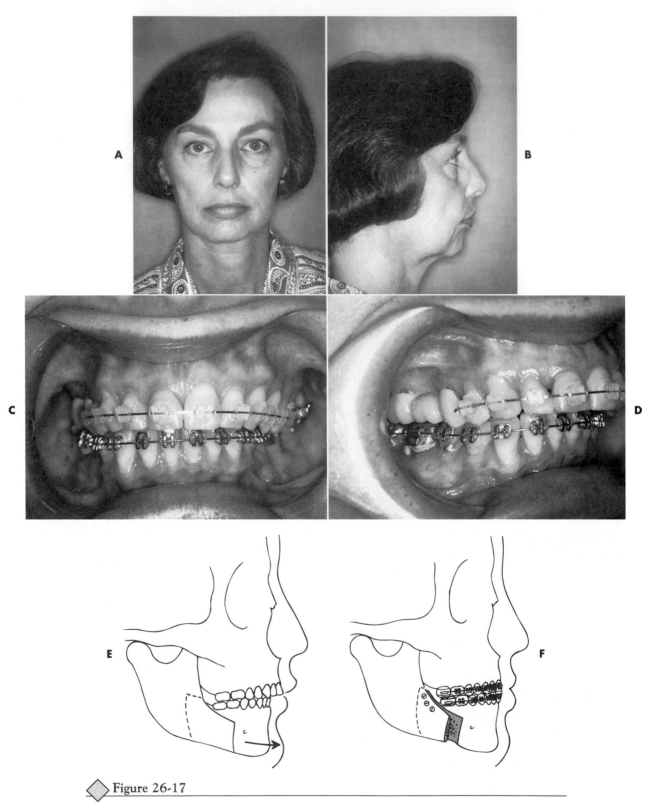

◇ Figure 26-17

Case report of mandibular advancement. **A** and **B,** Preoperative facial esthetics demonstrating clinical features of mandibular deficiency, **C** and **D,** Preoperative occlusion demonstrating class II relationship and overjet. **E** and **F,** Diagrammatic representation of bilateral sagittal split osteotomy with advancement of mandible.

Continued

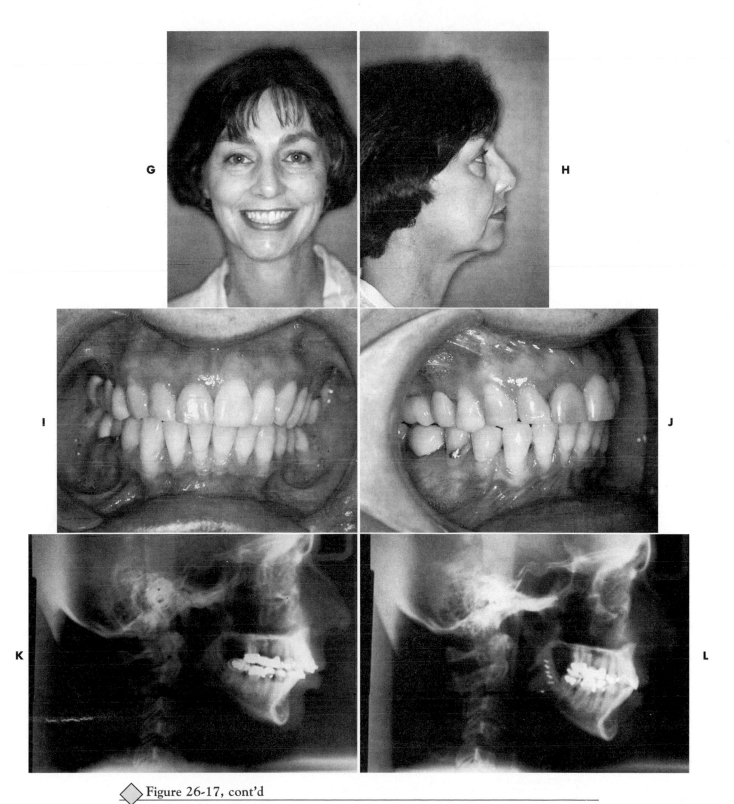

◇ Figure 26-17, cont'd

G and **H,** Postoperative facial appearance. **I** and **J,** Postoperative occlusion. **K** and **L,** Preoperative and postoperative radiographs.

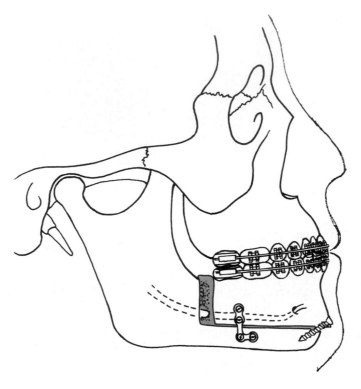

◇ **Figure 26-18**

Total subapical osteotomy. Dentoalveolar segment of mandible is moved anteriorly, allowing correction of class II malocclusion without increasing chin prominence.

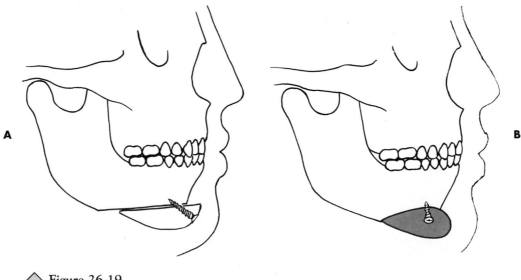

◇ **Figure 26-19**

Inferior border modification (genioplasty) techniques. **A,** Advancement of inferior border of mandible to increase chin projection. **B,** Diagram of implant used to augment anterior portion of chin, eliminating need for osteotomy in this area.   *Continued*

C 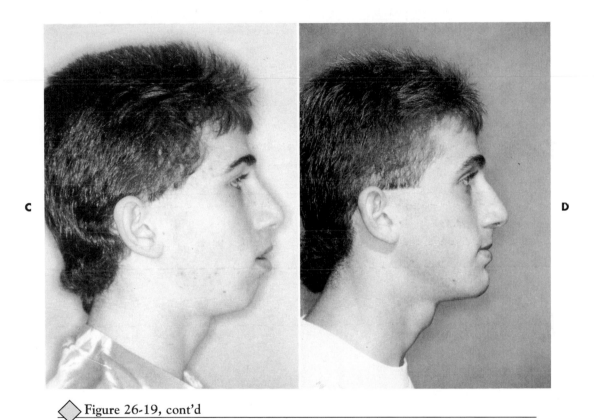 D

◇ Figure 26-19, cont'd

C, Clinical picture demonstrating significant chin deficiency. **D,** Postoperative photograph after advancement of inferior portion of anterior mandible.

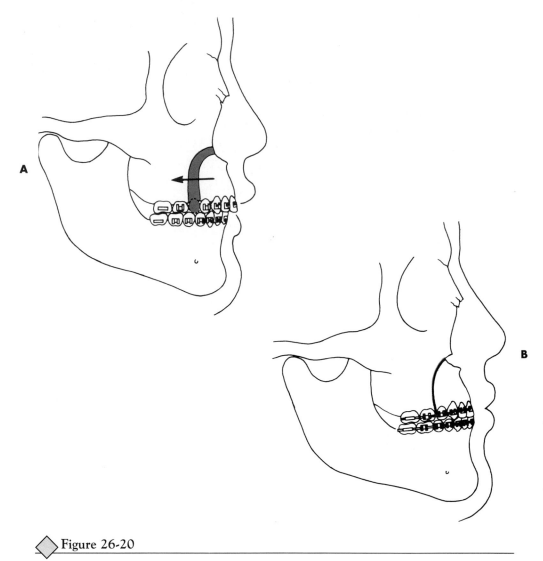

◇ Figure 26-20

Anterior maxillary osteotomy. **A,** Removal of premolar teeth and bone in extraction sites. **B,** Posterior positioning of anterior maxilla closes extraction spaces and corrects excessive anterior overjet relationship.

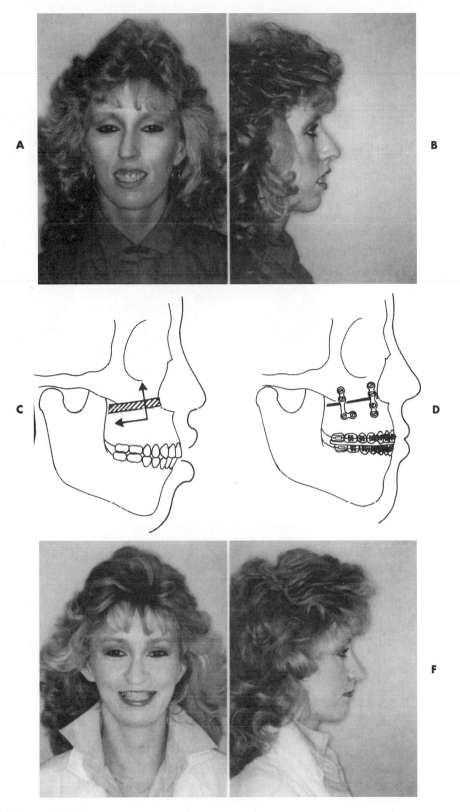

Figure 26-21

Typical clinical features of vertical maxillary excess. **A** and **B**, Full-face and profile views demonstrating elongation of lower third of face, lip incompetence, excessive gingival exposure, and narrow alar base width. **C** and **D**, Total maxillary osteotomy with superior repositioning. **E** and **F**, Postoperative full-face and profile views after total maxillary osteotomy with superior repositioning.

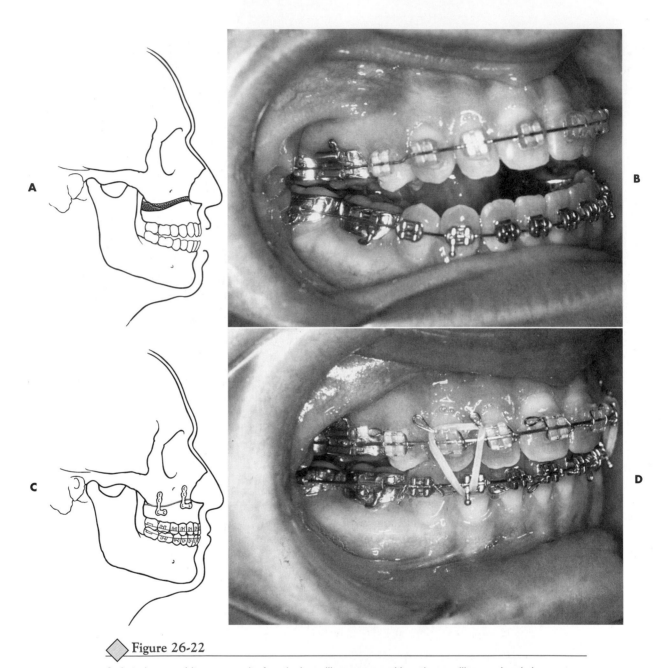

◆ Figure 26-22

A, Anterior open bite as a result of vertical maxillary excess with entire maxillary occlusal plane on one level. **B,** Presurgical occlusion. **C,** Surgical correction with superior repositioning of maxilla in one piece. **D,** Postoperative occlusion.   *Continued*

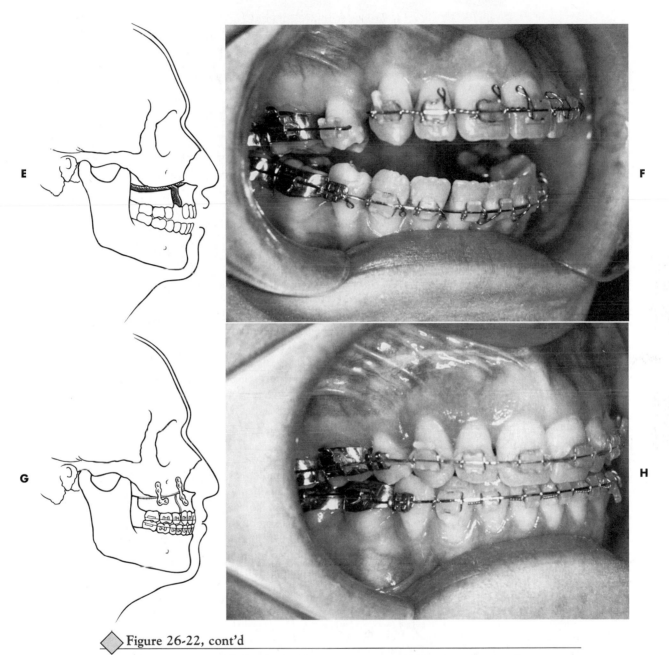

◇ **Figure 26-22, cont'd**

E, Open bite with maxillary occlusal plane on two levels. **F,** Presurgical occlusion. **G,** Segmental maxillary repositioning to close open bite and place segments on same plane of occlusion. **H,** Postoperative occlusion.

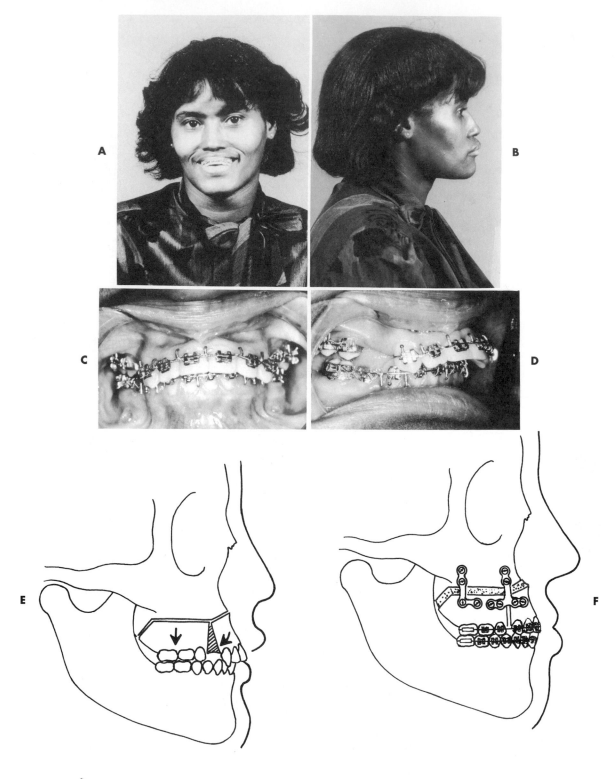

◇ Figure 26-23

Case report of segmental maxillary osteotomy. **A** and **B,** Preoperative facial appearance demonstrating extreme protrusion of anterior maxillary segment and upper lip, decreased nasolabial angle, and decreased lower face height as a result of maxillary vertical deficiency. **C** and **D,** Preoperative occlusion demonstrating protrusive maxillary incisors and extraction space remaining after removal of maxillary bicuspid tooth bilaterally. **E** and **F,** Segmental maxillary osteotomy with closure of bicuspid extraction space, retraction of anterior segment of maxilla, and placement of bone graft in posterior maxillary area.

Continued

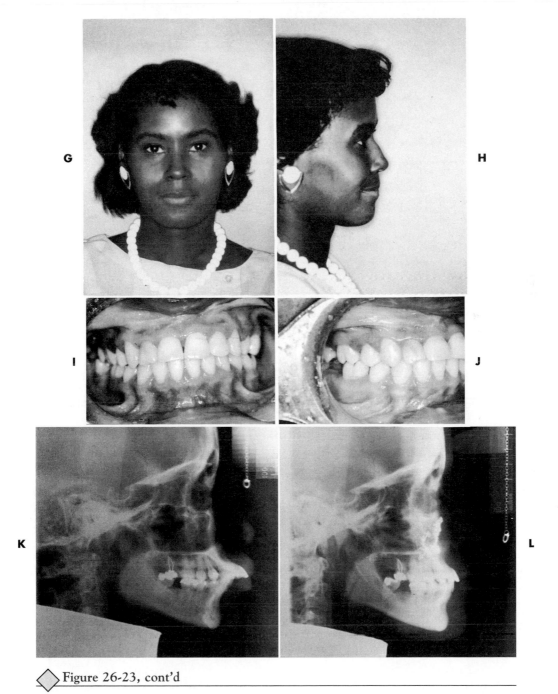

⬥ Figure 26-23, cont'd

G and **H,** Postoperative facial appearance. **I** and **J,** Postoperative occlusion. **K** and **L,** Preoperative and postoperative radiographs.

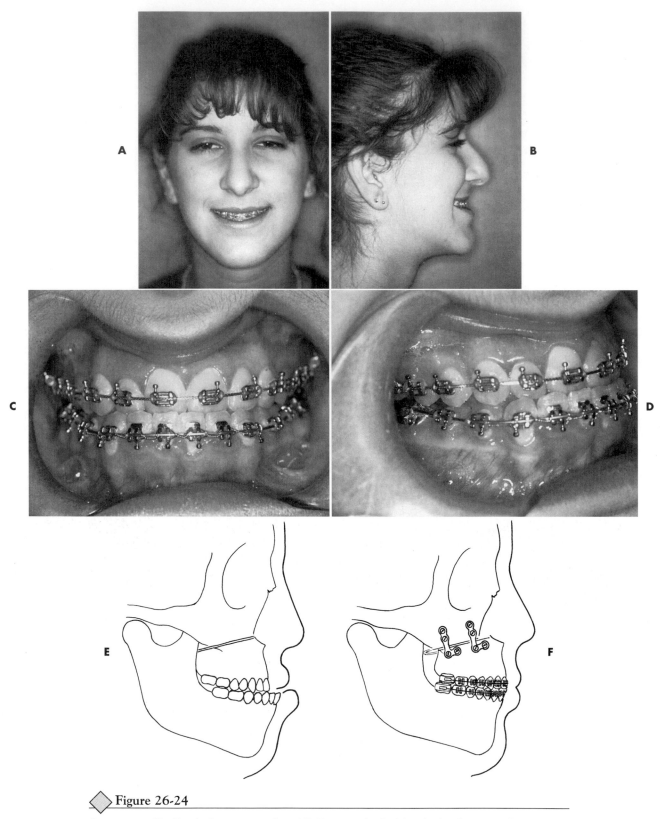

◇ Figure 26-24

Case report of Le Fort I advancement. **A** and **B,** Preoperative facial esthetics demonstrating maxillary deficiency evident by slight facial concavity and paranasal deficiency. **C** and **D,** Preoperative occlusion demonstrating class III relationship. **E** and **F,** Le Fort I osteotomy for maxillary advancement.

Continued

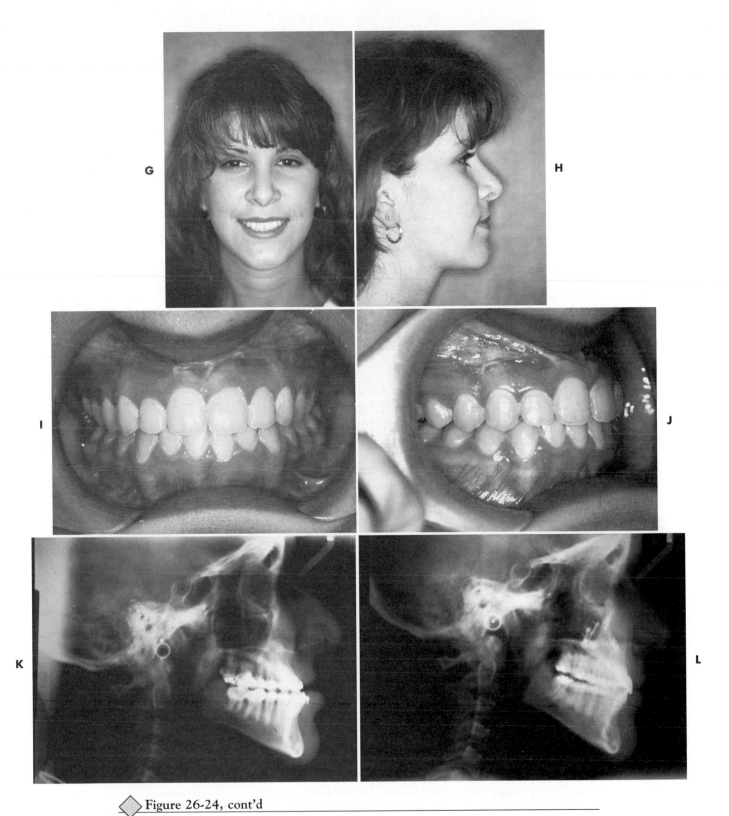

◇ **Figure 26-24, cont'd**

G and **H,** Postoperative facial appearance. (This patient also underwent a simultaneous rhinoplasty procedure.) **I** and **J,** Postoperative occlusion. **K** and **L,** Preoperative and postoperative radiographs.

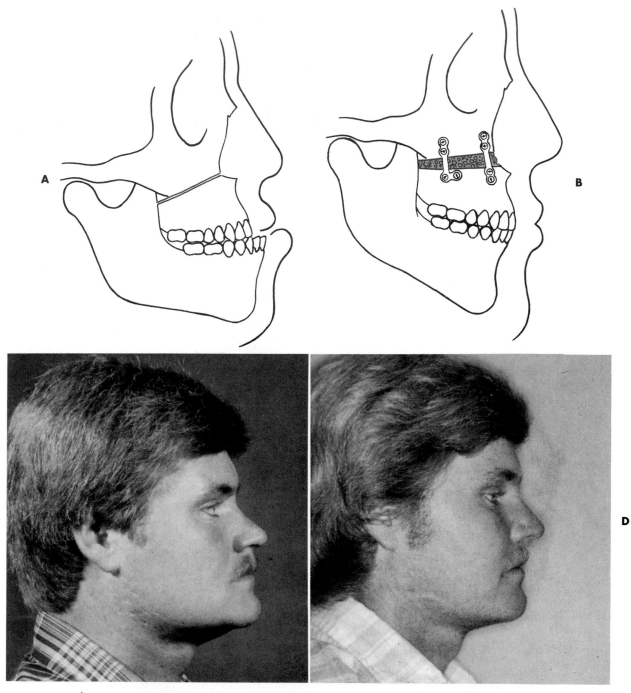

◇ Figure 26-25

A and **B,** Inferior repositioning of maxilla and interpositional bone grafting. **C,** Preoperative profile view demonstrating vertical deficiency of lower third of face and resulting appearance of relative mandibular excess. **D,** Postoperative view after inferior repositioning of maxilla. Note normal facial vertical and anteroposterior relationships.

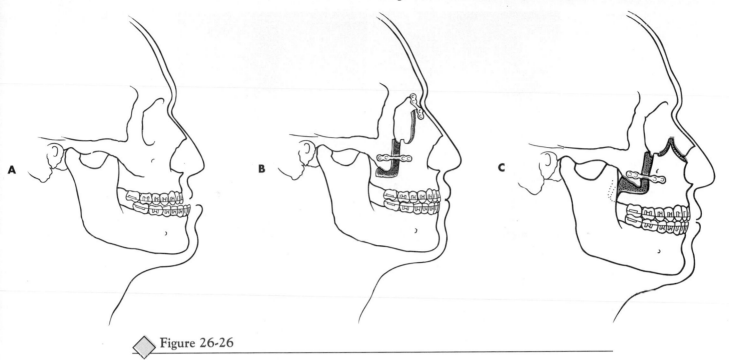

◆ Figure 26-26

A, Severe midface deficiency. **B**, Le Fort III advancement. **C**, Modified Le Fort III advancement.

MAXILLARY AND MIDFACE DEFICIENCY

Patients with maxillary deficiency commonly appear to have a retruded upper lip, deficiency of the paranasal and infraorbital rim areas, inadequate tooth exposure during smile, and a prominent chin relative to the middle third of the face. Maxillary deficiency may occur in the anteroposterior, vertical, and transverse planes. The patient's clinical appearance depends on the location and severity of the deformity. In addition to the abnormal facial features a class III malocclusion with reverse anterior overjet is frequently seen.

The primary technique for correction of maxillary deficiency is the Le Fort I osteotomy. This technique can be used for advancement of the maxilla to correct a class III malocclusion and associated facial abnormalities (Figure 26-24). Depending on the magnitude of advancement, bone grafting may be required to improve bone healing and postoperative stability. In the case of vertical maxillary deficiency, elongation of the lower third of the face can be accomplished by bone grafting the maxilla in an inferior position with the Le Fort I osteotomy technique (Figure 26-25). This technique improves overall facial proportion and normalizes exposure of the incisors during smiling.

In severe midface deformities with infraorbital rim and malar eminence deficiency, a Le Fort III or modified Le Fort III type of osteotomy is necessary. These procedures advance the maxilla and the malar bones and in some cases the anterior portion of the nasal bones. This type of treatment is commonly required in patients with craniofacial deformities such as Apert's or Crouzon's syndrome (Figure 26-26).

COMBINATION DEFORMITIES AND ASYMMETRIES

In many cases the facial deformity involves a combination of abnormalities in both the maxilla and the mandible. In these cases, treatment may require a combination of maxillary and mandibular osteotomies to achieve the best possible occlusal, functional, and esthetic result (Figures 26-27, 26-28, and 26-29). Treatment of asymmetry in more than two planes frequently requires maxillary surgery, mandibular surgery, and inferior border osteotomies, as well as recontouring or augmentation of other areas of the maxilla and mandible (Figure 26-30).

PERIOPERATIVE CARE OF THE ORTHOGNATHIC SURGICAL PATIENT ◇

Patients undergoing orthognathic surgery are usually admitted to the hospital on the day of surgery. Before surgery the medical history, complete physical examination, preoperative laboratory tests and radiographic examinations, and consultation with the anesthesiologist are completed. Orthognathic surgery is accomplished in the operating room with the patient under general anesthesia. After surgery the patient is taken to the postanesthesia care unit (recovery room) for an appropriate period, usually until alert, oriented, comfortable, and exhibiting stable vital signs, and is then returned to the

Text continued on p. 653

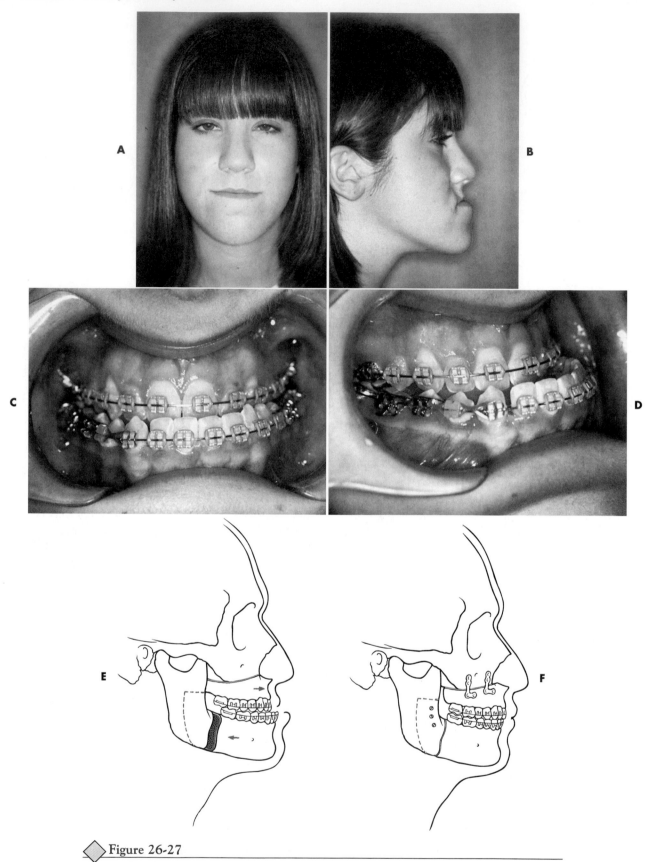

◈ Figure 26-27

Case report of maxillary advancement and mandibular setback. **A** and **B,** Preoperative facial esthetics demonstrating severe maxillary deficiency combined with mandibular excess. **C** and **D,** Preoperative occlusion demonstrating class III relationship. **E** and **F,** Le Fort I osteotomy for maxillary advancement and bilateral sagittal osteotomies for setback of the mandible.

Continued

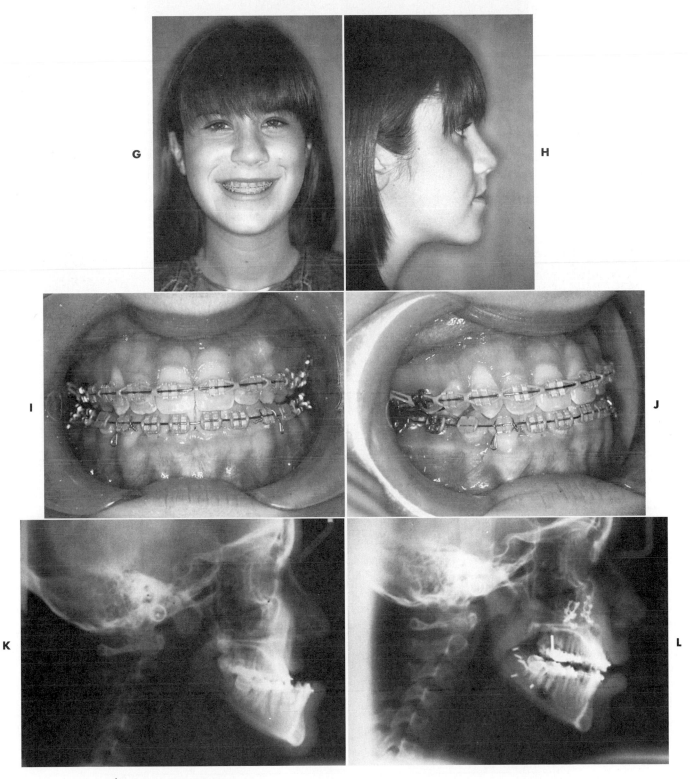

◇ Figure 26-27, cont'd

G and **H,** Postoperative facial appearance. **I** and **J,** Postoperative occlusion. **K** and **L,** Preoperative and postoperative radiographs.

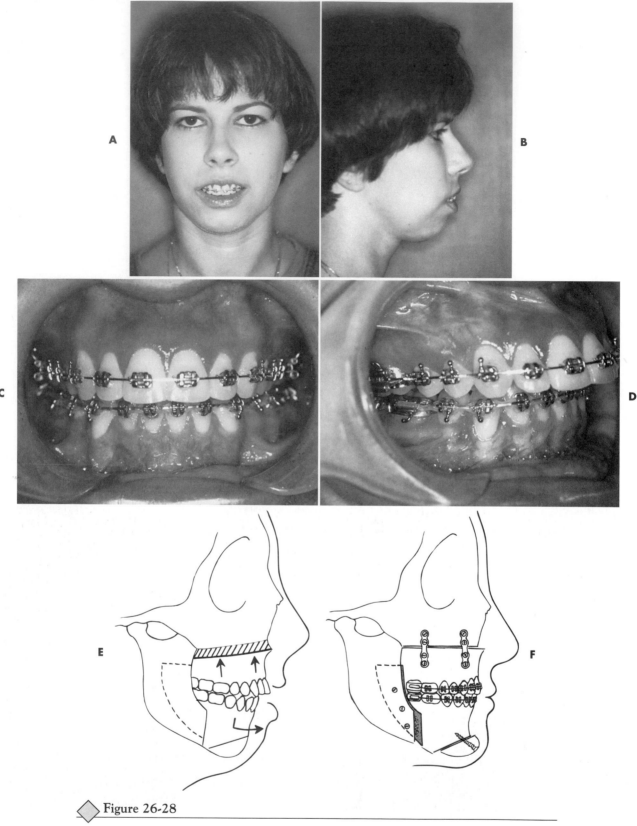

◇ **Figure 26-28**

Case report of superior maxillary repositioning, mandibular advancement, and genioplasty. **A** and **B,** Preoperative facial esthetics demonstrating typical appearance of vertical maxillary excess and mandibular deficiency, including excess incisor exposure, lip imcompetence, and lack of chin projection. **C** and **D,** Preoperative occlusion demonstrating class II malocclusion. **E** and **F,** Diagram of Le Fort I osteotomy with superior repositioning of maxilla, sagittal osteotomies of mandible for advancement, and advancement genioplasty.

Continued

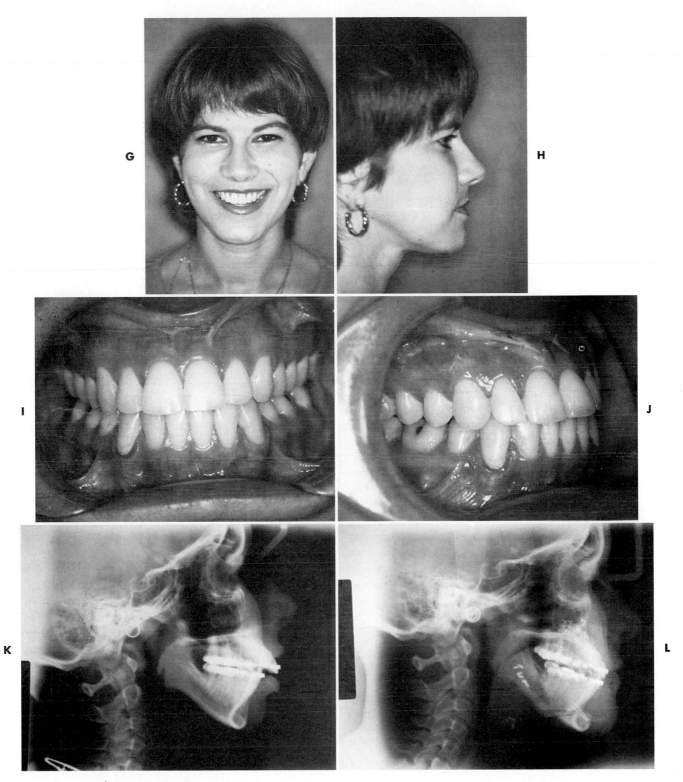

◇ Figure 26-28, cont'd

G and **H,** Postoperative facial appearance. **I** and **J,** Postoperative occlusion. **K** and **L,** Preoperative and postoperative radiographs.

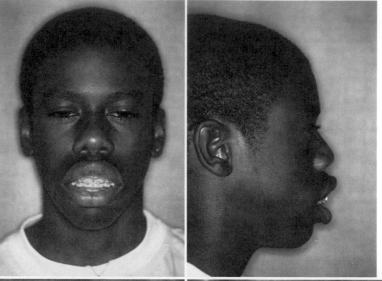

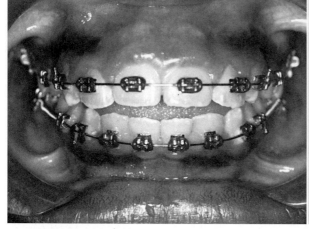

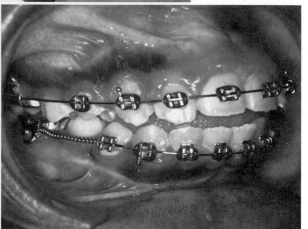

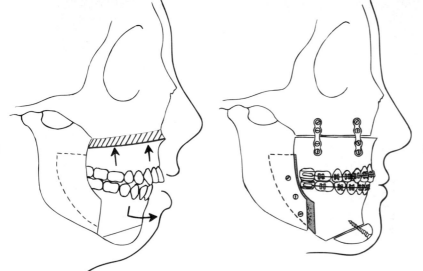

◇ **Figure 26-29**

Case report demonstrating vertical and antero-posterior excess of maxilla combined with protrusion of the dentoalveolar component (bimaxillary protrusion) and mandibular deficiency at the inferior border. **A** and **B,** Preoperative facial appearance demonstrating facial elongation, excess tooth and gingival exposure, extreme protrusion of anterior maxillary segment and upper lip, elongated lower face height as a result of maxillary vertical excess, and chin deficiency. **C** and **D,** Preoperative occlusion demonstrating protrusive maxillary and mandibular incisors. **E** and **F,** Segmental maxillary osteotomy with closure of bicuspid extraction space and superior repositioning. Removal of lower premolar teeth with anterior mandibular segmental osteotomy and advancement of the inferior border of the mandible (genioplasty). *Continued*

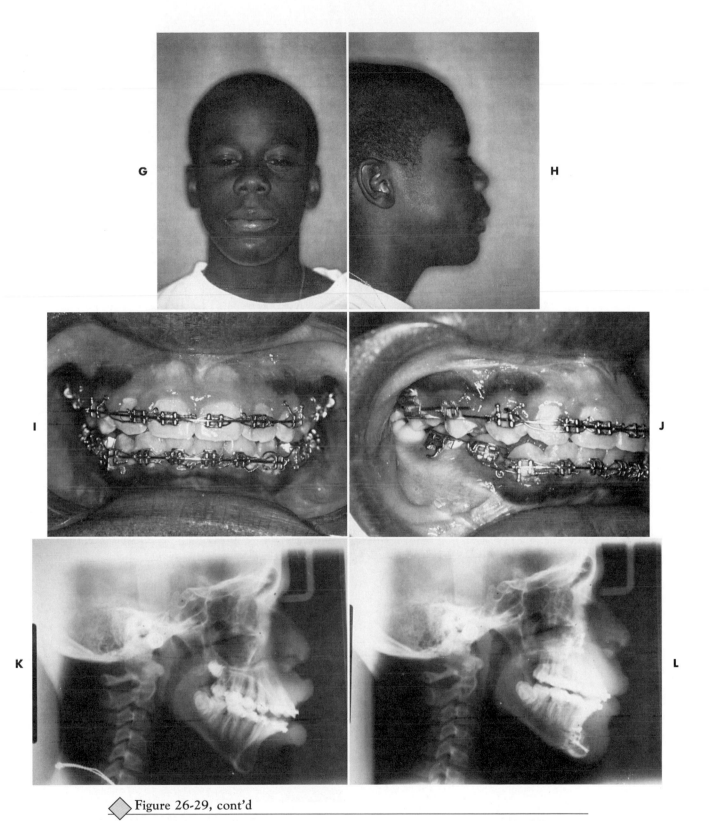

◇ Figure 26-29, cont'd

G and **H,** Postoperative facial appearance. **I** and **J,** Postoperative occlusion. **K** and **L,** Preoperative and postoperative radiographs.

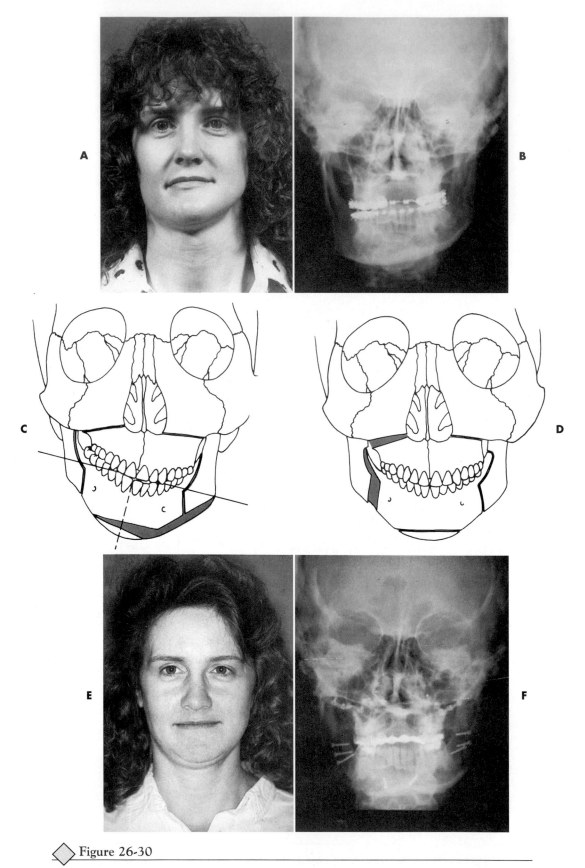

◇ **Figure 26-30**

Facial asymmetry requiring maxillary and mandibular osteotomies, genioplasty, and inferior border recontouring for correction. **A,** Preoperative facial esthetics. **B,** Preoperative radiograph. **C** and **D,** Diagrams of Le Fort I osteotomy with inferior repositioning on left side and superior repositioning on right, sagittal osteotomies of mandible with advancement on left side and setback/superior repositioning on right, asymmetric genioplasty, and right inferior border recontouring. **E,** Postoperative facial appearance. **F,** Postoperative radiograph.

hospital rooms. Postoperative progress is continually monitored by a nursing staff trained and experienced in the postoperative care of surgery patients. As soon as is feasible, postoperative radiographs are obtained to ensure that the predicted bone changes have taken place. The patient is discharged when feeling comfortable, taking food and fluid orally without difficulty, and ambulating well. The postsurgical hospital stay usually ranges from 1 to 4 days. Patients generally require only mild-to-moderate pain medication during this time and often require no analgesics after discharge.

The importance of postoperative nutrition should be discussed with patients and their families before the hospital admission for surgery. During the postoperative hospital stay, a member of the dietary staff should instruct the patient in methods of obtaining adequate nutrition during the period of IMF or limited jaw function. Special cookbooks designed for patients undergoing jaw surgery contain instructions for the preparation of diets in a blender.

In the past, one of the major considerations in the immediate postoperative period was the difficulty resulting from intermaxillary fixation (IMF; wiring of the jaws). When the jaws are wired together the patient has initial difficulties in obtaining adequate nutrition, performing necessary oral hygiene, and communicating verbally. The average IMF period ranges from 6 to 8 weeks.

During the past few years, several systems using small bone screws and bone plates have been developed to provide direct bony stabilization in the area of the osteotomies (Figure 26-31).[16,20] These systems allow for early release from or total elimination of IMF, which results in improved patient comfort, convenience of speech and oral hygiene, and improved postsurgical jaw stability and function.

At the time of surgery a small acrylic occlusal wafer is used to help position and stabilize the occlusion. When the IMF is released (usually in the operating room), the splint is wired to either the upper or lower jaw. Light elastics are then placed on the surgical wires, and the combination of the splint and elastics serves to guide the jaw into the new postsurgical occlusion (Figure 26-32). After an adequate accommodation period the occlusal splint is removed and the patient returned to the orthodontist's care.

Postsurgical Treatment Phase
Completion of Orthodontics

When satisfactory range of jaw motion and stability of the osteotomy sites are achieved, the orthodontic treatment can be finished. The heavy surgical arch wires are removed and replaced with light orthodontic wire. Final alignment and positioning of the teeth is accomplished, as is closure of any residual extraction space. The light vertical elastics are left in place at this time to override proprioceptive impulses from the teeth, which otherwise would cause the patient to seek a new position of maximal intercuspation. The settling process proceeds rapidly and rarely takes longer than 6 to 10 months.

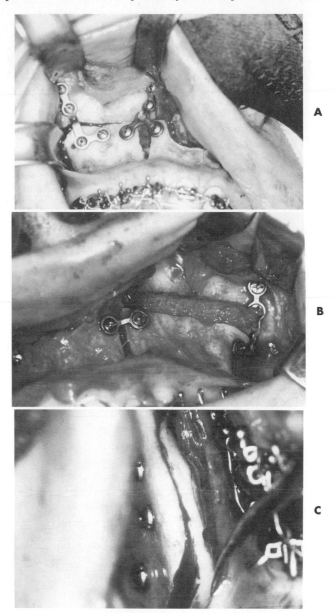

◇ **Figure 26-31**

A, Use of small bone plates for stabilization of maxillary osteotomy. **B,** Maxillary advancement and downgraft with iliac crest bone graft, stabilized with bone plates. **C,** Lag screws used to secure mandibular sagittal split osteotomy.

Retention after surgical orthodontics is no different than for other adult patients, and definitive periodontal and prosthetic treatment can be initiated immediately after the final occlusal relationships have been established.

Postsurgical Restorative and Prosthetic Considerations

When patients require complex final restorative treatment, it is important to establish stable, full-arch contact as soon after orthodontic debanding as possible. Posterior vertical contacts

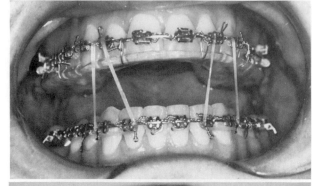

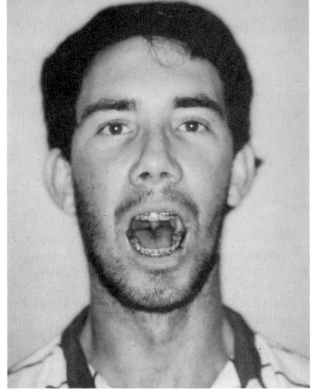

mouth deplaqued, and areas of inflammation or pocketing lightly instrumented. Frequent recall maintenance should continue during the remainder of orthodontic care when necessary. After the orthodontic appliances are removed, a thorough prophylaxis with a review of oral hygiene techniques is advisable. A thorough periodontal reevaluation 3 to 6 months after completion of the postsurgical orthodontics will determine future treatment needs. Periodontal surgery, including crown lengthening or regenerative procedures, should be performed after the inflammation associated with orthodontic appliances has resolved. Areas of hyperplastic tissue should be observed for 6 to 12 months after orthodontic therapy, unless esthetic or restorative considerations necessitate earlier tissue removal. Following completion of periodontal treatment, recall intervals should be adjusted to accommodate the individual patient's needs.

SUMMARY

The treatment of patients with dentofacial deformity involves the evaluation and treatment of many types of dental and skeletal problems. These problems require that all practitioners involved in patient care interact in a multidisciplinary team approach to treatment. This sequential, team approach yields the most satisfying results.

◇ Figure 26-32

A, Interocclusal splint wired to maxilla. Light elastics are used to help guide patient into new postoperative occlusion. **B,** Patient 7 days after maxillary and mandibular osteotomies. Note excellent early function.

REFERENCES

1. Bell WH, Dann JJ: Correction of dentofacial deformities by surgery in the anterior part of the jaws, *Am J Orthod* 64:162, 1973.
2. Bell WH et al: Bone healing and revascularization after total maxillary osteotomy, *J Oral Surg* 33:253, 1975.
3. Bell WH, Proffit WR, White RP: *Surgical correction of dentofacial deformities,* Philadelphia, 1980, WB Saunders.
4. Burstone CJ et al: Cephalometrics for orthognathic surgery, *J Oral Surg* 36:269, 1978.
5. Caldwell JB, Letterman GS: Vertical osteotomy in the mandibular rami for correction of prognathism, *J Oral Surg* 12:185, 1954.
6. Dalpont G: Retromolar osteotomy for the correction of prognathism, *J Oral Surg* 19:42, 1961.
7. Enlow DH: *Handbook of facial growth,* Philadelphia, 1975, WB Saunders.
8. Enlow DH: Wolff's law and factor of architectonic circumstance, *Am J Orthod* 54:803, 1968.
9. Epker BN: Modifications in the sagittal osteotomy of the mandible, *J Oral Surg* 35:157, 1977.
10. Hall HD, Chase DC, Payor LG: Evaluation and realignment of the intraoral vertical subcondylar osteotomy, *J Oral Surg* 33:333, 1975.
11. Hunsick EE: A modified intraoral sagittal splitting technique for mandibular prognathism, *J Oral Surg* 26:249, 1968.
12. Kufner J: Experience with a modified procedure for correction of open bite. In Walker RV, editor: *Transactions of the Third International Congress of Oral Surgery,* London, 1970, E & S Livingstone.
13. Moss ML: Facial growth: the functional matrix concept. In

are important in patients who have only anterior components of occlusion remaining. Well-fitting, temporary, removable partial dentures may suffice, and these appliances should be relined with tissue-conditioning materials as needed to maintain the posterior support during healing. When postsurgical orthodontics is complete, the remainder of restorative treatment can be accomplished in the same manner as for any nonsurgical patient.

POSTSURGICAL DENTAL AND PERIODONTAL CONSIDERATIONS

The patient should be seen for a maintenance dental and periodontal evaluation approximately 10 to 14 weeks postoperatively. The mucogingival status is reevaluated, the

Grabb WC et al, editors: *Cleft lip and palate,* Boston, 1971, Little, Brown.

14. Robinson M: Micrognathism corrected by vertical osteotomy of ascending ramus and iliac bone graft: new technique, *Oral Surg* 10:125, 1957.
15. Schuchardt K: Experiences with the surgical treatment of deformities of the jaws: prognathia, micrognathia, and open bite. In Wallace AG, editor: *Second Congress of International Society of Plastic Surgeons,* London, 1959, E & S Livingstone.
16. Spiessl B: *New concepts of maxillofacial bone surgery,* Berlin, 1975, Springer-Verlag.
17. Steiner CC: Cephalometrics in clinical practice angle, *Orthodontics* 28:8, 1959.
18. Trauner R, Obwegeser H: The surgical correction of mandibular prognathism and retrognathia with consideration of genioplasty, *Oral Surg* 10:677, 1957.
19. Tucker MR et al: Evaluation of treatment of patients with dentofacial deformities: a multidisciplinary approach, *NC Dent Rev* 3:13, 1985.
20. Tucker MR, White RP Jr: Maxillary orthognathic surgery. In Tucker MR et al, editors: *Rigid fixation for maxillofacial surgery,* Philadelphia, 1991, JB Lippincott.
21. Wassmund M: *Frakturen und Luxationen des Gesichtsschadels,* Berlin, 1927, H Meusser.
22. Wunderer S: Erfahrungen mitder operativen Behandlung hochgradiger Prognathien, *Dtsch Zahn-Mund-Keiferheilkd* 39:451, 1963.

MANAGEMENT OF PATIENTS WITH OROFACIAL CLEFTS

EDWARD ELLIS III

CHAPTER OUTLINE

A cleft is a congenital abnormal space or gap in the upper lip, alveolus, or palate. The colloquial term for this condition is *harelip*. The use of this term should be discouraged because it carries demeaning connotations of inferiority. The more appropriate terms are *cleft lip, cleft palate,* or *cleft lip and palate.*

Clefts of the lip and palate are the most common serious congenital anomalies to affect the orofacial region. Their initial appearance may be grotesque. Because they are deformities that can be seen, felt, and heard, they constitute a serious affliction to those who have them. Because of their location, they are deformities that involve the dental specialties throughout their protracted course of treatment. The general dentist will become involved in managing these patients' special dental needs, because they may have partial anodontia and supernumerary teeth. Malocclusion is usually present, and orthodontic therapy with or without corrective jaw surgery is frequently indicated.

The occurrence of a cleft deformity is a source of considerable shock to the parents of an afflicted baby, and the most appropriate approach to the parents is one of informed explanation and reassurance. They should be told that the defects are correctable and need not adversely affect the child's future. However, they should be prepared for a protracted course of therapy to correct the cleft deformities and to allow the individual to function with them.

The problems encountered in rehabilitation of patients with cleft deformities are unique. Treatment must address patient appearance, speech, hearing, mastication, and deglutition. Most children currently affected with orofacial clefts are managed by a team. Cleft teams are found in most cities of at least moderate size. These teams commonly comprise a general dentist or pedodontist, an orthodontist, a prosthodontist, an oral and maxillofacial surgeon and/or plastic surgeon, an audiologist, an otorhinolaryngologist, a pediatrician, a speech pathologist, a psychologist or psychiatrist, and a social worker. The number of specialists required reflects the number and complexity of the problems faced by individuals with orofacial clefts.

The occurrence of oral clefts in the United States has been estimated as 1 in 600 to 1000 live births.[1] Clefts exhibit interesting racial predilections, occurring less frequently in blacks but more so in Orientals. Boys are affected by orofacial clefts more often than girls, by a ratio of 3:2. Clefts of the lip are more frequent in boys, whereas isolated cleft palates are more common in girls.

Oral clefts commonly affect the lip, alveolar ridge, and hard

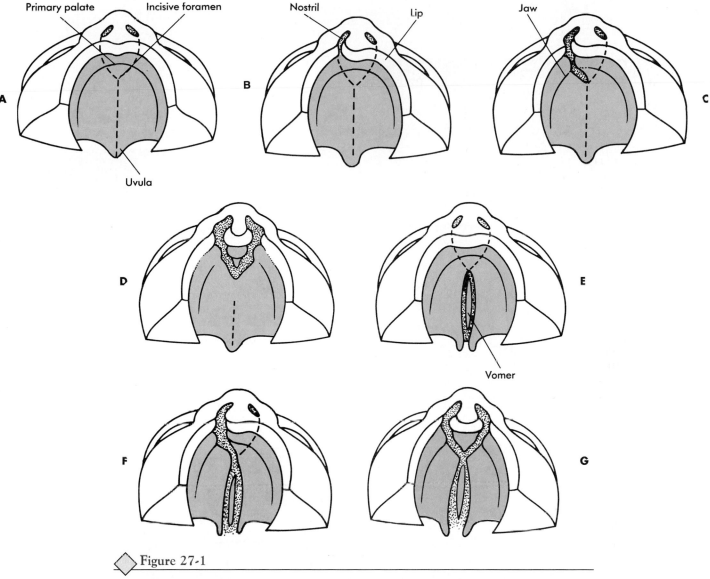

◇ Figure 27-1

Ventral view of palate, lip, and nose showing variability of cleft lip and palate deformity. **A,** Normal. **B,** Unilateral cleft lip extending into nose. **C,** Unilateral cleft involving lip and alveolus, extending to incisive foramen. **D,** Bilateral cleft involving lip and alveolus. **E,** Isolated cleft palate. **F,** Cleft palate combined with unilateral cleft of alveolus and lip. **G,** Bilateral complete cleft of lip and palate. *(From Langman J:* Medical embryology, *ed 3, Baltimore, 1975, Williams & Wilkins.)*

and soft palates. Three fourths are unilateral deformities; one fourth are bilateral. The left side is involved more frequently than the right when the defect is unilateral. The cleft may be incomplete, that is, it may not extend the entire distance from lip to soft palate. Cleft lip may occur without clefting of the palate, and isolated cleft palate may occur without clefting of the lip (Figure 27-1). A useful classification divides the anatomy into primary and secondary palates. The primary palate involves those structures anterior to the incisive foramen—the lip and alveolus; the secondary palate consists of those structures posterior to the incisive foramen—the hard and soft palates.[2] Thus an individual may have clefting of the primary palate, the secondary palate, or both (Figure 27-2).

Clefts of the lip may range from a minute notch on the edge of the vermilion border to a wide cleft that extends into the nasal cavity and thus divides the nasal floor. Clefts of the soft palate may also show wide variations from a bifid uvula to a wide inoperable cleft. The bifid uvula is the most minor form of cleft palate, in which only the uvula is clefted. Submucosal clefts of the soft palate are occasionally seen. These clefts are also called *occult* clefts, because they are not readily seen on cursory examination. The defect in such a cleft is a lack of continuity in the musculature of the soft palate. However, the nasal and oral mucosa are continuous and cover the muscular defect. To diagnose such a defect, the dentist inspects the soft palate while the patient says "ah." This action lifts the soft palate, and in individuals with submucosal palatal clefts a furrow in the midline is seen where the muscular discontinuity

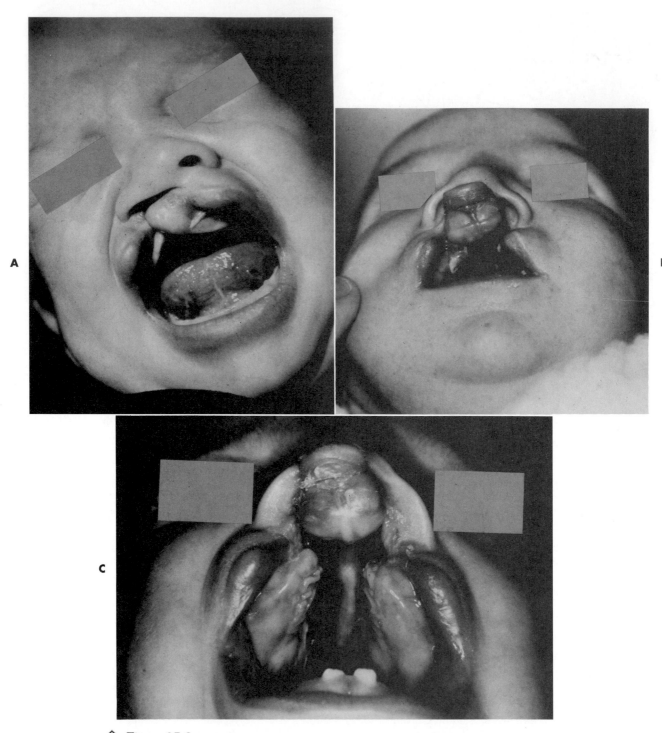

◇ **Figure 27-2**

Photographs of various types of cleft deformities. Nasal deformities are also apparent. **A,** Unilateral complete cleft of lip and palate. **B,** Bilateral complete cleft lip and palate. **C,** Palatal view of bilateral complete cleft lip and palate. Note that nasal septum is unattached to either palatal shelf.

Continued

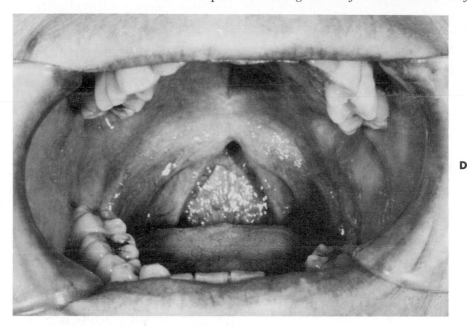

D

Figure 27-2, cont'd

D, Isolated cleft of soft palate.

is present. The dentist can also palpate the posterior aspect of the hard palate to detect the absence of the posterior nasal spine, which is characteristically absent in submucosal clefts. If a patient shows hypernasal speech without an obvious soft palatal cleft, the dentist should suspect a submucosal cleft of the soft palate.

EMBRYOLOGY

To understand the causes of oral clefts, a review of nose, lip, and palate embryology is necessary. The entire process takes place between the fifth and tenth weeks of fetal life.[3]

During the fifth week, two fast-growing ridges, the *lateral* and *medial nasal swellings,* surround the nasal vestige (Figure 27-3). The lateral swellings will form the alae of the nose; the medial swellings will give rise to (1) the middle portion of the nose, (2) the middle portion of the upper lip, (3) the middle portion of the maxilla, and (4) the entire *primary palate.* Simultaneously, the maxillary swellings will approach the medial and lateral nasal swellings but remain separated from them by well-marked grooves.

During the following 2 weeks, the appearance of the face changes considerably. The maxillary swellings continue to grow in a medial direction and compress the medial nasal swellings toward the midline. Subsequently, these swellings simultaneously merge with each other and with the maxillary swellings laterally. Hence the upper lip is formed by the two medial nasal swellings and the two maxillary swellings.

The two medial swellings merge not only at the surface but also at the deeper level. The structures formed by the two merged swellings are known together as the *intermaxillary segment* (Figure 27-4). It comprises (1) a labial component, which forms the philtrum of the upper lip; (2) an upper jaw component, which carries the four incisor teeth; and (3) a palatal component, which forms the triangular primary palate. Above, the intermaxillary segment is continuous with the nasal septum, which is formed by the frontal prominence.

The secondary palate is formed by two shelflike outgrowths from the maxillary swellings. These *palatine shelves* appear in the sixth week of development and are directed obliquely downward on either side of the tongue. In the seventh week, however, the palatine shelves ascend to attain a horizontal position above the tongue and fuse with each other, thereby forming the *secondary palate.* Anteriorly, the shelves fuse with the triangular primary palate, and the incisive foramen is formed at this junction. At the same time, the nasal septum grows down and joins the superior surface of the newly formed palate. The palatine shelves fuse with each other and with the primary palate between the seventh and tenth weeks of development.

Clefts of the primary palate result from a failure of mesoderm to penetrate into the grooves between the medial nasal and maxillary processes, which prohibits their merging with one another. Clefts of the secondary palate are caused by a failure of the palatine shelves to fuse with one another. The causes for this are speculative and include failure of the tongue to descend into the oral cavity.

ETIOLOGIC FACTORS

The etiologic factors of facial clefting have been extensively investigated. It was initially thought that heredity played a significant role in the causation of orofacial clefts. However, studies have been able to implicate genetics in only 20% to

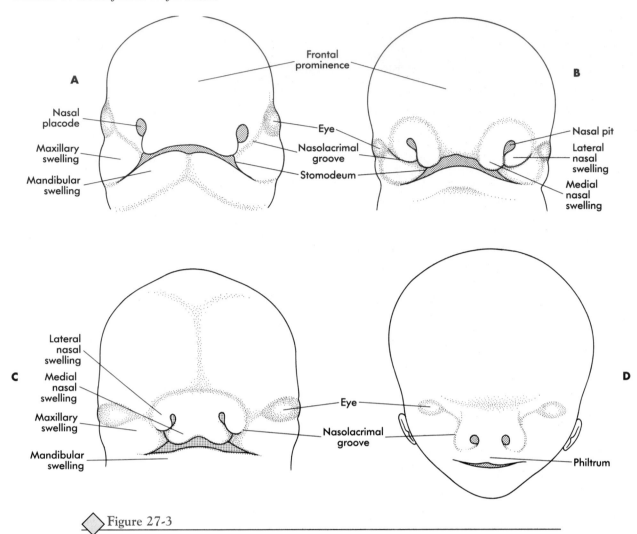

◇ Figure 27-3

Frontal aspect of face. **A,** Five-week-old embryo. **B,** Six-week-old embryo. Nasal swellings are gradually separated from maxillary swelling by deep furrows. At no time during *normal* development does this tissue break down. **C,** Seven-week-old embryo. **D,** Ten-week-old embryo. Maxillary swellings gradually merge with nasal folds, and furrows are filled with mesenchyme. *(From Langman J: Medical embryology, ed 3, Baltimore, 1975, Williams & Wilkins.)*

30% of cleft lip or palate patients. Even in those individuals whose genetic backgrounds may verify familial tendencies for facial clefting, the mode of inheritance is not completely understood. It is not a simple case of mendelian dominant or recessive inheritance but is multigenetic. However, if a person has a cleft, the chances are much higher when compared with the general population that one or more of his or her siblings will have a cleft. If a child is born with an orofacial cleft, the next child born of the same parents is at increased risk of developing a cleft (5%). If a parent and one child have clefts, the chances for another child having a cleft are much higher (15%). Genetic counselors may be consulted for parents of children with clefts or for people with clefts who would like to obtain more information on the relative risks for their offspring.

Environmental factors seem to play a contributory role at the critical time of embryologic development when the lip and palatal halves are fusing. A host of environmental factors have been shown in experimental animals to result in clefting. Nutritional deficiencies, radiation, several drugs, hypoxia, viruses, and vitamin excesses or deficiencies can produce clefting in certain situations.

In summary, orofacial clefts are produced by incompletely understood mechanisms, both genetic and environmental. With lack of complete knowledge of the causes, effective preventive measures are not available to prevent this deformity from developing other than the following of good prenatal practices, such as avoiding any medications that are not absolutely necessary.

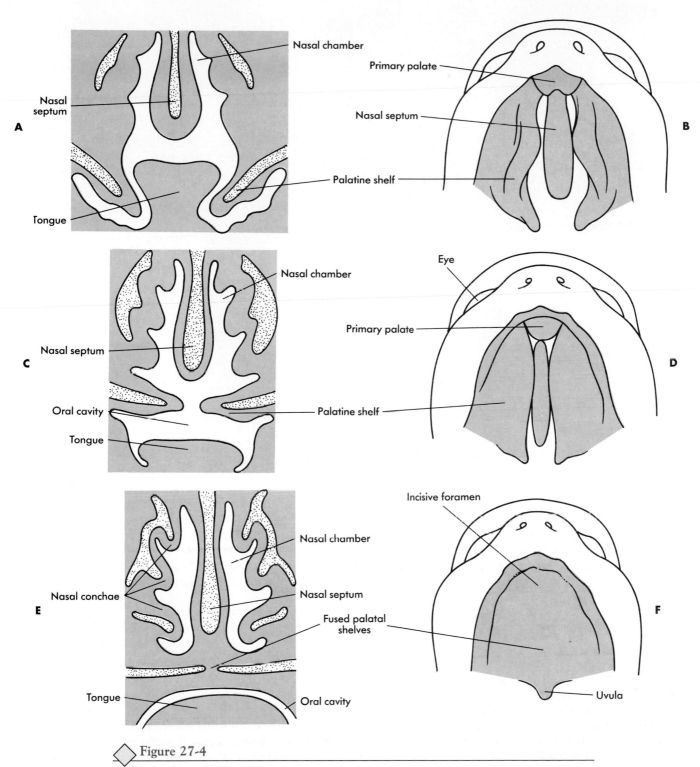

⬦ Figure 27-4

A, Frontal section through head of 6½-week-old embryo. Palatine shelves are located in vertical position on each side of tongue. **B,** Ventral view of same. Note clefts between primary triangular palate and palatine shelves, which are still in vertical position. **C,** Frontal section through head of 7½-week-old embryo. Tongue has moved downward, and palatine shelves have reached horizontal position. **D,** Ventral view of same. Shelves are in horizontal position. **E,** Frontal section through head of 10-week-old embryo. Two palatine shelves have fused with each other and with nasal septum. **F,** Ventral view of same. *(From Langman J: Medical embryology, ed 3, Baltimore, 1975, Williams & Wilkins.)*

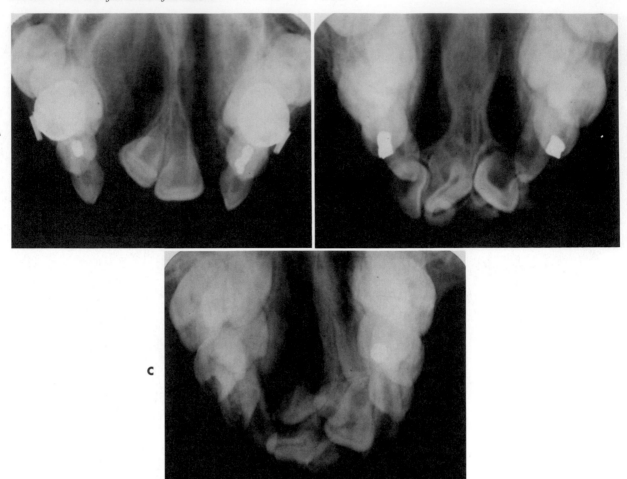

Figure 27-5

Occlusal radiographs from individuals with various types of cleft deformities. **A,** Bilateral complete cleft of alveolus and palate. Note absence of permanent lateral incisors. **B,** Bilateral complete cleft of alveolus and palate. Note absence of permanent lateral incisor on patient's left side. **C,** Unilateral complete cleft of alveolus and palate. Note supernumerary teeth.

PROBLEMS OF THE CLEFT-AFFLICTED INDIVIDUAL

DENTAL PROBLEMS

A cleft of the alveolus can often affect the development of the primary and permanent teeth and the jaw itself.[4] The most common problems may be related to congenital absence of teeth and, ironically, supernumerary teeth (Figure 27-5). The cleft usually extends between the lateral incisor and canine area. These teeth, because of their proximity to the cleft, may be absent; when present, they may be severely displaced, so that eruption into the cleft margin is common. These teeth may also be morphologically deformed or hypomineralized. Supernumerary teeth occur frequently, especially around the cleft margins. These teeth usually must be removed at some point during the child's development. However, they may be retained if they can furnish any useful function in the patient's overall dental rehabilitation. Frequently, supernumerary teeth

of the permanent dentition are left until 2 to 3 months before alveolar cleft bone grafting, because these teeth, although nonfunctional, maintain the surrounding alveolar bone. If extracted earlier, this bone may resorb, making the alveolar cleft larger.

MALOCCLUSION

Individuals affected with cleft deformities, especially those of the palate, show skeletal discrepancies between the size, shape, and position of their jaws. Class III malocclusion, seen in most cases, is caused by many factors. A common finding is mandibular prognathism, which is frequently relative and is caused more by the retrusion of the maxilla than by protrusion of the mandible (pseudoprognathism) (Figure 27-6). Missing or extra teeth may partially contribute to the malocclusion. However, retardation of maxillary growth is the factor most responsible for the malocclusion. Generally, the operative trauma of the cleft closure and the resultant fibrosis (scar contracture) severely limit the amount of maxillary growth

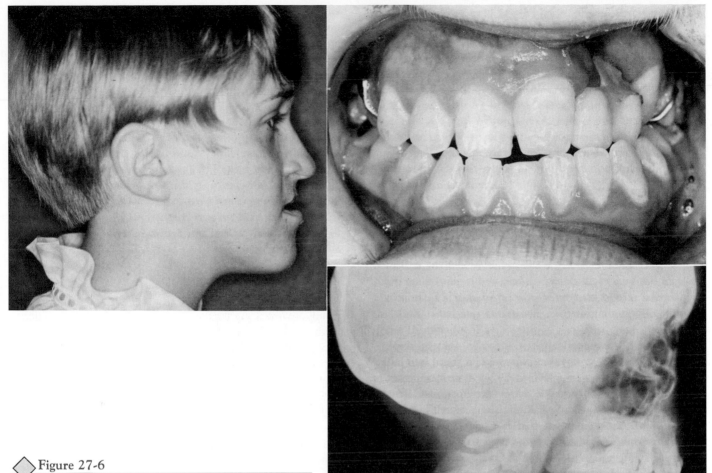

◇ Figure 27-6

A, Facial profile of typical cleft patient. Note pseudoprognathic appearance of mandible. **B,** Occlusal relationship of patient showing Angle's class III relationship with anterior cross bite. **C,** Lateral cephalogram showing maxillary skeletal sagittal deficiency contributing to class III occlusal relationship.

and development that can take place. The maxilla may be deficient in all three planes of space, with retrusion, constriction, and vertical underdevelopment common. Unilateral palatal clefts show collapse of the cleft side of the maxilla (the lesser segment) toward the center of the palate, which produces a narrow dental arch. Bilateral palatal clefts show collapse of all three segments or may have constriction of the posterior segments and protrusion of the anterior segment.

Orthodontic treatment may be necessary throughout the individual's childhood and adolescent years. Space maintenance and control is instituted during childhood. Appliances to maintain or increase the width of the dental arch are frequently used. This treatment is usually begun with the eruption of the first maxillary permanent molars. Comprehensive orthodontic care is deferred until later, when most of the permanent teeth have erupted. Consideration for orthognathic surgical intervention for correction of skeletal discrepancies and occlusal disharmonies is frequently necessary at this time.

NASAL DEFORMITY

Deformity of normal nasal architecture is commonly seen in individuals with cleft lips (see Figure 27-2). If the cleft extends into the floor of the nose, the alar cartilage on that side is flared, and the columella of the nose is pulled toward the noncleft side. There is also lack of underlying bony support to the base of the nose, which compounds the problem.

Surgical correction of nasal deformities should usually be deferred until all clefts and associated problems have been corrected, because correction of the alveolar cleft defect and the maxillary skeletal retrusion will alter the osseous foundation of the nose. Improved changes in the nasal form will therefore result from these osseous procedures. Thus nasal revision may be the last corrective surgical procedure the cleft-afflicted individual will undergo.

FEEDING

Babies with cleft palates can swallow normally once the material being fed reaches the hypopharynx but have extreme difficulty producing the necessary negative pressure in their mouth to allow sucking either breast or bottle milk. When a nipple is placed in the baby's mouth, he or she starts to suck just like any other newborn, because the sucking and swallowing reflexes are normal. However, the musculature is undeveloped or not properly oriented to allow the sucking to be effective. This problem is easily overcome through the use of specially designed nipples that are elongated and extend further into the baby's mouth. The opening should be enlarged, because the suck will not be as effective as in a normal baby. Other satisfactory methods are the use of eyedroppers or large syringes with rubber extension tubes connected to them. The tube is placed in the baby's mouth, and a small amount of solution is injected. These methods of feeding, while adequate for sustenance, require more time and care. Because the child will swallow a considerable amount of air when these feeding methods are used, the child is not usually fed while recumbent, and more frequent burping is necessary.

EAR PROBLEMS

Children afflicted with a cleft of the soft palate are predisposed to middle ear infections. The reason for this becomes clear on review of the anatomy of the soft palate musculature. The levator veli palatini and tensor veli palatini, which are normally inserted into the same muscles on the opposite side, are left unattached when the soft palate is cleft. These muscles have their origins either directly on or near the auditory tube. These muscles allow opening of the ostium of this tube into the nasopharynx. This action is demonstrated when middle ear pressures are equalized by swallowing during changes in atmospheric pressure, as when ascending or descending in an airplane. When this function is disrupted, the middle ear is essentially a closed space, without a drainage mechanism. Serous fluid may then accumulate and result in serous otitis media. Should bacteria find their way from the nasopharynx into the middle ear, an infection can develop (suppurative otitis media). To make matters worse the auditory tube in infants is at an angle that does not promote dependent drainage. With age this angulation changes and allows more dependent drainage of the middle ear. Children afflicted with cleft palate will frequently need to have their middle ear "vented." This is performed by the otorhinolaryngologist, who creates a hole through the inferior aspect of the tympanic membrane and inserts a small plastic tube, thus draining the ear to the outside instead of the nasopharynx.

Chronic serous otitis media is common among children with cleft palate, and multiple myringotomies are frequently necessary. Chronic serous otitis media presents a serious threat to hearing. Because of the chronic inflammation in the middle ear, hearing impairments are common in patients with cleft palate. The type of hearing loss experienced by the patient with cleft palate is conductive, meaning that the neural pathway to the brain continues to function normally. The defect in these instances is simply that sound cannot reach the auditory sensory organ as efficiently as it should because of the chronic inflammatory changes in the middle ear. However, if the problem is not corrected, permanent damage to the auditory sensory nerves (sensory neural loss) can also result. This type of damage is irreparable. The range of hearing impairment found in individuals with cleft palates is vast. The loss can be great enough so that normal-sounding speech is heard at less than one half of expected volume. Also, certain sounds of speech (called *phonemes*), such as the *s, sh,* and *t* sounds, may be heard poorly. Audiograms are useful tools and are performed repeatedly on patients with cleft palates, to monitor hearing ability and performance.

SPEECH DIFFICULTIES

Four speech problems are usually created by cleft lip and palate deformity. Retardation of consonant sounds (*p, b, t, d, k,* and *g*) is the most common finding. Because consonant sounds are necessary for the development of early vocabulary, much language activity is omitted. As a result, good sound discrimination is lacking by the time the palate is closed. Hypernasality is usual in the patient with a cleft of the soft palate and may remain after surgical correction. Dental malformation, malocclusion, and abnormal tongue placement may develop before the palate is closed and thus produce an articulation problem. Hearing problems contribute significantly to the many speech disorders common in patients with oral clefts.

In the normal individual, speech is created by the following scheme. Air is allowed to escape from the lungs, pass through the vocal cords, and enter the oral cavity. The position of the tongue, lips, lower jaw, and soft palate working together in a highly coordinated fashion results in the sounds of speech being produced. If the vocal cords are set into vibration while the airstream is passing between, then voice is superimposed on the speech sounds that result from the relationships of the oral structures. The soft palate is raised during speech production, preventing air from escaping through the nose.

For clear speech it is necessary for the individual to have complete control of the passage of air from the oropharynx to the nasopharynx. The hard palate provides the partition between the nasal and oral cavities. The soft palate functions as an important valve to control the distribution of escaping air between the oropharynx and nasopharynx (Figure 27-7). This is called the *velopharyngeal mechanism* (*velo* means soft palate). As the name implies, its two main components are the soft palate and pharyngeal walls. When passive the soft palate hangs downward toward the tongue, but during speech the muscles of the soft palate elevate it and draw it toward the posterior pharyngeal wall, which is what happens to the normal individual's soft palate when he or she is asked to say "ah." In normal speech this action takes place rapidly and with an unbelievable complexity, so that the valving mechanism can allow large amounts of air to escape into the nasopharynx or can limit the escape to none.

In individuals whose soft palate is cleft, the velopharyngeal

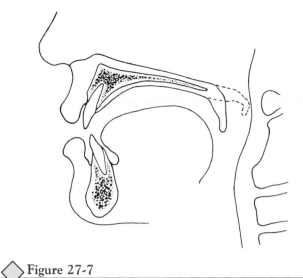

◇ **Figure 27-7**

Upward and backward movement of soft palate during normal speech. Note its contact with posterior pharyngeal wall.

mechanism cannot function because of the discontinuity of the musculature from one side to the other. The soft palate thus cannot elevate to make contact with the pharyngeal wall. The result of this constant escape of air into the nasal cavity is *hypernasal speech*.

Individuals with cleft palate develop compensatory velopharyngeal, tongue, and nasal mechanisms in an attempt to produce intelligible speech. The posterior and lateral pharyngeal walls obtain great mobility and attempt to narrow the passageway between the oropharynx and nasopharynx during speech. A muscular bulge of the pharyngeal wall actually develops during attempts at closure of the passageway in some individuals with cleft palate and is known as *Passavant's ridge* or *bar*. Individuals with cleft palates develop compensatory tongue postures and positions during speech to help valve the air coming from the larynx into the pharyngeal areas. Similarly, the superficial muscles around the nose involved in facial expression are recruited to help limit the amount of air escaping from the nasal cavity. In this instance the valving is at the other end of the nasal cavity than the velopharyngeal mechanism. However, in an uncorrected cleft of the soft palate, it is literally impossible for compensatory mechanisms to produce a satisfactory velopharyngeal mechanism. Unfortunately, in surgically corrected soft palates, velopharyngeal competence is not always achieved with one operation, and secondary procedures are frequently necessary.

Speech pathologists are well versed in assisting children with cleft deformities to develop normal articulation skills. The earlier in life speech training is started in patients with cleft deformities, the better the eventual outcome. The patient may need to undergo speech counseling for several years to produce acceptable speech.

When hearing problems are also present, the speech problems are compounded. Hearing loss at an early age is especially detrimental to the development of normal speech skills. The child who is unable to hear is unable to imitate normal speech. Thus the parents must be cognizant of their child's development and ensure that regular visits to the pediatrician are undertaken.

ASSOCIATED ANOMALIES

Although the child with an oral cleft is 20 times more likely to have another congenital anomaly than a normal child, no correlation is evident with specific anatomic zones of additional anomaly involvement.[2] Thirty-eight percent of children with isolated cleft palate and 21% of children with cleft lip, with or without cleft palate, have associated anomalies. In the overall cleft-afflicted population, approximately 30% have other anomalies in addition to the facial cleft, ranging from clubfoot to neurologic disturbances. Of the overall cleft-afflicted population, 10% have congenital heart disease, and 10% have some degree of mental retardation. Thus the child with a facial cleft may require additional care beyond the scope of the cleft team.

TREATMENT OF CLEFT LIP AND PALATE ◇

The aim of treatment of cleft lip and palate is to correct the cleft and associated problems surgically and thus hide the anomaly so that patients can lead normal lives. This correction involves surgically producing a face that does not attract attention, a vocal apparatus that permits intelligible speech, and a dentition that allows optimal function and esthetics. Operations begin early in life and may continue for several years. In view of the gross distortion of tissues surrounding the cleft, it is amazing that success is ever achieved. However, with modern anesthetic techniques, excellent pediatric care centers, and surgeons who have had a wealth of experience because of the frequency of the cleft deformity, acceptable results are commonplace.

TIMING OF SURGICAL REPAIR

The timing of the surgical repair has been and remains one of the most debated issues among surgeons, speech pathologists, audiologists, and orthodontists. It is tempting to correct all of the defects as soon as the baby is able to withstand the surgical procedure. The parents of a child born with a facial cleft would certainly desire this mode of treatment, eliminating all of the baby's clefts as early in life as possible. Indeed, the cleft lip is usually corrected as early as possible. Most surgeons adhere to the proven "rule of 10" as determining when an otherwise healthy baby is fit for surgery, that is, 10 weeks of age, 10 lb in body weight, and at least 10 g of hemoglobin per deciliter of blood. However, because surgical correction of the cleft is an elective procedure, if any other medical condition jeopardizes the health of the baby, the cleft surgery is postponed until medical risks are minimal.

Unfortunately, each possible advantage for closing a palatal cleft early in life has several possible disadvantages for the individual later in life. The advantages for early closure of palatal defects are (1) better palatal and pharyngeal muscle development once repaired, (2) ease of feeding, (3) better development of phonation skills, (4) better auditory tube function, (5) better hygiene when the oral and nasal partition is competent, and (6) improved psychologic state for parents and baby. The disadvantages of closing palatal clefts early in life are also several. The most important are (1) surgical correction is more difficult in younger children with small structures, and (2) scar formation resulting from the surgery causes maxillary growth restriction.

Although different cleft teams time the surgical repair differently, a widely accepted principle is compromise. The lip is corrected as early as is medically possible. The soft palatal cleft is closed between 18 and 24 months of age, leaving the hard palate cleft open. The hard palatal cleft is then closed in the preschool years, around age 4 or 5. Closure of the lip as early as possible is advantageous, because it performs a favorable "molding" action on the distorted alveolus. It also assists the child in feeding and is of psychologic benefit. The soft palatal cleft is closed next, to produce a functional velopharyngeal mechanism when or before speech skills are developing. The hard palatal cleft is left as long as possible so that maxillary growth will proceed as unimpeded as possible. Most surgeons feel that closure of the hard palatal cleft should be postponed at least until all of the deciduous dentition has erupted. This postponement facilitates the use of orthodontic appliances and allows more maxillary growth to occur before scarring from the surgery is induced. Because a significant portion of maxillary growth has already occurred by ages 4 to 5, closure of the hard palate at this time is usually performed before the child's enrollment in school. However, some cleft teams will wait to close the hard palate until maxillary growth is complete at ages 11 to 13. Removable palatal obturators can be fitted and worn in the meantime to partition the oral and nasal cavities.

The largest problem in evaluation of treatment regimens is the fact that the final results of surgical repair of clefts can only be judged conclusively when the individual's growth is complete. A surgical method employed today cannot be put to careful scrutiny for 10 to 20 years, which, unfortunately, may allow many individuals with cleft deformities to be treated with procedures that may later be discarded, when follow-up examinations and studies show unsatisfactory or poor effects.

CHEILORRHAPHY

Cheilorrhaphy is the surgical correction of the cleft lip deformity; this term is derived from *cheilo,* lip, and *rhaphy,* junction by a seam or suture. It is usually the earliest operative procedure used to correct cleft deformities and is undertaken as soon as medically possible.

The cleft of the upper lip disrupts the important circumoral orbicularis oris musculature. The lack of continuity of this muscle allows the developing parts of the maxilla to grow in an uncoordinated manner, so that the cleft in the alveolus is accentuated. At birth the alveolar process on the unaffected side may appear to protrude from the mouth. The lack of

sphincteric muscle control from the orbicularis oris will cause a bilateral cleft lip to exhibit a premaxilla that protrudes from the base of the nose and produces an unsightly appearance. Thus restoration of this muscular sphincter with lip repair has a favorable effect on the developing alveolar segments.

OBJECTIVES.   The objectives of cheilorrhaphy are two-fold: functional and esthetic. The cheilorrhaphy should restore the functional arrangement of the orbicularis oris musculature to reestablish the normal function of the upper lip. If muscle continuity is not restored across the area of the cleft, an esthetically unpleasing depression will result when the lip is brought into function. The second objective of cheilorrhaphy is to produce a lip that displays normal anatomic structures, such as a vermilion tubercle, cupid's bow, and philtrum. The lip must be symmetric, well contoured, soft, and supple and the scars must be inconspicuous. Another esthetic necessity is to correct (at least partially) the nasal deformity resulting from the cleft lip.

Despite the skill of the surgeon, these ideal objectives are rarely achieved. Hindrances are the poor quality of tissues in the cleft margins and the distortion of structures before surgical intervention. Several surgical techniques reproduce normal appearance immediately but do not maintain this appearance with growth. However, with careful selection of surgical technique, satisfactory results are obtainable.

SURGICAL TECHNIQUES.   As each cleft is unique, so must be the surgical procedure. There are countless techniques used for cheilorrhaphy, each designed to elongate the cleft margins to facilitate closure (Figures 27-8 and 27-9). In unilateral cases the unaffected side serves as a guide for lip length and symmetry. A key point in design is to break up lines of scar so that with fibrosis and contracture deformity of the lip will be minimized. In lips closed in a linear fashion, scar contracture causes a characteristic notching of the upper lip. Attention to reorienting and reuniting the musculature of the lip is of paramount importance if normal function is to be established.

Cheilorrhaphy procedures serve to restore symmetry not only to the lip but to the nasal tip, as well. With the cleft extending through the floor of the nose, the continuity of the nasal apparatus is disrupted. Without the bony foundation for the alar cartilage, a collapse of the lateral aspect of the nose occurs. When the lip is closed, it is necessary to advance this laterally displaced tissue toward the midline. Thus cheilorrhaphy is the first and one of the most important steps in correcting the nasal deformity so common in cleft patients.

PALATORRHAPHY

Palatorrhaphy may be performed in one operation or two. In two operations the soft palate closure (staphylorrhaphy) is usually performed first and the hard palate closure (uranorrhaphy) is performed second.

OBJECTIVES.   The primary purpose of the cleft palate repair is to create a mechanism capable of speech and

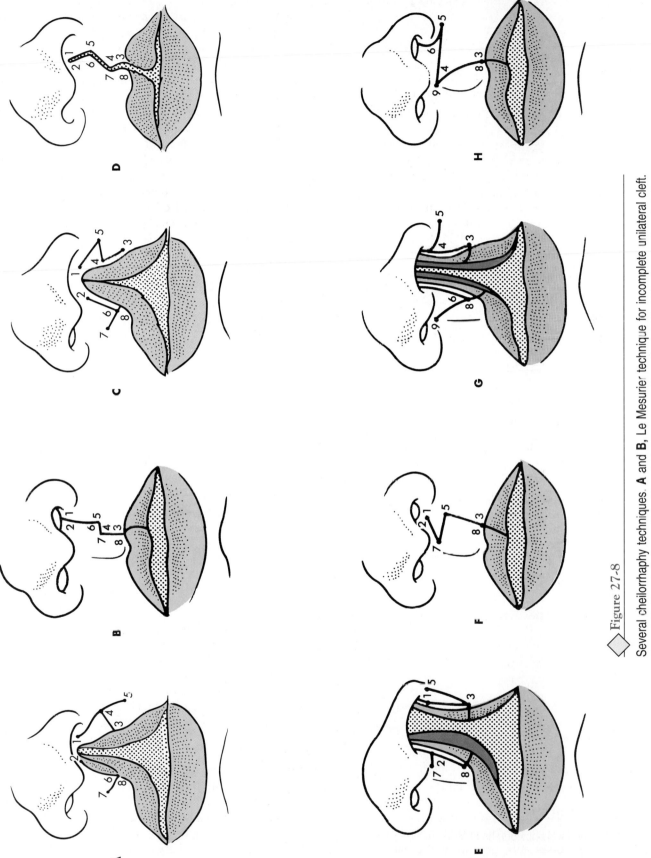

Figure 27-8

Several cheilorrhaphy techniques. **A** and **B**, Le Mesurier technique for incomplete unilateral cleft. **C** and **D**, Tennison operation. **E** and **F**, Wynn operation. **G** and **H**, Millard operation (rotation advancement technique).

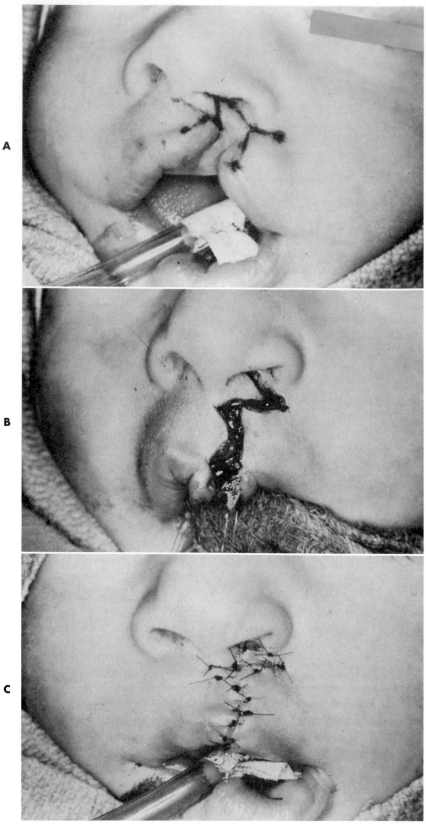

◇ **Figure 27-9**

Clinical photographs of Millard cheilorrhaphy technique. **A,** Incisions outlined. **B,** Flaps rotated and advanced into position. **C,** Closure.

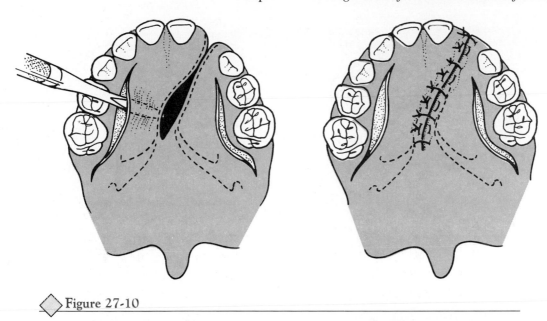

◇ Figure 27-10

Von Langenbeck operation for closure of hard palate using lateral releasing incisions. This technique is one-layer closure—nasal (superior) aspect of palatal flaps will epithelialize, as will denuded areas of palatal bone.

deglutition without significantly interfering with subsequent maxillary growth. Thus creation of a competent velopharyngeal mechanism and partitioning of the nasal and oral cavities are prerequisites to achieving these goals. The aim is to obtain a long and mobile soft palate capable of producing normal speech. Extensive stripping of soft tissues from bone will create more scar formation, which will adversely affect maxillary growth. The precarious nature of the problem indicates the complexity of the surgical procedures designed and the ages at which they are instituted.

SURGICAL TECHNIQUES. Operative procedures for palatorrhaphy are as varied as techniques for cleft lip repair. Each cleft of the palate is unique. They vary in width, completeness, amount of hard and soft tissue available, and palatal length. Thus the surgical techniques used to close cleft palate deformities are extremely varied, not just from one surgeon to another but from one patient to the next.

HARD PALATE CLOSURE. The hard palate is closed with soft tissues only. Usually no effort is made to create an osseous partition between the nasal and oral cavities. The soft tissues extending around the cleft margin vary in quality. Some are atrophic and not particularly useful. Others appear healthy and readily lend themselves to dissection and suture integrity. In the most basic sense the soft tissues are incised along the cleft margin and dissected from the palatal shelves until approximation over the cleft defect is possible. This procedure frequently necessitates the use of lateral relaxing incisions close to the dentition (Figure 27-10). The soft tissues are then sutured in a watertight manner over the cleft defect and allowed to heal. The areas of bone exposed by lateral

relaxing incisions are allowed to heal by secondary intention. The superior aspect of the palatal flaps will also reepithelialize with respiratory epithelium, because this surface is now the lining of the nasal floor. When possible, it is advisable to obtain a two-layer closure of the hard palatal cleft (Figure 27-11), which necessitates that the nasal mucosa from the floor, lateral wall, and septal areas of the nose be mobilized and sutured together before the oral closure.

When the vomer is long and attached to the palatal shelf opposite the cleft, a mucosal flap can be raised from it and sutured to the palatal tissues on the cleft side (Figure 27-12). This procedure (vomer flap technique) requires little stripping of palatal mucoperiosteum and produces minimal scar contraction. The denuded areas of vomer and the opposite sides of the flap where no epithelium is present will reepithelialize. The vomer flap technique is useful in clefts that are not wide and where the vomer is readily available for use. It is a one-layer closure.

SOFT PALATE CLOSURE. The closure of the soft palate is technically the most difficult of the operations yet discussed in the cleft-afflicted individual. Access is the largest problem, because the soft palate is toward the back of the oral cavity. The combination of difficulty with light, retraction, and the fact that the clinician can work only from the oral side yet must correct both the oral and nasal sides of the soft palate lead to difficulties. Also, the clinician may have to work with extremely thin, atrophic tissues yet produce a closure that will hold together under function while healing is progressing. To help accomplish this goal, the soft palate is always closed in three layers—nasal mucosa, muscle, and oral mucosa—in that order (Figure 27-13). The margins of the cleft are incised from

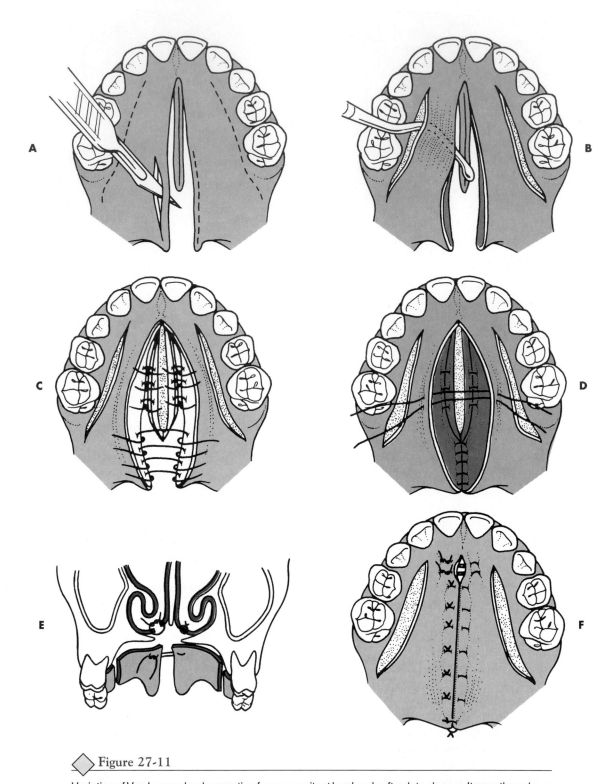

◇ Figure 27-11

Variation of Von Langenbeck operation for concomitant hard and soft palate closure. It uses three-layer closure for soft palate (nasal mucosa, muscle, oral mucosa) and two-layer closure for hard palate (flaps from vomer and nasal floor to produce nasal closure, palatal flaps for oral closure). **A,** Removing mucosa from margin of cleft. **B,** Mucoperiosteal flaps on hard palate are developed; note lateral releasing incisions. **C,** Sutures placed into nasal mucosa after development of nasal flaps from vomer and nasal floor. Sutures are placed so that knots will be on nasal side. **D,** Nasal mucosa has been closed. **E,** Frontal section showing repair of nasal mucosa. **F,** Closure of oral mucoperiosteum.

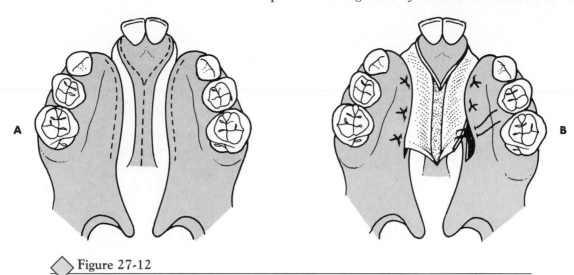

◇ Figure 27-12

Vomer flap technique for closure of hard palate cleft (bilateral in this case). **A,** Incisions through nasal mucosa on underside of nasal septum (vomer) and mucosa of cleft margins. **B,** Mucosa of nasal septum is dissected off nasal septum and inserted under palatal mucosa at margins of cleft. This is one-layer, nasal closure only. Connective tissue undersurface of nasal mucosa will epithelialize. This technique, because it does not require extensive elevation of palatal mucoperiosteum, produces less scarring with attendant growth restriction.

the posterior end of the hard palate to *at least* the distal end of the uvula (some surgeons carry the incision and closure down the palatopharyngeus fold to elongate the soft palate). The nasal mucosa is then dissected free from the underlying musculature and sutured to the nasal mucosa of the opposite side. The muscular layer requires special care. The musculature of the cleft soft palate is not inserted across to the opposite side but instead is inserted posteriorly and laterally along the margins of the hard palate. These muscular insertions must be released from their bony insertions and reapproximated to those of the other sides. Only then will the velopharyngeal mechanism have a chance to perform properly. If the quantity of muscular tissue is inadequate for approximation of the musculature in the midline, the pterygoid hamular processes can be infractured, thus releasing the tensor palatini muscles toward the midline. This maneuver is frequently necessary, especially in wide clefts.

Occasionally, the soft palate is found to be short, and articulation with the pharyngeal wall is impossible. This situation is especially prevalent in incomplete palatal clefts—those of the soft palate only. In these cases the palate can be closed in a manner that not only brings the two lateral halves together in the midline but that also gains palatal length (Figure 27-14). The so-called W-Y push-back procedure (Wardill) and U-shaped push-back procedure (Dorrance and Brown) are commonly used. The mucoperiosteum of the hard palate is incised and elevated in a manner that allows the entire soft tissue elements of the hard and soft palate to extend posteriorly, thus gaining palatal length.

ALVEOLAR CLEFT GRAFTS

The alveolar cleft defect is usually not corrected in the original surgical correction of either the cleft lip or the cleft palate (Figure 27-15). As a result, the cleft-afflicted individual may have residual oronasal fistulae in this area, and the maxillary alveolus will not be continuous because of the cleft. The problems that commonly occur because of the alveolar cleft and oronasal fistulae are (1) the escape of oral fluids into the nasal cavity, (2) the drainage of nasal secretion into the oral cavity, (3) eruption of teeth into the alveolar cleft, (4) collapse of the alveolar segments, and (5) if the cleft is large, speech that is adversely affected.

Alveolar cleft bone grafts provide several advantages. First, they unite the alveolar segments and help prevent collapse and constriction of the dental arch, which is especially important if the maxilla has been orthodontically expanded. Second, alveolar cleft bone grafts provide bone support for teeth adjacent to the cleft and for those that will erupt into the area of the cleft. Frequently, the bone support on the distal aspect of the central incisor is thin, and the height of the bone support varies. These teeth may show slight mobility because of this lack of bone support. Increasing the amount of alveolar bone for this tooth will help ensure its periodontal maintenance. The canine tends to erupt into the cleft site and with healthy bone placed into the cleft will maintain good periodontal support during eruption and thereafter. The third benefit of alveolar cleft grafts is closure of the oronasal fistula, which will partition the oral and nasal cavities and prevent escape of fluids between them. Augmen-

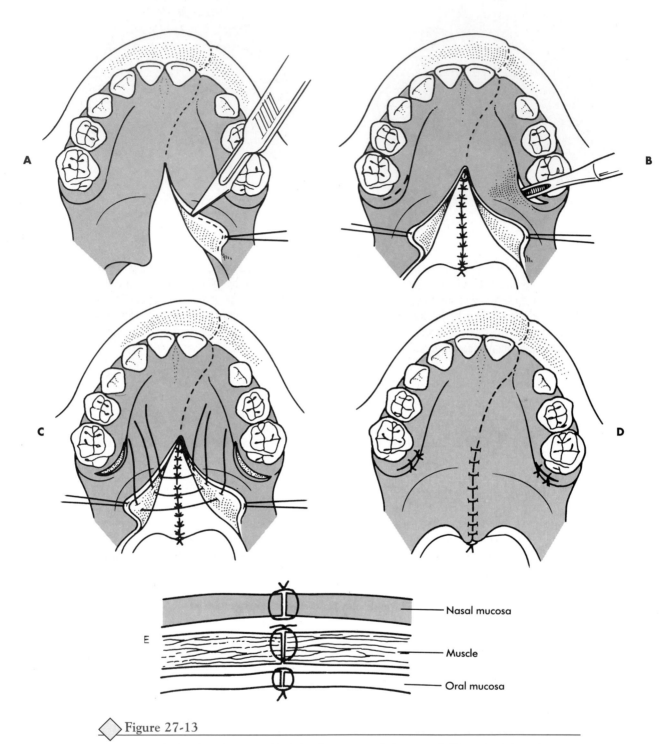

◇ Figure 27-13

Triple-layered soft palate closure. **A,** Excision of mucosa at cleft margin. **B,** Dissection of nasal mucosa from soft palate to facilitate closure. Nasal mucosa is sutured together with knots tied on nasal (superior) surface. Note small incision made to insert instrument for hamular process fracture. This maneuver releases tensor veli palatini and facilitates approximation in midline. **C,** Muscle is dissected from insertion into hard palate, and sutures are placed to approximate muscle in midline. **D,** Closure of oral mucosa is accomplished last. **E,** Layered closure of soft palate. *(From Hayward JR: Oral surgery, Springfield, Ill, 1976, Charles C Thomas.)*

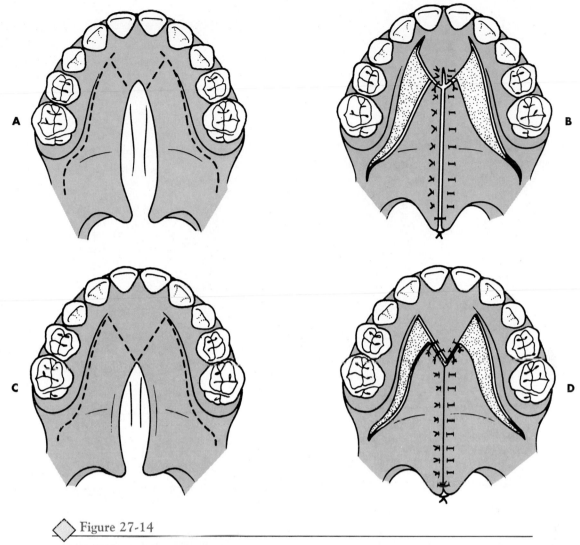

◇ Figure 27-14

The Wardill operations for palatal lengthening on closure. **A** and **B,** Four-flap operation for extensive cleft. **C** and **D,** Three-flap operation for shorter cleft. Note amount of denuded palatal bone left after these operations.

tation of the alveolar ridge in the area of the cleft is a fourth advantage, because it facilitates the use of dental prostheses by creating a more suitable supporting base. A fifth benefit is the creation of a solid foundation for the lip and alar base of the nose. It has become evident that the alveolar cleft grafting procedure itself creates a favorable change in the nasal structure, because the tissues at the base of the nose become supported after alveolar cleft grafting, whereas before the graft they had no solid osseous foundation. Therefore the alveolar graft should be performed before nasal revisions.

TIMING OF GRAFT PROCEDURE. The alveolar cleft graft is usually performed when the patient is between ages 7 and 10. By this time a major portion of maxillary growth has occurred, and the alveolar cleft surgery should not adversely affect the future growth of the maxilla. It is important to have the graft in place before the eruption of the permanent canines into the cleft, thus ensuring their periodontal support. Ideally,

the grafting procedure is performed when one half to two thirds of the unerupted canine root has formed.

Orthodontic expansion of the arch before or after the procedure is equally effective; however, some surgeons prefer to expand before bone grafting so that access into the cleft area is facilitated at surgery.

SURGICAL PROCEDURE. Bone grafts placed into the alveolar cleft must be covered by intact mucoperiosteal flaps on each side. This means that flaps of nasal mucosa, palatal mucosa, and labial mucosa must all be developed and sutured in a tension-free, watertight manner to prevent infection of the graft. The soft tissue incisions for alveolar cleft grafts vary, but in each procedure these conditions are met (Figure 27-16).

The bone placed into the alveolar cleft is usually obtained from the patient's ilium or cranium; however, allogeneic bone (homologous bone from another individual) is being used by some surgeons. The grafts are made into a particulate

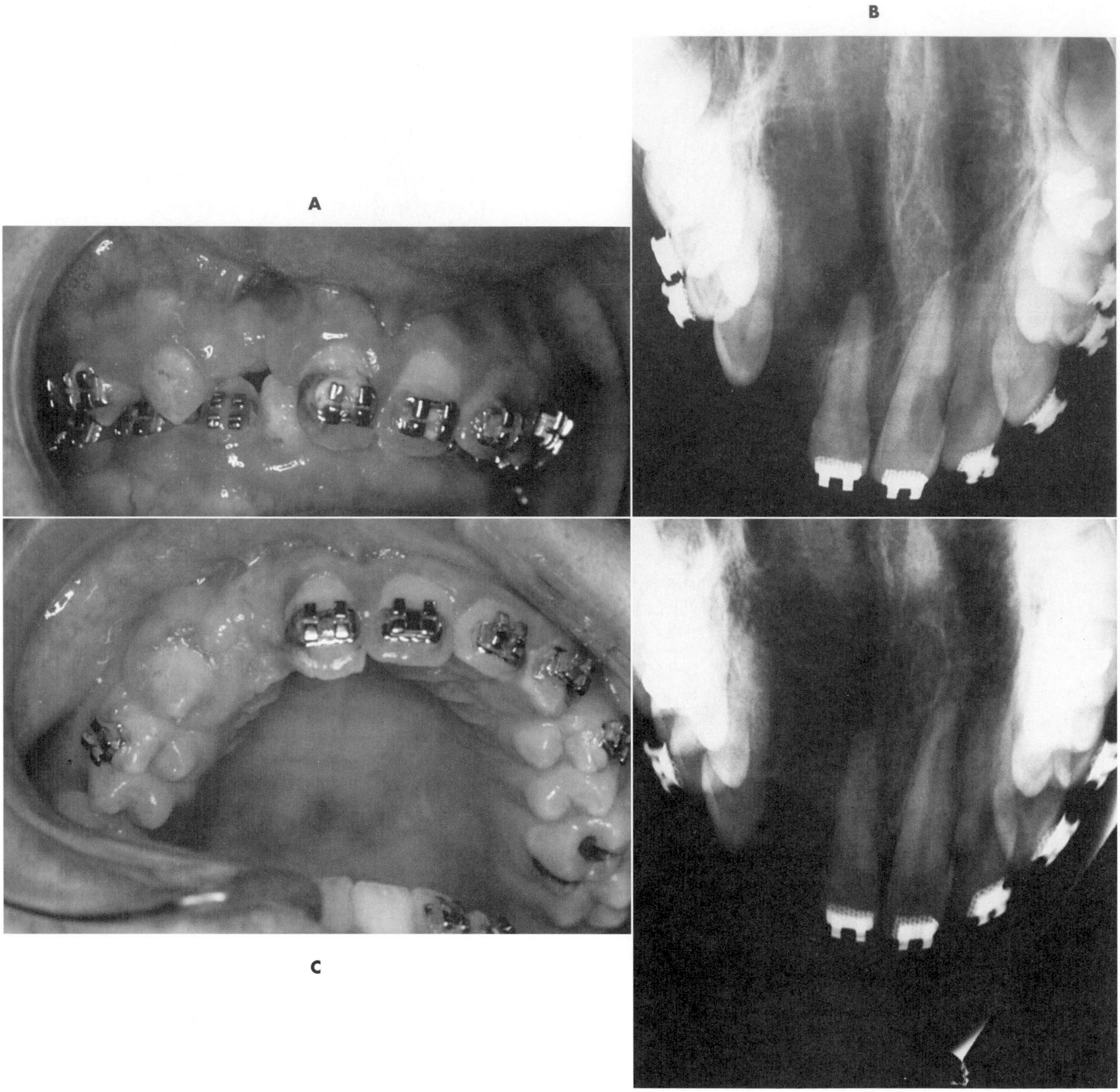

A

B

C

D

◇ **Figure 27-15**

A, Clinical photograph and **B,** radiograph of alveolar cleft. Note oronasal fistula and the lack of bone between the minor and major segments of the maxilla. **C,** Occlusal photograph and **D,** radiograph 6 months after surgery. Note the closure of the oronasal fistula and the bone continuity of the maxilla.

consistency and are packed into the defect once the nasal and palatal mucosa have been closed. The labial mucosa is then closed over the bone graft. In time these grafts are replaced by new bone that is indistinguishable from the surrounding alveolar process (see Figure 27-15). Orthodontic movement of teeth into the graft sites is possible, and eruption of teeth into them usually proceeds unimpeded.

CORRECTION OF MAXILLOMANDIBULAR DISHARMONIES

The individual with a cleft deformity will usually exhibit maxillary retrusion and a transverse maxillary constriction resulting from the cicatricial contraction of previous surgeries. In many instances the associated malocclusion is beyond the scope of orthodontic treatment alone. In these cases

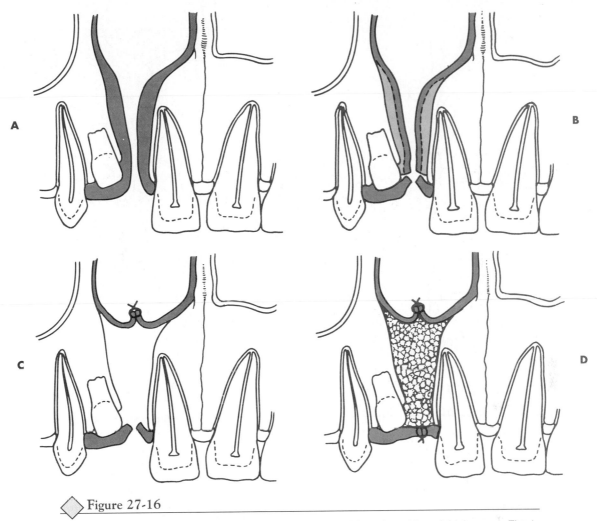

Figure 27-16

Technique for alveolar cleft bone grafting. **A,** Preoperative defect viewed from labial aspect. Fistula extends into nasal cavity. **B,** Incision divides mucosa fistula, which allows development of nasal and oral flaps. **C,** Mucosal flap developed from lining of fistula is turned inward, up into nasal cavity, and sutured in watertight manner. **D,** Bone graft material is packed into cleft, and oral mucosa is closed in watertight manner.

orthognathic surgery similar to the procedures outlined in Chapter 26 are indicated to correct the underlying skeletal malrelationships.

There are some differences, however, in the technical aspects of maxillary surgery because of the other deformities and scarring that are present in the maxillas of cleft-afflicted individuals. In general, total maxillary osteotomies are necessary to advance and sometimes widen the maxilla. Closure of some of the space in the alveolar cleft area by bringing the alveolus of the cleft side anteriorly is also performed in several instances. These latter procedures necessitate the segmentation of the maxilla, which, because of the cleft's nature, usually already has occurred. The differences between the cleft-afflicted patient and a non–cleft-afflicted patient, however, are the scar present across the palate and the decreased blood supply to the maxilla. Scarring from previous surgeries makes widening of the maxilla very difficult, and frequently excision of some of this tissue is

necessary. The clinician should try to be diligent and to maintain as much mucoperiosteum to the maxilla as possible because of the poor blood supply that the cleft maxilla receives. Care must also be taken not to create another oronasal fistula.

If the alveolar cleft had not been grafted previously, this can be done in the same operation. In bilateral clefts, however, the blood supply to the prolabial segment is very poor. It may be more prudent in these instances to perform the alveolar cleft grafts first and then perform a one-piece maxillary osteotomy after sufficient time has passed for revascularization of the prolabial segment.

One problem faced by the patient with a cleft palate when maxillary advancement procedures are planned is the effect this may have on the velopharyngeal mechanism. When the maxilla is brought forward, the soft palate is also drawn forward. A patient's preoperative marginal competence of the velopharyngeal mechanism may become incompetent in the

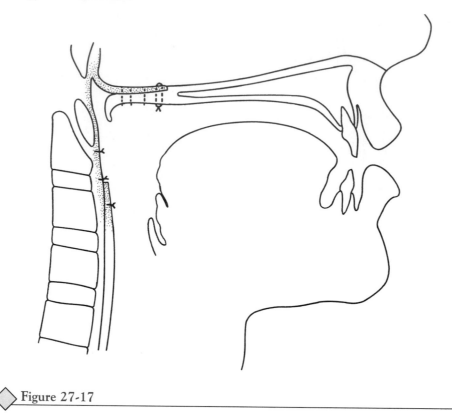

◇ Figure 27-17

Superiorly based pharyngeal flap. Flap is sutured to superior aspect of soft palate, thus partially partitioning oral and nasal cavities from one another. Only nasal airway remaining after this operation is two lateral openings on each side of flap.

postoperative period. It is very difficult to determine which patients will have this problem. Because of the possibility of this incompetence, however, secondary palatal and/or pharyngeal surgical procedures to increase velopharyngeal competence are discussed with the patient. These procedures can be performed later if necessary.

SECONDARY SURGICAL PROCEDURES

Secondary surgical procedures are procedures performed after the initial repair of the cleft defects in an effort to improve speech or correct residual defects. The most commonly employed technique to improve velopharyngeal competence secondarily is the pharyngeal flap procedure (Figure 27-17). In this procedure a wide vertical strip of pharyngeal mucosa and musculature is raised from the posterior pharyngeal wall and inserted into the superior aspect of the soft palate. These flaps are most often based superiorly. The defect left in the posterior pharyngeal wall from elevation of the pharyngeal flap can be closed primarily or left to heal by secondary intention. Once inserted into the soft palate, the pharynx and the soft palate are joined, leaving two lateral ports as the opening between the oropharynx and nasopharynx, which reduces the airstream between the oropharynx and nasopharynx. The velopharyngeal mechanism then consists of both raising the soft palate somewhat and medial constriction of the lateral pharyngeal walls.

Another technique that has recently had a resurgence of interest because of new biocompatible material is the placement of an implant behind the posterior pharyngeal wall to bring it anteriorly (Figure 27-18). Thus the soft palate has less distance to traverse to close off the nasopharynx. The major problems with this technique in the past have been migration of the implant and infection, which usually results in need for removal.

DENTAL NEEDS OF CLEFT-AFFLICTED INDIVIDUALS ◇

Dentists will have cleft-afflicted patients in their practice because of the relatively large number of people so affected. These patients should not pose any great problems, as their dental needs do not differ dramatically from those of other individuals. However, because of the presence of the cleft, either corrected or uncorrected, these individuals have a few special needs of which the dentist should be cognizant.

Because of the interdisciplinary approach that cleft-afflicted patients require, it behooves the dentist to be aware of the overall treatment plan formulated by the cleft team for the patient's management. Awareness of this plan precludes the performance of any irreversible or costly procedures on teeth that may be charted for extraction in the future. For

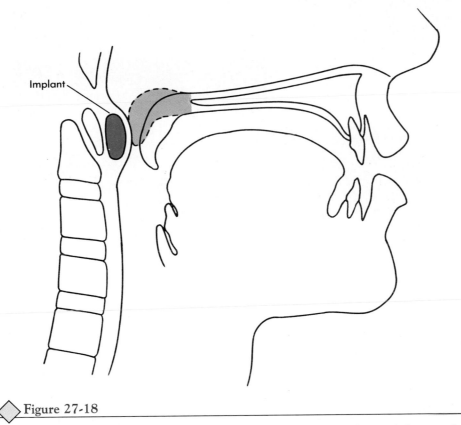

Implant

◇ **Figure 27-18**

Posterior pharyngeal wall implant. This makes distance between soft palate and pharyngeal wall smaller, so that velopharyngeal closure is facilitated.

instance, placing a bridge to replace a congenitally missing lateral incisor before alveolar bone grafting and orthodontic therapy is unwise. Similarly, extracting supernumerary teeth that may be temporarily retained to maintain alveolar bone support is also disadvantageous. All fixed bridgework should be delayed until after the orthodontic, orthognathic, and alveolar grafting procedures have been completed. Only then will the dentist be able to determine accurately the exact space and ridge form available for pontics. Furthermore, until the two halves of the maxillary arch have been united with bone grafts, the halves will move independently, and bridgework spanning the cleft margin may become loose. Therefore the dentist must communicate freely with the other professionals who are managing the patient's other cleft problems, and coordination of services is of paramount importance.

Teeth adjacent to the cleft margins not only may be malformed or absent, but those present may have poor periodontal support because of lack of bone and their position in the cleft margin. This situation predisposes them to periodontitis and early loss if not kept in an optimal state of health. Because teeth are frequently malaligned and rotated, oral hygienic measures may be more difficult; these individuals may need more frequent prophylaxis and special oral hygienic instructions with careful reinforcement. Otherwise, rampant caries with premature loss may occur, which is a special tragedy in the cleft-afflicted individual, because he or she may have fewer teeth to serve vital functions such as retaining orthodontic, orthopedic, or speech appliances.

PROSTHETIC SPEECH-AID APPLIANCES

Prosthetic care for the cleft patient may be necessary for two reasons. First, teeth that are so frequently missing in the cleft-afflicted patient should be replaced. Second, in patients who have failed to obtain velopharyngeal competence with surgical corrections, a speech-aid appliance can be made by the dentist to decrease hypernasal speech. A speech-aid appliance is an acrylic bulb attached to a tooth-born appliance in the maxilla (Figure 27-19). The bulb is fitted to project onto the undersurface of the soft palate and lifts the soft palate superiorly. If this bulb does not give adequate function, another projection of acrylic (bulb obturator) can be placed to extend to the posterior aspect of the palate. This narrows the pharyngeal isthmus, and the size can be adjusted for maximal effectiveness. The posterior pharyngeal wall then will contact this bulb in function. In many instances the size of the bulb can be reduced as the pharyngeal musculature becomes more active. This type of appliance is used in two instances. It can be used before a pharyngeal flap procedure to develop muscle action or if the secondary surgical procedures are not successful in producing velopharyngeal competence. The speech aid appliance is also useful concomitantly to hold prosthetic dental replacements, to cover hard palate defects,

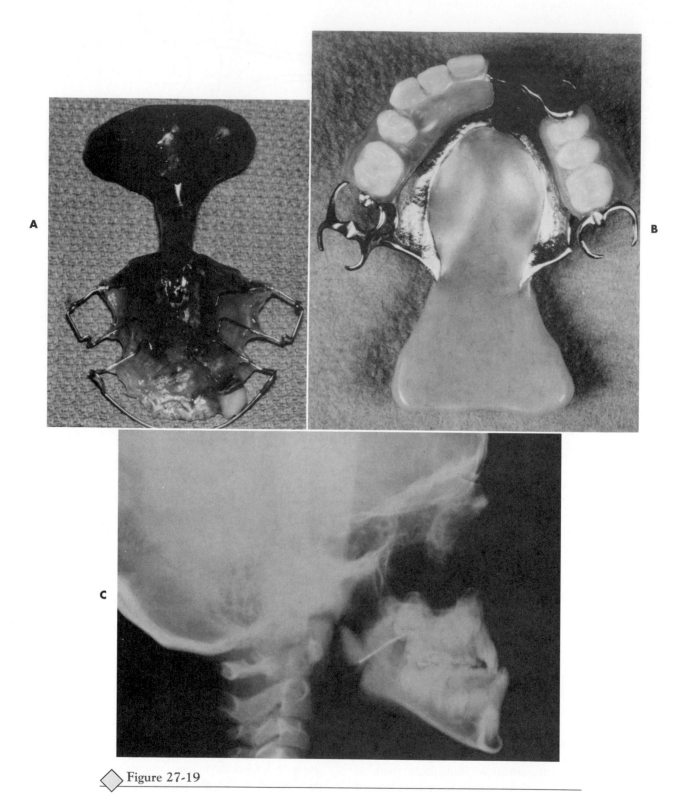

◇ Figure 27-19

Prosthetic speech-aid appliances. **A** and **B,** Appliances designed both to lift soft palate and to obturate oral and nasal cavities. **C,** Lateral cephalogram with appliance in place. Note acrylic bulb positioned between soft palate and posterior pharyngeal wall.

and to support deficient upper lips by a flange extending into the labial sulcus. Obviously, the maintenance of the residual dentition in an optimal state is prerequisite for successful speech-aid appliance therapy.

REFERENCES

1. Fogh-Anderson P: Incidence and aetiology. In Edwards M, Watson ACH, editors: *Advances in the management of cleft palate,* New York, 1980, Churchill Livingstone.

2. Hayward JR: Cleft lip and palate. In Hayward JR, editor: *Oral surgery,* Springfield, Ill, 1976, Charles C Thomas.

3. Langman J: *Medical embryology,* ed 3, Baltimore, 1975, Williams & Wilkins.

4. Ranta R: A review of tooth formation in children with cleft lip/palate, *Am J Orthod* 90:11, 1986.

5. Stark RB: The pathogenesis of harelip and cleft palate, *Plast Reconstr Surg* 13:20, 1954.

6. Stark RB, Ehrmann NA: The development of the center of the face with particular reference to surgical correction of bilateral cleft lip, *Plast Reconstr Surg* 21:177, 1958.

SURGICAL RECONSTRUCTION OF DEFECTS OF THE JAWS

EDWARD ELLIS III

CHAPTER OUTLINE

Defects of the facial bones, especially the jaws, have a variety of causes, such as eradication of pathologic conditions, trauma, infections, and congenital deformities. The size of the defects that are commonly reconstructed in the oral and maxillofacial region varies considerably from small alveolar clefts to mandibulectomy defects. Each defect poses a unique set of problems that reconstructive surgical intervention must address. In each of these instances, restoration of normal structure is usually possible, with resultant improvement in function and appearance.

When an osseous structure is defective either in size, shape, position, or amount, reconstructive surgery can be undertaken to replace the defective structure. The tissue most commonly used to replace lost osseous tissue is bone. Bone grafting has been attempted for centuries with varying degrees of success. Recent advancements in the understanding of bone physiology, immunologic concepts, tissue banking procedures, and surgical principles have made possible the successful reconstruction of most maxillofacial bony defects. As such, the biology and principles of transplantation of bone are presented in this chapter.

BIOLOGIC BASIS OF BONE RECONSTRUCTION

A tissue that is transplanted and expected to become a part of the host to which it is transplanted is known as a *graft*. There are several types of grafts available to the surgeon, which are discussed later. A basic understanding of how a bone heals when grafted from one place to another *in the same individual* (autotransplantation) is necessary to understand the benefits of the various types of bone grafts available.

The healing of bone and bone grafts is unique among connective tissues, because new bone formation arises from tissue regeneration rather than from simple tissue repair with scar formation.[6] This healing therefore requires both the element of cellular proliferation (that is, osteoblasts) and the element of collagen synthesis. When bone is transplanted from one area of the body to another, there are several processes that become active during the incorporation of the graft.

TWO-PHASE THEORY OF OSTEOGENESIS

There are two basic processes that occur on transplanting bone from one area to another in the same individual.[1-4,6] The first process that leads to bone regeneration arises initially from transplanted cells in the graft that proliferate and form new osteoid. The amount of bone regeneration during this phase depends on the amount of transplanted bone cells that survive the grafting procedure. Obviously, when the graft is first removed from the body, the blood supply has been severed. Thus the cells in the bone graft depend on diffusion of nutrients from the surrounding graft bed (the area where the graft is placed) for survival. A considerable amount of cell death occurs during the grafting procedure, and this first phase of bone regeneration may not lead to an impressive amount of bone regeneration when considered by itself. Still, this phase is responsible for the formation of most of the new bone. The more viable cells that can be successfully transplanted with the graft, the more bone that will form.

The graft bed also undergoes changes that lead to a second phase of bone regeneration beginning in the second week. Intense angiogenesis and fibroblastic proliferation from the graft bed begin on grafting, and osteogenesis from host connective tissues soon begins. Fibroblasts and other mesenchymal cells differentiate into osteoblasts and begin to lay down new bone. There is evidence that a protein or proteins found in the bone induces these reactions in the surrounding soft tissues of the graft bed.[7,8] This second phase is also responsible for the orderly incorporation of the graft into the host bed with continued resorption, replacement, and remodeling.

IMMUNE RESPONSE

When a tissue is transplanted from one site to another in the same individual, immunologic complications usually do not occur. The immune system is not triggered, because the tissue is recognized as "self." However, when a tissue is transplanted from one individual to another or from one species to another, the immune system may present a formidable obstacle to the success of the grafting procedure. If the graft is recognized as a foreign substance by the host, it will mount an intense response in an attempt to destroy the graft. The type of response the immune system mounts against "foreign" grafts is primarily a cell-mediated response by T lymphocytes. It may not occur immediately, however, and in the early period the incorporation of a bone graft into the host may appear to be progressing normally. The length of this latent period depends on the similarity between the host and the recipient. The more similar they are (antigenically), the longer an immunologic reaction may take to appear. This type of immunologic reaction is the most common reason for rejection of hearts, kidneys, and other organs transplanted to another individual. Tissue typing procedures, in which a donor and recipient are genetically compared for similarities before transplantation, are currently commonplace for organ transplantation but never for bone grafts.

Because of the immunologic rejection of transplants between individuals or between species, methods have been devised to improve the success of grafting procedures in these instances. Two basic approaches are used clinically. The first is the suppression of the host individual's immune response. Immunosuppression with various medications is most commonly used in organ transplant patients. This approach is not used routinely in oral and maxillofacial surgical bone grafting procedures because of the nature of the potential complications from immunosuppression.

Another approach that has been used extensively in oral and maxillofacial surgical procedures is the alteration of the antigenicity of the graft, so that the host's immune response will not be stimulated. Several methods of treating grafts have been used, including boiling, deproteinizing, merthiolating, freezing, freeze-drying, irradiating, and dry-heating. All of these methods, potentially helpful for use in bone grafts, are obviously not helpful in organ transplants.

TYPES OF GRAFTS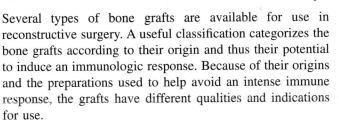

Several types of bone grafts are available for use in reconstructive surgery. A useful classification categorizes the bone grafts according to their origin and thus their potential to induce an immunologic response. Because of their origins and the preparations used to help avoid an intense immune response, the grafts have different qualities and indications for use.

AUTOGENOUS GRAFTS

Also known as *autografts* or *self-grafts*, autogenous grafts are composed of tissues from the same individual. Fresh autogenous bone is the most ideal bone graft material. It is unique among bone grafts in that it is the only type of bone graft to supply living, immunocompatible bone cells essential to phase I osteogenesis. The more living cells that are transplanted, the more osseous tissue that will be produced.

Autogenous bone is the type used most frequently in oral and maxillofacial surgery. It can be obtained from a host of sites in the body and can be taken in several forms. Block grafts are solid pieces of both cortical bone and underlying cancellous bone (Figure 28-1). The iliac crest is often used as a source for this type of graft. The entire thickness of the ilium can be obtained, or the ilium can be split to obtain a thinner piece of block graft. Ribs also constitute a form of block graft. Particulate marrow-cancellous bone grafts are obtained by harvesting the medullary bone and the associated endosteum and hematopoietic marrow. Particulate marrow-cancellous bone grafts produce the greatest concentration of osteogenic cells, and, because of the particulate nature, more cells survive transplantation because of the access they have to nutrients in the surrounding graft bed. The most common site for the procurement of this type of graft is the ilium. The iliac crest can be entered, and large volumes of particulate marrow-cancellous bone grafts can be obtained with large curettes. The diploic space of the cranial vault has recently been used as a site for obtaining this type of graft when small amounts of bone chips are needed (for example, alveolar cleft grafts).

Autogenous bone may also be transplanted while maintaining the blood supply to the graft. There are two methods by which this can be accomplished. The first involves the transfer of a bone graft pedicled to a muscular (or muscular and skin) pedicle. The bone is not stripped of its soft tissue pedicle, preserving some blood supply to the bone graft. Thus the amount of surviving osteogenic cells is potentially great.

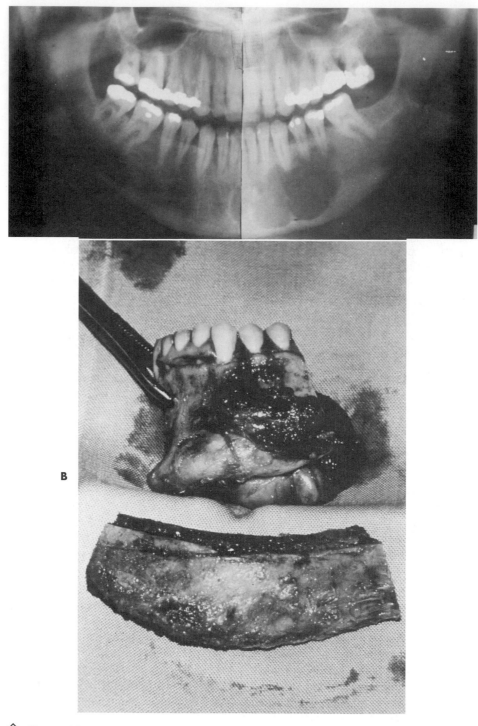

◇ Figure 28-1

Photographs illustrating use of autogenous block corticocancellous bone graft to replace defect in mandibular symphysis. Graft was placed immediately (at time of tumor removal) by transoral route. **A,** Preoperative radiograph of benign aggressive mandibular tumor. **B,** Sizing of graft with resected specimen used as guide.

Continued

An example of this type of autogenous graft is a segment of the clavicle transferred to the mandible, pedicled to the sternocleidomastoid muscle. The second method by which autogenous bone can be transplanted without losing blood supply is by the use of microsurgical techniques. A block of ilium, tibia, rib, or other suitable bone is removed along with the overlying soft tissues after dissecting free an artery and a vein that supply the tissue. An artery and a vein are also prepared in the recipient bed. Once the bone graft is secured in place, the artery and veins are reconnected using

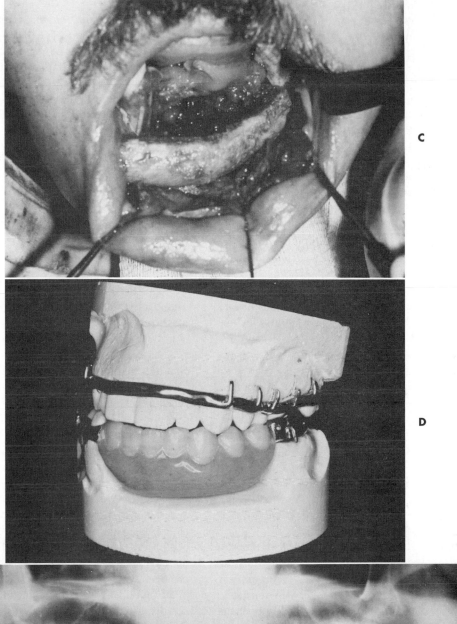

C

D

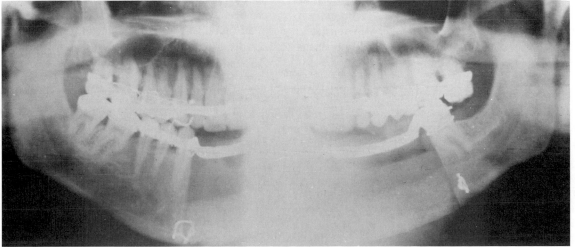

E

◇ Figure 28-1, cont'd

C, Bone graft has been inserted into defect and wired to residual mandibular skeleton bilaterally.
D, Prefabricated maxillary arch bar and mandibular splint, manufactured to place at time of surgery.
Mandibular splint served to maintain mandibular rami in their preoperative positions while healing
of graft took place. **E,** Postoperative radiograph showing result. Patient underwent 8 weeks of
intermaxillary fixation. Future procedures to increase height of alveolus were planned.

microvascular anastomoses. In this way the blood supply to the bone graft is maintained.

Both of these types of autogenous grafts are known as *composite grafts,* because they contain both soft tissue and osseous elements. The first type described, in which the bone maintains a muscular origin, is a pedicled composite graft. The pedicle is the soft tissue remaining on it, which supplies the vasculature. The second type of composite graft is a free composite graft, meaning that it is totally removed from the body and immediately replaced, and its blood supply is restored by reconnection of blood vessels. Although these types of grafts may seem ideal, they have serious shortcomings when used to restore defects of the jaws. Because the soft tissues attached to the bone graft maintain the blood supply, there can be minimal stripping of the soft tissue from the graft during procurement and placement. Thus the size and shape of the graft cannot be altered to any significant degree. Frequently, inadequate bulk of bone is provided when these grafts are used to restore mandibular continuity defects. Another problem is the morbidity to the donor site. Instead of just removing osseous tissue, soft tissues are also removed with composite grafts, which causes greater functional and cosmetic defects. Because of these problems and because of the success obtained without the use of composite grafts, the composite graft has not been used extensively in oral and maxillofacial surgery.

Advantages.   The advantages of autogenous bone are that it provides osteogenic cells for phase I bone formation, and no immunologic response occurs.

Disadvantages.   A disadvantage is that this procedure necessitates another site of operation for procurement of graft.

ALLOGENEIC GRAFTS

Also known as *allografts* or *homografts,* allogeneic grafts are grafts taken from another individual of the same species. Because the individuals are usually genetically dissimilar, treating the graft to reduce the antigenicity is routinely accomplished. Today the most commonly used allogeneic bone is freeze-dried. All of these treatments destroy any remaining osteogenic cells in the graft, and therefore allogeneic bone grafts cannot participate in phase I osteogenesis. The assistance of these grafts to osteogenesis is purely passive; they offer a hard tissue matrix for phase II induction. Thus the host must produce all of the essential elements in the graft bed for the allogeneic bone graft to become resorbed and replaced. Obviously, the health of the graft bed is much more important in this set of circumstances than it is if autogenous bone were to be used.

Advantages.   Advantages are that allogeneic grafts do not require another site of operation in the host and that a similar bone or a bone of similar shape to that being replaced can be obtained (for example, an allogeneic mandible can be used for reconstruction of a mandibulectomy defect).

Disadvantages.   The disadvantage is that an allogeneic graft does not provide viable cells for phase I osteogenesis.

XENOGENEIC GRAFTS

Also known as *xenografts* or *heterografts,* xenogeneic grafts are taken from one species and grafted to another. The antigenic dissimilarity of these grafts are greater than with allogeneic bone. The organic matrix of xenogenic bone is antigenically dissimilar to that of human bone, and therefore the graft must be treated more vigorously to prevent rapid rejection of the graft. Bone grafts of this variety are rarely used in oral and maxillofacial surgery.

Advantages.   Advantages are that xenografts do not require another site of operation in the host, and a large quantity of bone can be obtained.

Disadvantages.   Disadvantages are that xenografts do not provide viable cells for phase I osteogenesis and must be rigorously treated to reduce antigenicity.

COMBINATIONS OF GRAFTS

The ideal graft would have the structural characteristics of a block graft with the osteogenic potential of particulate marrow-cancellous bone grafts. However, a large block graft necessitates removal of a large portion of the patient's anatomy and does not provide the high concentration of osteogenic cells the particulate marrow-cancellous graft does. A technique that is commonly employed to reconstruct defects of the mandible uses the advantages of both autogenous and allogeneic bone grafts (Figure 28-2). An allogeneic block graft is obtained in the form of an ilium or mandible. This graft is used for its structural strength and protein, which induces phase II bone formation from the surrounding tissues. This graft is hollowed out until only the cortical plates remain. Autogenous particulate marrow-cancellous bone is then obtained and packed into the shell to provide the osteogenic cells necessary for phase I bone formation. In this way the ingredients necessary for both phases of osteogenesis are provided without necessitating the removal of a large portion of the individual's anatomy. The allogeneic portion of the graft acts as a biodegradable tray, which in time is completely replaced by host bone.

Advantages.   Advantages of this procedure are the same as those for both autogenous and allogeneic grafts.

Disadvantages.   The disadvantage is that this procedure necessitates a second site of operation in the host to obtain autogenous particulate marrow-cancellous graft.

ASSESSMENT OF PATIENT IN NEED OF RECONSTRUCTION ⟶◇

Patients who have defects of the jaws can usually be surgically treated to replace the lost portion. Each patient, however, must be thoroughly evaluated individually, because no two patients have the exact same problems. Analysis of the patient's

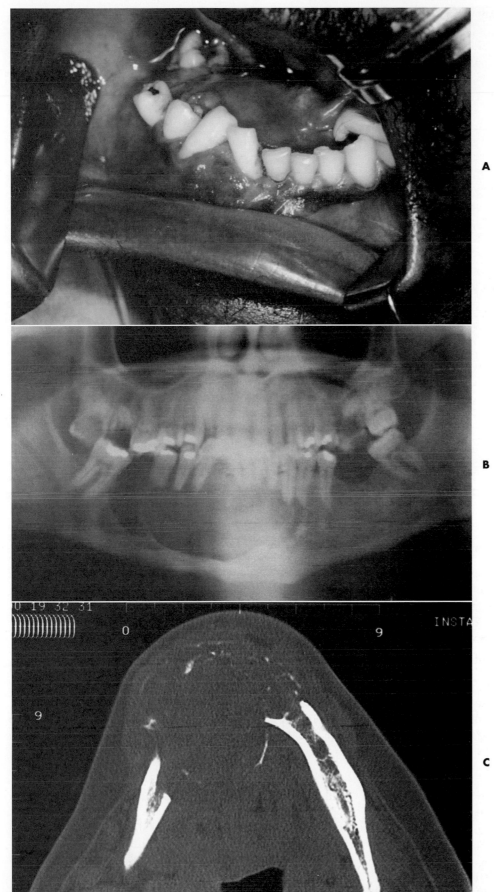

A

B

C

Figure 28-2

Photographs showing use of combination of allogeneic and autogenous bone grafts to reconstruct mandible after resection for ameloblastoma. **A,** Photograph of large expansile lesion of mandibular body and symphysis.
B, Panoramic radiograph of lesion.
C, Axial computed tomogram showing size of lesion. *Continued*

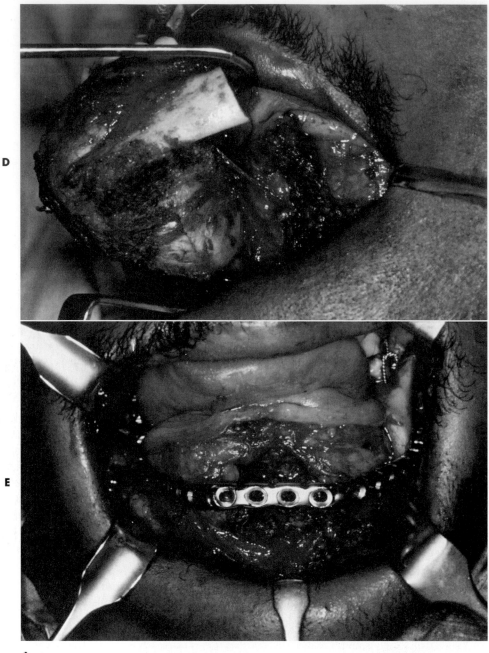

◇ Figure 28-2, cont'd

D, Resection of lesion via a transoral approach. **E,** Placement of large metal bone plate to reconstruct mandible after tumor resection. The plate is attached to both rami and provides support to the overlying soft tissues to prevent their contraction during the healing process. The tongue musculature is sutured to the bone plate to maintain its forward position, ensuring patency of the airway.

Continued

problem must take into consideration the hard tissue defect, any soft tissue defects, and any associated problems that will affect treatment.

HARD TISSUE DEFECT

Several factors concerning the actual osseous defect must be thoroughly assessed to help formulate a viable treatment plan. Adequate radiographs are necessary to evaluate the full extent of the osseous defect. The site of the defect may be just as important as the size of the defect when dealing with mandibular osseous problems. For example, if the mandibular condyle is missing, treatment is relatively more difficult. A residual portion of the ramus with the condyle still attached makes osseous reconstruction easier, because the temporomandibular articulation is difficult to restore.

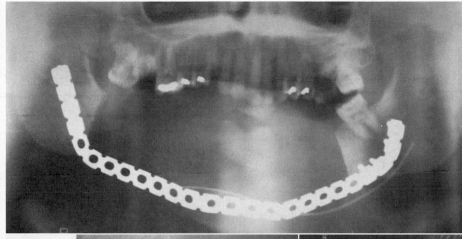

F

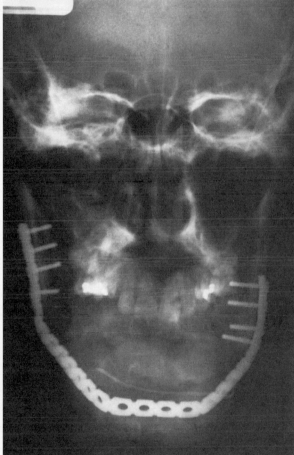

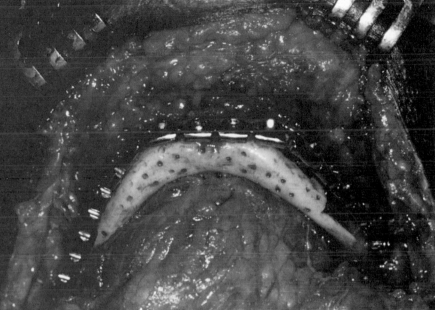

H

◇ **Figure 28-2, cont'd**

F, Panoramic and **G,** frontal radiographs showing bone plate in position. **H,** After healing of the intraoral soft tissues, an extraoral approach is used for bone graft reconstruction. An allogeneic mandible is hollowed out and secured to the bone plate with bone screws. Note the perforations of the mandible to promote revascularization.

Continued

The mandible has powerful muscles attached to it that usually direct functional movements. When the continuity of the mandible is broken, these muscles no longer work in harmony and may severely displace mandibular fragments into unnatural positions. Therefore the position of the residual mandibular fragments must be ascertained. For example, if a portion of the mandible in the area of the molars is missing, the muscles of mastication still attached to the mandibular ramus may rotate the ramus superiorly and medially, which may allow penetration into the oral cavity and compound the difficulty of planned treatment.

SOFT TISSUE DEFECT

Proper preparation of the soft tissue bed that is to receive the bone graft is just as important to the success of bone grafting as the bone graft material itself. The transplanted bone cells must survive initially by diffusion of nutrients from the surrounding soft tissues. Revascularization of the bone graft through the development of new blood vessels from the soft tissue bed must then occur. Thus an essential factor for the success of any bone-grafting procedure is the availability of an adequately vascularized soft tissue bed. Fortunately, this essential factor is usually obtainable in the lush vascular tissue

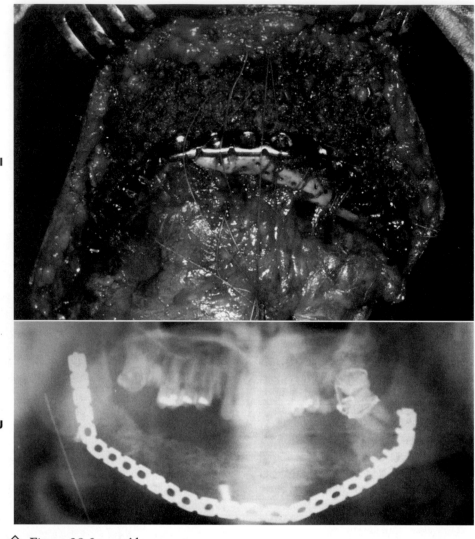

◇ Figure 28-2, cont'd

I, Particulate marrow-cancellous bone is packed within the allogenic mandible before closure.
J, Panoramic radiograph showing bone graft in place. The bone plate is left in situ.

of the head and neck region. There are, however, several instances when the soft tissue bed is not as desirable as it could be, such as after radiotherapy or excessive scarring from trauma or infection. Therefore a thorough assessment of the quantity and quality of the surrounding soft tissues is necessary before undertaking bone graft procedures.

The reason for the osseous void often provides important information on the amount and quality of soft tissues remaining. For example, if the patient lost a large portion of the mandible from a composite resection for a malignancy, the chances are that the patient will have deficiencies both in quantity and quality of soft tissues. During the initial surgery, many vital structures were probably removed, and denervation of the platysma will result in atrophy of the muscular fibers. An intraoral examination helps the clinician determine how much oral mucosa was removed with the mandibular fragment. Frequently, the tongue or floor of the mouth appears

to be sutured to the buccal mucosa, with no intervening alveolar ridge or buccal sulcus, because the gingiva is sacrificed with the osseous specimen.

If the patient received cancericidal doses of radiation to the area of the osseous defect, the clinician can assume that the patient's soft tissues have undergone extreme atrophy and scarring and will be nonpliable and fragile. The soft tissues in this instance will provide a poor bed for a bone graft, because the environment is hypovascular, hypoxic, and hypocellular.[6] Similarly, if the patient's defect was caused by a severe infection, it is likely that an excess of scar tissue formation occurred, which will result in nonpliable, poorly vascularized tissue.

After a thorough evaluation, a decision must be made about the adequacy of the soft tissues. If there is a deficient *quantity* of tissue, soft tissue flaps from the neck that contain muscle and skin can be used to enhance the amount of tissue available to close over the bone graft. If the soft tissues are deficient in *quality,* one of two basic methods can be used to reconstruct a patient's defects. The first is to supply an autogenous bone graft with its own blood supply in the form of a free or pedicled composite graft. However, as pointed out, this method has serious shortcomings. The second method is to improve the quality of the soft tissues already present by the use of hyperbaric oxygen (HBO). The HBO method improves tissue oxygenation by the administration of oxygen to the patient under higher-than-normal atmospheric pressures. Tissue oxygenation has been shown to improve to acceptable levels after 20 HBO treatments.[5] Following HBO treatment, bone-grafting procedures can be performed with good success. Another course of HBO treatment is then recommended after the bone-grafting procedure.[5]

ASSOCIATED PROBLEMS

The clinician must always remember that the cure should be less offensive to the patient than the disease process. In other words, if a reconstructive procedure will significantly risk the individual's life or is associated with a very high incidence of complications that may make life worse for the patient, it would probably be in the patient's best interest to forego the procedure. As with any type of therapy, significant factors must be assessed, such as the patient's age, health, psychologic state, and, most important perhaps, desires. Thorough understanding by the patient of the risks and benefits of any treatment recommendation is imperative so that an informed decision can be made.

GOALS AND PRINCIPLES OF MANDIBULAR RECONSTRUCTION ———◇

Marx and Sanders[6] have identified several major goals for mandibular reconstruction that should be strived for and achieved before any grafting procedure can be considered a success.

RESTORATION OF CONTINUITY

Because the mandible is a bone with two articulating ends acted on by muscles with opposing forces, restoration of continuity is the highest priority when reconstructing mandibular defects. Achieving this goal will provide the patient with better functional movements and improved facial esthetics by realigning any deviated mandibular segments.

RESTORATION OF ALVEOLAR BONE HEIGHT

The functional rehabilitation of the patient rests on the ability to masticate efficiently and comfortably. Prosthetic dental appliances are frequently necessary in patients who have lost a portion of their mandible. To facilitate prosthetic appliance usage, an adequate alveolar process must be provided during the reconstructive surgery. The ideal ridge form outlined in Chapter 13 for the edentulous patient applies equally to patients undergoing mandibular reconstructive surgery.

RESTORATION OF OSSEOUS BULK

Any bone-grafting procedure must provide enough osseous tissue to withstand normal function. If too thin an osseous strut is provided, fracture of the grafted area may occur.

SURGICAL PRINCIPLES OF MAXILLOFACIAL BONE-GRAFTING PROCEDURES ———◇

There are several important principles to be followed during any grafting procedure. They must be strictly adhered to if a successful outcome is desired. The following are a few that pertain to reconstructing mandibular defects.

1. *Control of residual mandibular segments.* When a continuity defect is present, the muscles of mastication attached to the residual mandibular fragments will distract them in different directions unless efforts were made to stabilize the remaining mandible in its normal position at the time of partial resection. Maintaining relationships of the remaining mandible fragments after resection of portions of the mandible is a key principle of mandibular reconstruction. This is important for both occlusal and temporomandibular joint positioning. When the residual fragments are left to drift, significant facial distortions can occur from deviation of the residual mandibular fragments (Figure 28-3). Metal bone plates inserted at the time of resection are useful for controlling the position of the mandibular fragments (Figure 28-2, *E*). They are of sufficient strength to obviate the need for maxillomandibular fixation, permitting active use of the mandible in the immediate postoperative period. In older individuals or those with significant medical compromise, this may be the final form of reconstruction. It provides soft tissue support to maintain facial symmetry. When the mandibular symphysis has been removed, the tongue can be sutured to the plate, maintaining its forward position to prevent airway obstruction (Figure 28-2, *E*). The bone plate can be left in place when the mandible is secondarily reconstructed with bone grafts, permitting mobility of the mandible during the bone graft's healing phase (Figure 28-2, *J*).

   When the position of the residual mandibular fragments have not been maintained during the resection, realignment is more difficult during the reconstructive surgery. Over time the muscles of mastication become atrophic, fibrotic, and nonpliable, which makes realignment of the fragments extremely difficult. During the reconstructive surgery, it may be necessary to strip several muscles off the mandibular fragments to release the bone from their adverse pull. A coronoidectomy is usually performed to remove the superior pull of the temporalis muscle. Before inserting a bone graft, the clinician must be sure to reach the desired position of the remaining mandibular frag-

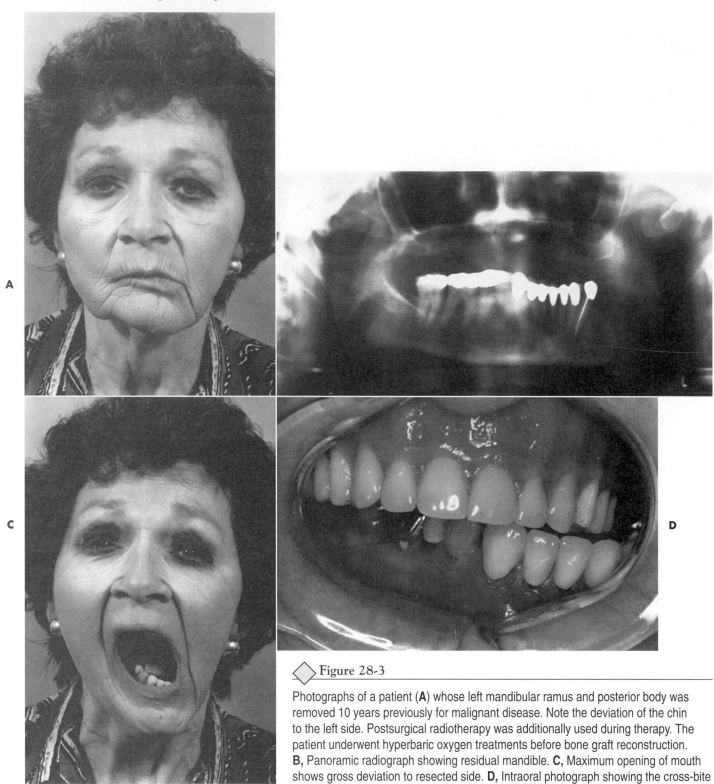

◇ Figure 28-3

Photographs of a patient (**A**) whose left mandibular ramus and posterior body was removed 10 years previously for malignant disease. Note the deviation of the chin to the left side. Postsurgical radiotherapy was additionally used during therapy. The patient underwent hyperbaric oxygen treatments before bone graft reconstruction. **B,** Panoramic radiograph showing residual mandible. **C,** Maximum opening of mouth shows gross deviation to resected side. **D,** Intraoral photograph showing the cross-bite relationship from the deviation of the mandible to the left side. *Continued*

ments, because what is achieved at surgery is what the patient must live with.

If the mandibular condyle has been resected or is unusable, reconstruction of the condyle with a costochondral junction of a rib or alloplastic condyle is necessary to maintain the forward position of the reconstructed mandible (Figure 28-3).

2. *Provide a good soft tissue bed for the bone graft.* All bone grafts must be covered on all sides by soft tissues to avoid contamination of the bone graft and to provide the vascularity necessary for revascularization of the graft. Areas of dense scar should be excised until healthy tissue is encountered. Incisions should be designed so that when the wound is closed, the incision will not be over the graft,

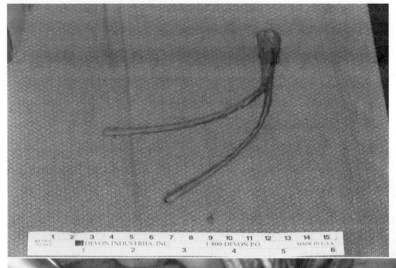

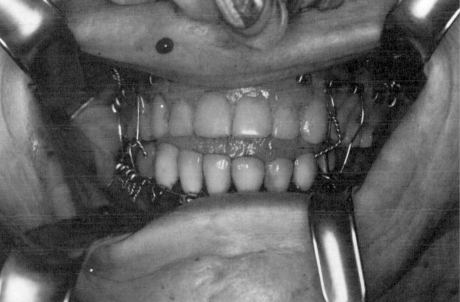

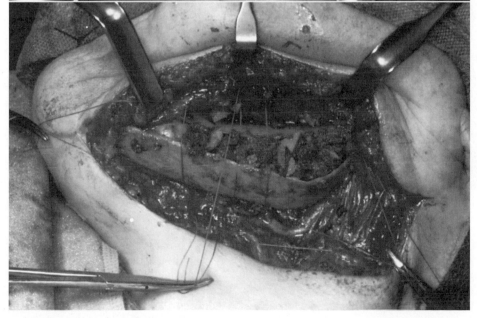

◇ **Figure 28-3, cont'd**

E, Splitting of the bony rib portion of a costochondral graft, leaving the cartilaginous tip to function as a mandibular condyle. **F,** During surgery, the maxillary denture is wired to the midface, and maxillomandibular fixation is used to hold the mandible into its proper position. **G,** Graft placed so that costochondral portion is in mandibular fossa and bony ends are secured to residual mandibular fragments. Iliac crest bone chips are then packed into the void between the two portions of the rib. *Continued*

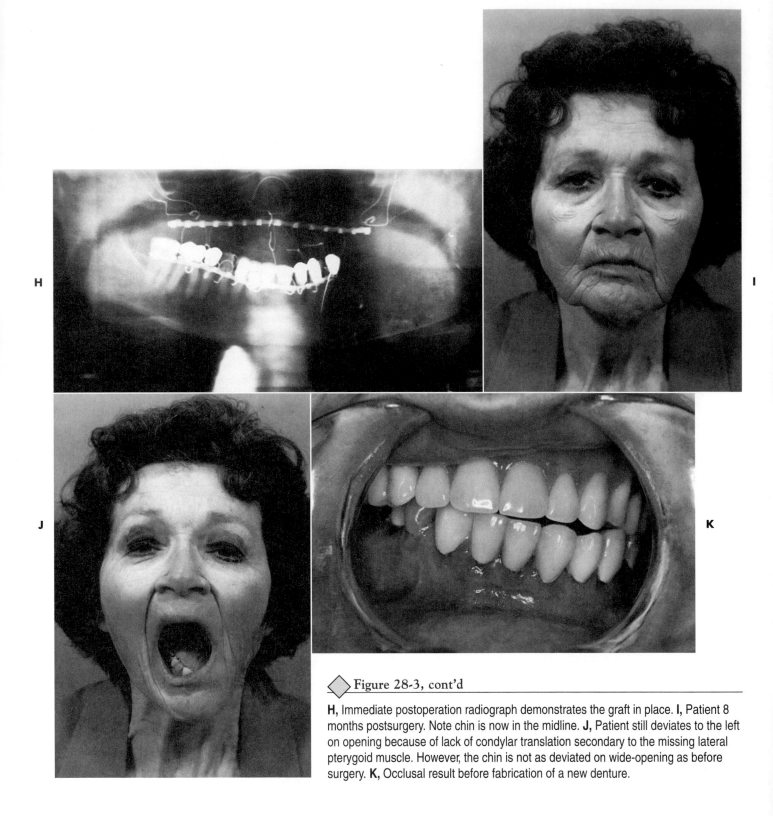

⬥ **Figure 28-3, cont'd**

H, Immediate postoperation radiograph demonstrates the graft in place. **I,** Patient 8 months postsurgery. Note chin is now in the midline. **J,** Patient still deviates to the left on opening because of lack of condylar translation secondary to the missing lateral pterygoid muscle. However, the chin is not as deviated on wide-opening as before surgery. **K,** Occlusal result before fabrication of a new denture.

which means that the initial incision may be very low in the neck (Figure 28-3, *G*). A multilayered soft tissue closure is performed to reduce any space that might allow collection of blood or serum and to provide a watertight closure.

3. *Immobilization of the graft.* Immobilization of bone is necessary for osseous healing to progress, which is why orthopedic surgeons apply a cast to a fractured extremity. In dealing with mandibular defects, the graft must be secured to remaining mandibular fragments, and these fragments must be rigidly immobilized to ensure that no movement exists between them. This immobilization is most often provided by the use of intermaxillary fixation,

in which the mandible is secured to the maxilla (Figure 28-3). However, several other methods are possible, such as using a bone plate between the residual bone fragments (Figure 28-2). Immobilization for 8 to 12 weeks is usually necessary for adequate healing between the graft and the residual mandibular fragments.

4. *Provide an aseptic environment.* Even when transplanting autogenous osseous tissue, the bone graft is basically avascular, which means that the graft has no way of fighting any amount of infection. Therefore a certain percentage of bone grafts become infected and must be removed. Several measures can be taken to improve the success of bone-grafting procedures. The first is to use an extraoral incision where possible. The skin is much easier to cleanse and disinfect than is the oral cavity. Bone grafts inserted through the mouth are exposed to the oral flora during the grafting procedure. Furthermore, the intraoral incision may dehisce and again expose the bone graft to the oral flora. Bone grafts placed through a skin incision are more successful than those inserted transorally. However, it is important that during the extraoral dissection the oral cavity is not inadvertently entered. Ideally, dissection to the level of the oral mucosa without perforation is preferred.

5. *Systemic antibiosis.* The use of prophylactic antibiotics may be indicated when transplanting osseous tissue. Their use may be beneficial in helping reduce the incidence of infection (see Chapter 16).

Because of the many muscles attaching to and providing mobility to the mandible, it is the facial bone most difficult to reconstruct. Other facial bones are reconstructed on similar principles.

REFERENCES

1. Axhausen W: The osteogenetic phases of regeneration of bone: a historical and experimental study, *J Bone Joint Surg* 38A:593, 1956.
2. Burwell RG: Studies in the transplantation of bone: the fresh composite homograft-autograft of cancellous bone, *J Bone Joint Surg* 46B:110, 1964.
3. Elves MW: Newer knowledge of immunology of bone and cartilage, *Clin Orthop* 120:232, 1976.
4. Gray JC, Elves M: Early osteogenesis in compact bone, *Tissue Int* 29:225, 1979.
5. Marx RE, Ames JR: The use of hyperbaric oxygen therapy in bony reconstruction of the irradiated and tissue-deficient patient, *J Oral Maxillofac Surg* 40:412, 1982.
6. Marx RE, Saunders TR: Reconstruction and rehabilitation of cancer patients. In Fonseca RJ, Davis WH, editors: *Reconstructive preprosthetic oral and maxillofacial surgery*. Philadelphia, 1986, WB Saunders.
7. Urist MR: Osteoinduction in undermineralized bone implants modified by chemical inhibitors of endogenous matrix enzymes, *Clin Orthop* 78:132, 1972.
8. Urist MR: The substratum for bone morphogenesis, *Dev Biol* 4(suppl):125, 1970.

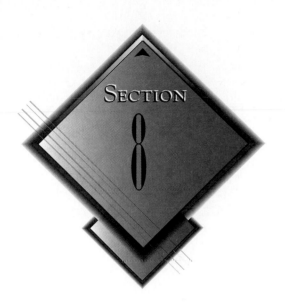

TEMPOROMANDIBULAR DISORDERS AND FACIAL PAIN

The dentist is commonly perceived as the health care provider with the most expertise in facial neuropathy, whether it is facial pain or altered nerve function, and disorders of the temporomandibular joints. Dentists receive extensive professional education in facial and temporomandibular joint anatomy, physiology, and pathologic conditions. Painful disorders of the maxillofacial region, whether neurologic or musculoskeletal in origin, are common reasons for obtaining a dental opinion. Therefore it is important for dentists to become knowledgeable about facial neuropathology and temporomandibular joint disorders.

Chapter 29 presents an overview of facial neuropathology. The neurophysiology of pain, differential diagnosis of facial pain disorders, and methods of managing various neurogenic facial pain problems are discussed. Then the evaluation and management of altered sensory nerve function are considered, including the rapidly advancing area of microneurosurgery.

Temporomandibular joint physiology and pathology is a broad topic, and entire, comprehensive books exist on this topic. Chapter 30 is a concise, up-to-date discussion of the ever-changing field of temporomandibular joint disorders from the viewpoint of oral and maxillofacial surgeons. The chapter is designed to provide the reader with knowledge of the evaluation and management of patients with functional disorders of the temporomandibular joint, including internal derangements, ankylosis, and immunogenic arthritides.

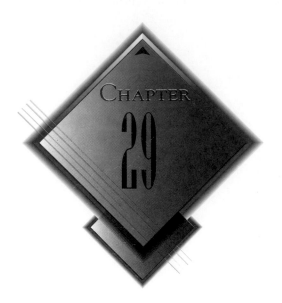

CHAPTER

29

FACIAL NEUROPATHOLOGY

JAMES R. HUPP

CHAPTER OUTLINE

Orofacial pain is a common reason for patients to consult a dentist. In many instances the dentist finds an odontogenic source of the patient's discomfort and successfully manages the disease process through dental therapy. However, nonodontogenic neurologic disorders are also frequent causes of orofacial pain. Therefore the ability to recognize and properly manage nonodontogenic sources of head and neck pain and nerve dysfunction are important skills for the dental practitioner.

This chapter discusses diagnosis and management of painful maxillofacial neurologic conditions caused by primary nerve dysfunction or vascular lesions. The evaluation and management of nerve dysfunction caused by nerve injuries are also discussed.

PAIN PHYSIOLOGY

Pain is a subjectively unpleasant sensory and emotional experience that is usually associated with tissue injury. Painful stimuli are thought to trigger nociceptors (1- to 5-mm diameter nerve fibers that are specifically stimulated to fire when exposed to noxious stimuli). Nociceptors are unmyelinated or thinly myelinated fibers of the relatively slowly conducting A-delta and C types (Table 29-1). According to the gate control theory, these fibers are believed to be capable of being inhibited by large A-alpha and beta nerves, which transmit

modulation from higher centers in the brain (Figure 29-1). The inhibitory fibers provide the means by which psychologic factors, such as emotion, personality, learned behavior, and psychopathology, can alter pain perception and a person's reaction to perceived pain.

EVALUATION OF FACIAL PAIN

The evaluation of the patient with facial pain, headache, or other sensory disturbance begins like any other diagnostic workup, with the dentist obtaining a concise chief complaint and history of the present problem. For pain problems this usually consists of learning the onset, course, intensity, and location of the pain, as well as other characteristics of the pain, such as whether it is continuous or intermittent, whether it occurs in relation to any other event (such as eating), what factors can precipitate or relieve it, and what other symptoms seem to be associated with it (for example, motor nerve dysfunction, nausea, or visual disturbances). A complete medical and dental history should be obtained with particular emphasis on systemic disorders, medications, psychologic problems, infections, and trauma history (Box 29-1).

 Table 29-1. Relationship between sensory nerve fiber size (diameter) and conduction velocity

Fiber type	Size (μ diameter)	Velocity (m/sec)
A-alpha	13-22	70-120
A-beta	8-13	40-70
A-gamma	4-8	15-40
A-delta	1-4	5-15
B	1-3	3-14
C	0.5-1	0.5-2

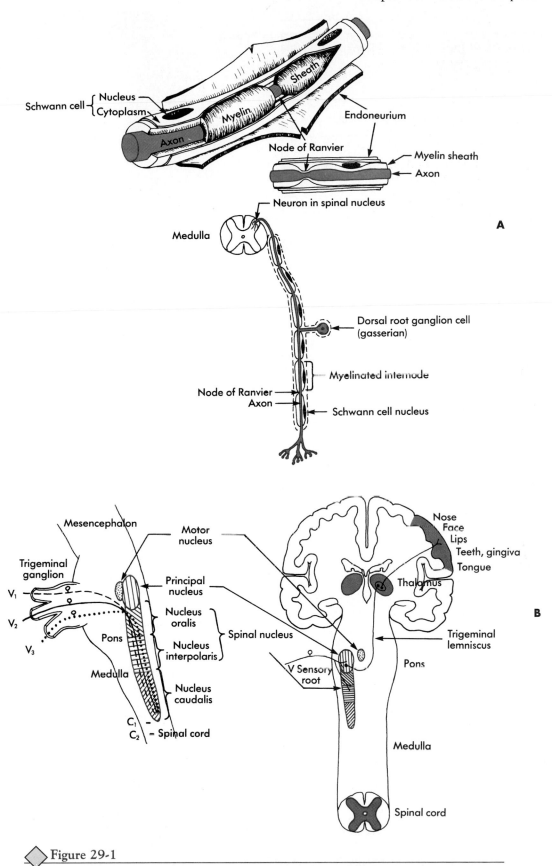

◇ Figure 29-1

A, Normal myelinated facial sensory nerve anatomy. **B,** Trigeminal nerve tracts and projections in central nervous system. *(Modified from Mumford JM:* Orofacial pain: aetiology, diagnosis, and treatment, *ed 3, Edinburgh, 1982, Churchill Livingstone.)*

◇ Box 29-1 ◇

Evaluation of maxillofacial pain or sensory dysfunction

I. History
   A. Chief complaint, describing pain
      1. Location (where it begins, size of affected area, referral pattern)
      2. Intensity
      3. Nature (for example, stabbing, burning, dull, throbbing)
      4. Duration (when pain is present)
      5. Influences (time of day, jaw motion, body position, cold, medications)
   B. History of pain problem
      1. Onset
      2. Suspected initiating factor(s)
      3. Symptom course (worsening, periods of remission, changes in quality)
      4. Previous therapy
   C. Medical history, with particular attention paid to:
      1. Systemic diseases (for example, diabetes, anemia, atherosclerosis)
      2. Medications
      3. Neurologic problems (including any chronic pain problems)
      4. Psychiatric problems
      5. Connective tissue or autoimmune diseases
      6. Maxillofacial inflammatory processes (for example, otitis, sinusitis)
      7. Maxillofacial trauma and/or surgery
   D. Review of systems with particular attention paid to:
      1. Constitutional symptoms (for example, fever, weight loss, fatigue)
      2. Head, ear, eye, nose, mouth, throat, neck
      3. Musculoskeletal system
      4. Skin
      5. Nervous system
      6. Psychiatric
II. Physical examination with particular attention paid to:
   A. General appearance
   B. Maxillofacial region (head, ear, eye, nose, mouth, throat, neck)
   C. Nervous system (cranial nerves, sympathetic and parasympathetic nerves, mental status)

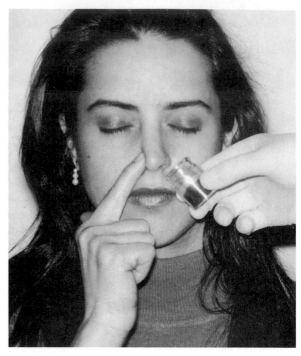

◇ Figure 29-2

Patient closes contralateral nostril and gently inhales. Clinician holds vial containing nonpungent but aromatic, easily recognizable substance, such as coffee, close to nostril. Failure to identify odor from only one side may indicate anterior nasal obstruction. Failure to identify odor from both sides may indicate problem involving olfactory nerve (cranial nerve I).

evaluation of cranial nerve function should be performed (Box 29-2). If an especially localized painful point is identified, its exact location should be precisely identified.

Finally, diagnostic nerve blocks can sometimes be used to help pinpoint the precise nerve involved in cases of neuritis or neuralgias (Figure 29-9). Although not commonly performed by dentists, electromyography and nerve conduction studies can be performed if the presence of a diseased motor nerve is suspected.

Many clinicians who manage facial pain problems routinely obtain testing by clinical psychologists, because of the common finding of mental disorders in patients with facial pain complaints. Occasionally, a chronic pain problem precipitates a psychopathologic condition. However, more often, mental disorders seem to predispose patients to pain problems.

Radiographic imaging is of limited value in the identification of facial neuropathology causing pain, except for excluding nonneurogenic pain problems.

The patient with decreased sensation in a portion of the maxillofacial region should have an evaluation similar to that of a patient complaining of pain. However, particular attention should be paid to sensory testing. The dentist should use a sharp, sterile needle to test sensory nerves grossly. If a problem is found, the patient can then be referred to an oral and maxillofacial surgeon for fine testing. This fine testing

Physical examination of the patient with facial pain that has no readily apparent etiology consists of a careful oral and maxillofacial examination, including a detailed neurologic examination of the head and neck region (Figures 29-2 through 29-8). This neurologic examination includes a gross assessment of level of consciousness and peripheral noncranial nerve function. In addition, a comprehensive

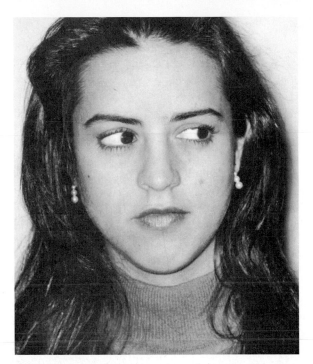

◇ **Figure 29-3**

Patient looks directly to one side and then to the other. Inability to move an eye toward nose (adduction) may indicate problem with oculomotor nerve (cranial nerve III). Inability to move an eye laterally (abduction) may indicate problem with abducent nerve (cranial nerve VI). Patient should also be asked to look at each of their shoulders. Inability to move an eye down and laterally may indicate a problem with the trochlear nerve (cranial nerve IV).

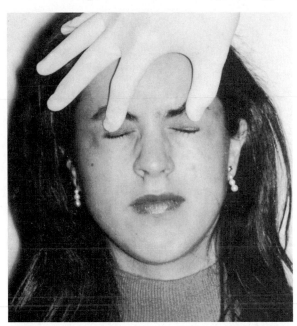

◇ **Figure 29-5**

Patient tries to keep eyes tightly closed. Clinician attempts to open upper eyelids. Ability of clinician to open eyelid may indicate problem with facial nerve (cranial nerve VII). Other branches of the facial nerve are tested by having patient try to raise eyebrows, pucker lips, and evert lower lip.

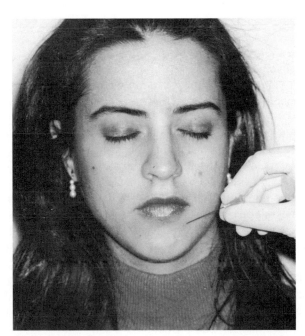

◇ **Figure 29-4**

Patient closes eyes, and clinician uses sterile needle to test patient's ability to discriminate sharp from dull stimuli. Needle tip used for sharp stimuli, and hub used for dull stimuli. Test areas in all three sensory divisions of trigeminal nerve. Inability to distinguish sharp from dull or a decreased sensibility to sharp stimuli may indicate a problem with the trigeminal nerve (cranial nerve V).

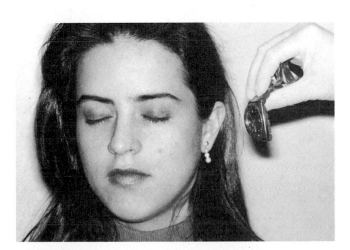

◇ **Figure 29-6**

Patient closes eyes and clinician slowly brings soft sound close to ear being tested. Distance from where patient first hears sound is recorded. Clinician can use himself or herself or other patients with normal hearing as standard for comparison. An ear for which sound must be brought closer than the standard may have problem with the acoustic nerve (cranial nerve VIII).

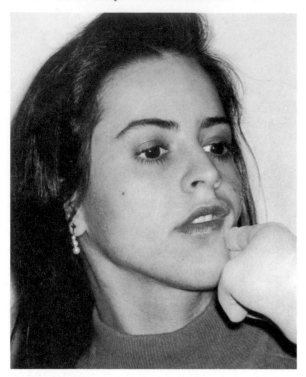

Patient attempts to move clinician's fingers, which are pushing patient's chin laterally. Weakness or inability to push fingers toward a shoulder may indicate problem with accessory nerve (cranial nerve XI).

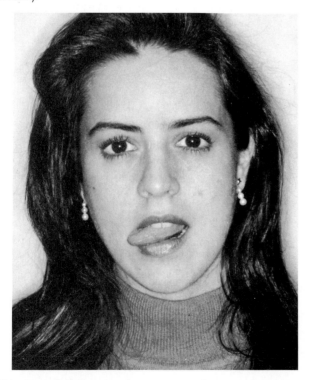

◇ **Figure 29-8**

Patient attempts to stick tongue straight out of mouth. Deviation of tongue to either side (simulated in this photograph) may indicate problem with hypoglossal nerve (cranial nerve XII) on side to which tongue deviates.

may include testing pain sensation with a sharp stimulus, temperature sensation with metal disks, light touch sensation with small filament hairs, and two-point discrimination with a double-pointed compass. Serial testing is then performed to document signs of nerve recovery.

Radiographs are of value for the patient with decreased facial sensation to help discern if a lesion is causing altered nerve function. If a lesion is suspected in the mandible or anterior maxilla, dental radiographs are useful. However, if a more proximal problem is thought to be present, more specialized imaging techniques, such as tomography, xerography, computerized tomographic or magnetic resonance scanning, may be indicated.

Several classification systems of facial sensory nerve disorders have been designed. Especially useful for making therapeutic decisions is categorizing facial sensory nerve problems as either traumatic or nontraumatic in origin. This classification will be used in this chapter when describing the most common facial sensory nerve disorders. A comprehensive discussion is beyond the scope of this chapter; detailed texts on facial neuropathology are provided in the reference list.

CLASSIFICATION ───◇
FACIAL NEUROPATHOLOGY OF NONTRAUMATIC ORIGIN

FACIAL NEURALGIAS

A neuralgia is a paroxysmal, intermittent intense pain usually confined to specific nerve branches and occurring most commonly in the maxillofacial region. Although not definitively proved, the cause may be the loss of a portion of the myelination that normally insulates sensory axons from each other. Lesions may be present anywhere from the peripheral nerve branches to the ganglion or posterior nerve roots.

A neuralgia should not be confused with a neuritis, which is an acute, usually reversible inflammation of a nerve that causes pain as a result of peripheral, nonneural pathologic conditions, such as pulpitis, sinusitis, or sialoadenitis. A neuritis can usually be cured by properly managing the nonneural pathologic condition. Therapy of a neuralgia, on the other hand, usually involves measures aimed directly at neural tissue.

TRIGEMINAL NEURALGIA. The best-known form of facial neuralgia is that of the sensory divisions of the fifth cranial nerve, called *trigeminal neuralgia,* or *tic douloureux.* This condition is characterized by extreme pain that is (1) described as "stabbing," "burning," or "shocking" lasting from several seconds to minutes; (2) able to be provoked by tactile or thermal stimulation over a trigger zone; (3) anatomically confined to the distribution of one or more divisions of the trigeminal nerve unilaterally; and (4) without objective motor or sensory nerve deficits in the affected area.

Trigeminal neuralgia is slightly more common in women, has its highest incidence in the sixth decade, and has a

◇ Box 29-2 ◇

Rapid cranial nerve (CN) examination for the general dentist

The examination begins with patient seated in the dental chair. The clinician asks if patient has any severe problems with seeing, hearing, or dizziness and observes patient for signs of visual or auditory problems, including whether the eyes move consensually. The clinician also checks for eyelid ptosis and mouth symmetry when patient smiles.

Next, the patient tries to hold eyelids tightly closed while the clinician tries to open them with his or her fingers. While the patient's eyes are closed the clinician holds coffee or cloves to the patient's nose and asks patient to identify the odor. The patient then opens the eyes widely while raising the eyebrows. The clinician shines a bright light into each eye individually and observes the reaction of the pupil. The patient looks directly left and right, then tries to look at each shoulder without moving his or her head.

The clinician then asks the patient to show his or her teeth, then pucker, and then evert the lower lip. Next, the patient clenches the jaw closed while the clinician palpates each masseter muscle. The patient then opens his or her mouth and sticks the tongue straight out. While the tongue is out, the clinician uses a cotton-tipped applicator to stroke each side of the uvula briefly. With the clinician's hands on the lateral aspects of the patient's chin, the patient then tries to push laterally against the hands.

Finally, the clinician rubs his or her fingers in front of each of the patient's ears and asks what the patient hears.

Interpretation of test

Cranial nerve (CN)	Abnormal test result
I-Olfactory	Unable to identify odor may indicate either nasal obstruction or CN I problem.
II-Optic	Failure of pupil to constrict or presence of nonconsensual gaze may indicate CN II problem.
III-Oculomotor	Failure of pupil to constrict or presence of ptosis may indicate CN III problem.
IV-Trochlear	Inability of eye to look to ipsilateral shoulder may indicate CN IV problem.
V-Trigeminal	Inability to feel light touch may indicate sensory CN V problem. Weakness of masseter may indicate motor CN V problem.
VI-Abducent	Inability of eye to look to ipsilateral side may indicate CN VI problem.
VII-Facial	Inability to raise eyebrows, hold eyelids closed, symmetrically smile, pucker, and evert lower lip may indicate CN VII problem.
VIII-Acoustic	Poor hearing or symptoms of vertigo may indicate CN VIII problem.
IX-Glossopharyngeal	Failure of uvula to elevate on stroked side may indicate CN IX problem.
X-Vagus	Failure of uvula to elevate on stroked side may indicate CN X problem.
XI-Accessory	Weakness in turning head against resistance may indicate CN XI problem.
XII-Hypoglossal	Deviation of tongue to one side may indicate CN XII problem on that side.

predilection for the right side. The problem is generally cyclic in nature, seeming to go into remission for several months, only to return with similar symptoms. Trigger zones can exist in any part of the trigeminal nerve distribution, and triggering events can include gentle touching of the trigger zone manually or during speech, mastication, or other facial movements or by the application of cold materials or air to the trigger zone. Patients commonly take exaggerated precautions to prevent trigger zone stimulation, including physically preventing touching of the trigger zone (Figure 29-10).

The diagnosis of trigeminal neuralgia relies on the demonstration of these clinical characteristics. In addition, the administration of a local anesthetic into the patient's trigger zone should temporarily eliminate all pain; if not, an atypical facial neuralgia should be considered (Table 29-2).

Therapy of trigeminal neuralgia usually begins with a trial administration of antiseizure medications, with carba-

mazepine (Tegretol) being the drug most commonly used. This medication frequently suppresses the pain problem, but only for as long as the patient continues taking it. Carbamazepine has toxicities, particularly bone marrow suppression, so it should be used only by clinicians willing and able to monitor this toxicity. Procedures such as chemical (alcohol) or surgical neurectomies, can be attempted to eliminate peripheral trigger effects, but their success is usually only temporary. (Figure 29-11.)

Recently, peripheral radiofrequency thermoneurolysis and radiofrequency thermogangliolysis have shown promise for the treatment of trigeminal neuralgia (see Figure 29-4).

Finally, microvascular nerve root decompression, a neurosurgical procedure involving the lifting of an aberrantly positioned superior cerebellar artery away from the trigeminal nerve root (Dandy-Janetta procedure), frequently relieves the pain without altering normal nerve function. However, long-term success of this procedure is still unproved.

VAGOGLOSSOPHARYNGEAL NEURALGIA. Vagoglossopharyngeal neuralgia, much less common than trigeminal neuralgia, affects cranial nerves IX and X. Pain in patients with this disorder is characteristically located in the base of the tongue, the tonsillar pillars, and occasionally in the soft palate and auditory canal. The process has no gender predilection, is more common on the left side, and its onset is usually in the fourth decade. Trigger zones may exist in the areas of oropharyngeal, vagal, or glossopharyngeal sensory innervation, with pain triggered by swallowing or touching the soft palate, tonsillar pillars, or base of the tongue. Tearing, vertigo, and involuntary movements of the pharynx with coughing and vomiting may occur (Table 29-2). The therapy of vagoglossopharyngeal neuralgia is similar to that for trigeminal neuralgia.

RAMSAY HUNT'S SYNDROME. Ramsay Hunt's syndrome, or intermedius (geniculate) neuralgia, is a rare facial pain problem that involves the sensory portion of cranial nerve VII. The severe pain of this disorder is felt in the medial portion of the external auditory canal, the auricle of the ear, and, occasionally, the soft palate. The process tends to occur in women in the third, fourth, and fifth decades. The pain is commonly not provokable and is associated with sialorrhea, rhinorrhea, tinnitus, vertigo, and dysgustia (abnormal taste).

Supplies
3 - 1cc syringes
3 - 25 gauge (or smaller) needles
Sterile normal saline
0.5% lidocaine without epinephrine
2.0% lidocaine without epinephrine
Several alcohol wipes

Technique

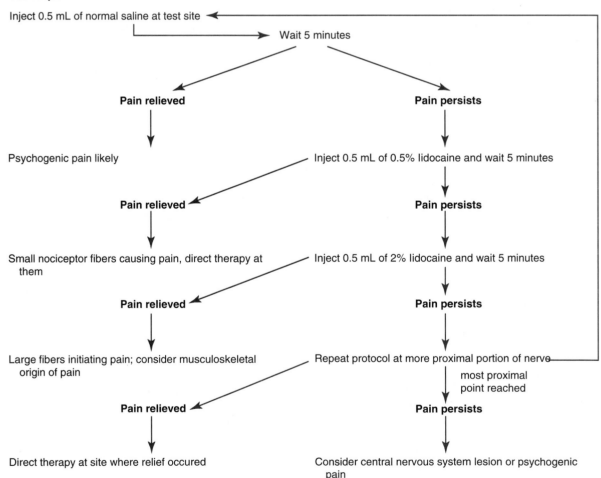

Always begin injections at surface site of pain and then move proximally, for example, pain perceived in lower left vermillion—inject lip, then mental nerve, then inferior alveolar nerve, then first division of the trigeminal nerve.

◇ Figure 29-9

Protocol for diagnostic nerve blocks.

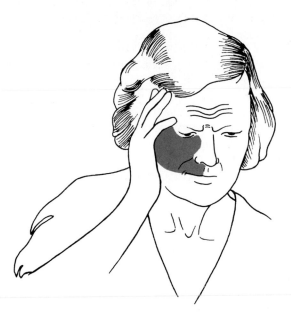

Typical clinical manifestations of patient during paroxysm of pain from trigeminal neuralgia. This late–middle-age woman has severe pain limited to anatomic distribution of one or two divisions of the trigeminal nerve. She raises arm to keep anything from touching trigger zone. Pain has stabbing, burning, or shocking quality and lasts several seconds to minutes. *(From Netter F:*CIBA-GEIGY, Clin Symp, *1981.)*

The diagnosis is based on the clinical signs of disease and can be confirmed by directed stimulation of the tympanic plexus and chorda tympanic nerves through the middle ear. Treatment involves peripheral neurectomy of these nerves (see Table 28-2).

POSTHERPETIC TRIGEMINAL NEURALGIA.   Herpes zoster, also termed *shingles,* represents the reactivation of a varicella viral infection of sensory nerve ganglia. The process can affect any sensory nerve but tends to confine itself to the distribution from a single ganglion. Although all cranial nerves with sensory fibers can be affected, the trigeminal nerve is by far the most common, with the ophthalmic division of cranial nerve V the most frequently affected site of the body.

A herpes zoster outbreak usually first manifests with pain in the affected area, soon followed by the appearance of vesicles. In some patients, after the skin lesions heal, the pain in the involved area remains and becomes chronic and is accompanied by an associated hypesthesia. It is usually a burning pain, and touching the region may exacerbate the pain (see Table 29-2).

Relief of the pain of postherpetic trigeminal neuralgia is difficult to obtain. Usually, trials of nonnarcotic analgesics and antiinflammatory medications are used in an attempt to find a drug that provides satisfactory pain control.

ATYPICAL FACIAL NEURALGIA.   Although many clinicians have used *atypical facial neuralgia* as a wastebasket

Table 29-2. Differential diagnosis and therapy of the most common facial neuralgias

	Trigeminal	Vagoglossopharyngeal	Ramsay Hunt's	Postherpetic	Atypical
Age at onset	≥Sixth decade	≥Fifth decade	Third to fifth decades	≥Sixth decade and all immunosuppressed patients	Third to fourth decades
Gender predilection	F > M*	M = F	F > M	F = M	M > F
Location of pain	Confined to one or more divisions of V; unilateral; R > L*	Base of tongue, tonsillar pillars, soft pallate; unilateral, L > R	External auditory canal, auricle of ear	Mostly confined to dermatome V	Retro-orbital and malar regions
Character of pain	Severe burning, stabbing, or shocking	Less severe than trigeminal neuralgia; burning or boring	Severe stabbing	Burning with hyperesthesia of area	Dull ache, throbbing
Duration of pain	Seconds to minutes	Seconds to minutes	Seconds to minutes	Chronic	30-90 min
Provoking factors	Tactile stimulation of trigger zone	Swallowing or touching affected areas	Not triggered	Not triggered	Not triggered
Other features	Paroxysms	Associated bradycardia, hypotension, and syncope	Associated sialorrhea, rhinorrhea, tinnitus, vertigo, dysgustia	Follows herpes zoster outbreak	Paroxysms
Therapy	Carbamazepine, peripheral neurectomy, microsurgery, Dandy-Janetta procedure	Carbamazepine, neurosurgery	Carbamazepine, neurosurgery	Analgesics, antiinflammatory drugs	Nerve blocks, medications (several), behavioral therapy

*F, Females; *M,* Males; *R,* right side; *L,* left side.

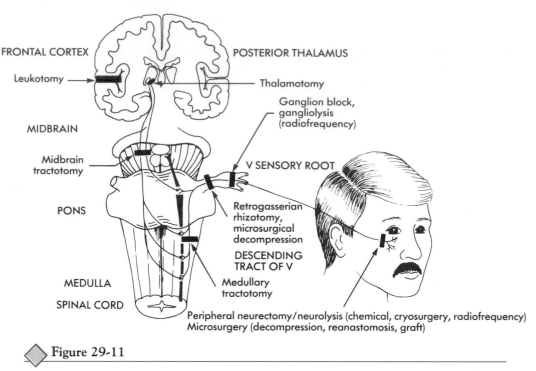

◇ **Figure 29-11**

Available sites for neurosurgical control of facial pain. *(Redrawn from Kruger GO:* Textbook of oral and maxillofacial surgery, *ed 6, St Louis, 1984, Mosby.)*

designation for pain problems that cannot be placed in one of the more specific categories, an accepted definition exists. Atypical facial neuralgia is a vascular syndrome that manifests with a dull throbbing in the retro-orbital and malar regions that is referred toward the ear, neck, and/or shoulder. The pain appears paroxysmally, lasting 30 to 90 minutes. It is not lancinating in quality and is not commonly provokable. The pain pattern does not tend to follow the anatomic boundaries of the trigeminal nerve. Atypical facial neuralgia is seen most commonly in young men with compulsive and/or depressive personalities (see Table 29-2).

Therapy of atypical facial neuralgia tends to be empiric with modalities such as sympathetic nerve blocks or the administration of antiseizure, vasodilatory, or antidepressant medications and behavioral therapies, bringing variable success. Treatment regimens that emphasize patient self-help have been the most effective therapeutic plans.

HEADACHE

Most individuals have experienced headache of one type or another, accept them as a fact of life, and usually initiate treatment without seeking the opinion of a health care provider. However, sometimes patients experience especially severe or frequent headaches or headaches coexisting with facial pain that prompts them to seek professional advice, often from their dentist. Although there is always a remote chance that a headache is a symptom of a life-threatening neuropathology, such as a tumor or intracranial bleeding, a headache in the absence of signs of increasing intracranial pressure is usually caused by less serious problems.

MUSCLE CONTRACTION HEADACHE. Most mildly or moderately painful headaches are commonly attributed to excessive skeletal muscle contractions in the head and neck. Although a cerebral vasodilatory component may be involved, these headaches are not thought to be caused primarily by vascular or inflammatory processes, which helps separate them from other headache types. These muscle contraction, or tension, headaches may be accompanied by facial, neck, shoulder, or back pain that is also of musculoskeletal origin. Muscle contraction headaches are anxiety and fatigue related and tend to occur when either is increased, such as near the end of a busy day or after a task requiring prolonged concentration (Table 29-3).

The muscle contraction headache tends to appear initially as a steady, nonpulsatile pressure sensation in either a caplike distribution or localized to the frontal, temporal, and/or occipital regions. The headache is usually increased with head movement or if pressure is placed on the involved muscles. The patient is commonly able to get relief by attempting to relax or sleep or by taking over-the-counter analgesics. The importance of muscle contraction headaches to the dentist is their common association with facial pain in etiology, pathophysiology, and therapy. Treatment for patients frequently troubled by these headaches should focus on the psychogenic basis of this process. Relaxation therapies, such as avocations, physical therapy, or anxiety-redirection activities (for example, daily periods of physical exertion), are often successful. More resistant forms of muscle contraction headaches may require the administration of low-dose tricyclic antidepressants by clinicians experienced in their use.

◇ Table 29-3. The features, differential diagnosis, and treatment of the most common types of headaches

Types of headaches	Age	Gender predilection	Location of pain	Character of pain	Pattern of pain	Provoking factors	Other features	Therapy
Muscle contraction	≥Second decade	M = F*	Generalized over head; bilateral	Tightness or pressure sensation; aching	Intermittent; generally near end of day	Tension; fatigue; hypoglycemia	Concurrent facial pain	Nonnarcotic analgesics; rest; relaxation
Migraine	Second to third decades	F:M = 3:2	Frontotemporal; may be unilateral or (less common) bilateral	Throbbing; dull ache	Intermittent; lasts 2–3 hr	Tension; noise; various foods; ethanol; fatigue; bright lights; hypoglycemia	Aura; nausea; photophobia; can be hereditary	Ergot alkyloids; antidepressants; beta or calcium channel blockers; antiemetics
Cluster	≥Second decade	M > F	Retro-orbital; temporal; unilateral	Intense, nonthrobbing	Usually in evening or during sleep	Occasionally ethanol	Ptosis; miosis; lacrimation; associated with cigarette smoking	Ergot alkyloids; tricyclic antidepressants; lithium
Giant cell (temporal) arteritis	≥Sixth decade	M = F	Occipital and/or temporal; unilateral	Steady burning or aching	Can be continuous or intermittent	Pressure on maxillofacial arteries	Visual disturbance; elevated sedimentation rate; rheumatologic problems; constitutional symptoms	Corticosteroids

*F, Female; M, male.

Fatigue-related muscle contraction headaches are best managed with increased hours of sleep, which sometimes requires the management of insomnia.

Many clinicians believe that myofascial pain and dysfunction (MPD) syndrome is actually a type of muscle contraction phenomenon occurring in the face and neck. The causes and treatment are in many ways similar to those for muscle contraction headaches.

HEADACHES OF VASCULAR ORIGIN.   Headaches of vascular origin include migrane headaches, cluster headaches, and giant cell arteritis.

Migraine headaches.   Migraine headache is second only to muscle contraction headache in frequency, although the incidence of migraine headache disorders is difficult to measure because of variations in clinical diagnostic criteria. Migraines are periodic, severe headaches that are (1) often preceded by an aura, (2) usually unilateral in distribution at the onset of the pain, and (3) often associated with irritability, photophobia, nausea, and vomiting.

Many forms of migraine have been described to account for the variability in clinical presentation, but the pathophysiology thought to be common to all migraine headaches is abnormal cerebral vasodilation, possibly preceded by an initial vasoconstriction. Migraine headaches are more common in females (3:2) and usually appear in the second and third decades of life. A family history of migraine disorders is frequently present.

The first clinical characteristic of classic migraine headaches is the aura, or prodrome, that occurs commonly. Examples of visual auras include scotomata (blind spots) or the appearance of a zigzag pattern, flashing lights, or hallucinations. Other sensory aura can occur but are less common. The headache follows the aura in 5 to 20 minutes and is typically unilateral, pulsating, and moderately severe. Patients become photophobic and nauseated. During a migraine headache the patient usually wants to lie motionless and attempt to sleep. The common migraine headache is similar to classic migraines, except for the absence of an aura (see Table 29-3).

Therapy of migraine headaches is usually best administered by a patient's primary care physician and often consists of the use of ergot alkaloids, antidepressants, beta-adrenergic blockers, or calcium slow-channel blockers. Patients are usually advised not to miss meals, and sleep and dietary restrictions are commonly prescribed.

Cluster headaches.   A second type of head pain of vascular origin is the cluster headache. As the name implies, the bouts of pain of this type of headache appear in closely spaced clusters of paroxysms.

Cluster headaches, in contrast to migraines, occur primarily in males (5:1). Although they can appear at any age, the majority occur in the third through the fifth decades and usually in those who smoke cigarettes heavily.

Typically, a cluster headache occurs without an aura. The pain usually has a burning quality and can be so severe that some patients contemplate suicide. The headache may last only a few minutes, but most commonly last 30 to 45 minutes. The pain always begins and remains unilateral during an attack and is located behind or around the orbit. Patients generally prefer to walk around during the headache, unlike migraine sufferers. Nausea and vomiting rarely occur. Associated signs of cluster headache include flushing of the involved area and eye signs, such as lacrimation, ptosis, and miosis (see Table 29-3).

Therapy of cluster headaches, generally provided by a physician, can be either prophylactic or therapeutic. Prophylactic measures include avoidance of vasoactive foods and the administration of ergot alkaloids, corticosteroids, and lithium carbonate. Therapy for the attacks includes administration of oxygen or ergot alkaloids and, rarely, surgery on the trigeminal root. Cluster headaches often spontaneously disappear with time.

Giant cell arteritis.   Head pain can be evoked by intravascular inflammatory processes. The most common form of vasculitis that causes headaches is giant cell, or temporal or cranial, arteritis in which vasculitis occurs in the branches of the external carotid artery. In this disease the endothelium of cranial arteries becomes inflamed, with the appearance of numerous giant cells that are seen when an affected vessel is examined histologically.

Patients are rarely affected with giant-cell arteritis before age 50. The incidence of giant-cell arteritis is equal in women and men and is extremely low in blacks.

Headaches are not invariably present in giant-cell arteritis, but when present the pain is severe, throbbing, and localized in the temporal and retro-orbital regions. Placing pressure on affected arteries, lying down, or masticating tends to worsen the pain. Skin over affected arteries becomes erythematous, and constitutional symptoms occur, including a low-grade fever. An ominous symptom of temporal arteritis is the occurrence of partial or complete loss of vision caused by involvement of the ophthalmic vessels.

The diagnosis of temporal arteritis depends on the characteristic clinical presentation, a markedly elevated erythrocyte sedimentation rate, and the positive demonstration of arteritis on a temporal artery biopsy (Table 29-3).

Therapy involves the administration of corticosteroids emergently in patients in whom visual symptoms have begun.

FACIAL NEUROPATHOLOGY OF TRAUMATIC ORIGIN

Injuries to sensory nerves of the maxillofacial region occasionally occur as the result of facial fractures, during the treatment of oral pathologic conditions, or when maxillofacial reconstructive surgery is performed. Fortunately, most injured nerves spontaneously recover. However, in the past little was done to treat persistent sensory nerve disorders. Recent advances in the understanding of how nerves heal and in the

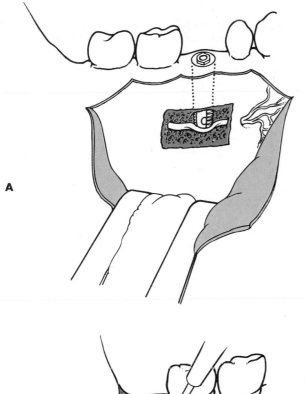

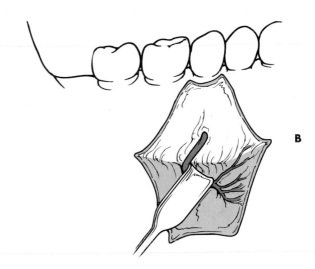

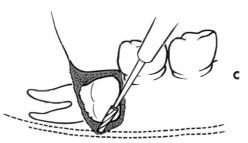

 Figure 29-12

Three types of peripheral nerve injury. **A,** Neurapraxia. Injury to nerve loses no continuity of axon or endoneurium. Example shown is implant placed in inferior alveolar canal, compressing the nerve. **B,** Axonotmesis. Injury to nerve causes loss of axonal continuity but preserves endoneurium. Example shown is overly aggressive retraction of mental nerve. **C,** Neurotmesis. Injury to nerve causes loss of both axonal and endoneurium continuity. Example is cutting of inferior alveolar nerve during removal of deeply impacted third molar.

surgical means of repairing peripheral nerves currently provide patients with the possibility of regaining normal nerve function.

The three branches of the trigeminal nerve injured most commonly, for which the altered sensation is clinically significant, are the inferior alveolar-mental nerve, the lingual nerve, and the infraorbital nerve. When the inferior alveolar-mental nerve is injured, the usual causes are the following:

1. Mandibular (body) fractures
2. Preprosthetic surgical procedures
3. Sagittal split osteotomy surgery
4. Mandibular resection for oral neoplasms
5. Removal of impacted lower third molars

Lingual nerve damage occurs in the course of surgery to remove oral malignancies or impacted third molars. Injury to the infraorbital nerve is most common during zygomaticomaxillary complex fractures.

CLASSIFICATION. Research and clinical experience have shown that surgical intervention to repair damaged nerves is more successful when performed soon after the injury has occurred. Thus an understanding of the various types of nerve damage, especially their prognoses, is important, for this enables the clinician to decide when referral for peripheral nerve surgery is warranted.

The three types of nerve injuries are neurapraxia, axonotmesis, and neurotmesis (Figure 29-12). Although a determination as to which type of nerve damage has occurred is usually made retrospectively, knowledge of the pathophysiology of each type is important for gaining an appreciation of nerve healing.

Neurapraxia, the least severe form of peripheral nerve injury, is a contusion of a nerve in which continuity of both the epineurial sheath and the axons is maintained. A neurapraxia can be produced by blunt trauma or traction (stretching) of a nerve, inflammation around a nerve, or local ischemia of a nerve. Because there has been no loss in axonal continuity, spontaneous full recovery of nerve function usually occurs in a few days or weeks.

Axonotmesis has occurred when the continuity of the axons but not the epineurial sheath is disrupted. This type of injury can be produced by severe blunt trauma, nerve crushing, or extreme traction of a nerve. Because the epineural sheath is still intact, axonal regeneration can (but does not always) occur with a resolution of nerve dysfunction in 2 to 6 months.

Neurotmesis, the most severe type of nerve injury, involves a complete loss of nerve continuity. This form of damage can be produced by badly displaced fractures, severance by bullets or knives during an assault, or by iatrogenic transection.

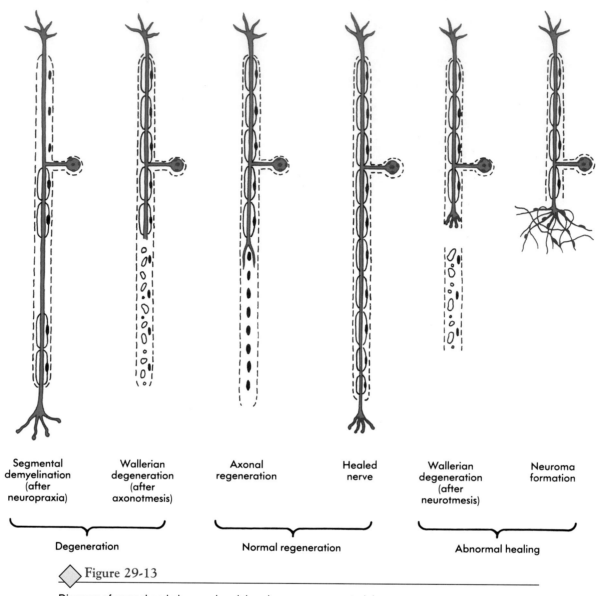

Segmental demyelination (after neuropraxia)

Wallerian degeneration (after axonotmesis)

Axonal regeneration

Healed nerve

Wallerian degeneration (after neurotmesis)

Neuroma formation

Degeneration

Normal regeneration

Abnormal healing

◇ Figure 29-13

Diagram of normal and abnormal peripheral nerve response to injury.

Prognosis for spontaneous recovery of nerves that have undergone neurotmesis is poor, except if the ends of the affected nerve have been left in close approximation and properly oriented.

NERVE HEALING.   Nerve healing usually has two phases: degeneration and regeneration.

Two types of degeneration can occur. The first is segmental demyelination, in which there is dissolution of the myelin sheath in isolated segments. This partial demyelination causes a slowing of conduction velocity and may prevent the transmission of some nerve impulses. Symptoms include paresthesia (a spontaneous and subjective altered sensation that a patient does not find painful), dysesthesia (a spontaneous and subjective altered sensation that a patient finds painful), hyperesthesia (excessive sensitivity of a nerve to stimulation), and hypesthesia (decreased sensitivity of a nerve

to stimulation). Segmental demyelination can occur after neurapraxic injuries or with vascular or connective tissue disorders (Figure 29-13).

Wallerian degeneration is the second type of degeneration occurring after nerve trauma. In this process the axons and myelin sheath of the nerve distal to (away from the central nervous system) the site of nerve trunk interruption undergo disintegration in their entirety. The axons proximal to (toward the central nervous system) the site of injury also undergo some degeneration, occasionally all the way to the cell body but generally just for a few nodes of Ranvier. Wallerian degeneration stops all nerve conduction distal to the proximal axonal stump. This type of degeneration follows nerve transsection and other destructive processes that affect peripheral nerves (Figure 29-13).

Regeneration of a peripheral nerve can begin almost immediately after nerve injury. Normally, the proximal nerve

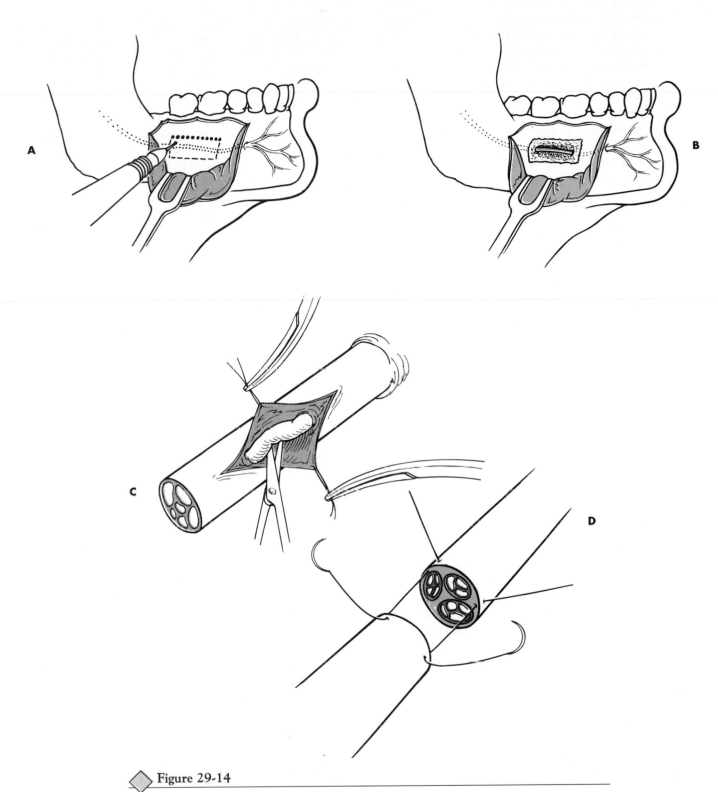

◆ Figure 29-14

A, Example of intraoral approach to inferior alveolar nerve for microneurosurgery. Area over portion of nerve to be exposed is scored to allow the overlying bone to be removed. **B,** Exposed nerve ready for surgical repair. **C,** Opening of nerve trunk to expose fascicles. In this illustration an individual fascicle is being dissected away from the others as part of a decompression procedure. **D,** Epineurial repair of sectioned nerve trunk. Note sutures being placed to reestablish continuity of epineurium.

stump sends out a group of new fibers (the growth cone) that grow down the remnant Schwann cell tube. Growth progresses at a rate of 1 to 1.5 mm per day and continues until the site innervated by the nerve is reached or growth is blocked by fibrous connective tissue or bone. During regeneration new myelin sheaths may form as the axons increase in diameter. As functional contacts are made the patient will experience altered sensations in the previously anesthetic area, which take the form of paresthesias or dysesthesias.

Problems can occur during regeneration that prevent normal nerve healing. If the continuity of the Schwann cell tube is disrupted, connective tissue may enter the tube while it is partially vacant. When the growth cone reaches the connective tissue obstruction, it may find a way around it and continue on, or it may form a mass of aimless nerve fibers that constitutes a traumatic neuroma subject to pain production when disturbed (see Figure 29-13).

NERVE INJURY SYNDROMES.   The loss of oral or facial sensory nerve function is frequently disturbing to patients because of the functional disturbances sometimes produced by lack of normal sensation. However, rarely, an injured nerve can be the source of pain syndromes, such as causalgia, anesthesia dolorosa, and phantom facial pain.

SURGICAL THERAPY OF TRAUMATIZED PERIPH-ERAL NERVES.   Peripheral nerves of the face that have undergone neurapraxia or axonotmesis generally spontaneously recover. However, the following three nerve injuries warrant treatment by an oral and maxillofacial surgeon trained in microneurosurgery:

1. External or internal nerve compression
2. Intentional or accidental severance of a nerve
3. Appearance of a traumatic neuroma and/or pain syndromes after nerve injury

External compression of a nerve trunk can result from impingement of bone, a tooth root, a dental implant, a broken instrument on a nerve, or the formation of constricting fibrous connective tissue. This external compression may be visible with special radiographic imaging techniques but frequently depends on exploratory surgery for establishing a diagnosis. Internal compression is usually caused by growth of scar tissue into the nerve trunk while it is regenerating. Surgical decompression (removal of the obstructing tissue or foreign material) is the treatment of choice for either external or internal nerve compression (Figure 29-14).

Transection of a nerve, whether complete or incomplete,

may be recognized at the time of occurrence or only after symptoms arise and exploratory surgery is performed. Nerves that are cleanly cut or that have been damaged for only a short distance can be microsurgically reanastomosed by an oral and maxillofacial surgeon. Under high magnification the individual fascicles and/or the epineurium is sutured together with 9-0 or 10-0 nylon suture. When a relatively long length of nerve is missing, nerve grafting is indicated. In this procedure the oral and maxillofacial surgeon harvests a nerve of suitable size, usually the sural nerve of the lower leg or the greater auricular nerve. The harvested nerve is sutured into the area of nerve discontinuity. In this case the patient is trading anesthesia of the donor nerve site for the potential return of sensation in the area supplied by the grafted nerve.

Several factors are known to affect the success of microsurgical nerve repairs. The prognosis is worse with advanced patient age, the presence of an avulsive or proximal nerve injury, delay in the timing of repair, and the presence of problems such as infection or excessive scar tissue. Microsurgery of peripheral nerves of the face is undergoing extensive research, with potential improvement in techniques likely to include the use of biocompatible tissue adhesives and biologic or synthesized conduit grafts.

The final condition for which microsurgical intervention may be necessary is nerve trauma with concomitant chronic pain problems, such as traumatic neuromas. Pharmacotherapy may be used for pain control, but, occasionally, nerve exploration is indicated. If on visualization of the nerve a neuroma is discovered, it can be resected and the nerve either reanastomosed or grafted.

BIBLIOGRAPHY

Bonica JJ: *The management of pain,* ed 2, Philadelphia, 1990, Lea & Febiger.

Dalessio DJ, Silberstein SD: *Wolff's headache and other head pain,* ed 6, New York, 1996, Oxford University.

Fricton JR, Dubner R: Orofacial pain and temporomandibular disorders. In Fricton JR, Dubner R, editors: *Advances in pain research and therapy,* vol 21, New York, 1995, Raven Press.

LaBanc JP, Gregg JM: Trigeminal nerve injury: diagnosis and management, *Oral Maxillofac Surg Clin North Am* 4:2, 1992.

Okeson JP: *Bell's orofacial pains,* ed 5, Carol Stream, Ill, 1995, Quintessence.

Weisenberg M: *Pain: clinical and experimental perspectives,* St Louis, 1975, Mosby.

CHAPTER 30

MANAGEMENT OF TEMPOROMANDIBULAR DISORDERS

MYRON R. TUCKER AND M. FRANKLIN DOLWICK

CHAPTER OUTLINE

Patients frequently consult a dentist because of pain or dysfunction in the temporomandibular (TM) region. The most common causes of temporomandibular dysfunctions (TMDs) are muscular disorders, which are commonly referred to as *myofascial pain and dysfunction.* These muscular disorders are generally managed well with a variety of reversible nonsurgical treatment methods.

Other causes of temporomandibular pain or dysfunction originate primarily within the temporomandibular joint (TMJ). These causes include internal derangement and osteoarthritis, rheumatoid arthritis, chronic recurrent dislocation, ankylosis, neoplasia, and infection. Although some of these disorders will respond to nonsurgical therapy, some cases may eventually require surgical treatment. Management of these patients requires a coordinated plan between the general dentist, oral and maxillofacial surgeon, and other health care services if a successful result is to be achieved.

EVALUATION

The evaluation of the patient with TM pain and/or dysfunction is like that in any other diagnostic workup. This evaluation should include a thorough history, a physical examination of the masticatory system, and some type of routine TMJ radiography. Special diagnostic studies should be performed only as indicated and not as routine studies.

INTERVIEW

The patient's history may be the most important part of the evaluation because it furnishes clues for the diagnosis. The history begins with the chief complaint, which is a statement of the patient's reasons for seeking consultation or treatment. The history of the present illness should be comprehensive, including an accurate description of the patient's symptoms, chronology of the symptoms, description of how the problem affects the patient, and information about any previous treatments (including the patient's response to those treatments).

EXAMINATION

The physical examination consists of an evaluation of the entire masticatory system. The head and neck should be inspected for soft tissue asymmetry or evidence of muscular hypertrophy. The patient should be observed for signs of jaw clenching or other habits. The masticatory muscles should be systematically examined. The muscles should be palpated for the presence of tenderness, fasciculations, spasm, or trigger points (Figure 30-1).

The TMJs are examined for tenderness and noise (Figure 30-2). The location of the joint tenderness (lateral/posterior) should be noted. If the joint is more painful during different areas of the opening cycle or with different types of functions, this should be recorded. The most common forms of joint noise are clicking (a distinct sound) and crepitus (multiple scraping or grating sounds). Many joint sounds can be easily heard without special instrumentation or can be felt during palpation of the joint. However in some cases auscultation with a stethoscope may allow less obvious joint sounds, such as mild crepitus, to be appreciated.

The mandibular range of motion should be determined. Normal range of movement of an adult's mandible is about 50 mm vertically (interincisally) and 10 mm protrusively and laterally (Figure 30-3). The normal movement is straight and symmetric. In some cases tenderness in the joint or muscle areas may prevent opening. The clinician should attempt to ascertain not only the painless voluntary opening but also the maximum opening that can be achieved with gentle digital pressure. In some cases the patient may appear to have a mechanical obstruction in the joint causing limited opening but with gentle pressure may actually be able to achieve near normal opening. This may suggest muscular rather than intracapsular problems.

The dental evaluation is also important. Odontogenic sources of pain should be eliminated. The teeth should be examined for wear facets, soreness, and mobility, which may be evidence of bruxism. Although the significance of occlusal abnormalities is controversial, the occlusal relationship should be evaluated and documented. Missing teeth should be noted, and dental and skeletal classification should be determined. The clinician should note any centric relation-centric occlusion discrepancy or significant posturing by the patient. The examination's findings can be summarized on a TMD evaluation form and included in the patient's chart (see below). In many cases a more detailed chart note may be necessary to adequately document all of the history and examination findings described above.

RADIOGRAPHIC EVALUATION

Radiographs of the TMJ are extremely helpful in the diagnosis of intraarticular, osseous, and soft tissue pathology. The use of radiographs in the evaluation of the patient with TMD should be based on the patient's signs and symptoms instead of routinely ordering a "standard" set of radiographs. In many cases the panoramic radiograph provides adequate information as a screening radiograph in evaluation of TMS. A variety of other radiographic techniques are available that may provide useful information in certain cases.

TRANSCRANIAL RADIOGRAPHS. A standard dental radiographic unit combined with a head-holding device can be used to produce a transcranial image of the TMJ. Although this view will not allow detailed examination of all aspects of the TMJ, excellent evaluation of the lateral pole of the condyle can be accomplished when the proper radiographic technique is used. Because bony pathology of the TMJ frequently extends to the lateral pole, this technique can be helpful in diagnosing bony internal joint pathology (Figure 30-4).[2]

PANORAMIC RADIOGRAPHY. One of the best overall radiographs for screening evaluation of the TMJs is the panoramic radiograph. This technique allows visualization of both TMJs on the same film. Because a panoramic technique provides a tomographic type of view of the TMJ, this can frequently provide a good assessment of the bony anatomy of the articulating surfaces of the mandibular condyle and glenoid fossa (Figure 30-5), and other areas, such as the coronoid process, can also be visualized. Many machines are equipped to provide special views of the mandible, focusing primarily on the area of the TMJs. These radiographs can often be completed in both the open and closed position.

TOMOGRAMS. The tomographic technique allows a more detailed view of the TMJ.[1] This technique allows radiographic sectioning of the joint at different levels of the condyle fossa complex, which provides individual views visualizing the joint in "slices" from the medial to the lateral pole (Figure 30-6). These views eliminate bony supraimposition and overlap and provide a relatively clear picture of the bony anatomy of the joint (Figure 30-6).

TMJ ARTHROGRAPHY. This imaging method was the first technique available that allowed visualization (indirect) of the intraarticular disk. Arthrography involves the injection of contrast material into the inferior and/or superior spaces of a joint, followed by radiography of the joint.[4] Evaluation of the configuration of the dye in the joint spaces allows evaluation of the position and morphology of the articular disk (Figure 30-7). This technique also demonstrates the presence of perforations and adhesions of the disk or its attachments. With the availability of more advanced, less invasive techniques arthrography is used less frequently.

COMPUTERIZED TOMOGRAPHY. Computerized tomographs (CTs) provide a combination of tomographic views of the joint, combined with computer enhancement of hard and soft tissue images.[6] This technique allows evaluation of a variety of hard and soft tissue pathology in the joint. CT images provide the most accurate radiographic assessment of the bony components of the joint (Figure 30-8). CT scan

Text continued on p. 716

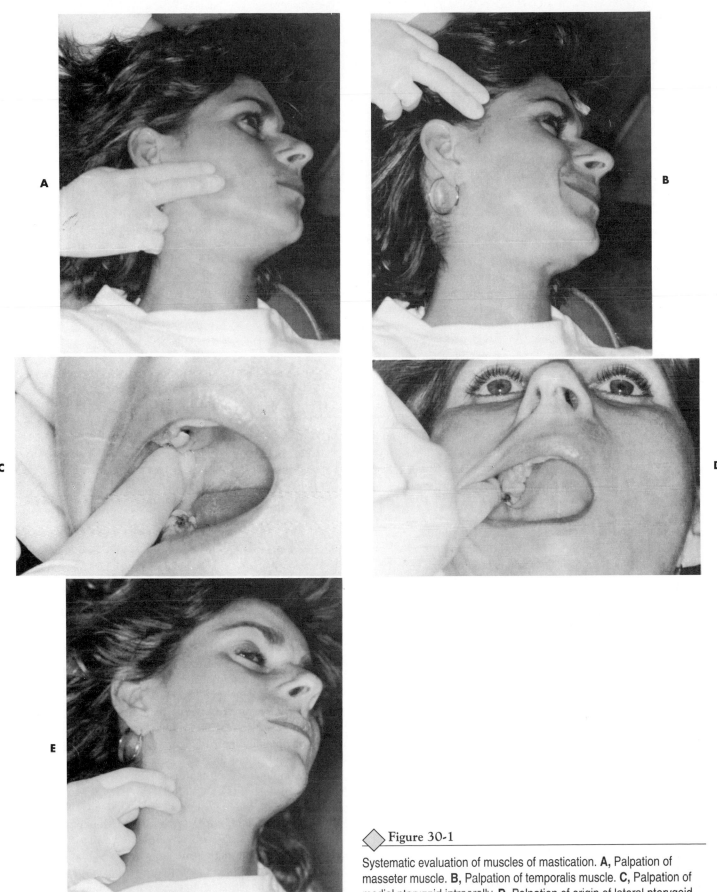

Figure 30-1

Systematic evaluation of muscles of mastication. **A,** Palpation of masseter muscle. **B,** Palpation of temporalis muscle. **C,** Palpation of medial pterygoid intraorally. **D,** Palpation of origin of lateral pterygoid. **E,** Palpation of sternocleidomastoid muscle.

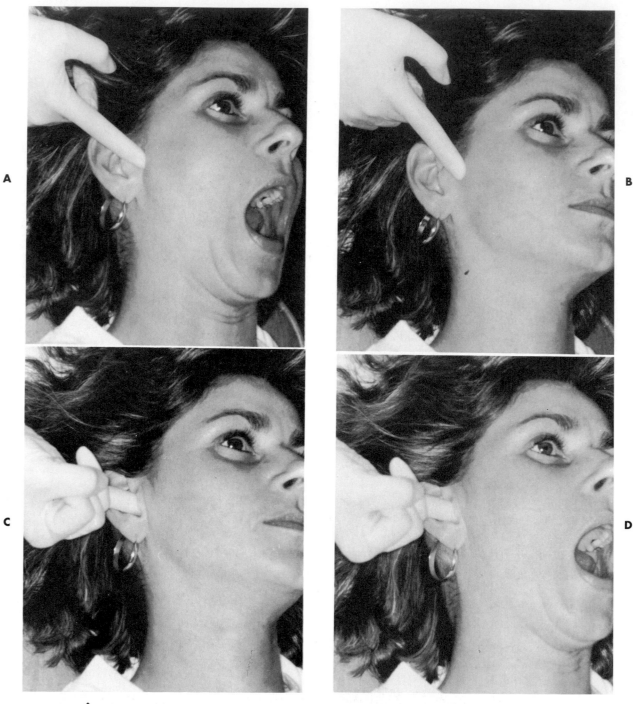

◇ Figure 30-2

Evaluation of TMJ for tenderness and noise. Joint is palpated laterally in closed position (**A**) and open position (**B**) and through the external auditory canal in the closed position (**C**) and open position (**D**).

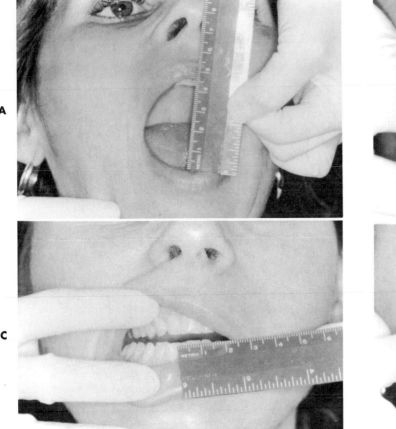
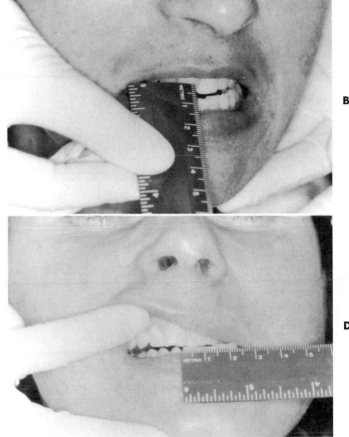
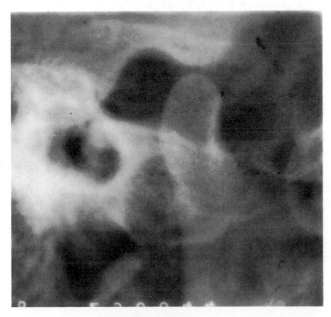
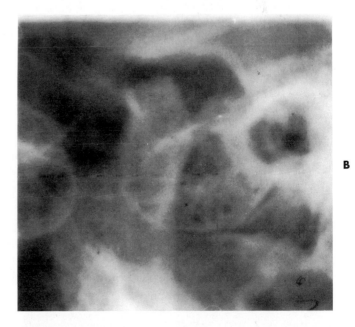

◇ Figure 30-3

Measurement of range of jaw motion. **A,** Maximum voluntary vertical opening (should be 45 mm or greater). **B,** Protrusion (should be approximately 10 mm). **C** and **D,** Left and right lateral excursions (should be approximately 10 mm).

◇ Figure 30-4

Examples of transcranial radiographs. **A,** Radiograph of right side shows normal anatomy of fossa and condyle. **B,** Left side view demonstrates degenerative changes of condyle.

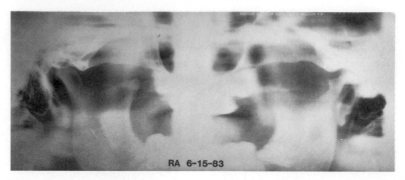

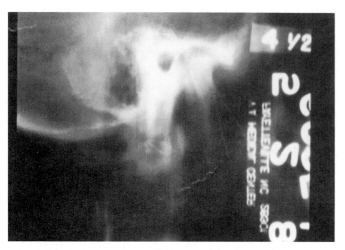

◇ **Figure 30-5**

Modified panoramic view demonstrating normal anatomy of right condyle and degenerative changes of left condyle. (This is modified panoramic radiographic technique showing increased detail of posterior ramus and condyle area while eliminating anterior mandible from radiographic image.)

◇ **Figure 30-6**

Tomographic projection of temporomandibular joint demonstrating typical degenerative changes with loss of well-defined joint space, absence of cortical outline of condylar, and anterior condylar lipping.

reconstruction capabilities allow images obtained in one plane of space to be reconstructed so that the images can be evaluated from a different view. Thus evaluation of the joint from a variety of perspectives can be made from a single radiation exposure.

MAGNETIC RESONANCE IMAGING. The most effective diagnostic imaging technique to evaluate TMJ soft tissues is magnetic resonance imaging (MRI) (Figure 30-9).[12] This technique allows excellent images of intraarticular soft tissue, making MRI a valuable technique for evaluating disk morphology and position. The fact that this technique does not use ionizing radiation is a significant advantage.

NUCLEAR IMAGING. This technique involves injection of ⁹⁹Tc, a gamma-emitting isotope that is concentrated in areas of active bone metabolism. Approximately 3 hours after injection of the isotope, images are obtained using a gamma camera. Single photon emission computerized tomography (SPECT) images can then be used to determine active areas of bone metabolism (Figure 30-10).[17] Although this technique is extremely sensitive, the information obtained may be somewhat difficult to interpret. Because bone changes, such as degeneration, may appear identical to repair or regeneration, this technique must be evaluated cautiously and in combination with clinical findings.

PSYCHOLOGIC EVALUATION

Many patients with TM pain and dysfunction of long-standing duration develop manifestations of chronic pain syndrome behavior. This complex may include gross exaggeration of symptoms and clinical depression.[23] To evaluate possible behavioral changes associated with pain and dysfunction, the history should include questions regarding functional limitation that results from the patient's symptoms. If the functional limitation appears to be excessive when compared with the patient's clinical signs or if the patient appears to be clinically depressed, further psychologic evaluation may be warranted.[21]

CLASSIFICATION OF TEMPOROMANDIBULAR DISORDERS

MYOFASCIAL PAIN

Myofascial pain and dysfunction (MPD) is the most common cause of masticatory pain and limited function for which patients seek dental consultation and treatment. The source of the pain and dysfunction is muscular, with masticatory muscles developing tenderness and pain as a result of abnormal muscular function or hyperactivity. This abnormal muscular function is frequently but not always associated with daytime clenching or nocturnal bruxism. The cause of MPD is controversial, although it is generally considered to be multifactorial.[10] One of the most commonly accepted causes

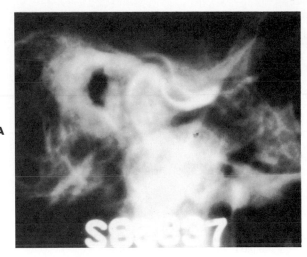
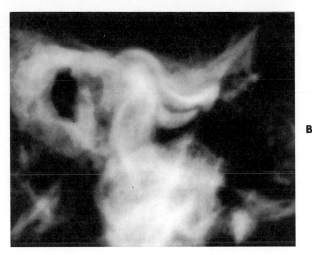

◆ **Figure 30-7**

Arthrogram showing dye in inferior and superior joint spaces. Anatomy and location of disk is indirectly interpreted from dye pattern seen after injection of joint spaces above and below disk. This demonstrates anterior disk displacement without reduction. **A,** Closed position. **B,** Open position.

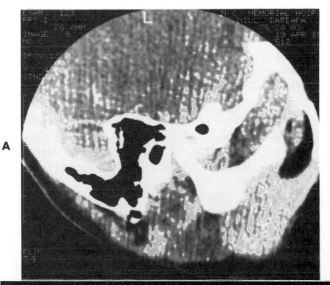
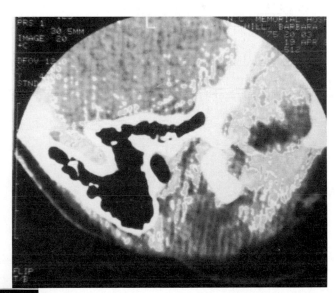
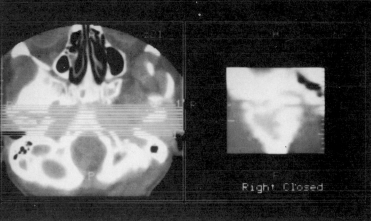

◆ **Figure 30-8**

Computerized tomogram showing disk displacement with reduction. **A,** Condyle in closed position with disk anteriorly displaced. **B,** Maximum opening position (after click) with disk in reduced position. **C,** Coronal reconstruction of axially produced computerized tomogram. This illustrates degenerative joint disease resulting from alloplastic implant replacement of disk tissue.

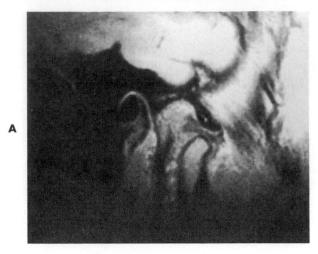
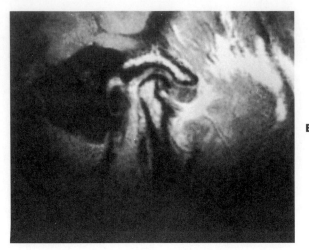

◇ Figure 30-9

Magnetic resonance imaging. **A,** This view shows normal disk-condyle relationship in open position. **B,** Image demonstrating anterior disk displacement and slight bone changes on articulating surface of condyle.

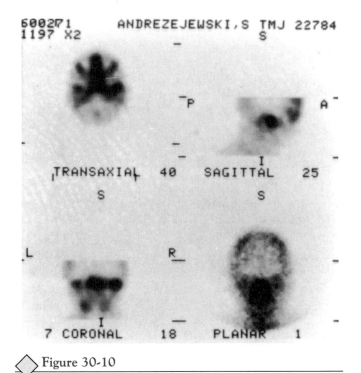

◇ Figure 30-10

Single photon emission CT (bone scan). Area of increased activity is apparent in both TMVs.

of MPD is bruxism secondary to stress and anxiety, with occlusion being a modifying or aggravating factor. MPD may also occur secondary to internal joint problems, such as disk displacement disorders or DJD.

Patients presenting with MPD generally complain of diffuse, poorly localized, preauricular pain that may also involve other muscles of mastication, such as the temporalis and medial pterygoid muscles. In patients with nocturnal bruxism the pain is frequently more severe in the morning.

Patients generally describe decreased jaw opening with pain during functions such as chewing. Headaches, usually bitemporal in location, may also be associated with these symptoms. Because of the role of stress, the pain is often more severe during periods of tension and anxiety.

Examination of the patient reveals diffuse tenderness of the masticatory muscles. The TMJs are frequently nontender to palpation. In isolated MPD, joint noises are usually not present. However, as mentioned previously, MPD may be associated with a variety of other joint problems that may produce other TMJ signs and symptoms. The range of mandibular movement in MPD patients may be decreased and is associated with deviation of the mandible toward the affected side. The teeth frequently have wear facets. However, the absence of such facets does not eliminate bruxism as a cause of the problem.

Radiographs of the TMJ's are usually normal. Some patients have evidence of degenerative changes, such as altered surface contours, erosion, or osteophytes. These changes, however, may be secondary to or unassociated with the MPD problem.

DISK DISPLACEMENT DISORDERS

In a normally functioning TMJ the condyle functions in both a hinge and a sliding fashion. During full opening the condyle not only rotates on a hinge axis but translates forward to a position near the most inferior portion of the articular eminence (Figure 30-11). During function the biconcave disk remains interpositioned between the condyle and fossa, with the condyle remaining against the thin intermediate zone during all phases of opening and closing.

ANTERIOR DISK DISPLACEMENT WITH REDUCTION.
In anterior disk displacement the disk is positioned anterior and medial to the condyle in the closed position.

A   B   C

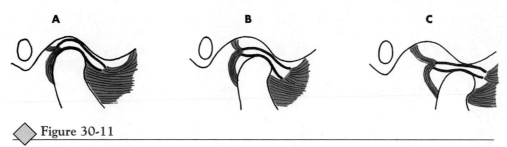

◈ Figure 30-11

Diagram of normal disk-condyle relationship. **A,** Biconcave disk is interpositioned between fossa and condyle in closed position. **B,** As condyle translates forward, thin intermediate zone stays in consistent relationship with condyle. **C,** Maximum open position.

A   B   C

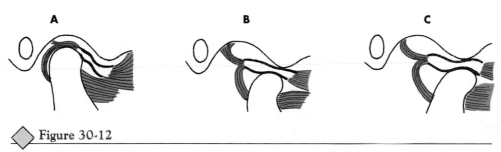

◈ Figure 30-12

Anterior disk displacement with reduction. **A,** Biconcave disk is situated anterior to articulating surface of condyle. As condyle translates forward, it eventually passes over thickened posterior band of disk, creating clicking noise. **B,** After click occurs, disk remains in appropriate relationship with condyle through remainder of opening cycle. **C,** Maximum opening position. As mandible closes, condyle and disk relationship will return to position shown in **A.**

During opening the condyle moves over the posterior band of the disk and eventually returns to the normal condyle-disk relationship, resting on the thin intermediate zone. During closing the condyle then slips posteriorly and rests on the retrodiscal tissue, with the disk returning to the anterior, medially displaced position (Figure 30-12).

Examination of the patient usually reveals joint tenderness, and muscle tenderness may also exist. Joint noise (clicking) is commonly heard with opening as the condyle moves from the area posterior to the disk into the thin concave area in the middle of the disk. In some cases clicking can be heard or palpated during the closing cycle. Maximal opening can be normal or slightly limited, with the click occurring during the opening movement. Anatomically, the opening click corresponds to the disk reducing to a more normal position. The closing click (reciprocal click) corresponds to the disk failing to maintain its normal position between the condylar head and the articular eminence and slipping forward to the anteriorly displaced position. Crepitus may be present and is usually a result of articular movement across irregular surfaces.

The images obtained from plane TMJ radiography in patients with anterior disk displacement may be normal or may demonstrate slight bone abnormalities. TMJ arthrography, CT scans, or MRI images can be used to document anterior displacement of the disk.

ANTERIOR DISK DISPLACEMENT WITHOUT REDUCTION.

In this type of internal derangement the disk displacement cannot be reduced, and thus the condyle is unable to translate to its full anterior extent, which prevents maximal opening and causes deviation of the mandible to the affected side (Figure 30-13).

In these patients no clicking occurs, because they are unable to translate the condyle over the posterior aspect of the disk. This lack of translation results in restricted opening and deviation. Lateral excursions to the contralateral side are also limited.

Radiographic evaluation of disk displacement without reduction is similar to findings in anterior disk displacement with reduction. Plain TMJ radiography may appear normal, whereas arthrography, CT scans, and MR images generally demonstrate anteriomedial disk displacement. However, in this disorder, images taken in the maximal open position continue to show anterior disk displacement within the open position.

DEGENERATIVE JOINT DISEASE (ARTHROSIS, OSTEOARTHRITIS)

Degenerative joint disease (DJD) includes a variety of anatomic findings, including irregular, perforated, or severely damaged disks in association with articular surface abnor-

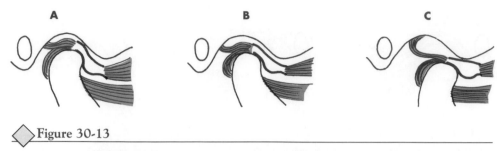

Figure 30-13

Anterior disk displacement without reduction. **A,** Disk that has been chronically anteriorly displaced now has amorphous shape rather than distinct biconcave structure. **B,** As condyle begins to translate forward, disk remains anterior to condyle. **C,** In maximum open position, disk tissue continues to remain anterior to condyle, with posterior attachment tissue interposed between condyle and fossa.

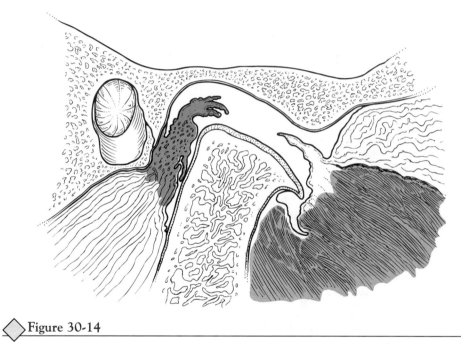

Figure 30-14

Diagram of degenerative joint disease demonstrating large perforation of disk tissue and erosion and flattening of articulating surfaces of both condyle and fossa.

malities, such as articular surface flattening, erosions, or osteophyte formation (Figure 30-14). DJD may be a result of a variety of causes, including repetitive microtrauma or macrotrauma, myofascial pain, or a progression from disk displacement with reduction to disk displacement with perforation, followed by bone changes. Recent information suggests that there may be several biochemical factors involved in osteoarthritis.[7,8,19] These factors may include substances such as neuropeptides, proteoglycans, and prostaglandins. These compounds not only have a role in the disease process but may also serve as biologic markers that may help to diagnose and eventually treat joint pathology. It must be emphasized that it is impossible to predict the progression of joint pathology. It is also important to note that there is not necessarily a precise correlation of pathology to clinical signs and symptoms, particularly in regard to pain.

Patients with DJD frequently present with pain associated with clicking or crepitus, located directly over the TMJ. Usually, an obvious limitation of opening is present, and symptoms usually increase with function. Radiographic findings are variable but generally exhibit decreased joint space, surface erosions, osteophytes, and flattening of the condylar head. Irregularities in the fossa and articular eminence may also be present.

SYSTEMIC ARTHRITIC CONDITIONS

A variety of systemic arthritic conditions are known to affect the TMJ. The most common of these is rheumatoid arthritis. Other processes, such as systemic lupus, can also affect the TMJ. In these cases symptoms are rarely isolated to the TMJs, and several other signs and symptoms of arthritis are usually present in other areas of the body.

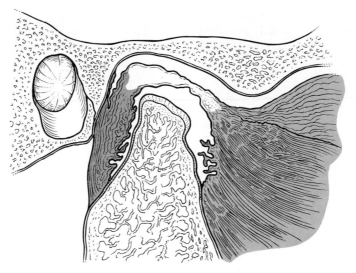

◆ Figure 30-15

Diagram of changes seen in rheumatoid arthritis of TMJ. These changes include proliferation of synovial tissue, creating resorption in anterior and posterior areas of condyle. Irregularities of disk tissue and articulating surface of condyle eventually occur.

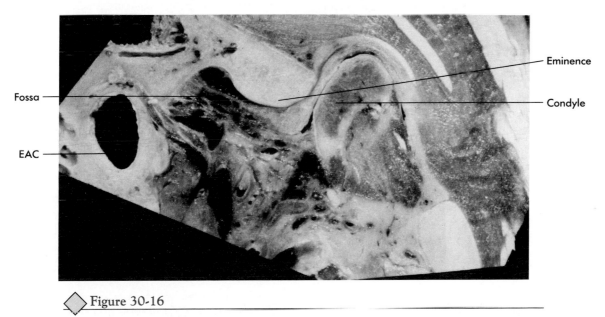

◆ Figure 30-16

Anatomic specimen demonstrating dislocation of condyle in front of eminence.

In the case of rheumatoid arthritis, an inflammatory process results in abnormal proliferation of synovial tissue in a so-called pannus formation (Figure 30-15).

TMJ symptoms that result from rheumatoid arthritis may occur at an earlier age than those associated with DJD. As opposed to DJD, which is usually unilateral, rheumatoid arthritis (and other systemic conditions) usually affect the TMJs bilaterally. Radiographic findings of the TMJ initially show erosive changes in the anterior and posterior aspects of the condylar heads. These changes may progress to large eroded areas that leave the appearance of a small, pointed condyle in a large fossa. Eventually the entire condyle and condylar neck may be destroyed. Laboratory tests, such as rheumatoid factor and erythrocyte sedimentation rate, may be helpful in confirming the diagnosis of rheumatoid arthritis.

CHRONIC RECURRENT DISLOCATION

Dislocation of the TMJ occurs frequently and is caused by mandibular hypermobility. Subluxation is a displacement of the condyle, which is self-reducing and generally requires no medical management. A more serious condition occurs when the mandibular condyle translates anteriorly in front of the articular eminence and becomes locked in that position (Figure 30-16). Dislocation may be unilateral or bilateral and may occur spontaneously after opening the mouth widely, such as during a yawn, eating, or a dental procedure. Dislocation of the mandibular condyle that persists for more than a few seconds generally becomes painful and is often associated with severe muscular spasms.

Dislocations should be reduced as soon as possible. This reduction is accomplished by applying downward pressure on the posterior teeth and upward pressure on the chin, accompanied by posterior displacement of the mandible. Usually, reduction is not difficult. However, muscular spasms may prevent simple reduction, particularly when the dislocation cannot be reduced immediately. In these cases, anesthesia of the auricular temporal nerve and the muscles of mastication may be necessary. Sedation to reduce patient anxiety and provide muscular relaxation may also be required. Following reduction the patient should be instructed to restrict mandibular opening for 2 to 4 weeks. Moist heat and nonsteroidal antiinflammatory drugs are also helpful in controlling pain and inflammation.

ANKYLOSIS

INTRACAPSULAR ANKYLOSIS. Intracapsular ankylosis, or fusion of the joint, leads to reduced mandibular opening that ranges from partial reduction in function to complete immobility of the jaw. Intracapsular ankylosis results from a fusion of the condyle, disk, and fossa complex, as a result of the formation of fibrous tissue, bone fusion, or a combination of the two (Figure 30-17). The most common cause of ankylosis involves macrotrauma, most frequently associated with condylar fractures. Other causes of ankylosis include previous surgical treatment that resulted in scarring and, in very rare cases, infections.

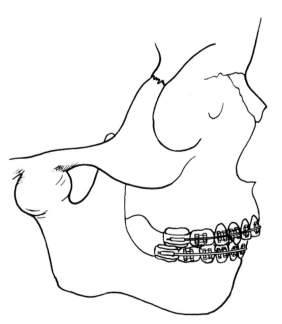

◇ Figure 30-17

Bony ankylosis. Diagram represents complete bone fusion of condyle process and glenoid fossa area.

Evaluation of the patient reveals severe restriction of maximal opening, deviation to the affected side, and decreased lateral excursions to the contralateral side. If the ankylosis is the result primarily of fibrous tissue, jaw mobility will be greater than if the ankylosis is a result of bone fusion.

Radiographic evaluation reveals irregular articular surfaces of the condyle and fossa, with varying degrees of calcified connection between these articulating surfaces.

EXTRACAPSULAR ANKYLOSIS. This type of ankylosis usually involves the coronoid process and temporalis muscle. Frequent causes of extracapsular ankylosis are coronoid process enlargement, or hyperplasia, and trauma to the zygomatic arch area. Infection around the temporalis muscle may also produce extracapsular ankylosis.

Patients initially have limitation of opening and deviation to the affected side. In these cases, complete restriction of opening is extremely rare. Although limited lateral and protrusive movements can usually be performed, indicating that there is no intracapsular ankylosis, panoramic radiography generally demonstrates the elongation of a coronoid process. A submental vertex radiograph may be useful in demonstrating impingement caused by a fractured zygomatic arch or zygomaticomaxillary complex.

NEOPLASIA

Neoplasms in the TMJ are extremely rare. They can occasionally result in restriction of opening and joint pain. Tumors within the TMJ may result in an abnormal condyle fossa relationship or an intracapsular ankylosis. A complete discussion of the neoplastic processes known to occur in the TMJ area is beyond the scope of this chapter.

INFECTIONS

Infections in the TMJ area are extremely rare, even in the case of trauma or surgical intervention in this area. In Third World countries where antibiotic therapy of middle ear infections is not available, extension of infectious processes may occasionally involve the TMJ and result in intracapsular ankylosis.

REVERSIBLE TREATMENT ——◇

Although the cause of TM pain and dysfunction can arise from several different sources, initial treatment is frequently aimed at nonsurgical methods of reducing pain and discomfort, decreasing inflammation in muscles and joints, and improving jaw function. In some cases, such as ankylosis or severe joint degeneration, surgical treatment may be the preferred initial course of therapy. However, in most cases, including MPD, disk displacement disorders, and degenerative and systemic arthritic disorders, a nonsurgical, reversible treatment phase may provide significant reduction in pain and improvement in function. In fact, most patients with MPD and internal derangements do extremely well without any type of long-term or invasive treatment. In the case of anterior disk displacement without reduction (closed lock) most patients experience a gradual progression of increased opening and decreased discomfort without extensive treatment. This is apparently the result of physiologic and anatomic adaptation of tissue within the joint. It appears that in many patients the posterior attachment tissue undergoes fibrous adaptation and adequately serves as interpositioning tissue between the condyle and fossa.[3] This is often termed *pseudodisk adaptation* (Figure 30-18). This pseudodisk formation combined with other normal healing capabilities of joints is most likely responsible for clinical improvement in many patients.

PATIENT EDUCATION

The first step in involving patients in their own treatment is to make them aware of the pathology producing their pain and dysfunction and to describe the prognosis or possible progression of their pain and dysfunction. Many problems of masticatory pain and dysfunction stabilize or improve with conservative therapy, despite patients' concerns that they may be on a continually deteriorating course. In the case of a patient with MPD a precise, confident explanation should attempt to assure the patient that muscular pain usually improves with minimal treatment and that even though symptoms may recur on occasion, they generally can be controlled with the treatment described later in this chapter.

In some cases, such as DJD, the patient should be made aware of the long-term spectrum of outcomes of this problem. Warning signs of further deterioration, including increased pain, limitation of motion, and increased joint noise, should be emphasized to the patient.

Patients who have an awareness of the factors associated with their pain and dysfunction can actively participate in their own improvement. Myofascial pain often results from parafunctional habits or muscular hyperactivity secondary to stress and anxiety. Patients who are aware of these factors are often able to control their activity and thereby reduce discomfort and improve function. Biofeedback devices provide information to patients to help them control their muscular activity. For example, the output from surface electrodes over the masseter or temporalis muscle can be used to indicate clenching or grinding during daytime activity (Figure 30-19).[20] EMG recordings can also be useful in evaluating nocturnal bruxism and associated pain and can be used to monitor the effectiveness of splint therapy and medication to control muscular hyperactivity. Other forms of stress control, such as physical exercise, reducing exposure to stressful situations, and psychologic counseling, can also be explored. When the patient becomes aware of the relationship between his or her own actions and the symptoms of pain and dysfunction, behavior modification can follow.

Modification of diet and home exercise routines are also an important part of the patient's educational process. The patients who experience TM pain or dysfunction frequently find that it is most apparent when chewing hard food. Temporary alteration of the diet with nonchew, blenderized food may result in a significant reduction in symptoms. A gradual progression to a more normal diet over a period of 6 weeks may be sufficient to reduce joint or muscle symptoms.

Although the patient is generally encouraged to reduce the functional load placed on the joint and muscles, it is important to remember that maximizing range of motion is also an important aspect of treatment of all TM disorders. Home exercises may be helpful in maintaining normal function. These exercises include gentle stretching exercises done to pain tolerance through passive opening or active exercise routines. In some cases, patients can obtain simple appliances that provide easy and efficient methods for improving jaw mobility (Figure 30-20).

MEDICATION

Four types of medication are generally useful in the treatment of TM disorders. These include nonsteroidal antiinflammatory drugs, occasional use of stronger analgesics, muscular relaxants, and tricyclic antidepressants.

Nonsteroidal antiinflammatory drugs (NSAIDs) not only reduce inflammation but also serve as an excellent analgesic. Some examples of NSAIDs are naproxen (Naprosyn), ibuprofen (Motrin), diflunisal (Dolobid), and piroxicam (Feldene). These medications can be effective in reducing inflammation in both muscles and joints and in most cases provide satisfactory pain relief. These drugs are not associated with severe addiction problems, and their use as an analgesic is strongly preferred over narcotic medications. It is important to remember that these medications work best when administered on a timetable rather than on a pain-dependent schedule. Patients should be instructed to take the medicine on a regular basis, obtaining an adequate blood level that should then be maintained for a minimum of 14 to 21 days. Discontinuation or tapering of the medicine can then be attempted.

Analgesic medicines for TMJ patients may range from acetaminophen to potent narcotics. One important principle of treatment for all pain and dysfunction patients is to remember that the problem may be chronic and that medication could produce long-term addiction. Because of the sedative and depressive effects of narcotics and their potential for addic-

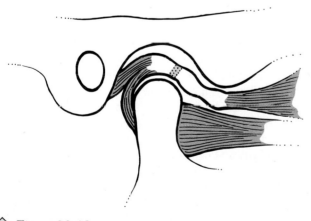

◇ Figure 30-18

Pseudodisk adaptation. When disk becomes anteriorly displaced, retrodiskal tissue undergoes fibrous adaptation, producing functional, although anatomically different, interpositional disk.

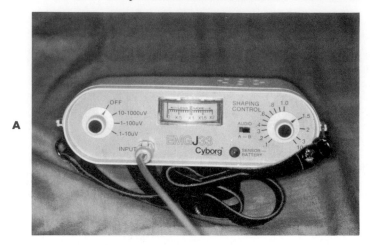

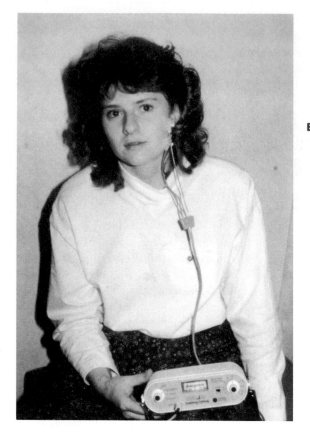

Figure 30-19

EMG biofeedback monitor. **A,** This instrument provides audio and visual (meter) output (**B**), allowing patient to hear and see increased muscle activity. Various treatments, such as physical therapy, splint therapy, and medication, can then be used to reduce muscle activity.

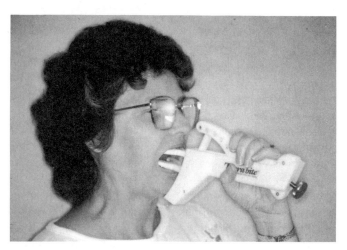

Figure 30-20

Jaw exercising device. Therabite appliance can be used by patient to increase range of jaw motion.

tion, these medications should be restricted to short-term use in patients with severe, acute pain. In such instances, medications such as acetaminophen with codeine should be sufficient. This medication should not be used for longer than 10 days to 2 weeks.

Muscle relaxants may provide significant improvement in jaw function and relief of masticatory pain. However, muscle relaxants have a significant potential for depression and sedation and can produce long-term addiction. In many patients with acute pain or exacerbation of muscular hyperactivity, muscle relaxants can be considered for short periods, such as 10 days to 2 weeks. The lowest effective dose should be used. Diazepam (Valium) 2 to 5 mg or cyclobenzaprine (Flexeril) 10 mg generally provides adequate relief of muscular symptoms in patients with TMJ.

Tricyclic antidepressants in low doses appear to be useful in the management of patients with chronic pain. Tricyclic antidepressants prevent the reuptake of amine neurotransmitters, such as serotonin and norepinephrine, causing an inhibition of pain transmission. Recently, anecdotal evidence has suggested that these antidepressants may be effective in decreasing nocturnal bruxism. It appears that nighttime bruxing may be in part a result of disruption of normal sleep patterns. The use of amitriptyline (Elavil) in small doses (10 to 25 mg at bedtime) may improve sleep patterns, decrease bruxism, and result in decreased joint and muscle pain.

PHYSICAL THERAPY

Physical therapy can be extremely useful in the management of patients with TM pain and dysfunction. The most common modalities used include electromyographic (EMG) biofeedback and relaxation training, ultrasound, spray and stretch, and pressure massage.

Relaxation training, although perhaps not physical therapy in the strictest sense, can be extremely effective in reducing symptoms caused by muscular pain and hyperactivity. During the educational phase, patients are made aware of the contribution of stress and muscular hyperactivity to pain.

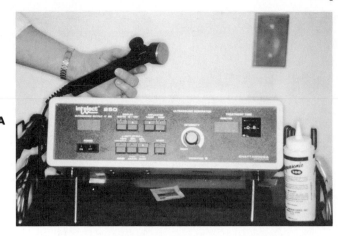 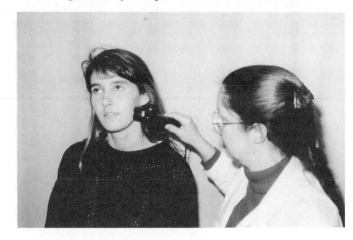

A

B

◇ Figure 30-21

A, Ultrasound unit for TM joint/facial pain physical therapy. **B,** Application of ultrasound to masseter muscle area.

Relaxation techniques can be used to reduce the effects of stress on muscle and joint pain. EMG monitoring of the patient's muscular activity can be used as an effective teaching tool by providing instant feedback demonstrating relaxation therapy, reduction of muscular hyperactivity, and the resultant improvement in symptoms of pain.

Ultrasound is an effective way to produce tissue heating with the use of ultrasonic waves, which alter blood flow and metabolic activity at a deeper level than that provided by simple surface moist-heat applications.[5] The effect of ultrasonic tissue heating is theoretically related to increase in tissue temperature, increase in circulation, increase in uptake of painful metabolic byproducts, and disruption of collagen cross-linking, which may affect adhesion formation. All of these effects may result in a more comfortable manipulation of muscles and a wider range of motion. In addition, intraarticular inflammation may also be reduced with ultrasonic applications. Ultrasonic treatments are usually provided by a physical therapist in combination with other treatment modalities. The typical routine for application of ultrasound is the use of 0.7 to 1 watts per cm^2 applied for approximately 10 minutes over the affected areas (i.e., temporalis and masseter muscles and TM joint) (Figure 30-21). Ultrasonic treatments are most effective when repeated every other day or every third day for several consecutive treatments.

Spray and stretch is an effective method for improving range of motion. The theory behind spray and stretch is the concept that stimulating large cutaneous nerve fibers can produce an inhibitory or overriding effect on pain input from smaller fibers that originate in the muscles and joints.[24] By spraying a vapocoolant material, such as fluormethane, over the lateral surface of the face, the muscles of mastication can be passively or actively stretched with a reduced level of pain because of the inhibitory input from cold stimulation to cutaneous fibers (Figure 30-22).

Friction massage involves the use of firm cutaneous pressure sufficient to produce a temporary degree of ischemia.

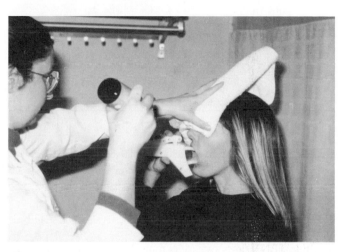

◇ Figure 30-22

Spray and stretch technique. Vapocoolant is applied while patient performs increased range-of-motion exercises using Therabite appliance.

This ischemia and the resultant hyperemia have been described as a method for inactivation of trigger points, which are areas responsible for pain referred to muscles in the head and neck area.[24] More frequently, this technique may be useful in disrupting small fibrous connective tissue adhesions that may develop within the muscles during healing after surgery and injury or as a result of prolonged muscular shortening from restricted motion.

Transcutaneous electronic nerve stimulation (TENS) is sometimes used by physical therapists and other practitioners to provide pain relief for chronic pain patients when other techniques have been unable to eliminate or reduce pain symptoms (Figure 30-23). This technique is based on the concept that stimulation of superficial nerve fiber with transcutaneous electronic stimulation may be responsible for overriding pain input from structures such as mastica-

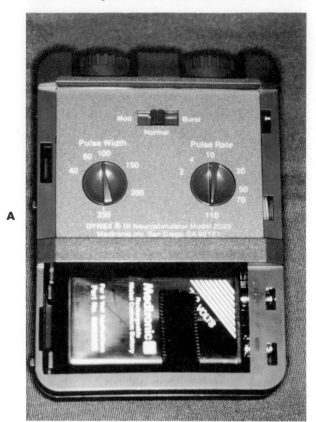

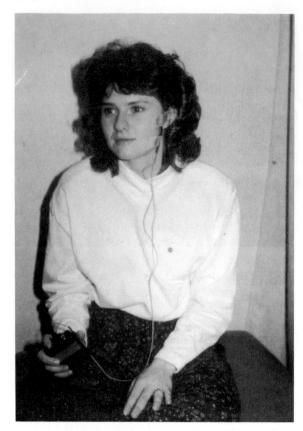

◇ **Figure 30-23**

TENS (*t*ranscutaneous *e*lectronic *n*erve *s*timulation). **A,** Unit used for applying electrical stimulation to face. **B,** Placement of electrodes over masseter muscle area for application of electric stimulus.

tory muscles and the TMJs. Interestingly, many patients who use TENS units experience pain relief that is longer in duration than the time during which the unit is actually applied. This may be a result of the release of endogenous endorphin compounds that can provide extended periods of decreased pain.

Each of the physical therapy modalities may be extremely useful in initial attempts to reduce TMJ pain and increase range of motion. The low cost of physical therapy compared with other medical treatment, the likelihood that some benefit will occur, and the minimal risk associated with these techniques are strong arguments for frequent use of physical therapy in the management of patients with TMD.

SPLINTS

Occlusal splints are generally considered a part of the reversible or conservative treatment phase in the management of TMD patients. There are many variations on splint designs; however, most splints can be classified into two distinct groups, autorepositioning splints and anterior repositioning splints.

AUTOREPOSITIONAL SPLINTS. The autorepositioning splints, also called *anterior guidance splints, superior repo-*sitioning splints, or *muscle splints,* are most frequently used to treat muscle problems or eliminate TMJ pain when no specific internal derangement or other obvious pathology can be identified. However, these splints may be used in some cases, such as anterior disk displacement or DJD, in an attempt to unload or reduce the force placed directly on the TMJ area. The splint is usually designed to provide full-arch contact without working or balancing interferences and without ramps or deep interdigitation, which would force the mandible to function in one specific occlusal position (Figure 30-24). This splint allows the patient to seek a comfortable muscle and joint position without excessive influence of the occlusion. An example of this type of splint would be in a patient with a class II malocclusion and significant overjet who continually postures forward to obtain incisor contact during mastication. Many of these patients complain of muscular symptoms and describe a feeling that they do not have a consistent, repeatable bite relationship. Wearing an autorepositional splint allows full-arch dental contact with the condyles in a more posterior retruded position, which frequently results in reduction in muscle and joint symptoms.

ANTERIOR REPOSITIONING SPLINT. The anterior repositioning splint is constructed so that there is an anterior

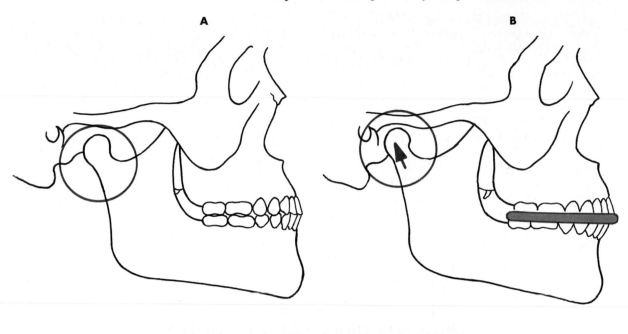

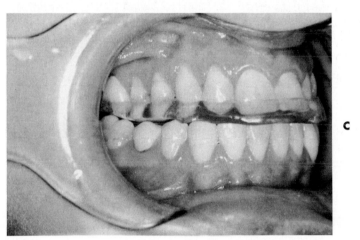

◇ Figure 30-24

Autorepositioning splint. **A,** Diagram representing maximum interdigitation obtained with condyle slightly down and forward. **B,** Repositioning of mandible by eliminating forced interdigitation of teeth results in posterior and superior repositioning of condyle. **C,** Clinical photograph of autorepositioning splint.

ramping effect forcing the mandible to function in a protruded position (Figure 30-25). This splint is most useful in providing temporary relief and, in some cases, a long-term cure for anterior disk displacement with reduction. In these cases the anterior position is determined by protrusion of the mandible necessary to produce the proper disk-condyle relationships (after the protruding or opening click has occurred). The splint is usually worn 24 hours a day for several months. Theoretically, after the disk is repositioned for a long period, the posterior ligaments may shorten and maintain the disk in proper relationship to the condyle. These splints are generally ineffective in producing permanent reduction of disk displacement. However, even when the splints are not curative, they often provide significant relief of discomfort in the acute stages of TMJ dysfunction.

PERMANENT OCCLUSION MODIFICATION ◇

After completion of a course of reversible treatment many patients may be candidates for permanent modification of the occlusion. This permanent modification appears to be most appropriate when patients have had significant improvement in masticatory function and reduction in pain as a result of temporary alteration of occlusal position with splint therapy.

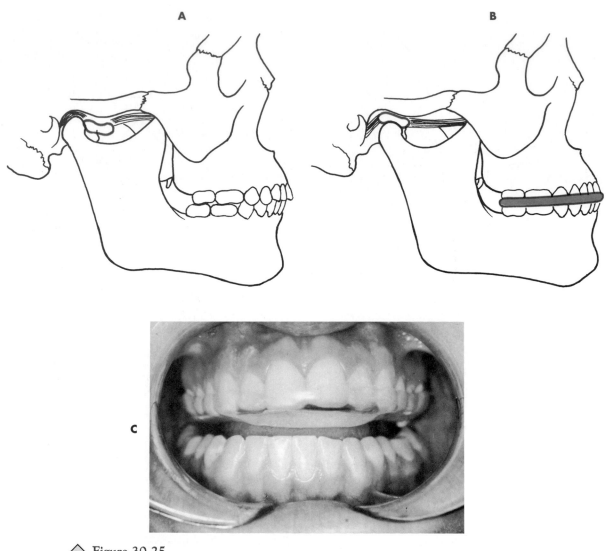

◇ **Figure 30-25**

Anterior repositioning splint. **A,** Diagram of anteriorly displaced disk. **B,** Disk interposition between condyle and articular eminence, with anterior repositioning splint in place. Anterior position of mandible allows function with condyle in appropriate condyle-disk relationship. **C,** Clinical photograph of anterior repositioning splint.

Permanent occlusion modification may include occlusal equilibration, prosthetic restoration, orthodontics, and orthognathic surgery. Although the relationship between occlusion abnormalities and TMD is unclear, it does appear that permanent modification of the occlusion in indicated patients may provide long-term improvement in symptoms of pain and dysfunction.

TEMPOROMANDIBULAR JOINT SURGERY ◇

Despite the fact that many patients with internal joint pathology will improve with reversible nonsurgical treatment, some patients will eventually require surgical intervention to improve masticatory function and decrease pain. Several techniques are currently available for correction of a variety of TMJ derangements.

ARTHROCENTESIS

Arthrocentesis involves placing needles into the temporomandibular joint and therefore is not actually a surgical procedure. However, because it is somewhat invasive and generally performed by oral and maxillofacial surgeons it is discussed here.

Most patients undergoing arthrocentesis do so with local anesthesia and intravenous sedation. Several techniques have been described for TMJ arthrocentesis.[16] The most common method involves initially placing one needle into the superior joint space. A small amount of lactated Ringers solution is

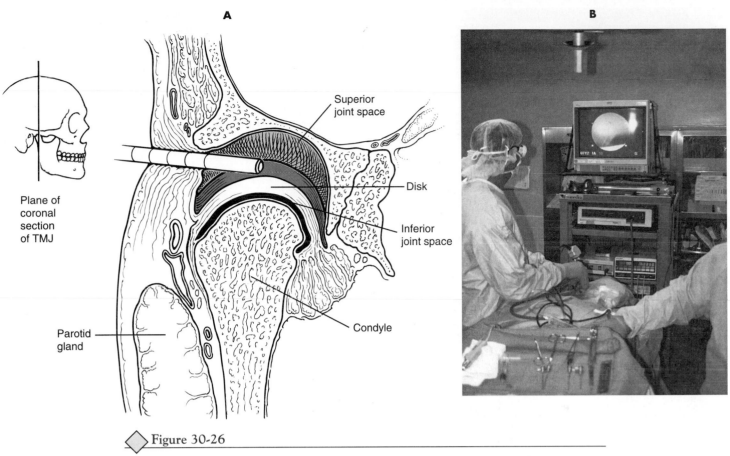

Continued

A, Diagram of arthroscope placed in superior joint space. **B,** Operating room setup for arthroscopy.

injected to distend the joint space and can then be withdrawn and evaluated for diagnostic purposes if desired. The joint is redistended, and a second needle is placed into the superior joint space. This allows larger amounts of fluid (approximately 200 mL) to lavage the joint. During the arthrocentesis the jaw can be gently manipulated. At the conclusion of the procedure steroids, local anesthesia, or a combination of both can be injected into the joint space before the needles are withdrawn. Discomfort after the procedure is managed with mild analgesics or NSAIDs. Some type of exercise regimen or physical therapy is accomplished during the recovery period.

Many types of internal joint pathology appears to respond well to arthrocentesis. The most common use appears to be in patients with anterior disk displacement without reduction. Treatment appears to be very effective, with results similar to other types of arthroscopic and open surgical procedures. Nitzan[15] compiled the results from three centers treating 68 patients and found interincisal opening increasing from 25 mm before arthrocentesis to 43 mm after treatment. These patients also experienced a significant reduction in pain symptoms.

There are several potential explanations for the success seen with arthrocentesis. When disk displacement occurs, negative pressure may develop within the joint, causing a 'suction cup' effect between the disk and fossa. Distending the joint obviously eliminates the negative pressure. In some cases of more chronic disk displacement, some adhesion may develop between the disk and fossa. With arthrocentesis the distension under pressure can release these adhesions. Capsular constriction may occur as a result of joint hypomobility and can be stretched with pressure distension. Finally, there may be an accumulation of some of the chemical mediators described above. The simple flushing action in the joint may eliminate or decrease biochemical factors contributing to inflammation and pain.

ARTHROSCOPY

Arthroscopic surgery has become one of the most popular and effective methods of diagnosing and treating TMJ disorders.[22] This technique involves placement of a small cannula into the superior joint space. An arthroscope with light source is then inserted through the cannula into the superior joint space (Figure 30-26). The arthroscope is then connected to a TV camera and video monitor, which allow excellent visualization of all aspects of the glenoid fossa and superior aspect of the disk. Initial arthroscopic techniques are limited primarily to visualization of the joint for diagnostic purposes and lysis of fibrous joint adhesions, combined with lavage of the joint.

More sophisticated arthroscopic operative techniques have been developed, increasing the ability of the surgeon to correct

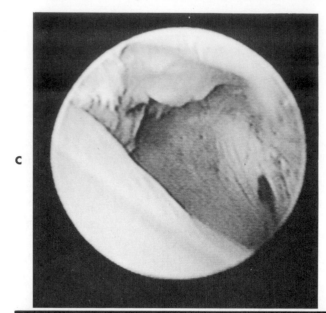

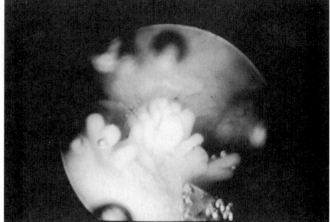

Figure 30-26, cont'd

C, View of superior joint space. Inferiorly, disk tissue can be clearly visualized. Superiorly, fibrous tissue covering fossa is disrupted as result of separation of adhesions with arthroscopic surgical techniques. **D,** Close-up view of synovial tissue hypertrophy.   *Continued*

a variety of intracapsular disorders. Current surgical techniques usually involve the placement of at least two cannulas into the superior joint space. One cannula is used for visualization of the procedure with the arthroscope while instruments are placed through the other cannula, allowing instrumentation in the joint (Figure 30-26, *E* through *G*). Instrumentation used through the arthroscope includes forceps, scissors, sutures, medication needles, cautery probes, and motorized instrumentation, such as burs and shavers. Laser fibers can also be used to eliminate adhesions and inflamed tissue and incise tissue within the joint. Disk manipulation, disk attachment release, posterior band cautery, and suture techniques have been developed in an attempt to reposition or stabilize displaced disks.[13] Although it appears that attempts to reposition displaced disks do not result in anatomic restoration of normal disk position, patients under-

going this type of treatment appear to have significant clinical improvement after arthroscopic surgery.[14]

Arthroscopic surgery has been advocated for treatment of a variety of TMJ disorders, including internal derangements, hypomobility as a result of fibrosis or adhesions, DJD, and hypermobility. The efficacy of arthroscopic treatment appears to be very similar to that of open joint procedures, with the advantage of less surgical morbidity and fewer and less severe complications.[13,14,22]

As with most TMJ surgical procedures, patients are placed on some type of physical therapy regimen following surgical treatment.

DISK REPOSITIONING SURGERY

During the late 1970s and 1980s one of the most commonly performed TMJ surgical procedures was disk repositioning and plication. The indication for this procedure is anterior disk displacement that has not responded to nonsurgical treatment and that most frequently results in persistent painful clicking joints or closed locking (i.e., anterior disk displacement with or without reduction). Although these disorders are more frequently managed surgically with arthrocentesis or arthroscopy, many surgeons still prefer this type of surgical correction. In this operation the displaced disk is identified and repositioned into a more normal position by removing a wedge of tissue from the posterior attachment of the disk and suturing the disk back to the correct anatomic position (Figure 30-27). In some cases this procedure is combined with recontouring of the disk, articular eminence, and mandibular condyle. Following surgery, patients generally begin a nonchew diet for several weeks, progressing to a relatively normal diet in 3 to 6 months. A progressive regimen of jaw exercises is also instituted in an attempt to obtain normal jaw motion within 6 to 8 weeks after surgery.

In general, the results of open arthroplasty have been good, with 80% to 90% of the patients having less pain and improved jaw function. Approximately 50% of the patients are totally pain free postsurgically. In addition, another 35% have significant decrease in pain and improvement in function. Unfortunately, this surgery does not produce improvement in all patients, with 10% to 15% of patients describing no improvement or a worsening of the condition.

DISK REPAIR OR REMOVAL

In advanced internal joint pathology, the disk may be severely damaged. In some cases the disk may be perforated but may have adequate remaining disk tissue so that a repair or patch procedure can be accomplished (Figure 30-28). A variety of autogenous tissue sources have been used for disk repair, including grafts of dermal or fascial tissue.

In some cases the disk is so severely damaged that the remnants of disk tissue must be removed. Until recently the disk was usually replaced with alloplastic implant material. However, significant failures have been seen with many of these implant materials, including implant fragmentation, foreign body reaction, synovitis, and gross erosion of bony articular surfaces. These problems have led to a renewed

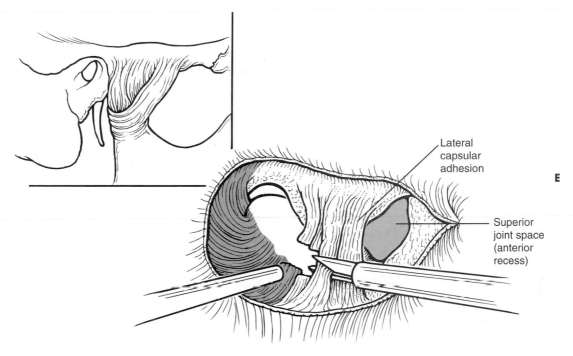

Lateral capsular adhesion

Superior joint space (anterior recess)

E

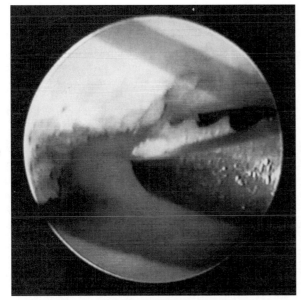

F

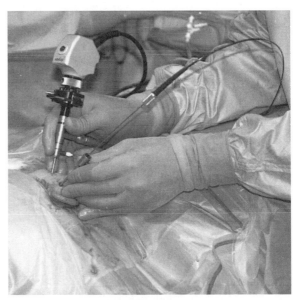

G

◇ Figure 30-26, cont'd

E, Diagram of arthroscope and working cannula using surgical microscissors placed through cannula to cut fibrous band. **F,** View through arthroscope of motorized shaver used to remove fibrous tissue from articular surface. **G,** Arthroscopic surgery using laser fiber inserted through working cannula.

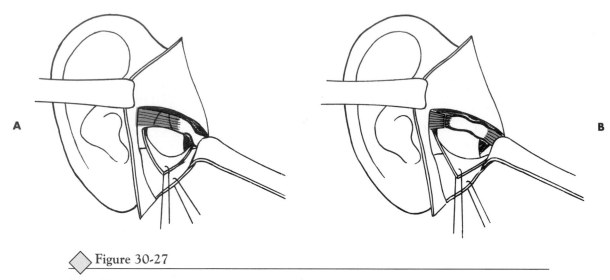

◆ Figure 30-27

Open TMJ surgical procedure to replace displaced disk. **A,** Preauricular incision through skin subcutaneous tissue and TMJ capsule, exposing anteriorly displaced disk. **B,** Wedge of tissue is removed from posterior attachment area, and disk is repositioned and sutured into its correct position.

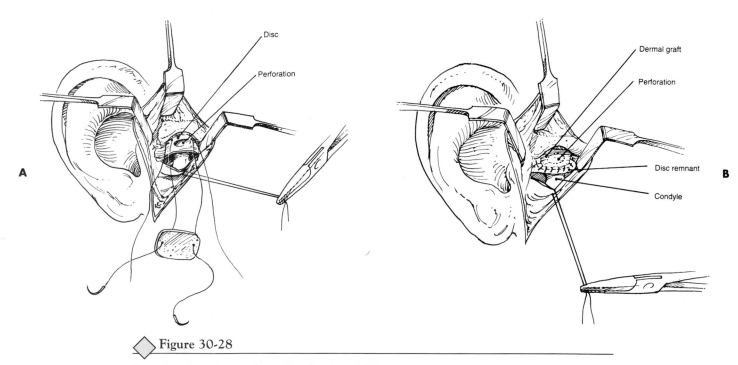

◆ Figure 30-28

Dermal graft used to patch small perforation of disk.

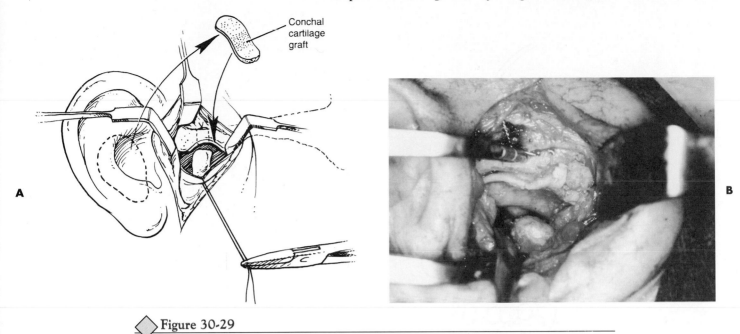

◇ **Figure 30-29**

A, Diagram of auricular cartilage harvested from inferior portion of ear, used as a graft material in TMJ following removal of disk tissue. **B,** Clinical photograph.

interest in autogenous tissue replacement following disk removal. Autogenous grafting techniques include the use of auricular cartilage, temporalis fascia, and the combination of muscle and fascial flaps (Figure 30-29).[27] Many surgeons advocate removal of the disk without use of any interpositioning tissue as a replacement material. The use of silastic as a temporary replacement has also been advocated.[26] This technique uses a thin sheet of silastic placed between the condyle and fossa to eliminate connective tissue adhesions following surgery. The piece of silastic is then removed in a minor office procedure 8 to 12 weeks following the open-joint surgery. Although long-term results of each of these techniques are limited, most patients realize significant improvement in pain and function following these procedures.

CONDYLOTOMY FOR TREATMENT OF TMJ DISORDERS

The condylotomy is an osteotomy completed in a manner identical to the vertical ramus osteotomy described in Chapter 26. When used for treatment of TMJ problems the osteotomy is completed, but no wire or screw fixation is placed, and the patient is placed into intermaxillary fixation for a period ranging from 2 to 6 weeks. The theory behind this operation is that muscles attached to the proximal segment (segment attached to the condyle) will passively reposition the condyle, resulting in a more favorable relationship between the condyle, disk, and fossa.[18]

This technique has been advocated primarily for treatment of disk displacement with or without reduction. DJD and subluxation or dislocation have also been suggested as possible indications for use of this technique. Although this method of surgical treatment has been somewhat controver-

sial, it appears to provide significant clinical improvement in a variety of TMJ disorders.

ARTHROPLASTY FOR ANKYLOSIS

One absolute indication for open-joint arthroplasty is in cases of bony intracapsular ankylosis. In these cases a surgical procedure is the only method available for improving jaw function. The surgery involves an arthroplasty to separate the condyle and fossa at the point of fusion. After the ankylosis is released, recontouring of the condyle and fossa is completed. Coronoidectomy on the affected side may also then be performed to release the possible influence of muscular restriction on opening. The surgical gap created is then maintained, usually with the use of an alloplastic material, such as silastic. Tissue grafts may be used in isolation or in combination with a silastic interpositioning material to maintain bone separation. Problems associated with foreign body reactions to material such as silastic have caused some concern regarding placement of alloplastic materials within the joint. However, in many cases this remains one of few options available. When ankylosis and/or surgical release result in significant loss of bony tissue, joint replacement techniques may be indicated, as described below. Following arthroplasty and coronoid release, vigorous jaw manipulation is usually completed intraoperatively.

TOTAL JOINT REPLACEMENT

In some cases, joint pathology results in destruction of joint structures, so that reconstruction or replacement of components of the TMJ is necessary (Figure 30-30, *A*). Examples of such situations include severe degenerative or rheumatoid arthritic disorders, severe cases of ankylosis, neoplastic

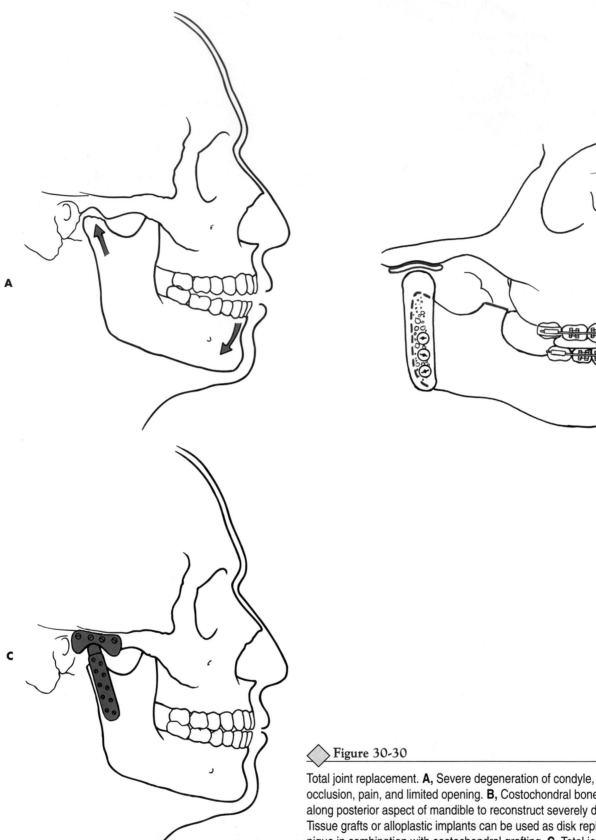

◆ Figure 30-30

Total joint replacement. **A,** Severe degeneration of condyle, resulting in mal-occlusion, pain, and limited opening. **B,** Costochondral bone graft placed along posterior aspect of mandible to reconstruct severely damaged condyle. Tissue grafts or alloplastic implants can be used as disk replacement technique in combination with costochondral grafting. **C,** Total joint reconstruction with prosthetic replacement of both condyle and fossa components.

pathology, and posttraumatic destruction of joint components. Surgical techniques may involve replacement of the condyle or fossa or both elements. One common method of joint reconstruction involves grafting autogenous tissue using a costochondral bone graft.[11] These grafts are most frequently used in growing individuals but also can be used effectively in the treatment of a variety of adult disorders. Figure 30-30, *B* shows the use of a costochondral graft for replacement of a severely degenerated mandibular condyle. In this situation the graft replaces only the condylar portion of the joint and does not address significant abnormalities of the fossa.

In the past, several types of prosthetic joint replacement have been available.[9] However, long-term results of prosthetic joint replacements have been somewhat disappointing because of a variety of technique and biologic problems. However, for many patients with significant destruction of TMJ structures who have had poor results from other surgical treatment, there are no other viable surgical options. In these cases the joint destruction results in severe pain, limited motion or complete ankylosis, and severe malocclusions (Figure 30-30, *C*). Total joint replacement can replace the condyle and fossa, resulting in improved jaw motion, decreased pain, and correction of the occlusal relationship.[18,25]

REFERENCES

1. Blair GS et al: Circular tomography of the temporomandibular joint, *Oral Surg Oral Med Oral Pathol* 35:416, 1973.
2. Blaschke DD, White SC: Radiolog. In Sarnat BG, Laskin DM, editors: *The temporomandibular joint: biological diagnosis and treatment,* ed 3, Springfield, Ill, 1980, Charles C Thomas.
3. Blaustein D, Scappino RP: Remodelling of the temporomandibular joint disk and posterior attachment in disk displacement specimens in relation to glycosaminoglycan content, *Plast Reconstr Surg* 78:756, 1986.
4. Dolwick MF et al: Arthrotomographic evaluation of the temporomandibular joint, *J Oral Surg* 37:793, 1979.
5. Griffin JE, Karselis GD, Terrence C: *Ultrasonic energy in physical agents for physical therapists,* Springield, Ill, 1979, Charles C Thomas.
6. Helms CA et al: Computed tomography of the temporomandibular joint: preliminary observations, *Radiology* 145:719, 1982.
7. Holmlund A et al: Concentrations of neuropeptide substance P, meruokinin A, calcitonin gene-related peptide, neuropeptide Y, and vasoactive intestinal polypeptide in synovial fluid of human temporomandibular joint: a correlation with symptoms, signs, and arthroscopic findings, *Int J Oral Maxillofac Surg* 20:228, 1991.
8. Israel HA, Saed-Nejad R, Ratliffe A: Early diagnosis of osteoarthrosis of the temporomandibular joint: correlation between arthroscopic diagnosis and keratan sulfate levels in the synovial fluid, *J Oral Maxillofac Surg* 49:708, 1991.
9. Kent JN et al: Temporomandibular joint condylar prosthesis: a ten-year report, *J Oral Maxillofac Surg* 41:245, 1983.
10. Laskin DM: Etiology of the pain-dysfunction syndrome, *J Am Dent Assoc* 79:147, 1969.
11. Lindqvist C et al: Adaptation of autogenous costocondylar grafts used for temporomandibular joint reconstruction, *J Oral Maxillofac Surg* 46:465, 1988.
12. Manzione JV et al: Magnetic resonance imaging of the temporomandibular joint, *J Am Dent Assoc* 3:398, 1986.
13. McCain J, Podrasky A, Zabiegalskin NA: Arthroscopic disc repositioning and suturing: a preliminary report, *J Oral Maxillofac Surg* 50:568, 1992.
14. Moses J et al: The effect of arthroscopic surgical lysis and lavage of the superior joint space on TMJ disk position and mobility, *J Oral Maxillofac Surg* 47:674, 1989.
15. Nitzan DW: Arthrocentesis for management of severe closed lock of the temporomandibular joint: current controversies in surgery for internal derangement of the temporomandibular joint, *Oral Maxillofac Surg Clin North Am* 6:245, 1994.
16. Nitzan DW, Dolwick MF, Martinez GA: Temporomandibular joint arthrocentesis: a simplified treatment for severe limited mouth opening, *J Oral Maxillofac Surg* 48:163, 1991.
17. Oesterreich FU et al: Semi-quantitative SPECT imaging for assessment of bone reaction to internal derangements of the temporomandibular joint, *J Oral Maxillofac Surg* 45:1022, 1987.
18. *Proceedings of the symposium on current concepts of TMJ total joint replacement,* University of New Jersey School of Medicine and Dentistry, Health Science Center, Newark, Mar 20, 1992.
19. Quinn JH, Bazan NG: Identification of prostaglandin E_2 and leukotriene BA_4 in the synovial fluid of painful dysfunctional temporomandibular joints, *J Oral Maxillofac Surg* 48:968, 1990.
20. Riggs RR, Rugh JD, Borghi W: Muscle activity of MPD and TMJ patients and nonpatients, *J Dent Res* 61:277, 1982 (abstract).
21. Rugh JD, Solberg WK: Psychological implications in temporomandibular pain and dysfunction, *Oral Sci Rev* 7:3, 1976.
22. Sanders B, Buoncristiani R: Diagnostic and surgical arthroscopy of the temporomandibular joint: clinical experience with 137 procedures over a two year period, *J Craniomandib Disord* 1:202, 1987.
23. Sternback RA: Varieties of pain games. In Bonica JJ, editor: *Advances in neurology: international symposium on pain,* vol 4, New York, 1973, Raven.
24. Travell JG, Simons DJ: *Myofacial muscles in myofascial pain and dysfunction: the trigger point manual,* Baltimore, 1983, Williams & Wilkins.
25. Tucker MR, Proffit WR: Temporomandibular dysfunction: considerations in the surgical orthodontic patient. In Proffit WR, White RP Jr, editors: *Surgical-orthodontic treatment,* St Louis, 1990, Mosby.
26. Tucker MR, Watzke IM: Autogenous auricular cartilage graft for temporomandibular joint repair: a comparison of techniques with and without temporary silastic implantation, *J Craniomaxillofac Surg* 19:99, 1991.
27. Tucker MR, Jacoway JR, White RP Jr: Use of autogenous dermal graft for repair of TMJ meniscus perforations, *J Oral Maxillofac Surg* 44:781, 1986.
28. Zeitler D, Porter B: A retrospective study comparing arthroscopic surgery with arthrotomy and disc repositioning. In Clark G, Sanders B, Bertolami C, editors: *Advances in diagnostic and surgical arthroscopy of the temporomandibular joint,* Philadelphia, 1993, WB Saunders.

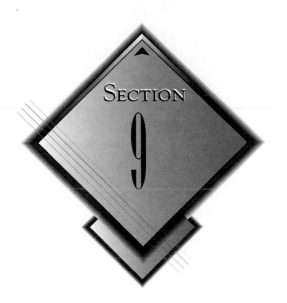

MANAGEMENT OF THE HOSPITALIZED PATIENT

The willingness and ability of a dental practitioner to manage hospitalized patients can be both a fulfilling experience for the dentist and a tremendous service to the dentist's patients and community. Patients with serious medical problems requiring dental care sometimes need the facilities and staff support available only in a hospital. Institutionalized patients frequently find hospitals the only setting in which dental care can be provided. Patients hospitalized for nondental reasons occasionally develop dental problems for which definitive care cannot be deferred until they are discharged. Finally, patients with dental emergencies or facial trauma commonly go to hospital emergency departments and immediately require someone with dental expertise to provide proper evaluation and therapy.

Effective dental practice in a hospital requires more than common sense. Although each hospital is unique, there are common administrative concepts that must be learned to effectively practice in a hospital. Chapter 31 is designed to inform the reader of the common protocols used in hospitals to facilitate communication among care providers and between health care providers and agencies outside of the hospital. The chapter also describes some of the basic problems hospitalized patients may experience.

MANAGEMENT OF THE HOSPITALIZED PATIENT

JAMES R. HUPP

Most dentists find they can practice without hospital facilities, but the ability to care for patients in a hospital setting adds a stimulating dimension to a dentist's professional life. As a vital member of a community's health care team, the hospital-affiliated dentist is consulted about the dental needs of patients in the emergency room and of those admitted to the hospital by other doctors or the dentist himself or herself. Dentists who join a hospital medical staff will not only be in a position to perform dental consultations for hospitalized patients but will also be allowed to bring patients to the hospital to perform procedures best done there.

HOSPITAL GOVERNANCE ⬦
ADMINISTRATIVE ORGANIZATION
Hospital organization varies from institution to institution, but most are based on standards of the Joint Commission for the Accreditation of Healthcare Organizations (JCAHO). This national body's mission is to set standards for hospitals and ambulatory care clinics, to monitor these facilities to ensure that those standards are being met, and then to accredit hospitals and clinics meeting the standards.

Most general, acute care community hospitals have a board of trustees made up of community leaders who form the highest governing body of the institution. They are advised in health matters by a joint conference committee, which is a liaison group that includes members from hospital management, the medical staff, and the board of trustees. The hospital's chief executive officer (CEO) is in charge of the daily operation of the hospital and reports to the board of trustees. Hospital governance from this point is divided into two major organizational bodies: the medical staff and the hospital administration.

The medical staff includes all the health care professionals who work at the hospital. The chief of staff is the most senior governing member of the medical staff. He or she reports to the hospital president and joint conference committee and chairs the medical board. The medical board or executive committee commonly includes the chiefs of all the medical departments of the hospital and sometimes includes representatives from nursing and hospital administration. Dentists who become members of the medical staff are members of the dental department or division. Although at some large hospitals dentistry is on equal footing with other major departments, such as psychiatry or pediatrics, it is more often made a division, or section, of the department of surgery, similar to other surgical specialties, such as urology and neurosurgery. As a member of the medical staff, a dentist is usually asked to serve on committees in which dental expertise is needed, such as those on infection control and pharmacy and therapeutics.

Hospital administration is managed by the hospital CEO, who has several vice presidents or assistant directors to direct various areas of hospital operations, such as nursing, support services, and finance (Figure 31-1).

MEDICAL STAFF MEMBERSHIP
Membership on a hospital medical staff is not usually gained by simple request. The hospital's credentials committee,

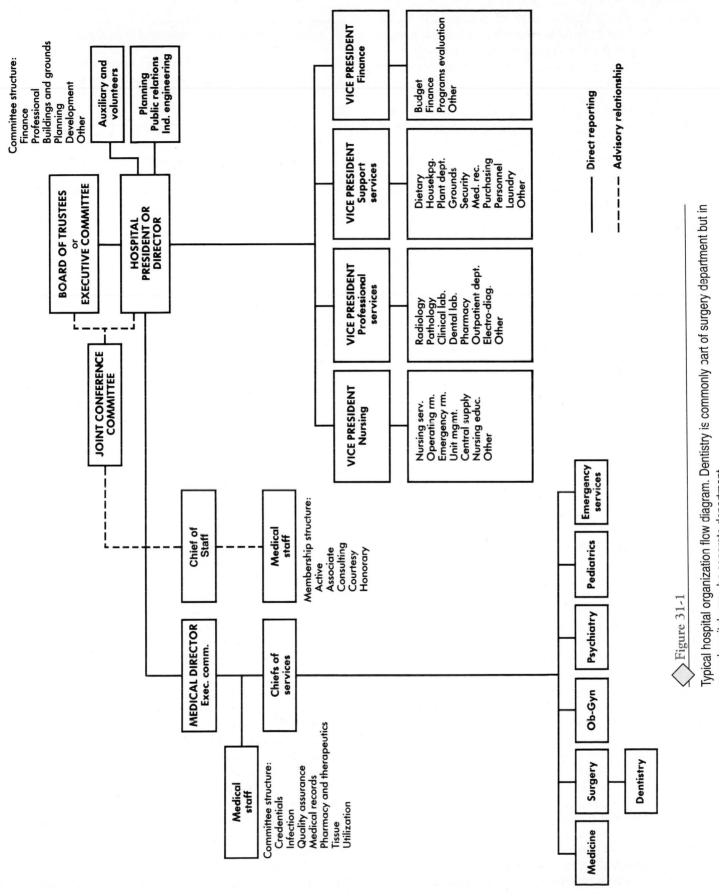

◊ Figure 31-1

Typical hospital organization flow diagram. Dentistry is commonly part of surgery department but in some hospitals may be separate department.

consisting of physicians and dentists on the medical staff, carefully reviews the qualifications of doctors applying for staff membership to ensure that individuals granted privileges are competent to practice in the hospital environment.

Various levels of medical staff membership exist (for example, active, associate, or courtesy), each carrying certain privileges and restrictions. Staff membership, however, never automatically gives the dentist the privilege to admit patients to the hospital or to use the operating room facilities. These privileges are granted based on a review of the applying dentist's education and experience. Dentists who have completed a general practice residency or dental specialty training that provided hospital experience usually have little difficulty gaining medical staff membership and some admitting privileges. However, because of hospital regulations, most dental patients admitted to a hospital by dentists other than oral and maxillofacial surgeons will require a physician's participation in the admission process.

HOSPITAL DENTISTRY
CONSULTATIONS

The request for consultation carries different connotations among health professionals. To some, the consultant is only expected to render an opinion and not to begin implementing any advice until given permission by the patient's admitting physician or, in the case of the emergency room, by the physician designated as the patient's primary care provider. However, many physicians allow consultants to perform any test or procedure necessary to act on their opinion. The dental consultant, therefore, must clarify with the requesting doctor before seeing the patient if only an opinion is being sought or if the dentist can proceed to order tests and render treatment. In some cases, the consultation request form provides a section in which the requesting doctor can indicate the type of consultation desired.

EMERGENCY ROOM CONSULTATIONS. Emergency room consultations are usually requested verbally because of the urgency of the situation. The dentist should make use of any history and physical examination, laboratory, and radiographic results already available, to avoid excessive duplication. However, the dentist should do a careful, comprehensive history and physical examination of the oral and maxillofacial region and order special radiographs as necessary to allow a complete, well-organized assessment of the patient's dentofacial problems. All of this information is then recorded in the medical record. A recommendation should be offered that considers other medical problems, acute or long-standing, and the urgency of the treatment. Guidelines for answering consultations are shown in Box 31-1, and a sample of a written emergency suite dental consultation is shown in Figure 31-2.

There is great variability in how well emergency suites are equipped for dental therapy. If the dentist cannot offer high-quality care in the emergency setting, the problem should be temporized and an appointment made for definitive care in the dental office. Dentists who are frequently called to hospital

---

◇ Box 31-1 ◇

Guidelines for answering consultations

1. State reason for consultation in opening sentence.
2. State that chart has been reviewed and patient examined.
3. Be brief but thorough, particularly with dentofacial portion of the examination.
4. Be specific with recommendations.
5. Provide contingency plans.
6. Follow up written consultation with verbal contact with requesting doctor.
7. Follow patient's progress until dental problem is resolved.

---

emergency rooms sometimes find it useful to carry in their car a set of instruments and supplies necessary for providing emergency dental care.

If more than one dentist serves as a dental consultant to an emergency room, a call schedule is usually established to designate, on a daily or weekly basis, which dentist is expected to be available in case of an emergency. The on-call dentist should make certain that the hospital is kept aware of how she or he can be quickly contacted if needed.

INPATIENT CONSULTATIONS. Dental consultation for a hospitalized patient is similar to consultations for emergency patients: the dentist is expected to evaluate the oral and maxillofacial region, offer an assessment, and formulate a treatment plan that considers the overall clinical situation. Dental consultation requests should be written on standard hospital consultation forms on which the requesting physician states the question(s) to be answered by the dental consultant. The requesting doctor should also provide a brief statement of other active problems the patient may have. If a dentist receives an unwritten or unclearly written consultation request, he or she should make an effort to clarify what is desired. The dentist should make every attempt to answer all consultation requests within 24 hours.

Written consultations should be sufficiently complete to document all significant findings (both positive and negative). The assessment should read as a concise dental problem list, and the treatment plan should be clearly written, with an indication of the priority and urgency of any necessary care. The terms used should be those a physician can understand, not technical dental terms. Excessive verbiage should be avoided. If the dentist finds it impossible to finish the evaluation without additional tests, arrangements should be made to obtain necessary tests in the near future, and a preliminary consultation note should be made to inform the requesting physician of the findings and preliminary recommendations. After seeing the patient, it is good practice to call the physician who requested the consultation to inform him or her of findings and recommendations. However, it is still necessary to record a formal answer directly on the consultation form or on a progress note, with an indication on the

CONSULTATION REPORT

Patient Identification

NORTHSIDE GENERAL HOSPITAL

TO: (Consultant and/or Service)	FROM: (Physician and/or Service)	Date Requested
Dr. Brown – Dental	Dr. Scott – ER	12/8/98

Summary and Reason for Request:

9 year old boy hit in face with ball today. Please evaluate and treat dental injuries. Thank You.

James Scott M.D.

CONSULTANT: Findings and Recommendations:

Consultation Date
12/8/98

Thank you for asking me to provide a dental consultation for this unfortunate 9 year old male baseball pitcher who was struck in the nasal area by a line-drive about two hours ago. His parents state that he fell to the ground striking the back of his head and had a 4-5 second long loss of consciousness but the patient claims he remembers being hit by the ball. Epistaxis occurred initially, but spontaneously ceased in about 10 minutes. Since the accident, the patient has been alert and seemed to his parents to be fully oriented. The patient now complains of pain in the nose and upper lip as well as a mild generalized headache.

The patient has no pertinent medical, family or social history. Patient received last tetanus booster 5 yrs. ago. He last saw his dentist 2 months ago.

The patient denies any occlusal change or oral bleeding but thinks both of his maxillary central incisors are loose. He denies any visual disturbance, problems breathing through either nasal passage, or neck pain.

My H & N exam reveals a 2x2 cm abrasion in the occipital region of his scalp. There are no palpable steps or areas of ecchymosis in the facial bones but he is tender to palpation of the nasal tip and upper lip. Inspection of the nasal septum reveals no hematoma but a fresh blood clot is present on the anterior septum of the right nares.

Use one side only: For additional space, use 2nd sheet

CONSULTATION REPORT (continued next page) M.D.

◇ Figure 31-2

Example of dental consultation form written for patient who suffered sports injury to face and whom dentist was asked to see in hospital emergency department.   *Continued*

CONSULTATION REPORT

Patient Identification

NORTHSIDE GENERAL HOSPITAL

TO: (Consultant and/or Service)	FROM: (Physician and/or Service)	Date Requested

Summary and Reason for Request:

_____ M.D.

CONSULTANT: Findings and Recommendations:	Consultation Date

Intraorally the occlusion is class I and all teeth are stable except #8 & 9 which are in good alignment but can be moved slightly in an A-P direction but cannot be intruded or rotated with gentle pressure. The inside of the upper lip has a 1cm long superficial laceration of the mucosa and the upper lip is mildly edematous. The crowns of all teeth and restorations appear intact. Neck was normal to exam.

I obtained an oblique occlusal film of the maxillary anterior teeth that shows mild enlargement of the periodontal ligament space around teeth #8 & 9 but no root fractures are visible.

Impression: ① Subluxation teeth #8&9
② Small laceration mucosal upper lip
③ Contusion upper lip and nose
④ Abrasion scalp
⑤ ? Concussion

Recommendations: ① Avoid biting anything with front teeth
② Intraoral laceration this size doesn't require repair, but pt. should rinse c̄ NS p̄ meals and NS vigorously
③ Shave hair in area of scalp abrasion. Clean c̄ betadine scrub. Keep scalp clean
④ Tetanus booster
⑤ See family dentist within 5 days
⑥ Advise parents & pt. that injured teeth may eventually require endodontic care.

Use one side only: For additional space, use 2nd sheet

CONSULTATION REPORT   *John Brown* D. M.D.

Note: I have gone ahead and carried out these recommendations and will let you make the discharge decision.

◇ **Figure 31-2, cont'd**

For legend see p. 741.

consultation form of where the answer has been written. An example of a dental consultation form is presented in Figure 31-3.

REQUESTING A CONSULTATION.   When a patient has a problem the dentist does not feel qualified to evaluate or manage alone, a formal consultation request can be made. When requesting a medical consultation, the dentist should indicate whether the consultant is free to order necessary tests and to proceed with any necessary treatment. Preferably, the requesting dentist should personally call to ask the consultant for an opinion. Alternatively, an order can be written directing a hospital clerk to call the consultant's office.

A consultant's recommendations should be viewed as an educated opinion. A doctor is under no obligation to follow a consultant's advice in its entirety or at all. The patient's attending doctor must make the final decision of which diagnostic tests to perform and what care the patient will receive.

HOSPITALIZING A PATIENT FOR DENTAL CARE

DECIDING ON HOSPITALIZATION.   The vast majority of patients needing routine dental care, including oral and maxillofacial surgery, can be safely managed in the dental office. However, occasionally there are patients who require that their dental care be provided in a hospital environment.

There are several reasons why a patient may be better treated in a hospital setting. One of the most common reasons is behavioral management. Patients unable to cooperate (for example, because of mental retardation), unwilling to cooperate (for example, uncontrollable children), or who refuse dental care while awake can be deeply sedated or placed under general anesthesia; this allows routine dental care to be delivered to these individuals quickly and safely. An operating room setting for dental treatment may also be necessary for the physically handicapped patient who is either unable to gain access to a dental office or is unable to remain relatively motionless during procedures. An operating room is also needed to provide dental care for patients with high-risk medical conditions, such as patients requiring care that cannot be delayed until the medical condition can be alleviated or improved or patients requiring emergency dental care shortly after a myocardial infarction. In some cases a patient's physician may be able to provide guidance as to the safety of office-based dental care. A final reason for planning a procedure in an operating room facility is for patients in whom acceptable local anesthesia cannot be attained, such as those requiring care on teeth in an area of severe infection. Usually these patients are best referred to an oral and maxillofacial surgeon, but hospitalization may be an alternative if the dentist feels capable of managing the surgical problem.

DAY SURGERY FACILITIES.   In the past, operating room facilities were available only in hospitals, and patients had to be admitted the day before dental surgery and remain in the hospital until the dentist believed discharge was indicated,

commonly 1 to 2 days postoperatively. However, changes have occurred in methods of delivering operating room care. Free-standing surgical centers now exist that offer staffed operating and recovery rooms, which include anesthesiologists, for patients not needing preoperative or postoperative hospitalization. Many hospitals also offer the use of their operating room and staff, without requiring hospital admission. A dentist may find that many patients unable to be cared for in the dental office can be effectively treated in day surgery facilities without hospitalization.

PREOPERATIVE PATIENT EVALUATION.   Once the decision to use an operating room facility has been made, several steps must be taken before the operation. The operating room staff must be contacted and the operating time scheduled. Most facilities need some biographic information about the patient, the reason for the procedure, the procedure planned, who will perform the procedure, how long the operating room will be in use, the type of anesthesia required (that is, sedation only or general anesthesia), and whether special equipment will be required. A hospital-based operating room must also know if the patient will be admitted; patients to be admitted must have a room reservation made and an estimated length of stay.

All operating room facilities require that a medical history and physical examination be performed before the operation. See Appendix I for guidelines for recording the history and physical examination results in the medical record. This recording can be performed either by the patient's physician before the day of the operation or, in some facilities, by the anesthesiologist during the preanesthetic consultation. Most facilities also require that any medically indicated laboratory tests, radiographs, or electrocardiograms be done at a time proximate to the surgery. Requirements vary from place to place, but the usual minimal testing necessary is a hematocrit.

"Doctor's orders" communicate patient care instructions to nurses and other hospital staff members. The dentist's orders should be accurate, clearly written, and comprehensive.

Preoperative orders are necessary for patients being admitted to a hospital or scheduled to be treated in an operating room setting without hospital admission. Orders are best written by the dentist, but may be given to nurses over the telephone. However, even telephone orders must eventually be signed by the dentist. An example of admission and preoperative orders is given in Figure 31-4. See a list of commonly used medical abbreviations in Appendix X.

Before surgery the operating dentist should place a note in the patient's record that briefly describes the nature of the patient's medical and dental problems and the expected operating room and hospital course. This note can then be used by the hospital staff to familiarize themselves with the patient's general condition and reason for admission (Figure 31-5).

CARE OF THE HOSPITALIZED PATIENT

OPERATING ROOM PROTOCOLS.   The patient's operating dentist bears the ultimate responsibility for any mishaps that occur in the operating room. Therefore the dentist must

---

CONSULTATION REPORT

Patient Identification

NORTHSIDE GENERAL HOSPITAL

TO: (Consultant and/or Service)	FROM: (Physician and/or Service)	Date Requested
Dr. Cole - Dental	Dr. Smith - Heme - Oncology	7/3/98

Summary and Reason for Request:

Right-sided oral pain for past 3 days. Patient presently receiving chemotherapy for leukemia. Please evaluate and recommend treatment.

Drew Smith M.D.

CONSULTANT: Findings and Recommendations:

Consultation Date 7/3/98

Thank you for asking me to see this seriously ill 19 year old leukemic who has a three day history of pain in the area of his lower right posterior teeth. The patient denies any previous problems in this area until a dull pain began 3 nights ago. The pain has gradually worsened and now requires narcotic analgesics for relief. The pain is well localized in the molar region, worsened by chewing, and radiates to his ear. Robert has had a metallic taste in his mouth for 2 days and reports that his gums bleed during brushing. On examination I found the dentition to be well restored but the lower right 3rd molar is only partly erupted. The tissue over-lying that tooth appears inflamed but I was unable to express pus from it on palpation. The opposing tooth tends to impinge on the inflamed tissue when Robert bites. The patient has moderate trismus and I note that although his WBC is only 500, that he is afebrile.

Impression: I believe Mr. Miller has a severe pericoronitis (inflammation of soft tissue over an impacted tooth) which is exacerbated by his immunodeficient state and trauma from the opposing tooth.

Recommendations:
① Panarex radiograph to examine entire tooth and local anatomy.
② Coagulation screen including platelet count and bleeding time
③ Oral Hygiene with 50:50 mix of NS and H_2O_2
④ Hold antibiotics unless patient becomes febrile
⑤ If coagulation studies OK, extract tooth #1 under local anesthesia
⑥ Defer removal of involved lower 3rd molar until inflammation resolves

Use one side only: For additional space, use 2nd sheet

CONSULTATION REPORT Neal Cole D.M.D.

and pts. general condition improves. Thank you for letting me see this poor young gentlemen. Please let me know if you want me to carry out my recommendations.

◇ **Figure 31-3**

Example of dental consultation form for hospital inpatient on hematology-oncology service, whom dentist was asked to see for problem with pericoronitis.

ORDER SHEET

Patient Identification

NORTHSIDE GENERAL HOSPITAL

USE BALLPOINT PEN. BEAR DOWN.
You are making up to four copies.

Unless an order is specifically noted, authorization is hereby given for the dispensing of drugs by non-proprietary nomenclature as set forth by The Pharmacy and Therapeutics Committee.

AUTOMATIC STOP ORDERS   Narcotics and anticoagulants must be rewritten within 48 hours of original order; all other drugs within 7 days.

DATE AND TIME	ORDERS	SIGNATURE	TRANSCRIBED BY
10/7/98	Admission / Preoperative Orders		
	① Admit to 6th floor – Dental Service		
	Dr. Brown: attending		
	Office # 555-2427		
	② Cond – Good		
	③ Dx – Impacted third molars		
	Cerebral palsy		
	Penicillin allergy please label chart		
	④ NPO		
	⑤ Med: Lorazepam 2mg PO @ 6:30 c̄		
	small sip of H₂O		
	⑥ Void on call to OR		
	⑦ Ambulate c̄ asst only p̄ pre med given		
	⑧ Solumedrol 125mg on chart to OR with		
	patient		
	Thank You		
	Dr. John Brown		

ORIGINAL — CHART COPY   ORDER SHEET

◇ Figure 31-4

Example of admission preoperative physician's orders written for patient with cerebral palsy admitted to hospital on day of third molar surgery. Note that because patient is coming to hospital on day of surgery, admission orders and preoperative orders can be combined.

CLINICAL RECORD—IN-PATIENT   Patient Identification

NORTHSIDE GENERAL HOSPITAL

DATE TIME	DOCTOR'S NOTES	ALL OTHER NOTES BEGIN	ALL ENTRIES MUST BE SIGNED AND POSITION NOTED
10/7/98	◄ BEGIN HERE	◄ HERE Admission note	
0730		This is the third admission to this hospital for this 22 yr. old cerebral palsy victim for elective surgical removal of four impacted 3rd. molars in the operating room this morning. Performance in OR found necessary due to patients inability to stay relatively immobile for the surgery without general anesthesia. Patient has penicillin allergy but no other medical problems. Patient and parents advised in lay terms of reasons for potential problems including infection, nerve damage, bleeding, mandibular fracture, damage to other teeth, and dry socket and they consent to my plans	
		Dr. John Brown	

CLINICAL RECORD IN-PATIENT

◇ Figure 31-5

Example of hospital admission note that attending surgeon uses to document (in record) reason for hospitalization and projected hospital course.

be meticulous in monitoring all that is done to the patient and should take charge if anything is done that may harm the patient.

The operating team usually consists of the operating surgeon and an assistant. The assistant should have sufficient familiarity with the planned procedure to help the dentist by suctioning, retracting, and cutting sutures. Many hospitals allow the dentist to bring one of his or her own office assistants to assist in the operating suite. Anesthesia may be provided by an anesthesiologist (a medical doctor) or by an anesthetist (a nurse with special training in anesthesiology who must work under an anesthesiologist's supervision). A scrub nurse is available, who is sterilely gowned and gloved, who passes instruments to the surgeon during the procedure and, among other duties, keeps track of the sponges and needles used. The circulating nurse remains unsterile and assists in setting up equipment, retrieving supplies, and completing records of the operation.

The dentist should try to see the patient in the preoperative area before anesthetic premedication to help clarify any final questions the patient may have, to learn who the patient wants notified at the completion of the operation, and to give emotional support to the patient.

During final preanesthetic patient preparation, the dentist should review the operative plans with the anesthesiologist. These plans include surgical site, length of procedure, oral hazards (such as loose teeth or restricted opening), route of intubation desired, and whether the patient will be admitted to the hospital. The dentist should remain near the patient's head during intubation to assist if necessary.

Once the patient is under general anesthesia, the dentist should ensure that steps are taken to prevent accidental injuries. Dental patients are usually operated on in a supine position, with the head end of the operating table raised about 15 degrees. The extremities must be placed in physiologic positions (that is, positions patients would find comfortable for long periods if they were not anesthetized). Proper positioning helps prevent nerve injuries and excess loading of any part of the anatomy. In addition, padding should be placed in any area of pressure concentration, such as under heels and around elbows, particularly if the dental procedure is likely to last longer than an hour. Most hospitals currently place all patients on foam or gel-filled cushions or air mattresses during surgery to help prevent pressure sores. The head should be placed on a contoured cushion to help prevent excessive movement of the head during surgery.

Patient protection during anesthesia is also provided by several other means. If the procedure is expected to last more than 4 hours, a urinary (Foley) catheter should be placed, to prevent overdistention of the bladder. The anesthesiologist may want this done even for shorter operations for monitoring urinary output. If an electrocautery unit will be used, a grounding pad must be placed. Eyes should be protected by applying a lubricating ointment and taping the eyelids closed. Patients who are intubated nasally require close attention to proper tube stabilization; tubes that place excess pressure on the nasal alar cartilage can easily cause pressure sores that result in an unsightly deformity (Figure 31-6).

The final step before surgery is preparation of the patient's operative site. If necessary, any facial hair can be shaved. Then the skin in the maxillofacial and anterior neck regions should be prepared by scrubbing with a soap-containing solution, followed by painting with a disinfecting solution, such as iodophor. The patient can then be draped with two layers of linen material or one layer of waterproof paper material to cover all portions of the body except the operative site. The oral cavity is prepared for the procedure by first gently suctioning the pharynx, placing a moist throat pack, and using large volumes of irrigation solution to help decrease the bacterial count by dilution. The use of a sterile toothbrush and chlorhexidine improves the effectiveness of oral cavity preparation. The anesthesiologist and circulating nurse should be asked to make a note that the throat has been packed so they can help remind the surgeon to remove the pack after the surgery is complete.

Dental surgeon and assistant preparation. The dental surgeon prepares for surgery by first checking that all instruments and patient records required to perform the surgery successfully are available. This preparation should be done before the day of surgery, in case any necessary equipment or records must be brought from the surgeon's office on the day of surgery.

Before entering the operating room suite, the surgical team changes from street clothes into surgical scrub uniforms. Shoes worn outside of the operating suite are covered with shoe covers. Scalp hair is covered with a cap. Members of the surgical team with long beards should wear head covers that extend across the chin and anterior neck. All jewelry, including watches, rings, necklaces, and earrings, should be removed before scrubbing. A mask that covers the nose and mouth should be tied in place before the surgeon enters the operating area. Before the surgical scrub, the surgeon should check the patient's records, place radiographs on the viewbox, adjust overhead lights, check the patient's position, apply defogging solution to eyeglasses, adjust his or her headlight, and so on.

The surgical hand and arm scrub is then performed to lessen the chance of contaminating a patient's wound. Although sterile gloves are worn, gloves are frequently torn during oral and maxillofacial surgical procedures, thereby exposing the patient to the surgeon's hands. By proper scrubbing with antiseptic solutions, the hand and arm bacterial level is reduced.

There are several acceptable methods of performing a surgical hand and arm scrub. Most hospitals have a surgical scrub protocol that should be followed when doing surgery there. Standard in most techniques is the use of an antiseptic soap solution, a moderately stiff brush, and a fingernail cleaner. The hands and forearms are wetted in a scrub sink, keeping the hands above the level of the elbows until the hands and arms are dried. A copious amount of antiseptic soap from

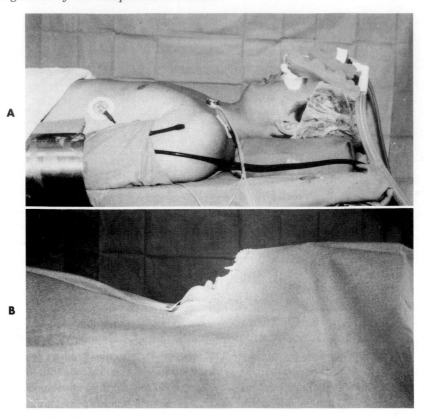

◇ **Figure 31-6**

Patient prepared for operating room oral and maxillofacial surgery. **A,** Patient before draping, with padding of pressure points. Nasoendotracheal tube is supported to prevent alar damage, eye pads are placed to protect eyes, and antiseptic solution is applied on face to reduce number of bacteria not indigenous to patient's facial region. **B,** Same patient after draping is completed. Only operative site is exposed.

wall dispensers or antiseptic-impregnated scrub brushes is applied to the hands and arms up to the elbows. The antiseptic soap is allowed to remain on the arms, while all visible debris is removed from underneath each fingernail tip with the sharp-tipped fingernail cleaner. Then more antiseptic soap is applied and scrubbing begun using repeated firm strokes of the scrub brush on every surface of the hands and arms, stopping about 5 cm below the elbow (Figure 31-7). Scrub techniques based on the number of strokes to each surface rather than a set time for scrubbing are more reliable. An individual's scrub technique should follow a set routine designed to ensure that all forearm and hand surfaces are properly prepared. However, scrubbing too long and too firmly can be as detrimental as inadequate scrubbing, because skin that is excessively traumatized by scrubbing develops a much higher resident bacterial flora. Once scrubbing is completed, the hands and forearms should be rinsed free of soap solution under running water, moving the arm through the stream from fingertips to elbow. The hands must be kept higher than the elbows during the entire scrub and rinse to allow all excess fluid to drip off the arm at the elbow.

Once the surgeon completes scrubbing, he or she should enter the operating room, taking care to avoid contaminating scrubbed hands and arms. Drying commences with a sterile towel handed to the surgeon by the scrub nurse. The towel is held in one hand to dry the other hand, advancing up the forearm and stopping short of the elbow. The towel is then transferred to the dry hand, and the process is repeated on the wet hand with an unused portion of the towel. The sterile surgical gown is then fully opened by the scrub nurse, and the surgeon introduces his or her hands into the openings for the arms of the gown. While the scrub nurse helps push the gown up the surgeon's arm, the circulating nurse pulls the gown on from the rear of the surgeon and ties it securely (Figure 31-8). The scrub nurse then holds the surgical gloves open while the surgeon places her or his hand into each glove. The glove should completely cover the hand and wrist and completely overlap the cuff of the surgical gown (Figure 31-9). Once the gloves are on, the surgeon should use a moist towel to remove any powder from the surface of the gloves. The surgeon must not allow his or her hands to fall beneath waist level from this point until ungowning (Figure 31-10).

Text continued on p. 753

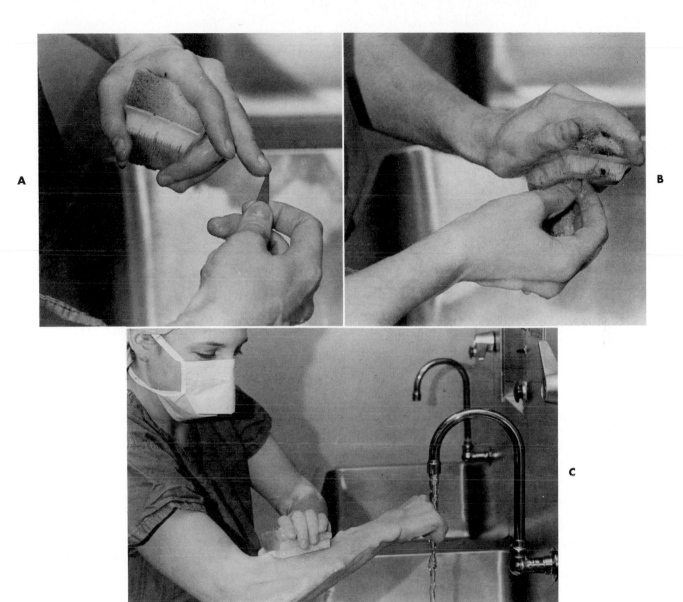

◇ Figure 31-7

Technique of hand scrub used before gowning and gloving for operating room procedure. **A,** Scrub sink is turned on. Then disposable scrub brush and nail cleaner are taken out of package, and hands are wetted in scrub sink. Brush is wetted, and, if brush is not preimpregnated, antiseptic soap is absorbed into sponge side of brush. While holding scrub brush in one hand, surgeon uses nail cleaner under each fingernail. Nail cleaner is then discarded, and scrubbing commences. **B and C,** Both arms are lathered with antiseptic soap from fingers to area about 5 cm below elbows. Scrub brush is then used to scrub all surfaces of hands and forearms thoroughly, with most brush strokes on each surface of each hand (20 per surface) and fewer strokes on each surface of forearms (10 per surface). Note that during scrubbing and rinsing, forearms are not allowed to fall below level of elbow.

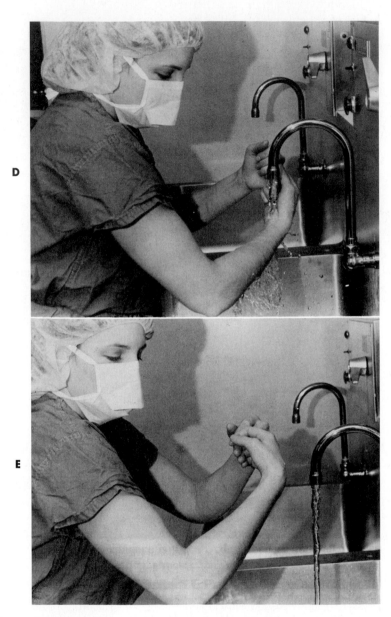

⬥ Figure 31-7, cont'd

D, After scrubbing is completed, brush is discarded and arms rinsed completely. During rinsing, arm is put through the water, starting at fingertips, then pushing through to elbow. **E,** Arms are then allowed to drain for several seconds over scrub sink. Again, forearms are kept raised above level of elbows.

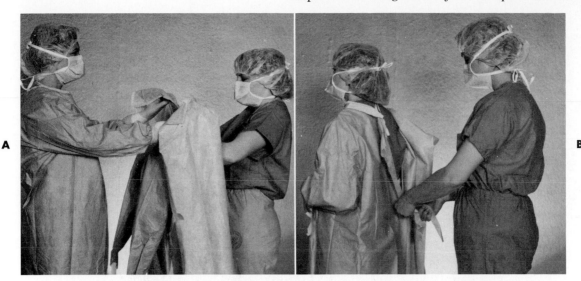

◆ Figure 31-8

Gowning for operating room surgery. **A,** Scrub nurse on left holds sterile gown open for surgeon to place her arms into sleeves. Note that scrub nurse has her hands on front side of gown to prevent possibility of accidentally touching ungowned surgeon. Surgeon pushes her arms into sleeves of gown, taking care not to thrust through cuff of gown, potentially contaminating scrub nurse. While surgeon is placing her arms into sleeves, scrub nurse is pushing gown onto surgeon. **B,** Unsterile circulating nurse then ties back of surgeon's gown, taking care to touch only inside surfaces of gown.

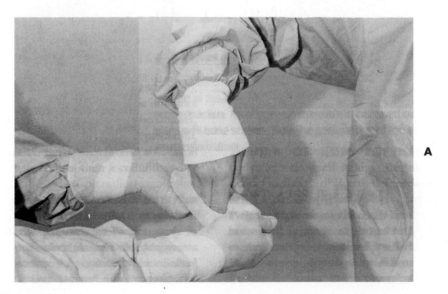

◆ Figure 31-9

Gloving for operating room surgery. **A,** Scrub nurse holds open first glove to allow surgeon to insert hand into glove while surgeon's wrist is in flexion. Surgeon pushes hand into glove with fingers adducted, while nurse pulls glove onto surgeon's hand.   *Continued*

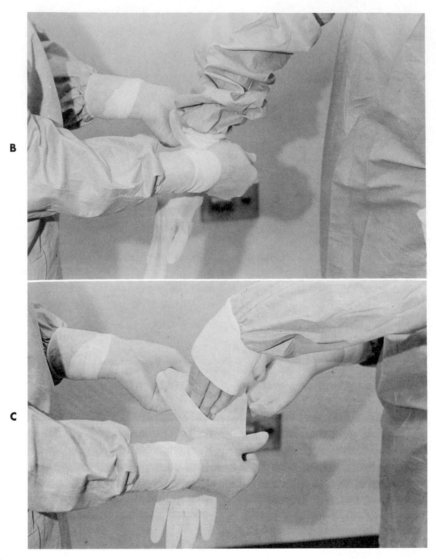

◆ Figure 31-9, cont'd

B, Once surgeon's hand is into palm region of glove, fingers are partially abducted and slipped into appropriate finger holes. Nurse continues to pull glove on until cuff of glove is above cuff of surgeon's gown. Nurse then releases glove. No further adjustments of first glove are made at this time. **C,** Scrub nurse then holds second glove open in same manner that first glove was presented to surgeon. Surgeon can now help hold cuff of glove open while inserting other hand. Hand being gloved is pushed into glove while other hand assists nurse in pulling glove into place. Once both gloves are in place, they can be used to adjust each other, pulling all slack out of area of fingertips.

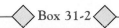

Box 31-2

Principle components of postoperative orders

1. Diagnosis (or diagnoses) and surgical procedure
2. Condition
3. Allergies
4. Instructions for monitoring vital signs
5. Activity and positioning
6. Diet
7. Medications
8. Intravenous fluids
9. Wound care
10. Parameters for notification of physician or dentist
11. Special instructions (for example, ice packs, lip protection, and hygiene instructions)

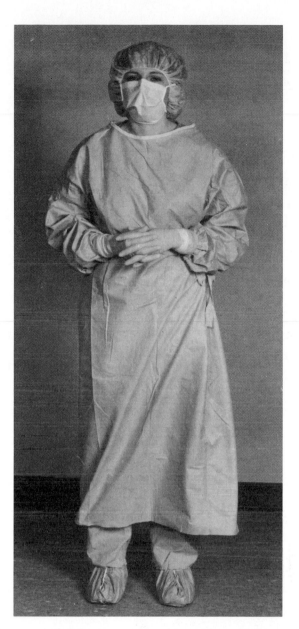

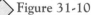

Figure 31-10

Surgeon ready for operating room surgery. Hands should not be allowed to fall below waist level from this point until the surgery is completed and all surgical wounds are closed and dressed.

Postoperative responsibilities. Once the operative procedure is completed, the oral cavity is again irrigated and suctioned clear of accumulated fluids. Before throat pack removal, the scrub nurse should be asked if all sponges and needles used during the surgery are accounted for; if they are not, a search must be made to find them. If necessary, intraoral gauze packs should be placed for hemostasis, and the packs should have long ends that trail out of the mouth for easy retrieval.

Many of the immediate postoperative decisions are made in the postanesthesia care unit by nurses under the supervision of the anesthesiologists. However, the dentist should write

postoperative orders immediately after the completion of surgery, to ensure that any special instructions can be initiated in the postanesthesia care unit.

Postoperative orders should include statements of the diagnosis, procedure performed, patient allergies, and general condition of the patient after surgery. Nursing actions, such as vital sign monitoring, wound care, and medication administration schedule, should be clearly spelled out. The patient's diet, activity level, bed positioning, and allowable personal hygiene should be delineated. Finally, parameters should be outlined for which, if violated, immediate notification of the dentist or physician is mandatory. An outline for postoperative orders is listed in Box 31-2; a sample of postoperative orders is shown in Figure 31-11.

Shortly after the surgical procedure is completed, a brief operative note should be placed in the patient's record. This note is usually in a relatively standard format that includes listing the preoperative and postoperative diagnoses, the names of the procedures performed during surgery, the name(s) of the surgeon(s), the type of anesthesia, the placement of any drains, the estimated blood loss, and whether any specimens were sent for pathologic examination. This note is used by hospital staff members to quickly learn general information about the operative procedure. Additionally, before leaving the operating suite a full report of the operation should be dictated, using the designated format of the facility at which the surgery was performed. The general outlines and examples of a brief operative note and transcribed operative report are shown in Boxes 31-3 and 31-4 and in Figure 31-12.

Patients generally remain in the postanesthesia care unit until they are sufficiently alert and unlikely to injure themselves and until vital signs are stable within acceptable limits. An anesthesiologist usually makes the decision about discharge to a hospital room or home, unless the dentist specifies that he or she will make that decision. The discharged patient should be placed directly under the care of a competent adult and should not be allowed to go home unescorted.

ORDER SHEET   Patient Identification

NORTHSIDE GENERAL HOSPITAL

USE BALLPOINT PEN. BEAR DOWN.   Unless an order is specifically noted, authorization is hereby given
You are making up to four copies.   for the dispensing of drugs by non-proprietary nomenclature as set
                                        forth by The Pharmacy and Therapeutics Committee.

AUTOMATIC STOP ORDERS   Narcotics and anticoagulants must be rewritten within 48
                        hours of original order; all other drugs within 7 days.

DATE AND TIME	ORDERS	SIGNATURE	TRANSCRIBED BY
10/7/98 9:20	Post op orders		
	① S/p Surgical extraction 4 third molars		
	② Condition: Good		
	③ Allergy: Penicillin, please label chart		
	④ Vital signs: q 15 min until stable then q 1° x2, then q 4° Oral Temps q 4° w/a		
	⑤ HOB at least 30°, OOB c̄ assistance only		
	⑥ Ice packs to face if patient desires, please inquire		
	⑦ Diet: clear cool liquids, advance to full cool liquids as tolerated		
	⑧ I & O q shift		
	⑨ Meds:		
	ⓐ M.S. 4 mg & Phenergan 50 mg IM q 4° prn mod-severe pain or		
	ⓑ Tylox T po q 4° prn mod-severe pain		
	ⓒ Acetaminophen 500 mg po q 3° prn mild pain		
	ⓓ Decadron 0.75 mg PO 3ID		
	ⓔ Compazine 5 mg IM prn N or V. May repeat in 30 min. x1. Call surgeon if nausea persists thereafter.		
	ⓕ Medihaler II puffs q 4° prn wheezing		
	⑩ IV: D5¼NS @ 100 cc/hr Change to Hep lock when PO >400 cc/8hr		
	⑪ Bite on moistened 4x4 gauze placed over op sites continuously for 45 min prn bleeding		
	⑫ Keep lips thinly coated with Vaseline		
	⑬ Call surgeon — office 674-1212, home - 525-6666 if BP > ¹⁸⁰/₁₀ < ⁹⁰/₆₀, P > 120 < 55, T > 101°; uncontrollable bleeding, wheezing or if pt. fails to void by 1700.		
	Thank You Dr. John Brown		

ORIGINAL — CHART COPY   ORDER SHEET

◇ Figure 31-11

Example of postoperative orders written after removal of third molars in operating room.

◇ Box 31-3 ◇

Common format for recording brief operative note

1. Preoperative diagnosis
2. Postoperative diagnosis
3. Procedure
4. Surgeon(s)
5. Type of anesthesia
6. Unusual, unexpected, or significant findings at surgery
7. Fluid status, including estimated fluid loss and amount of fluid administered to patient
8. Description of anything left in operative site, such as drains or packing
9. Specimens (Was a specimen sent to the pathology laboratory?)

◇ Box 31-4 ◇

Common format for dictating operative note

1. Identify dictator
2. State that operative note is being dictated
3. State patient's name, spelling out last name
4. State patient's medical record (hospital) number
5. State date of operation
6. State preoperative diagnosis
7. State postoperative diagnosis
8. Give name of procedure performed
9. Give name of surgeon and any surgical assistants
10. Completely describe surgical procedure, including how the patient was anesthetized and prepared for surgery in the operating room
11. Reidentify dictator
12. State to whom copies of the dictation should be sent

Hospital rounds (patient visits) give the surgeon the opportunity to check the patient's postoperative recovery personally and to revise orders as necessary. Unstable hospitalized patients require frequent visits; stable patients are usually seen twice a day during the first week after surgery and once daily thereafter. Each patient visit by the surgeon warrants a brief notation (progress note) in the record, which documents the patient's progress and any new plans for further care. Notes are usually written in the problem-oriented medical record format. This format includes a brief description of how the patient is progressing *subjectively* and *objectively,* an *assessment* of the patient's condition, and a *plan* for further care *(SOAP).* Figure 31-13 shows a typical postoperative progress notation in the SOAP format.

Discharge planning should begin as soon as the surgical procedure is completed and includes making arrangements for any necessary patient education, such as oral hygiene, wound care, and dietary instructions. Also, the patient should be told of acceptable activity levels and plans for follow-up office visits. Necessary prescriptions for medications should be provided, as well as instructions on how to contact the appropriate physician or dentist should problems arise. A written discharge note should be included in the progress note section of the medical record (Figure 31-14 and Box 31-5).

A dictated discharge summary is necessary for hospitalized patients, whereas surgical centers generally accept a written discharge summary on a special form. The dictated summary should include a brief narrative, including the reason for hospital admission and the pertinent history that led to admission. The significant positive and negative findings of the history and physical examination should be described, including any laboratory results. The hospital course, including the name of the operative procedure, should be in the summary. Finally, discharge instructions, prescriptions, and follow-up appointments should be detailed in the report. Arrangements should be made to send copies of the discharge summary to other doctors who may find the information useful, including the patient's family physician (Figure 31-15 and Box 31-6).

MANAGEMENT OF POSTOPERATIVE PROBLEMS

POSTOPERATIVE AIRWAY PROBLEMS. Routine dentoalveolar surgery is unlikely to cause airway compromise unless a condition such as Ludwig's angina is present. However, patients in whom an endotracheal tube has been placed during general anesthesia are at risk for airway narrowing or obstruction after extubation, which is caused by trauma to mucosal lining of the upper respiratory tract that produces edema. The narrowest portion of the upper respiratory tract is the region of the vocal cords through which the endotracheal tube must be passed and on which the tube rests during anesthesia. The amount of respiratory tract mucosal injury depends on the patient's anatomy, the size of tube used, the type of tube, and care used during placement. Injuries caused by tube type have been lessened by the use of tubes with high-volume, low-pressure cuff designs. Patients generally do well after extubation, except for mild-to-moderate throat discomfort during swallowing for 1 to 2 days. However, occasionally, laryngeal edema of sufficient severity to compromise the patient's ability to breathe will be produced. The first symptom is usually a crowing sound during attempts to inspire and expire. The patient may also need to use accessory muscles of respiration to force air past the cords.

Prevention of airway trauma is the best form of care. If trauma is known to have occurred during intubation or extubation or in patients having prolonged intubation, postoperative orders should include the delivery of cooled, humidified air or oxygen, administration of racemic epinephrine through an aerosol, and placement of tracheotomy equipment near the patient's bed. These patients should be closely monitored, preferably under close supervision by an anesthesiologist, until the dentist is comfortable that airway problems are under control.

Text continued on p. 761

CLINICAL RECORD—IN-PATIENT   Patient Identification

NORTHSIDE GENERAL HOSPITAL

DATE / TIME	DOCTOR'S NOTES ◄ BEGIN HERE	ALL OTHER NOTES BEGIN ◄ HERE	ALL ENTRIES MUST BE SIGNED AND POSITION NOTED
10/7/98 9:30		Brief Op Note :	
		Pre-op dx: 4 impacted 3rd molars	
		Post op dx: same	
		Procedure: Surgical removal of 4 complicated 3rd molars	
		Surgeon: Brown Asst: Jones	
		Anes: Nitrous – Narcotic – Ethrane	
		Findings: Impacted teeth c̄ follicles associated with maxillary impactions	
		EBL : <100 mL	
		Fluids : 800 mL D5 ⅓ NS	
		Drains or Packs : None	
		Specimen: Teeth and follicles to pathology.	
		Dr. John Brown	

A

CLINICAL RECORD
IN-PATIENT

◆ Figure 31-12

A, Example of brief operative note used for quick documentation in hospital record of what was performed, whether in operating room or elsewhere in hospital.   *Continued*

NORTHSIDE GENERAL HOSPITAL

OPERATIVE REPORT

NAME: SCHULTZ, Carl
UNIT NUMBER: X00012345
OPERATIVE DATE: 10-07-98
DOB: 06-06-76

PREOPERATIVE DIAGNOSIS: Full bony impacted teeth Nos. 1, 16
                          Partial bony impacted teeth Nos. 17, 32
POSTOPERATIVE DIAGNOSIS: Same
SURGEON: John Brown, D.M.D.
ASSISTANT SURGEON: William Jones, D.D.S.
OPERATIONS: Surgical extraction of impacted third molars
                          Nos. 1, 16, 17, and 32

PROCEDURE: The patient was brought to the operating room without premedication
and placed onto the operating table in the supine position. After attaching
monitoring equipment and checking the vital signs the patient was placed under
general anesthesia induced by a combination of inhalational and intravenous
agents. A right nasal endotracheal intubation was performed and the tube
secured into position after good breath sounds were heard bilaterally on
auscultation. The operating table was placed into a 15-degree head-up position, and then the patient was prepped and draped in the usual fashion for
intraoral oral surgery.

The oral cavity was inspected and suctioned free of gross secretions, and a
moist throat pack was placed. 0.5% Marcaine with 1:200,000 epinephrine was infiltrated in the maxillary posterior buccal vestibules, the greater palatine
nerve regions, and the inferior alveolar, lingual, and buccal nerves were
blocked bilaterally with a total of 45 mg of Marcaine and 0.045 mg of epinephrine. The oral cavity was then irrigated with copious amounts of normal saline
irrigation and suctioned free of gross liquid. A medium sized rubber bite
block was carefully placed between the arches on the left side. Attention was
first directed to the right retromolar region of the mandible, where a No. 15
blade was used to make an incision beginning in the lower fourth of the external oblique ridge of the mandible, bringing the incision forward to the distal
line angle of tooth No. 31. The incision was then continued in the buccal
gingival sulcus to the distal aspect of tooth No. 30. A No. 9 dental periosteal elevator was then used to create a full-thickness mucoperiosteal envelope
type of flap, exposing the buccal aspect of the retromandibular region of the
mandible. A right angle retractor was placed into the depth of the envelope
flap to protect it, and the assistant used a tongue retractor to protect the
tongue. The mesio-angularly impacted tooth No. 32 was identified, and a
straight tissue burr in an air-driven handpiece under continuous saline irrigation was used to remove sufficient bone on the buccal and distal aspects of
tooth No. 32 to expose the height of contour. The burr was then used to section the tooth along its long axis through the furcation. A large, straight

B

◇ Figure 31-12, cont'd

B, Example of dictated operative note to describe in detail exact procedure performed in operating
room.   *Continued*

dental elevator was used to complete the tooth sectioning. The Crane pick was then used to remove the distal aspect of the tooth, and a small straight dental elevator was used to remove the mesial aspect. The roots of both tooth segments appeared intact. A dental curette was used to gently remove the small remnant of dental follicle remaining in the socket. A bone rasp was used to smooth the bone in regions where elevators had been used, and the sockets and areas under the flaps were irrigated with copious amounts of saline irrigation. Little bleeding was present at that time, so half a capsule of tetracycline was poured into the socket, and the flap was reapproximated with two 4-0 black silk sutures.

Attention was next directed to the right maxillary tuberosity region, where a new No. 15 blade was used to create a crestal incision beginning on the distosuperior aspect of the tuberosity, continuing the incision anteriorly to the posterior aspect of tooth No. 2. The incision was then continued in the buccal gingival sulcus anteriorly to the distal line angle of tooth No. 3. A No. 9 dental periosteal elevator was then used to create a full-thickness mucoperiosteal flap on the buccal aspect of the tuberosity. The Minnesota retractor was used to remove a small amount of thin bone overlying the full bony impacted tooth No. 1. A Potts elevator was used to elevate tooth No. 1 out of the socket along with the attached dental follicle. The root of the tooth appeared to be intact. The socket was inspected and then irrigated with normal saline. The flap was then reapproximated with two 4-0 black silk sutures. A large gauze was then placed over the fresh extraction sites, and attention was directed to the left side of the mouth, where teeth Nos. 16 and 17 were extracted in an identical fashion to teeth Nos. 1 and 32.

The oral cavity was then suctioned free of all gross fluids, and the throatpack was removed. The hypopharynx was then suctioned with a tonsil suction. The patient was extubated in the operating room and taken to the post-anesthesia care unit in good condition for recovery.

ESTIMATED BLOOD LOSS: 50 mL
FLUIDS RECEIVED: 1,200 mls Dextrose 5%/Lactated Ringers
DRAINS: None
DRESSINGS: Bilateral oral packs that trailed out of the mouth
COMPLICATIONS: None

John Brown D.M.D.
John Brown, D.M.D.
Attending Surgeon

cc: Dr. William Jones

◇ Figure 31-12, cont'd

B, For legend see previous page.

CLINICAL RECORD—IN-PATIENT

Patient Identification

NORTHSIDE GENERAL HOSPITAL

DATE TIME	DOCTOR'S NOTES	ALL OTHER NOTES BEGIN · ALL ENTRIES MUST BE SIGNED AND POSITION NOTED
10/7/98	◄ BEGIN HERE	◄ HERE
20:00		Post-op check
	S-	Pt. feels drowsy. Moderate pain well controlled with oral narcotic. Denies nausea
	O-	Vital signs WNL & stable
		Mild facial edema
		Operative sites show slight ooze
		Chest clear to auscultation
		IV site benign
		Intake last 8 hrs. ~ 1450 mL (250 mL PO)
		Ambulated to BR with assistance
		Voided 600 mL
	A-	Doing well, needs to increase PO intake
	P-	Encourage PO intake
		Slow IV rate to 75 mL/hr
		Bite on moistened gauze if bleeding increases during the night
		John Brown DMD

CLINICAL RECORD IN-PATIENT

◆ Figure 31-13

Example of hospital progress note made to document patient's course in hospital and to inform others of future plans for patient. Note SOAP format used: *S* is any comments made by patient (subjective); *O* is objective findings by dentist; *A* is assessment by dentist of how patient is doing; *P* is plans for future care.

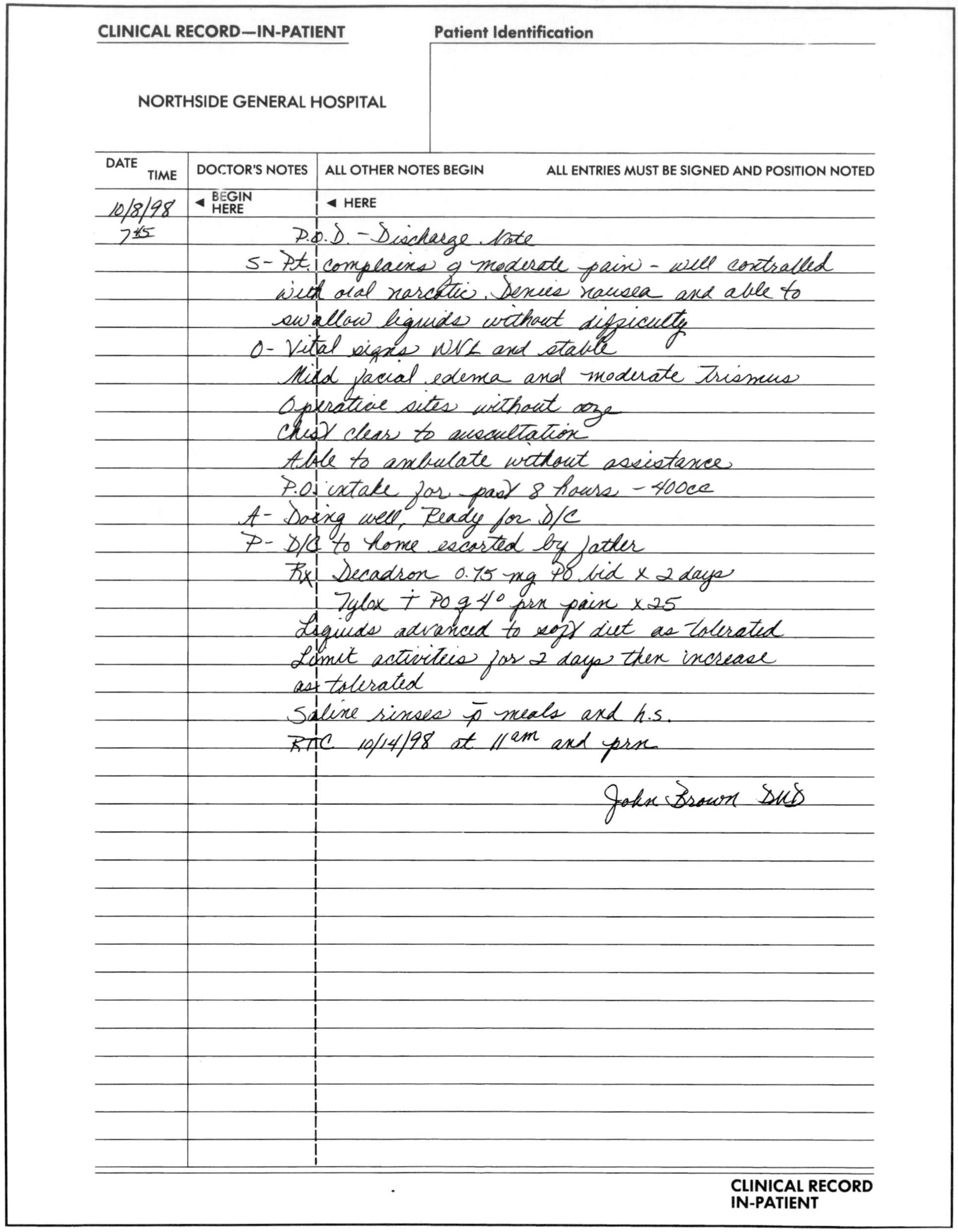

CLINICAL RECORD—IN-PATIENT　　　**Patient Identification**

NORTHSIDE GENERAL HOSPITAL

DATE / TIME	DOCTOR'S NOTES	ALL OTHER NOTES BEGIN	ALL ENTRIES MUST BE SIGNED AND POSITION NOTED
10/8/98	◄ BEGIN HERE	◄ HERE	

7⁴⁵　　P.O.D. – Discharge Note

S – Pt. complains of moderate pain – well controlled with oral narcotic. Denies nausea and able to swallow liquids without difficulty

O – Vital signs WNL and stable
　　Mild facial edema and moderate Trismus
　　Operative sites without ooze
　　Chest clear to auscultation
　　Able to ambulate without assistance
　　P.O. intake for past 8 hours – 400cc

A – Doing well, Ready for D/C

P – D/C to home escorted by father
　　Rx Decadron 0.75 mg PO bid x 2 days
　　　　Tylox ī PO q 4° prn pain x 25
　　Liquids advanced to soft diet as tolerated
　　Limit activities for 2 days then increase as tolerated
　　Saline rinses p̄ meals and h.s.
　　RTC 10/14/98 at 11ᵃᵐ and prn

　　　　　　　　　　　John Brown DMD

CLINICAL RECORD IN-PATIENT

◆ Figure 31-14

Example of written discharge note in SOAP format to document patient's progress. Discharge instructions are documented under *P*.

◇ Box 31-5 ◇

**General information to include
in written discharge note**

A. Complete a standard SOAP progress note
B. Under *P* (plans) section, include the following:
1. Deposition (to where and with whom patient will be discharged)
2. List of medications that the patient is prescribed or instructed to take, including drug name, dosing regimen, and instructions for use
3. Dietary instructions
4. Activity instructions
5. Hygiene instructions
6. Follow-up appointment

NAUSEA AND VOMITING. Nausea and vomiting occur commonly after general anesthesia, which is part of the rationale for fasting patients preoperatively. The symptoms are primarily related to anesthetic drugs and occasionally to excessive air that might have been forced into the stomach during induction of anesthesia. Nausea and vomiting usually resolve with time but can be a serious problem if the patient is not fully in control of laryngeal reflexes, is in intermaxillary fixation, or is unable to begin taking needed medications and sustenance orally.

Vomiting in a patient with depressed reflexes is best handled by placing the patient in a horizontal position on one side until reflexes are recovered. Patients in intermaxillary fixation but with normal airway reflexes should be able to eliminate any vomitus through the nose and mouth, because postoperative stomach contents should be of liquid consistency. Even so, constant retching can disrupt a properly set facial fracture or a delicate wound repair, so awake patients in or out of fixation may need to receive antiemetic medications to relieve nausea. However, before giving antiemetic agents, the possibility of depressed gastrointestinal motility or brain injury should be ruled out. If a patient develops airway problems while in intermaxillary fixation, an instrument capable of releasing fixation should be readily available. Many dentists have a pair of wire cutters taped to the head of a patient's bed.

FEVER. Fever is generally defined as an oral temperature of greater than 99° F (37.2° C) or rectal temperature higher than 99.8° F (38° C). The variety of factors that may produce a postoperative fever is large. However, there are a few common reasons to account for a fever after surgery that are differentiated based partially on when in the postoperative period they occur. Fever the night after surgery is usually attributed to bacteremias resulting from organisms in surgical wounds. Fevers occurring in the first or second postoperative day after general anesthesia or major surgery are generally attributed to insufficient depth of breathing, which produces

atelectasis (collapse of terminal lung alveoli), or, less commonly, to dehydration. Fever 2 days after surgery can be an early sign of a wound infection or, if the patient had his or her bladder catheterized or has prolonged atelectasis, it may be caused by a bladder infection or pneumonia.

No matter when a fever arises, an investigation should be undertaken to discover the cause. The patient should be questioned about wound pain, swelling, foul taste, productive cough, and dysuria. On examination, particular reference to the surgical wound, sites of intravenous catheters, and lungs should be made. Studies such as a white blood cell count, urinalysis, and chest radiographs may be useful in determining an explanation for a postoperative fever, if clinically indicated. A medical consultation may be necessary if a cause for a persistent fever remains obscure. Once it is documented that a fever exists, the patient's symptoms and increased metabolic expenditure from the fever can be lessened by administration of acetaminophen.

ATELECTASIS. Atelectasis is a common problem in patients who have undergone abdominal surgery and fail to fill their lungs to normal capacity because of the incisional pain provoked by deep breathing. In patients who have had dentoalveolar surgery under general anesthesia, atelectasis can result from (1) inactivity that allows the patient to breathe without filling the lungs to normal capacity; (2) postoperative narcotic analgesics that depress the sigh reflex, which normally functions to prevent atelectasis; or (3) an endotracheal tube misplaced, so that only one lung was aerated during surgery.

Prolonged atelectasis can lead to pneumonia; thus prevention of atelectasis is important. Instructing patients to take deep sustained inspirations periodically during the postoperative period and to begin ambulation as soon as possible after surgery lessen the possibility of developing atelectasis. Limiting the use of unnecessarily large doses of narcotic analgesics can also prevent atelectasis.

FLUIDS AND ELECTROLYTES. Hypovolemia can be found in patients after surgery because of insufficient fluid intake to match fluid loss. Fluids are lost through the obvious routes of urination, vomiting, and nasogastric suctioning and by insensible routes, such as expired air and perspiration. The primary source of replacement fluids is normally oral ingestion. However, postoperative patients who are unable or unwilling to maintain necessary fluid intake orally require intravenous supplementation until oral fluid intake resumes. The usual volume of fluid intake necessary (combination of oral and intravenous) for a nonfebrile adult in the postoperative period is between 2500 and 3000 mL daily, with a higher volume for patients with higher-than-normal fluid loss and a lower volume for patients susceptible to fluid overloading, such as those with renal or myocardial insufficiency.

The choice of intravenous fluid type is based on the knowledge that human serum must have certain electrolytes kept within a narrow range to maintain vital physiologic functions. Sodium, potassium, and chloride are the three

```
NORTHSIDE GENERAL HOSPITAL          Schultz, Carl
                                    X00012345   DOB: 6/6/78

Discharge Summary

Admitted: 10/7/98        Discharged: 10/8/98

       This  was  the  third  admission  at Northside General for  this
20  year  old male with cerebral palsy.    Elective admission  was
necessary  for  surgical  removal  of  four  impacted  third  molars
which  had  recently  become  symptomatic  necessitating  extraction
under general anesthesia.
       PMH: Hospitalizations: 1986-restorative dentistry under GA
                             1990-appendectomy without problems
                             1994-restorative dentistry under GA
            Illnesses: Cerebral palsy due to birth anoxia
                       Asthma, never needed hospitalization
            Medications: Medi-inhaler as needed.
            Allergies: Penicillin
            Social: Lives at home with parents
       Past  medical,  family  and  social  history  otherwise
unremarkable.

       ROS:  Pertinent findings-Intermittent pain and swelling around
partially  erupted  lower  third  molars.    Denies  other  oral
discomfort.  Patient claims inability to maintain upright posture
without the use of body brace.  Weakness in leg asnd back muscles
bilaterally.  ROS otherwise unremarkable.
       PE: Pertinent findings-
       HEENT- nasal  airways patent,  Class I occlusion with well-
restored dentition,  no mucosal lesions. No adenopathy. All teeth
except #1 and 16 visible. Teeth #17 and 32 partially erupted with
operculums present.
       Chest- Clear  to  percussion  and  auscultation  without
wheezes  or  rales.   Heart had regular rate and  rhythm  without
murmurs or extra sounds present.

Hospital  course:   On  morning of admission patient  was  placed
under  general anesthesia in  the operating room and had surgical
removal of 4 third molars.  Surgery and anesthesia tolerated well
and  patient was discharged to home on the  first  post-operative
day in good condition.

Discharge instructions:
       Rx-Decadron 0.75mg PO bid for 2 days
       Rx-Tylox 1 PO q4hr prn pain X 25
       Cool liquid advanced to soft diet as tolerated
       Warm saline rinses after meals and hs
       Restrict normal activities for 2 days
       Return to office on 10/14/98 at 11am.

                                        John Brown D.M.D.
                                        John Brown, D.M.D.
                                        Attending Surgeon
```

◇ Figure 31-15

Example of dictated hospital discharge summary.

electrolytes considered when choosing an intravenous solution. Three standard intravenous crystalloid solutions are available for use either individually or in combination. Dextrose 5% in water (D_5W) is a 5% glucose solution that provides free water, a source of calories in a fluid that is isotonic with plasma, and no electrolytes. Normal saline, or 0.9% sodium chloride solution, provides 154 mEq each of sodium and chloride per liter of water, which makes the solution roughly isotonic but actually functioning to draw interstitial fluid into the intravascular compartment.* Lactated Ringer's solution contains generally physiologic electrolyte concentrations (Na^+–130 mEq; Cl^-–109 mEq; K^+–4 mEq;

---

*Saline is commonly available in several dilutions (0.9%. [normal], 0.45%, 0.33%, and 0.25%).

◇ Box 31-6 ◇

Common format for dictating the hospital discharge summary

A. Identify dictator
B. State that discharge summary is being dictated
C. State patient's name, spelling out last name
D. Give patient's medical record (hospital) number
E. State date of hospital admission and discharge
F. State final diagnosis
G. Give patient's chief complaint on admission
H. Describe history of illness or problem requiring surgery
I. List any significant findings on history and on physical, radiographic, and laboratory examination
J. Briefly describe hospital course, including the following:
  1. Description of all therapy rendered
  2. Any complications that occurred
  3. Outcome of any therapy provided
K. Describe discharge instructions given to the patient, including the following:
  1. Disposition (to where and with whom the patient is being discharged)
  2. Medications
  3. Activity
  4. Diet
  5. Hygiene
  6. Follow-up plans
L. Describe patient's condition on discharge
M. Reidentify dictator
N. State to whom copies of the summary should be sent

Ca^{++}–3 mEq) and lactate, which buffers serum acidity by providing a substrate that can be metabolized into bicarbonate.

In general, after dentoalveolar surgery the otherwise healthy patient requires a relatively physiologic intravenous solution with some calories during and after surgery, which can be provided by combination crystalloid solutions such as 5% dextrose in a 0.45% sodium chloride solution to which 20 mEq of potassium chloride per liter have been added. Patients with special medical problems likely to cause electrolyte abnormalities, such as those on potassium-wasting diuretics or prolonged intravenous fluids, will need their serum electrolytes monitored to guide intravenous fluid choice.

BLOOD COMPONENT TRANSFUSION.   Blood transfusions are rarely required after dentoalveolar surgery, which is fortunate because of the potential for spread of infectious diseases in the course of transfusions and the risk of incompatibility reactions. The primary reason why transfusions are unnecessary is the nature of oral surgery, which, if properly performed, is unlikely to allow significant blood loss. In addition, placement of patients in reverse Trendelenburg position* and the use of hypotension anesthetic techniques have further lessened blood loss.

Occasionally, circumstances arise in which blood components are necessary, such as for trauma patients who have lost blood from serious injuries or patients with thrombocytopenia. In the past, patients requiring transfusions were given whole blood; however, modern blood banks currently separate donated blood into its various components, that is, plasma, red blood cells, platelets, and white blood cells. Patients with a low hematocrit and therefore lowered oxygen-carrying capacity of the blood can be given only the portion of blood that they require—packed red blood cells. Similarly, patients who are thrombocytopenic from chemotherapy but require emergency oral surgery can be given platelet concentrates.

Another means of transfusion therapy—autogenous blood transfusion—is available in most centers. This technique is used when it is suspected that an intraoperative blood transfusion may be required. Patients can donate a unit or two of their own blood before surgery. The blood is then stored and made available for the patient's use during surgery.

Various criteria exist to help determine when red cell or platelet transfusions are necessary. In general, a healthy patient with normal red cell mass can tolerate an acute fall in hematocrit of 25% to 30% without suffering significant ill effects. A chronically anemic patient can tolerate an even lower concentration of red blood cells. Dentists managing patients with thrombocytopenia should seek the advice of a hematologist when deciding if platelet transfusion is warranted.

---

*Patient is supine on operating table, with the head end of the table raised.

BIBLIOGRAPHY

Atkinson LJ: *Berry & Kohn's Operating room technique,* ed 8, St Louis, 1996, Mosby.

Donoff RB: *Manual of oral and maxillofacial surgery,* ed 3, St Louis, 1997, Mosby.

Goldman L, Rudd P, Lee T: Ten commandments for effective consultations, *Arch Intern Med* 143:1753, 1983.

Kwon PH, Laskin DM: *Clinician's manual of oral and maxillofacial surgery,* ed 2, Chicago, 1996, Quintessence.

Zambito RF, Black H, Tesch LB: *Hospital dentistry,* St Louis, 1997, Mosby.

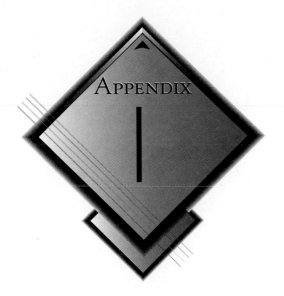

COMPONENTS OF STANDARD HISTORY AND PHYSICAL EXAMINATION

A. Patient's name, age, gender, and, if not of legal age or competent to make own decisions, guardian

B. Source of historical information and reliability of source if not the patient

C. Patient's chief complaint

D. History of the chief complaint (present illness)

E. Medical history
   1. Hospitalization and surgeries
   2. Serious medical illnesses
   3. Medications (both those that patient regularly uses or is supposed to be using)
   4. Allergies (particularly to medications or substances such as latex)
   5. Health-related habits—smoking, ethanol intake, exercise, diet
   6. Approximate date of last medical check-up, name of family physician

F. Review of systems
   1. Constitutional (for example, fevers, weight change, malaise)
   2. Head, ears, eyes, nose, mouth, throat, neck
   3. Respiratory
   4. Cardiovascular
   5. Gastrointestinal

   6. Genitourinary
   7. Endocrine
   8. Neurologic
   9. Musculoskeletal and dermatologic

G. Physical examination
   1. Vital signs
   2. General appearance
   3. Head, ears, eyes, nose, mouth, throat, neck
   4. Thoracic
   5. Abdomen
   6. Extremities
   7. Skin
   8. Back
   9. Neurologic
   10. Mental status

H. Diagnostic test results
   1. Diagnostic images (for example, radiographs)
   2. Clinical laboratories (for example, hematocrit)
   3. Special tests (for example, electrocardiogram)

I. Problem list (listed in order of priority of management)

J. Treatment plans

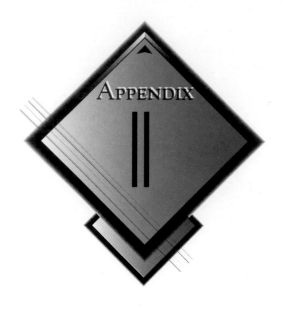

Normal Laboratory Values

Hematology

Hematocrit

Males = 47 ± 2%

Females = 42 ± 2%

Hemoglobin

Males = 16 g/dL ± 2

Females = 14 g/dL ± 2

White blood count—7000/mL ± 3000

Mean corpuscular volume (MCV)—90 ± 7mm^3

Mean corpuscular hemoglobin (MCH)—29 ± 2 pg/cell

Mean corpuscular hemoglobin concentration (MCHC)—34 ± 2 g/dL

Coagulation

Template bleeding time—(9-mm wound) 1 to 9 minutes

Prothrombin time (PT)—control + 1 s

International normalized ratio (INR)—1

Partial thromboplastin time (PTT)—activated, 32 to 46 seconds (compared with normal control)

Platelets—140,000 to 440,000/mL

Blood chemistry

Arterial blood gases

HCO_3 = 18 to 21 mEq/L

P_{CO_2} = 35 to 45 mmHg

pH = 7.38 to 7.44

pO_2 = 80 to 100 mmHg

Calcium—9 to 11 mg/dL

Carbon dioxide—21 to 30 mEq/L

Chloride—98 to 106 mEq/L

Cholesterol

Total—180 to 240 mg/dL

Esters—100 to 180 mg/dL

Creatinine—1 to 1.5 mg/dL

Glucose—75 to 105 mg (fasting)

Osmolality—280 to 300 mOsm/L

Phosphatase

Acid—0.2 to 1.8 international units

Alkaline—21 to 91 international units

Phosphorus—3 to 4.5 mg/dL, 1 to 1.5 mEq/L

Potassium—3.5 to 5 mEq/L

Protein—5.5 to 8 g/dL

Sodium—136 to 145 mEq/L

Urea nitrogen—10 to 20 mg/dL

Urine

pH 6.0 (4.7-8.0)

Specific gravity—1.005 to 1.025

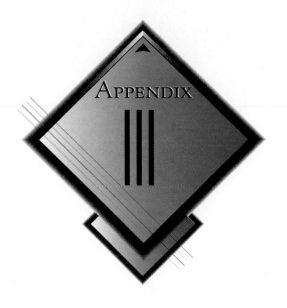

INSTRUMENT LIST AND TYPICAL RETAIL PRICES (1997)

Basic tray

Local anesthesia syringe	$ 30.00
Woodson elevator	20.00
Periapical curette	33.00
Small straight elevator	40.00
Large straight elevator	41.00
College pliers	17.00
Curved hemostat	26.00
Towel clip	23.00
Austin retractor	33.00
Suction	23.00
TOTAL	**$286.00**

Forceps

No. 150 upper universal	$100.00
No. 151 lower universal	100.00
No. 53L upper molar	101.00
No. 53R upper molar	101.00
No. 23 lower cowhorn	101.00
No. 17 lower molar	101.00
No. 286 root	101.00
TOTAL	**$705.00**

Surgical tray

Needle holder	$ 62.00
Suture	1.73
Suture scissor	43.00
Periosteal elevator	34.00
No. 3 blade handle	11.00
No. 15 blade	.31
Adson tissue forceps	27.00
Bone file	45.00
Tongue retractor	41.00
Root tip pick	28.00
Russian tissue forceps	37.00
Cryer elevator R	43.00
Cryer elevator L	43.00
Rongeur	155.00
TOTAL	**$571.04**

Biopsy tray

No. 3 blade handle	$ 11.00
No. 15 blade	.31
Needle holder	65.00
Suture	1.73
Suture scissors	43.00
Metzenbaum scissors	51.00
Allis tissue forceps	40.00
Adson tissue forceps	27.00
Curved hemostat	26.00
TOTAL	**$ 265.04**

Postoperative tray

Suture scissors	$ 43.00
College pliers	17.00
Suction	30.00
TOTAL	**$ 90.00**

Miscellaneous

Molt mouth prop	$ 145.00
Rubber bite block	23.00
Minnesota retractor	21.00
TOTAL	**$ 189.00**
GRAND TOTAL	**$2106.08**

The above prices are average prices from 1997 catalogs from the following companies: Walter Lorenz Surgical Instruments Inc, Jacksonville, FL; Hu-Friedy, Chicago, Ill; G. Hartzell & Son, Banning, CA; KLS Martin, Jacksonville, FL.

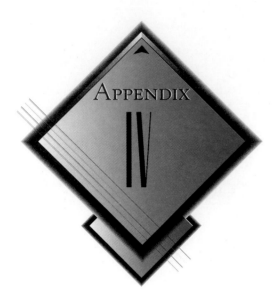

POSTVISIT NOTE (OFFICE RECORD)

COMPONENT PARTS

1. Date
2. Patient ID
3. Diagnosis
4. Review of medical history, medications, and vital signs
5. Oral examination
6. Anesthesia—mg and block technique used
7. Procedure, including statement of progress of procedure and complications
8. Discharge instructions
9. Medications prescribed (drug and amount or copy of prescription)
10. Return appointment—scheduling
11. Signature—(legible or printed underneath)

ORAL SURGERY NOTE
Example:

DATE: July 1, 1997

ID & DX: This 52 y.o. w. m. presents for extraction of mandibular left 2nd premolar and 1st molar. Both teeth are nonrestorable because of extensive caries.

MEDICAL HISTORY: Patient has chronic hypertension for which he takes a thiazide diuretic. Remainder of history is unremarkable. Pulse 84; BP 130/85.

ORAL EXAM: Soft tissue of cheeks, lips, tongue, floor of mouth, and palate are WNL. No palpable nodes or masses.

ANESTHESIA: Lidocaine 36 mg with 0.018 mg epinephrine via mandibular and long buccal blocks.

PROCEDURE: Routine forceps extraction. Distal root of 1st molar fractured—retrieved with Cryer elevator. No flap required. Patient tolerated procedure without difficulty.

DISCHARGE: Copy of routine postop instructions given and reviewed.

MEDICATIONS: Tylenol #3—24 caps. 1 or 2 caps q4h prn pain.

RETURN: One week for postop check

John Jay Jones

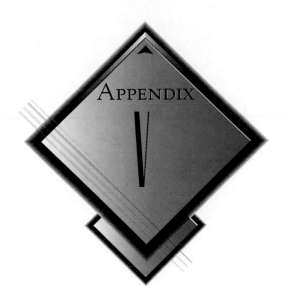

DRUG ENFORCEMENT ADMINISTRATION SCHEDULE OF DRUGS AND EXAMPLES

A. Schedule I drugs

These drugs are not available for clinical use in the United States.

EXAMPLES: Heroin, marijuana, LSD

B. Schedule II drugs

These drugs have high abuse liability. Require written prescription and DEA number. Prescription cannot be refilled without a new prescription.

EXAMPLES: Morphine, meperidine, plain codeine, oxycodone compounds, pentobarbital

C. Schedule III drugs

These drugs have lower abuse potential. Prescriptions may be phoned in to pharmacy, but require DEA number. The prescription can be refilled up to 5 times in 6 months.

EXAMPLES: Codeine compounds, hydrocodone compounds, dihydrocodeine compounds, pentazocine

D. Schedule IV drugs

Nonnarcotic drugs with lower abuse potential. DEA number required.

EXAMPLES: Chloral hydrate, diazepam

E. Schedule V drugs

These drugs are in low-dosage preparation for over-the-counter sales. Primarily for cough syrups and antidiarrheal purposes.

Note: Nonsteroidal antiinflammatory analgesics are not scheduled drugs.

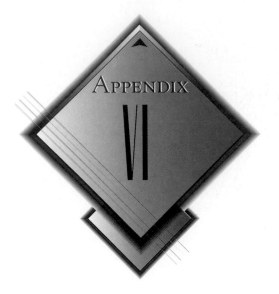

EXAMPLES OF USEFUL PRESCRIPTIONS

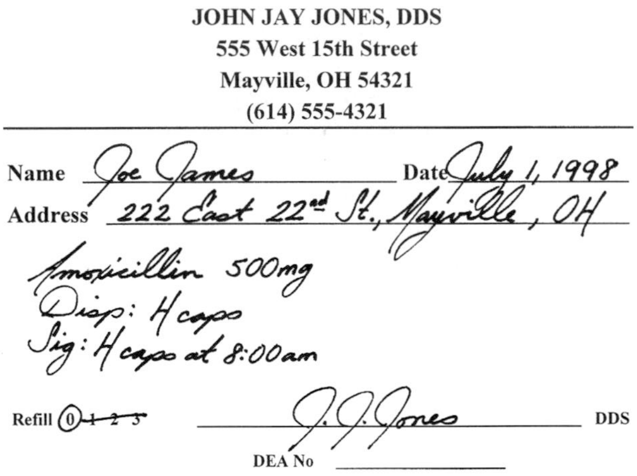

JOHN JAY JONES, DDS
555 West 15th Street
Mayville, OH 54321
(614) 555-4321

Name *Joe James* Date *July 1, 1998*

Address *222 East 22nd St., Mayville, OH*

Amoxicillin 500mg
Disp: 4 caps
Sig: 4 caps at 8:00am

Refill ⓪ 1 2 3 *J.J. Jones* DDS

DEA No _____

◆ Figure A-1

Prescription for oral subacute bacterial endocarditis prophylaxis with amoxicillin.

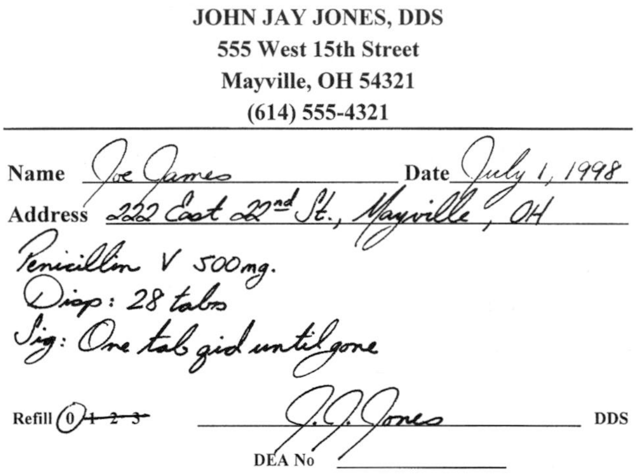

JOHN JAY JONES, DDS
555 West 15th Street
Mayville, OH 54321
(614) 555-4321

Name *Joe James* Date *July 1, 1998*

Address *222 East 22nd St., Mayville, OH*

Penicillin V 500mg.
Disp: 28 tabs
Sig: One tab qid until gone

Refill ⓪ 1 2 3 *J.J. Jones* DDS

DEA No _____

◆ Figure A-2

Prescription for oral penicillin therapy of odontogenic infection.

JOHN JAY JONES, DDS
555 West 15th Street
Mayville, OH 54321
(614) 555-4321

Name _Joe James_   Date _July 1, 1998_
Address _222 East 22nd St., Mayville, OH_

Erythromycin 250 mg
Disp: 28
Sig: One tab qid until gone

Refill (0) 1 2 3   _J.J. Jones_   DDS
DEA No _____

◇ Figure A-3

Prescription for treatment of odontogenic infection with erythromycin.

JOHN JAY JONES, DDS
555 West 15th Street
Mayville, OH 54321
(614) 555-4321

Name _Joe James_   Date _July 1, 1998_
Address _222 East 22nd St., Mayville, OH_

Aspirin 325 mg c̄ 5 mg Oxycodone
Disp: 12 (twelve) tabs
Sig: One tab q 4 h prn pain

Refill (0) 1 2 3   _J.J. Jones_   DDS
DEA No _AJxxxxxxx_

◇ Figure A-6

Prescription for aspirin with oxycodone. This prescription must have DEA number and cannot be phoned in.

JOHN JAY JONES, DDS
555 West 15th Street
Mayville, OH 54321
(614) 555-4321

Name _Joe James_   Date _July 1, 1998_
Address _222 East 22nd St., Mayville, OH_

Ibuprofen 400mg
Disp: 15 tabs
Sig: One tab q 4 h, prn pain

Refill 0 (1) 2 3   _J.J. Jones_   DDS
DEA No _____

◇ Figure A-4

Prescription for nonsteroidal antiinflammatory drug analgesic. No Drug Enforcement Administration (DEA) number required.

JOHN JAY JONES, DDS
555 West 15th Street
Mayville, OH 54321
(614) 555-4321

Name _Joe James_   Date _July 1, 1998_
Address _222 East 22nd St., Mayville, OH_

Tylenol #3
Disp: 18 (eighteen) caps
Sig: One cap q 4 h prn pain

Refill 0 (1) 2 3   _J.J. Jones_   DDS
DEA No _AJ xxxxxxx_

◇ Figure A-7

Typical brand name prescription. This compound has 650 mg of acetaminophen and 30 mg of codeine.

JOHN JAY JONES, DDS
555 West 15th Street
Mayville, OH 54321
(614) 555-4321

Name _Joe James_   Date _July 1, 1998_
Address _222 East 22nd St., Mayville, OH_

Acetaminophen 325 mg c̄ 15 mg
Codeine
Disp: 30 (thirty) caps
Sig: One or two caps q 4 h.
     prn pain
Refill 0 (1) 2 3   _J.J. Jones_   DDS
DEA No _AJxxxxxxx_

◇ Figure A-5

Prescription for analgesic with 325 mg acetaminophen and 15 mg codeine. Normal dose is two capsules. This prescription requires DEA number but can be phoned in.

JOHN JAY JONES, DDS
555 West 15th Street
Mayville, OH 54321
(614) 555-4321

Name _Joe James_   Date _July 1, 1998_
Address _222 East 22nd St., Mayville, OH_

Duracef 500 mg
Disp: 15 caps
Sig: One cap bid until gone

Refill (0) 1 2 3   _J.J. Jones_   DDS
DEA No _____

◇ Figure A-8

Typical brand name prescription for an oral cephalosporin.

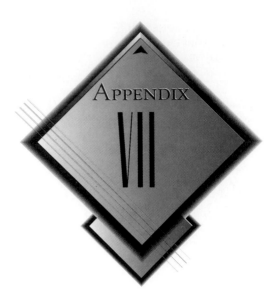

POSTOPERATIVE INSTRUCTIONS

A. Wound care
1. Bite firmly on gauze pack that has been placed, until you arrive home, then remove it gently.
2. Do not smoke for at least 12 hours, because this will promote bleeding and interfere with healing.

B. Bleeding
1. Some blood will ooze from the area of surgery and is normal. You may find a blood stain on your pillow in the morning, so it is advisable to use an old pillowcase the first night.
2. Do not spit or suck thick fluids through a straw, because this promotes bleeding.
3. If bleeding begins again, place a small damp gauze pack directly over the tooth socket and bite firmly for 30 minutes.
4. Keep your head elevated with several pillows or sit in a lounge chair.

C. Discomfort
1. Some discomfort is normal after surgery. It can be controlled but not eliminated by taking the pain pills your dentist has prescribed.
2. Take your pain pills with a whole glass of water and with a small amount of food if the pills cause nausea.
3. Do not drive or drink alcohol if you take prescription pain pills.

D. Diet
1. It is important to drink a large volume of fluids. Do not drink thick fluids through a straw, because this may promote bleeding.
2. Eat normal regular meals as soon as possible after surgery. Cold, soft food such as ice cream or yogurt may be the most comfortable for the first day.

E. Oral hygiene
1. Do not rinse your mouth or brush your teeth for the first 8 hours after surgery.

2. After that, rinse gently with warm salt water (½ teaspoon of salt in 8 oz of warm water) every 4 hours.
3. Brush your teeth gently, but avoid the area of surgery.

F. Swelling
1. Swelling after surgery is a normal body reaction. It reaches its maximum about 48 hours after surgery and usually lasts 4 to 6 days.
2. Applying ice packs over the area of surgery for the first 12 hours helps control swelling and may help the area to be more comfortable.

G. Rest
1. Avoid strenuous activity for 12 hours after your surgery.

H. Bruising
1. You may experience some mild bruising in the area of your surgery. This is a normal response in some persons and should not be a cause for alarm. It will disappear in 7 to 14 days.

I. Stiffness
1. After surgery you may experience jaw muscle stiffness and limited opening of your mouth. This is normal and will improve in 5 to 10 days.

J. Stitches
1. If stitches have been placed in the area of your surgery, you will need to have them removed in about 1 week.

K. Call the office if:
1. You experience excessive discomfort that you cannot control with your pain pills.
2. You have bleeding that you cannot control by biting on gauze.
3. You have increased swelling after the third day following your surgery.
4. You feel that you have a fever.
5. You have any questions.

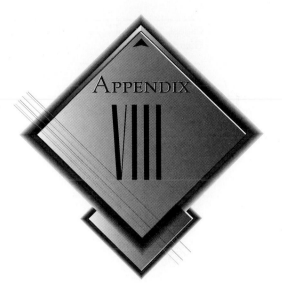

INFORMED CONSENT

_____ This is my consent for Dr. _____ and/or any dentist who is working with him/her to perform the following treatment/procedure/surgery: _____

_____

_____

as previously explained to me, or other procedures deemed necessary to complete the planned operation.

_____ I understand that the purpose of the procedure/surgery is to treat and possibly correct my diseased oral tissues. The doctor has advised me that if this condition persists without treatment or surgery, my present oral condition will probably worsen in time, and the risks to my health may include, but are not limited to, the following: swelling, pain, infection, cyst formation, periodontal (gum) diseases, dental decay, malocclusion, pathologic fracture of jaw, premature loss of teeth, and/or premature loss of bone. I have been informed of possible alternative methods of treatment, if any.

Dr. _____ has explained to me that there are certain inherent and potential risks in any treatment plan or procedure, and that in this specific instance such operative risks include but are not limited to the following:

(Check items applicable)

_____ 1. Postoperative discomfort and swelling that may necessitate several days of home recuperation

_____ 2. Heavy bleeding that may be prolonged

_____ 3. Injury to adjacent teeth, caps, or fillings

_____ 4. Postoperative infection requiring additional treatment

_____ 5. Stretching of the corners of the mouth, with resultant cracking and bruising

_____ 6. Restricted mouth opening for several days or weeks

_____ 7. Decision to leave a small piece of root in the jaw when its removal would require extensive surgery

_____ 8. Breakage of the jaw

_____ 9. Injury to the nerve underlying the teeth, resulting in numbness or tingling of the lip, chin, gums, cheek, teeth, and/or tongue on the operated side; this may persist for several weeks, months, or, in remote instances, permanently

_____ 10. Opening of the sinus (a normal cavity situated above the upper teeth), requiring additional surgery

_____ 11. Other _____

_____

_____

Medications, drugs, anesthetics, and prescriptions may cause drowsiness and lack of awareness and coordination, which can be increased by the use of alcohol or other drugs; thus I have been advised not to work or operate any vehicle, automobile, or hazardous device while taking medications and/or drugs, or until fully recovered from the effects of same. I understand and agree not to operate any vehicle or hazardous device for at least 24 hours after my release from surgery or until further recovered from the effects of the anesthetic medication and drugs that may have been given to me in the office or hospital for my care. I agree not to drive myself home after surgery and will have a responsible adult drive me or accompany me home after my discharge from surgery.

_____ If any unforeseen condition should arise in the course of the operation, calling for the doctor's judgment or for procedures in addition to or different from those now contemplated, I request and authorize the doctor to do whatever (s)he may deem advisable.

_____ No guarantee or assurance has been given to me that the proposed treatment will be curative and/or successful to my complete satisfaction. Because of individual patient differences, there exists a risk of failure, relapse, selective retreatment, or worsening of my present condition despite the care provided. However, it is the doctor's opinion that therapy would be helpful and that a worsening of my condition would occur sooner without the recommended treatment.

_____ I have had an opportunity to discuss with the surgeon my medical and health history, including any serious problems and/or injuries.

_____ I agree to cooperate completely with the recommendations of Dr. _____ while I am under his/her care, realizing that any lack of same could result in a less-than-optimal result.

I CERTIFY THAT I HAVE HAD AN OPPORTUNITY TO READ AND FULLY UNDERSTAND THE TERMS AND WORDS WITHIN THE ABOVE CONSENT TO THE OPERATION AND THE EXPLANATION REFERRED TO OR MADE, AND THAT ALL BLANKS OR STATEMENTS REQUIRING INSERTION OR COMPLETION WERE FILLED IN AND INAPPLICABLE PARAGRAPHS, IF ANY, WERE STRICKEN BEFORE I SIGNED. I ALSO STATE THAT I READ AND WRITE ENGLISH.

—————————————   —————————————   —————
Witness   Patient, Parent, or   Date
                                 Guardian

—————————————   —————————————
Witness   Doctor

———————————————————————————————

Modified from *Informed consent: important considerations for the oral and maxillofacial surgeon*, Chicago, 1986, American Association of the Oral and Maxillofacial Surgeons.

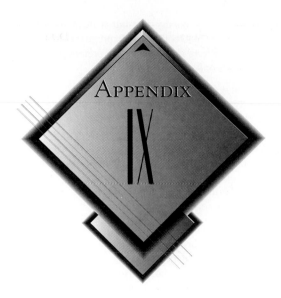

ANTIBIOTIC OVERVIEW

I. AMINOGLYCOSIDES

Aminoglycosides are broad-spectrum antibiotics that are useful for infections caused by gram-negative organisms. They are also active against some gram-positive organisms, such as staphylococci, but they are ineffective against streptococci and anaerobic bacteria. The most popular aminoglycoside is currently gentamicin, with amikacin and tobramycin being held in reserve for gram-negative organisms that are resistant to gentamicin. The major toxicities of the aminoglycosides are renal and cranial nerve VIII toxicity. They are rarely useful for odontogenic infections.

II. CEPHALOSPORINS

The cephalosporins are a group of β-lactam antibiotics that are effective against gram-positive cocci and many gram-negative rods. A large number of cephalosporins are available and are roughly divided into three generations, based on their activity against gram-negative organisms. The first-generation antibiotics have a similar activity, including activity against gram-positive cocci, *Escherichia coli, Klebsiella* organisms, and *Proteus mirabilis.*

The second-generation cephalosporins have broader activity against gram-negative bacteria and increased activity against the anaerobic bacteria. They have less activity against the gram-positive cocci than the first generation.

The third-generation cephalosporins are much more active against enteric gram-negative rods but are decidedly less active than first- and second-generation cephalosporins against gram-positive cocci.

There are two useful oral cephalosporins that are effective in odontogenic infections:

Cephalexin (Keflex)

Cefadroxil (Duricef)

Although neither of these are the drug of first choice for odontogenic infections, they may be useful in certain situations in which a bactericidal antibiotic is necessary.

The toxicity of the cephalosporin group is primarily related to allergy. Patients who are allergic to penicillin drugs should be given the cephalosporin antibiotics *with caution.* Patients who have had anaphylactic reactions to penicillin should *not* be given the cephalosporins.

III. CLINDAMYCIN

The antibacterial spectrum of clindamycin includes the gram-positive cocci and almost all anaerobic bacteria. It is effective for streptococci, staphylococci, and anaerobic infections. It is more expensive than penicillin and erythromycin and may have increased gastrointestinal toxicity in susceptible patients. For odontogenic infections, it should be considered as a second-line drug to be used when less expensive drugs are contraindicated.

IV. ERYTHROMYCIN

Erythromycin has a spectrum similar to that of penicillin in that it is effective against gram-positive cocci and oral anaerobic bacteria. The major adverse effect is mild gastrointestinal disturbance that increases with increased dosages. Oral erythromycin is useful in mild odontogenic infections but should not be used for serious infections. It is a bacteriostatic antibiotic and should usually not be used for the patient with depressed defenses.

V. IMIPENEM

Imipenem is a parenteral β-lactam antibiotic with an extremely broad antibacterial spectrum. It should be reserved for serious infections in which complex groups of bacteria are involved.

VI. METRONIDAZOLE

Metronidazole is an antibiotic that is effective *only* for anaerobic bacteria. It has no effect on aerobic bacteria, such as streptococci. It is primarily used in periodontal disease therapy but may also be useful in the management of anaerobic odontogenic infections alone or in combination with antiaerobic antibiotics, such as penicillin.

VII. PENICILLIN

Penicillin is the drug of choice for odontogenic infections, because its antibacterial spectrum includes the gram-positive cocci (except staphylococci) and oral anaerobes. Penicillin G is the form given parenterally, and penicillin V is preferred for oral administration. Penicillin has little toxicity except for allergic reactions, which occur in about 3% of the population.

Penicillinase-resistant penicillins are a group of drugs that are useful for penicillinase-producing staphylococci. Dicloxacillin is the preferred penicillinase-resistant penicillin for oral use. These drugs should be used only for culture-documented infection caused by staphylococci.

There are several extended-spectrum penicillins. The ampicillin-amoxicillin group are effective against more gram-negative rods than penicillin. Amoxicillin is absorbed better from the gastrointestinal tract than ampicillin and is thus preferred when the drug is given orally. Amoxicillin is the drug of choice for prevention of bacterial endocarditis because of its excellent GI absorption and slow elimination through the kidney.

VIII.   TETRACYCLINES

The tetracyclines are available for oral and parenteral administration and are generally considered to be broad-spectrum antibiotics. However, there is common bacterial resistance to these drugs. At this time, tetracyclines are useful only against anaerobic bacteria, which forms the basis for their use in odotongenic infections.

Their toxicities are generally low but include staining of developing teeth if given to children or to pregnant or lactating women. Minocycline and doxycycline are preferred, because they need be taken only once or twice daily.

IX.   FLUOROQUINOLONES

This recently introduced family of antibiotics includes Ciprofloxacin (Cipro) and Ofloxacin (Floxin). The antibiotics are broad-spectrum, bactericidal, orally taken antibiotics. Unfortunately they are only marginally effective against streptococci and have little or no effect against anaerobic bacteria. Therefore their usefulness in odontogenic infections is quite low. They should rarely, if ever, be used empirically for a patient with an odontogenic infection.

X.   ANTIFUNGAL DRUGS

Mucosal candidosis, or oral thrush, should be treated with the topical application of antifungal agents. The two drugs of choice are nystatin and clotrimazole. Both drugs are available as lozenges that are held in the mouth until they dissolve. The patient should use one lozenge 4 times daily for 10 days for effective control and to prevent relapse of the candidosis.

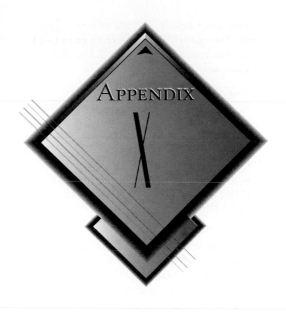

APPENDIX

COMMON MEDICAL ABBREVIATIONS

ABBREVIATION	MEANING
ad	up to
bid	twice a day
Bx	biopsy
c̄	with
CA	carcinoma
CBC	complete blood count
CC	chief complaint
cc	cubic centimeter (milliliter)
c/o	complaining of
Dx	diagnosis
Fx	fracture
gtt	drops
h	hour
h/o	history of
hs	at bedtime
Hx	history
I&D	incision and drainage
I&O	intake and output
IM	intramuscular
IV	intravenous
NPO	nothing by mouth
NS	normal saline
OOB	out of bed
p̄	after

ABBREVIATION	MEANING
P&A	percussion and auscultation
PI	present illness
PO	by mouth
prn	as necessary
pt	patient
q	every
qd	every day
qh	every hour
q3h	every 3 hours
qid	4 times a day
R/O	rule out
ROS	review of systems
Rx	prescription
s̄	without
sig	let it be labeled
s/p	status post
SQ	subcutaneously
stat	immediately
tab	tablet
tid	3 times a day
VS	vital signs
WNL	within normal limits
y/o	years old

INDEX ⸺⬦

Page numbers in italics indicate illustrations: *t* indicates tables.